Vascular and Endovascular Opportunities

Vascular and Endovascular Opportunities

Edited by

RM GREENHALGH MA MD MChir FRCS

Professor of Surgery
Head of Department of Vascular Surgery

JT POWELL MD PhD

Professor of Vascular Biology

AW MITCHELL MBBS FRCS FRCR

Consultant Radiologist
Imperial College School of Medicine
Charing Cross Hospital
London

2000

W B SAUNDERS

London · Edinburgh · New York · Philadelphia · Toronto · St Louis · Sydney · Tokyo

WB SAUNDERS
An imprint of Harcourt Publishers Limited

First published 2000

ISBN 0-7020-2610-7

British Library Cataloguing in Publication Data

A catalogue record for this book is available from the British Library

Library of Congress Cataloging in Publication Data

A catalog record for this book is available from the Library of Congress

Note
Medical knowledge is constantly changing. As new information becomes available, changes in treatment, procedures, equipment and the use of drugs become necessary. The editors/authors/contributors and the publishers have, as far as it is possible, taken care to ensure that the information given in this text is accurate and up to date. However, readers are strongly advised to confirm that the information, especially with regard to drug usage, complies with the latest legislation and standards of practice.

Editorial and Production Services by Jane Duncan
10 Barley Mow Passage, London W4 4PH

Typeset by Phoenix Photosetting, Chatham, Kent
Printed in Great Britain at the University Press, Cambridge

The Publisher's policy is to use **paper manufactured from sustainable forests**

Contents

PERIPHERAL ARTERIAL OPPORTUNITIES
Intermittent claudication issues

PERIPHERAL ARTERIAL OPPORTUNITIES
Newer techniques

RENAL ARTERY STENOSIS OPPORTUNITIES

Contributors

Dr Georg-Wilhelm Albrecht-Fruh, MD
Deutsche Gesellschaft fur Angiologie
Krankenhaus Porz a Rhein
Urbacher Weg 19
51149 Koln
Germany

Dr Ale Algra, MD PhD
Julius Center for Patient Oriented Research
and Department of Neurology
PO Box 85500
3508 GA Utrecht
The Netherlands

Professor Jens-Rainer Allenberg, MD PhD
Head of Department of Vascular Surgery
Rupert-Karls University, Heidelberg
Im Neuerhauer Feld 110
D-69120 Heidelberg
Germany

Dr Max Amor, MD
Interventional Cardiologist, Co-Director
UCCI Polyclinique
Polyclinique d'Essey
7 rue Parmentier
54270 Essey les Nancy
France

Mr M P Armon, DM FRCS
Specialist Registrar
Department of Vascular and Endovascular Surgery
E16, University Hospital
Queens Medical Centre
Nottingham NG7 2UH, UK

Dr Ray Ashleigh, MD
Consultant Vascular Radiologist
Department of Radiology
South Manchester University Hospital
Nell Lane
West Didsbury
Manchester M20 2LR, UK

Dr Syed Babar, MB BS FCPS (Radiology) FRCR
Specialist Registrar in Radiology
Department of Radiology
Royal Free Hospital NHS Trust
Pond Street
London NW3, UK

Evy Bashiardes, Mphil
Cyprus Institute of Neurology and Genetics
Nicosia

Dr Trevor Bayston, MD
Department of Vascular Surgery
Imperial College School of Medicine
Charing Cross Hospital
Fulham Palace Road
London W6 8RF, UK

Mr Jonathan D Beard, ChM FRCS
Consultant Vascular Surgeon
Sheffield Vascular Institute
Northern General Hospital
Herries Road
Sheffield S5 7AU, UK

Professor Jean-Pierre Becquemin, MD
Department of Vascular Surgery
Henri Mondor Hospital
AP/HP Paris
University Paris Val de Marne
Creteil
94010 France

Professor Jill J F Belch, MD FRCP
Section of Vascular Biology and Medicine
Ninewells Hospital and Medical School
University of Dundee
Ninewells
Dundee DD1 9SY
Scotland, UK

Professor Peter R F Bell, MD FRCS
Department of Surgery
University of Leicester
Robert Kilpatrick Building
Leicester LE2 7LX, UK

Dr Jocelyn Bell, MD
Trial Co-ordinator
Vascular Surgery Unit
University Department of Surgery
Birmingham Heartlands Hospital,
Bordesley Green East,
Birmingham B9 5SS, UK

Dr Anna-Maria Belli, MD
Consultant in Vascular Interventional Radiology
Department of Radiology
St George's Hospital
Blackshaw Road
London SW17 0QT, UK

Professor David Bergqvist, MD PhD
Professor of Vascular Surgery
Department of Surgery
University Hospital
S-75185 Uppsala
Sweden

Dr Jan D Blankensteijn, MD
Chief, Division of Vascular Surgery G.04.232
University Hospital Utrecht
PO Box 85500
3508 GA Utrecht
The Netherlands

Dr Amman Bolia, FRCR
Department of Radiology
Leicester Royal Infirmary NHS Trust
Leicester LE1 5WW, UK

Scott A Bovard, MS
Center for Vascular Intervention, Division of Vascular Surgery
Union Memorial Hospital/MedStar Health
330 North Calvert St
Suite 570
Baltimore, MD 2128
USA

Professor Andrew W Bradbury
Department of Vascular Surgery
Birmingham Heartlands Hospital,
Bordesley Green East,
Birmingham B9 5SS, UK

Anthony R Brady, MSc
Research Fellow
Hammersmith Hospital
150 Du Cane Road
London W12 0HS, UK

Louise Brown, MSc
Department of Vascular Surgery
Imperial College School of Medicine
Charing Cross Hospital
Fulham Palace Road
London W6 8RF, UK

Professor T M Buckenham, MD
Department of Medical Radiology
The Royal Infirmary of Edinburgh
Lauriston Place
Edinburgh Eh3 9YW
Scotland, UK

Dr Ahn Bui, PhD
Advanced Fluid Dynamics Laboratory
CSIRO/BCE
Highett
Victoria
Australia

Professor Kevin G Burnand, MS FRCS
Professor of Surgery
Academic Department of Surgery
St Thomas' Hospital
Lambeth Palace Road
London SE1 7EH, UK

Mr Bruce Campbell, MS FRCP FRCS
Consultant Surgeon
Department of Surgery
Royal Devon and Exeter Hospital
Barrack Road
Exeter EX2 5DW, UK

Dr Marios Cariolou, PhD
Director
Molecular Genetics Unit B
Cyprus Institute of Neurology and Genetics
Nicosia
Cyprus

Mr N Cheshire, MD FRCS FACS (Ed)
Consultant Vascular Surgeon, Honorary Senior Lecturer
Regional Vascular Unit
St Mary's Hospital
Praed Street
Paddington
London W2 1NY, UK

Mr Patrick Chong, MBBS FRCS
Clinical Research Fellow
Department of Vascular Surgery
Imperial College School of Medicine
Charing Cross Hospital
Fulham Palace Road
London W6 8RF, UK

Dr Frank J Criado, MD
Director, Center for Vascular Intervention
Chief, Division of Vascular Surgery
Union Memorial Hospital/MedStar Health
3333 North Calvert St
Suite 67
Baltimore, MD 2128
USA

Dr Alexandre D'audiffret, MD
Service de Chirurgie Vasculaire
Hôpital Henri Mondor
51 Ave du Marechal
de Lattre de Tassigny
94010 Creteil
France

Professor A Darzi, MD FRCS FRCSI FACS
Professor of Surgery
St Mary's Hospital
Praed Street
London W2 1NY, UK

Dr Ian R Davidson, FRCSI FRCR
Consultant Vascular Radiologist
Department of Diagnostic Imaging, B Floor
University College Hospital Nottingham
Queens Medical Centre
Derby Road
Nottingham NG7 2UH, UK

Mr Alun H Davies, MA DM FRCS
Reader and Honorary Consultant in Surgery
Department of Vascular Surgery
Imperial College School of Medicine
Charing Cross Hospital
Fulham Palace Road
London W6 8RF, UK

Dr David H Deaton, MD
Department of Thoracic and Vascular Surgery
Anne Arundel Medical Center
64 Franklyn Street
Annapolis
MD 21401
USA

Surinder Dhanjil, AVT RVT MSc
Chief Vascular Ultrasonographer
Irvine Laboratory for Cardiovascular Investigation and Research
Imperial College School of Medicine at St Mary's Hospital
Department of Vascular Surgery
QEQM Wing, 10th Floor
London W2 1NY, UK

Mr Simon R Dodds, MA MS FRCS(sen)
Consultant General and Vascular Surgeon
Department of Surgery
Good Hope Hospital NHS Trust
Rectory Road
Sutton Coldfield
West Midlands B75 7RR, UK

Professor Bert C Eikelboom, MD PhD
Division of Vascular Surgery G 04 232
University Hospital Utrecht
Heidelberglaan 100
3584 CX Utrecht
The Netherlands

Dr Tarek S El-Atrozy, MD
Vascular Surgery Research Fellow
Irvine Laboratory for Cardiovascular Investigation and Research
Imperial College School of Medicine at St Mary's Hospital
Department of Vascular Surgery
QEQM Wing, 10th Floor
London W2 1NY, UK

Dr Duncan Ettles, MD
Consultant Cardiovascular Radiologist
Department of Radiology
Royal Hull Hospitals
Hull Royal Infirmary
Anlaby Road
Hull HU3 2JZ, UK

Dr Tor Flørenes, MD
Consultant
Centre for Vascular Surgery in Oslo
Aker Hospital
University of Oslo
0514 Oslo
Norway

Professor F G R Fowkes, PhD FRCPE FFPHM
Professor of Epidemiology and Director
Wolfson Unit for Prevention of Peripheral Vascular Diseases
Department of Public Health Sciences
University of Edinburgh
Teviot Place
Edinburgh EH8 9AG
Scotland, UK

Mr Ian J Franklin, FRCS
Department of Surgery
Imperial College School of Medicine
Charing Cross Hospital
Fulham Palace Road
London W6 8RF, UK

Dr Peter A Gaines, MRCP FRCR
Consultant Vascular Radiologist
Department of Radiology, Sheffield Vascular Institute
Northern General Hospital
Herries Road
Sheffield S5 7AU, UK

Dr Andrew Garratt, BA MsC PhD
Co-Director
National Centre for Health Outcomes Development
Unit of Health-Care Epidemiology
Division of Public Health and Primary Health Care
Institute of Health Sciences
University of Oxford
Oxford, UK

Dr W Gedroyc, MD
Consultant Radiologist, Medical Director of MR Scanning
Department of Radiology
St Mary's Hospital
Praed Street
Paddington
London W2, UK

Mr George Geroulakos, MD PhD FRCS
Senior Lecturer and Honorary Consultant Surgeon
Imperial College School of Medicine
Department of Vascular Surgery
Charing Cross Hospital
Fulham Palace Road
London W6 8RF, UK

Dr Hari Gnanaserkeram, MS
Division of Vascular Surgery
Union Memorial Hospital/Helix Health
3333 North Calvert St
Suite 570
Baltimore, MD 2128
USA

Mr John Golledge, MA MChiR FRCS
Department of Vascular Surgery
Imperial College School of Medicine
Charing Cross Hospital
Fulham Palace Road
London W6 8RF, UK

Professor Roger M Greenhalgh, MA MD Mchir FRCS
Professor of Surgery
Head of Department of Vascular Surgery
Imperial College School of Medicine
Charing Cross Hospital
Fulham Palace Road
London W6 8RF, UK

Maura Griffin, MSc
Research Fellow
Department of Vascular Surgery
Irvine Laboratory for Cardiovascular Investigation and Research
Imperial College School of Medicine at St Mary's Hospital
QEQM Wing, 10th Floor
London W2 1NY, UK

Dr Marie-Louise M Grønholdt, PhD
Research Fellow
Department of Vascular Surgery RK
Rigshospitalet 3111
University of Copenhagen
Blegdamsvej 9
DK2100 Copenhagen
Denmark

Mr Peter L Harris, MD FRCS
Consultant Vascular Surgeon
Director for Vascular and Transplant Services
Regional Vascular Unit, 8c Link
Royal Liverpool University Hospital
Prescott St
Liverpool L7 8XP, UK

Dr David E Hartley, FIR
Endovascular Unit
Royal Perth Hospital
Perth
Western Australia

Dr Staal Hatlinghus, MD
Consultant Radiologist
Department of Radiology
University Hospital of Trondheim
N-7006 Trondheim
Norway

Mr Adriano M Henney, PhD
Section and Project Manager
CVGI Research Department
AstraZeneca Pharmaceuticals
Alderley House
Alderley Park
Macclesfield
Cheshire SK10 4TF, UK

Dr Isabelle Henry, MD
Interventional Cardiologist
Polyclinique d'Essey, UCCI Polyclinique
7 rue Parmentier
54270 Essey les Nancy
France

Dr Michel Henry, MD
Interventional Cardiologist
Co-Director, Polyclinique d'Essey
UCCI Polyclinique
7 rue Parmentier
54270 Essey les Nancy
France

Dr Gwan H Ho, MD
Department of Surgery
St Antonius Hospital
Koekoekslaan 1
3435 CM Nieuwegien
The Netherlands

Professor Brian R Hopkinson, ChM FRCS
Professor and Head of Department
Department of Vascular Surgery
E16, University Hospital
Queens Medical Centre
Nottingham NG7 2UH, UK

Professor Svante Horsch, MD
Krankenhaus Porz a Rhein
Urbacher Weg 19
51149 Koln
Germany

Michele Hugel, RN
Registered Nurse
Polyclinique d'Essey, UCCI Polyclinique
7 rue Parmentier
54270 Essey les Nancy
France

Dr Allan Irvine, MRCP FRCR
Consultant Radiologist
Academic Department of Radiology
St Thomas' Hospital
Lambeth Palace Road
London SE1 7EH, UK

Dr Krassi Ivancev, MD
Department of Diagnostic Radiology
Malmo University Hospital
S-205 02 Malmo
Sweden

Dr Ralph Jackson, MD
Department of Radiology
The Freeman Hospital
High Heaton
Newcastle upon Tyne, NE7 7DN, UK

Dr M K W Johnston, MB BS BSc MRCS
Specialist Registrar in Radiology
Department of Radiology
Royal Free Hospital NHS Trust
Pond Street
London NW3, UK

Dr Sadettin Karacagil, MD PhD
Associate Professor of Surgery
Department of Surgery
University Hospital
S-75185 Uppsala
Sweden

Mr D C Kinsella, FRCR
Consultant Radiologist
Department of Radiology
Royal Devon and Exeter NHS Trust
Barrack Road
Exeter EX2 5DW, UK

Dr Christos Klonaris, MD
Vascular Surgeon
Polyclinique d'Essey, UCCI Polyclinique
7 rue Parmentier
54270 Essey les Nancy
France

Professor Andries J Kroese, MD PhD
Centre for Vascular Surgery in Oslo
Aker Hospital
University of Oslo
0514 Oslo
Norway

Dr Kiriakos Ktenidis, MD
Deutsche Gesellschaft fur Angiologie
Krankenhaus Porz a Rhein
Urbacher Weg 19
51149 Koln
Germany

Mr Michael MD Lawrence-Brown, FRACS
Consultant Vascular Surgeon
Endovascular Unit
Royal Perth Hospital
Perth
Western Australia

Dr James A Lawson, MD PhD
Department of Surgery
Hospital Amstelveen
Laan van de Helende Meesters 8
1186 AM Amstelveen
The Netherlands

Mr Tim A Lees, FRCS
Consultant Vascular Surgeon
The Freeman Hospital
High Heaton
Newcastle upon Tyne NE7 7DN, UK

Dr Gillian C Leng, MD MFPHM
Royal Free and University College Medical School
Department of Primary Care and Population Sciences
Royal Free Campus
Rowland Hill Street
London NW3 2PF, UK

Dr Kurt Liffman, PhD
Advanced Fluid Dynamics Laboratory
CSIRO/BCE
Highett
Victoria Australia

Dr Bengt Lindblad, MD PhD
Department of Vascular Surgery
Malmo University Hospital, Lund University
S-205 02 Malmö
Sweden

Dr Mats Lindh, MD
Department of Diagnostic Radiology
Malmö University Hospital, Lund University
S-205 02 Malmö
Sweden

Dr Christer Ljungman, MD PhD
Associate Professor of Surgery
Department of Surgery
University Hospital
S-75185 Uppsala
Sweden

Dr Anne-Marie Lofberg, MD PhD
Consultant of Radiology
Department of Surgery
University of Hospital
S-75185 Uppsala
Sweden

Professor N J M London, MD FRCS
Department of Surgery
Leicester Royal Infirmary NHS Trust
Leicester LE1 5WW, UK

Dr Jan Lundbom, MD
Consultant Vascular Surgeon
Department of Surgery
University Hospital of Trondheim
N-7006 Trondheim
Norway

Jennifer A Martin, MS
Center for Vascular Intervention, Division of Vascular Surgery
Union Memorial Hospital/MedStar Health
330 North Calvert St
Suite 570
Baltimore, MD 2128
USA

Dr Matthew B Matson, MRCP FRCR
Fellow in Interventional Radiology
Department of Radiology
St George's Hospital
Blackshaw Road
London SW17 0QT, UK

Heather Maxwell, BA
Cochrane Review Group on Peripheral Vascular Diseases
Public Health Sciences
Medical School
Teviot Place
Edinburgh EH8 9AB, Scotland, UK

Professor Charles McCollum, MB BS FRCS MD
Professor of Surgery, Honorary Consultant Surgeon
Department of Surgery
South Manchester University Hospital
Nell Lane
West Didsbury
Manchester M20 2LR, UK

Adam W Mitchell, MB BS FRCS FRCR
Consultant Radiologist, Imperial College of Medicine
Charing Cross Hospital
Fulham Palace Road
London W6 8RF, UK

Dr Frans L Moll, MD PhD
Department of Surgery
St Antonius Hospital
Koekoeslaan 1
3435 CM Nieuwegein
The Netherlands

Professor Hans O Myhre, MD PhD
Professor of Surgery
Department of Surgery
University Hospital of Trondheim
N-7006 Trondheim
Norway

Dr P Nafteux, MD
Department of Surgery
Royal Devon and Exeter NHS Trust
Barrack Road
Exeter EX2 5DW, UK

Dr Anthony Nicholson, BSc MSc FRCR
President, British Society of Interventional Radiologists
Consultant Cardiovascular Radiologist
Department of Radiology
Hull and East Yorkshire Hospitals Trust
Anlaby Road
Kingston upon Hull HU3 2JZ, UK

Professor Andrew N Nicolaides, MS FRCS FRCSE
Professor of Vascular Surgery
Director
Irvine Laboratory for Cardiovascular Investigation and Research
Imperial College School of Medicine at St Mary's Hospital
QEQM Wing, 10th Floor
London W2 1NV, UK

Dr Laszio Papp, MD
Research Fellow
Vascular Surgery Unit
University Department of Clinical and Surgical Sciences
The Royal Infirmary
Edinburgh EH3 9YW, Scotland, UK

Snehal C Patel, MS
Division of Vascular Surgery
Union Memorial Hospital/MedStar Health
3333 North Calvert St
Suite 570
Baltimore, MD 2128
USA

Mr Jeremy M T Perkins, MD FRCS
Clinical Vascular Fellow
Vascular Surgical Unit
St Mary's Hospital
Praed Street
Paddington
London W2 1NY, UK

Dr Andrew D Platts, MB FRCS(ed) FRCS FRCR
Consultant Radiologist
Department of Radiology
Royal Free Hospital NHS Trust
Pond Street
London NW3 2QG, UK

Professor Janet T Powell, MD PhD
Professor of Vascular Biology
Department of Vascular Surgery
Imperial College School of Medicine
Charing Cross Hospital
Fulham Palace Road
London W6 8RF, UK

Dr Rubeena Razzaq, MB ChB MRCP FRCR
Consultant Radiologist
Department of Radiology
South Manchester University Hospital
Nell Lane
West Didsbury
Manchester M20 2LR, UK

Dr Timothy Resch, MD PhD
Department of Surgery
Malmö University Hospital, Lund University
S-205 02 Malmö
Sweden

Mr Graham Riding, BSc MBCHB FRCS
Lecturer in Surgery (Research)
Department of Surgery
South Manchester University Hospital
Nell Lane
West Didsbury
Manchester M20 2LR, UK

Dr John D G Rose, MD
Consultant Radiologist
The Freeman Hospital
High Heaton
Newcastle upon Tyne NE7 7DN, UK

Dr Murray Rudman, PhD
Advanced Fluid Dynamics Laboratory
CSIRO/BCE
Highett
Victoria
Australia

Professor Ian Russell, PhD FSS FRCCP FRCPEdin
Founding Professor of Health Sciences
Department of Health Sciences
University of York
Alcuin College
Heslington
York YO10 5DD, UK

Dr Michael M Sabetai, MD
Vascular Surgery Research Fellow
Department of Vascular Surgery
Irvine Laboratory for Cardiovascular Investigation and Research
Imperial College School of Medicine at St Mary's Hospital
QEQM Wing, 10th Floor
London W2 1NY, UK

Dr Marc R H M van Sambeek, MD PhD
Deaprtment of Vascular Surgery
Erasmus University Medical Center Rotterdam
PO Box 2040
3000 CA Rotterdam
The Netherlands

Professor Torben V Schroeder, DMSc
Consultant Vascular Surgeon
Department of Vascular Surgery RK
Rigshospitalet 3111
University of Copenhagen
Blegdamsvej 9
DK2100 Copenhagen
Denmark

Dr Hardy Schumacher, MD
Vascular Surgeon
Department of Vascular Surgery
Rupert-Karls University, Heidelberg
Im Neuerhauer Feld 110
D-69120 Heidelberg
Germany

Dr James B Semmens, PhD
Research Fellow
Centre for Health Services Research
Department of Public Health
The University of Western Australia
Nedlands
Western Australia

Dr Henrik H Sillesen, DMSc
Gentofte
University of Copenhagen
Copenhagen, Denmark

Professor Carl Erik Slagsvold, MD PhD
Consultant
Centre for Vascular Surgery in Oslo
Aker Hospital
University of Oslo
0514 Oslo
Norway

Mr Jason Smith, FRCS
Specialist Registrar
Department of Vascular Surgery
Imperial College School of Medicine
Charing Cross Hospital
Fulham Palace Road
London W6 8RF, UK

Dr Sunita Srivastava, MD
Department of Diagnostic Radiology
Malmö University Hospital, Lund University
S-205 20 Malmö
Sweden

Mr Brendan M Stanley, FRACS
Consultant Vascular Surgeon
Endovascular Unit
Royal Perth Hospital
Perth
Western Australia

Dr Marco J D Tangelder, MD
Department of Vascular Surgery G 04 232
University Hospital Utrecht
Heidelberglaan 100
3584 CX Utrecht
The Netherlands

Dr Thomas J Tegos, MD
Neurologist
Department of Vascular Surgery
Irvine Laboratory for Cardiovascular Investigation and Research
Imperial College School of Medicine at St Mary's Hospital
QEQM Wing, 10th Floor
London W2 1NY, UK

Mr John F Thompson, MS FRCS(ed) FRCS
Department of Surgery
Royal Devon and Exeter NHS Trust
Barrack Road
Exeter EX2 5DW, UK

Dr Petr Uher, MD
Department of Diagnostic Radiology
Malmö University Hospital, Lund University
S-205 02 Malmö
Sweden

Dr A Tulga Ulus, MD
Research Fellow
Department of Surgery
University Hospital
S-75185 Uppsala
Sweden

Professor Hero van Urk, MD PhD FRCSEd
Professor of Surgery
Erasmus University Medical Center
Vascular Surgery Unit
PO Box 2040
3000 CA Rotterdam
The Netherlands

Dr Marc R H M van Sambeek, MD PhD
Senior Lecturer in Surgery
Department of Vascular Surgery
Erasmus University Medical Center Rotterdam
PO Box 2040
3000 CA Rotterdam
The Netherlands

Mr Matthew Waltham, MA FRCS
Clinical Lecturer
Academic Department of Surgery
St Thomas' Hospital
Lambeth Palace Road
London SE1 7EH, UK

Dr Lesley Walton, MD
Department of Vascular Surgery
Imperial College School of Medicine
Charing Cross Hospital
Fulham Palace Road
London W6 8RF, UK

Dr A Watkinson, MBBS FRCS FRCR
Consultant and Honorary Senior Lecturer in Radiology
Department of Radiology
Royal Free Hospital NHS Trust
Pond Street
London NW3, UK

Dr Jarlis Wesche, MD PhD
Assistant Professor of Surgery
Department of Surgery
University Hospital of Trondheim
N-7006 Trondheim
Norway

Dr Rodney A White, MD
Chief Vascular Surgery Associate Chair
Department of Surgery
University of California
Harbor UCLA Medical Center
1000 West Carson St
Torrance, CA 90502
USA

Dr Eric P Wilson, MD
Associate Director Center for Vascular Intervention
Division of Vascular Surgery
Union Memorial Hospital/MedStar Health
3333 North Calvert St
Suite 570
Baltimore, MD 2128
USA

Mr John H N Wolfe, MS FRCS
Consultant Vascular Surgeon
Regional Vascular Unit
St Mary's Hospital
Praed Street
Paddington
London W2 1NY, UK

Mr Michael G Wyatt, FRCS
Consultant Vascular Surgeon
The Freeman Hospital
High Heaton
Newcastle upon Tyne NE7 7DN, UK

Preface

Management in vascular disease is undergoing rapid change. The first chapters have been grouped under the heading 'The wind of change' in vascular management, a phrase used by Harold Macmillan about Africa in the 1960s. Currently, some management is by standard vascular surgery using significant incisions. The tendency is for as many procedures as possible to be managed by smaller incisions using endovascular techniques, or even by the percutaneous route. The trend of surgery has always been from larger procedures to smaller ones. This is only part of the story because at the same time scientists are seeking the cause of vascular disease and trying to understand the underlying abnormality with a view to treating the patients by medical means. The ultimate is neither surgery, interventional radiology or medicine, but prevention in the community.

During this 'wind of change' there are threats but there are also opportunities. The threats are the threats of the turf. It is natural for vascular surgeons, radiologists and physicians to question who should dominate the management of a patient. Whichever is seen to be in the ascendant at any one time will not necessarily be a year later or a year after that. Therefore humility is appropriate. Most patients would prefer to have no operation at all or a smaller rather than a larger procedure, but it is reasonable to expect that there is proof that a minimal procedure or medical management is at least as good and as durable as the standard surgical procedure. There are opportunities for collaboration between the disciplines in the new millennium.

The opportunities present themselves around the management of carotid artery disease, aortic aneurysm, and peripheral arterial disease. Thrombolytic therapy is being used more than ever before and the management of renal artery stenosis is controversial and involves radiologists, surgeons and physicians at the present time.

The levels of evidence are not always understood by vascular specialists but it is important that they should be understood. It is important to grasp what is not known and how strongly we can believe what we are told. The chapter by Gillian Leng on this matter is therefore of key importance in relation to the other chapters.

At all stages we have tried to stress the opportunities for collaboration particularly between the vascular surgeon and the vascular radiologist, but also with the vascular biologist and vascular physician and therefore these subjects appear in each of the parts of the book and are edited by a vascular surgeon [RMG], a vascular radiologist [AWM], and a vascular biologist [JTP].

RM Greenhalgh
AW Mitchell
JT Powell

THE WIND OF CHANGE IN VASCULAR MANAGEMENT

Open surgery has not had its day

Peter RF Bell

INTRODUCTION

The inexorable increase in the use of endovascular techniques to treat almost any condition where occlusion or dilatation of the arteries has occurred, has led to the suggestion that open surgery has had its day and soon everything will be done intraluminally.[1] Do young vascular surgeons need therefore to change their name or retrain as radiologists or physicians? The answer is of course NO. However, it is fair to say that many intraluminal procedures are gaining ground and may, without at present much evidence that they are better, eventually replace open surgery – although not, I suspect, completely.

The arterial operation which is perhaps done most often these days is carotid endarterectomy. This is the staple diet of most vascular surgeons and until recently appeared to be a preserve which could not be breached. Things have changed, however, with the introduction of carotid angioplasty and the proposition that this can replace and be as safe as surgery in most patients.[2,3] What is the evidence for this suggestion? The answer is that very little, if any, evidence exists to support this view.

The only randomized multicentre trial so far performed, the CAVATAS study [as yet unpublished] found a risk of >10% of stroke [major or minor] and death after angioplasty or surgery and concluded that angioplasty was as safe as surgery. These results of course conveniently ignore the fact that most reasonable centres can now achieve stroke and death rates of around 2% with appropriate quality control measures[4] and with local anaesthesia gaining ground even this figure may improve further.[5]

The only randomized trial so far carried out on the intention to treat basis showed that angioplasty and stenting was dangerous[6] and could not be recommended at present. This trial was different from all others in that no exclusion criteria were allowed. All patients satisfied the criteria for surgery, i.e. they were symptomatic and had severe stenoses >70% and were randomized at that time. This was done because of the impossibility at present of deciding which patients are at risk of embolization or other problems during or immediately after angioplasty. The only patients not randomized were those who had an occluded internal carotid artery. This study showed clearly that embolization from the plaque is a major problem and cannot be ignored. At present, therefore, there is no evidence that angioplasty can produce results equivalent to or better than surgery in specialized centres, and surgery remains the gold standard.

Embolization occurs during all phases of the procedure[7] from wire manipulation, flushing with saline (Fig. 1), inflating the balloon, deflating the balloon and inserting the stent and can reach very large numbers, as occurred in our own study (Table 1). The advent of a number of techniques to protect the patient against inevitable

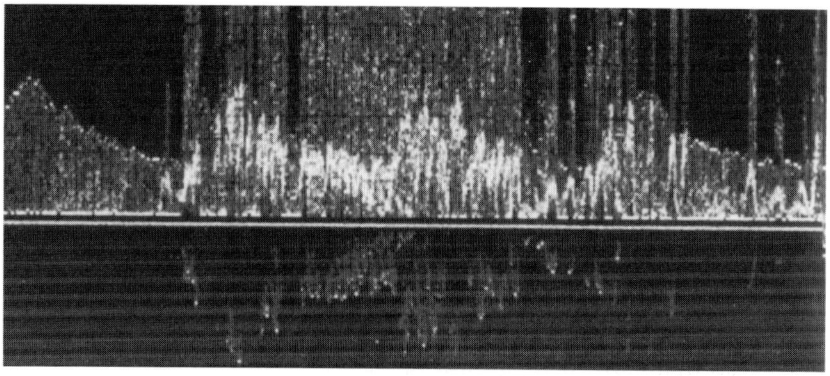

Fig. 1. Transcranial Doppler tracing during saline flush. Many air and particulate emboli are seen.

Table 1. Number of emboli detected during carotid angioplasty and consequences

	Number of emboli						
Time of detection of emboli	*Case 1*	*Case 2*	*Case 3*	*Case 4*	*Case 5*	*Case 6*	*Case 7*
Manipulation of wire across stenosis	29	20	115	50	71	158	115
Balloon predilatation	0	56	21	0	60	42	1
Stent deployment	125	90	110	65	159	76	115
Balloon inflation	1	28	23	14	29	0	0
Balloon deflation	26	81	101	22	60	86	53
Total emboli	181	275	370	151	379	362	284
OHS stroke score at 30 days	No CVA	No CVA	3	0	2	3	3

OHS: Oxfordshire Health Study.
CVA: Cerebrovascular accident.

embolization that occurs during angioplasty may eventually lead to a reduction in the number of carotid endarterectomies being performed. These techniques, the results of which have not yet been extensively published, include:

1. the use of a thin (0.14) guidewire which incorporates a balloon which can avoid distal embolization during the procedure [PercuSurg];
2. various filter devices which can be extended beyond the stenosis and trap debris which can then be withdrawn [Angioguard];
3. various techniques to encourage retrograde flow during the procedure and therefore prevent embolization occurring.

All of these need to be validated and the results obtained before they can be used generally. However, the initial results from personal communication appear to be promising. The important point will be to ensure that the initial passage of a wire does not cause significant embolization. Of all these techniques the one where retrograde flow is induced seems to be the most promising, if a patient can tolerate occlusion of the common and external carotid arteries while this is taking place, although approximately 10% will not be able to do so. Even if these techniques do produce better results I cannot see them replacing surgery completely.

The problem with carotid endarterectomy is that we know that only about 30% of patients who are symptomatic actually need treatment.[8,9] What we should be doing is trying to find out who these patients are; only then can we do a comparative trial on similar patients. I strongly suspect, however, that angioplasty, with or without protective devices, will not be able to replace endarterectomy as the safest option in patients with severe (>90%) symptomatic carotid stenosis. It may be useful in those with lesser lesions, but these patients probably do not need treatment anyway. I therefore believe that carotid surgery will still be here for some time to come. One possible note of caution is risk factor modification using statins and possibly other drugs such as doxycycline which may stabilize plaques. This could lead to the need for treatment being abolished altogether or angioplasty again becoming safer with smoother lesions. Even then angioplasty will have to compete with the excellent long-term result of removing the plaque completely rather than simply compressing it. Restenosis following angioplasty or stent insertion due to intimal hyperplasia[10] is a problem which is not at present soluble, though local irradiation[11] or growth factor inhibition may eventually solve this. The other difficulty is stent compression or distortion in places such as the neck where a lot of movement occurs. This needs to be resolved. I suspect that severely stenosed lesions (>90%) will still be best and most safely dealt with by surgery for the foreseeable future.

The recent upsurge in the use of stent graft combinations to treat aortic aneurysms also suggests that surgery for this condition is doomed.[12] Let us look at the facts at the present time. In spite of a number of exaggerated claims, it is the case that only about 40% or so of abdominal aortic aneurysms can be dealt with by endovascular techniques.[13] Restrictions on the use of endografts relate to two areas, the first is the neck, where currently between 1–1.5 cm clearance between the renal arteries and the sac is advised. The exact length of this area needed to promote a good seal is not based on any data but appears to have evolved as time has gone by. Attempts to use shorter and shorter necks without these data has resulted in an illogical extension of uncovered stents into the aorta above the renal arteries. I am not sure how this migration of a stent in a cephalad direction is going to allow aneurysms with shorter and shorter necks to be treated. The vital question is how much of a neck is necessary to avoid leakage and allow a better seal – not how far up the aorta can the stent extend. I suspect, therefore, that attempts to deal with the problem of a short neck in this way will simply lead to increasing levels of endoleakage and surgical treatment of aneurysms with a short neck will continue to be the better option for some time to come. Other problems which include the possibility of neck enlargment, what size neck we should start treating at, etc all remain unresolved and this area is one where open surgery will continue to be pre-eminent. The other area where problems arise is in the iliac arteries where at present the majority view is that the internal iliac artery should be revascularized. With this in mind any iliac artery which is larger than about 16mm in diameter is difficult to treat, particularly if the aneurysm extends into the bifurcation area. In this situation the only solution is to use a uni-iliac graft with a crossover as an alternative to open surgery.[14,15] This may be the solution to the problem and can allow up to 70% of patients to be treated in this way. However its long-term complication rate and durability remains to be proven.

Let us not forget that at the present time the endoleak [Fig. 2] rate in patients treated by endovascular repair is about 10%[16] and a number of stent-graft combinations are dislocating because of sac shrinkage.[17] Material is also breaking and metal stents disintegrating.[18] The recently started UK trial to compare fit and unfit patients with open surgery or best medical treatment may provide the answer to many of these questions including the question of costs. At present the cost of these devices is such that open surgery is an attractive alternative. For all of these reasons, I suspect that open surgery for aneurysms has a long way to run yet. Eventually it may become the case that about half of these lesions will be dealt with by endocascular means and the rest by open surgery.

Suprarenal and thoracoabdominal aneurysms may also be dealt with by endovascular techniques. It is true tha aneurysms of the descending thoracic aorta are easily treated by endovascular means. The rates of paraplegia, other complications and mortality are reduced compared with open repair[19] but the long-term performance of these grafts remains unknown. Type 2 thoracic aneurysms have a high mortality and complication rate and endovascular repair may turn out to be better here. Type 4 lesions are best treated surgically but ingenuity in the production of grafts with branches which may fit into the visceral arteries could happen but not I suspect in the foreseeable future and surgery will remain the mainstay here. More than half of the aneurysmal lesions we see will, therefore, still need open repair for the foreseeable future. The problem is going to be how to ensure that enough surgeons are trained properly to deal with the remaining open procedures because

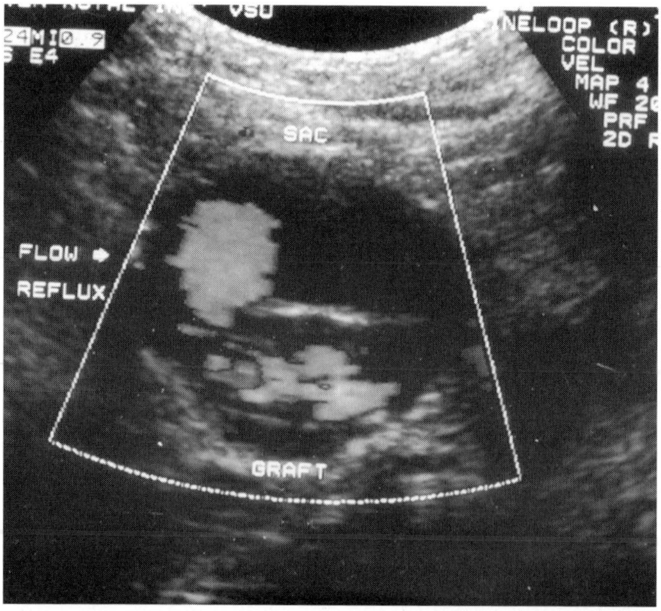

Fig. 2. Duplex examination of a stent graft showing an endoleak.

the number of cases needing surgery will be reduced and therefore the training opportunities will be fewer.

No one knows whether renal artery disease is worth treating at all, although there are thousands of stents inserted[20] and angioplasties performed every year. Whether these do any good for the patient in terms of improvement in renal function or hypertension remains unknown. There are a number of complex lesions of the aorta and renal artery involvement which are better treated by surgical techniques and will continue to be dealt with in this way. However, the number of operations needing to be done will inevitably be reduced and it will be particularly important to establish centres where operations are done by surgeons dealing with large numbers of cases rather than the occasional operation being done locally.

If we now turn to the lower limb which is the source of a good deal of our work, endovascular techniques have not in general proved to be useful in treating such patients. With the exception of the iliac arteries, angioplasty of stenoses or occlusions of <5cm in length are effective for a short time[21] but most of these patients would not have an operation in any case because of mild claudication. For longer occlusions [Fig. 3] the use of stent-graft combinations in above-knee occlusions has proved uncertain with relatively poor primary and secondary patency rates compared with femoropopliteal grafting.[22,23] This is partly because of intimal hyperplasia which might be solved in the future but the technique in any case remains very expensive. Distal disease involving the crural arteries is so far not treatable by stent-graft techniques. The one thing that is a threat to open surgery is subintimal angioplasty [Fig. 4]. This technique can be used successfully in the femoropopliteal[24] and crural vessels.[25] At present a number of centres do not seem to be able to use this technique

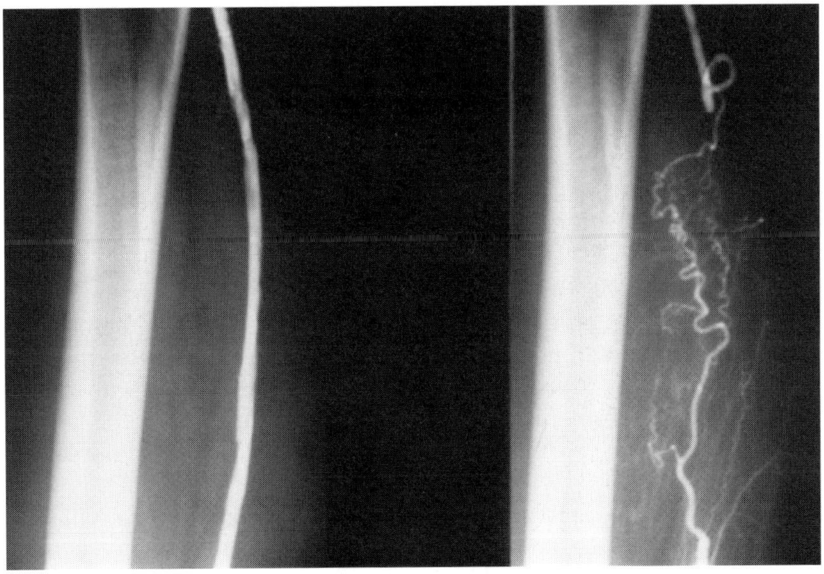

Fig. 3. A long occlusion unsuitable for intraluminal angioplasty before and after subintimal angioplasty.

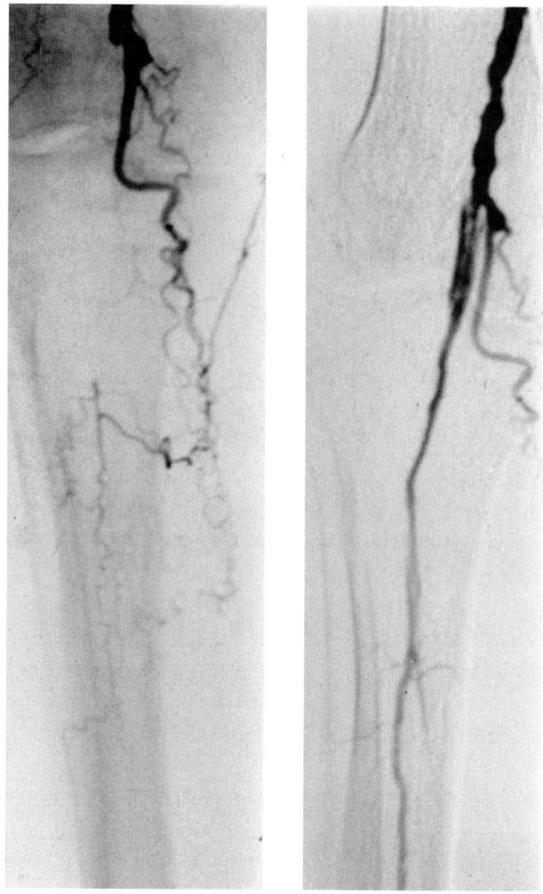

(a) (b)

Fig. 4. Subintimal angioplasty of a crural occlusion (a) before and (b) after treatment.

successfully but for those that do it has reduced the incidence of femorodistal grafting by 60%.[26] However, even in those centres there still remains a significant number of patients who will need femorodistal grafting. Again the question of how to train surgeons to do the procedure adequately when the numbers needing surgery are reducing remains a problem. Operative surgery in this area of the leg will remain with us for a long time, particularly as the exact place of angioplasty remains unresolved and comparisons with surgery have not been made.

For those who may be depressed by the fact that open surgery will probably be reduced by half, it is important to remember the thoracic outlet syndrome and cervical or first rib removal [Fig. 5]. There are surgeons both in this country and abroad who have made this into a specialty and as far as I can tell, there is no way at present of replacing this with endovascular techniques. I suspect there will be an

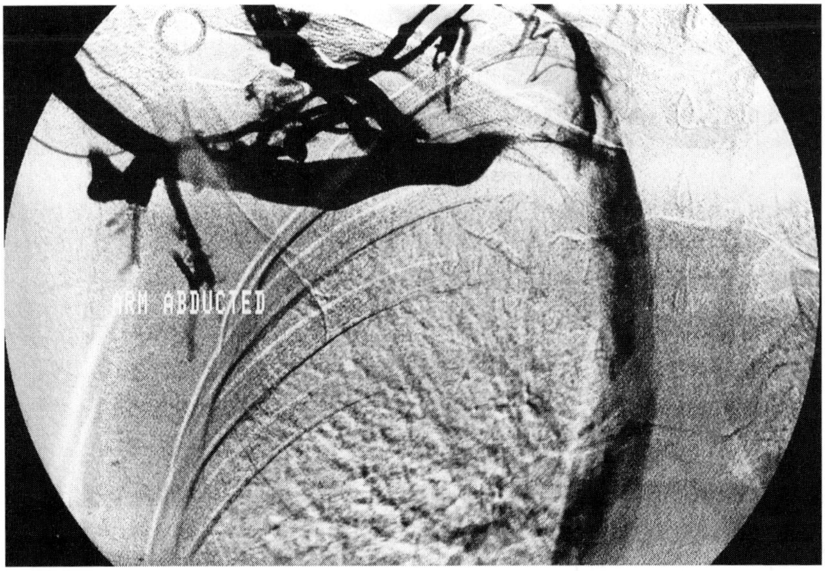

Fig. 5. Thoracic outlet syndrome. Abduction of the arm causing venous compression.

increase in the number of ribs being removed in this way; at present I think we are undertreating this condition.

On the plus side, we should not forget the emergence of laparoscopic vascular surgery.[27] Although this has few obvious applications at present, it is an area which needs to be expanded and could be used in association with endovascular techniques to achieve better results. It could, for example, be used to place grafts between the thoracic aorta and the groins in certain patients. It might be useful to reduce endoleaks or allow clips to be placed on lumbar arteries. It may perform better when compared with endovascular techniques in proper trails and be expanded in the future. I suspect it will become a direct competitor to endovascular surgery in the fullness of time. Any young vascular surgeon would be well advised to become trained in this area.

What about varicose veins? These will surely remain the backbone of vascular surgery. This is not necessarily the case and minimally invasive techniques which cauterize the vein rather than removing it are becoming more commonly practised. Whether these are better or worse than existing techniques remains to be proven. I suspect, however, the best technique will remain removal of these veins using smaller and smaller instruments and creating smaller and smaller scars with better imaging and localization of the veins which need to be removed. The treatment of deep vein problems remains a huge untapped area. Research into adequate venous replacement grafts and valves needs to be intensified in future.

Open surgery is therefore very much alive and kicking and will go on being necessary for many years to come. Endovascular procedures do go wrong and open operations are needed to salvage the situation. There are many patients who will outlive their endovascular operations and then require an open procedure thereafter. The problem is that these operations will be more difficult and the number of simple cases available to train surgeons will be less, making life difficult indeed. One other thing that should not be forgotten is that few if any of these techniques have been proven to be better than open surgery. We must become involved in more trails to show that surgery is as good as, better, or more cost-effective than endovascular techniques or the reverse. The era of unproved highly advertised untried techniques being used extensively should be brought to an end by proper trials.

REFERENCES

1. Earnshaw JJ: The endovascular revolution. *Ann Roy Coll Surg Eng* **79:** 308–309, 1997
2. Dietrich EB, Ndiayer M, Reid DM *et al.*: Stenting in the carotid artery: initial experience in 110 patients. *J Endovasc Surg* **3:** 42–62, 1996
3. Theron J, Curtheoux P, Alach F *et al.*: A new triple catheter system for carotid angioplasty with cerebral protection. *Am J Neuroradiol* **11:** 69–74, 1990
4. Naylor AR, Gaunt ME: Quality control during carotid endarterectomy. *Vasc Med* **1:** 125–132, 1996
5. Shah DM, Darling C III, Chenby B *et al.*: Carotid endarterectomy in awake patients, safety acceptability and outcome. *J Vasc Surg* **19:** 1015–1020, 1994
6. Naylor AR, Bolia A, Abbott R *et al.*: Randomised study of carotid angioplasty and stenting versus carotid endarterectomy. A stopped trial. *J Vasc Surg* **28:** 326–334, 1998
7. Otiki T, Marvin ML, Lyon RT *et al.*: *Ex vivo* lumen carotid bifurcation stenting: correlation of lesion characteristics with embolic potential. *J Vasc Surg* **3:** 467–471, 1998
8. North American Symptomatic Carotid Endarterectomy Trial Collaborators: Beneficial effect of carotid endarterectomy in symptomatic patients with high graft carotid stenosis. *New Engl J Med* **325:** 445–453, 1991
9. European Carotid Surgery Trialists Collaborative Group: MRC European Carotid Surgery Trial. Interim results for symptomatic patients with severe [70–90%] or mild [0–29%] carotid stenosis. *Lancet* **337:** 1235–1243, 1991
10. Gray BH, Sullivan TM, Childs MB: High incidence of restenosis/reocclusion of stents in the percutaneous treatment of long segment superficial femoral artery disease after suboptimal angioplasty. *J Vasc Surg* **25:** 74–83, 1997
11. Gillette EL, Powers BE, McChesney SL *et al.*: Response of aorta and branch arteries to experimental intraoperative irradiation. *Int J Radiat Oncol Biol Phys* **17:** 1247–1255, 1989
12. Mialhe C, Amicabile C, Becquemin JP *et al.*: Endovascular treatment of infra-renal abdominal aneurysms by the stentor system. Preliminary results of 79 cases. *J Vasc Surg* **26:** 199–209, 1997
13. Armon MP, Yusuf W, Latief K *et al.*: Anatomical suitability of abdominal aortic aneurysm for endovascular repair. *Br J Surg* **84:** 178–180, 1997
14. Ivancev K, Malina M, Lindblad B *et al.*: Abdominal aortic aneurysms: experience with the Ivancev–Malmo endovascular system for aortomonoiliac stent grafts. *J Endovasc Surg* **4:** 242–251, 1997
15. Thompson MM, Hartshorn T, Maltzeos C *et al.*: Comparison of computed tomography and duplex imaging in assessing aortic morphology following endovascular aneurysm repair. *Br J Surg* **85:** 346–350, 1998
16. Matsumura JS, Moore WS: Clinical consequences of periprosthetic leak after endovascular repair of abdominal aortic aneurysm. *J Vasc Surg* **27:** 606–613, 1998
17. Harris PL, Dimitri S: Predicting failure of endovascular aneurysm repair. *Eur J Vasc Endovasc Surg* **17:** 1–2, 1999

18. Riepe G, Heilberger P, Umscheid T *et al.*: Frame dislocation of body rings in endovascular stent tube grafts. *Eur J Vasc Endovasc Surg* **17:** 28–34, 1999
19. Dake MD, Miller DC, Semba CP *et al.*: Transluminal placement of endovascular stent grafts for the treatment of descending thoracic aortic aneurysms. *New Engl J Med* **331:** 1729–1734, 1994
20. Pattison JM, Reidy JF, Rafferty MJ *et al.*: Percutaneous transluminal renal angioplasty in patients with renal failure. *Q J Med* **85:** 883–888, 1992
21. Stanley B, Teague B, Raptis S *et al.*: Efficacy of balloon angioplasty of the superficial femoral artery and popliteal artery in the relief of leg ischaemia. *J Vasc Surg* **23:** 679–685, 1996
22. Spoelstra H, Casselman F, Lesceu O *et al.*: Balloon expandable endobypass for femoropopoliteal atherosclerotic occlusive disease. A preliminary evaluation of 55 patients. *J Vasc Surg* **24:** 647–654, 1996
23. Ho GH, Moll FL, Hederman PH *et al.*: Endovascular remote endarterectomy in femoropopliteal occlusive disease: one year clinical experience with a ring strip cutter device. *Eur J Vasc Endovasc Surg* **12:** 105–112, 1996
24. Bolia A, Miles KA, Brennan J *et al.*: Percutaneous transluminal angioplasty of occlusions of the femoral and popliteal arteries by subcutaneous dissection. *Cardiovasc Intervent Radiol* **13:** 357–363, 1990
25. London NJM, Srinivasan R, Varty K *et al.*: Infrapopliteal angioplasty. A safe and successful procedure. *Br J Surg* **80:** 530–532, 1993
26. Varty K, Nydahl S, Butterworth P *et al.*: Changes in the management of critical limb ischaemia. *Br J Surg* **83:** 953–956, 1996
27. Said Samir, Moll J, Frank R: Laparoscopic aortofemoral bypass grafting: human cadaveric and initial clinical experience. *J Vasc Surg* **29:** 639–649, 1999

Endovascular first, please

Krassi Ivancev, Sunita Srivastava, Timothy Resch, Petr Uher, Mats Lindh, Bengt Lindblad

INTRODUCTION

During the last decade vascular surgery has undergone fundamental changes. These gradual and seemingly inevitable changes have resulted in a rapid transformation of the 'classical open' vascular surgery to endovascular treatment for a growing number of vascular diseases. The cause for this transformation has been the introduction of an angiographic technique, previously used mainly as a preoperative diagnostic tool, today employed as a therapeutic method for treatment of occlusive as well as aneurysmatic conditions. With all the changes this new technique has brought in the management of vascular patients, it is a little surprising that it has been met with reservation and questioning with regard to its effectiveness and safety. However, there is a growing body of evidence to suggest that this new treatment modality is associated with not only less trauma to the patient but also provides results competitive with open vascular surgery. Similar to laparoscopic surgery, the development of the endovascular technique has been driven by the need for reducing costs and suffering for the patient. This chapter will cover those fields in which endovascular treatment has been shown, in our opinion, to offer clear advantages over the open surgical alternative to be worthy of consideration as the first option of treatment.

STENT TREATMENT OF OCCLUSIVE AORTOILIAC ATHEROSCLEROTIC DISEASE CAUSING SEVERE CLAUDICATION

Traditionally, claudication caused by occlusive aortoiliac disease has been treated by exercise and platelet aggregation inhibitors. When these measures have been shown to be insufficient, these patients have been offered surgically placed aortobifemoral grafts or femorofemoral bypasses. Though patency rates for these procedures have been excellent at 5-year follow-up, i.e. in the range of 85–90% for aortobifemoral grafts and 75–80% for femorofemoral bypasses, the morbidity and mortality associated with this treatment has not been negligible.

When stents were introduced approximately 10 years ago, it became obvious that not only was it useful to supplement failed percutaneous transluminal angioplasty (PTA) with stents but that they could be used for recanalization of complex lesions and occlusions in the aortoiliac segment as primary treatment. Since then an increasing number of reports have been published in the literature showing that stent treatment in this region provides results comparable with open surgery and associated with less morbidity and mortality.[1-7]

We started using stents routinely in occlusive aortoiliac lesions in claudicants in 1992. Since then we have treated 206 patients with 262 limbs at risk until 1998. The treatment was performed by four vascular radiologists. The patients were 163 men and 99 women of mean age of 65 years (range 42–85 years). The indication for treatment was claudication at the following distances: less than 50 m – 81 limbs, between 50 and 200 m – 143 limbs and more than 200 m – 34 limbs. In four limbs, stents were placed in the contralateral common iliac artery without symptoms for technical reasons. Among the symptomatic limbs there were five limbs presenting with 'blue toe' syndrome as an evidence of microembolization. Stenting was performed secondary to occlusions in 84 limbs, complex stenoses in 154 limbs, failed PTA in 19 limbs, and restenoses after previous PTA in five limbs. The main reasons for primary stenting in the majority of the lesions have been because of the advantages offered by the stents over simple PTA, especially with respect to recanalization of long, complex stenoses and occlusions. These advantages include improved end result along with equal trauma when employing the current technology of balloons, stents, stent-grafts and introducer sheaths. The stented arteries were as follows: common iliac artery 129 limbs, external iliac artery 92 limbs and a combination of common iliac artery and external iliac artery 41 limbs.

The aortic bifurcation was reconstructed on 50 occasions. The stents used evolved over time but, in general, balloon-expandable stents – Palmaz (Johnson & Johnson Interventional Systems Co, Warren, NJ, USA) in the beginning and Jomed subsequently – were used for precision placement, while self-expandable stents – i.e. Wallstents (Scheider [Europe] AG, Bülach, Switzerland) initially and Memotherm (Angiomed GmbH, Karlsruhe, Germany) stents later – were used for long lesions to cover long distances. Occasionally a combination of stents was applied.

There was one technical failure and no 30-day perioperative mortality. Only one minor complication occurred involving transitory microembolization which improved without treatment. There were major complications, requiring treatment or prolonging hospital stay, occurring in 10 of 206 treated patients (or 5%). These included haematoma requiring surgery (n = 4), pseudoaneurysm (n = 2), thrombosis requiring thrombolysis (n = 1), surgical embolectomy (n = 1), rupture treated with stent-graft (n = 1), and moderate renal function impairment (n = 1). All complications were successfully managed. The patients were evaluated clinically and with ankle brachial index measurements prior to intervention, at discharge and 1, 3 and 12 months after intervention.

During the first year of follow-up there were nine patients who required reinterventions, including redo PTA in five patients, new stent placement in three patients and thrombolysis followed by stent placement in one patient (Fig. 1). In addition there were 15 of 262 limbs (5.7%) in which the stented vessels occluded, which in turn required additional surgical procedures. There were 34 limbs lost to follow-up and another 54 limbs waiting to be evaluated. This has resulted in 153 limbs available for evaluation at 1-year follow-up. The primary and secondary patency rates at 1-year follow-up were 89% and 94% respectively. The corresponding condition of the limbs included improvement in 134 limbs (markedly 50, moderately 41, and minimally 43 limbs) whereas an unchanged condition was observed in ten limbs and worsening condition occurred in nine limbs (mildly four, moderately four, and markedly worse in one limb).

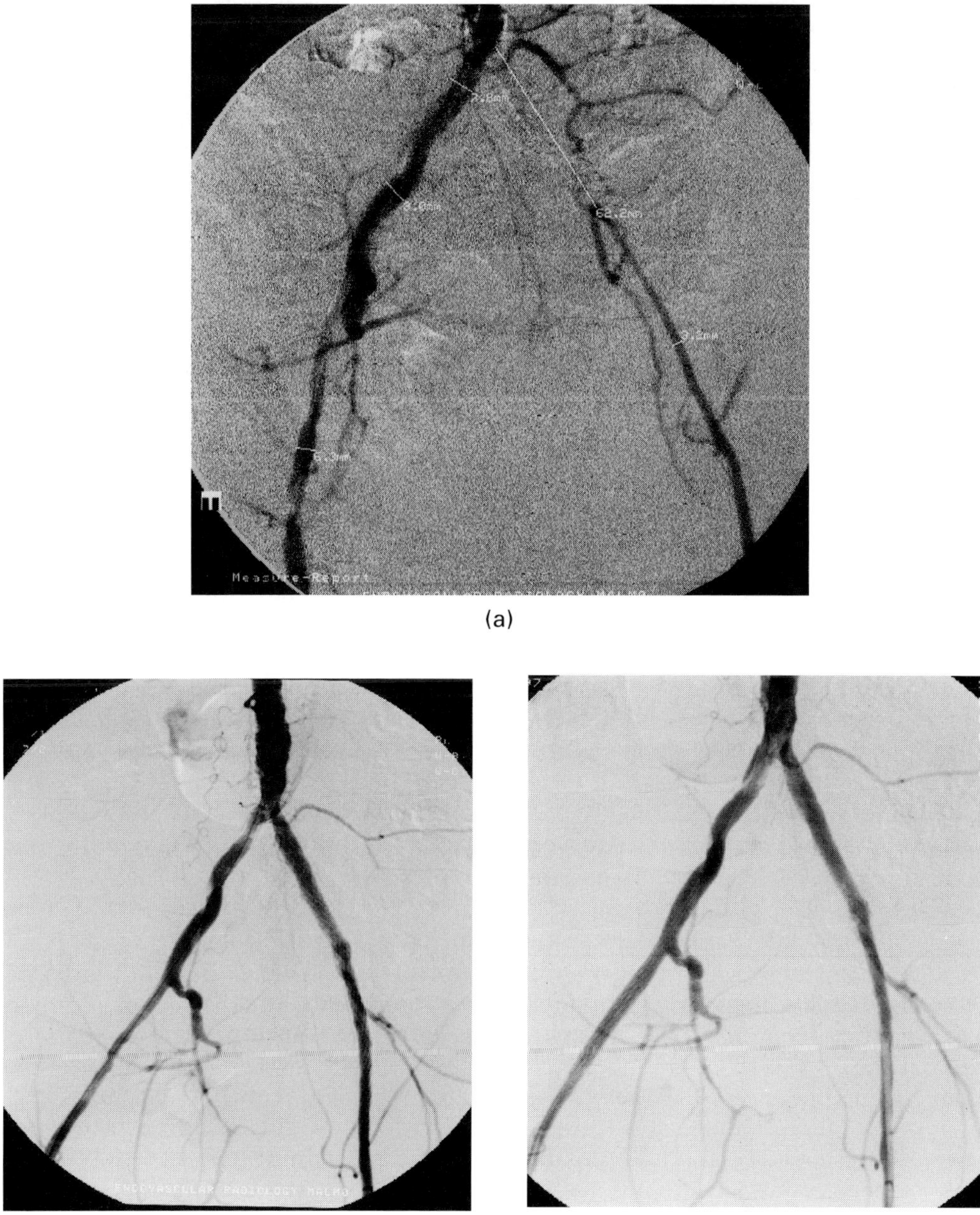

(a)

(b) (c)

Fig. 1. A 68-year-old female presented with renal insufficiency and previous lung transplantation with severe left lower extremity claudication caused by left common iliac occlusion. Angiography was performed with CO_2 (a). Six months after left common iliac stent placement, the patient developed moderate right lower extremity claudication. Stenoses are noted in previously stented common iliac artery and also in external iliac artery (b) which responded to PTA of the common iliac and stenting of the external iliac lesion (c).

In conclusion, the presented results are in strong agreement with those previously published.[1–7] This has led us to consider primary stenting of occlusive lesions in the aortoiliac segment causing intractable claudication to be the first choice of treatment for these patients (Fig. 1). Similar lesions causing critical ischaemia may also be treated by primary stenting. However, this group of patients is usually in a more advanced stage of occlusive atherosclerotic disease and therefore often in need of additional open surgical procedures.

SYMPTOMATIC CHRONIC VENOUS OCCLUSIONS IN THE ILIOFEMORAL AND INFERIOR VENA CAVA VEINS TREATED BY STENT RECANALIZATION

Chronic occlusions of the inferior vena cava and the iliofemoral veins may cause symptoms depending on the degree of development of collaterals. When symptoms developed they presented as either acute deep venous thrombosis in the legs, i.e. below the level of the occluded veins or as chronic ones. The symptoms include a combination of severe leg oedema, non-healing ulcers, claudication and rest pain. They are often worsened by coexisting post-thrombotic changes in the leg veins from previous deep venous thrombosis. Traditionally, conservative management consisting of chronic anticoagulation therapy and manoeuvers to relieve symptoms has been the main treatment offered to these patients. Little has been done to address the underlying causes. Surgical reconstruction of the inferior vena cava and the iliac veins has proven to be difficult and frustrating. Though recent improvements have been made in surgical techniques and conduits, the overall results are disappointing. Therefore, primary recanalization with stents of central chronic venous occlusions has become an attractive option.[8–13]

Since 1994 we have treated 33 patients with symptomatic chronic venous occlusions in the iliofemoral and inferior vena cava veins by stent recanalization. There were 15 men and 18 women with a median age of 40 years (range 19–69 years). Fourteen patients presented with acute deep venous thrombosis of the legs requiring initial thrombolysis. Seventeen patients had chronic symptoms from a post-thrombotic syndrome and presented with the following symptoms: severe claudication (n = 2), venous ulcers (n = 6), severe oedema (n = 22), pain (n = 13) and phlegmasia (n = 4). In the remaining two patients, one presented with ascites due to Budd–Chiari syndrome whereas the other had malfunctioning kidney transplant due to stenotic common iliac vein. The most frequently used stent was Wallstent (n = 36), followed by Palmaz (n=10) and Memotherm stent (n = 4). The most commonly stented sites were the left iliac veins, performed in 18 patients. In nine patients, the inferior vena cava was either partially (n = 7) or completely recanalized with stents (n = 2) due to occlusion or incomplete spontaneous recanalization (Fig. 2). In the remaining six patients, the right iliac veins were stented. Notably, in 13 patients it was necessary to place the stents under the inguinal ligament in order to secure adequate inflow (Fig. 2). Prestent placement venogram with pressure measurements and duplex were used to confirm clinical diagnosis. In selected cases computed tomography was performed to identify the underlying venous anatomy in the abdomen.

The follow-up consisted of clinical evaluation and duplex at 1, 3, 6 months and

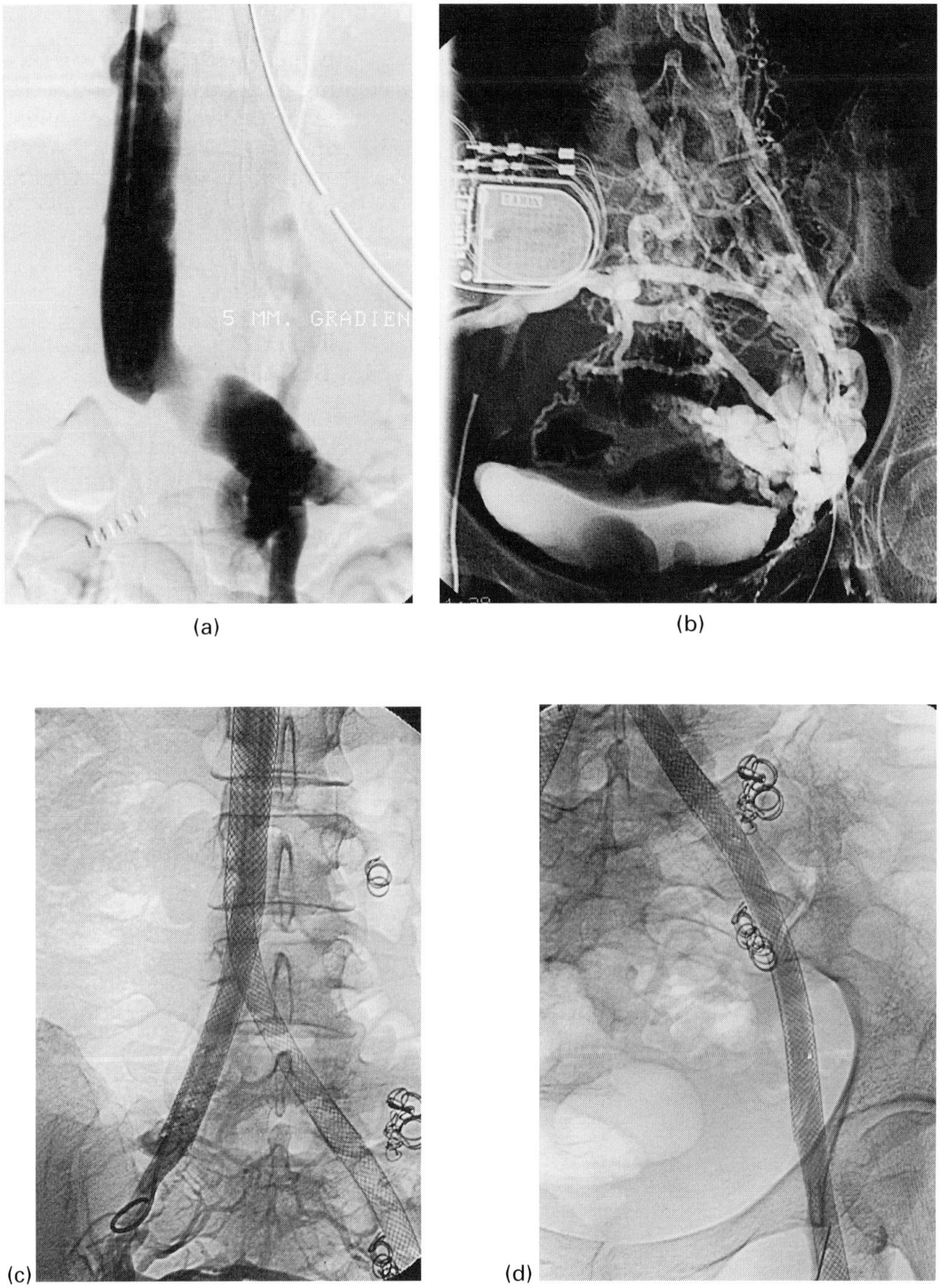

Fig. 2. A 36-year-old female after right nephrectomy for Wilms' tumour. Total occlusion of infrarenal inferior vena cava and bilateral iliac veins (a and b). One-year follow-up after ovarian vein coil embolization and stent recanalization; there is unimpeded flow throughout the reconstructed inferior vena cava and iliac veins (c and d).

annually thereafter. Venogram with pressure measurements was performed at 6-months follow-up and whenever clinically indicated. The mean follow-up was 17.3 months (range 0.5–60 months). The primary patency rate was 70% (23 patients of 33) and secondary patency was 88% (29 patients of 33). In the remaining four patients (12%) the stents thrombosed. However, no further attempts were made to recanalize them because the patients' symptoms were not considered severe enough to justify associated risks with additional thrombolysis and reinterventions. With respect to symptom improvement, there were eight patients who made complete recovery, 16 patients who experienced considerable improvement, five patients whose improvement was only moderate and four patients whose symptoms remained unchanged. There was only one complication consisting of a retroperitoneal haemorrhage requiring blood transfusion in one patient who was undergoing thrombolysis.

In conclusion, recanalization of chronic venous occlusions appears feasible and safe. This is the only treatment modality which provides improvement of symptoms in the majority of patients. It seems that the degree of improvement is dependent on the extent and severity of post-thrombotic changes which exist in the veins below the occlusions. In light of the fact that complete cure was achieved only in patients with presentation of acute symptomatic deep venous thrombosis, an aggressive and early approach including thrombolysis and adjunctive stenting may be justified in young patients with symptomatic deep venous thrombosis.

RENAL ARTERY INTERVENTIONS

Various methods of renal artery reconstruction have been described, ranging from endarterectomy to bypasses.[14–16] The operative mortality overall ranges from 1.4 to 5.6%.[15–16] with higher mortality in those reconstructions involving the aorta (8.1–13%). Overall patency in 5 years has ranged from 81 to 96% in most series.[15–17]

Percutaneous renal angioplasty (PTRA) has been successfully applied in several pathological states, namely, non-ostial lesions, lesions secondary to fibromuscular dysplasia and multiple stenotic lesions. Our own centre has reported excellent results with a procedural success rate of 85% and primary patency of 50%.[18–19] The initial complication rate, however, was high at 20% in 101 PTRA from 1979 to 1984.[18] The ensuing years have resulted in more experience, improvements in catheters and wires, with a resultant decrease in major complications. In most series, the complication rate from PTRA is now 3–4%.

The first prospective randomized study was reported by our institution in 1993, which compared PTRA with operative reconstruction among 58 patients during 1984–1990.[20] The primary patency for the operative group was 90% and in the PTRA group was 70%. The morbidity and mortality for both groups were not statistically different. Secondary patency over 24 months, however, was 95% in the operative group and 90% in the PTRA group. We have since continued to follow our patients and report 5-year results as follows: Among 86 patients who underwent operative procedure, 18 have required re-operation (21%) while 50 of 197 PTRA treated patients (25%) have required re-intervention. Thus, patency and the need for re-intervention have been the same although less invasive methods are needed with PTRA.

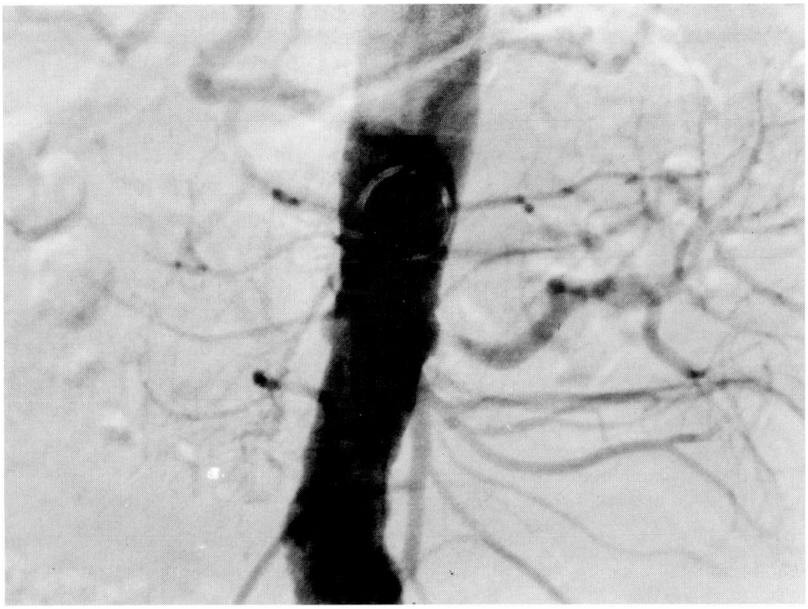

(a)

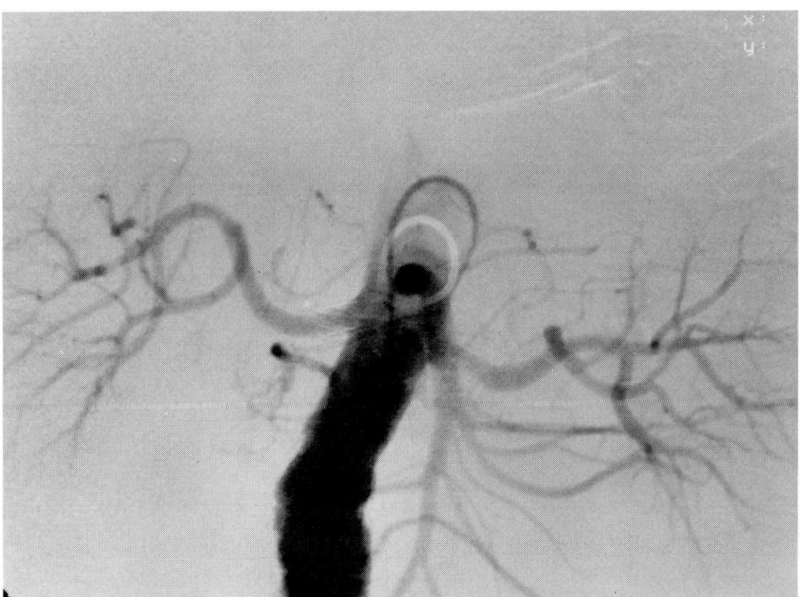

(b)

Fig. 3. A 70-year-old male with uncontrolled hypertension and moderately elevated creatinine. The angiogram shows occlusion of the right renal artery and moderate stenosis of the left renal artery without a pressure gradient (a). Angiogram at 6 months following recanalization of occluded right renal artery with bilateral well perfused kidneys (b).

Renal artery stents have been shown to be the treatment of choice in the settings of ostial lesions, failed angioplasty with residual stenosis or gradient, restenosis after PTRA and certainly in the treatment of PTRA complications such as dissection and thrombosis.[21–25] The complication rate for stenting remains low at 3% with experienced operators and its patency rates are clearly equal to surgery.[21–22, 24] Improvements in guiding catheters, wires and experience have led to satisfactory results with renal stents.

Our institution has examined 136 patients in 1994–1996 and identified a 25% rate of restenosis after PTRA and 16% rate of restenosis after PTRA and stent placement. We have found that in those patients with a good radiographic result and without a pressure gradient, the risk of restenosis after PTRA is low. If there is a residual 4–5 mmHg mean pressure gradient after PTRA, the risk of restenosis was two to three times higher.

The third group of patients that we have treated non-operatively includes those with renal artery occlusions. In the past, these patients were only offered a surgical option. In the last 3 years, we have recanalized 12 patients with renal artery occlusions with success in all but one patient. The long-term results are yet to be evaluated (Fig. 3). The improvement in sheaths and various wire options have allowed us to use aggressive endovascular manoeuvers for this patient population.

The treatment of renal artery stenosis has changed drastically in the last decade. With the advent of percutaneous techniques and improved equipment, renal artery angioplasty and stent have become the preferred approach. The procedural success rate and patency are comparable with surgical repair while the morbidity and mortality are lower. This impacts favourably on the length of hospital stay and costs of procedure. These treatment modalities do not jeopardize further surgical intervention if needed at a later date. Thus, the endovascular treatment is the optimal and first line approach to renal artery stenosis.

ENDOVASCULAR STENT GRAFTING OF ABDOMINAL AORTIC ANEURYSMS

In Malmö, we treated our first abdominal aortic aneurysm endograft patient in November 1993. Initially we, like many others, used stent-grafts designed with conventional aortic grafts in mind. The grafts (conventional Dacron fabric) were unsupported in their main portion and fixated in the proximal and distal ends by self-expanding Gianturco Z stents (COOK Europe, Bjaeverskov, Denmark). To improve fixation at the proximal attachment site four pairs of hooks and barbs were added to the stent. In the beginning, we developed a custom-made uni-iliac device that was combined with an occluder device in the contralateral iliac artery and a conventional femorofemoral crossover graft, known as the Ivancev–Malmö stent-graft.[26] Early on we also used a bifurcated stent-graft designed by Dr Chuter that, besides being bifurcated, shared many features of our own device.[27]

After overcoming some early technical difficulties, short-term results were promising and over 110 patients were successfully treated. However, during follow-up, problems started emerging.[28] The first complication was kinking of stent-graft limbs. This was the result of two factors: distal migration of the stent-graft and the

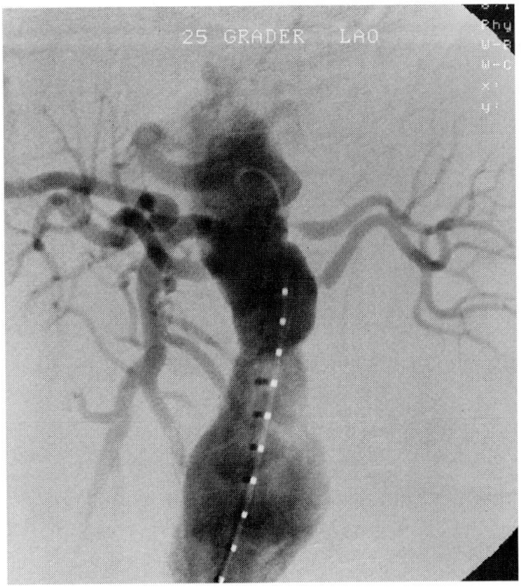

(a)

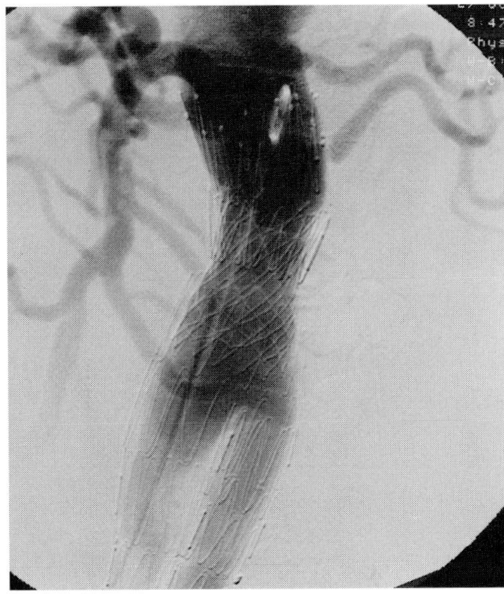

(b)

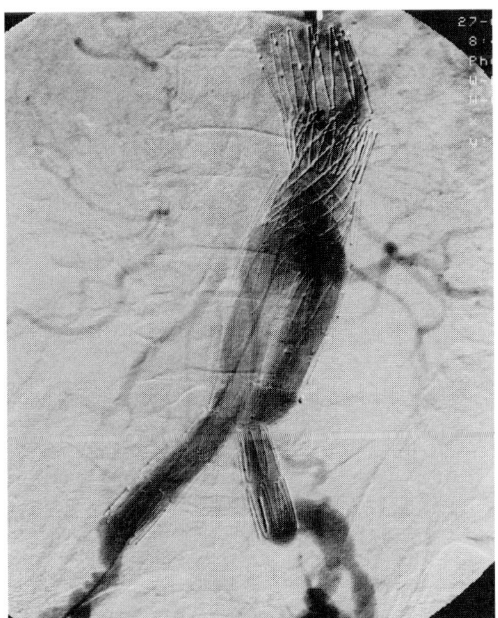

(c)

Fig. 4. Infrarenal abdominal aortic aneurysm with left renal artery stenosis (arrow) found on diagnostic angiogram in patient with uncontrolled hypertension (a). PTA performed in same setting. One year following successful endovascular repair of aneurysm demonstrating excluded aneurysm and patent left renal artery following PTA (b and c).

lack of columnar support. Whereas the kinks were often easily treated by placement of additional stents, the underlying problem of migration was more difficult to treat and prevent. The cause of migration seemed to be multifactorial and dependent on the stent-graft design and also on the dilating tendencies of the aortic neck.[29] In ten cases the migration was total, leaving the aneurysm sac unprotected from systemic pressure and necessitating late open conversion. Another major problem was endoleaks. In our early experience, the occluder device caused many endoleaks. Other graft-related endoleaks were seldom encountered because of careful patient selection and workup.[30]

These problems and the lessons that we have learned from them have made us develop and improve the stent-graft design. Experimental work suggested that reinforcement of the hooks and barbs on the proximal stent would improve fixation significantly.[31–32] Several studies indicated that transrenal stent-graft placement was safe and might improve fixation.[33] The high incidence of kinks and migration also made us use fully supported stent-grafts, which we have since proven to be important experimentally (M Malina *et al.* submitted ms). Finally, we have become more persistent in treating small intraoperative problems such as minor kinks or flow disturbances because we know these can cause major problems later on.

Since late 1997 we have been using our new device. It is a fully supported stent graft (multiple Z stents interconnected by a spiral wire) with the option of having the top stent uncovered for transrenal placement. The proximal stent carries eight sets of hooks and barbs that are longer and stronger than on the previous stent-grafts. In addition to this graft, we have been using the COOK Zenith stent-graft (COOK Europe, Bjaeverskov, Denmark) more frequently (Fig. 4). This graft utilizes the same principles that we have found clinically and experimentally to be important for good durability and, in addition, it is bifurcated and modular, which allows for vast customization. Our early results are promising:) 39 patients (11 custom-made device, 28 Zenith) have been treated. After a mean of 9 months follow-up (range 1–29 months) we have had no 30-day mortality and no immediate or late conversions. One proximal graft-related endoleak occurred, which was treated by placement of a giant Palmaz stent (Cordis/Johnson & Johnson). The incidence of perfusion endoleaks has been decreased to 10% compared with 20–25% in our previous series.

In conclusion, the introduction of fully stented stent-grafts with reinforced appendages on the proximal stent designed for suprarenal placement demonstrates very promising results. Further development in stent-graft fixation is bound to make this very rapidly evolving technique an option replacing open repair in 60–70% of all treatment for abdominal aortic aneurysms.

CONCLUSION

In our opinion, endovascular treatment offers clear advantages over open surgery, particularly with regard to treating symptomatic occlusive disease in the aortoiliac segment, renal arteries, as well as chronic venous occlusions. Regarding endovascular exclusion of abdominal aortic aneurysms the recent significant improvement of technology has resulted in outcomes which also suggest that for these patients the endovascular approach is the preferable modality of treatment.

REFERENCES

1. Vworek D, Gunther RW, Churmann K *et al.*: Aortic and iliac stenoses: Follow up results of stent placement after insufficient balloon angioplasty in 118 cases. *Radiology* **198:** 45–48, 1996
2. Palmaz J, Laborde JC, Rivera FJ *et al.*: Stenting of the iliac arteries with the Palmaz stent: Experience from a multicenter trial. *Cardiovasc Intervent Radiol* **15:** 291–297, 1992
3. Hausegger KA, Lammer J, Hagen B *et al.*: Iliac artery stenting – clinical experience with the Palmaz stent, Wallstent and Strecker stent. *Acta Radiologica* **33:** 292–296, 1992
4. Henry M, Amor M, Ethevenot G *et al.*: Palmaz stent placement in iliac and femoropopliteal arteries: Primary and secondary patency in 310 patients with 2–4 year follow up. *Radiology* **197:** 167–174, 1995
5. Murphy TP, Webb MS, Lambiase RE *et al.*: Percutaneous revascularization of complex iliac artery stenoses and occlusions with use of Wallstent: three year experience. *J Vasc Intervent Radiol* **7:** 21–27, 1996
6. Bergqvist D, Jendteg S, Johansen L *et al.*: Cost of long term complications of deep venous thrombosis of the lower extremities: An analysis of a defined patient population in Sweden. *Annl Intern Med* **126:** 454–457, 1997
7. Rilinger N, Gorich J, Mickley V *et al.*: Endovascular stenting in patients with iliac compression syndrome. *Invest Radiol* **31:** 729–733, 1996
8. Alimi YS, DiMauro P, Fabre D *et al.*: Iliac vein reconstructions to treat acute and chronic venous occlusive disease. *J Vasc Surg* **11:** 373–381, 1990
9. Irving JD, Dondelinger RF, Reidy JF *et al.*: Gianturco self expanding stents: Clinical experience in the vena cava and large veins. *Cardiovasc Intervent Radiol* **15:** 328–333, 1992
10. Elson JD, Becker GJ, Wholey MH *et al.*: Vena caval and central venous stenoses: Management with Palmaz balloon expandable intraluminal stents. *J Vasc Intervent Radiol* **2:** 215–223, 1991
11. Trerotola SO, Lund GB, Samphilipo MA *et al.*: Palmaz stent in the treatment of central venous stenosis: Safety and efficacy of redilation. *Radiology* **190:** 379–385, 1994
12. Åkesson H, Lindh M, Ivancev K *et al.*: Venous stents in chronic iliac vein occlusions. *Eur J Vasc Endovasc Surg* **13:** 334–336, 1997
13. Lakin PC, Rösch J: Stenting for the treatment of venous disease: Indications and results. *J Endovasc Surg* **2:** 396–397, 1995
14. Bergentz SE, Ericsson BF, Husberg B: Technique and complications in the surgical treatment of renovascular hypertension. *Acta Chir Scand* **145:** 143–147, 1979
15. Stanley JC, Whitehouse WM, Graham LM *et al.*: Operative therapy of renovascular hypertension. *Br J Surg* **69**(Suppl): S63–66, 1982
16. Cambria R, Brewster DC, L'Italien GJ *et al.*: Renal artery reconstruction for the preservation of renal function. *J Vasc Surg* **24:** 371–382, 1996
17. Erdoes LS, Berman SS, Hunter GC *et al.*: Comparative analysis of PTA and operation for renal revascularization. *Am J Kidney Dis* **27:** 496–503, 1996
18. Weibull H, Bergqvist D, Jonsson K *et al.*: Analysis of complication after percutaneous transluminal angioplasty of renal artery stenoses. *Eur J Vasc Surg* **1:** 77–84, 1987
19. Weibull H, Bergqvist D, Jonsson K *et al.*: Long term results after percutaneous transluminal angioplasty of atherosclerotic renal artery stenosis. The importance of intensive follow up. *Eur J Vasc Surg* **5:** 291–301, 1991
20. Weibull H, Bergqvist D, Bergentz SE *et al.*: Percutaneous transluminal renal angioplasty versus surgical reconstruction of atherosclerotic renal artery stenosis: A prospective randomized study. *J Vasc Surg* **18:** 841–852, 1993
21. Dorros G, Jaff M, Mathiak L *et al.*: Four year follow up of Palmaz stent revascularization as treatment for atherosclerotic renal artery stenosis. *Circulation* **98:** 642–647, 1998
22. Blum U, Krumme B, Flugel P *et al.*: Treatment of ostial renal artery stenoses with vascular endoprosthesis after unsuccessful balloon angioplasty. *New Engl J Med* **336:** 459–465, 1997
23. Fiala L, Jackson M, Gillespie D *et al.*: Primary stenting of atherosclerotic renal artery ostial stenosis. *Ann Vasc Surg* **12:** 128–133, 1998

24. Rees C: Stents for atherosclerotic renovascular disease. *J Vasc Intervent Radiol* **10:** 689–705, 1999
25. van de Ven PJ, Kaatee R, Beutler JJ *et al.*: Arterial stenting and balloon angioplasty in ostial atherosclerotic renovascular disease: a randomised trial. *Lancet* **353:** 282–286, 1999
26. Ivancev K, Malina M, Lindblad B *et al.*: Abdominal aortic aneurysms: experience with the Ivancev–Malmö endovascular system for aortomonoiliac stent-grafts. *J Endovasc Surg* **4:** 242–251, 1997
27. Chuter T, Wendt G, Hopkinson B *et al.*: European experience with a system for bifurcated stent-graft insertion. *J Endovasc Surg* **4:** 13–22, 1997
28. Ivancev K, Resch T, Brunkwall J *et al.*: Endoluminal repair of abdominal aortic aneurysms – a critical reappraisal after a three and a half year experience. *Semin Intervent Radiol* **15:** 97–108, 1998
29. Resch T, Ivancev K, Brunkwall J *et al.*: Distal migration of stent-grafts after endovascular repair of abdominal aortic aneurysms. *J Vasc Intervent Radiol* **10:** 257–264, 1999
30. Resch T, Ivancev K, Brunkwall J *et al.*: Mid-term changes in aortic aneurysm morphology after endovascular repair. *J Endovasc Surg* (in press).
31. Resch T, Malina M, Lindblad B *et al.*: The impact of stent-design on proximal stent-graft fixation in the abdominal aorta. An experimental study. *Eur J Vasc Endovasc Surg* (in press).
32. Malina M, Lindblad B, Ivancev K *et al.*: Will stents with hooks and barbs prevent stent-graft migration? *J Endovasc Surg* **5:** 310–317, 1998
33. Malina M, Brunkwall J, Lindblad B *et al.*: Endovascular management of the juxtarenal aortic aneurysm: can uncovered stents safely cross the renal arteries? *Semin Vasc Surg* **12:** 182–191, 1999

The need for patient-assessed measures of health outcome

Ian Russell, Andrew Garratt

INTRODUCTION

This chapter is a guide for those new to the measurement of health outcome and health-related quality of life. We begin by defining health outcomes and discussing the need to measure patients' perceptions of their health. We then consider different approaches to the measurement of health outcome and their potential applications. We conclude by describing the desirable attributes of outcome measures suitable for clinical evaluation and similar tasks.

Donabedian[1] defines a health outcome as a change in current or future health status that can be attributed to antecedent health care. This definition is useful but perhaps too narrow, for two reasons. First, merely to stabilize health often represents a good outcome. Second, health care is only one of many influences on health status. Others include cultural, social, economic and environmental factors.

Traditionally the outcomes of health care have been assessed within the biomedical model where outcome is defined in terms of the presence or absence of disease. At the individual level the consequences of disease are measured using objective biomedical measures that focus on disease and how it affects the body. At the population level the consequences of disease are defined in terms of mortality and the incidence and prevalence of morbidity. Sustained improvements in living standards and health technology have changed perceptions of health, reducing the validity of these measures of health outcome.[2]

In the first half of the twentieth century the test of advances in medical science lay in prolonging life. The change in emphasis from acute disease to chronic means that evaluation no longer compares active treatment with none, but new treatment with old. This has called into question the relevance of the biomedical model as a basis for measuring health. Dichotomous health outcomes like survival or death are limited in assessing chronic conditions like asthma or diabetes. Health care does not cure these conditions but aims to limit their consequences for the patient.[3] Traditional clinical, laboratory and radiological measures are less appropriate as measures of health outcome.[4–6] This change of emphasis has been reflected in changing definitions of the goals of health care – to give patients a more effective life[7] or to preserve functioning and well-being.[8,9]

As new technologies become available, the marginal benefits in health outcome diminish. This has created a demand for instruments that can detect the differences between alternative methods for treating patients. Clinical judgement is giving way to a more sensitive basis for assessing the effects of health care. Measures of health outcome must address these changing goals and be responsive to the improvements in health and quality of life that health care aims to provide. So traditional objective measures for assessing health need the complement of patients' subjective perceptions of their health.

The use of subjective perceptions to measure health has had limited recognition until recently. [10, 11] The measurement of these subjective perceptions is grounded in the belief that patients are the best judges of their health and can report these perceptions with accuracy.[12] There is a growing body of research to support this case.[13] Empirical research increasingly demonstrates the limitations of objective biomedical measurement and the contribution that subjective health perceptions can make to the evaluation of health care.[4,14,15] This trend coincided with developments in sampling and data analysis.[2,16] These methodological developments have played an increasing role in the development of measures of functional disability and handicap, of psychological well-being and, more recently, of general health and health-related quality of life.[2,17,18]

The World Health Organization [WHO][19] defined health as 'physical, psychological and social well-being'. This was originally criticised as being difficult to measure. More recently, however, the concept of health-related quality of life (HRQL) has addressed the WHO definition by covering health status and social well-being. It draws on theories from disciplines like economics, psychology and sociology.[20] By measuring patients' perceptions of health outcome it distinguishes the effects of health on quality of life from those of work and the environment.[21]

The measurement of HRQL is now recognized as a core component in the assessment of health outcome.[10,13] The rising importance of this activity is highlighted by the rapid increase in articles using the keywords 'quality of life'.[22] In the United Kingdom and the United States of America research into HRQL has been given further impetus through health care reforms. If managed competition is to be more than a cost containment strategy, evaluation must include the measurement of health outcome.

TAXONOMY OF HEALTH OUTCOME MEASURES

There are two main approaches to measuring patients' perceptions of their health – generic instruments that summarize their HRQL and specific instruments that focus on a particular disease or client group. Both approaches have strengths and weaknesses. Several groups have stressed the advantages from using the two in conjunction.[23–26]

Generic instruments cover many, if not all, conditions. Thus they can measure broad effects and co-morbidity. They can compare different groups of patients with general or disease-free populations.[27] In addition they can detect the side-effects of interventions that restricted specific instruments may not detect. This makes them useful for assessing new health care technologies whose effects are uncertain.

There are two main types of generic instrument – health profiles and health indices. Health profiles measure HRQL across distinct dimensions. Patients' responses to individual questions are scored and summed to measure their position on these dimensions. For example the Short-Form 36-item Health Survey [SF-36][11] measures health along eight dimensions – physical functioning, social functioning, role limitations due to physical and emotional problems, mental health, vitality, pain and general health. Responses to the 36 items are summed to produce eight scores between 0 and 100, where 0 is the worst possible and 100 is the best possible. The broad focus of such profiles permits comparisons across different conditions.[16,28] This is useful for some, but not all, forms of economic evaluation. For example cost-effectiveness analysis compares treatments by measuring their effects along one or more scales. The dimensions of a health profile can provide those scales.

In contrast cost-utility analysis focuses on the value or utility ascribed to individual health states. These utilities can be estimated either directly or indirectly. In direct estimation patients assess and value their current health state. There are many possible techniques for doing this, including the standard gamble and the time trade-off.[29] Both of these techniques need patients to imagine that there is a new treatment that can cure their condition. Both ask patients how much they would be prepared to sacrifice to receive this treatment. The standard gamble specifies that the treatment carries a risk R that patients will die immediately, and thus a probability (1-R) that they will revert to perfect health. In contrast the time trade-off specifies that the new treatment shortens patients' lives by a proportion T and leaves them with proportionately less time (1-T) in perfect health. Patients must judge how large R or T should be for them to be indifferent between accepting their current health state and accepting the new treatment and its associated risk or loss of longevity. Then the estimated utility of their health state is (1-R) or (1-T) respectively, where 1 is the utility of perfect health and 0 is the utility of death.

Indirect estimation initially resembles health profile measurement. Patients' responses to individual questions are scored and summed to measure their position on one or more scales and thus their current health status. These scores are converted into utilities using values estimated from independent surveys, typically of the

Table 1. The European Quality of Life Scale (EQ-5D)

Item	*No. of levels*	*Lowest response*	*Highest response*
Mobility	3	I have no problems in walking about	I am confined to bod
Self-care	3	I have no problems with self-care	I am unable to wash or dress myself
Usual activities (e.g. work, study, housework, family, leisure)	3	I have no problems with performing my usual activities	I am unable to perform my usual activities
Pain or discomfort	3	I have no pain or discomfort	I have extreme pain or discomfort
Anxiety or depression	3	I am not anxious or depressed	I am extremely anxious or depressed

Source: Ref. 30

Table 2. The Aberdeen Varicose Veins Scale

Item	*No. of levels*	*Lowest response*	*Highest response*
Please draw your varicose veins in the diagrams below	128[a]	None at all	Legs completely covered with veins
In the last 2 weeks for how many days did your varicose veins cause you pain or ache?	4 for each leg	None at all	More than 10 days
In the last 2 weeks at what *time* of day were your varicose veins usually *most* painful or aching?	5	Not painful at all	At night
In the last 2 weeks on how many days did you take pain-killing tablets for your varicose veins?	4	None at all	More than 10 days
In the last 2 weeks how much ankle swelling have you had?	4	None at all	Severe ankle swelling
In the last 2 weeks have you worn support stockings or tights?	4 for each leg	No	Yes – those prescribed which I wear every day
Do you take 'water tablets' for ankle swelling?	2	No	Yes
In the last 2 weeks have you had any itching in association with your varicose veins?	4 for each leg	No	Both above and below the knee
Do you have purple discoloration (caused by areas of tiny blood vessels in the skin) in association with your varicose veins?	2 for each leg	No	Yes

Do you have a rash or eczema in the area of your ankle?	3 for each leg	No	Yes – requires treatment from my doctor or nurse
Do you have a skin ulcer associated with your varicose veins?	2 for each leg	No	Yes
Does the appearance of your varicose veins cause you concern?	4	No	Yes – a great deal of concern
Does the appearance of your varicose veins influence your choice of clothes including tights?	4	No	Always
In the last 2 weeks have your varicose veins interfered with your work or other daily activities?	4	No	Yes – prevented from working for 1 day or more
In the last 2 weeks have your varicose veins interfered with your leisure activities (including sport, hobbies and social life)?	4	No	Yes – prevented from any leisure activities

Source: Ref. 38

[a] Assessed by a grid with 64 squares for each leg.

general public. For example the European Quality of Life Scale (EQ-5D) includes five three-point items covering mobility, self-care, usual activities, pain or discomfort, and anxiety or depression (Table 1). The general public has previously valued all 243 possible combinations of responses or states of health using the time trade-off technique mentioned above.[30] Whether health utilities are estimated indirectly by the EQ-5D or directly, they can be combined with data about the time that patients spend in each state of health to estimate the Quality Adjusted Life Years (QALYs) generated by the procedure being evaluated.[31]

In theory the narrow focus of specific instruments makes them more responsive or sensitive to clinically important changes in health. They can relate to a specific condition, disease, function, problem or population.[26,32] The wide range of conditions and diseases with specific instruments include asthma,[33] back pain,[34] end-stage renal disease,[35] rheumatoid arthritis,[36] rhinoconjunctivitis[37] and varicose veins[38] (Table 2). Functions and problems with specific instruments include daily living activities,[39] sexual functioning[40] and pain.[41] Populations with specific instruments include children[42] and the frail elderly.[32]

APPLICATION OF HEALTH OUTCOME MEASURES

There are three main reasons for measuring patients' health – discrimination, prediction and evaluation.[43] Only the last is concerned with health outcome in the sense in which we have defined it. Discriminatory instruments are used in cross-sectional studies to distinguish between different groups of patients, notably in diagnosis. For example the Hospital Anxiety and Depression Scale was designed to detect the presence of mood disorder in non-psychiatric hospital patients.[44] It has since been found useful in identifying similar patients in general practice.[45] Discriminatory instruments can also estimate the prevalence of disease in populations. For example the Nottingham Health Profile was proposed as a tool for assessing the health of populations.[46] However, criticism has focused on its inability to detect low levels of morbidity.[47] Predictive instruments are used in longitudinal studies to distinguish between different groups of patients, notably in screening. For example to improve the criteria for selecting patients for upper gastrointestinal endoscopy, Naji *et al.*[48] selected those variables that had the greatest power in predicting a 'useful' procedure.

This chapter focuses mainly on evaluative instruments, intended to measure health outcome in the assessment of policies, procedures or practice. Although they are used mainly within clinical trials, there are other useful applications. These include medical audit, patient monitoring especially in chronic disease, population studies, and resource allocation and policy decisions.[49,50] In principle, generic instruments are more appropriate for these wider functions because they can compare defined patient groups with population norms. Provided they are sensitive to differences, therefore, generic instruments are the most versatile.

The application of health outcomes has been predominantly in randomized trials.[12] These trials allocate patients at random, either to the experimental group who receive the treatment that is being evaluated, or to the control group who receive a comparable treatment. Both groups complete health outcome measures before and after treatment. Comparing the resulting changes in scores following treatment between the two groups assesses the relative effectiveness of the treatments. Although the need to include such measures in trial design is increasingly recognized, there is still scope for a much greater emphasis on these measures.[51,52]

DEVELOPMENT OF HEALTH OUTCOME MEASURES

The development of health profiles and specific health instruments generally follows the same sequence – item definition, response definition, item selection, combining items to form a scale, and testing empirically whether the scale fulfils methodological and practical criteria. These issues are discussed within both the psychometric literature[53] and that on health measurement.[54]

Streiner and Norman[54] offer several possible sources for items – clinical observation, expert opinion, interviews (with health professionals, patients and healthy people) and literature review. In addition novel concepts like the time trade-off technique need considerable developmental research. Some health profiles have used explicit definitions as a conceptual base. For example the McMaster Health Index Questionnaire[55] elaborates on the WHO definition of health.[19]

After identifying a pool of items comes the difficult task of defining the potential responses. The basic choice lies between binary, categorical, ordinal, interval and continuous responses. Other choices include the number of categories and the method of labelling these categories. The scales in Tables 1 and 2 both label all possible responses. The EQ-5D in Table 1 offers three responses for all five items. The Aberdeen Varicose Veins Scale in Table 2 offers 2, 3, 4 or 5 points depending on the nature of the item. Another common method is Likert scaling, in which respondents rate agreement with statements like 'my varicose veins restrict my social activities' on a scale with 5, 7, 9 or even 11 points ranging from 'strongly agree' to 'strongly disagree'. Also useful is semantic differential scaling, in which respondents rate their condition, for example varicose veins, on a scale in which the extreme points are labelled by two contrasting adjectives, for example from 'painful' to 'painless'.

Specific instruments usually select items derived in these ways to cover the entire range of concerns relevant to the particular condition.[34,37] If they are used alongside generic instruments, however, there may be replication. Other approaches to deriving specific instruments include modifying and supplementing generic instruments.[26] Modified generic instruments adapt relevant items to make them specific and remove irrelevant items.[56,57,58] Specific supplements to generic instruments take account of the generic domains and add domains of specific concern. These last two approaches avoid replicating items and reduce the burden on respondents.

All health outcome measures use some form of weighting in their construction. Weights are either explicit statements of relative value or else implicit in the combination of items. Explicit weights are typical of health indices and less common in other measures. While profiles and most specific instruments regard HRQL as a multidimensional concept, indices have to weight these dimensions to create a single utility. Direct estimation of weights is founded in decision analysis or economic theory. Indirect estimation uses the same principles to derive single indices from health profiles (e.g. Table 1). Approaches to implicit weighting, not mutually exclusive, include: clinical judgement; equal weighting of Likert or semantic differential items; psychometric techniques like factor analysis; and psychological theory like latent trait theory.[54,59]

To be useful, outcome measures must satisfy four main criteria – validity, reliability, responsiveness and practicality. Validity is the ability to measure what is intended. Reliability is the ability to measure consistently. Responsiveness is the ability to detect clinically important changes in health. Finally instruments must be practical – easy to administer and simple for patients to complete. Instruments for research should satisfy more rigorous methodological criteria but less stringent practical criteria than instruments for routine use.

RELIABILITY

Reliability assesses whether health outcome scores can be reproduced, for example on different occasions or by different observers.[54] There are two broad approaches to assessing reliability – internal consistency and test-retest. Tests of internal consistency are appropriate for scales that comprise many related items, namely most specific instruments and the individual dimensions of health profiles. These tests assess reliability at a single time by measuring the extent to which these items yield consistent scores. Item-total correlations achieve this by estimating the correlation between individual items and the remainder of the scale. Cronbach's Alpha averages these correlations across all the items in the scale. However internal consistency should not be the sole criterion of reliability because it cannot take account of variation over time in patients whose health has not changed.[43,54]

Test-retest reliability is designed to take account of variation over time. It assesses the level of agreement between two sets of scores derived from the same group of patients on two separate occasions. The design of test-retest studies raises three issues: the choice of interval between test and retest; the procedure for patients who actually change over that interval; and the correct method of statistical analysis. The shorter the interval between test and retest, the less likely that patients' health will have changed. However, there is a danger that responses to the first test will influence responses to the retest.[46] Researchers therefore extend the interval and try to identify patients who do not change, both indirectly through clinical judgement or laboratory tests and directly through explicit questions. These questions usually consist of a single item that assesses whether there has been any change in the health dimension in question.

The traditional method of quantifying test-retest reliability is to correlate scores from successive administrations and quote Pearson's correlation coefficient. However, this is theoretically inferior to the intra-class correlation coefficient, which takes account of other sources of variation.[60] Fortunately these two methods usually result in similar estimates of reliability.[54] Standards for either of these reliability coefficients vary. For decisions about groups of patients, Helmstadter[61] recommends a reliability coefficient of at least 0.5 while Nunnally[62] recommends 0.7. Decisions about individual patients require a greater level of reliability than decisions about groups. Streiner and Norman[54] therefore recommend 0.95.

VALIDITY

Establishing an instrument's reliability or reproducibility is necessary, but not sufficient, to assess its usefulness. Differences in scores on a health outcome measure may be reliable but do not necessarily reflect differences in health. While consistency with theory or expert opinion is an important aspect of validity, empirical testing is essential.[62] New instruments, refined instruments and instruments that are being used in a new context all need empirical tests of validity.

There are three main approaches to validation – content, criterion and construct.[54] Content validity measures the adequacy of the sample of items included in the instrument in spanning the entire range of concerns relevant to the particular condition. It is simply assessed: the more representative of the domain of interest is the sample of items, the stronger the inferences that can be drawn.

Criterion validity compares the instrument directly with a criterion variable or 'gold standard'. It is known as concurrent validity when the criterion is available at the same time as the instrument, for example when a measure is being shortened to reduce completion times and respondent burden. It is known as predictive validity when this criterion will become available in future, for example when an instrument to measure cardiovascular risk is compared with subsequent cardiovascular events. Tests of criterion validity are rare in the measurement of health outcomes because gold standards are themselves rare.

Instead validity is usually assessed by examining the relationship between the instrument and relevant, but not directly observable, variables known as 'constructs'. Such a relationship does not need to be as strong as that with a criterion variable. Instead one is testing whether the instrument is consistent with established theories. Thus construct validity rests not on a single powerful experiment but on a series of experiments that lend validity to the instrument. There are three main methods of establishing construct validity – extreme groups, and convergent and discriminant validity. The method of extreme groups is used when theory suggests that one subgroup of patients possesses more or less of the attribute in question. In assessing the SF-36 scale of mental health, for example, Anderson *et al.*[63] showed that patients with mental illness had a significantly lower mean score than those who were free from mental illness. Convergent validity occurs when two instruments that measure a similar, but not the same, attribute are positively related. Discriminant validity occurs when instruments that measure different or unrelated attributes are related negatively or not at all.

RESPONSIVENESS

Responsiveness is the ability of an instrument to detect clinically important changes in health.[64,65] Until recently research into health outcome measurement has focused on validity and reliability and given little attention to responsiveness.[66] Furthermore there is no standard method of assessing responsiveness.[52,60] It is helpful to group the available methods according to the design for studying responsiveness, and the statistical technique for quantifying responsiveness.

There are two main types of study design – using external variables to characterize changes in patients' health, and giving patients an intervention of known efficacy. External variables have themselves been used in two ways. First, changes in the scores generated by the instrument under review have been correlated with changes in external variables in tests of 'longitudinal validity'.[43] Second, external criteria discriminate between patients whose health changes or remains the same over time. For example patients or clinicians judge whether their health has changed over a given interval – a valid way of identifying patients for whom responsiveness is relevant.[67] This approach has successfully assessed the responsiveness of several instruments.[64,68,69]

The alternative approach to assessing responsiveness is to administer instruments to patients undergoing an intervention known to improve health.[70,71] For example Liang *et al.*[72] compared the responsiveness of generic and specific instruments in 38 patients with end-stage arthritis undergoing total joint arthroplasty. Patients completed instruments before the intervention and at 3 and 12 months thereafter.

Methods proposed for quantifying the responsiveness of outcome measures include: receiver operating characteristic (ROC) curves,[69] the index of responsiveness,[65] mean differences and significance levels,[73] standardized response means,[72] and effect sizes.[74] The relative merits of these different approaches are still not fully understood.[60]

ROC curves assess the ability of quantitative scales to predict an external dichotomous criterion by plotting their sensitivity and specificity as the corresponding internal criterion changes. They normally assess diagnostic tests. However, Deyo and Inui[68] used ROC curves to assess the ability of the Sickness Impact Profile (SIP)[75,76] and the American Rheumatism Association functional classification to predict clinicians' and patients' judgements whether their health had changed. Although this approach allows statistical comparisons of responsiveness across instruments, it requires that patients fall into two groups – those who change and those who do not. Hence it cannot compare instruments in terms of responsiveness to the size of change.

Guyatt *et al.*[73] used mean differences and associated significance levels to assess the responsiveness of instruments in assessing patients with inflammatory bowel disease. Their external criterion was 'global' in the sense that it considered patients' *general* health. Nevertheless the smallest significance levels, and thus the highest responsiveness, arose from a condition-specific instrument rather than measures of physical and emotional function. This approach is also limited by its use of significance levels, which are difficult to interpret.

The effect size is equal to the mean change in scores divided by the standard deviation of the baseline scores. Fitzpatrick *et al.*[77] used effect sizes to compare generic and specific instruments in a study of patients with rheumatoid arthritis. Their external criterion was 'specific' in the sense that patients rated whether their *disease* had changed. A more sophisticated variant of this approach is Guyatt and colleagues'[65] index of responsiveness. This uses the same numerator but takes as denominator the standard deviation of score changes among stable patients. A compromise between the effect size and the index of responsiveness is the standardized response mean (SRM).[72] This takes as denominator the standard deviation of score changes across all patients. Katz *et al.*[71] used SRMs to compare the responsiveness of short and long instruments in patients undergoing total hip arthroplasty. The improvements in health expected from the arthroplasty provided the criterion for judging the responsiveness of different instruments.

PRACTICALITY

Practicality is important in selecting instruments for particular applications. Many generic measures are too long for clinical settings, where patients are sicker than the general population and time is limited.[28] For example the SIP consists of 136 items and takes 30 minutes to complete.[75] Long instruments also suffer from reduced response rates and reliability. Stewart *et al.*[28] therefore recommended that generic instruments should describe a wide range of general functioning and well-being, achieve high standards of reliability and validity, and be simple and easy to use. In response three short multi-item measures suitable for self-completion – the Duke Health Profile,[78] the SF-36,[11] and the SF-12[79] – were derived from longer measures. They aim to retain the original levels of validity and reliability despite the constraints associated with large studies in clinical settings. Such measures also increase the scope for using complementary specific instruments, which are more responsive to changes in health, at least in theory.

Practicality also depends on the mode of administration. Health outcome measures can be completed in three basic ways – by patients themselves or by interview over the telephone or face to face. Self-completion generally achieves lower response rates than both types of interview. Nevertheless the substantial reduction in cost makes it the most practical approach to health outcome measurement for most purposes.[17] Furthermore instruments suitable for self-completion can be given to patients or distributed by post; and patients can still be followed by postal survey after treatment is complete. Even so self-completion may not be suitable if the instrument is complex or patients are unable to complete it themselves through illness or cognitive problems. In deciding between different modes of administration, one should therefore appraise the benefits and costs of each.

Some patients are too ill, confused or young to complete instruments even through an interviewer. Rather than ignore these patients and incur the risk of drawing invalid conclusions, one can seek information on their health outcomes by proxy from their carers or families. Such proxy measures must still be reliable, valid and responsive. Sprangers and Aaronson's review[80] of the use of proxy responders identified many outstanding methodological issues.

The measurement of health outcomes in children and the elderly presents special problems.[59,81] There are several measures of child health outcome that can be extended to younger children by using parents as proxies.[42,82,83] There is also a need for measures that focus on subgroups.[84] Most measures for children have yet to be assessed for reliability, validity and responsiveness across different conditions. Although generic instruments have been used with some success in elderly general populations,[85] the relevance of these instruments to the elderly and the interpretation of the resulting scores still needs rigorous research. There is also a need for measures that are specific to subgroups such as the frail or chronically ill.[32]

SUMMARY

Patients' assessments of their own health is an important component in the evaluation of the effectiveness of health care. Traditional measures like mortality rates in populations and biomedical measures in individuals fail to take account of the effect of health care on functioning or health-related quality of life. This change of emphasis has come at a time when health care budgets are coming under closer scrutiny. If the recent reorganizations of health care in the UK and the USA are to achieve efficient resource allocation rather than mere cost containment, then information about health outcomes is essential.

There are two approaches to measuring health outcomes – generic instruments that cover most if not all patients and specific instruments that focus on particular conditions or patient groups. Generic instruments have more potential to detect unexpected or side-effects of treatment and to contribute to economic evaluation. Specific instruments are more likely to detect small but important changes in health. These two approaches are most effective in combination.

To be useful a health outcome measure must be reliable, valid, responsive and practical. Validity and reliability have received most attention. They are necessary but not sufficient for a measure to be suitable for health care evaluation. Such measures also need to be responsive to important changes in health. They should be practical, cost-effective and acceptable to patients. Fortunately there is an increasing number of short responsive measures that can be used in clinical settings.

REFERENCES

1. Donabedian A: *Explorations in Quality Assessment and Monitoring* Vol 3. Ann Arbor, Michigan: Health Administration Press, 1985
2. McDowell I, Newell C: *Measuring Health: a Guide to Rating Scales and Questionnaires.* Oxford: Oxford University Press, 1987
3. Ebbs SR, Fallowfield LJ, Fraser SCA, Baum M: Treatment outcomes and quality of life. *Int J Technol Assess Hlth Care* **5:** 391–400, 1989
4. Garrett JW, Drossman DA: Health status in inflammatory bowel disease: biological and behavioural considerations. *Gastroenterology* **99:** 90–96, 1990
5. MacKeigan LD, Pathak DS: Overview of health-related quality of life measures. *Am J Hosp Pharm* **49:** 2236–2245, 1992

6. Tarlov AR: Foreword. In: Stewart AL, Ware JE (Eds), *Measuring Functioning and Well-being*. Durham, North Carolina: Duke University Press, 1992
7. McDermott W: Absence of indicators of the influence of its physicians on society's health. *Am J Med* **70:** 833–843, 1981
8. Tarlov AR: The increasing supply of physicians, the changing structure of the health services system, and the future practice of medicine. *New Engl J Med* **308:** 1235–1422, 1983
9. Ellwood P: Outcomes management: a technology of patient experience. *New Engl J Med* **318:** 1549–1556, 1988
10. Geigle R, Jones SB: Outcomes measurement: a report from the front. *Inquiry* **27:** 7–13, 1990
11. Ware JE, Sherbourne CD: The MOS 36-item Short-Form Health Survey (SF-36) I: conceptual framework and item selection. *Med Care* **30:** 473–483, 1992
12. Fitzpatrick R: Applications of health status measures. In: Jenkinson C (Ed), *Measuring Health and Medical Outcomes*. London: UCL Press, 1994
13. Albrecht GL: Subjective health assessment. In: Jenkinson C (Ed), *Measuring Health and Medical Outcomes*. London: UCL Press, 1994
14. Norton PA, MacDonald LD, Sedgwick PM, Stanton SL: Distress and delay associated with urinary incontinence, frequency and urgency in women. *Br Med J* **297:** 1187–1189, 1988
15. Williams SJ. *Chronic Respiratory Disease*. London: Routledge, 1993
16. Ware JE, Snow KK, Kosinski M, Gandek B: *SF-36 Health Survey Manual and Interpretation Guide*. Boston: Nimrod Press, 1993
17. Wilkin D, Hallam L, Doggett MA: *Measures of Need and Outcome for Primary Health Care*. Oxford: Oxford University Press, 1992
18. Bowling A: *Measuring Health: A Review of Quality of Life Measurement Scales*. Milton Keynes: Open University Press, 1991
19. World Health Organization: *Constitution*. Geneva: WHO, 1947
20. Patrick DL, Erickson PE: *Health Status and Health Policy: Allocating Resources to Health Care*. Oxford: Oxford University Press, 1993
21. Guyatt GH, Feeny DH, Patrick DL: Measuring health-related quality of life. *Ann Intern Med* **118:** 622–629, 1993
22. Ruta DA, Garratt AM: From health status measurement to quality of life. In: Jenkinson C (Ed), *Measuring Health and Medical Outcomes*. London: UCL Press, 1994
23. Laupacis A, Wong C, Churchill D, Canadian Erythropoietin Study Group: The use of generic and specific quality of life measures in haemodialysis patients treated with erythropoietin. *Contr Clin Trials* **12** (Suppl)**:** 168S–179S, 1991
24. Wiklund I, Karlberg J: Evaluation of quality of life in clinical trials: selecting quality of life measures. *Contr Clin Trials* **12** (Suppl)**:** 204S–216S, 1991
25. Parkerson GR, Connis RT, Broadhead WE *et al.*: Disease-specific versus generic measurement of health-related quality of life in insulin-dependent diabetic patients. *Med Care* **31:** 629–639, 1993
26. Patrick DL, Deyo RA: Generic and disease-specific measures in assessing health status and quality of life. *Med Care* **27** (Suppl)**:** S217–S232, 1989
27. Stewart AL, Greenfield S, Hays RD *et al.*: Functional status and well-being of patients with chronic conditions: results from the Medical Outcomes Study. *J Am Med Assoc*, **262:** 907–913, 1989
28. Stewart AL, Hays RD, Ware JE: The MOS Short Form General Health Survey: reliability and validity in a patient population. *Med Care* **26:** 724–733, 1988
29. Torrance GW: Measurement of heath state utilities for economic appraisal: a review. *J Hlth Econ* **5:** 31–61, 1986
30. EuroQol Group: EuroQol – a new facility for the measurement of health related quality of life. *Hlth Policy* **16:** 199–208, 1990
31. Williams AH: Economics of coronary artery bypass grafting. *Br Med J* **291:** 326–329, 1985
32. Guyatt GH, Eagle DJ, Sackett B *et al.*: Measuring quality of life in the frail elderly. *J Clin Epidemiol* **46:** 1433–1444, 1993
33. Juniper EF, Guyatt GH, Epstein RS: Evaluation of impairment in health related quality of life in asthma: development of a questionnaire for use in clinical trials. *Thorax* **47:** 76–83, 1992

34. Ruta DA, Garratt AM, Wardlaw D, Russell IT: Developing a valid and reliable measure of health outcome for patients with low back pain. *Spine* **19:** 1887–1896, 1994
35. Parfrey PS, Vasasour H, Bullock M *et al.*: Development of a health questionnaire for end-stage renal disease. *Nephron* **52:** 20–28, 1989
36. Meenan RF, Gertman PM, Mason JH: Measuring health status in arthritis: the Arthritis Impact Measurement Scales. *Arthr Rheum* **25:** 1048–1053, 1980
37. Juniper EF, Guyatt GH: Development of a new measure of health status for clinical trials in rhinoconjunctivitis. *Clin Expl All* **21:** 77–83, 1991
38. Garratt AM, MacDonald LM, Ruta DA *et al.*: Towards the measurement of outcome for patients with varicose veins. *Qual Hlth Care* **2:** 5–10, 1993
39. Kerner JE, Alexander J: Activities of daily living: reliability and validity of gross versus specific ratings. *Arch Phys Med Rehab* **62:** 161–166, 1981
40. Fedor-Freybergh P: The influence of estrogens on wellbeing and mental performance in clinacteric and postmenopausal women. *Acta Obstet Gyn Scand* **64** (Suppl)**:** 1–68, 1977
41. Tursky B, Jamner LD, Friedman R: The Pain Perception Profile: a psychophysical approach to the assessment of pain report. *Behav Ther* **13:** 376–394, 1982
42. Landgraf JM, Aberz L, Ware JE, Maunsell E: French-Canadian, German and United Kingdom translations of the Child Health Questionnaire (CHQ-PF50): methodology and preliminary item scaling results. *J Clin Epidemiol* **49:** 1996
43. Kirshner B, Guyatt G: A methodological framework for assessing health indices. *J Chron Dis* **38:** 27–36, 1985
44. Zigmund AS, Snaith RP: The Hospital Anxiety and Depression Scale. *Acta Psychiat Scand* **67:** 361–370, 1983
45. Wilkinson MJB, Barczak P: Psychiatric screening in general practice: comparison of the General Health Questionnaire and the Hospital Anxiety and Depression Scale. *J Roy Coll Gen Pract* **38:** 311–313, 1988
46. Hunt SM, McEwen J, McKenna SP: Measuring health: a new tool for clinicians and epidemiologists. *J Roy Coll Gen Pract* **35:** 185–188, 1985
47. Kind P, Carr-Hill R. The Nottingham Health Profile: a useful tool for epidemiologists? *Social Sci Med* **25:** 905–910, 1987
48. Naji SA, Brunt PW, Hagen S *et al.*: Improving the selection of patients for upper gastrointestinal endoscopy. *Gut* **34:** 187–191, 1993
49. Fitzpatrick R, Fletcher A, Gore S *et al.*: Quality of life measures in health care I: applications and issues in assessment. *Br Med J* **305:** 1074–1077, 1992
50. Ware JE: Measures for a new era of health assessment. In: Stewart AL, Ware JE (Eds), *Measuring Functioning and Well-being*. Durham, North Carolina: Duke University Press, 1992
51. Guyatt G, Feeny D, Patrick D: Issues in quality of life measurement in clinical trials. *Contr Clin Trials* **12** (Suppl)**:** 81S–90S, 1991
52. Pocock SJ: A perspective on the role of quality of life assessment in clinical trials. *Controlled Clin Trials* **12** (Suppl)**:** 257S–265S, 1991
53. Nunnally JC, Bernstein IH: *Psychometric Theory* 3rd edn. New York: McGraw-Hill, 1994
54. Streiner GL, Norman RD: *Health Measurement Scales: a Practical Guide to their Development and Use*. Oxford: Oxford University Press, 1989
55. Chambers LW: The McMaster Health Index Questionnaire: methodologic documentation and report of the second generation of investigations. Hamilton, Ontario, Department of Clinical Epidemiology and Biostatistics, McMaster University, 1982
56. Roland M, Morris R: A study of the natural history of back pain I: development of a reliable and sensitive measure of disability in low back pain. *Spine* 141–144, 1983
57. Temkin NR, Dikmen S, Machamer J, Mclean A: General versus disease-specific measures: further work on the Sickness Impact Profile for head injury. *Med Care* **27** (Suppl)**:** S44–S53, 1989
58. Kantz ME, Harris WJ, Levitsky K *et al.*: Methods for assessing condition-specific and generic functional status outcomes after total knee replacement. *Med Care* **30** (Suppl)**:** S240–S252, 1992

59. Patrick DL, Bergner M: Measurement of health status in the 1990s. *Ann Rev Publ Hlth* **11:** 165–183, 1990
60. Deyo RA, Diehr P, Patrick DL: Reproducibility and responsiveness of health status measures: statistics and strategies for evaluation. *Contr Clin Trials* **12** (Suppl): 142S–158S, 1991
61. Helmstadter GC: *Principles of Psychological Measurement*. New York: Appleton-Century-Crofts, 1964
62. Nunnally JC: *Psychometric Theory* 2nd edn. New York: McGraw-Hill, 1978
63. Anderson J St C, Sullivan F, Usherwood TP: The Medical Outcomes Study Instrument – use of a new health status measure in Britain. *Family Practice* **7:** 203–218, 1990
64. Deyo RA, Centor RM: Assessing the responsiveness of functional scales to clinical change: an analogy of diagnostic test performance. *J Chron Dis* **39:** 897–906, 1986
65. Guyatt G, Walter S, Norman G: Measuring change over time: assessing the usefulness of evaluative instruments. *J Chron Dis* **40:** 171–178, 1987
66. Tuley MR, Mulrow CD, McMahan CA: Estimating and testing an index of responsiveness and the relationship of the index to power. *J Clin Epidemiol* **44:** 417–421, 1991
67. Fitzpatrick R, Ziebland S, Jenkinson C *et al.*: Transition questions to assess outcomes in rheumatoid arthritis. *Br J Rheumatol* **32:** 807–811, 1993a
68. Deyo RA, Inui TS: Towards clinical applications of health status measures: sensitivity of scales to clinically important changes. *Hlth Services Res* **19:** 275–289, 1984
69. MacKenzie CR, Charlson ME, DiGioia D, Kelley K: Can the Sickness Impact Profile measure change? an example of scale assessment. *J Chron Dis* **39:** 429–438, 1986
70. Kazis LE Anderson JJ, Meenan RF: Effect sizes for interpreting changes in health status. *Med Care* **27** (Suppl): S178–S189, 1989
71. Katz JN, Larson MG, Phillips CB *et al.*: Comparative measurement sensitivity of short and longer form health status instruments. *Med Care* **30:** 917–925, 1992
72. Liang MH, Fossel AH, Larson MG: Comparisons of five health status instruments for orthopedic evaluation. *Med Care* **28:** 632–642, 1990
73. Guyatt G, Mitchell A, Irvine EJ *et al.*: A new measure of health status for clinical trials in inflammatory bowel disease. *Gastroenterology* **96:** 804–810, 1989
74. Fitzpatrick R, Ziebland S, Jenkinson C *et al.*: Importance of sensitivity to change as a criterion for selecting health status measures. *Qual Hlth Care* **1:** 89–93, 1992
75. Bergner M, Bobbitt RA, Pollard WE *et al.*: The Sickness Impact Profile: validation of a health status measure. *Med Care* **14:** 57–67, 1976
76. Bergner M, Bobbitt RA, Carter WB, Gilson BS: The Sickness Impact Profile: development and final revision of a health status measure. *Med Care* **19:** 787–805, 1981
77. Fitzpatrick R, Ziebland S, Jenkinson C *et al.*: A comparison of the sensitivity to change of several health status instruments in rheumatoid arthritis. *J Rheumatol* **20:** 429–436, 1993
78. Parkerson GR, Broadhead WE, Chiu-Kit JT: The Duke Health Profile: a 17-item measure of health and dysfunction. *Med Care* **28:** 1056–1072, 1990
79. Ware JE, Kosinski M, Keller SD: A 12-Item Short-Form Health Survey (SF-12): construction of scales and preliminary tests of reliability and validity. *Med Care* **34:** 220–233, 1996
80. Sprangers MAG, Aaronson NK: The role of health care providers and significant others in evaluating the quality of life of patients with chronic disease: a review. *J Clini Epidemiol* **45:** 743–760, 1992
81. Kutner NG, Ory MG, Baker DI *et al.*: Measuring the quality of life of the elderly in health promotion intervention clincal trials. *Publ Hlth Rep* **107:** 530–539, 1992
82. Eisen M, Ware JE, Donald CA, Brook RH: Measuring components of children's health status. *Med Care* **17:** 902–921, 1979
83. Stein REK, Jessop DJ: Functional Status II(R): a measure of child health status. *Med Care* **28:** 1041–1055, 1990
84. Wiklund I, Wiren L, Erling A *et al.*: A new self-assessment questionnaire to measure well-being in children, particularly those of a short stature. *Qual Life Res* **3:** 449–455, 1994
85. Lyons RA, Lo SV, Littlepage BN: Comparative health status of patients with 11 common illnesses in Wales. *J Epidemiol Commun Hlth* **48:** 388–390, 1994

Prevention of vascular disease is the endpoint

FGR Fowkes

SCOPE FOR PREVENTION

The prevention of disease can occur at all stages of the disease process from intervening in healthy individuals through to reducing complications in those with established disease. The term 'primary prevention' is used traditionally in clinical practice to describe strategies used prior to the occurrence of recognizable clinical disease; 'secondary prevention' is used to describe interventions applied to those with established disease (Fig. 1).

In the primary prevention of cardiovascular disease, community lifestyle programmes, multiple risk factor screening and health promotion in general practice have generally been disappointing;[1] a major problem would appear to be that people find it difficult to change their lifestyles. However, some trials of single risk factor screening followed by medical treatment, rather than lifestyle changes, have shown a significant effect in preventing vascular events. For example, in the West of Scotland Coronary Prevention Study, screening and treating high serum cholesterol concentrations in 45- to 64-year-old men led to a 31% reduction in cardiovascular events.[2] Likewise, casefinding and treatment of hypertension in primary care is considered to be an effective preventive measure.[1]

The prime focus of primary prevention is usually coronary heart disease and stroke. Very few, if any, studies have measured the extent of peripheral arterial disease in the legs as an endpoint. Given that the risk factors for coronary heart disease and peripheral arterial disease are similar,[3] it would be surprising if successful primary preventive efforts against coronary heart disease did not also

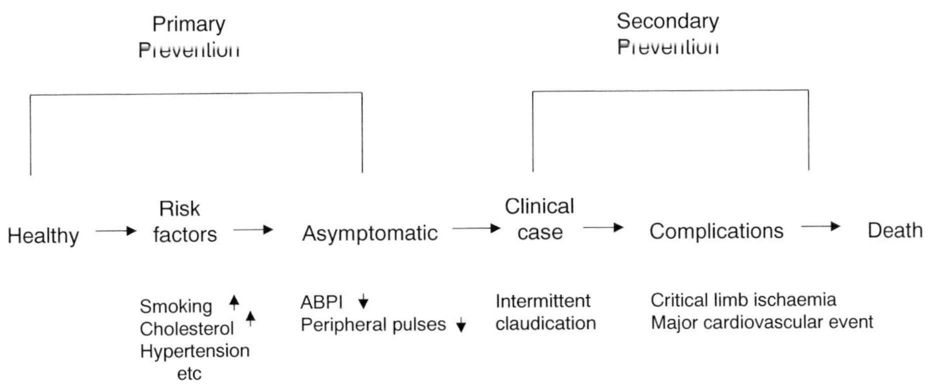

Fig. 1. Prevention and stages of peripheral arterial disease.

reduce the development of peripheral atherosclerosis. However, the net effect in the community might not be a reduction in the prevalence of peripheral arterial disease because some individuals, who in previous years would have died of coronary heart disease, might now survive and develop peripheral arterial disease in later life. Thus, paradoxically, primary prevention of cardiovascular disease might lead to a greater burden of peripheral arterial disease in the general population.

In recent years, individuals in the general population with a low ankle brachial pressure index (ABPI) have been shown to be at increased risk of developing intermittent claudication as well as major cardiovascular events.[4] Thus the ABPI has the potential to act as a screening tool for those at high risk. In the UK, two trials are currently in progress in which the ABPI is being used for this purpose. In the Aspirin for Asymptomatic Atherosclerosis (AAA) trial, healthy individuals in the general population with an ABPI less than 0.95 are being randomly allocated to aspirin or placebo; in the Prevention of Progression of Asymptomatic Diabetic Arterial Disease (POPADAD) study, diabetics with a low ABPI are being randomly allocated to aspirin and/or antioxidant. The main endpoints in these trials are major cardiovascular and cerebrovascular events, but information on peripheral arterial disease is also being collected.

Undoubtedly, the greatest opportunity for the prevention of vascular disease in relation to peripheral vascular disease is the secondary prevention of coronary heart disease and stroke in claudicants. There is now good information on the cardiovascular and cerebrovascular risks in subjects with peripheral arterial disease.

RISKS OF CORONARY HEART DISEASE AND STROKE

Non-fatal events

Patients with intermittent claudication are at increased risk of non-fatal coronary heart disease. In the Edinburgh Artery Study of claudicants in the general population, approximately 8% experienced a myocardial infarction over a 5-year follow-up period[4] (Table 1). Similarly in the Basel Study of pharmaceutical workers,[5] 16% of those with evidence of arterial disease had a non-fatal cardiac event after 11 years. Likewise, in a hospital-based series, 7% of claudicants had a non-fatal infarction after 10 years[6]. Interestingly, in a study in Malmo[7] the cardiac event rate was 21.2 per 1000 person years for those with only evidence of leg arterial disease, but for those who had leg arterial disease and evidence of coronary heart disease and/or carotid stenosis, the event rate was no higher, emphasizing that arterial disease in the legs is a serious indicator of risk. As well as an increased risk of acute coronary events, claudicants have an increased risk of developing angina compared with subjects without lower limb arterial disease.[4]

Non-fatal stroke occurs more commonly in patients with lower limb disease than in normal subjects, but generally less frequently than for coronary heart disease events. In the Edinburgh Artery Study, the 5-year incidence was almost 7% (Table 1). In the Basel Study the 11-year incidence of cerebrovascular complications was 12% compared with 16% for coronary heart disease.[5] A follow-up study of 400 hospital claudicants in England found that over a 5-year period approximately 5% developed a non-fatal

Table 1. 5-Year incidence of non-fatal cardiovascular events in a random sample of the general population aged 55–74 years at baseline: Edinburgh Artery Study

	Events %		
	Claudicants at baseline (n=73)	*Normal patients[a] at baseline (n=1080)*	*Relative risk (95% CI) of events in claudicants*
Myocardial infarction	8.2	6.7	1.20 (0.52–2.76)
New angina	9.6	5.3	2.31[b] (1.04–5.10)
Stroke or transient ischaemic attack	6.8	2.8	2.00 (0.80–4.99)
Others	4.1	1.5	1.70 (0.53–5.42)

Source: Ref 4.
[a] No intermittent claudication or asymptomatic leg arterial disease.
[b] $p<0.05$.

stroke compared with 14% having a non-fatal cardiac event.[8] Overall, the risk of a claudicant having a non-fatal stroke would appear to be about 1% per annum.[9]

Fatal events

The risk of death, mostly from coronary heart disease and stroke, is also high in claudicants. Among males with intermittent claudication followed up in population studies, 5-year cumulative mortality rates have ranged between approximately 10% and 20%.[4,10,11] As would be expected, 5-year mortality rates tend to be higher in intermittent claudication patients referred to hospital, although part of this difference can be attributed to the older age groups in hospital studies.[12] Indeed, the relative risks are not noticeably higher in hospital studies; overall the risk of dying within 5 years is about two or three times that of an age- and sex-matched population. Mortality rates are invariably higher in men than in women[6,13] but the relative risks of death are similar. Although mortality rates increase with age, the relative risks of death fall with increasing age.[6,13,14]

Coronary heart disease is the commonest cause of mortality in subjects with intermittent claudication contributing to between 35% and 60% of deaths; stroke causes between 7% and 17% and other vascular diseases about 8% of deaths.[3,6,13] Very few deaths are due directly to peripheral arterial disease except for the operative mortality associated with vascular reconstruction and amputations. Population follow-up studies have shown that the relative risk of death from ischaemic heart disease is approximately three times that in comparable populations without intermittent claudication[10,11] and the risk of death from stroke is twice as high.[15]

Survival is adversely affected by the presence of concomitant coronary or cerebrovascular disease.[10,14] Indeed in the Framingham study, survival rates with intermittent claudication and no evidence of coronary or cerebrovascular disease were similar to the general population free of such cardiovascular impairments.[11] Multiple logistic analysis of prognostic factors on death in a Finnish study suggested that most, but not all, of the excess mortality in subjects with intermittent claudication was due to other concomitant cardiovascular disease.[10]

Risk factors

Certain risk factors have been shown in many studies over the years to be associated in claudicants with an increased incidence of cardiovascular events and death. These factors have included cigarette smoking,[10,14,16,17] blood pressure,[10,13,18] serum cholesterol[10] and diabetes mellitus.[16] There is little doubt that smoking has a profound effect with relative risks of between 1.5 and 3.0 for smokers compared with non-smokers[10] and improved survival among subjects who stop smoking.[16] But increased risks have not been found to be universally associated with blood pressure,[14] serum cholesterol[17] and diabetes mellitus.[13,14] However, the inconsistency of results may partly relate to inadequacies of study design and lack of statistical power. The balance of evidence would suggest that these factors are likely to have an impact on the risk of coronary heart disease and stroke, and that control of these factors must be seriously considered in patients with intermittent claudication.

RISK FACTOR MANAGEMENT

Stopping smoking

Given that cigarette smoking is related to the development of peripheral arterial disease and to a worse prognosis,[19] smoking cessation would be expected to be beneficial.[20] Randomized controlled trials of the effectiveness of smoking cessation are not available because of the difficulties of ensuring patient compliance. However, two large follow-up studies of patients with intermittent claudication referred to hospital indicate probable benefits.[21,22] In one of these[21] 11% and in the other[22] 27% of the patients complied with the advice to stop smoking.

After 10 years 53% of persistent smokers suffered a myocardial infarction compared with only 11% of stopped smokers; 54% of persistent smokers died compared with 18% of stopped smokers[21] (Fig. 2). In a recent comprehensive review of the literature, abstinence from smoking was found to be associated consistently with improved survival in claudicants.[23]

The National Health Service Centre for Review and Dissemination has recently produced a brief report on smoking cessation and concluded that the most effective interventions that the health service can provide are advice from a health professional, and nicotine replacement therapy.[24] This accords with findings of the US Agency for Health Care Policy and Research.[25] Brief advice to stop smoking given by health professionals, and taking around 3 minutes, achieves a 2% reduction in the number of smokers. This may be increased to up to 5% by lengthening the duration of advice and follow-up.[25,26] Meta-analysis of trials on the efficacy of nicotine replacement therapies indicate that, when accompanied by advice or counselling, around a 20% quit rate over a minimum period of 6 months can be achieved.[27] All modes of nicotine replacement therapy (gum, patches, sprays and inhalers) appear to be effective although there is some evidence that higher dose gum may be more effective in heavily dependent smokers – a common category of smoker in those with peripheral arterial disease.[28] Such smoking cessation interventions are considered to be cost-effective in saving lives and reducing morbidity.[24]

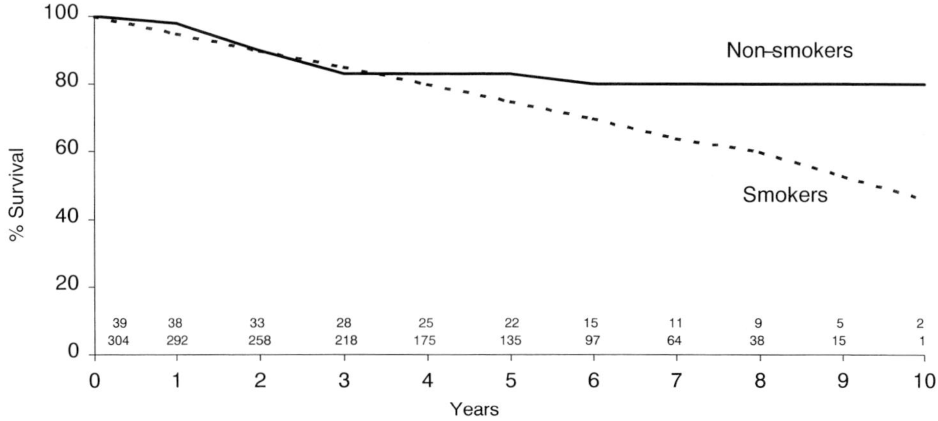

Fig. 2. Cumulative survival among smoking and non-smoking claudicants (p=0.076). (Source: Ref. 21.)

Little information is available on the effectiveness of smoking cessation programmes in patients with peripheral arterial disease[23] but the assumption is that the measures shown to be effective in the general population also work in the diseased population, although the level of effectiveness may differ. Fortunately, nicotine replacement therapy has been shown to be safe in patients with cardiovascular disease.[29,30] An increase in angina, palpitations or adverse events was not found in patients with coronary heart disease. In these studies, about one-third of patients had peripheral arterial disease. Thus, nicotine replacement therapy, along with advice on smoking cessation, can be recommended for patients with peripheral arterial disease.

Exercise programmes

Moderate or stenuous exercise, particularly in middle-aged male smokers, may decrease the risk of developing peripheral arterial disease in later life (Fig. 3). For patients with established disease, the effectiveness of exercise programmes has been investigated in a Cochrane systematic review.[31] Exercise therapy significantly improved maximal walking distance by approximately 150%. However, the long-term effects of exercise in patients with peripheral arterial disease on the incidence of fatal and non-fatal cardiovascular events has not been investigated. In the population as a whole, those who exercise on a regular basis have half the cardiovascular mortality of those who are inactive, and the benefits occur in those who take either moderate or intense exercise.[32] The National Institutes of Health Consensus Conference on physical activity and health concluded that individuals should ideally have 30 minutes of moderate exercise, such as walking, each day.[33] It is likely that patients with peripheral arterial disease would also enjoy longer term benefits from regular exercise.

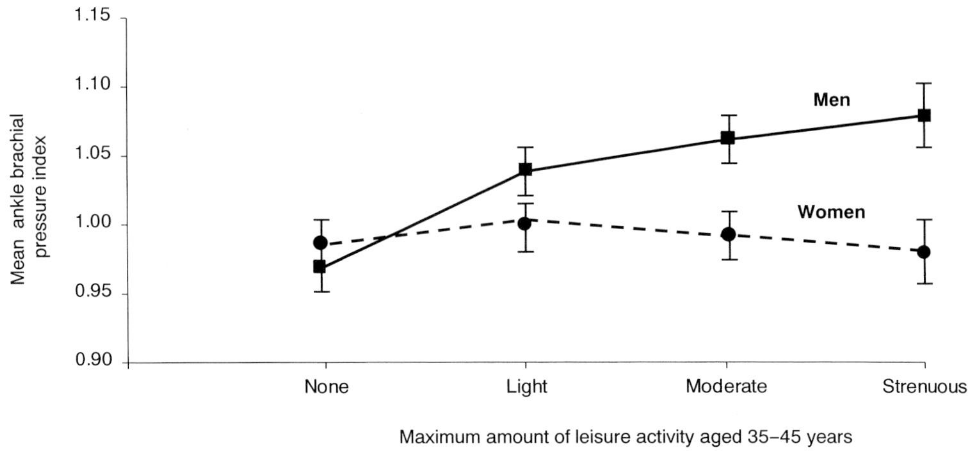

Fig. 3. Ankle brachial pressure index (mean ± 2 SEM) in relation to earlier leisure activity in men and women aged 55–74 years. (Source: Ref. 49.)

Lipid lowering therapy

A Cochrane systematic review has been carried out of lipid lowering therapy in peripheral arterial disease.[34] The conclusion of the review was that lipid lowering may improve leg symptoms but the variation in the trials was such that firm conclusions could not be drawn. The review also found evidence that lipid lowering therapy might reduce mortality in patients with peripheral arterial disease (OR 0.21, 95% CI 0.03–1.17) but with little change in non-fatal cardiovascular events (OR 1.21, 95% CI 0.80–1.83).[34] However, these results need to be interpreted with caution because of the relatively small numbers of events in the studies. On the other hand, the benefits of lipid lowering therapy, especially with the statin group of drugs, in the secondary prevention of cardiovascular events have been demonstrated in large randomized controlled trials.[35,36] Statins result in a risk reduction of about one-third for fatal and non-fatal myocardial infarction and total mortality in patients with coronary heart disease.[35,36] The relative risk reductions are consistent, irrespective of baseline cholesterol, so that the largest absolute benefits are in patients with high risk of cardiovascular events. Since patients with peripheral arterial disease are at high risk, the case for treating such patients with a statin is as strong as the case for treating survivors of myocardial infarction,[37] although a trial in patients with peripheral arterial disease *per se* has not been carried out. In the light of this evidence, key messages on lipid lowering in claudicants have recently been proposed by an expert group in the UK (Davies *et al.*, unpublished information).

- Measure non-fasting serum cholesterol.
- Provide dietary advice if cholesterol > 5.2 mmol/litre.
- Prescribe statin if under 70 years of age and cholesterol over 5.2 mmol/litre despite dietary measures.

Blood pressure reduction

Randomized controlled trials have demonstrated that in patients with hypertension, reducing blood pressure decreases morbidity and mortality from cardiovascular and cerebrovascular disease. Guidelines based on the best available evidence on the management of hypertension are readily available.[38,39] Trials on the long-term cardiovascular effects of controlling blood pressure in patients with peripheral arterial disease have not been carried out. However, in such patients at high risk of future cardiovascular events, the control of blood pressure, including the use of antihypertensive drugs, is considered to be more beneficial than in low-risk patients.[38] Indeed the cost-effectiveness of treatment is greater in elderly patients and in those with established cardiovascular disease.[38]

Although control of blood pressure in patients with peripheral arterial disease is warranted, the treatment requires special care because lowering systolic pressure can decrease local perfusion pressure and blood flow to ischaemic muscle and skin. The type of antihypertensive may be important[40] and the reduction in blood pressure needs to be carried out slowly and monitored carefully, particularly in patients with critical ischaemia.[40]

Control of diabetes mellitus

Although there is some limited evidence from follow-up studies of patients with peripheral arterial disease that those with diabetes have a higher mortality,[3,19] the extent to which glycaemic control might affect prognosis has not been determined. In diabetics as a whole, good control is likely to reduce the development of microvascular complications, especially retinopathy[41] and nephropathy.[42] However, only borderline support exists for a comparable reduction in macrovascular outcomes, such as myocardial infarction, in both type I diabetes[43] and type II (as shown in the UK Prospective Diabetes Study[44]). There is no reason to believe that these findings would not be relevant to diabetics with peripheral arterial disease. Thus, despite the lack of firm evidence in peripheral arterial disease, good diabetic control, at least to prevent microvascular complications, can be recommended, as specified in European guidelines based on expert consensus.[45]

Antiplatelet therapy

A comprehensive meta-analysis of the effect of aspirin, and other antiplatelet drugs, in reducing the risk of fatal and non-fatal vascular events in patients with various manifestations of atherosclerosis was published in 1994 by the Antiplatelet Trialists' Collaboration.[46] Overall, antiplatelets reduced the risk of myocardial infarction, stroke and death by about 25%. In patients with intermittent claudication, the reduction was not quite statistically significant, but the consistency of results suggest that there is probably a similar effect in this group. A Scottish Intercollegiate Guideline Network (SIGN) expert group on the treatment of peripheral arterial disease concluded therefore that 'Patients with intermittent claudication should receive aspirin long-term as prophylaxis against cardiovascular events'.[47] Recently a large multinational trial has shown that clopidogrel, a new antiplatelet agent, has a significant improvement (8.7%) over aspirin in overall efficacy and has fewer side-effects.[48]

IMPLICATIONS FOR CLINICAL PRACTICE

The prevention of coronary heart disease and stroke in patients with peripheral arterial disease needs to be given a high priority by surgeons, radiologists, general practitioners and others involved in their care. Attention has to be given to smoking cessation, exercise programmes, lipid lowering therapy, blood pressure reduction, diabetic control and antiplatelet therapy. In some countries these aspects of care have not traditionally been the concern of the surgeon nor have primary care physicians taken responsibility for risk factor management. Thus, for secondary prevention to succeed, clinicians may have to broaden their therapeutic approach or give more emphasis to the involvement of multidisciplinary teams in the management of patients with peripheral arterial disease. Also, the division of responsibilities between the primary and secondary care sectors needs to be clarified and guidelines and protocols drawn up for the secondary prevention of cardiovascular disease.

REFERENCES

1. National Heart Forum: *Preventing Coronary Heart Disease in Primary Care. The Way Forward.* London: Her Majesty's Stationery Office, 1995
2. Shepherd J, Cobbe SM, Ford I *et al.*: Prevention of coronary heart disease with pravastatin in men with hypercholesterolaemia. *New Engl J Med* **333:** 1301–1307, 1995
3. Fowkes FGR: Epidemiology of atherosclerotic arterial disease in the lower limbs. *Eur J Vasc Surg* **2:** 283–291, 1988
4. Leng GC, Lee AJ, Fowkes FGR *et al.*: Incidence, natural history and cardiovascular events in symptomatic and asymptomatic peripheral arterial disease in the general population. *Int J Epidemiol* **25:** 1172–1181, 1996
5. Widmer LK, Biland L, Zemp E, Da Silva A: Course of occlusive peripheral artery disease in early detected patients. *Proceedings of 14th World Congress of International Union of Angiology*, pp 13–15, Munich, 1986
6. Kallero KS: Mortality and morbidity in patients with intermittent claudication as defined by venous occlusion plethysmography. A ten year follow-up study. *J Chron Dis* **34:** 455–462, 1981
7. Ogren M, Hedblad B, Isaccson S-O *et al.*: Non-invasively detected carotid stenosis and ischaemic heart disease in men with leg arteriosclerosis. *Lancet* **342:** 1138–1141, 1993
8. Gilliland EL, Llewellyn CD, Gors DE *et al.*: The morbidity and mortality of claudicants. Results of five year follow-up. Presented at: *2nd International Vascular Symposium*, 1986
9. Dormandy JA, Murray GD: The fate of the claudicant: a prospective study of 1969 claudicants. *Eur J Vasc Surg* 5: 131–133, 1991
10. Reunanen A, Takkunen H, Aromaa A: Prevalence of intermittent claudication and its effect on mortality. *Acta Med Scand* **211:** 249–256, 1982
11. Kannel WB, Shurtleff D: The natural history of arteriosclerosis obliterans. *Cardiovasc Clin* **3:** 37–52, 1971
12. Smith FB, Fowkes FGR: Life expectancy for intermittent claudicants (peripheral vascular disease). In: Greenhalgh RM (Ed) *The Durability of Vascular and Endovascular Surgery* pp. 149–162. London: WB Saunders, 1999

13. Jelnes R, Gaardsting O, Hougaard Jensen K *et al.*: Fate in intermittent claudication – outcome and risk factors. *Br Med J* **293:** 1137–1140, 1986
14. Hughson WG, Mann JI, Tibbs DJ *et al.*: Intermittent claudication: factors determining outcome. *Br Med J* **1:** 1377–1379, 1978
15. Bowlin SJ, Medalie JH, Flocke SA *et al.*: Intermittent claudication in 8343 men and 21 year specific mortality follow-up. *Ann Epidemiol* **7:** 180–187, 1997
16. Silbert S, Zazeela H: Prognosis in arteriosclerotic peripheral vascular disease. *J Am Med Assoc* **166:** 1816–1821, 1958
17. Juergens JL, Barker NW, Hines EA: Arteriosclerosis obliterans: a review of 520 cases with special reference to pathogenic and prognostic factors. *Circulation* **21:** 188–195, 1960
18. Begg TB, Richards RL: The prognosis of intermittent claudication. *Scot Med J* **7:** 341–352, 1962
19. Leng GC, Fowkes FGR: The epidemiology of peripheral arterial disease. *Vasc Med Rev* **4:** 5–18, 1993
20. Housley E: Treating claudication in five words. *Br Med J* **296:** 1483, 1988
21. Jonason T, Bergstrom R: Cessation of smoking in patients with intermittent claudication. *Acta Med Scand* **221:** 253–260, 1987
22. Smith I, Franks PJ, Greenhalgh RM *et al.*: The influence of smoking cessation and hypertriglyceridaemia on the progression of peripheral arterial disease and the onset of critical ischaemia. *Eur J Vasc Endovasc Surg* **11:** 402–408, 1996
23. Hirsch AT, Treat-Jacobson D, Lando HA, Hatsukami DK: The role of tobacco cessation, antiplatelet and lipid loweing therapies in the treatment of peripheral arterial disease. *Vasc Med* **2:** 243–251, 1997
24. NHS: *Effectiveness Matters. Smoking Cessation: What the Health Service Can Do.* York: NHS Centre for Reviews and Dissemination, 1998
25. Smoking Cessation Clinical Practice Guidelines Panel and Staff: Consensus statement: Agency for Health Care Policy and Research Smoking Cessation Clinical Practice Guidelines. *J Am Med Assoc* **275:** 1270–1280, 1996
26. Law M, Ling Tang J: An analysis of the effectiveness of interventions intended to help people stop smoking. *Arch Intern Med* **155:** 1933–1941, 1995
27. Silagy C, Mant D, Fowler G, Lodge M: Meta-analysis on efficacy of nicotine replacement therapies in smoking cessation. *Lancet* **343:** 139–142, 1994
28. Ling Tang J, Law M, Wald N: How effective is nicotine replacement therapy in helping people to stop smoking. *Br Med J* **308:** 21–26, 1994
29. Transdermal Nicotine Working Group: Nicotine replacement therapy for patients with coronary artery disease. *Arch Intern Med* **154:** 989–995, 1994
30. Joseph AM, Norman S, Ferry L *et al.*: Safety of transdermal nicotine therapy in patients with cardiac disease: a randomised controlled trial. *New Engl J Med* **335:** 1792–1798, 1996
31. Leng GC, Fowler N, Ernst E: Exercise for intermittent claudication (Cochrane Review). In: *The Cochrane Library, Issue 4.* Oxford: Update Software, 1998
32. Powell KE, Pratt M: Physical activity and health. *Br Med J* **313:** 126–127, 1996
33. NIH Consensus Development Panel on Physical Activity and Cardiovascular Health: Physical activity and health. National Institutes of Health Consensus Conference. *J Am Med Assoc* **267:** 241–246, 1996
34. Leng GC, Price JF, Jepson RG: Lipid lowering therapy in lower limb atherosclerosis (Cochrane Review). In: *The Cochrane Library, Issue 4.* Oxford: Update Software, 1998
35. Sacks FM, Pfeffer MA, Moye LA *et al.*: for Cholesterol and Recurrent Events Trial Investigators. The effect of pravastatin on coronary events after myocardial infarction in patients with average cholesterol levels. *New Engl J Med* **335:** 1001–1009, 1996
36. Scandinavian Simavastatin Survival Study Group: Randomised trial of cholesterol lowering in 4444 patients with coronary heart disease: the Scandinavian Simavastatin Survival Study (4S). *Lancet* **344:** 1383–1389, 1994
37. Haq IU, Yeo WW, Hackson PR, Ramsay LE: The case for cholesterol reduction in peripheral vascular disease. *Critical Ischaemia* **7:** 15–22, 1997
38. Subcommittee of WHO/ISH Mild Hypertension Liaison Committee: Summary of 1993

World Health Organisation – International Society of Hypertension guidelines for the management of mild hypertension. *Br Med J* **307:** 1541–1546, 1993

39. Sever P, Beevers G, Bulpitt C *et al.*: Management guidelines in essential hypertension: report of the second working party of the British Hypertension Society. *Br Med J* **306:** 983–987, 1993
40. Clement DL, Verhaeghe R: Atherosclerosis and other occlusive arterial diseases. In Clement DL, Shepherd JT (Eds), *Vascular Diseases in the Limbs. Mechanisms and Principles of Treatment* pp. 81–82. St Louis: Mosby Year Book, 1993
41. Brinchmann-Hansen O, Dahl-Jorgensen K, Sandvik L, Hanssen KF: Blood glucose concentrations and progression of diabetic retinopathy: the seven year results of the Oslo study. *Br Med J* **304:** 19–22, 1992
42. Feldt-Rasmussen B, Mathieson ER, Deckert T: Effect of two years strict metabolic control on progression of incipient nephthropathy in insulin-dependent diabetes. *Lancet* **ii:** 1300–1304, 1986
43. DCCT Research Group: The effect of intensive diabetes treatment on the development and progression of long term complications in insulin-dependent diabetes mellitus. The Diabetes Control and Complications Trial. *New Engl J Med* **329:** 978–986, 1993
44. UK Prospective Diabetes Study (UKPDS) Group: Intensive blood-glucose control with sulphonylureas or insulin compared with conventional treatment and risk of complications in patients with type 2 diabetes (UKPDS 33). *Lancet* **352:** 837–853, 1998
45. European IDDM Policy Group: Consensus guidelines for the management of insulin-dependent (Type 1) diabetes. *Diabet Med* **10:** 990–1005, 1993
46. Antiplatelet Trialists' Collaboration: Collaborative overview of randomised trials of antiplatelet therapy. 1. Prevention of death, myocardial infarction, and stroke by prolonged antiplatelet therapy in various categories of patients. *Br Med J* **308:** 81–106, 1994
47. Scottish Intercollegiate Guidelines Network: *Drug Therapy for Peripheral Vascular Disease.* SIGN Publication No 27. Edinburgh: SIGN Secretariat, 1998
48. CAPRIE Steering Committee: A randomised, blinded trial of clopidogrel versus aspirin in patients at risk of ischaemic events (CAPRIE). *Lancet* **348:** 1329–1339, 1996
49. Housley E, Leng GC, Donnan PT, Fowkes FGR: Physical activity and risk of peripheral arterial disease in the general population: Edinburgh Artery Study. *J Epidemiol Commun Hlth* **47:** 475–480, 1993

Training the future vascular surgeon

Simon R Dodds, Jason Smith

INTRODUCTION

The last 30 years has seen the emergence of endovascular surgery as the dominant primary treatment strategy for patients with vascular disease. Following the early pioneers, a long period of research and development has created a mature philosophy based on evidence and implemented increasingly through consensus guidelines and protocols. The emphasis is switching to effective and efficient patient-centred care delivered by competent teams and monitored through local and national audit. The challenge of delivering a high quality, cost-effective, maximum benefit, minimum risk clinical service requires collaboration. Effective collaboration requires shared values, common objectives and good communication. The main obstacles to collaboration are the natural human resistance to change and the desire to protect vested interests. Change is a natural part of life and managing change is as important a part of a consultant's role as providing clinical judgment and technical expertise. The working life of a future vascular surgical consultant will continue to evolve and in order to maintain and develop skills training will be need to continue throughout the working career. Such training will need to address all major influences on modern clinical practice, e.g. information technology, and be integrated into the provision of the clinical service. These requirements imply adopting novel approaches to continued professional development.

Planning future service provision requires attracting a sufficient number of competent staff to do the work and this requires designing roles with the appropriate balance of challenge and reward. One model based loosely on the Maslovian hierarchy of needs ranks the tasks under the headings of Service, Training, Audit, and Research (STAR). Achieving a 'higher' level requires achieving a challenge/ reward balance at the 'lower' level first. In a smaller unit these tasks may fall within the role of one individual, in a larger unit they may need to be more separated. Assessing if an individual is competent to perform a specified role implies knowing what skills, knowledge, attitudes and judgment are required as well as a robust method of assessment. Training for a consultant role requires providing an environment in which the necessary knowledge, skills and attitude are developed incrementally. Training the consultant vascular surgeon of the future requires educating the vascular surgeons of the present about modern teaching methods and assessment tools: i.e. training the trainers.

THE FUTURE VASCULAR SURGICAL UNIT

Current recommendations are that elective and emergency endovascular surgery is delivered through a minimum unit consisting of a team of vascular surgeons, interventional radiologists and vascular technicians.[1] A typical blueprint which is being promoted is a four-person vascular surgical team working with at least two vascular radiologists, a non-invasive vascular laboratory and providing a 24-hour emergency vascular service for a population of between 300000 and 600000 depending on the degree of vascular surgical specialization. Such a unit would be capable of managing the majority of arterial, venous, lymphatic and other vascular conditions and provide a comprehensive training opportunity including the common level III procedures. Such units would have an integrated audit system as part of a national vascular audit programme and could contribute to multicentre clinical research studies. Larger academic/teaching units would be needed to provide the necessary infrastructure to support the more complex vascular procedures, specialist training, coordination of multicentre trials, development of new techniques and basic vascular biology research. Strategic planning must be based on international, national and regional consensus of what services can be offered, how the service should be delivered, and the evidence to support why specific procedures are justified. Tactical planning based on local and regional consensus and resources focuses on who will deliver the service, where it is delivered and when. The essential flavours of a vascular unit will be a comprehensive consultant-led service; training and audit closely integrated into the clinical service; a culture of continuous education of everyone involved in the care of vascular patients and the inclusion of essential non-medical team members such as vascular technicians and nurse specialists. Within this wider framework the delivery of treatment covers a continuum from simple advice through an increasing variety of minimally invasive endovascular procedures to the major open vascular surgical procedures, and often a combination of several modalities. The rapidly developing armamentarium of endovascular procedures that are being developed and tested in centres of excellence around the world will ultimately devolve in a mature form to the intermediate vascular units that will provide the majority of the clinical service. Individuals should be able to identify and work towards a role within this framework that suits their personal abilities and aspirations, balancing the challenge/reward equation and providing both a high quality service and, to borrow a Maslovian term, achieve self-actualization.

TRAINING THE FUTURE VASCULAR SURGEON

If the utopian view expressed above is accepted in principle then the training needs of a future endovascular surgeon can be defined, at least in broad terms. Assuming that the basic medical and surgical training continues as now, the individuals who express a desire to follow a career in vascular surgery will require further specialist training and assessment that includes:

- in-depth knowledge of vascular epidemiology, biology and medicine;
- theoretical knowledge and practical skills in open and endovascular procedures;
- direct clinical experience of a broad range of vascular conditions;
- critical appraisal of research evidence;
- clinical management skills (self management, team working, teaching, research);
- service management skills (audit, information technology, service planning).

The wide range and diverse nature of the knowledge and skills that a future vascular surgeon will need imply that a range of training and assessment techniques will need to be adopted, each suited to the particular skill required. Close parallels can be drawn between this specialist surgical training and the training of other professionals such as pilots or even astronauts. Lessons can be learned from what has been proven with experience in these other disciplines, and technology can be borrowed and adapted for vascular surgical training and assessment. For example, it is clearly inappropriate for all trainees to learn all their knowledge and develop their skills on residential courses, just as it is impossible to learn the whole of vascular medicine and surgery from a single mentor. A combination of techniques will be required that represent different combinations of the following:

- structured or informal training;
- live or simulated scenarios;
- local, regional and national training courses;
- local or distance self-learning tools;
- individual, small and large group working;
- formative or summative assessment;
- qualification, proficiency, refresher and 'as-required' training.

The strengths and weaknesses of existing training can only be identified if some form of explicit analysis is attempted and based on the above there appear to be a number of issues which stand out. The first is the need for improved communication and team management skills for all health care workers, including doctors, nurses and managers. The increasing reliance on information technology (IT), its rapid pace of development and the length of medical and surgical training imply that clinicians are often deficient in even basic IT skills. Such skills once mastered can make dramatic improvements in individual and team effectiveness. However, to be familiar with and make the best of IT requires a continuous programme of cascaded education at all levels. Every clinician should be able to operate a desktop computer, browse the Internet, use a word processor, send and receive electronic mail, create and deliver an electronic presentation and use their local hospital information system (HIS). Mastering these basic IT skills opens the opportunity to use and develop computer-based distance learning tools. Typical examples include remote access to electronic structured training and education programmes (STEP), virtual 'grand rounds' using store and forward technology (an extended form of electronic mail), video conferencing and live interactive video demonstrations. Modern Internet browser technology can readily be adapted to support both formative and summative assessment of core knowledge and such tools naturally fill the gap between the existing cheap, local, informal training and the expensive, residential, structured courses. Development of distance learning material should be coordinated centrally but be collaborative and made widely available at reasonable cost.

THE FUTURE OF ENDOVASCULAR TRAINING

The recommendation of an invasive vascular treatment is the outcome of a decision chain that includes general knowledge of vascular conditions, specific patient information, clinical management decisions and the ability to provide the treatment option. It is no longer possible to separate the contributions made to this process by vascular technologists, radiologists and surgeons (Table 1). Future trends are towards the direction of greater use of non-invasive investigation (duplex, magnetic resonance angiography), minimally invasive endovascular therapeutic procedures (angioplasty, stent, stent-graft) and complex open procedures that are performed only by appropriately trained and accredited vascular surgeons. The modern digital

Table 1. Examples of the contribution made by vascular technicians, radiologists and surgeons to the investigation and treatment of the most common vascular conditions

Clinical problem	*Investigation*	*Treatment*
Carotid stenosis/transient ischaemic attack	Duplex (MRA)	**Endarterectomy** (Angioplasty)
Aortic aneurysm	Ultrasound CT	**Open surgery** (Endovascular graft)
Aortoliac occlusive	Duplex Angiography (MRA)	Angioplasty (Endovascular stent) **Bypass graft** **Amputation**
Femoropopliteal occlusive	Duplex Angiography (MRA)	Angioplasty **Bypass graft** **Amputation**
Femorodistal occlusive	Angiography Duplex (MRA)	**Bypass graft** (Subintimal angioplasty) **Amputation**
Acute limb ischaemia	Emergency angiography	Thrombolysis **Embolectomy** **Emergency bypass** **Amputation**
Chronic venous insufficiency	Duplex venography	**Superficial venous surgery** **(SEPS)** **Skin grafting** **Amputation**

Bold type represents open surgical procedures and items (in parentheses) represent evolving techniques. MRA: magnetic resonance angiography; SEPS: subfascial endoscopic perforator surgery.

angiography suite is evolving into a primary therapeutic rather than diagnostic resource. Endovascular stent-grafts are likely to mature into an established treatment modality for a number of conditions that are difficult or high risk for open surgery and can be deployed in the angiography suite or an appropriately equipped vascular operating theatre. Endovascular stent-grafting may include infrarenal aortic aneurysms once the durability of the procedure is proven and trials have established that it is both clinically- and cost-effective. Thus an increasing proportion of the vascular surgical workload will move into the grey area between interventional radiology and vascular surgery and this trend is highly significant when put in the context of current changes in clinical accountability, governance and accreditation. There is no practical reason why endovascular procedures cannot be performed by any vascular specialist with the appropriate training and experience. The logistical problems with providing a comprehensive emergency vascular service at a district general hospital level leads naturally to the development of some degree of cross-training for the basic vascular and endovascular procedures by dedicated vascular radiologists and surgeons.

A recent Internet-based survey of senior vascular trainees in the UK has shown that the majority expect to work in a district general hospital as a general surgeon with a major vascular interest (Figs 1, 2). The general consensus is that vascular surgeons need to master the basic endovascular skills and should leave the more complex and less commonly performed procedures to the interventional vascular radiologists (Fig. 3). While only 33% of vascular surgical trainees have been exposed to some degree of endovascular skill training, more than 75% feel that such training should be provided (Fig. 4). In addition, it was felt among surgeons that interventional vascular radiologists should master the basic vascular surgical skills of femoral and brachial artery exposure but should leave the more complex open procedures to experienced vascular surgeons. The findings of this survey provide grass-roots support for the concept of common basic skills training for those vascular surgeons and radiologists who wish to work closely with each other. There was, however, a minority of vascular surgical trainees (25%) who felt that endovascular skills should remain solely with radiologists and who expressed no interest in

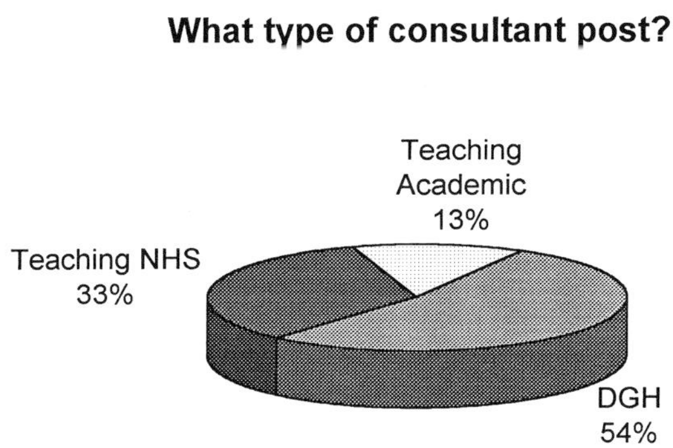

Fig. 1. Intended consultant vascular surgical post type from a survey of UK senior vascular trainees (n = 15). DGH: District general hospital.

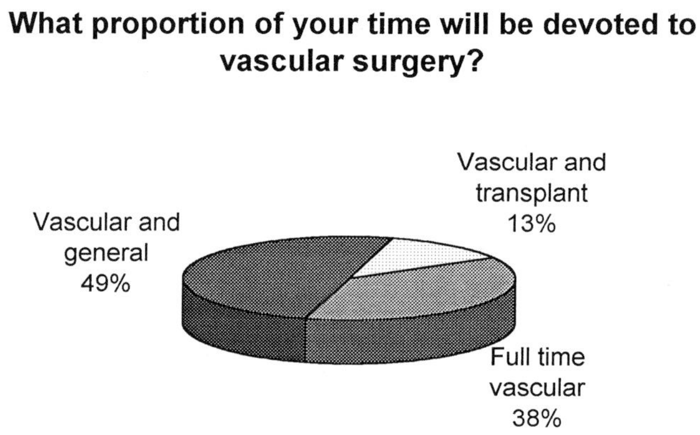

Fig. 2. Intended degree of specialization in vascular surgery from survey of UK senior vascular trainees (n = 24).

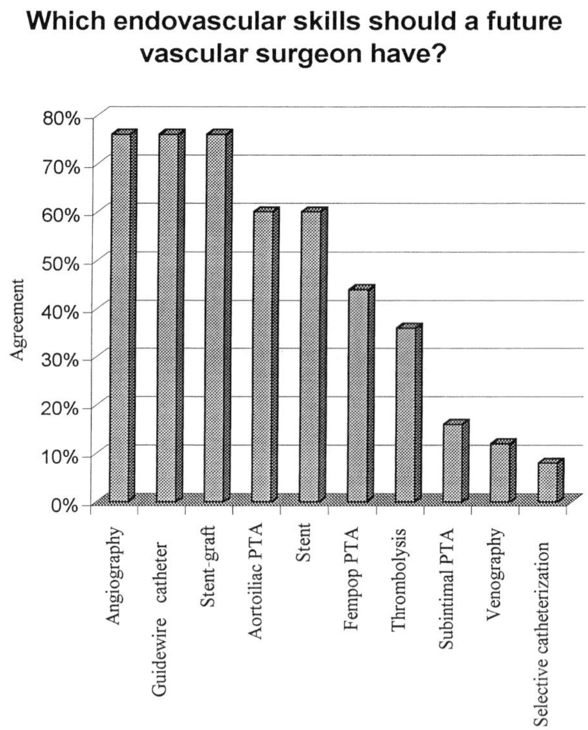

Fig. 3. Recommended endovascular skills required by a future vascular surgeon from a survey of UK senior vascular trainees (n = 25). PTA: Percutaneous transluminal angioplasty.

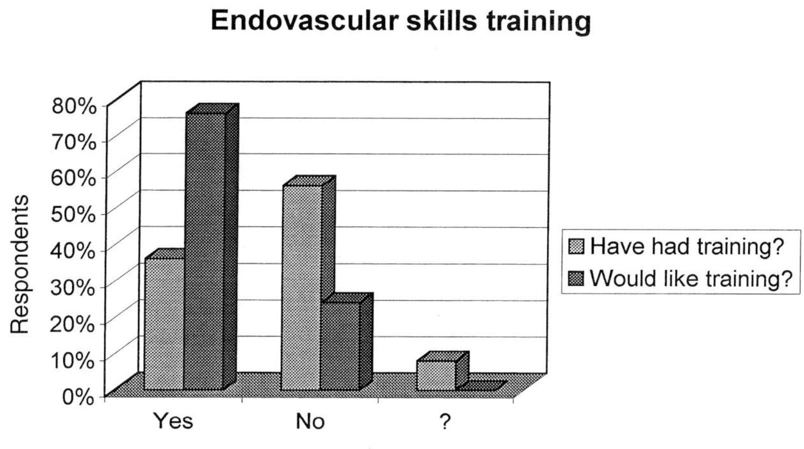

Fig. 4. Comparison between actual and desired endovascular skill training from survey of UK senior vascular trainees (n = 25).

contributing to a combined emergency service. A typical district general hospital with four vascular surgeons sharing a separate vascular rota is unlikely to be supported by four vascular radiologists. If two of the surgeons are trained in basic endovascular skills it would allow a full 24-hour vascular emergency cover to be offered without overloading either the radiologists or the surgeons. In the survey of UK trainees, the majority would only wish to provide an emergency endovascular service if already on call for vascular surgery. Given the move towards consultant-led clinical services and continued professional development for consultants, such endovascular skills training could take place at any time during the working life of a vascular surgeon or radiologist but should be mandatory before undertaking independent practice in that area. Endovascular skills training has been proven to be feasible as part of general/vascular surgical training[2] but such skills need to be maintained and developed. The survey of UK vascular trainees showed that the majority who expressed an interest felt that one session per week in the angiography suite would be acceptable to maintain basic endovascular skills that could be used in the vascular operating theatre and as part of an emergency vascular service.

SUMMARY

The vascular surgeons of the future will require knowledge and skills in general surgery, vascular medicine, endovascular techniques, information technology and team management in order to be competent to coordinate interventional treatment of vascular patients as part of multidisciplinary, evidence-based, patient-centred care. Changes to the existing educational philosophy of both trainees and consultants, together with adoption of new technology will be needed to keep both service and training objectives within realistic limits. Structured education programmes, distance computer-based learning, and interdisciplinary hands-on training are some of the methods that could be used to support future training and competence assessment. Despite the advances in vascular biology there is unlikely to be a shortage of patients who need treatment and the future vascular surgeon will need to work as part of an efficient and effective team to provide high quality care to as many patients as possible.

REFERENCES

1. Vascular Advisory Committee of the Vascular Surgical Society of Great Britain and Ireland: *The Provision of Vascular Services*. Revised Edition October 1998
2. Dodds SR, Birch SJ, Chant ADB: Integrated vascular surgical and interventional radiological training. *Br J Surg* **83:** 569, 1996

Where does this leave the trainee? – the future vascular radiologist

Ian Robert Davidson

INTRODUCTION

Vascular radiology can trace its origins back to the 1920s with the first arteriograms and venograms performed on humans in 1923[1] and the first femoral angiogram in 1924.[2] Catheter angiography was first described by Farinas in 1941.[3] It wasn't until 1953 when, Sven-Ivar Seldinger described his technique of percutaneous catheterization that modern interventional vascular radiology was born.[4] Dotter first described transluminal angioplasty in 1964[5] but it was only in 1984 when Gruntzig described his technique of balloon angioplasty that this technique became widely applied to the vascular tree.[6] In 1975 Cesare Gianturco described his technique for coil embolization.[7] Gianturco went on to describe the bird's nest inferior vena caval filter[8] and the Gianturco self-expanding endovascular stent.[9]

As we move forward in the next millennium vascular radiology has come of age. There has never been a more exciting time in which to embark on a career in vascular radiology. Our profile has increased dramatically in the last two decades with several significant developments such as improved balloon catheters, catheter directed thrombolysis, improved embolization techniques, microcatheters, vascular stents and stent-grafts. Over the last 5 years vascular radiology has reached to new heights with the development of endovascular stentgrafts for the treatment of abdominal aortic aneurysms. This new technique has perhaps more than any other procedure done more to raise the profile of the vascular radiologist. The vascular radiologist has an essential role to play in this new procedure, being of critical importance in the preoperative imaging, procedural planning, stent-graft deployment, postoperative surveillance and finally the treatment of postoperative complications.

The achievements of vascular radiology have neither gone unrecognized nor unappreciated. The Vascular Surgical Society of Great Britain and Ireland has put on record that they consider 'the relationship between vascular surgeon and vascular radiologist to be of prime importance' and go on to affirm that the interventional vascular radiologist is an 'integral member' of the vascular team, providing both diagnostic services and endovascular treatments. Regarding the provisions for vascular radiology they have stated 'for every vascular surgeon there should be a vascular radiologist delivering state of the art endovascular treatment 24 hours a day 365 days of the year'.[10]

Whilst peripheral vascular disease will continue for some time to be the main indication for patient referral, there are, however, many other new techniques which are likely to have as significant an impact on our workload such as uterine artery embolization for the treatment of uterine fibroids. This new procedure expanded so rapidly that it is estimated that there have been some 4165 such procedures performed in the USA as of September 1999.[11] The vascular radiologist of the future will not only be at the heart of any successful 'vascular team' but will also be at the centre of a much wider sphere of influence. We will continue working closely with vascular surgeons but also general surgeons, gynaecologists, haematologists, oncologists, hepatobiliary specialists, urologists, renal physicians, endocrinologists, pulmonary specialists, trauma specialists and as well as experts in a wide range of other specialties. It is a testimony to the success of our specialty that others are now looking to our work with keen interest. As vascular radiology impacts on other specialties it is not too surprising that some of our non-radiological colleagues feel threatened. In most instances, however, it is unlikely that these fears will be realized. Whilst it is true that the role of the vascular radiologist is expanding at what seems almost an exponential rate, specialties such as vascular surgery have nothing to fear from us. In fact vascular surgery has itself benefited from the close links with vascular radiology and the two specialties have evolved together as has our understanding of vascular disease. Developments such as catheter directed thrombolysis and aortic stent-grafts have progressed as a direct result of the close collaboration and cooperation between surgeons and radiologists.

As we move to meet new challenges it is time to take stock and ask some questions about the future of vascular radiology, our relationship with other specialties, our response to change, how we will adapt to the rapid rate of change that we are already experiencing, and perhaps most importantly how are we going to train future vascular radiologists.

WHAT IS INTERVENTIONAL VASCULAR RADIOLOGY?

Interventional vascular radiology is a medical specialty that uses image-guided, minimally invasive diagnostic and therapeutic techniques. These techniques may be an alternative or a complement to both minimally invasive surgery or conventional surgery. Interventional radiologists are trained in medical imaging modalities, radiation safety and are skilled in the performance of minimally invasive image guide procedures. They have a thorough understanding of modern patient care and management.

HOW DOES ONE TRAIN TO BECOME AN INTERVENTIONAL RADIOLOGIST?

The Educational Board of the Faculty of Clinical Radiology at the Royal College of Radiologists (RCR)[12] has recently published its training recommendations. These recommendations mirror training requirements laid down in the USA and throughout much of Europe. Trainees entering an accredited training programme should have a minimum of 2 years of appropriate clinical experience. Whilst 1 year of this may be preregistration many trainees have gone on to obtain higher medical or surgical qualifications prior to commencing their radiology training. The minimum period of radiology training is 5 years from time of entry.

In the first year basic sciences such as clinical and radiological anatomy and medical physics (including radiation safety and protection) are taught. Training is also undertaken in the principles of imaging modalities and of radiological techniques. Trainees are exposed to image interpretation and given practical experience in radiological procedures. This knowledge and experience also forms the basis of the FRCR part 1 examination in physics, radiological anatomy and radiological procedures.

Trainees are subsequently, over the next 36 months of their training, given practical experience in a wide range of procedural and interpretative skills in all required specialties. The Final FRCR, which comprises part A (MCQ) and part B (Viva and reporting) is usually completed by the end of this period. During the final 12 months of their development trainees are encouraged to expand and cultivate at least one or possibly two subspecialty interests. At this stage additional subspecialty training is then undertaken for those who wish to specialize in interventional radiology. The curriculum for this subspecialty training has recently been spelt out by the RCR.[13]

Trainees are given credit for any interventional experience gained in their first 4 years. Distinction should be made between vascular and non-vascular intervention. Emphasis is given to practical, hands-on experience based on a graded supervision. The RCR has set down minimum number of procedures to which trainees should be exposed with at least 50% of these procedures being performed with the trainee as the lead interventionist. They are expected to maintain an up-to-date logbook and undertake both research and audit projects, and have a good clinical awareness. The development of close links with vascular, surgical and medical teams is encouraged. Training centres should promote such an environment of multidisciplinary cooperation and foster the communication skills of its trainees. Training in patient analgesia and sedation together with knowledge of monitoring procedures and equipment is recommended. An appreciation of indications, complications, hazards and relative risks together with knowledge of national and local guidelines for informed consent is essential. Trainees who wish to go on to become full-time interventional vascular radiologists should spend a total of at least 2 years in vascular intervention. In this instance a 6th year is recommended so that training in more complex procedures can be undertaken.

HOW CAN THIS TRAINING BE IMPROVED?

There is no doubt that the current system described above is capable of producing highly skilled and talented vascular radiologists. With time it will be necessary to raise the standard of this training to a higher level as the role of the vascular radiologist continues to develop. In the long term this will take the form of a specialist examination in interventional vascular radiology. The introduction of such an 'exit' examination is probably some time off, as its introduction would most likely act as a disincentive to trainees entering the specialty. As such examinations become more widely accepted in other specialties (such as surgery and medicine) and as clinical radiology becomes increasingly subspecialized (breast screening, neuro-radiology, musculoskeletal and gastrointestinal radiology) then there will be a demand from patients and semi-professional bodies for formal accreditation with a measurable standard.

HOW WILL TRAINEES KEEP UP WITH NEW DEVELOPMENTS?

Apart from reading standard texts, and keeping up to date with recent publications, trainees should be encouraged to attend regional and national meetings. In the UK it would be desirable that trainees join and are encouraged to become active members of the British Society of Interventional Radiologists (BSIR). Membership of the Cardiovascular and Interventional Radiological Society of Europe (CIRSE) and other societies should also be advocated as a platform for keeping abreast of new developments and techniques. These associations and others throughout the world should encourage membership and the active participation of the trainee vascular radiologist. Training centres and those responsible for training should promote the benefit of association with other interventional radiologists. Workshops and panel discussions are frequently more informative than textbooks, which by their nature are soon out of date. We have already entered the generation of the vascular radiologists who must, in order to sharpen their axe, undertake continued medical education as part of a life-long learning programme.

WILL NON-INVASIVE IMAGING TECHNIQUES IMPACT ON TRAINING?

There is no doubt that the diagnostic angiogram as a technique for the investigation of limb ischaemia is in decline. Intravenous digital subtraction angiography has been superseded by contrast-enhanced magnetic resonance angiography. New and improved imaging modalities such as colour flow Doppler, magnetic resonance angiography, contrast-enhanced magnetic resonance angiography, direct thrombus imaging (using magnetic resonance imaging)[14] and computed tomography angiography have all reduced the need for diagnostic catheter angiography. This move towards non-invasive imaging is to the benefit of the patients provided it can be delivered promptly when required. Whilst some of these techniques are only available in larger centres it is just a matter of time before they gain wider acceptance. Colour flow Doppler is now widely available both in radiology departments and also in vascular laboratories. Contrast-enhanced magnetic resonance angiography is less widely available but it has distinct advantages in imaging the main branches of the thoracic and abdominal aorta[15] and the small vessels of the feet[16] which are difficult to access with ultrasound. This trend towards non-invasive imaging will increase and will impact on the vascular radiological trainee.

First, it will become increasingly important that trainees are familiar and proficient with these new imaging modalities. Second, there will be fewer diagnostic angiograms performed in the radiology departments of the future and consequently fewer situation in which to gain the necessary dexterity and experience to become an interventional vascular radiologist. There are two solutions to this problem. The length of time to train an interventional vascular radiologist may need to be increased. Alternatively, experience might be gained elsewhere. This might include centres that do not have access to these new imaging modalities. It has been suggested that, in the future, we will need to find a suitable animal model (such as the pig) in order to train the next generation of vascular radiologists.[17] Others have suggested that simulators including virtual reality techniques will become necessary.[18]

WHERE SHALL WE FIND THE NEXT GENERATION OF TRAINEES?

As with many other specialties there is currently a manpower crisis in the field of interventional vascular radiology. This situation will only improve if we can find the way to first attract and subsequently train new junior doctors into our specialty. If we are to meet with the recommendations of the Vascular Surgical Society of Great Britain and Ireland that 'for every vascular surgeon there should be a vascular radiologist delivering state of the art endovascular treatment 24 hours a day 365 days of the year'[10] then we must take the issue of recruitment seriously. There is no doubt that many observe our specialty with jealous eyes. We are fortunate to be in a specialty at the cutting edge of new technologies. Our dependence on high-tech image guidance means that the one thing that we can rely on is change. To some this may be daunting to others it will be refreshing. There is no doubt that junior doctors looking for a career that is rewarding, stimulating and exciting will need to consider interventional vascular radiology. I have no doubt that many current medical and surgical specialist registrars trainees will be attracted to our specialty. I do, however, feel that we will have to increase our profile if we are to succeed in attracting sufficient numbers into our specialty.

SHOULD WE BE TRAINING ENDOVASCULAR SURGICAL SPECIALISTS OR INTERVENTIONAL VASCULAR RADIOLOGISTS?

With the advent of endovascular stent-grafts for the treatment of aortic aneurysms there has been some suggestion that there will be a new role: that of the 'endovascular specialist'.[19] This model is certainly beginning to appear in the USA. The motivation for this development is not necessarily the advancement of patient care. These 'specialists' are likely to focus primarily on the endovascular treatment of aortic aneurysms and peripheral vascular disease. This takes no account of considerable vascular intervention performed by vascular radiologists outside the influence of the vascular surgeon. Unconditional merger of the two specialties would necessarily involve the creation of an all-encompassing role. Some models of merging vascular surgery and radiology have been to the detriment of vascular surgery.[20] In this model the number of vascular surgical procedures fell after the merger (–9.3%; historical trend [HT], +4.7%). By contrast, the number of interventional radiology procedures rose (+56.1%; HT, +15.2%), as did the number of non-invasive testing (+9.2%; HT, +3.5%). In concordance with the number of procedures, the gross revenue of vascular surgery fell (–23.7%; HT, +1.1%) and that of interventional radiology rose (+53.5%; HT, +46.0%).

Such a specialist might conceivably evolve from a vascular surgeon who goes on to complete an accredited radiological training scheme or by a vascular radiologist who goes on to complete an accredited vascular surgical training programme. It is worth noting that in the UK there are far more radiologists with higher surgical qualifications than there are surgeons with higher radiological training. In the era of clinical governance and self-regulation it is clear that vascular surgery should continue to be done by those individuals who can demonstrate that they consistently deliver the best results with the least complications. Similarly vascular radiology should continue to be done by those individuals who can demonstrate that they consistently deliver the best results with the least complications. It is therefore in the interest of both vascular surgeons and vascular radiologists to first put their own house in order. With this in place both specialties have nothing to fear from each other and everything to gain by closer association.

We must be proactive in our pursuit of excellence. One way to achieve this is by setting minimum standards of performance. Such minimum standards were published for the first time by the Royal College of Radiologists in 1999.[21] Each individual must maintain a database of their own cases, recording complications and outcomes. Specialists should be able to stand by their results and have them subject to scrutiny. Those individuals who appear to be falling below recommended standards should be allowed to address this and given the opportunity to retrain if necessary. By strengthening each other's camp we have an opportunity to advance our science and improve patient care.

There is no doubt that where hospitals have 'vascular teams' there is a range in the degree of cooperation and collaboration between vascular surgery and vascular radiology. In centres where there is little or no cooperation it will be increasingly important to build bridges. If both specialties are to evolve then cooperation must be fostered and encouraged.

Over the last 18 months I have been privileged to be part of a training team, (comprising both radiologists and surgeons) responsible for training surgical and radiological colleagues in the endovascular repair of abdominal aortic aneurysms in the UK and in Europe. I have gained some insight of what components go to making a successful endovascular team. In my opinion there is no doubt that a high degree of close collaboration between radiologist and surgeons is fundamental to this success. Vascular radiologists and vascular surgeons will need to be skilled communicators. Tolerance, respect for each other's point of view and sensitivity for each other's egos will, I feel, be necessary if we are to avoid destructive territorial battles. In the words of Francis Bacon 'Whoever is out of patience is out of possession of his soul. Men must not turn themselves into bees, and kill themselves in stinging others'.

There will be some convergence between the two specialties as time goes on but both specialties will, I believe, retain their distinctive character in that the vascular surgeon will have his basis in surgical training. It will be these surgical skills that will make the vascular surgeon an indispensable member of the vascular team. The vascular radiologist will have his foundation in the ever-expanding field of diagnostic imaging. It will be this knowledge of diagnostic imaging together with the years of training, gaining expertise in manual dexterity, that the vascular radiologist will bring to the vascular team. Both vascular surgery and vascular radiology will continue to be in demand into the next century. Vascular surgeons will continue to train the next generation of vascular surgeons and vascular radiologist have a responsibility to train those fortunate to be among the next generation of vascular radiologists.

REFERENCES

1. Berberich J, Hirsch S: Die roentegographische Dartellung der Arterien und Venun am Lebenden. *Munchen Klin Wochenschr* **49:** 2226, 1923
2. Brooks B: Intraarterial injection of sodium iodide. *J Am Med Assoc* **82:** 1016, 1924
3. Farinas PL: A new technique for the arteriographic examination of the abdominal aorta and its branches. *Am J Roent* **46:** 641, 1941
4. Seldinger S: Catheter replacement of Needle in percutaneous angiography: a new technique. *Acta Radiol* **39:** 368–376, 1953
5. Dotter CT, Judkins MP: Transluminal treatment of arteriosclerotic obstruction: description of a new technique and a preliminary report of its application. *Circulation* **30:** 654–670, 1964
6. Gruntzig A, Hopff M: Perkutane Recanalisation chronischer arterieller Verschlusse mit einem neuen Dilatationskatheter: Modifikation der Dotter-Technique. *Dtsch Med Wochenschr* **99:** 2052–2055, 1974
7. Gianturco C, Anderson JH, Wallace S: Mechanical devices for arterial occlusion. *Am J Roent* **124:** 428, 1975
8. Roemm JOF, Gianturco C, Barth MH: The bird's nest inferior vena caval filter. *Radiology* **150:** 225–257, 1984
9. Wright KC, Wallace S, Carnsangavej C *et al.*: Percutaneous endovascular stents: an experimental evaluation. *Radiology* **156:** 69–72, 1985
10. Vascular advisory committee of the Vascular Surgical Society of Great Britain and Ireland: *Provisions of Vascular Services* October 1998
11. Society of Cardiovascular and Interventional Radiology survey results: www.scvir.org/uae_surv_res.htm.
12. The Royal College of Radiologists: *Structured Training in Clinical Radiology* 2nd edn. London: The Royal College of Radiologists EBFCR(99)1, 1999
13. The Royal College of Radiologists: *Structured Training in Clinical Radiology* 2nd edn. *Appendix: Curricula for Subspecialty Training.* London: The Royal College of Radiologists EBFCR(99)1, 1999
14. Moody AR, Pollock JG, O'Connor AR, Bagnall M: Lower-limb deep venous thrombosis: direct MR imaging of the thrombus. *Radiology* **209:** 349–355, 1998
15. Prince MR, Narasimham DL, Stanley JC *et al.*: Breath-hold gadolinium-enhanced MR angiography of the abdominal aorta and its major branches. *Radiology* **197:** 785–792, 1995
16. Velázquez OC, Baum RA, Carpenter JP: Magnetic resonance angiography of lower extremity arterial disease. *Surg Clin North Am* **78:** 519–537, 1998
17. Dondelinger RF, Ghysels MP, Brisbois D *et al.*: *Eur Radiol* **8:** 1254–1273, 1998
18. Barnes SZ, Morr DR, Oggero E *et al.*: The realization of a haptic (force feedback) interface device for the purpose of angioplasty surgery simulation. *Biomed Sci Instrum* **33:** 19–24, 1997
19. Criado FJ: The surgeon as an endovascular interventionist. Why and how? *J Cardiovasc Surg (Torino)* **37** (Suppl 1): 17–25, 1996
20. Ouriel K, Green RM, Waldman D *et al.*: A model for merging vascular surgery and interventional radiology: clinical and economical implications. *J Vasc Surg* **28:** 1006–1010, 1998
21. London: The Royal College of Radiologists: *Standards in Vascular Radiology* BFCR **(99)9,** 1999

Levels of evidence: Vascular Cochrane review

Gillian C Leng, Heather Maxwell

INTRODUCTION

Recent years have seen a phenomenal increase in the amount of published medical research, and consequently in the number of medical journals on the shelves. There has been a similar increase in randomized controlled trials conducted in patients with peripheral arterial disease, and the number published in the last 10 years has more than doubled (Fig. 1). This vast array of literature makes it impossible for the busy clinician to read all the relevant new studies, despite increasing pressure for all practice to be evidence-based. It is therefore important that those with limited time can focus on the studies that provide the best evidence.

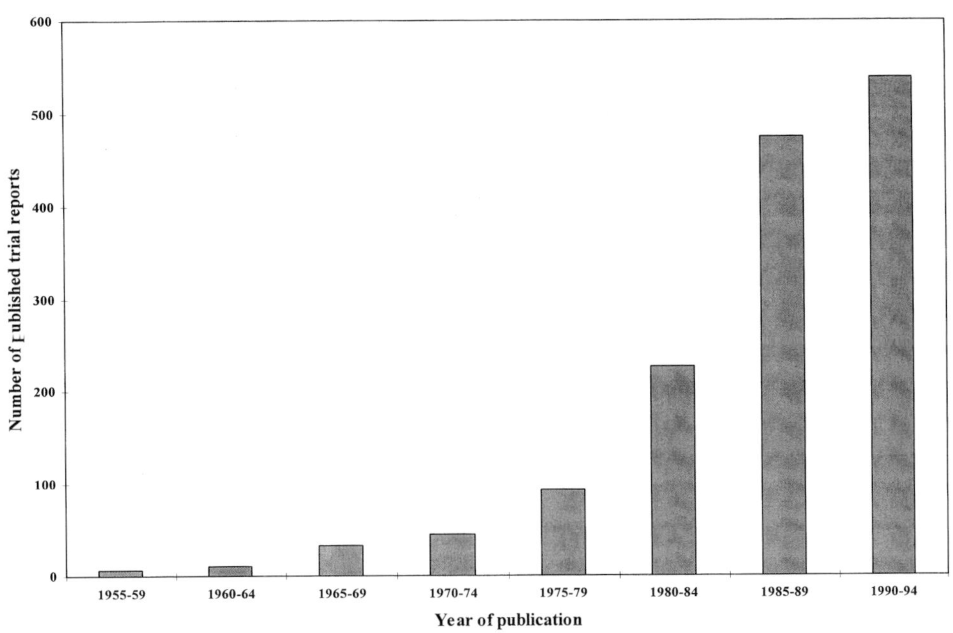

Fig. 1. Randomized controlled trials in patients with lower limb arterial disease and abdominal aortic aneurysm, by year of publication. Data from the Cochrane Review Group on Peripheral Vascular Diseases' Specialist Register of trials.

LEVELS OF EVIDENCE

The United States Agency for Health Care Policy and Research has defined four levels of evidence for therapeutic interventions[1] (Table 1), which are now widely used to produce guidelines and recommendations for patient management. Levels of evidence have also been developed for other areas, including prognosis, diagnosis and economic analysis. In all cases, the highest level is a systematic review of the best primary research, and the lowest level is expert opinion. For therapeutic interventions, the best evidence is based on the randomized controlled trial, or a meta-analysis of randomized controlled trials. The rest of this chapter focuses on these two highest levels of evidence.

Table 1. Levels of evidence for therapeutic interventions

Level	*Sources of evidence*
Ia	Meta-analysis of randomized controlled trials
Ib	At least one randomized controlled trial
IIa	At least one well-designed controlled study without randomization
IIb	At least one other type of well-designed quasi-experimental study
III	Well-designed non-experimental descriptive studies, such as comparative studies, correlation studies and case studies
IV	Expert committee reports or opinions and/or clinical experiences of respected authorities, where there is no explicit critical appraisal

THE RANDOMIZED CONTROLLED TRIAL

The randomized controlled trial was established as a key piece of medical research primarily as a result of the efforts of Sir Austen Bradford Hill. One of the first ever randomized controlled trials was published in 1952 by Daniels and Hill, describing chemotherapy for tuberculosis.[2] It was not until the 1970s, however, that randomized controlled trials began to increase in popularity, a trend reflected in the publication of trials relating to peripheral arterial disease (Fig. 1). A randomized controlled trial is now recognized as the most scientific way of demonstrating the benefits of a treatment regimen. As with any piece of research, however, quality can vary, and it is therefore important to be able to distinguish a good trial from one which is likely to be biased.

Assessing the validity of a randomized controlled trial

When assessing a trial, it is important to consider not only the factors influencing its validity, but also to assess the applicability of the results (Table 2). The most important factors in determining validity are randomization, concealment of allocation, intention to treat analysis and blinding.

Table 2. Questions to ask when reading a trial report[3]

1 *Are these trial results valid?*

Key questions to ask:
- Were participants randomly assigned to a given intervention, and was the randomization list concealed *(concealment of allocation)*?
- Were all participants accounted for at the end of the trial, and were they analysed in the groups to which they were randomized *(intention to treat)*?

Minor points:
- Were the participants and those administering the treatments kept 'blind' to which intervention was being received *(double blind)*?
- Were the groups treated equally apart from the intervention under study?
- Were the groups similar at the start of the trial, i.e. was the randomization effective?

2 *If this is a valid trial:*

What are the results?
- Is there a quantitative result that is clinically meaningful?
- How precise is that result?

Are the results applicable to your patients?
- Are your patients so different from the study participants that the trial results are unlikely to be helpful?
- Were all clinically relevant benefits and side-effects reported?

Randomization

The first and most important feature to check in any trial is that the treatment and control groups were established using a bone fide method of randomization, such as random number tables or computer-generated numbers. Randomization ensures that groups of patients at the start of the trial are as identical as possible, and that any differences in outcome events at the end of the trial are likely to be due to differences in the treatment received. Randomization therefore balances factors such as age or disease severity that may be important in prognosis, plus other factors that might not yet be known.

Concealment of allocation

In addition to simply being randomized, it is also important that the randomization was concealed. Concealment of allocation ensures that the clinician who is entering subjects into a trial is unaware of which treatment the next patient entering the trial will receive, and therefore cannot either deliberately or unconsciously alter the balance between the two groups. If randomization is not adequately concealed, more patients with favourable prognoses tend to be given the experimental treatment. This exaggerates the apparent benefits of therapy and may even lead to a false-positive conclusion that the treatment was effective when it was not. Concealment of allocation is often classified into the following groups:

A *Concealment of allocation was clearly achieved:* e.g. randomization by telephone or a computer system at some distance from where patients were being entered into the trial. Other methods such as sealed opaque envelopes are also acceptable.
B *Unclear:* e.g. the trial report states that the allocation was 'random' but gives no additional information. In this case it is usually recommended to write to the authors of the trial.
C *Allocation was not concealed:* e.g. clear envelopes containing the treatment group, or open lists of random number tables, or allocation by alternation or days of the week. Many systematic reviews of randomized controlled trials will exclude trials where allocation was not concealed.

Intention to treat analysis

All patients entered into the trial should have been accounted for at its conclusion, and been analysed in the groups to which they were originally randomized. To be sure of a trial's conclusions, it should be possible to take all patients lost to follow-up and assign them the 'worst-case' outcomes (that is, assume everyone lost from the group fared worse), and still be able to support the original conclusion.[3] It is unlikely that any trial could withstand a worst-case analysis if more than 20% of its patients had been lost to follow-up.

An intention-to-treat analysis should also be performed, in which patients are analysed according to the groups into which they were randomized, even those who failed to comply with treatment. This is an essential pre-requisite for valid evidence about the effects of therapy. It has repeatedly been shown that patients who do and don't take their medicine have very different outcomes, even when the study medicine they were prescribed was a placebo.[4]

Blinding

It is important that the groups in any trial were treated equally in all respects other than the intervention being tested. One important way of preventing such bias is by keeping those involved in the trial 'blind' to the allocation. Increasingly this is being extended beyond the traditional 'double blind' trial, in which the treating clinician and the patient are unaware of the treatment assignment, to also include blinding of measurement technicians and those undertaking the statistical analysis. In some situations, however, it is impossible for a trial to fulfil all these criteria. In a trial of exercise therapy, for example, it is impossible to mask either doctor or patients, although those performing the outcome assessment and the statistical analysis could be made unaware of the treatment allocation.

Practical relevance

Having established that a trial is of high quality, the next step is to determine whether it holds any relevant messages for your own practice. It is therefore important to establish that the trial report provides a clinically meaningful result, and that all clinically relevant benefits and harms are stated. Finally, check that the participants in the trial were not so different from those in your care that the trial results are not applicable to you.

THE SYSTEMATIC REVIEW AND META-ANALYSIS

A systematic review differs from a more traditional literature review by following a more structured approach using predefined criteria. An important first step in preparing a systematic review is to formulate a well focused question relevant to patient care, as this enables selection criteria to be defined for the inclusion of primary studies in the review.[5] To avoid bias, it is important that these criteria are stipulated at the outset, for example the types of participants involved, treatment, control group, outcomes and study design.

A meta-analysis is a systematic review that uses quantitative statistical methods to evaluate information from the studies included for review.[6] A meta-analysis is especially useful when results from several studies lack statistical significance, but appear to have effects in the same direction. The principal aims of performing a meta-analysis[7] are therefore to:

- Provide a quantitative estimate of the current state of knowledge concerning a treatment effect.
- Improve the precision of an estimated measure of treatment effect.
- Obtain sufficient power to test the statistical significance of a treatment effect.
- Resolve controversy when studies appear to disagree.
- Answer new questions that have not been posed in individual studies, and which the existing studies individually may not have sufficient precision or power to answer.

One of the benefits of combining small studies in a statistical meta-analysis was illustrated in a recent review of angioplasty for intermittent claudication published in the *Cochrane Library*.[8] This review included the only two trials that have compared the effect of angioplasty with conservative management, one based in Edinburgh[9,10] and the other in Oxford.[11,12] After 6 months, both trials showed a significant improvement in the ankle brachial pressure index (ABPI), but combining the results in a meta-analysis increased the precision of the estimate (Fig. 2).

Study	Expt (n)	Expt Mean (SD)	Control (n)	Control Mean (SD)	WMD (95%CI)	Weight (%)
Edinburgh	29	0.88 (0.16)	30	0.74 (0.16)		65
Oxford	20	0.85 (0.18)	16	0.62 (0.16)		35
Total (95% CI)	49		46			100
Chi-square 1.63 (df=1) Z= 5.1						

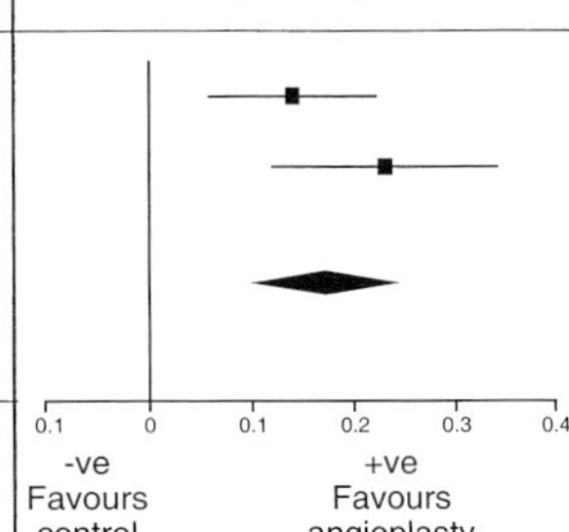

Fig. 2. Meta-analysis of angioplasty for intermittent claudication: angioplasty (Expt) compared with non-surgical management (Ctrl). Outcome was assessed after 6 months using the ankle brachial pressure index. WMD = weighted mean difference.

Stages in performing a systematic review

In the course of preparing a systematic review, seven key stages can be identified (Fig.3). The first stage relates to stating the objectives of the review, as described above, and the final stage is preparing the report. The most time-consuming stages involve identifying trials and then extracting relevant information and data. Delays may result from difficulties obtaining hard copies of trial reports, contacting trialists to obtain additional information, and performing data extraction in duplicate to reduce errors. If there are sufficient data from trials with similar characteristics, these can be pooled in a statistical meta-analysis, otherwise the details of the individual trials must be reported without additional analysis.

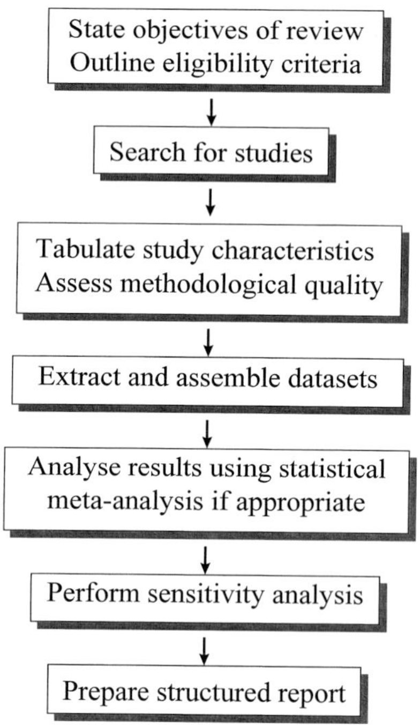

Fig. 3. Stages in preparing a systematic review, as described by the Cochrane Collaboration.

Potential problems with systematic reviewing

Publication bias

A systematic review can be only as good as the evidence on which it is based, and one potential problem is lack of evidence due to publication bias. This is particularly likely to affect trials with inconclusive or negative findings, which are less likely to be published than trials with positive benefits.[13] Several strategies should therefore be employed to reduce the impact of potential publication bias, including locating as many trials as possible. A wide search strategy will include scouring grey literature such as conference proceedings and theses, searching electronic databases and writing to trialists and pharmaceutical companies. It is also important to hand search journals, as up to 30% of trials may be incorrectly indexed on electronic databases.[14]

Once all possible trials have been located, statistical methods can be employed to determine whether any trials are still potentially missing because of publication bias. The most usual method is to perform a funnel plot, in which sample size (on the x-axis) is plotted against effect size, e.g. the odds ratio (on the y-axis). As sample size increases, the effect size should converge in a funnel shape. Publication bias should be suspected if points are missing from one side of the 'funnel', typically smaller trials with negative results.

It is generally agreed that the best method to minimize publication bias is to introduce prospective registration of trials. This will ensure that all planned trials are recorded at the planning stage, independent of subsequent publication. Unfortunately, although there has been some progress in this area, systematic registration of trials is unlikely to occur in the near future.

Trial size

It has been argued that a meta-analysis of several small trials introduces so much variation that the conclusions are not consistent with a single large trial.[15] To determine if this were indeed the case, the results of large clinical trials in pregnancy and childbirth were compared with the findings produced by pooling all the available small trials. This evaluation concluded that results were usually compatible, but some differences occurred even when the diversity among both small and large trials was taken into account.[16] If there are no large trials available, however, a well-conducted meta-analysis represents the best available evidence. It remains unclear whether this is sufficient or whether a large trial will ultimately be required.

Heterogeneity between trials

Significant differences between trials is another potential problem in statistical meta-analysis, often described as summing 'apples and oranges'. Meta-analysis should be performed only if the data being summed are similar or at least comparable, including treatment, patients and outcome measures.[17] The presence of possible heterogeneity should therefore be carefully assessed prior to performing a meta-analysis, both subjectively by clinical judgement and by a statistical test.

How to assess a systematic review

Although in general a systematic review of results from randomized controlled trials constitutes the highest level of evidence, such a review may not always have been carried out to the highest standards. As with any piece of published research, a systematic review should be assessed for quality (Table 3). If the methods of the review have not been clearly stated, and the numbers in the review are not easily accessible then, at the very least, the reviewer has done the reader a disservice.

Table 3. Questions to ask when reading a systematic review [3]

1 Are the results of this systematic review valid?

Were the following steps addressed?

- Objectives of the review clearly stated.
- Comprehensive methods used to identify relevant studies.
- Explicit criteria applied to determine which studies were included.
- Methodological quality assessment of included studies.
- Adequate explanation given for any difference in study results.
- Results combined appropriately.

2 If the results are valid:

Are the results important?

- Conclusions supported by the data given in the review.
- Numerical results which are clinically meaningful

THE COCHRANE REVIEW GROUP ON PERIPHERAL VASCULAR DISEASE

The Cochrane Collaboration

The Cochrane Collaboration was established in 1992 with the broad aims of 'preparing, maintaining and disseminating systematic reviews of the effects of health care'. The Collaboration is named after the British epidemiologist, Professor Archie Cochrane, whose experiences as a prisoner of war inspired him to ensure that all forms of health care would be critically evaluated, thus enabling really effective treatments to be distinguished from those which are of no benefit. In a statement made in 1979,[18] Archie Cochrane reminded the medical profession of the need to obtain reliable evidence about the effects of the treatment it was offering:

> It is surely a great criticism of our profession that we have not organised a critical summary, by specialty or subspecialty, adapted periodically, of all relevant randomised controlled trials.

The Cochrane Review Group on Peripheral Vascular Diseases

To evaluate the evidence relating to peripheral vascular disease, a Cochrane Review Group was established in 1995, based in Edinburgh. The Group now has around 100 active members in 20 countries, largely comprising medical and surgical specialists, but also including hospital administrators and policy makers. Its scope includes varicose veins, chronic venous insufficiency and thromboembolism, lower limb arterial disease, abdominal aortic aneurysm and vasospasm. The Review Group has two main functions: 1) to establish a comprehensive database of all trials relating to peripheral vascular disease; and 2) to produce systematic reviews of the evidence relating to peripheral vascular disease.

Trials relating to peripheral vascular disease

The Review Group has performed extensive searches of electronic databases and hand-searched relevant journals and grey literature to produce a comprehensive database of relevant trials. This Specialist Register of Trials is now one of the best sources of information in the peripheral vascular field and is used by the Review Group as a primary source of trial evidence for reviewers. It is also included in the Register of Trials published in the *Cochrane Library*. The majority of trials in arterial disease involve patients with intermittent claudication (Fig. 4), although many trials relating to aneurysm and critical limb ischaemia have also been published. In venous disease, the vast majority of trials (72%) relate to deep vein thrombosis and thromboembolism.

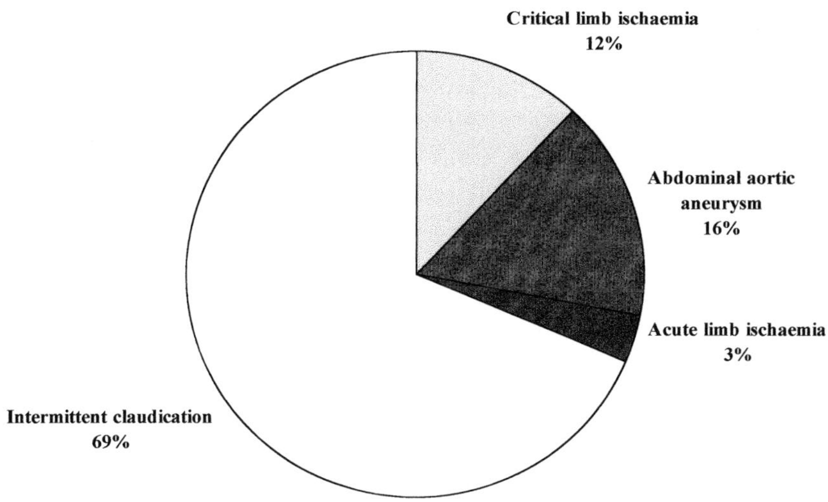

Fig. 4. Trials in arterial disease: breakdown by disease category.

Systematic reviews relating to peripheral arterial disease

The Review Group on Peripheral Vascular Diseases works with reviewers to produce systematic reviews for publication in the *Cochrane Library*. A fundamental aim of the Group is to prepare reviews of all treatments relevant to peripheral vascular disease. This involves reviewing all randomized controlled trials in the field of peripheral vascular disease, and anyone prepared to contribute both time and intellectual effort is welcome to contribute. There are currently over 40 reviews either written or underway, but many more are required. Anyone interested in writing a review is asked to inform the editorial base of the area they wish to review, and assistance is given in terms of software support and identification of trials. Training workshops are also held by the Collaboration at regular intervals. Once a reviewer is ready to start work, they are expected to deliver a draft review within 15 months of registering a title.

CONCLUSIONS

Randomized controlled trials and systematic reviews provide the highest levels of evidence on which to base clinical practice. The number of published trials has increased sharply since the 1960s, and currently over 3000 trials relating to peripheral vascular disease have been identified. There have been relatively few systematic reviews performed in this area, however, and many more are required, particularly in relation to amputation, rehabilitation and radiological interventions. Vascular surgeons and policy makers need to work together to ensure the available evidence is used to produce real improvements in the quality, effectiveness and cost-effectiveness of health care.

REFERENCES

1. US Department of Health and Human Services, Public Health Service, Agency for Health Care Policy and Research: *Acute Pain Management: Operative of Medical Procedures and Trauma*. Agency for Health Care Policy and Research Publications, Rockville, MD, (AHCPR Pub 92-0038), 1992
2. Daniels M, Hill AB: Chemotherapy of pulmonary tuberculosis in young adults. An analysis of the combined results of three Medical Research Council trials. *Br Med J* **i:** 1162, 1952
3. Sackett DL, Richardson WS, Rosenberg W, Hayes RB: *Evidence-based Medicine: How to Practise and Teach EBM. London*: Churchill Livingstone, 1997
4. Murphy J, Coster G: Issues in patients compliance. *Drugs* **54:** 797–800, 1997
5. Counsell C: Formulating questions and locating primary studies for inclusion in systematic reviews. *Annl Intern Med* **127:** 380–387, 1997
6. D'Agostino RB, Weintraub M: Meta-analysis: a method for synthesizing research. *Clin Pharmacol Ther* **58:** 605–616, 1995
7. Mulrow CD: Rationale for systematic reviews. *Br Med J* **309:** 597–599, 1994
8. Fowkes FGR, Gillespie IN: Angioplasty (versus non surgical management) for intermittent claudication (Cochrane Review). In: *The Cochrane Library,* Issue 3, Oxford: Update Software, 1999
9. Whyman MR, Fowkes FGR, Kerracher EMG *et al.*: Randomised controlled trial of percutaneous transluminal angioplasty for intermittent claudication. *Eur J Vasc Endovasc Surg* **12:** 167–172, 1996
10. Whyman MR, Fowkes FGR, Kerracher EMG *et al.*: Is intermittent claudication improved by percutaneous transluminal angioplasty? A randomised controlled trial. *J Vasc Surg* **26:** 551–557, 1997
11. Creasy TS, McMillan PJ, Fletcher EWL *et al.*: Is percutaneous transluminal angioplasty better than exercise for claudication? – preliminary results of a prospective randomised trial. *Eur J Vasc Surg* **4:** 135–140, 1990
12. Perkins JMT, Collin J, Creasy TS *et al.*: Exercise training versus angioplasty for stable claudication. Long and medium term results of a prospective, randomised trial. *Eur J Vasc Endovasc Surg* **11:** 409–413, 1996
13. Dickersin K, Min Y-I, Meinhart CL: Factors influencing publication of research results: follow-up of applications submitted to two institutional review boards. *J Am Med Assoc* **267:** 374–378, 1992
14. Dickersin K, Scheer R, Lefebvre C: Identifying relevant studies for systematic reviews. *Br Med J* **309:** 1286–1291, 1994
15. Borzak S, Ridker PM: Discordance between meta-analyses and large scale randomised controlled trials. *Annl Intern Med* **123:** 873–877, 1995

16. Cappelleri JC, Ioannidis JPA, Schmid CH *et al.*: Large trials vs meta-analysis of smaller trials. How do their results compare? *J Am Med Assoc* **276:** 1332–1338, 1996
17. Eysenck HJ: Meta-analysis and its problems. *Br Med J* **309:** 789–792, 1994
18. Cochrane AL: 1931–1971: a critical review, with particular reference to the medical profession. In: *Medicines for the Year 2000* pp. 1–11. London, Office of Health Economics, 1979

CAROTID OPPORTUNITIES

The unstable carotid plaque: lipid lowering and platelet inhibitory therapy

Marie-Louise M Grønholdt, Henrik H Sillesen, Torben V Schroeder

INTRODUCTION

What triggers a stable carotid atherosclerotic plaque to become unstable, rupture and lead to thrombosis/ cerebral embolism? This question is still largely unanswered, despite years of effort to prevent the outcome, an ischaemic stroke. Whether a surgical or medical approach is taken, cost-effectiveness has to be considered for carotid patients as a group and for every single patient. It has emerged, that plaque vulnerability and thrombogenicity may be more important than plaque size and stenosis severity for event-free survival, at least in coronary arteries.[1] The morphology of the carotid plaque, as evaluated with ultrasound B-mode imaging, has been found to be associated with presence of previous neurological symptoms[2–8] as well as with the risk of development of new neurological symptoms.[9–15] The morphology of a carotid plaque as well as risk factors for atherosclerosis should potentially be considered along with the degree of stenosis, in the determination of which patient will benefit from a carotid endarterectomy and especially which patient will not benefit.

CHARACTERISTICS OF A RUPTURE-PRONE ATHEROSCLEROTIC PLAQUE

Histologically, the most dangerous, rupture-prone plaques causing neurological events are thought to consist of an atheromatous, lipid-rich core covered by a thin fibrous cap.[1] The stability of an atherosclerotic plaque depends on many factors: 1) the thickness and collagen content of the fibrous cap covering an atheromatous core; 2) inflammation with macrophages, T-cells and mast cell infiltration, and repair within the fibrous cap; 3) the size and consistency of the core.[1] Patients with symptomatic carotid disease tend to have more frequent plaque rupture, macrophage foam cell infiltration, and thinning of the fibrous cap than asymptomatic patients.[16] Patients with an echolucent and heterogeneous plaque as assessed by ultrasound – subjectively or computer-assisted – have a higher risk of developing neurological events or infarction on computed tomography (CT) scans than patients with homogeneous, echo-rich plaques (Figs 1,2).[9–15] Furthermore, echolucent plaques are associated with a higher content of lipid and haemorrhage, whereas echo-rich plaques contain more calcification and fibrous tissue.[17–25]

The consistency of the core as well as the inflammation within the fibrous cap may be positively influenced by lipid lowering diet and statins.

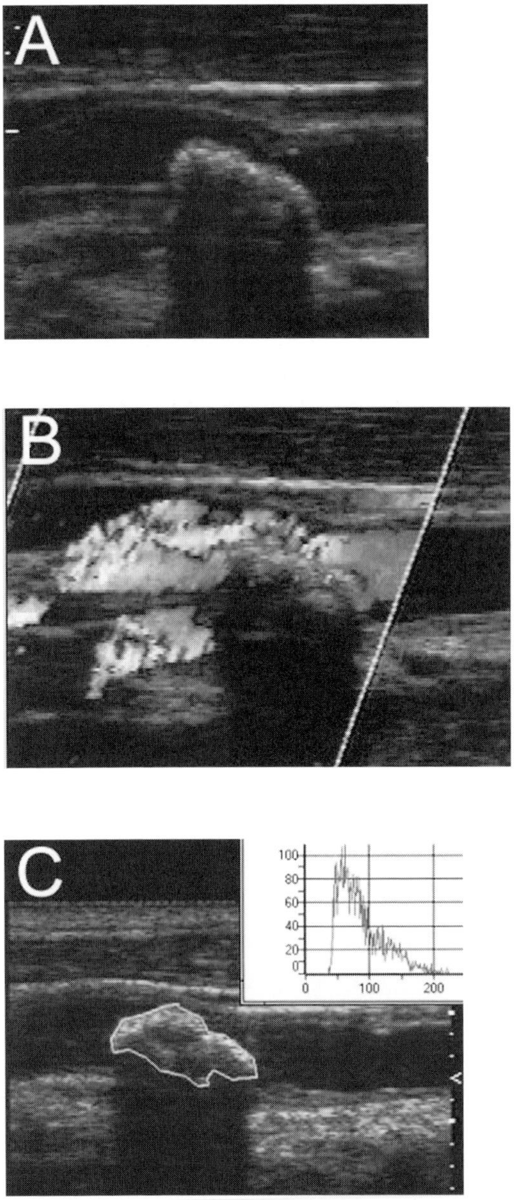

Fig. 1. An echogeneous plaque.

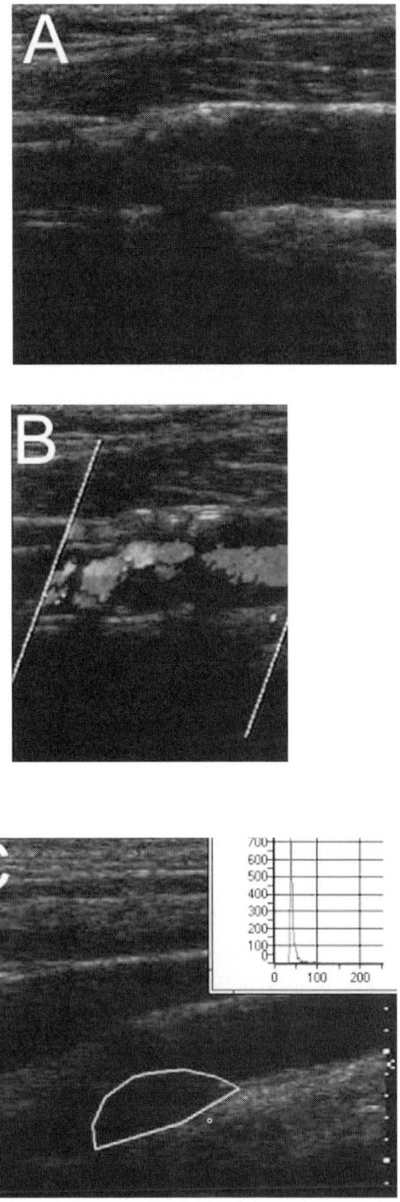

Fig. 2. An echolucent plaque.

LIPID LOWERING IN STROKE PREVENTION

Plasma concentration of lipoproteins is important in the development of atherosclerosis.[26–29] Whereas the associations of cerebrovascular atherosclerosis and infarction and lipoproteins are still under debate, the presence of high levels of low density lipoprotein and low levels of high density lipoprotein cholesterol in plasma is an accepted risk factor for coronary artery disease.[30] Still, more than 10 years ago a meta-analysis of 26 studies on extent and severity of cerebrovascular disease concluded, that similar lipoprotein associations were seen.[31] Most pathogenetic studies on plaque morphology have been performed on coronary arteries, where overlying thrombosis on a ruptured plaque is by far the most common reason for myocardial infarction.[1] In contrast, ischaemic stroke has numerous precursors. Though coronary-type rupture of an unstable plaque is the usual cause of fatal carotid artery occlusion at the bifurcation,[32] the majority of cerebral ischaemic events are thought to be due to embolism from the carotid artery, the heart, or the aorta. In addition, other causes usually underlie intracranial carotid occlusion, including inflammatory arterial disease and small vessel disease in the brain.

It is assumed that the atherosclerotic process and the cells involved are the same in coronary disease as in carotid disease.[33] There is a time delay of about a decade in developing neurological compared with coronary symptoms. This could, in part, be due to the greater blood flow and lumen of the carotid artery. Continuous intimal accumulation of lipoproteins derived from the lumen leads to plaque formation and increasing vulnerability. Tissue lipoproteins are trapped and retained extracellularly or taken up by macrophage foam cells, contributing to core formation and enlargement.[34,35] Low density liprotein cholesterol either derives from the lumen in an oxidized form[36] or is oxidized, mainly by endothelial cells, within the plaque, prior to uptake via macrophage scavenger receptors.[37] Exposure to the cytotoxic effect of oxidized low density liprotein leads to death of the macrophage, thereby releasing proteolytic enzymes like matrix metalloproteinases and subsequent weakening of the fibrous cap and necrosis of the plaque, predisposing it to its rupture.[38,39]

The collagen secreted by smooth muscle cells probably stabilizes plaques, whereas the soft atheromatous 'gruel' destabilizes plaques, making them vulnerable to rupture with high risk of subsequent thrombus formation.[1] An atheromatous core 'gruel' lacks supporting collagen,[40] is rich in extracellular lipids (cholesterol and its esters),[41,42] temperature-dependent (very soft at body-temperature),[41,42] avascular[43,44] and hypocellular. The lipid composition influences the consistency: liquid cholesterol esters soften while crystalline cholesterol stiffens the 'gruel'.[41,42] Lipid-lowering therapy is expected to influence the relative amount of these two lipid-components. The cholesterol esters are depleted, resulting in a stiffer and more stable plaque, but not necessarily a decreased volume of the plaque.[45] However, lowering plasma and low density liprotein cholesterol levels has been shown to reduce progression or even to cause regression of atherosclerotic disease in carotid (intima-media thickness),[46–49] femoral,[50] and coronary[51] arteries, along with a reduced incidence of cerebrovascular events[52–54] myocardial infarction[50] and death[54] in patients with elevated cholesterol levels, as well as in patients with average or below-average cholesterol levels.[55]

Recently, lipid lowering by diet[56] or statins[57–59] was found to have anti-inflammatory actions reducing macrophage accumulation, oxidized low density liprotein, cell death, and matrix metalloproteinase activity and increasing collagen accumulation in the fibrous cap, thereby probably stabilizing the plaques. Statins probably also exert anti-thrombotic effects by inhibition of platelet aggregation and maintenance of a favourable balance between prothrombotic and fibrinolytic mechanisms.[59] This explains the beneficial effects of statins on cardio- and cerebrovascular events, beyond the observed effects on baseline and treated low density liprotein cholesterol level.

Five major interventional studies have shown the beneficial effect on coronary morbidity and mortality of lowering low density liprotein cholesterol by statins.[60–64] Although stroke morbidity was reduced in three of the trials,[60,62,64] this was not a predefined *a priori* end-point and the treated patients had no history of cerebral events nor demonstrated carotid disease. Also, the risk reduction was in fractions of a percent requiring hundreds of patient treatment years to prevent one stroke. Though meta-analyses indicate an effect,[52–54] no single study today has demonstrated convincing evidence that lipid-lowering will reduce the morbidity in patients with carotid atherosclerosis although this would seem logical. It must be noted that cholesterol seems to be a less potent risk factor for ischaemic stroke than for coronary heart disease.[65] Larger reductions in cholesterol or a higher number of patient-years of observation may therefore be required to prove the benefits of statins in ischaemic cerebrovascular disease.

Plasma triglyceride-rich lipoproteins are transferred and selectively retained by macrophages in the arterial intima without prior oxidation, in contrast to low density liproteins. The importance to atherogenesis in some individuals is assumed to be the accumulation, reduced clearance, prolonged exposure of the endothelial surface of these dietary triglyceride-rich particles.[27] Postprandial triglyceride-rich lipoproteins and their remnants and reduced levels of high density liprotein cholesterol are independent predictors of carotid intima-media thickness,[65–67] echolucency[68,69] and coronary artery disease.[32,70–72] The relation of triglycerides to total[73] and ischaemic stroke[74,75] has been found to be positively associated in some studies, but not in others.[76–78] Lately, the controversial role of triglyceride-rich lipoproteins has been stressed in three intervention trials finding a beneficial effect on progression of coronary atherosclerosis[79] and coronary events,[80,81] when reducing triglycerides in plasma. However, no influence was found on carotid atherosclerosis and cerebral events.

In addition to the stabilization of the atherosclerotic plaques in the carotid artery or aorta, there is accumulationg evidence, that statins have an important direct effect during cerebral ischaemia and reperfusion.[82] This potentially neuroprotective effect seems to be cholesterol independent.

In summary, it seems that statin treatment is gaining increasing importance by lowering lipoproteins in plasma as well as decreasing the inflammatory activity and vulnerability in coronary and carotid plaques. However, some individuals are not responding and have thereby no or only limited benefit of statin treatment. Unfortunately, at present, statins are expensive and the magnitude of costs, even if only secondary prevention was applied, might reach the limit of reason if all patients at risk should receive treatment.

ANTIPLATELET THERAPY IN STROKE PREVENTION

Antiplatelet therapy is widely recognized as having the potential to reduce the incidence of stroke, as well as heart attacks and death in patients with symptomatic atherosclerotic disease. Platelet inhibition may be obtained by several methods of action, depending on which part of the complicated process of platelet activation and aggregation is blocked.[83] After vessel injury, i.e. rupture of an atherosclerotic plaque, platelets adhere to the exposed subendothelial structures where they become activated. Upon activation additional platelets are recruited into the growing thrombus by three parallel and coordinated mechanisms. First, aggregated platelets release thromboxane A2; second they release adenosine diphosphate (ADP), both of which stimulate additional platelets; third the activated platelet promotes activation of clotting factors, thereby amplifying thrombin generation (Fig. 3). The last step involves activation of glycoprotein IIb/IIIa, the platelet receptor for fibrinogen.[84] The most well known platelet inhibitor, aspirin, produces its antithrombotic effect by blocking the synthesis of thromboxane A2, whereas ticlopidine and clopidogrel inhibit ADP-induced aggregation. In contrast, glycoprotein IIb/IIIa antagonists block response to all agonists by preventing cross-linkage of fibrinogen to

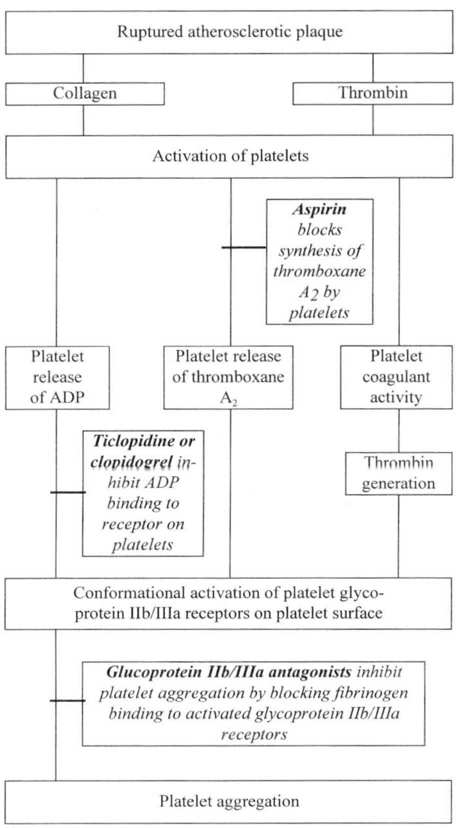

Fig. 3. Sites of action of platelet inhibitors. (Redrawn from Ref. 83.)

platelets.[84,85] These latter antagonists are beyond the scope of this presentation, and will therefore only be mentioned briefly. The glycoprotein IIa/IIIb receptor may be blocked by antibodies (abciximab/ReoPro) or by synthetic inhibitors (eptifibatide or tirofiban). Both types have been effective in studies of acute myocardial ischaemia and/or patients who undergo coronary intervention.[86–89] Abciximab is under evaluation in patients with acute stroke.[83]

Aspirin

Since the Canadian Cooperative Study Group first published their data in 1978, showing effect of aspirin in patients at risk of stroke,[90] multiple randomized, controlled clinical trials have shown benefits of aspirin in decreasing cardiovascular morbidity in general and cerebrovascular morbidity specifically.[91,92] In 1994 the Antiplatelet Trialists concluded that no other antiplatelet regimen was more effective than aspirin alone in preventing recurrent myocardial infarction, stroke, or vascular death.[93] This was based on a large volume of data involving meta-analyses of 142 trials, including more than 70000 patients, in which aspirin was assessed against placebo as well as versus other antiplatelet drugs. Aspirin has been tested at a wide range of doses.[94] Many of the early studies used high doses, i.e. 0.5–1.5 g daily. There is no definitive evidence that a specific dose of aspirin is more clinically effective than another. Therefore, lower doses, i.e. 50 to 300 mg daily, are to be preferred, though opinions differ.[95] An additional argument in favour of the lower doses, is that side-effects – gastrointestinal discomfort, gastric erosion and bleeding – are dose and duration dependent.[96] The American Food and Drug Administration (FDA) now recommends the use of 50–325 mg of aspirin once a day for the prevention of ischaemic stroke and transient ischaemic attack.[94] There is also some evidence to suggest, that the effectiveness of aspirin depends on the "inflammatory status of the patient.[97]

Though an effect on stroke and other peripheral atherothrombotic events have been demonstrated for aspirin, the effectiveness is limited, because it fails to block platelet activation by other agonists such as shear stress, thrombin, collagen, and ADP. It could also be speculated, whether simultaneous intervention with several drugs that act on different targets, will reduce the incidence of vascular events more effectively than monotherapy.

Ticlopidine and Clopidogrel

Ticlopidine and the newer derivate, clopidogrel act through inhibition of one of the complementary pathways of platelet aggregation – the ADP-induced platelet activation.[98–101] More than 10 years ago it was established that ticlopidine could reduce the risk of serious vascular events, i.e. stroke, myocardial infarction and death, in patients with symptomatic atherosclerosis.[99,100,102] More recently it was shown that ticlopidine improved patency after infrainguinal bypass surgery as well as the number of patients who were alive with a patent graft.[103] Most studies compared ticlopidine with placebo and only one study used 'head-to-head' comparison with aspirin.[100] This latter study indicated that ticlopidine was slightly superior to aspirin in terms of stroke prevention and cumulative event rates.

More recently, clopidogrel has been developed as a non-toxic alternative to ticlopidine, known for a 2–3% risk of neutropenia, in which some cases have been fatal.[98–100] For the same reason the authorities in a number of countries, e.g. Denmark, have withdrawn ticlopidine. The clinical efficacy of clopidogrel in secondary prevention has been demonstrated in the CAPRIE study.[101] This trial enrolled 19185 patients, evenly distributed between three high-risk groups: patients with a recent myocardial infarction, a recent stroke, or significant peripheral arterial disease. Data from all three groups were combined for an overall annual event rate of 5.83% in the aspirin-treated group vs 5.32% in the clopidogrel-treated group (9% relative risk reduction; $p<0.05$). The absolute risk reduction of only five events per 1000 patient years questions whether this difference is clinically meaningful. However, the other conclusion to draw is that clopidogrel is at least as effective as aspirin in prevention of recurrent atherothrombotic events. Interestingly, in the subgroup of 6452 patients who were entered into the CAPRIE study due to peripheral arterial disease, clopidogrel significantly reduced, by 24%, the relative risk of vascular events compared with aspirin. In 1997, the FDA approved clopidogrel for use in secondary prevention of heart attacks and stroke. The marked cost difference, i.e. 0.25 Danish krone (DKK) vs 18.75 DKK per day, makes clopidogrel a less attractive overall regimen. However, it should be considered for the stroke patient who does not benefit from or tolerate aspirin[94] or in whom monotherapy with aspirin is considered insufficient.

Combined therapy

Since the antiplatelet agents block different sites, of which some are complementary, combinations of antiplatelet drugs may produce synergistic effects, increasing the antithrombotic effect. This option is of particular interest in situations of increased activation of haemostasis, as for instance during vascular or endovascular procedures. In contrast to the large number of studies on monotherapy, the documentation on combinations of antiplatelet agents is limited, but ticlopidine in combination with aspirin has resulted in higher platelet inhibition than aspirin alone.[104,105] Similarly *in vivo* studies have identified a substantial enhancement by the addition of aspirin to clopidogrel in baboon models.[106] The European Stroke Prevention Study showed combining dipyramidole and aspirin for secondary prophylaxis in patients who had suffered transient ischaemic attack or stroke resulted in an additive effect; the combined therapy resulted in approximately twice the risk reduction (37%) when considering the risk of stroke, compared with either aspirin or dipyramidole alone.[107] Thus, many physicians are recommending the combined regimen although debate is still ongoing. Glycoprotein IIa/IIIb inhibitors block another site. Accordingly, abciximab plus aspirin has been shown more effective than aspirin alone and the addition of abciximab to aspirin and ticlopidine is more effective than aspirin and ticlopidine, at least in patients with myocardial ischaemia.[86,87] Additional clinical research should be directed towards the potential for added benefit with combination therapy in carotid patients.

In summary, a large base of clinical trial experience exists demonstrating that aspirin is effective in the prevention of recurrent thromboembolic events in stroke and myocardial infarction patients. Clopidogrel appears to be a viable alternative to aspirin. The relative cost of aspirin treatment favours its use over clopidogrel.

Recent data indicating a synergistic effect in patients using both aspirin and an ADP-binding inhibitor or dipyridamole suggest increased protection with combination therapy.

REFERENCES

1. Falk E, Shah PK, Fuster V: Coronary plaque disruption. *Circulation* **92:** 657–671, 1995
2. Matalanis G, Lusby RJ: Is there still a place for carotid endarterectomy? *Clin Exp Neurol* **25:** 17–26, 1988
3. European Carotid Surgery Trialists Collaborative Group: Interim results for symptomatic patients with severe (70–99%) and mild (0–29%) stenosis. *Lancet* **325:** 1235–1243, 1991
4. Leahy AL, McCollum PT, Feeley TM *et al.*: Duplex ultrasonography and the selection of patients for carotid endarterectomy: plaque morphology or luminal narrowing? *J Vasc Surg* **8:** 558–562, 1988
5. Steffen CM, Gray-Weale AC, Byrne KE *et al.*: Carotid artery atheroma: ultrasound appearance in symptomatic and asymptomatic vessels. *Aust N Z J Surg* **59:** 529–534, 1989
6. Geroulakos G, Ramaswami G, Nicolaides A *et al.*: Characterization of symptomatic and asymptomatic carotid plaques using high-resolution real-time ultrasonography. *Br J Surg* **80:** 1274–1277, 1993
7. Holdsworth RJ, McCollum PT, Bryce JS *et al.*: Symptoms, stenosis and carotid plaque morphology. Is plaque morphology relevant? *Eur J Vasc Endovasc Surg* **9:** 80–85, 1995
8. Iannuzzi A, Wilcosky T, Mercuri M *et al.*: Ultrasonic correlates of carotid atherosclerosis in transient ischemic attack and stroke. *Stroke* **26:** 614–619, 1995
9. Cave EM, Pugh ND, Wilson RJ *et al.*: Carotid artery duplex scanning: does plaque echogenicity correlate with patient symptoms? *Eur J Vasc Endovasc Surg* **10:** 77–81, 1995
10. O'Holleran LW, Kennelly MM, McClurken M *et al.*: Natural history of asymptomatic carotid plaque. *Am J Surg* **154:** 659–661, 1987
11. Sterpetti AV, Schultz RD, Feldhaus RJ *et al.*: Ultrasonographic features of carotid plaque and the risk of subsequent neurologic deficits. *Surgery* **104:** 652–660, 1988
12. Giannoni MF, Speziale F, Faraglia V *et al.*: Minor asymptomatic carotid stenosis contralateral to carotid endarterctomy (CEA): our experience. *Eur J Vasc Endovasc Surg* **5:** 237–245, 1991
13. Bock RW, Gray-Weale AC, Mock PA *et al.*: The natural history of asymptomatic carotid artery disease. *J Vasc Surg* **17:** 160–169, 1993
14. Belcaro G, Laurora G, Cesarone MR *et al.*: Ultrasonic classification of carotid plaques causing less than 60% stenosis according to ultrasound morphology and events. *J Cardiovasc Surg* **34:** 287–294, 1993
15. Polak JF, Shemanski L, O'Leary DH *et al.*: Hypoechoic plaque at US of the carotid artery: an independent risk factor for incident stroke in adults aged 65 years or older. Cardiovascular Health Study. *Radiology* **208:** 649–654, 1998
16. Carr S, Farb A, Pearce WH *et al.*: Atherosclerotic plaque rupture in symptomatic carotid artery stenosis. *J Vasc Surg* **23:** 755–766, 1996
17. Reilly LM, Lusby RJ, Hughes L *et al.*: Carotid plaque histology using real-time ultrasonography. Clinical and therapeutic implications. *Am J Surg* **146:** 188–193, 1983
18. European Carotid Plaque Study Group: Carotid artery plaque composition – relationship to clinical presentation and ultrasound B-mode imaging. *Eur J Vasc Endovasc Surg* **10:** 23–30, 1995
19. Grønholdt MLM, Wiebe BM, Laursen H *et al.*: Lipid-rich carotid artery plaques may appear echolucent on ultrasound B-mode images and may be associated with intraplaque haemorrhage. *Eur J Vasc Endovasc Surg* **14:** 439–445, 1997
20. Ratliff DA, Gallagher PJ, Hames TK *et al.*: Characterisation of carotid artery disease: comparison of duplex scanning with histology. *Ultrasound Med Biol* **11:** 835–840, 1985

21. O'Donnell TF, Erdoes L, Mackey WC *et al.*: Correlation of B-mode ultrasound imaging and arteriography with pathology findings at carotid endarterectomy. *Arch Surg* **120:** 443–449, 1985
22. Gray-Weale AC, Graham JC, Burnett JR *et al.*: Carotid artery atheroma: comparison of preoperative B-mode ultrasound appearance with carotid endarterectomy specimen pathology. *J Cardiovasc Surg* **29:** 676–681, 1988
23. Spagnoli LG, Mauriello A, Bonanno E *et al.*: Echodensitometry: a methodologic approach to the non-invasive diagnosis of carotid atherosclerotic plaques. *Int Angiol* **8:** 216–223, 1989
24. Feeley TM, Leen EJ, Colgan MP *et al.*: Histologic characteristics of carotid artery plaque. *J Vasc Surg* **13:** 719–724, 1991
25. Widder B, Paulat K, Hachspacher J *et al.*: Morphological characterization of carotid artery stenoses by ultrasound duplex scanning. *Ultrasound Med Biol* **16:** 349–354, 1990
26. Davies MJ, Bland JM, Hangartner JRW *et al.*: Factors influencing the presence or absence of acute coronary artery thrombi in sudden ischaemic death. *Eur Heart J* **10:** 203–208, 1989
27. Zilversmit DB: Atherogenic nature of triglycerides, postprandial lipidemia, and triglyceride-rich remnant lipoproteins. *Clin Chem* **41:** 153–158, 1995
28. Cohn JS: Postprandial lipid metabolism. *Curr Opin Lipidol* **5:** 185–190, 1994
29. Nordestgaard BG, Nielsen LB: Atherosclerosis and arterial influx of lipoproteins. *Curr Opin Lipidol* **5:** 252–257, 1994
30. The American Heart Association and The National Heart, Lung and Blood Institute: The cholesterol facts. A summary of the evidence relating dietary fats, serum cholesterol, and coronary heart disease. *Circulation* **81:** 1721–1733, 1990
31. Tell GS, Crouse JR, Furberg CD: Relation between blood lipids, lipoproteins, and cerebrovascular atherosclerosis. A review. *Stroke* **19:** 423–430, 1988
32. Lammie GA, Sandercock PA, Dennis MS: Recently occluded intracranial and extracranial carotid arteries. Relevance of the unstable atherosclerotic plaque. *Stroke* **30:** 1319–1325, 1999
33. Karpe F, Steiner G, Uffelman K *et al.*: Postprandial lipoproteins and progression of coronary atherosclerosis. *Atherosclerosis* **106:** 83–97, 1994
34. Wight TN: Cell biology of arterial proteoglycans. *Arteriosclerosis* **9:** 1–20, 1989
35. Guyton JR, Klemp KF: Development of the atherosclerotic core region: chemical and ultrastructural analysis of microdissected atherosclerotic lesions from human aorta. *Arterioscler Thromb* **14:** 1305–1314, 1994
36. Palinski W, Horkko S, Miller E *et al.*: Cloning of monoclonal autoantibodies to epitopes of oxidized lipoproteins from apolipoprotein E-deficient mice. Demonstration of epitopes of oxidized low density lipoprotein in human plasma. *J Clin Invest* **98:** 800–814, 1996
37. Steinberg D and Workshop Participants: Antioxidants in the prevention of human atherosclerosis. *Circulation* **85:** 23–38, 1992
38. Matrisian LM: The matrix degrading metalloproteinases. *Bioessays* **14:** 455–463, 1992
39. Shah PK, Falk E, Badimon JJ *et al.*: Human monocyte-derived macrophages induce collagen breakdown in fibrous caps of atherosclerotic plaques. Potential role of matrix-degrading metalloproteinases and implications for plaque rupture. *Circulation* **92:** 1565–1569, 1995
40. Davies MJ: A macro and micro view of coronary vascular insult in ischemic heart disease. *Circulation* **82**(Suppl II): 38–46, 1990
41. Small DM: Progression and regression of atherosclerotic lesions. Insights from lipid physical biochemistry. *Arteriosclerosis.* **8:** 103–129, 1988
42. Lundberg B: Chemical composition and physical state of lipid deposits in atherosclerosis. *Atherosclerosis* **56:** 93–110, 1985
43. Gertz SD, Roberts WC: Hemodynamic shear force in rupture of coronary arterial atherosclerotic plaques. *Am J Cardiol* **66:** 1368–1372, 1990
44. Friedman M: The coronary thrombus: Its origin and fate. *Hum Pathol* **2:** 81–128, 1971
45. Brown BG, Zhao XQ, Sacco DE *et al.*: Lipid lowering and plaque regression: new insights into prevention of plaque disruption and clinical events in coronary disease. *Circulation* **87:** 1781–1791, 1993

46. Blankenhorn DH, Selzer RH, Crawford DW *et al.*: Beneficial effects of colestipol-niacin therapy on the common carotid artery. Two- and four-year reduction of intima-media thickness measured by ultrasound. *Circulation* **88:** 20–28, 1993
47. Furberg CD, Adams HP, Applegate WB *et al.* for the Asymptomatic Carotid Artery Progression Study (ACAPS) Research Group: Effects of lovastatin on early carotid atherosclerosis and cardiovascular events. *Circulation* **90:** 1679–1687, 1994
48. Crouse JR 3rd, Byington RP, Bond MG *et al.*: Pravastatin, lipids, and atherosclerosis in the carotid arteries (PLAC-II). *Am J Cardiol* **75:** 455–459, 1995
49. Salonen R, Nyyssönen K, Porkkala E *et al.*: Kuopio Atherosclerosis Prevention Study (KAPS). A population-based primary preventive trial of the effect of LDL lowering on atherosclerotic progression in carotid and femoral arteries. *Circulation* **92:** 1758–1764, 1995
50. Blankenhorn DH, Azen SP, Crawford DW *et al.*: Effects of colestipol-niacin therapy on human femoral atherosclerosis. *Circulation* **83:** 438–447, 1991
51. Bjelajac A, Goo AKY, Weart CW: Prevention and regression of atherosclerosis: effects of HMG-CoA reductase inhibitors. *Ann Pharmacother* **30:** 1304–1315, 1996
52. Blauw GJ, Lagaay AM, Smelt AHM *et al.*: Stroke, statins, and cholesterol. A meta-analysis of randomized, placebo-controlled, double-blind trials with HMG-CoA Reductase Inhibitors. *Stroke* **28:** 946–950, 1997
53. Crouse JR, Byington RP, Hoen HM *et al.*: Reductase inhibitor monotherapy and stroke prevention. *Arch Intern Med* **57:** 1305–1310, 1997
54. Hebert PR, Gaziano JM Chan KS *et al.*: Cholesterol lowering with statin drugs, risk of stroke, and total mortality. *J Am Med Assoc* 278: 313–321, 1997
55. MacMahon S, Sharpe N, Gamble G *et al.*: Effects of lowering average or below-average cholesterol levels on the progression of carotid atherosclerosis. Results of the LIPID atherosclerosis substudy. *Circulation* **97:** 1784–1790, 1998
56. Aikawa M, Rabkin E, Okada Y *et al.*: Lipid lowering by diet reduces matrix metalloproteinase activity and increases collagen content of rabbit atheroma. A potential mechanism of lesion stabilization. *Circulation* **97:** 2433–2444, 1998
57. Williams JK, Sukhova GK, Herrington DM *et al.*: Pravastatin has cholesterol-lowering independent effects on the artery wall of atherosclerotic monkeys. *J Am Coll Cardiol* **31:** 684–691, 1998
58. Weber C, Erl W, Weber KS *et al.*: HMG-CoA reductase inhibitors decrease CD11b expression and CD11b-dependent adhesion of monocytes to endothelium and reduce increased adhesiveness of monocytes isolated from patients with hypercholesterolemia. *J Am Coll Cardiol* **30:** 1212–1217, 1997
59. Rosenson RS, Tangney CC: Antiatherothrombotic properties of statins. Implications for cardiovascular event reduction. *J Am Med Assoc* **279:** 1643–1650, 1998
60. Scandinavian Simvastatin Survival Study Group: Randomised trial of cholesterol lowering in 4444 patients with coronary heart disease: the Scandinavian Simvastatin Survival Study (4S). *Lancet* **344:** 1383–1389, 1994
61. Shephard J, Cobbe SM, Ford I *et al.* for the West of Scotland Coronary Prevention Study Group: Prevention of coronary heart disease with pravastatin in men with hypercholesterolemia. *New Engl J Med* **333:** 1301–1307, 1995
62. Sacks FM, Pfeffer MA, Moye LA *et al.*: The effect of pravastatin on coronary events after myocardial infarction in patients with average cholesterol levels. *New Engl J Med* **335:** 1001–1009, 1996
63. Downs JR, Clearfield M, Weis S *et al.*: Primary prevention of acute coronary events with lovastatin in men and women with average cholesterol levels. Results of the AFCAPS. *J Am Med Assoc* **279:** 1615–1622, 1998
64. The Long-Term Intervention with Pravastatin in Ischaemic Disease (LIPID) Study Group: Prevention of cardiovascular events and death with pravastatin in patients with coronary heart disease and a broad range of initial cholesterol levels. *New Engl J Med* **339:** 1349–1357, 1998
65. Iso H, Jacobs DR Jr, Wentworth D *et al.*: Serum cholesterol levels and six-year mortality from stroke in 350 977 men screened for the multiple risk factor intervention trial. *New Engl J Med* **320:** 904–910, 1989

66. Sharrett AR, Patsch W, Sorlie PD *et al.*: for the ARIC Investigators. Associations of lipoprotein cholesterols, apolipoproteins A-I and B, and triglycerides with carotid atherosclerosis and coronary heart disease. *Arterioscler Thromb* **14:** 1098–1104, 1994
67. Hodis HN, Mack WJ, Dunn M *et al.*: Intermediate-density lipoproteins and progression of carotid arterial wall intima-media thickness. *Circulation* **95:** 2022–2026, 1997
68. Grønholdt MLM, Nordestgaard B, Nielsen TG *et al.*: Echolucent carotid artery plaques are associated with elevated levels of fasting and postprandial triglyceride-rich lipoproteins. *Stroke* **27:** 2166–2172, 1996
69. Grønholdt MLM, Nordestgaard BG, Wiebe BM *et al.*: Echolucency of computerized ultrasound images of carotid atherosclerotic plaques are associated with increased levels of triglyceride-rich lipoproteins as well as increased plaque lipid content. *Circulation* **97:** 34–40, 1998
70. Simons LA, Dwyer T, Simons J *et al.*: Chylomicrons and chylomicron remnants in coronary artery disease: a case-control study. *Atherosclerosis* **65:** 181–189, 1987
71. Simpson HS, Williamson CM, Olivacrona T *et al.*: Postprandial lipemia, fenofibrate and coronary artery disease. *Arteriosclerosis* **85:** 193–202, 1990
72. Uiterwaal CSPM, Grobbee DE, Witteman JCM *et al.*: Postprandial triglyceride response in young adult men and familial risk for coronary atherosclerosis. *Annl Intern Med* **121:** 576–583, 1994
73. Nubiola AR, Masana L, Masdeu S *et al.*: High-density lipoprotein cholesterol in cerebrovascular disease. *Arch Neurol* **38:** 468, 1981
74. Quiziblash N, Jones L, Warlow C, Mann J: Fibrinogen and lipid concentrations as risk factors for transient ischaemic attacks and minor ischaemic strokes. *Br Med J* **303:** 605–609, 1991
75. Lindenstrøm E, Boysen G, Nyboe J: Influence of total cholesterol, high density lipoprotein cholesterol, and triglycerides on risk of cerebrovascular disease: the Copenhagen city heart study. *Br Med J* **309:** 11–15, 1994
76. Wolf PA, Kannel WB: Reduction of stroke through risk factor modification. *Semin Neurol* **6:** 243–253, 1986
77. Sidharam R: Risk factors for ischemic stroke: a case control analysis. *Neuroepidemiology* **11:** 24–30, 1992
78. Aronow WS, Gutstein H, Lee NH *et al.*: Three-year follow-up of risk factors correlated with new atherothrombotic brain infarction in 708 elderly patients. *Angiology* **39:** 563–566, 1988
79. Ericsson CG, Hamsten A, Nilsson J *et al.*: Angiographic assessment of effects of bezafibrate on progression of coronary artery disease in young male postinfarction patients. *Lancet* **347:** 849–853, 1996
80. Manninen V, Elo MO, Frick MH *et al.*: Lipid alterations and decline in the incidence of coronary heart disease in the Helsinki Heart Study. *J Am Med Assoc* **260:** 641–651, 1988
81. Carlson LA, Rosenhamer G: Reduction of mortality in the Stockholm Ischemic Heart Disease Prevention Study by combined treatment with clofibrate and nicotinic acid. *Acta Med Scand* **223:** 405–418, 1988
82. Vaughan CJ, Delanty N: Neuroprotective properties of statins in cerebral ischaemia and stroke. *Stroke* **30:** 1969–1973, 1999
83. Hirsh J, Weitz: Thrombosis: New antithrombotic agents. *Lancet* **353:** 1431–1436, 1999
84. Coller BS: Platelet IIa/IIIb antagonists: the first anti-integrin receptor therapeutics. *J Clin Invest* **99:** 1467–1471, 1997
85. Topol EJ, Byzova TV, Plow EF: Platelet IIa/IIIb blockers. *Lancet* **353:** 223–227, 1999
86. EPIC investigators use of monoclonal antibody directed against the platelet glycoprotein IIa/IIIb receptor in high risk coronary angioplasty. *New Engl J Med* **330:** 956–961, 1994
87. EPISTENT investigators: Randomised placebo controlled and balloon angioplasty controlled trial to assess safety of coronary stenting with use of platelet glycoprotein IIa/IIIb blockade. *Lancet* **352:** 87–92, 1998
88. The PURSUIT Trials Investigators: Inhibition of platelet glycoprotein IIa/IIIb with eptifibatide in patients with acute coronary syndromes. *New Engl J Med* **339:** 436–443, 1998

89. The platelet receptor inhibition in ischaemic syndrome management in patients limited by unstable signs and symptoms (PRISM-PLUS). Study investigators. Inhibition of the platelet glycoprotein IIa/IIIb receptor with tirofiban in unstable angina and non-Q wave myocardial infarction. *New Engl J Med* **338:** 1488–1496, 1998
90. Canadian Cooperative Study Group: A randomised trial of aspirin and sulfapyrazone in threatened stroke. *New Engl J Med* **299:** 53–59, 1978
91. The SALT Collaborative Group: Swedish aspirin low-dose trial of 75 mg aspirin as secondary prophylaxis after cerebrovascular ischaemic events. *Lancet* **338:** 1345–1349, 1991
92. UK-TIA Study Group: The United Kingdom transient ischaemic attack (UK-TIA) aspirin trial: final results. *J Neurol Neurosurg Psychiat* **54:** 1044–1054, 1991
93. Antiplatelet Trialists´ Collaboration: Collaborative overview of randomized trials of antiplatelet therapy. I: prevention of death, myocardial infarction, and stroke by prolonged antiplatelet therapy in various categories of patients. *Br Med J* **308:** 81–106, 1994
94. Gorelick PB, Born GVR, D´Agostino RB *et al.*: Therapeutic benefit. Aspirin revisited in the light of the introduction of clopidogrel. *Stroke* **30:** 1716–1721, 1999
95. Barnett HJM, Kaste M, Meldrum H, Eliasziw M: Aspirin dose in stroke prevention. Beautiful hypotheses slain by ugly facts. *Stroke* **27:** 588–592, 1996
96. He J, Whelton PK, Vy B, Klag MJ: Aspirin and risk of hemorrhagic stroke: a meta-analysis of randomised controlled trials. *J Am Med Assoc* **280:** 1930–1935, 1999
97. Ridker PM, Cushman M, Stampfer MJ *et al.*: Inflammation, aspirin, and the risk of cerebrovascular disease in apparently healthy men. *New Engl J Med* **336:** 973–979, 1997
98. Ito MK, Smith AR, Lee ML: Ticlopidine: a new platelet aggregation inhibitor. *Clin Pharm* **11:** 603–617, 1992
99. Gent M, Blakely JA, Easton JD *et al.* and the CATS Group: The Canadian American ticlopidine study (CATS) in thromboembolic stroke. *Lancet* **i:** 1215–1220, 1989
100. Hass WK, Easton JD, Adams HP *et al.*: A randomised trial comparing ticlopidine hydrocloride with aspirin for the prevention of stroke in high-risk patients. *New Engl J Med* **321:** 501–507, 1989
101. Caprie Steering Committee: A randomised double blinded trial of clopidogrel versus aspirin in patients at risk of ischaemic events (CAPRIE). *Lancet* **348:** 1329–1339, 1996
102. Janzon L, Bergqvist D, Boberg J *et al.*: Prevention of myocardial infarction and stroke in patients with intermittent claudication: effects of ticlopidine. Results from STIMS, the Swedish ticlopidine multicentre study. *J Intern Med* **227:** 301–308, 1990
103. Becquemin J-P: Effect of ticlopidine on the long-term patency of saphenous vein bypass grafts in the legs. *New Engl J Med* **337:** 1726–1731, 1997
104. Bossavy JP, Thalamas C, Sagnard L *et al.*: A double blind randomised comparison of combined aspirin and ticlopidine therapy vs. aspirin or ticlopidine alone on experimental arterial thrombosis in humans. *Blood* **92:** 12518–12525, 1998
105. Gregorini L, Marco J, Fajadet J *et al.*: Ticlopidin and aspirin pretreatment reduces coagulation and platelet activation during coronary dilation. *J Am Coll Cardioil* **29:** 13–20, 1997
106. Harker LA, Marzec UM, Kelly AB: Clopidogrel inhibitiion of stent, graft and vascular thrombogenesis with antithrombotic enhancement by aspirin in nonhuman primates. *Circulation* **98:** 2461–2469, 1998
107. Diener HC, Cunha L, Forbes C *et al.*: European Stroke Prevention Study, 2: dipyridamole and acetylsalicylic acid in the secondary prevention of stroke. *J Neurol Sci* **143:** 1–13, 1996

Vascular ultrasound, genetic epidemiology and molecular biology: can we bridge the gap?

Andrew N Nicolaides, Michael M Sabetai, Thomas J Tegos, Maura Griffin, George Geroulakos, Surinder Dhanjil, Tarek S El-Atrozy, Marios Cariolou, Evy Bashiardes

INTRODUCTION

Atherosclerotic arterial plaques are responsible for two types of clinical manifestation: (a) chronic ischaemia producing angina, intermittent claudication or asymptomatic bruit and (b) acute syndromes such as myocardial infarction, acute lower limb ischaemia and amaurosis fugax, transient ischaemic attacks or stroke. Chronic ischaemia is the result of decreased blood flow due to arterial stenosis and acute ischaemia is that of plaque erosion or rupture with subsequent thrombosis producing occlusion or embolization.[1,2]

The realization that plaque rupture is a key mechanism underlying acute events is a product of research performed in recent years, particularly of the multidisciplinary approach combining angiography, thrombolytic therapy, plaque pathology, coagulation studies and more recently molecular biology.

Atherosclerotic plaques consist of a lipid-rich core and a fibrous cap separating the core from the lumen. The lipid-rich core contains lipid-laden macrophages (foam cells) derived from blood monocytes.[3] Foam cells produce tissue factor which stimulates thrombus formation when in contact with blood. Macrophages produce metalloproteinases (stromelysins, collagenases and gelatinases) which digest collagen and other extracellular matrix components. In addition, T cells and macrophages produce other substances such as interferon-γ which suppress the production of collagen by smooth muscle cells.[4]

Rupture-prone plaques tend to have a large lipid core, a thin fibrous cap, few smooth muscle cells and an abundance of macrophages.[5] Ruptured plaques heal or enlarge by incorporating the thrombus formed on their surface. Some thrombi grow and occlude the lumen or embolize. Whether a thrombus will occur or enlarge depends on the local blood flow and the hypercoagulable (thrombophilic) state. The latter is under genetic control.

The realization that atherosclerosis and its natural history depend not only on exogenous risk factors, but also on a number of genes with beneficial or detrimental polymorphisms has resulted in the new field of genetic epidemiology. For a long time the study of atherosclerotic disease has been confined to clinical symptomatology and angiography, both of which have inherent disadvantages. Symptoms and clinical events (e.g. stroke) can be the result of different mechanisms (e.g. stroke from large vessel occlusion, small vessel disease or lacunae). Angiography is invasive, cannot be repeated frequently and provides little information on plaque structure. The development of high resolution ultrasound vascular imaging in the last few years has enabled us to study the onset, rate of progression or regression of plaques and most importantly their consistency. The ultrasonic characteristics of unstable (vulnerable) plaques have been determined and populations or individuals at increased risk of cardiovascular events can now be identified.[6] In addition, high resolution ultrasound has enabled us to identify the different ultrasonic characteristics of unstable carotid plaques associated with amaurosis fugax, transient ischaemic attacks, stroke and different patterns of computed tomography (CT)-brain infarcts.[7,8] This provides new insight into the pathophysiology of the different clinical manifestations of extracranial atherosclerotic cerebrovascular disease using a non-invasive method. The success or failure of percutaneous transluminal angioplasty (PTA) in peripheral arteries can be predicted on the basis of the pre-PTA ultrasonic evaluation of the plaque. A group of patients who have an 80% incidence of restenosis after PTA has now been identified.[9] This type of information could not have been obtained by angiography.

The aim of this chapter is to highlight the importance of the multidisciplinary approach and the value of high resolution ultrasound in genetic epidemiology with emphasis on the implications and opportunities for the vascular physician and surgeon.

PLAQUE CHARACTERIZATION – THE NEED FOR UNIFORM TERMINOLOGY

High resolution ultrasound provides *in vivo* information not only on the degree of stenosis but also on the arterial wall characteristics including the size and consistency of the atherosclerotic plaque. Different classifications have been proposed in the literature, according to plaque consistency, resulting in considerable confusion. Plaques containing medium or high-level echoes were classified as homogenous by Reilly *et al.*[10] and correspond closely to Johnson's dense and calcified plaques,[11] to Gray-Weale's type 3 and 4[12] and to Widder's type I and II plaques[13] (i.e. echogenic or hyperechoic). A recent consensus on carotid plaque characterization has suggested that echodensity measurements should be used to reflect the overall brightness of the plaque with the term hyperechoic referring to echogenic and the term hypoechoic referring to echolucent plaques.[14] The reference structure to which plaque echodensity should be compared, is for hypoechoic plaques, blood; for the isoechoic, the sternomastoid muscle; and for the hyperechoic ones, the bone of the adjacent cervical vertebrae.

Measurements of texture should not be confused with measurements of echodensity. With the term homogenous we should refer to plaques of uniform consistency irrespective of whether they are predominantly hypoechoic or hyperechoic (Fig.1). The term heterogenous should be used for plaques of non-uniform consistency, i.e. having both hypoechoic and hyperechoic areas (Fig.2). Although this may seem a relatively simplistic view, it is the foundation for a uniform classification of carotid plaques based on high resolution ultrasound.

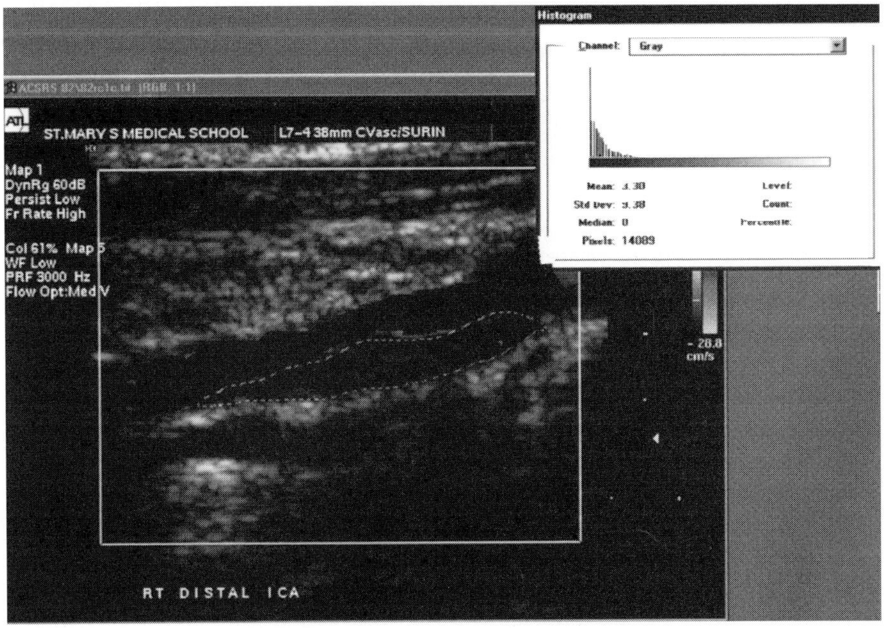

Fig. 1. Hypoechoic plaque (GSM=0) and homogenous (uniform consistency). Note the narrow range of the frequency distribution of the grey tones of the pixels within the

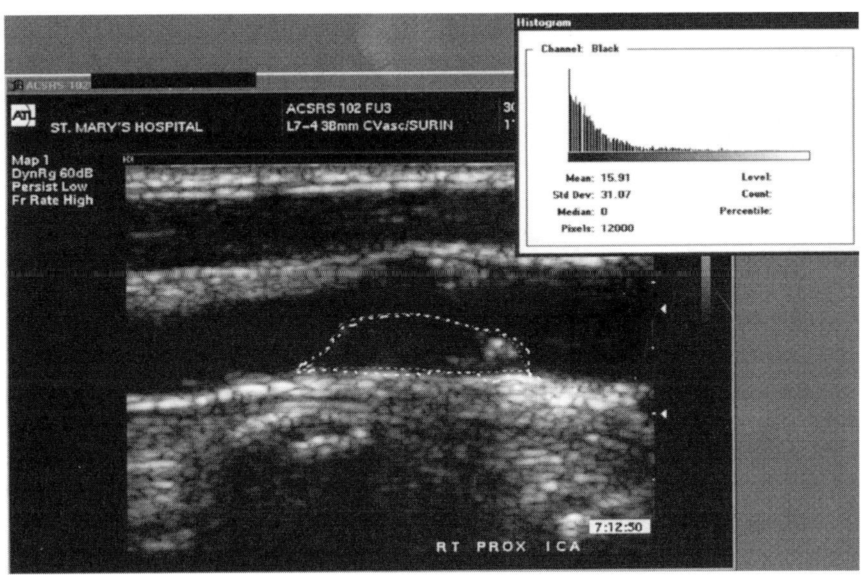

Fig. 2. Hypoechoic (GSM=0) and heterogenous (non-uniform consistency) plaque. Note the wider range of the frequency distribution of the grey tones of the pixels within the outlined area of interest (plaque).

The association between stroke and internal carotid artery plaque echodensity has been investigated recently by Polak *et al.*[15] in 4886 individuals with asymptomatic carotid stenosis who were followed up prospectively for 48 months. In this study plaques were characterized subjectively as hypoechoic, isoechoic or hyperechoic in relation to the surrounding soft tissues. The stroke rate for hypoechoic plaques was 4.2% per annum and 1.2% per annum for both isoechoic and hyperechoic plaques. In addition, hypoechoic plaques causing stenoses of 50–100% were associated with a significantly higher incidence of ipsilateral, non-fatal stroke than iso- or hyperechoic plaques of the same degree of stenosis (relative risk 2.78 and 3.08 respectively). The authors of this study suggested that quantitative methods of grading carotid plaque echomorphology such as computer-assisted plaque characterization may be more precise in determining the association between hypoechoic (echolucent) plaques and the incidence of stroke.

COMPUTER-ASSISTED CAROTID PLAQUE CHARACTERIZATION – THE NEED FOR B-MODE IMAGE NORMALIZATION

Computer-assisted plaque characterization is a recent development. Digitized B-mode images of plaques are taken from a duplex scanner with fixed instrument settings including gain and time gain control. The median of the frequency distribution of grey values of the pixels within the plaque (grey scale median – GSM, scale 0–255, 0=black, 255=white) is used as the measurement of echodensity. Plaques with a GSM of less than 32, i.e echolucent plaques (have been found to have a five-fold increase in the prevalence of silent brain infarcts on CT-brain scans.[16] Similar results for echolucent plaques have been obtained by another team[17] but the cut-off point for the GSM was 50 instead of 32. Their images were brighter because of different instrument settings and it became apparent that what was needed was ultrasonic image normalization, so that images captured under different instrument settings, from different scanners, by different operators and through different peripherals such as video or magneto-optical disk can be compared.

As a result a method has been developed to normalize images by means of digital image processing[18] and using blood and adventitia as the two reference points. A grey scale median of 0–5 is assigned to blood and 185–195 to adventitia using algebraic (linear) scaling (grey scale range: 0–255, black=0, white=255). The brightness of all pixels in the image including those of the plaque are adjusted according to the two reference points. This has resulted in a significant improvement in the comparability of the ultrasonic tissue characteristics.

REPRODUCIBILITY STUDIES

In order to assess the significance of image normalization on the reduction of variability introduced by two different scanners (ATL 3000 and ATL UM9) the same carotid plaque was scanned using the two scanners on the same day. The mean GSM difference before image normalization was 20.6 and was reduced to 6.1 after image

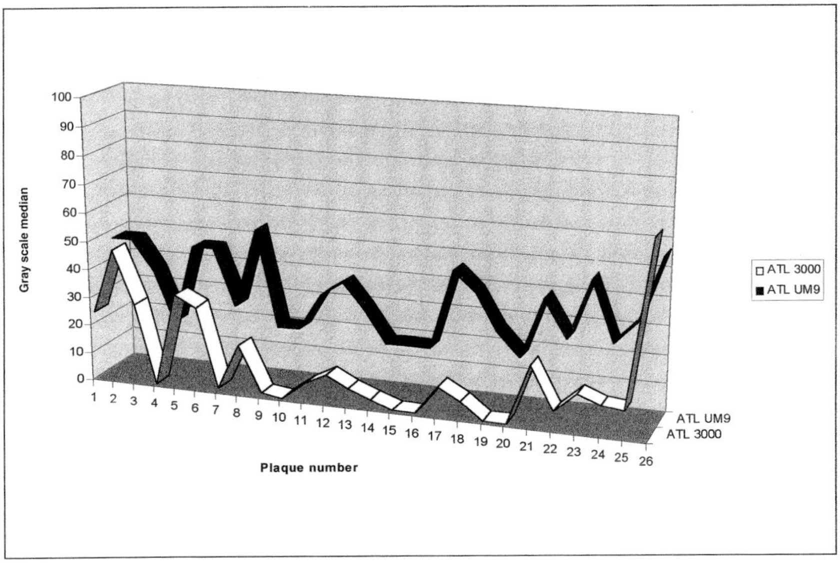

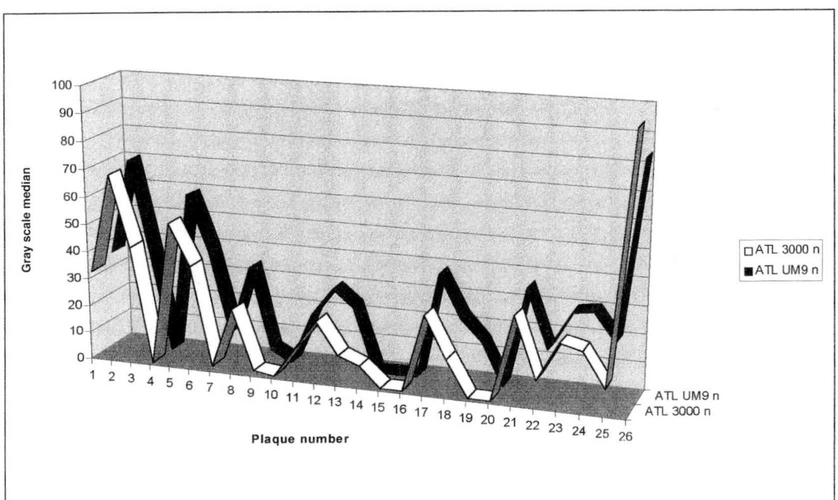

Fig. 3. The effect of ultrasonic image normalization when two different scanners are used (ATL HDI 3000 and ATL UM9).

normalization (t-test, $p<0.001$) (Fig.3). The same carotid plaque B-mode images obtained using the ATL 3000 scanner were stored on videotape and magneto-optical disk, which are the most frequently used storage media. The mean GSM difference before normalization was -14.5 and was reduced to -0.1 after image normalization (t-test, $p<0.001$). In addition, the effect of image normalization on B-mode images obtained using two different multi-frequency linear array probes (7^{-4} MHz and 10^{-5}

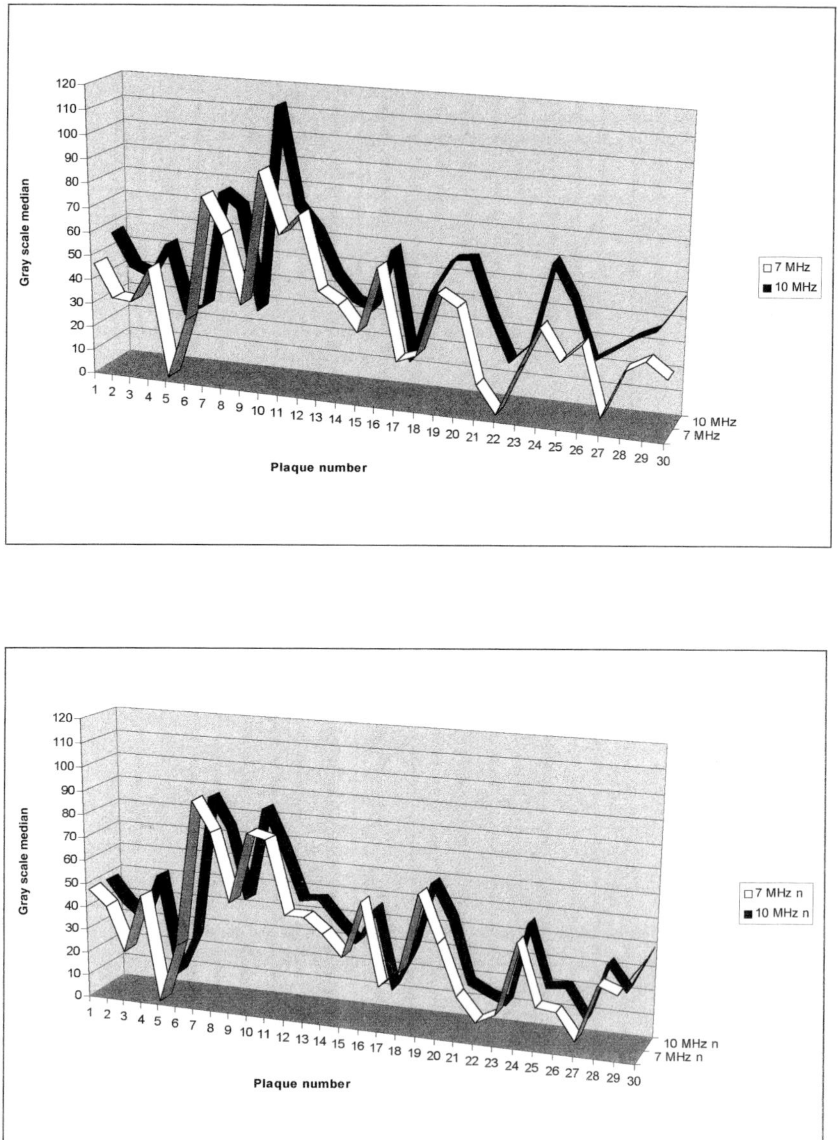

Fig. 4. The effect of ultrasonic image normalization when two different linear probes are used (7^{-4}MHz and 10^{-5}MHz – ATL HDI 3000).

MHz) revealed a mean GSM difference before and after normalization of –8.3 and –0.7, respectively (t-test, p<0.001) (Fig.4). Interobserver variability in normalizing B-mode images obtained from a single scanner (ATL 3000) revealed a mean GSM difference of –1±6.3 (limits of agreement by the Bland and Altman method ± 2SD = 12.6) (Fig.5). This has enabled us to define the limits of experimental error and to use this method to identify real changes in the echodensity of the atherosclerotic plaques in longitudinal studies using high resolution ultrasound.

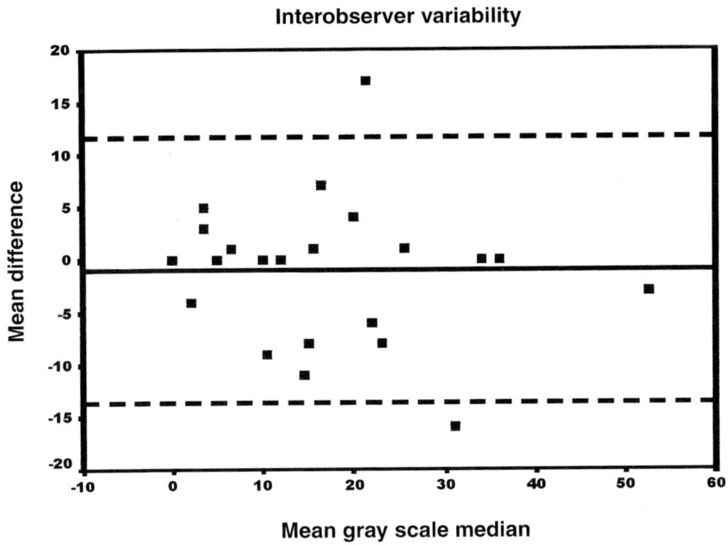

Fig. 5. Interobserver variability in measuring GSM of B-mode carotid plaque images. Limits of agreement are expressed as two standard plot deviations of the mean difference (25D = 12.6) (Bland and Altman plot).

CAROTID PLAQUE ECHODENSITY AND HEMISPHERIC SYMPTOMS

The application of the above method has resulted in the identification of differences in carotid plaque structure – in terms of echodensity and the degree of stenosis – not only between symptomatic and asymptomatic plaques but also between plaques associated with retinal and hemispheric symptoms.[7] In all, 264 patients with 295 carotid bifurcation plaques (146 symptomatic, 149 asymptomatic) causing 50–99% stenosis underwent a carotid duplex scan. Thirty-six plaques were related to amaurosis fugax, 68 to transient ischaemic attacks and 42 to stroke. Plaques associated with symptoms were significantly more hypoechoic, with higher degrees of stenosis than those not associated with any symptoms (mean GSM = 13.3 versus 30.5 and mean degree of stenosis = 80.5% versus 72.2%). Furthermore, plaques associated with amaurosis fugax were hypoechoic (mean GSM = 7.4) and severely stenotic (mean degree of stenosis = 85.6%). Plaques associated with transient ischaemic attacks and stroke had the same echodensity and the same degree of stenosis (mean GSM = 14.9 versus 15.8 and mean degree of stenosis = 79.3% versus 78.1%). These findings confirm previous reports which show that hypoechoic plaques are more likely to cause symptoms.[16–19] In addition, they support the hypothesis that amaurosis fugax has a different pathophysiological mechanism to that of transient ischaemic attacks and stroke.

Indeed, in patients with severe carotid stenosis who present with amaurosis fugax the ipsilateral stroke risk at 2 years is 16.6%, which is significantly lower than the

43.5% risk for those who present with transient ischaemic attacks.[20] Other studies have suggested a more favourable outcome after carotid endarterectomy for those patients who present with amaurosis fugax.[21,22] Holdsworth *et al.*,[23] in a cross-sectional study of individuals with 20–99% internal carotid artery stenosis found only amaurosis fugax to be associated with hypoechoic plaques, although overall the degree of stenosis was more predictive of the development of future neurological events.

The role of biomechanical forces in the induction of plaque fatigue has been emphasized.[24–26] In our group of patients, the carotid plaques associated with amaurosis fugax were hypoechoic and were associated with very high grade stenoses. It may be that these plaques which are hypoechoic and homogenous, undergo low internal stresses and therefore tend to rupture at a later stage (higher degrees of stenosis) producing small platelet aggregates in the post-stenotic cul-de-sac which interfere with the perfusion of the sensitive retina. On the other hand, plaques associated with transient ischaemic attack or stroke were less hypoechoic and less stenotic than those associated with amaurosis fugax. These plaques are hypoechoic but more heterogenous and therefore may tend to rupture at an earlier stage (lower degrees of strenosis), producing larger particle debris (plaque constituents or thrombi) that deprive large areas of the brain of adequate perfusion.

CAROTID PLAQUE ECHODENSITY AND SILENT CT-BRAIN INFARCTS

In patients presenting with hemispheric symptoms, the presence of brain infarcts on CT-scan is of significant prognostic value for the development of future neurological events,[27] shorter survival time[28] and higher neurological morbidity and mortality after carotid endarterectomy.[29,30] In patients undergoing carotid endarterectomy for asymptomatic carotid stenosis the presence of silent CT-brain infarcts is predictive of poor neurological outcome.[31] It has also been suggested that asymptomatic hypoechoic carotid plaques are associated with a higher risk for the development of future neurological events.[15]

We studied 273 asymptomatic carotid plaques (218 patients) causing 50–99% stenosis.[32] Plaque echodensity was expressed by means of the GSM. Every patient had a brain CT scan and the presence of silent infarcts in the ipsilateral anterior and middle cerebral artery territory was noted. Brain infarctions identified on CT scan were classified into the following groups according to their pathophysiological mechanism: group A (discrete subcortical, large and small cortical – related to carotid bifurcation plaques only, probable embologenic mechanism) group B (diffuse white matter lesions, basal ganglia infarcts and lacunae – not related to carotid bifurcation plaques only, cerebral small vessel disease)[33–36] and normal CT scans. The median GSM of plaques related to group A silent CT brain infarcts was 14, of plaques related to group B, 36 and of those not related to any infarcts, 28 ($p=0.004$, Kruskal–Wallis test). The median degree of stenosis for the three groups of plaques was 80%, 70% and 75%, respectively ($p=0.1$, Kruskal–Wallis test).

In this study we have shown that hypoechoic plaques (low GSM) are associated with silent infarcts, that are probably the result of atherothrombotic embolism. On the other hand, hyperechoic plaques are associated with normal CT scans or with silent infarcts that are less dependent (basal ganglia infarcts) or independent (diffuse white matter lesions and lacunae) of the presence of carotid bifurcation plaques. These results emphasize the embolic potential of asymptomatic hypoechoic plaques and show an association between asymptomatic hyperechoic plaques (carotid atherosclerosis) and cerebral small vessel disease. This is in accordance with preliminary results from our team which have shown that hypoechoic plaques are associated with higher embolic counts on transcranial Doppler in the ipsilateral middle cerebral artery than hyperechoic ones.[37] In addition, carotid plaques related to high embolic counts are associated with a higher prevalence of group A CT-brain infarcts.[8]

THE ACSRS STUDY AND THE ICAROS REGISTRY

Are carotid plaque echomorphology and the presence of silent brain infarcts important in identifying a subgroup of patients with asymptomatic carotid stenosis at increased risk of stroke? The methodology of computer-assisted carotid plaque characterization with B-mode image normalization and the aforementioned classification of silent brain infarcts are now being applied in a prospective multicentre international natural history study of asymptomatic carotid stenosis with stroke as the primary end-point.

The aim of the Asymptomatic Carotid Stenosis and Risk of Stroke study is to identify a high risk subgroup that has an ipsilateral stroke rate greater than 4% (ideally greater than 7%), based on risk factors and the findings of the non-invasive investigations (mainly ultrasonic carotid plaque characterization, ultrasonic morphometric measurements such as maximum plaque thickness and lipid core area and silent CT brain infarcts related to carotid bifurcation plaques).[38] In addition, a low risk subgroup with an ipsilateral stroke rate of less than 1% will be identified. This study will provide evidence about the importance of ultrasonic carotid plaque characterization and the different patterns of silent CT brain infarctions associated with cerebrovascular events (stroke, transient ischaemic attack, amaurosis fugax).

Ultrasonic carotid plaque characterization can provide useful information for the endovascular specialist who is likely to use it to select patients for carotid angioplasty and stenting.[39] It would be interesting to compare the outcome after carotid angioplasty and stenting between plaques of varying degrees of echodensity as assessed by computer-assisted plaque characterization. If such a correlation exists then plaque echodensity may prove to be an index of the risk of embolization during carotid angioplasty and stenting. As a result, the ICAROS registry was set up (Imaging: Carotid Angioplasty and Risk Of Stroke) in order to test the above hypothesis.[40]

RESTENOSIS FOLLOWING BALLOON ANGIOPLASTY

Recent work by our team has demonstrated that high resolution ultrasound can be used to study restenosis in peripheral arteries following angioplasty. A number of observations have important implications for future practice and research.

Echolucent plaques (GSM under 25) tend to be associated with successful angioplasty producing a large lumen. In contrast, echogenic plaques are associated with a smaller lumen and recoil producing restenosis. Plaque growth can be measured weekly or monthly and is associated with restenosis if such growth is seen on both the anterior and posterior wall of the artery. It is not associated with restenosis if it occurs on the anterior wall proximal to the lesion and on the posterior wall distal to the lesion.[41] Finally, by means of the GSM before PTA a subgroup has been identified that has an 80% incidence of restenosis.[8]

These observations provide a unique opportunity for obtaining information on restenosis not available with angiography. The effect of drugs on plaque growth should be studied with ultrasound rather than relying on angiographic stenosis. Also, the subgroup with the highest incidence of restenosis should be the ideal population for randomized studies on PTA versus stenting.

GENETIC EPIDEMIOLOGY OF VASCULAR DISEASE

Case-control studies have indicated that a number of gene polymorphisms are associated with atherosclerotic disease. However, the current literature is difficult and confusing. This is for the following reasons:

1. Atherosclerosis, as in many other forms of vascular disease is polygenic.
2. Gene expression is variable in different cells and even in the same type of cell (e.g endothelial cells) in different organs.
3. Some genetic mutations have incomplete penetrance. Expression is modulated by external factors and other genes. Endogenous risk factors which can be adverse (e.g. raised low density lipoprotein (LDL)) or protective (e.g. raised high density lipoprotein (HDL)) are often the result of gene polymorphisms and exogenous factors which can also be adverse or protective. Thus, the effect of each endogenous risk factor (e.g. blood level and type of fibrinogen) is often the result of an interaction between different gene polymorphisms and exogenous risk factors (Fig. 6). Also, the effect of each exogenous risk factor (e.g. smoking) is often modified by a number of genes depending on the individual's genotype. For example, the relative risk of myocardial infarction is 2 in smokers of RQ353 and QQ353 genotypes of factor VII polymorphism, but it is 6 in RR353 genotype.[42]
4. Our endpoints of disease are ill-defined. Too often we rely on angiography or clinical events. Unfortunately clinical events (e.g. stroke) can be the result of different pathophysiological mechanisms.

One of the earliest identified and studied genes is the apolipoprotein E. ApoE which plays a central role in the regulation of lipid metabolism by mediating the binding of lipoprotein particles to the LDL receptor and ApoE(remnant) receptor. The ApoE gene has three alleles; E2, E3 and E4. These alleles interact differently with lipoprotein receptors and alter circulating lipid levels. Although 60% of variation in plasma cholesterol is genetically determined, ApoE polymorphism accounts for only 14% of this. This illustrates the important effect of other genes in lipid metabolism.

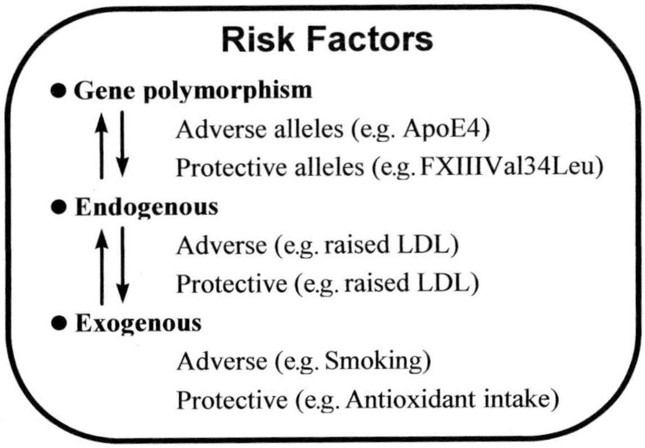

Fig. 6.

The frequency of the ApoE alleles in the European populations is as follows: E3 80%, E2 8% and E4 12%. The E2 allele is associated with low LDL, high triglycerides and low HDL. The E4 allele is associated with high LDL, high triglycerides and low HDL. Kinetic studies have shown that E4 allows the accumulation of LDL and E2 the accumulation of triglycerides. The presence of an E4 allele increases the risk of coronary heart disease and the genotype E3/E4 is associated with myocardial infarction at an early age.[43] In young men, under 40 years, undergoing coronary angioplasty the E4/E4 genotype was 16 times more common than in the general population.[44] The frequency of the E4 allele is increased in patients with ischaemic cerebrovascular disease[45] and in a recent case control study the E2 allele was associated with protection from stroke at age 70–79 but not in those over 80 years. Individuals not carrying an E2 allele had a relative risk of 2.6 for stroke.[45]

Another recent case control study has investigated the frequency of the ApoE and beta-fibrinogen G/A-455 polymorphisms in ischaemic stroke.[47] After excluding intracranial haemorrhage, 277 patients with focal cerebral ischaemia were compared with 277 normal controls. There was no difference in the allele frequency between the groups but when stroke was classified according to type, the E4 allele and the A allele of the beta-fibrinogen genes were more frequent in those with stroke (n=70) due to large vessel disease. The key message is that clinical end-points can be the result of different pathologies and future studies should use end-points that are appropriate for the genes studied.

Figure 7 shows a number of exogenous risk factors and genes with known polymorphisms, some beneficial and some adverse, influencing lipid metabolism. Lipid metabolism exogenous factors and a large number of genes with known polymorphisms interact to determine the development and progression of atherosclerotic disease (Fig. 7). It has been indicated earlier on in this chapter that atherosclerotic plaques are of different types and go through several stages before they produce local complications leading to the developments of symptoms. Plaque

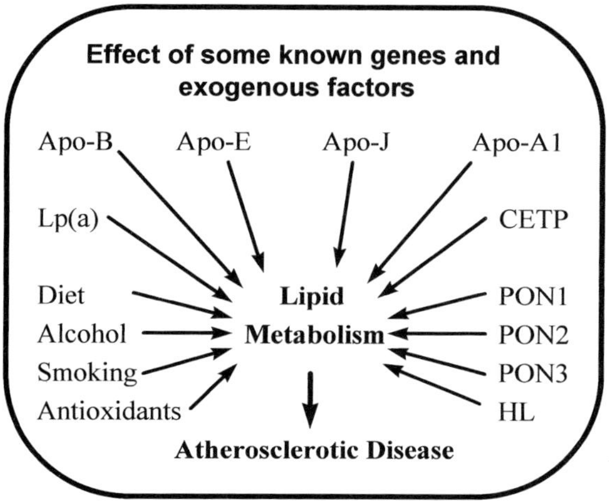

Fig. 7.

formation occurs early or late in life and growth can be slow or rapid. Plaques can be stable or unstable the latter being prone to rupture. Ruptured plaques may heal or develop intravascular thrombosis. Whether such thrombosis may be limited (become part of plaque growth) or extensive will depend on local flow and the coagulation and fibrinolytic systems. Some of the above stages can be determined and measured by ultrasound. The underlying mechanisms are influenced and controlled by different genes. Figure 8 shows the most likely actions of different exogenous and endogenous risk factors and cardiovascular genes in plaque development and progression according to the current literature. In contrast to clinical endpoints and angiography which provide little information about the consistency of plaques, ultrasound does. It is foreseen that ultrasound will become a major tool in the hands of genetic epidemiologists. Understanding the precise mechanism of gene/risk factor interaction will lead to novel therapeutic and prophylactic methods. For example, over-expression of specific beneficial genes could 'trap' the deleterious factors and can be used as part of gene therapy. Plaque stabilization by medication is now becoming a reality and ultrasound can be used in the development and monitoring of the effects of new therapeutic strategies.

Restenosis following balloon angioplasty is a major unsolved problem facing the vascular physician, surgeon and interventional radiologist. Prophylactic studies developed in animals do not work in humans. They need to be studied in humans and for this reason a 'human restenosis model' has been developed by our team. As indicated above restenosis occurs in 30–40% of patients and can be the results of inadequate dilatation, adventitial wall recoil or smooth muscle proliferation. Angiotensin II is a critical modulator of smooth muscle proliferation. However, several studies have failed to show an association between the angiotensin converting enzyme ACE I/D polymorphism and restenosis after conventional balloon angioplasty.

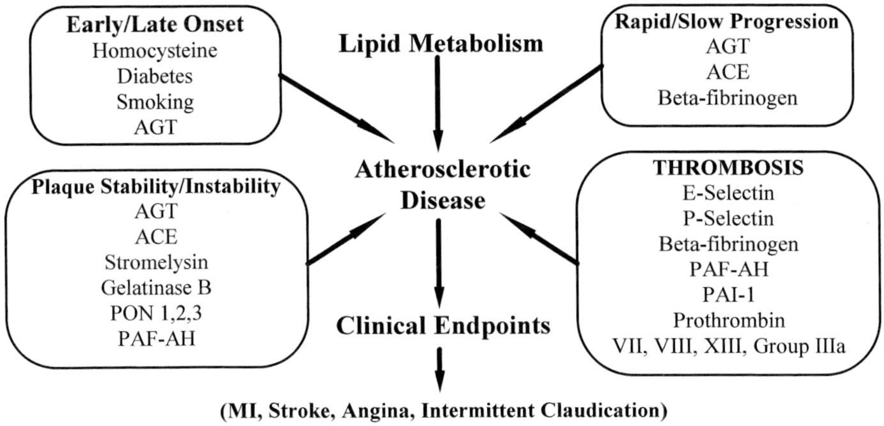

Fig. 8. Effect of known genes and exogenous factors.

A recent study of 146 patients who underwent successful implantation of a coronary stent and had repeat angiography at 6 months has shown that the minimal luminal diameter (MLD) was related to the ACE genotype. At 6 months the MLD was 1.65 (±0.71)mm for the DD genotype, 1.84(±0.60)mm for the ID genotype and 2.05 (±0.61)mm for the II genotype. The relative risk of restenosis (over 50% diameter stenosis at follow-up) was 2.00 (95% CI,1.03 to 3.88, $p<0.04$) per number of D alleles. The authors have argued that in this particular study restenosis was the result of smooth muscle proliferation in all cases since other causes of restenosis were eliminated by the stent.[48] These results have been confirmed by subsequent studies.[49,50]

Similar studies should be performed in patients undergoing peripheral angioplasty. The availability of ultrasound and its ability to measure plaque growth from smooth muscle proliferation and distinguish it from recoil or inadequate dilatation should be an asset.

CONCLUSION: THE PLACE OF VASCULAR ULTRASOUND

High resolution vascular ultrasound is a powerful new tool. Although it was initially developed as a diagnostic method it has already found applications in other related fields especially in epidemiology and in the study of the natural history of atherosclerosis. It should prove valuable in genetic epidemiology and in monitoring the results of the emerging vascular gene therapy. In the immediate future, information useful for the surgeon will emerge from the identification of high risk patients, better selection of patients for surgery and of those who would benefit most from primary peripheral artery stenting or angioplasty alone.

REFERENCES

1. Gutstein DE, Fuster V: Pathophysiology and clinical significance of atherosclerotic plaque rupture. *Cardiovasc Res* **41**: 323–333, 1999
2. Zukowski AJ, Nicolaides AN, Lewis RT *et al.*: The correlation between carotid plaque ulceration and cerebral infarction seen on CT scan. *J Vasc Surg* **1**: 782, 1984
3. Libby P: Molecular basis of acute coronary syndromes. *Circulation* **91**: 2844–2850, 1995
4. Clinton S, Underwood R, Sherman M *et al.*: Macrophage-colony stimulating factor gene expression in vascular cells and human atherosclerosis. *Am J Pathol* **140**: 301–316, 1992
5. Davies MJ, Richardson PD, Woolf N *et al.*: Risk of thrombosis in human atherosclerotic plaques: role of extracellular lipid, macrophage and smooth muscle cell content. *Br Hear J* **69**: 377–381, 1993
6. Belcaro G, Nicolaides AN, Lauroroa G *et al.*: Ultrasound morphology classification of the arterial wall and cardiovascular events in a 6-year follow-up study. *Arterioscler Thromb Vasc Biol* **16**: 851–856, 1996
7. Sabetai MM, Tegos TJ, Nicolaides AN *et al.*: Hemispheric symptoms and carotid plaque echomorphology. *J Vasc Surg* (in press), January 2000
8. Tegos TJ, Sabetai MM, Ramaswami G, Nicolaides AN: Clinical correlates of embolic events on transcranial Doppler. *Br J Surg* **85**(Suppl. 2): 161, 1998
9. Ramaswami G, Tegos T, Nicolaides AN *et al.*: Ultrasonic plaque character and outcome after lower limb angioplasty. *J Vasc Surg* **29**: 110–21, 1999
10. Reilly LM, Lusby RJ, Hughes L *et al.*: Carotid plaque histology using real-time ultrasonography: clinical and therapeutic implications. *Am J Surg* **146**: 188–193, 1983
11. Johnson JM, Kennelly MM, Decesare D *et al.*: Natural history of asymptomatic carotid plaque. *Arch Surg* **120**: 1010–1012, 1985
12. Gray-Weale AC, Graham JC, Burnett JR *et al.*: Carotid artery atheroma: comparison of preoperative B-mode ultrasound appearance with carotid endarterectomy specimen pathology. *J Cardiovasc Surg* **29**: 676–681, 1988
13. Widder B, Paulat K, Hachpacher J *et al.*: Morphological characterisation of carotid artery stenoses by ultrasound duplex scanning. *Ultrasound Med Biol* **16**: 349–354, 1990
14. deBray JM, Baud JM, Dauzat M for the Consensus Conference: Consensus concerning the morphology and the risk of carotid plaques. *Cerebrovasc Dis* **7**: 289–296, 1997
15. Polak JF, Shemanski L, O'Leary DH *et al.*: for the Cardiovascular Health Study. Hypoechoic plaque at ultrasound of the carotid artery: An independent risk factor in adults aged 65 years or older. *Radiology* **208**: 649–654, 1998
16. El-Barghouty NM, Nicolaides A, Bahal V *et al.*: The identification of high risk carotid plaque. *Eur J Vasc Surg* **11**: 470–478, 1996
17. Biasi GM, Sampaolo A, Mingazzini P *et al.*: Computer analysis of ultrasonic plaque echolucency in identifying high risk carotid bifurcation lesions. *Eur J Vasc Endovasc Surg* **17**: 476–479, 1999
18. El-Atrozy T, Nicolaides A, Tegos T *et al.*: The effect of B-mode image standardisation on the echodensity of symptomatic and asymptomatic carotid bifurcation plaques. *Int Angiol* **17**: 179–186, 1998
19. Geroulakos G, Ramaswami G, Nicolaides A *et al.*: Characterisation of symptomatic and asymptomatic carotid plaques using high-resolution real-time ultrasonography. *Br J Surg* **80**: 1274–1277, 1993
20. Streifler JY, Eliaziw M, Benavente OR *et al.*: for the North American Symptomatic Carotid Endarterectomy Trial. The risk of stroke in patients with first-ever retinal versus hemispheric transient ischemic attacks and high-grade carotid stenosis. *Arch Neurol* **52**: 246–249, 1995
21. Golledge J, Cuming R, Beattie DK *et al.*: Influence of patient-related variables on the outcome of carotid endarterectomy. *J Vasc Surg* **24**: 120–126, 1996
22. Blohme L, Sandstrom V, Hellstrom G *et al.*: Complications in carotid endarterectomy are predicted by qualifying symptoms and preoperative CT findings. *Eur J Vasc Endovasc Surg* **17**: 213–218, 1999

23. Holdsworth RJ, McCollum PT, Bryce JS, Harrison DK: Symptoms, stenosis and carotid plaque morphology. Is plaque morphology relevant? *Eur J Vasc Endovasc Surg* **9**: 80–85, 1995
24. Richardson PD, Davies MJ, Born GVR: Influence of plaque configuration and stress distribution and fissuring of coronary atherosclerotic plaque. *Lancet* **ii**: 941–944, 1989
25. Ku DN, McCord BN: Cyclic stress causes rupture of the atherosclerotic plaque cap. *Circulation* **88** (Suppl): 1362, 1993
26. Glagov S, Bassiouny HS, Sakaguchi CA *et al.*: Mechanical determinants of plaque modeling, remodeling and disruption. *Atherosclerosis* **131** Suppl.: S13–S14, 1997
27. The Dutch TIA Trial Study Group. Predictors of major vascular events in patients with transient ischemic attack or nondisabling stroke. *Stroke* **24**: 527–531, 1993
28. Evans GW, Howard G, Murros KE *et al.*: Cerebral infarction verified by cranial computed tomography and prognosis for survival following transient ischemic attack. *Stroke* **22**: 431–436, 1991
29. Cao P, Giordano G, De Rango P *et al.*: Computerised tomography findings as a risk factor in carotid endarterectomy: early and late results. *Eur J Vasc Endovasc Surg* **12**: 37–45, 1996
30. Blohme L, Sandstrom V, Hellstrom G *et al.*: Complications in carotid endarterectomy are predicted by qualifying symptoms and preoperative CT findings. *Eur J Vasc Endovasc Surg* **17**: 213–218, 1999
31. Cao P, Zannetti S, Giordano G *et al.*: Cerebral tomographic findings in patients undergoing carotid endarterectomy for asymptomatic carotid stenosis: short-term and long-term implications. *J Vasc Surg* **29**: 995–1005, 1999
32. Sabetai MM, Tegos TJ, Dhanjil S *et al.*: Carotid plaque structure and silent CT-brain infarcts. Presented at the 13th Annual Meeting of the European Society for Vascular Surgery, Copenhagen 1999.
33. Bogousslavsky J: The plurality of subcortical infarction. *Stroke* **23**: 629–631, 1992
34. Norrving B, Cronqvist S: Clinical and radiologic features of lacunar versus nonlacunar minor stroke. *Stroke* **20**: 59–64, 1989
35. Caplan LR: Silent brain infarcts. *Cerebrovasc Dis* **49**(Suppl. 1): 32–39, 1994
36. Nicolaides A, Kalodiki E, Ramaswami G *et al.*: The significance of cerebral infarcts on CT scans in patients with transient ischaemic attacks. In: Bernstein EF, Callow AD, Nicolaides AN, Shifrin EG (Eds), *Cerebral Revascularisation* pp. 159–178. London: Med-Orion; 1993
37. Tegos TJ, Guang M, Daskalopoulos M *et al.*: The identification of unstable carotid plaque. The value of TCD. *Int Angiol* **16**, S79, 1997
38. Nicolaides AN: Asymptomatic carotid stenosis and risk of stroke. Identification of a high risk group (ACSRS). *Int Angiol* **14**: 21–23, 1995
39. Reid DB. Carotid plaque characterisation: Helpful to endarterectomy and endovascular surgeons. *J Endovasc Surg* **5**: 247–250, 1998
40. Biasi GM, Mingazzini PM: Computerised assessment of the carotid plaque structure correlated with the severity of the disease. In: Branchereau A, Jacobs M (Eds), *New Trends and Developments in Carotid Artery Disease* pp. 53–59. Armonk, NY: Futura Publishing Co., 1998
41. Ramaswami G, Dhanjil S, Nicolaides AN *et al.*: Restenosis after percutaneous transluminal angioplasty: a human model. *Am J Surg* **176**: 102–108, 1998
42. Iacoviello L, DiCastelnuovo C, D'Orazio A, Donash MB: Cigarette smoking doubles the risk of myocardial infarction in carriers of a protective polymorphism in the blood coagulation factor VII gene. *Thromb Hemost* **81**: 658–659, 1999
43. Vauhkonen I, Niskanen L, Ryynanen M *et al.*: Divergent association of apolipoprotein E polymorphism with vascular disease in patients with NIDDM and control subjects. *Diabet Med* **14**: 748–756, 1997
44. van Bockxmeer FM, Mamotte CD: Apolipoprotein epsilon 4 homozygocity in young men with coronary heart disease. *Lancet* **340**: 879–880, 1992
45. Pedro-Botet S, Senti M, Nogues X *et al.*: Lipoprotein and apolipoprotein profile in men with ischemic stroke: role of lipoprotein (a), trigyceride-rich lipoproteins and apolipoprotein E polymorphism. *Stroke* **23**: 1556–1562, 1992

46. Ferrucci L, Guralnik JM, Pahor M *et al.*: Apolipoprotein E, E2 allele and risk of stroke in the older population. *Stroke* **28**: 2410–2416, 1997
47. Kessler C, Spitzer C, Stauske D *et al.*: The apolipoprotein E and beta-fibrinogen G/A-455 gene polymorphisms are associated with ischaemic stroke involving large vessel disease. *Arterioscler Thromb Vasc Biol* **17**: 2880–2884, 1997
48. Amant C, Bauters C, Lablanche JM *et al.*: D allele of the angiotensin I-converting enzyme is a major risk factor for restenosis after coronary stenting. *Circulation* **96**: 56–60, 1997
49. Ribichini F, Steffenino G, Dellavalle A *et al.*: Plasma activity and insertion/deletion polymorphism of angiotensin I-converting enzyme: a major risk factor and a marker of risk for coronary stent restenosis. *Circulation* **97**: 147–154, 1998
50. Guarda E, Fajuri A, Marchant E *et al.*: D/D genotype of the gene for angiotensin converting enzyme as a risk factor for post-stent coronary restenosis. *Rev Esp Cardiol* **52**: 475–480, 1999

New cerebral protection techniques for carotid angioplasty

Michel Henry, Christos Klonaris, Max Amor, Isabelle Henry, Michele Hugel

INTRODUCTION

Carotid endarterectomy has been the 'gold standard' for the treatment of carotid stenosis for the past 40 years. Large randomized trials have proved its efficacy for severe extracranial carotid artery disease and its superiority over medical treatment. However, the benefits of carotid endarterectomy are critically dependent on the rate of perioperative complications. If perioperative morbidity and mortality exceed 3% in asymptomatic and 6% in symptomatic patients the benefits of surgery are quickly lost.[1]

Despite well trained surgeons and strict inclusion criteria, stroke and death rates were 5.8% in the North American Symptomatic Carotid Endarterectomy Trial (NASCET), 7.5% in the European Carotid Surgery Trial (ECST) and 2.3% in the Asymptomatic Carotid Surgery Study (ACAS) studies.[2–4] It is important to recognize that in everyday clinical practice there is a large number of high-risk patients who do not meet the inclusion criteria set in these studies and for whom the indications and risks of carotid endarterectomy are not yet established. The mortality rate in the NASCET trial was 0.6%; however, among Medicare beneficiaries undergoing it, it was 3% during the same period.[5]

Based on the encouraging results obtained in coronary and peripheral circulation with angioplasty and stenting, a natural evolutionary step was the application of these techniques at the cerebrovascular level. Several series have been reported suggesting that carotid angioplasty and stenting can be performed with an acceptable perioperative combined stroke and death rate of 5.3–8.2%.[6–10] Nevertheless, even with the most meticulous techniques and experienced operators, embolic stroke during the procedure remains an unpredictable event and represents its major drawback. Indeed the majority of the reported neurological complications are due to the intracerebral embolism of plaque fragments or thrombus.

THE PROBLEM: GENERATION OF EMBOLIC PARTICLES

Many studies demonstrated the frequency of plaque fragments and debris embolic migration during the endovascular procedure. Theron[11] analysed the aspirated blood after carotid angioplasty under cerebral protection and found in 17 of 21 cases cholesterol crystals ranging from 600 to 1300 μ in length. Martin[12] studied samples taken during *in vitro* carotid stenting and found two types of plaque debris: cholesterol crystals, ranging from 3.7 to 500 μ and lipoid masses with a size ranging from 26 to 600 μ. Ohki[13] utilized human carotid artery specimens obtained from patients undergoing standard carotid endarterectomy and found that *ex vivo* balloon angioplasty and stenting produced embolic particles consisted of atherosclerotic debris, organized thrombus and calcified material. Echolucent plaques and lesions associated with stenosis more than 90% produced a higher number of embolic particles.

Jordan[14] analysing microemboli detected by transcranial Doppler after carotid endarterectomy and after carotid angioplasty and stenting reported that interventional procedures were associated with more than eight times the rate of microemboli seen during carotid endarterectomy.

Embolism may occur at different steps of a carotid angioplasty procedure. Placement of the guiding catheter in the common carotid artery which may be challenging in tortuous arteries and dilated atheromatous aortic arch. Crossing the lesion, balloon dilation, stent implantation and postdilation, all include a risk. In a small study with transcranial Doppler monitoring the majority of emboli occurred during catheter manipulation and carotid balloon deflation.[15] However, we believe that the risk of embolization is even higher during post-dilatation after stent deployment, because the struts of the stent are enlarged and are moving relatively to the vessel wall with a risk of producing embolic debris by cutting off fragments of the plaque surface.

The clinical significance of the number of emboli particles generated after balloon angioplasty and stenting is not clear but patients among whom balloon angioplasty and stenting produced a higher number of particles would be expected to have a higher periinterventional stroke rate than patients among whom fewer particles or smaller particles are produced.[13] Particle sizes vary from 50 μ to more than 1000 μ, with the majority being within the 100–500 μ range. Particles less than 200 μ are probably of no major significance but this has yet to be proved.

THE SOLUTION: ELIMINATING THE EMBOLIC RISK

Several possibilities may be considered:

Choice of the patients and of the lesion

Neurological complications are highly dependent on patient selection. Mathur[16] found that advanced age, lesion severity and long or multiple stenoses were independent predictors of procedural stroke. In contrast, sex, presence of coronary disease, diabetes, hyperlipidaemia, smoking, prior endarterectomy, bilateral lesions, contralateral carotid occlusion, plaque ulceration, type of stents, and the number of produced embolic particles were not correlated with perioperative events.

Ohki[13] showed by multivariate analysis that plaques with a high degree of stenosis and low echogenicity were independent risk factors for the generation of embolic particles. Therefore, these lesions may be less suitable for balloon angioplasty and stenting. He found no correlation between sex, diameters of the carotid artery, plaque ulceration or calcification and the number of embolic particles with perioperative symptoms. In our experience, we have aspirated particles in all cases even in the presence of lesions with theoretically low risk of cerebral embolism such as echogenic plaques, concentric lesions or restenoses.

The procedure

For all interventionists the learning curve plays an crucial role. In our single-centre experience with 315 carotid angioplasties, the neurological complication rate during the first 60 procedures was 8% versus 3.1% in the more recent cases ($p<0.05$).

From a technical point of view, it is important to perform the procedure as atraumatically as possible. The use of coronary techniques has reduced the risk of cerebral embolization. The introduction of stents has practically ruled out technical complications like dissections but the stent itself is not a sufficient protection against embolic events. In all series on carotid angioplasty and stenting the embolic risk remains regardless of the implantation techniques and stent characteristics.

The benefit of antiplatelet drugs has been well demonstrated for patients undergoing a carotid angioplasty procedure. The use of fibrinolytic drugs and abciximab may be considered in certain cases, in the presence of particularly thrombogenic lesions.

Cerebral protection

Certainly, wide application of carotid angioplasty is limited by the embolic potential. It has become evident that traditional techniques are insufficient to eliminate the debris generated by the procedure. In 1984 Vitec reported a case of successful angioplasty in a 55-year old patient with innominate artery stenosis and right subclavian steal.[15] He used a second balloon catheter to occlude the origin of the right common carotid artery during the procedure in order to reduce the risk of cerebral embolization. To our knowledge this was the first use of a protection mechanism in brachiocephalic interventions. Consequently several sophisticated techniques have been proposed to protect the cerebral circulation from embolic events.

Balloon occlusion of the internal carotid artery

This technique was first proposed by Theron[17] in 1990 and consists of occluding the internal carotid artery above the lesion prior to the procedure with a balloon inflated at low pressure. Thus the blood flow is oriented towards the external carotid artery. The brain is therefore protected from any embolic event and the generated debris is then removed by aspiration and flushing. Protection techniques using balloon devices are based on this concept.

Theron's technique. The technique consists of using a triple coaxial catheter that occludes the internal carotid artery with the use of a latex balloon incorporated at its tip. The lesion is directly crossed by the microcatheter without guidewire. The technique seems efficient and attractive; however, in our view it has some limitations: the system is not available on the market, has poor radiopacity, only peripheral balloons can be used, and most importantly the microcatheter is not steerable. In addition, there is no guidewire to help crossing the stenosis. Thus at least 10% of the lesions, such as tight stenoses or tortuous vessels, cannot be crossed. In these cases Theron proposed a simplified protection technique where, similar to current non-protected habits, the procedural steps of pre-dilatation and stent implantation are performed with a steerable guidewire but the post-dilatation is carried out under protection utilizing the microcatheter and occlusion balloon. This technique may shorten the occlusion time, but does not totally eliminate the risk of embolism during the first procedural steps.

We have used Theron's technique to treat 47 lesions, five of them with the simplified method, but we were unable to avoid four neurological complications and subsequently we abandoned it.

The PercuSurge Guardwire™ device. This recently developed emboli containment system was first tested experimentally[18] followed by clinical use in 27 aortocoronary saphenous vein graft angioplasties.[19] It has been shown that the system is compatible with routine angioplasty procedures and capable of containing and retrieving atherosclerotic and thrombotic debris and may aid in the prevention of distal embolization. The device has been proposed for cerebral protection during carotid angioplasty.

Description of the device

The PercuSurge GuardWire™ System (PercuSurge Inc., Sunnyvale, CA, USA) consists of three main components:

1. The GuardWire temporary occlusion catheter is a 0.014 inch or 0.018 inch angioplasty wire constructed of hollow nitinol hypotube. Incorporated into its distal segment is an inflatable elastomeric balloon capable of occluding vessel outflow. A marker shows the location of the balloon. The diameter of the balloon (5 or 6 mm) is chosen depending on the diameter of the artery. The terminal part of the wire is 3.5 cm long, floppy, shapeable to cross the lesion much like coronary wires. The wire is available in 2 lengths, 190 and 300 cm allowing 'monorail' or 'over the wire' techniques for balloon dilatation and stenting.
2. The proximal end of the hypotube wire incorporates a Microseal™ allowing inflation and deflation of the distal occlusion balloon utilizing a Microseal™ adapter. The Microseal™ keeps the elastomeric balloon inflated while allowing catheter exchange at the proximal end, similar to commonly used guidewires.
3. The Export™ aspiration catheter is placed over the shaft of the GuardWire™ to aspirate the debris generated by the procedure. It also may be used to flush the internal carotid artery.

Protected angioplasty and stenting technique (Figs 1–6)

An 8 or 9F guiding catheter is initially placed into the common carotid artery using the femoral approach. The GuardWire™ is then gently advanced through the guiding catheter. The lesion is crossed and the marker of the balloon was placed 2 or 3 cm beyond it. The MicroSeal™ adapter is then attached and the occlusion balloon slowly inflated with a fixed volume of dilute contrast, occluding the internal carotid and deriving vessel outflow towards the external carotid artery. On detaching the Microseal™ adapter, the occlusion balloon remains inflated. Angioplasty and stenting are then performed under protection. Any debris generated is removed from the internal carotid artery using aspiration and/or flushing techniques.

The occlusion balloon usually remains inflated during both stages of the procedure, i.e. pre-dilatation of the stenosis and stent implantation. In this case aspiration and flushing are performed only once after stent dilatation. Alternatively the balloon can be deflated between the two stages to restore the cerebral flow. Consequently aspiration and flushing are performed both after pre-dilatation and stent dilatation. The choice of the technique used depended on the tolerance of the occlusion, the cerebral collateral vascularization, the state of the contralateral artery, the duration of the procedure, and the technical problems encountered.

In both scenarios the Export™ catheter is advanced over the wire into the dilated area and a 20-cc syringe is connected to it to retrieve any debris by aspiration. Additionally, a lavage of the dilated and treated area can be performed using saline injections through the guiding catheter after removal of the aspiration catheter. By this technique, the particles are 'driven' towards the external carotid artery.

Once aspiration and flushing are complete, the Microseal™ adapter is reattached to the GuardWire™ and the distal occlusion balloon is then deflated, allowing normal vessel flow. In the presence of satisfactory angiographic result the device is removed.

Our experience

We have been using this device for cerebral protection for the last 21 months. So far 111 internal carotid artery stenoses in 100 eligible patients have been treated with this technique. Fifty seven lesions (51%) were associated with symptoms in the ipsilateral hemisphere. Twenty-five patients presented with a contralateral internal carotid stenosis, four had a total occlusion. One patients with contralateral total occlusion also had bilateral subclavian artery stenoses, one artery was dilated and stented before carotid angioplasty. We estimated that 71% of this population would have been excluded definitely or temporarily from NASCET or ACAS studies. The majority of lesions were atherosclerotic in origin. According to the NASCET criteria[2] the mean percent stenosis was 80.9 ± 9.5%.

Immediate technical success was 99.1%. (Figs 7, 8) In one patient it was impossible to cross the lesion with the Guardwire™ due to important tortuosities of the common and internal carotid arterial. The procedure was performed without cerebral protection. Deflation of the balloon and restoration of cerebral flow between pre-dilatation and stent implantation was used for 25 lesions; 84 lesions were treated with the balloon inflated during the total procedure. The

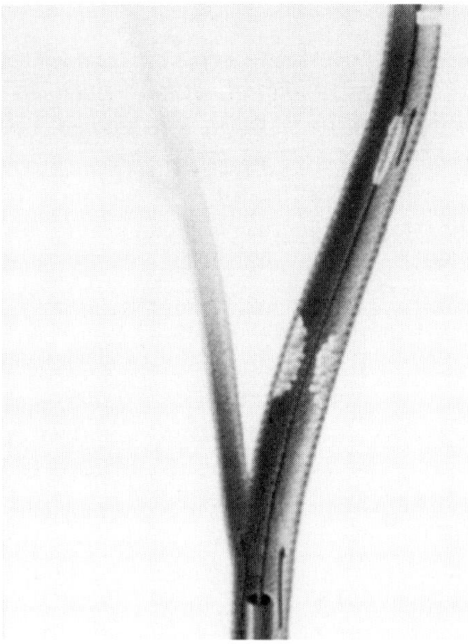

Fig. 1. A guide catheter is placed at the common carotid artery. The lesion is crossed by the GuardWire™ and the occlusion balloon is placed 2–3 cm distally.

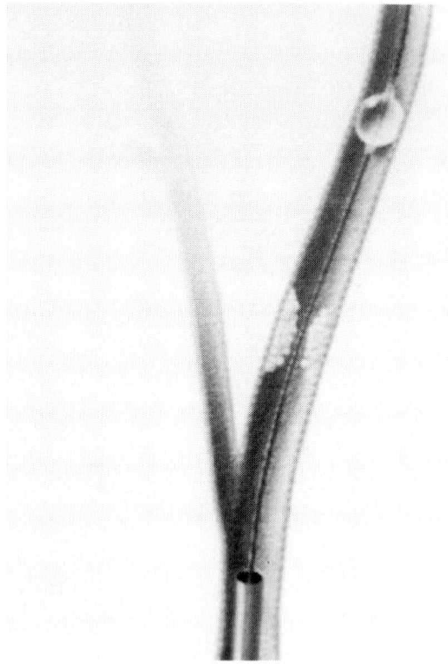

Fig. 2. The Guardwire™ balloon is inflated.

(a)

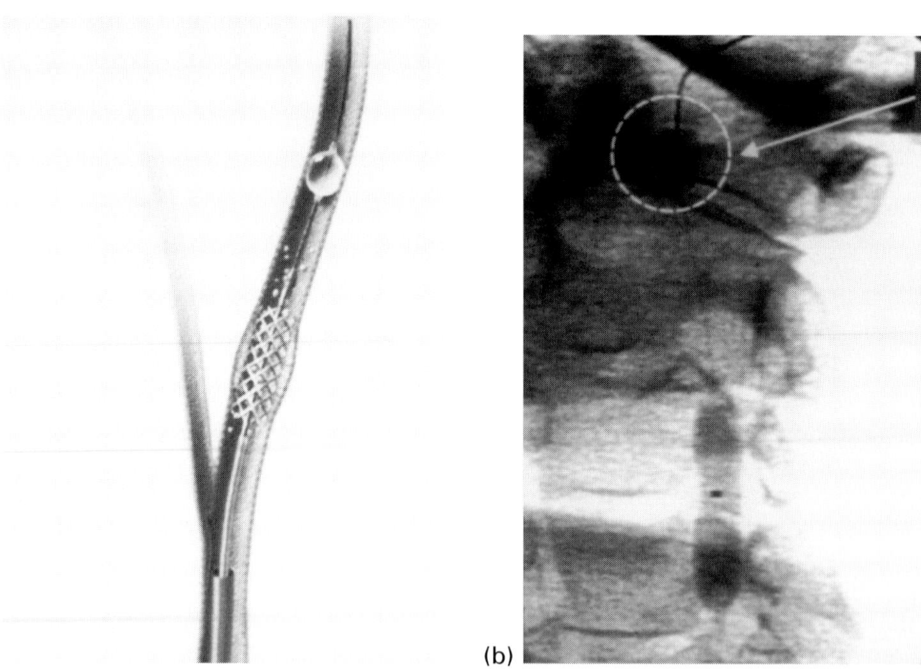

(b)

Fig. 3a, b. Angioplasty and stenting are performed under protection (arrow: protection balloon), the Guardwire™ is used as a standard guidewire.

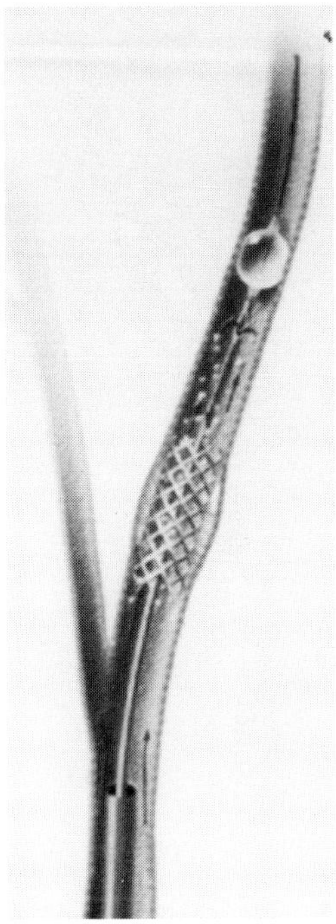

(a)

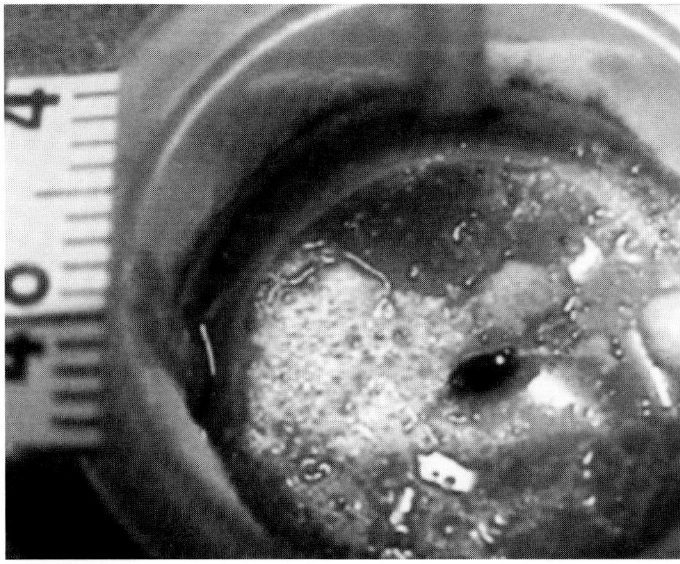

(b)

Fig. 4a, b. Generated debris is aspirated with the Export™ aspiration catheter.

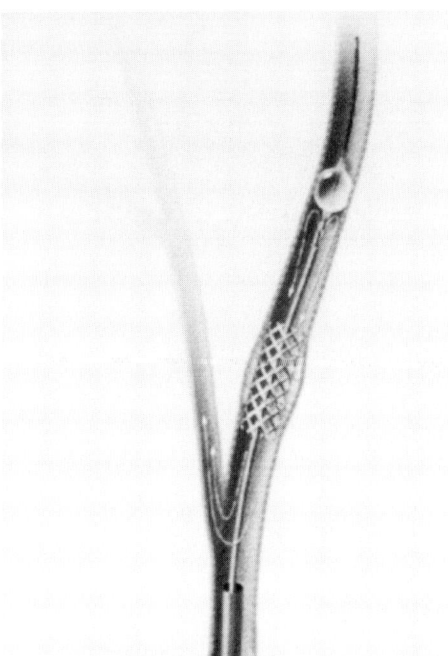

Fig. 5. Flushing of the debris to the external carotid artery can be performed after aspiration.

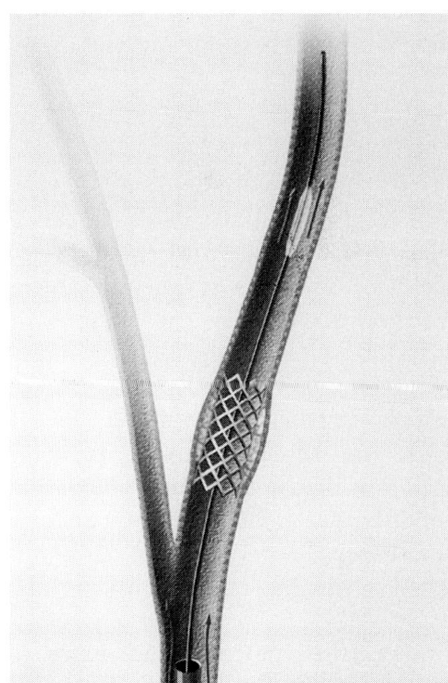

Fig. 6. The protection balloon is deflated re-establishing cerebral flow.

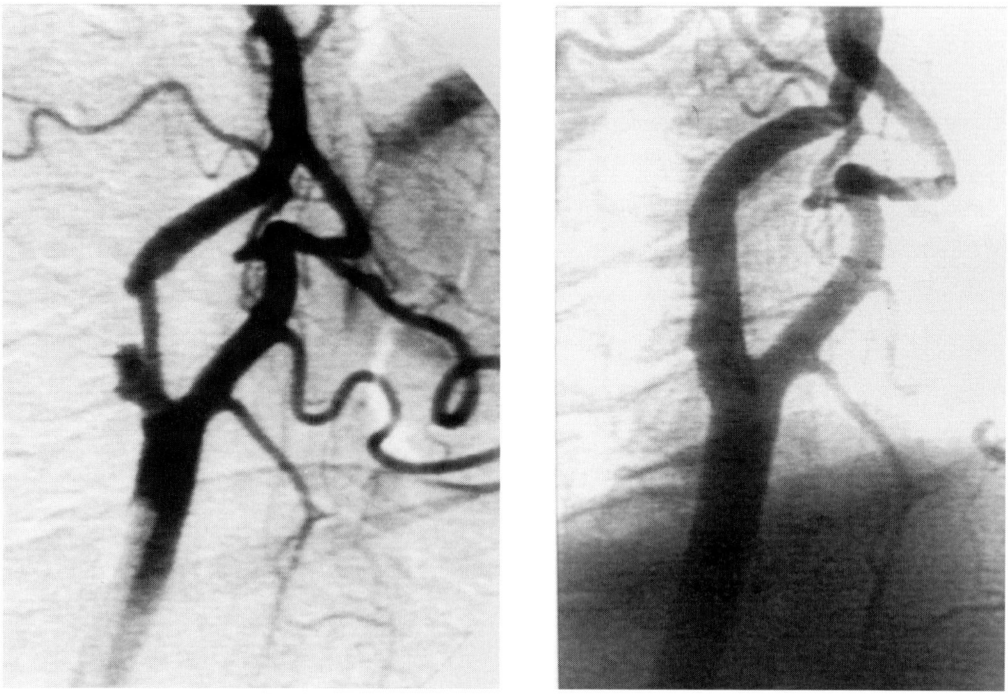

(a) (b)

Fig. 7. (a) Long ulcerated stenosis of the right internal carotid artery. (b) Result after protected angioplasty and stenting.

mean occlusion time for all patients was 470 ± 220 seconds. The occlusion was well tolerated in 104 cases (95%). Two types of intolerance were encountered due to cerebral ischaemia created by the balloon: one patient with contralateral occlusion had loss of consciousness and seizures, very soon after balloon inflation. We had to deflate the balloon and the procedure was finished successfully without cerebral protection. The patient completely recovered. Five patients developed a transient intolerance 2 to 3 minutes after balloon inflation with agitation or brief loss of consciousness, lasting less than 1 minute. The procedures could be finished under protection and all patients recovered fully before deflation of the protection balloon. We can speculate that the intolerance in these patients was related to poor collateral circulation and persisted until the collateral blood supply became sufficient. Two of them had a hypotensive episode with bradycardia as response to angioplasty which could also serve as a precipitating factor.

Also, three patients had spasm of the internal carotid artery at the location of the protection balloon, which rapidly resolved after injection of vasodilators.

Only one neurological ischaemic complication was observed. This patient was treated with a Wallstent stent for a tight calcified stenosis, and a thrombosis developed during the procedure, was seen after protection balloon deflation. The

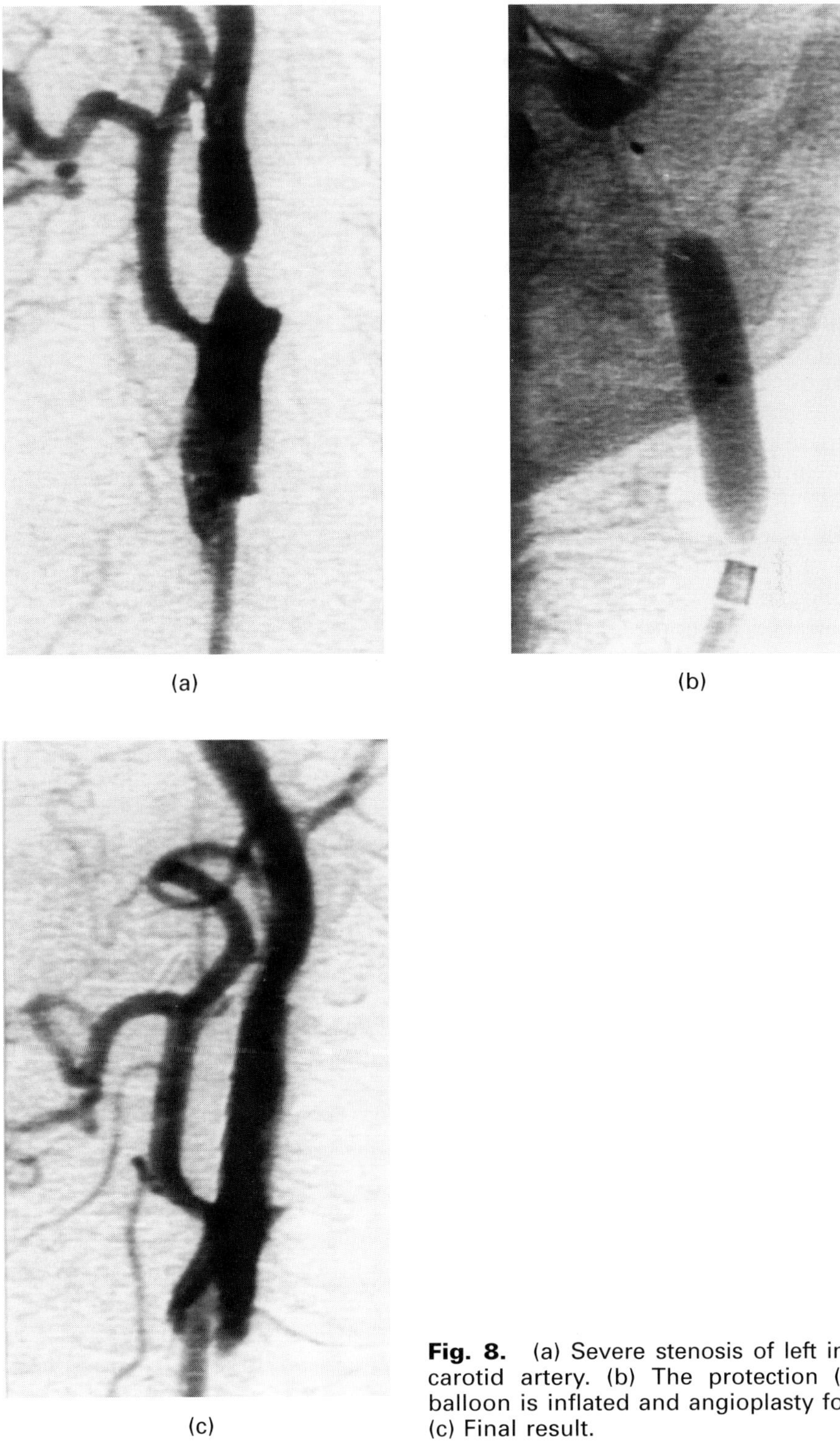

Fig. 8. (a) Severe stenosis of left internal carotid artery. (b) The protection (distal) balloon is inflated and angioplasty follows. (c) Final result.

balloon was quickly reinflated and abciximab was injected. Aspiration and flushing were performed again 10 minutes later. After flushing, the patient developed an amaurosis. Angiography showed no residual thrombus inside the stent and a communication between external carotid artery and ophthalmic circulation. Additionally a haemorreagic episode manifested with hemiparesis was seen in a patient with a tight stenosis in whom abciximab was given empirically during and after the intervention. This patient recovered 2 months later. One patient died 3 weeks following the procedure from acute cardiac failure.

We found the PercuSurge system easy to use. The GuardWire™ provides adequate support to advance the dilatation balloon and the stent. The deflation time of the occlusion balloon was fast, approximately 15 seconds. In one patient, after completion of the procedure, deflation of the balloon was impossible due to kinking of the GuardWire™. The deformed section of the wire, at the proximal end, was cut using scissors and the balloon was deflated immediately.

Microscopic analysis of the aspirated blood showed different types of particles: atheromatous plaques, cholesterol crystals, necrotic cores, fibrin, thrombi, platelets, macrophage foam cells. Their mean diameter was 0.8 μ (56–2652 μ); their number ranged between 7 and 145 per procedure.

One of the advantages of the technique is that the device behaves similarly to a steerable coronary guidewire which allows crossing of the stenosis more easily and decreases technical failures.

Some important points related with this device have to be discussed here.

Tolerance of occlusion

Before any carotid angioplasty procedure, anatomic knowledge of an efficient collateral supply through an intact Circle of Willis, and a fully functional vertebrobasilar and contralateral carotid circulation are favourable factors to tolerate the balloon occlusion. For patients with congenital absence or acquired disease of these structures, balloon occlusion may not be well tolerated. Complete angiographic assessment of the four supra-aortic vessels is crucial in this setting. In our practice, occlusion of the internal carotid artery was well tolerated in the majority of the cases, and the balloon could remain inflated during several minutes without discomfort. One patient developed rapid intolerance to occlusion and we had to deflate the occlusion balloon. In the remaining cases clinical symptoms started when the procedure was already well advanced. We believe that in this scenario, one has to complete the procedure quickly, with aspiration and reestablishment of the cerebral flow. These steps can be done within 2 minutes, thus keeping the benefits of the protection. This particular problem should be familiar to the users of balloon protection devices.

Is flushing safe?

Following aspiration, remaining debris may be flushed towards the external carotid artery territory. However, this manoeuver may be risky in the presence of collateral pathways between external and internal carotid arterial or vertebral artery territories, e.g. anatomic variations with blood supply of the ophthalmic artery from the middle meningeal artery or anastomotic channels connecting the occipital and the vertebral artery. Again, it is mandatory to carefully evaluate the preliminary diagnostic angiography including visualization of the external carotid artery branches to diagnose these particularities. In this case the flushing step should be ruled out and the technique should then be limited to aspiration. The only embolic complication we observed was after a flushing manoeuver. Currently, we hesitate to use it and we perform aspiration alone to remove any debris. Flushing performed too vigorously during the cleaning procedure may lead to reflux of the debris down to the origin of the common carotid artery and spread the debris in other aortic arch branches. This may be more critical on the right side since the average length of the right common carotid artery is shorter than the left. The flush rate should not exceed 2 ml/s to allow acceptance and to avoid that complication.

The Medicorp, Henry-Amor-Frid-Rüfenacht (HAFR) device

We have developed a new cerebral protection device that consists of a long haemostatic valve sheath which is placed into the common carotid artery, a microcatheter with a compliant protection balloon fixed at its tip, with markers on its centre for good opacification. The microcatheter is mounted over a steerable 0.014 inch coronary guidewire which is placed in the internal carotid artery and maintained there during the whole procedure providing a maximum of safety for all potential balloon exchanges. Next a dilatation balloon is advanced over the microcatheter and placed after inflation of the protection balloon. A balloon-expandable stent is placed over the dilatation balloon. If the stent is self-expandable, it is directly advanced over the microcatheter, without lesion predilatation. Angioplasty and stenting are performed under cerebral protection. Debris and particles generated are flushed towards the external carotid artery and/or aspirated. The advantage of this technique is that any coronary steerable or hydrophilic guidewire may be used. The device is well radiopaque, thus avoiding certain problems encountered with Theron's technique. We have started the first clinical study and treated ten patients with success. It seems to have the same advantages as the PercuSurge device.

Kachel's technique

Kachel[20] reported a coaxial balloon angioplasty technique consisting of a guide catheter with an occlusion balloon at its tip and a dilatation catheter. After dilatation of the lesion but before balloon deflation, the occluding balloon of the guide catheter is inflated to stop antegrade flow. After dilatation, balloon deflation and removal, blood is aspirated from the internal carotid artery to remove detached material. When this is completed the occlusion balloon is deflated. This technique seems easy, but it is our opinion that it does not offer sufficient security since there is no occlusion or debris collection device distal to the lesion. Kachel reported a complication rate of 4.3% which is not different from the results reported in series without cerebral protection.

Filters

Filters are currently under investigation or early clinical use; no available data exist to support their efficacy in embolism prevention or their superiority over balloon protection devices. The primary advantage of a filter based system is that it could hold detached embolic particles without ceasing blood flow to the brain because it does not occlude the vessel. However, as debris accumulates the filter may become clogged interrupting the flow. The size of filter pores is 100 mm, but there is no evidence that this is a safe cut-off level. The size of particles that have to be necessarily trapped is still to be determined. In order to pass the lesion a filter should be in a compressed form and by design it is partially enclosed within an outer catheter. Consequently the system, due to its increased thickness lacks the flexibility and steerability of the commonly used 0.018 inch or 0.014 inch coronary wires, or the PercuSurge Guardwire. This may lead to difficulties in crossing tight or tortuous lesions. Finally there is a possibility for late reactions due to injury induced by contact of the arterial wall with the nitinol frame of the filter.

CONCLUSION

Several published series on unprotected carotid angioplasty have shown an encouraging perioperative stroke/death rate, comparable with that following carotid endarterectomy. Most of the neurological complications are due to intracerebral embolism during the steps of the procedure. The stent itself is not sufficient to avoid cerebral embolism, occasionally it could be responsible for this complication. Thus, there is a need for a brain protection device. We believe that the future of the procedure mainly depends on finding ways to eliminate its Achilles heel, that is its embolic potential. The effectiveness of cerebral protection techniques in reducing the stroke rates may widen the indications of carotid angioplasty. Based on our experience of over 300 carotid interventional procedures with both unprotected and protected techniques we have been convinced that cerebral protection should become routine in all carotid angioplasty procedures. We would hardly advocate initiation of randomized studies of angioplasty without protection versus surgery at this time, since cerebral protection may lead to different results.

REFERENCES

1. Grotta J: Elective stenting of extracranial carotid arteries. *Circulation* **95:** 303–305, 1997
2. North American Symptomatic Carotid Endarterectomy Trial collaborators: Beneficial effect of carotid endarterectomy in symptomatic patients with high-grade carotid stenosis. *New Engl J Med* **325:** 445–453, 1991
3. European Carotid Surgery Trialists' Collaborative Group: MRC European Carotid Surgery Trial: Interim results for symptomatic patients with severe (70–99%) or with mild (0–29%) carotid stenosis. *Lancet* **337:** 1235–1243, 1991
4. The Executive Committee for the Asymptomatic Carotid Atherosclerosis Study: Endarterectomy for asymptomatic carotid stenosis. *J Am Med Assoc* **273:** 1421–1428, 1995
5. Hasi DC, Kroshat M, Mmosos LM: Epedimiology of carotid endarterectomies among Medicare beneficiaries. *J Vasc Surg* **16:** 201–208, 1992
6. Henry M, Amor M, Masson I *et al.*: Angioplasty and stenting of the extracranial carotid arteries. *J Endovasc Surg* **6:** 293–304, 1998
7. Yadav JS, Roubin GS, Iyer SS *et al.*: Elective stenting of the extracranial carotid arteries. *Circulation* **95:** 376–381, 1997

8. Diethrich EB, Ndiaye M, Reid DB: Stenting in the carotid artery: initial experience in 100 patients. *J Endovasc Surg* **3:** 42–62, 1996
9. Bergeron P, Chambran P, Hartung O *et al.*: Cervical carotid artery stenosis: which technique, balloon angioplasty or surgery? *J Cardiovasc Surg* **37**(Suppl I–5): 73–75, 1996
10. Roubin GS, Yadav S, Iyer S *et al.*: Carotid-stent supported angioplasty: a neurovascular intervention to prevent stroke. *Am J Cardiol* **78:** 8–12, 1996
11. Theron J, Payelle G, Coskun O *et al.*: Carotid artery stenoses: treatment with protected balloon angioplasty and stent placement. *Radiology* **201:** 627–636, 1996
12. Martin JB, Gailloud P, Sugiu K *et al.*: *In vitro* models of human carotid atheromatous disease. In: Henry M, Amor M (Eds), *Ninth International Course Book of Peripheral Vascular Intervention* pp. 541–546. Toulouse, France: Europa Editions 1998
13. Ohki T, Marin ML, Lyon RT *et al.*: *Ex vivo* human carotid artery bifurcation stenting: correlation of lesion characteristics with embolic potential. *J Vasc Surg* **27:** 463–471, 1998
14. Jordan WD, Voellinger DC, Doblar DD *et al.*: Microemboli detected by transcranial Doppler monitoring in patients during carotid angioplasty versus carotid endarterectomy. *Cardiovasc Surg* **7:** 33–38, 1999.
15. Vitek JJ, Raymon BC, Oh SJ: Innominate artery angioplasty. *Am J Neuroradiol* **5:** 113–114, 1984
16. Mathur A, Roubin G, Iyer S *et al.*: Predictors of stroke complicating carotid artery stenting. *Circulation* **97:** 1239–1245, 1998
17. Theron J, Courtheoux P, Alachkar F *et al.*: New triple coaxial catheter system of carotid angioplasty with cerebral protection. *Am J Neuroradiol* **11:** 869–874, 1990
18. Oesterle SN, Hayase M, Baim DS *et al.*: An embolization containment device. *Catheter Cardiovasc Interv* **47:** 243–250, 1999
19. Webb JG, Carere RG, Virmani R *et al.*: Retrieval and analysis of particulate debris after saphenous vein graft intervention. *J Am Coll Cardiol* **34:** 468–475, 1999
20. Kachel R: Results of balloon angioplasty in carotid arteries. *J Endovasc Surg* **3:** 22–30, 1996

The EUROCAST Registry of carotid stenting

Marc RHM van Sambeek on behalf of the EUROCAST Registry Steering Committee*

INTRODUCTION

Carotid endarterectomy

High-grade symptomatic atherothrombotic lesions of the carotid bifurcation are a frequent clinical problem and are associated with an increased risk of ipsilateral ischaemic stroke. This risk can be lowered in some groups of patients by an intervention. Two randomized controled trials of carotid endarterectomy with 'best medical treatment' with aspirin compared with best medical treatment with aspirin alone, produced clear benefits in favour of carotid endarterectomy in combination with aspirin medication in patients with recent (less than 6 months) cerebrovascular events.[1,2] The European Carotid Surgery Trial (ECST) and the North American Symptomatic Carotid Endarterectomy Trial (NASCET) showed a significant decrease in risk of ipsilateral stroke in operated patients with recently symptomatic severe (70–99%) carotid stenosis. ECST showed that surgery is harmful in patients with less than 30% stenosis, whereas NASCET showed no benefit in patients with 30–49% stenosis but did show a small benefit in those with 50–69% stenosis. The risk of procedure-related stroke and death with surgical endarterectomy was 7.0% in the ECST and 5.8% in the NASCET. With this knowledge carotid endarterectomy has become the preferred method for treatment of symptomatic patients with high-grade carotid stenosis.

Carotid stenting

In the effort to minimize invasive interventions, during the last several years carotid angioplasty and stenting has been recommended by some physicians as an alternative to carotid endarterectomy for patients with symptomatic extracranial carotid obstructive disease. At present carotid stenting is evolving as a therapeutic alternative to carotid endarterectomy. Compared with surgery, carotid stenting is less invasive and less traumatic for the patient. As it avoids a dissection of the neck and exposure of the artery, the procedure is faster and less painful. In addition carotid stenting avoids peripheral nerve damage and the anaesthetic risks of a surgical procedure.

*The EUROCAST Steering Committee consists of: Patrice Bergeron MD, Vascular Surgeon, Marseille, France; Prof. Peter RF Bell MD, Vascular Surgeon, Leicester, UK; Peter A Gaines MD, Interventional Radiologist, Sheffield, UK; Michel Henry MD, Interventional Cardiologist, Essey-les-Nancy, France; Marc RHM van Sambeek MD, Vascular Surgeon, Rotterdam, The Netherlands; Prof. Hero van Urk MD, Vascular Surgeon, Rotterdam, The Netherlands.

In the last decade many articles on this subject have appeared in several journals. A variety of catheter-based techniques have been reported concerning series of varying patient numbers. Many reports are available only in abstract form. Generally, the number of patients treated is small and the clinical data are often incomplete. The major problem with these reports is the tendency to group together patients with different types of lesions and dissimilar natural history or stroke risks.[3] Only few reports objectively assessed results.[4–8] The results from these series are not excellent, yet promising. In recent years the feasibility of carotid angioplasty – with or without stenting – has gained widespread acceptance, in particular for patients with obvious major contraindications for surgical correction like high cardiopulmonary risk or 'hostile neck'. Patients with radiation arteritis of the carotid arteries, with very high cervical lesions, or patients after radical neck dissection or with a permanent tracheostomy form a group for whom any type of surgical approach is not attractive. With the increased endovascular experience and equipment at hand, the move to endovascular repair is probably a very logical step in these cases. Encouraged by the rather successful experiences, carotid angioplasty has also been performed based on a wider range of indications, including 'low-risk' patients and even asymptomatic patients.

The Lennox Hill Heart and Vascular Institute has recently presented its last consecutive series of 249 carotid interventions with no deaths, 0.8% major strokes and 3.6% minor strokes (Current issues and new techniques in interventional radiology, New York, 16–19 November, 1999). Despite the improvements in technical skills, embolic stroke remains a major and unpredictable clinical event. During carotid angioplasty and stenting, different steps in the procedure may dislodge embolic particles. Several authors have reported evidence of an increased amount of embolic particles in the brain during carotid intervention.[9–11] Therefore, cerebral protection might play an important role in the prevention of these emboli. Theron[9] has been the pioneer in the field of cerebral protection and his results were convincing that cerebral protection could reduce the risk of embolization and consequently widen the indications for carotid angioplasty and stenting. Protection devices such as balloons and carotid filters are currently undergoing clinical evaluation and seem to show promise in reducing the incidence of embolic events to the less than 2% range.

RANDOMIZED TRIALS

Rationale and currently performed trials

The obvious question, that is not answered by the selected series, is: 'what is the safety and efficacy of carotid stenting compared with the gold standard of carotid endarterectomy?' The final answer to questions like this one can only be given by well designed prospectively controlled randomized clinical trials, preferably multicentre trials. Emergence of a position of clinical equipoise on the equivalent value of carotid endarterectomy and carotid angioplasty and stenting in symptomatic patients, has already resulted in the initiation of two randomized trials in the United Kingdom comparing the efficacy of the alternatives.[12,13] In the Carotid and Vertebral Artery Transluminal Angioplasty Study (CAVATAS) 504 patients were randomized. There was no statistical difference in the numbers of disabling stroke and death up to 3 years from entry to the study (surgery: 9.9% and angioplasty and stenting: 10.0%) Improvement of the technology bypassed the CAVATAS study between the design stage and its inception because it became apparent that carotid stenting had potential advantages over standard angioplasty alone (stenting was optional in CAVATAS).

Another randomized study from Leicester in the UK had to be abandoned because of the unacceptable mortality and morbidity in the balloon angioplasty group.[14]

In the United States of America the Carotid Revascularization Endarterectomy vs Stent Trial (CREST) has recently been approved for funding by the National Institute of Neurological Disease and Stroke (NINDS) and the National Institute of Health (NIH). The total enrollment in this well designed study will be 2500 patients from 60 centres and this study will start inclusion in the beginning of the year 2000.

Pitfalls and drawbacks of randomized studies

There is concern about the desirability of such studies. In particular in the world of vascular surgery a genuine concern has been raised and expressed about the potential danger and negative effects of untimely randomized trials. Is it not too early for such trials? Do we really know enough about the morbidity and mortality rates that are to be expected when multicentre trials – even in selected centres – will be undertaken? With the current level of knowledge and understanding of the new procedures, is it ethically justified to randomize patients for standard operation or balloon angioplasty and stenting?

Another concern about the randomized trials is the risk that the study will be bypassed by the improvements in technology as happened with the CAVATAS study. Initially the CREST will start randomization at a time that protective devices are not yet available in the USA, and the study will be carried out, using one (dedicated) stent uniquely. During a recent concensus meeting in New York in November 1999 (results will be published soon) the opinion of the majority of 17 experts in the field was that the current technique of carotid stenting is appropriate at the time, but the ideal stent is not available. In the opinion of many interventionalists a covered stent might solve some of the pitfalls of the technique, but the currently available covered stents have the disadvantage of a too large profile. Also the technique of cerebral protection is in the midst of its evolution.

Although it should be acknowledged that well-designed prospectively controlled randomized clinical trials will be of paramount importance for the future of carotid stenting and will give an answer to many of the uncertainties, the question is raised: is this the right time to do it?

EUROCAST REGISTRY

Rationale for a registry

One theme is becoming alarmingly clear: the medical profession is in need of a database for the clinical results of every physician (vascular surgeon, interventional cardiologist and interventional radiologist) who is working in the field and who is currently performing carotid stenting. There is a need for a European registry on carotid interventions, similar to the one so successfully created for endovascular treatment of abdominal aortic aneurysm, namely the EUROSTAR Registry.

The EUROCAST Registry is designed as an ongoing registration of carotid procedures so that the results of newer techniques and new devices can be immediately analysed. This will give an opportunity to compare the different results as the technique evolves.

Drawbacks and pitfalls

One of the possible drawbacks of a registry is that not all centres will include their procedures and that some centres might not include all their procedures in the registry. This consequently includes the risk of a registration of only selected series of carotid interventions, leading to an overexpression of favourable results.

Design of the EUROCAST Registry

It is probably too early to take a stand on the issue whether carotid stenting should be considered as standard care, simply by lack of sufficient and reliable information on 'what is happening where?' and 'how good or how bad is it really?'. If we are to bring this kind of information together, it should be the effort and responsibility of all doctors in the field, disregarding their background.

The Steering Committee of the EUROCAST Registry consists of interventionalists, representing the three disciplines involved. This committee has taken up the challenge of organizing a registry of carotid angioplasty and stenting that is now called EUROCAST.

The committee intends to approach and encourage all endovascular therapists, to submit their data to this databank assuming that a high degree of confidentiality and professional standards can be reached in the field of endovascular treatment of carotid disease.

Participants of the registry are requested to send in a pre-inclusion/pre-procedural fax to the EUROCAST office in an effort to ensure assessment reliable data and to minimize the risk of leaving unfavourable results outside the registry.

After discharge of the patient the participants are requested to fill out the case reply forms and send these forms to the office. The inclusion form consists of three pages that will take no more than 5–10 minutes to complete (Appendix I). The follow-up form is composed of two pages (Appendix II). It will also be possible to send in the data through the web (www.euro-cast.com).

Another effort to achieve the highest reliability of the data is the installation of a monitor. The monitor will visit one of the participating centres at random to complete and check the data.

Further information can be obtained at the administrative centre for EUROCAST: EUROCAST Registry, P/o Nathalie Fontant, 41, Rue Docteur Morucci, 13006 Marseille France (*Phone*: + 33 4 91 37 65 65; *Fax*: + 33 4 91 37 40).

It is not what we have done in the past that will decide where our future lies, it is how we apply lessons learned in the past to our current work which will pave the way to the future.

We hope you will join us.

REFERENCES

1. European Carotid Surgery Trialists' Collaborative Group: Randomised trial of endarterectomy for recently symptomatic carotid stenosis: final results of the MRC European Carotid Surgery trial (ECST). *Lancet* **351:** 1379–1387, 1998
2. North American Symptomatic Carotid Endarterectomy Trialists' Collaborative Group: The final results of the NASCET trial. *New Engl J Med* **339:** 1415–1425, 1998
3. Beebe HG: Scientific evidence demonstrating the safety of carotid angioplasty and stenting: do we have enough to draw conclusions yet? *J Vasc Surg* **27:** 788–790, 1998
4. Dietrich EB, Ndiaye M, Reid DB: Stenting in the carotid artery: initial experience in 110 patients. *J Endovasc Surg* **3:** 42–62, 1996
5. Yadav JS, Roubin GS, Iyer SS *et al.*: Elective stenting of the extracranial carotid arteries. *Circulation* **95:** 376–381, 1997
6. Mathur A, Roubin GS, Iyer SS *et al.*: Predictors of stroke complicating carotid artery stenting. *Circulation* **97:** 1239–1245, 1998
7. Henry M, Amor M, Masson I *et al.*: Angioplasty and stenting of extracranial carotid arteries. *J Endovasc Surg* **5:** 293–304, 1998
8. Bergeron P, Becquemin JP, Jausseran JM *et al.*: Percutaneous stenting of the internal carotid artery: The European CAST I study. *J Endovasc Surg* **6:** 155–159, 1999
9. Theron J, Payelle G, Goskun O *et al.*: Carotid artery stenoses: treatment with protected balloon angioplasty and stent placement. *Radiology* **201:** 627–636, 1996
10. Ohki T, Marin ML, Lyon RT *et al.*: *Ex vivo* human carotid artery bifurcation stenting: Correlation of lesion characteristics with embolic potential. *J Vasc Surg* **27:** 463–471, 1998
11. Jordan WD, Voellinger DC, Doblar DD *et al.*: Microemboli detected by transcranial Doppler monitoring in patients during carotid angioplasty versus carotid endarterectomy. *Cardiovasc Surg* **7:** 33–38, 1999
12. Freedman B: Equipoise and ethics of clinical research. *New Engl J Med* **317:** 141–145, 1987
13. Brown M: Balloon angioplasty for cerebrovascular disease. *Neurological Res* **14**(Suppl): 159–163, 1992
14. Naylor AR, Bolia A, Abbot RJ *et al.*: Randomised study of carotid angioplasty and stenting versus carotid endarterectomy: a stopped trial. *J Vasc Surg* **28:** 326–334, 1998

APPENDIX I

EUROCAST

Hospital:. . . . . Investigator name: . . . .
Patient name: . . . . Date of birth (D/M/Y): . . . . . /. . . . . /. . . . .
Date of intervention: . . . .

PREOPERATIVE EVALUATION

RISK FACTORS • smoking • hypertension • hyperlipidaemia • diabetes

COMORBIDITY • cardiac disease • pulmonary disease • renal failure

NEUROLOGICAL SYMPTOMS

- asymptomatic
- amaurosis fuga
- transient ischaemic attack
- minimal stroke
- major stroke

Independent neurological evaluation
- yes
- no

LESION

- de novo
- recurrent
- radiation
- other

LOCALIZATION

- right
- left

- Common caratid artery
- bifurcation
- Internal caratid artery: surgical inaccessible
  - yes
  - no

COMPUTED TOMOGRAPHY SCAN

- normal
- lacunar infarction
- ipsilateral infarction
- contralateral infarction

ARTERIOGRAPHY STENOSIS ipsilateral:. . . . .% contralateral:. . . . .%

EVALUATION WILLIS CIRCLE

- duplex • transcranial Doppler • arteriography
- magnetic resonance imaging
- intact
- deficient

PROCEDURE

ACCESS

- femoral
- cervical
- brachial

PROCEDURE

- percutaneous transluminal angioplasty
- percutaneous transluminal angioplasty + stent
- primary stenting

  Pre-dilatation
  - yes
  - no

STENT

type:.................................. . ...

number:...

post-treatment diameter:...

length :..............mm

:..............mm

PROTECTION DEVICE USED

- yes please specify: ....
- no

RESULT

- optimal
- residual stenosis
- dissection
- failure

ADDITIONAL INTERVENTION

- no
- second balloon inflation
- additional stent
- conversion

PROCEDURAL COMPLICATIONS

- bradycardia
- hypotension
- spasm
- neurological symptoms

POSTOPERATIVE EVALUATION

NEUROLOGICAL COMPLICATIONS

- no
- amaurosis fugax
- transient ischaemic attack
- minor stroke
- major stroke

- independent neurological evaluation
  - yes
  - no

POSTOPERATIVE COMPUTED TOMOGRAPHY SCAN

- no alteration
- worsening of pre-existent lesion
- new lesion

POSTOPERATIVE CAROTID ULTRASOUND

- no residual stenosis
- residual stenosis
- inside stent
- outside stent

percentage residual stenosis:..............%

COMPLICATIONS AT ACCESS SITE

- haematoma
- bleeding
- infection
- false aneurysm

COMMENTS: ....
....
....

APPENDIX II

EUROCAST
FOLLOW-UP

Hospital:............................ Investigator name: ....
Patient name: .... Date of birth (D/M/Y): ...../...../.....
Date of follow-up: ..../...../..... • M1 • M6 • Y1 • Y2 • Y3

NEUROLOGICAL SYMPTOMS

- asymptomatic
- amaurosis fugax
- transient ischaemic attack
- minimal stroke
- major stroke
- symptoms contralateral hemisphere
- patient died

INDEPENDANT NEUROLOGICAL EVALUATION

- yes
- no

CEREBRAL COMPUTED TOMOGRAPHIC SCAN

- no changes/normal
- new lesion ipsilateral side
- new lesion contralateral

CAROTID ULTRASOUND

- normal
- restenosis
- inside stent
- outside stent

  percentage stenosis: ....%
- occlusion

CONVENTIONAL ARTERIOGRAPHY OR THREE-DIMENSIONAL COMPUTED TOMOGRAPHY SCAN

- normal
- restenosis
- inside stent
- outside stent
  percentage stenosis: ....%
- occlusion

STENT MORPHOLOGY

- normal
- deformation
- migration

REINTERVENTION

- no
- yes
- surgery
- endovascular intervention

COMMENTS: ....

....

....

Endarterectomy versus angioplasty: the EVA trial

Jean-Pierre Becquemin on behalf of the EVA trialists

INTRODUCTION

Carotid surgery has proved its safety and long-term efficacy for the prevention of stroke in symptomatic patients with more than 60% stenosis.[1,2] In the North American Symptomatic Carotid Endarterectomy Trial (NASCET) study the rate of ipsilateral cerebral infarct after 2 years was 26% in the medical arm vs 9% in the surgical group, which represents a 65% reduction of the stroke risk.[1] Although less marked, similar beneficial results have been reported in asymptomatic patients.[3] On the whole, excellent results are currently obtained with carotid surgery, with a mortality/severe morbidity rate in the range of 5% in the symptomatic group and 3% in the asymptomatic group. In a systematic review of reports published after 1990, which included 17000 operations, the combined mortality and major stroke rate was 5.64% at 30 days following surgery.[4] However, these studies were not controlled by independent observers, which may underestimate the real risk of surgery.

Carotid angioplasty is a new therapeutic option, which is appealing for several reasons.

The most obvious advantage is that it does not require a cervical incision, avoiding the hazard of cervical nerve injuries and wound complications.

Other advantages of the technique are more dubious and can be questioned. Carotid angioplasty requires local anaesthesia, but surgery can also be performed using a cervical block. It avoids cervical haematoma, but with the need of full anticoagulation, groin haematoma are not infrequent with angioplasty. It reduces the time of carotid clamping, but neurological complications due to the reduction of brain perfusion, which occurred in 5–10% of carotid endarterectomies, have become very rare with the selective or systematic use of a shunt. The argument is all the more debatable as the new technical evolution of carotid angioplasty includes protective devices such as the PercuSurg Guardwire™ device which are aimed at preventing emboli but have induced a clamping time similar to that needed for a carotid endarterectomy. Proximal or distal lesions are more amenable to angioplasty. This is true for common carotid lesions particularly those which are close to the aortic arch, which were approached directly through a sternotomy. This is also applicable to distal lesions at the basis of the skull, but they are not so frequent. Patients at local risk because of expected anatomical difficulties such as radiation-induced stenosis or restenosis following a first carotid endarterectomy may benefit from carotid angioplasty, yet it remains unproven. Patients at general risk with severe coronary or pulmonary diseases may also benefit from angioplasty rather than endarterectomy.

On the other hand angioplasty of lesions located at the carotid bifurcation may provoke severe haemodynamic instability with hyper- or hypotension, severe bradycardia and even asystole, the consequences of which may be deleterious in those patients.

Apart from those medical arguments, the reasons for the enthusiasm for this new technology may come from the combined efforts of medical specialties which were not involved so far in the treatment of this pathology, namely cardiologists, and companies looking for a new market. In 1997, the French Agence Nationale pour l'Accreditation et l'Evaluation en Santé (ANAES) recommended that carotid angioplasty should not be performed outside trials, and as a result, neither the procedure nor the material are reimbursed by the Social Security.

The only way to overcome all the doubts, uncertainties, and second thoughts, is to evaluate the new technique vs the current gold standard treatment, carotid surgery. Results of open studies with selected patients in selected centres have shown that it was not unethical to start a randomized trial. Recent publications of carotid angioplasty with stent has shown that the one month combined mortality and all strokes rate was between 4.6% and 6.9%. However, when only mortality and major stroke are considered, the total rate is half these figures.[5–10] As far as long term is concerned, the recurrence of restenosis after carotid angioplasty and stent appears to be in the same range as after carotid surgery. In our own series, of 70 patients with various stents, the cumulative life-survival free of symptoms and restenosis was close to 98% at 12 months. However, as opposed to surgery[11,12] large long-term follow-up studies are not available so far. Randomized studies have already been completed. The randomized trial from the Leicester group was stopped after 20 inclusions due to the high complication rate in the angioplasty group.[13] However, patients were unselected, stents were not used and, experience with carotid angioplasty was low, even if the interventions were performed by well-trained interventionists in peripheral angioplasty. This study is worthy of analysis since it provides indications for avoiding the pitfalls in a new randomized trial. The Carotid and Vertebral Artery Transluminal Angioplasty Study (CAVATAS) trial was started in 1993, but has not been published yet. Whatever the results, important methodological flaws are already underlined: symptomatic and asymptomatic patients were enrolled, grade and site of lesions were not predetermined, and finally the techniques of angioplasty have considerably improved over the last years. Thus the start of a new randomized trial is appropriate.

The EVA trial was designed by a neurologist, Professor Mas, and a methodologist Professor Chatelier. Involved in the steering committee are physicians from different specialties, mainly vascular surgeons, interventional radiologists, neuroradiologists, and neurologists. A grant application has been fulfilled for the PHRC (Program Hospitalier de Recherche Clinique, section of the Ministry of Health), and finally accepted. The grant will pay for the monitoring of the study.

The main objective of the trial is to test the hypothesis that equivalent results may be obtained by carotid angioplasty and by surgery in symptomatic patients with more than 70% stenosis of the internal carotid artery.

The population studied will be patients of both sexes, older than 18 years, with ipsilateral reversible or with mild ischaemic neurological sequelae or ocular symptoms, and an atherosclerotic stenosis greater than 70% of the carotid artery, proximal, distal or at the level of the carotid bifurcation. The delay between symptoms and inclusion should be less than 120 days. The grade of stenosis will be determined by angiography with biplane views, according to the NASCET criteria. The features of lesions, calcification, ulcer, irregularity, will be recorded, but will not influence the randomization. However, both treatments should be technically feasible.

Excluded from the randomization will be patients with asymptomatic stenosis, or with severe sequaela (Rankin score >2), with non-atherosclerotic lesions, with associated cardiopathy which may be a source of emboli such as atrial fibrillation, intraventricular thrombus, patients with previous ipsilateral carotid surgery, proximal or distal severe stenosis, severe tortuosity precluding the advance of the catheter, long lesions precluding the insertion of the stent, or presence of a floating thrombus.

The preoperative evaluation will consist of analysis of symptoms by a neurologist, duplex scan of carotid arteries, computed tomography scan of the brain less than 30 days before the procedure, arteriogram with biplane views and intracerebral views.

Patients will have to sign an informed consent, and to agree to the burden of follow-up studies.

The treatment will be allocated in each centre, in real time, with a centralized randomization.

The procedures should be performed within 15 days of randomization. The surgical procedures may include all different types of surgery including endarterectomy with or without patch, eversion-endartectomy, or bypass according to the surgeon's preferences. As well, the different types of anaesthesia and cerebral monitoring will be left to the discretion of the surgeon and anaesthesiologist. Carotid angioplasty will be performed under local anaesthesia, using the femoral approach, with insertion of a self-expandable stent, either as a primary procedure or following a pre-dilation. Protective devices with balloons or filters are recommended.

The primary endpoints will be the mortality/severe stroke rate within the 30 days post-procedure and the mortality/severe stroke rate within the 2 years of follow-up. The secondary endpoint will be all complications occurring within the first 30 days and all transient ischaemic events within the 2 years of follow-up, restenosis and stent integrity judged by duplex scan and cervical X-rays, and total duration of hospitalization. Follow-up in each centre will be done by independent neurologists.

The hypothesis for the statistical analysis is equivalence.[14,15] The estimated rate of primary endpoints for surgery is 5.6% and for angioplasty somewhere between 3% and 5%. Thus according to the Blackwelder method[16] with a unilateral risk of 5% and a bilateral risk of 20% a median number of 900 patients should be required. This number enables testing the equivalence at 30 days with a power of 80% and the long-term equivalence with a power of 70% as long as the yearly incidence of ischaemic events is 1% in each group. There is thus a need for 30 centres with a recruitment of ten patients per year and per centre.

GENERAL ORGANIZATION

The scientific committee is responsible for the general organization, the writing of the trial, the final approval of centres and devices, the survey of the study, and the relationship with the scientific community.

Since results of the trial will be highly affected by the results obtained in each centre, only selected centres will be involved in the study. For the surgical group, centres should justify the performance of at least 25 carotid endarterectomies per year with a combined mortality/severe stroke rate of less than 5% for symptomatic patients during the last 3 years. The data will be provided on a voluntary basis by each centre and controlled by external audit, or by the consultation of PMSI data base, which is a mandatory computerized national registry of medical information of all hospitalized patients. The problem with carotid angioplasty arm is more complex since only a few centres are currently familiar with the technique. Centres will be selected if they fulfill the following criteria: proven performance of at least 25 carotid angioplasties, or routine performance of selective supra-aortic angiogram and peripheral angioplasty and stents. A training programme will be set up at the same time for physicians who have the potential for recruitment but who have not yet performed carotid angioplasty and stenting. They will have to attend and participate in ten procedures in already trained centres, and will be monitored for their very first cases. Material for carotid angioplasty will also be selected. Since the technology will probably improve during the on-going of the study, the choice is not definitively fixed. However, balloon, guidewire, and cerebral protection devices should have the CE (European Community approval) mark. Stents must be self-expandable and have the CE mark for the specific indication of carotid stenting. At present only two stents fulfill these requirements.

All data will be collected, centralized, and analysed by independent experts. Also, angiogram and duplex scan will be centralized and reviewed by a core lab.

The study should start by January 2000. A safety committee will review the data after the first 200 patients and the first 25 events. It will give advice to the scientific committee for the decision to go on with the trial, to stop it or to modify the planning of the trial.

REFERENCES

1. North American Symptomatic Carotid Endarterectomy Trial Collaborators: Beneficial effect of carotid endarterectomy in symptomatic patients with high-grade carotid stenosis. *New Engl J Med* **325:** 445–453, 1991
2. European Carotid Surgery Trialists' Collaborative Group: MRC European Carotid Surgery Trial: interim results for symptomatic patients with severe (70–99%) or with mild (0–29%) carotid stenosis. *Lancet* **337:** 1235–1243, 1991
3. Asymptomatic Carotid Atherosclerosis Study Group: Carotid endarterectomy for patients with asymptomatic internal carotid artery stenosis. *J Am Med Assoc* **273:** 1421–1428, 1995
4. Rothwell PM, Slattery J, Warlow CP: A systematic review of the risk of stroke and death due to endarterectomy for symptomatic carotid stenosis. *Stroke* **27:** 260–267, 1996
5. Eckert B, Zanella FE, Thie A *et al.*: Angioplasty of the internal carotid artery: results, complications and follow-up in 61 cases. *Cerebrovasc Dis* **6:** 97–105, 1996
6. Gil-Peralta A, Mayol A, Gonzalez Marcos JR *et al.*: Pecutaneous transluminal angioplasty of the symptomatic atherosclerotic carotid arteries. Results, complications, and follow-up. *Stroke* **27:** 2271–2273, 1996
7. Kachel R: Results of balloon angioplasty in carotid arteries. *J Endovasc Surg* **3:** 22–30, 1996

8. Diethrich EB, Mouhamadou N, Reid DB: Stenting in the carotid artery : initial experience in 110 patients. *J Endovasc Surg* **3:** 42–62, 1996
9. Théron J, Payelle G, Coskun O, Buet H: Carotid artery stenosis: treatment with protected balloon angioplasty and stent placement. *Neuroradiology* **201:** 627–636, 1996
10. Yadav JS, Roubin GS, Iyer S *et al.*: Elective stenting of the extracranial carotid arteries. *Circulation* **95:** 376–381, 1997
11. Zierler RE, Brandyk DF, Thiele BL, Strandness ED: Carotid artery stenosis following endarterectomy. *Arch Surg* **117:** 1408–1415, 1982
12. Edwards WHJ, Edwards WHS, Mulherin JLJ, Martin RS: Recurrent carotid artery stenosis. *Ann Surg* **209:** 662–669, 1989
13. Naylor AR, Bolia A, Abbott RJ *et al.*: Randomized study of carotid angioplasty and stenting versus carotid endarterectomy : a stopped trial. *J Vasc Surg* **28:** 326–34, 1998
14. Ware JH, Antman EM: Equivalence trials. *New Engl J Med* **337:** 1159–1161, 1997
15. Dunnet CW, Gent M: Significance testing to establish equivalence between treatments, with special reference to data in the form of 2 × 2 tables. *Biometrics* **33:** 593–602, 1977
16. Blackwelder WC: 'Proving the null hypothesis' in clinical trials. *Controlled Clin Trials* **3:** 345–353, 1982

Management of carotid restenosis

Graham Riding, Rubeena Razzaq, Ray Ashleigh, Charles McCollum

INTRODUCTION

Surgery for carotid restenosis is technically more demanding than for primary disease due to scarring, dense adhesions and the difficulty identifying surrounding anatomy. The morbidity of surgery for recurrent disease is reported to be up to four times that of primary endarterectomy.[1] Much of the reported morbidity can be avoided by careful surgery but there is no doubt that the procedure is more difficult and cranial nerve injury more likely.[2,3]

Over 3000 patients, in two large randomized controlled trials, were required to demonstrate the clear benefit of primary carotid surgery in patients with symptomatic severe carotid stenosis.[4,5] However, risk of stroke associated with severe primary carotid disease probably has little relevance to the management of postoperative stenosis, which is frequently due to pseudointimal hyperplasia. As restenosis is relatively infrequent, there is no adequate evidence to guide practice. In the context of the rapid development of vascular surgery and radiology, it is hardly surprising that no consensus exists on its treatment.

DIAGNOSIS

The definition of 'restenosis' has never been agreed; here we will describe stenosis and restenosis in terms of percentage diameter reduction. In most recent series, restenosis is defined as a 50% or greater stenosis on duplex ultrasound imaging.[6] The clinical relevance of determining this outcome is unclear; it is unlikely patients with restenosis between 50 and 70% will undergo reintervention. In our unit, we use carotid duplex peak velocity greater than 210cm/s (previously peak systolic frequency greater than 7kHz) checked against real-time B-mode imaging and colour flow, to define an internal carotid diameter reduction greater than 70%. These criteria have been prospectively validated against angiography for preoperative disease only.[7,8] Duplex ultrasonography correlates more closely with *ex vivo* measurement of carotid stenosis than does carotid angiography[9,10] and has the additional advantages of being non-invasive and less expensive.

Early postoperative carotid imaging is required to distinguish failures of the primary procedure from restenosis but their management is unlikely to be different. An apparent regression in the severity of restenosis may be seen in a small proportion of patients but this is infrequent in severe stenosis and its effect on stroke risk is not known.[11,12] The diagnosis of regression has usually been based on a fall in peak velocity on duplex imaging, which could be explained by the development of collaterals supplying the circle of Willis rather than reversal of the disease process.

There are no published criteria for external carotid stenosis. The external carotid supplies a vascular bed of higher and more variable resistance and tends to have a higher peak systolic velocity at any apparent severity of stenosis on imaging. A duplex velocity of more than 210cm/s was also used to define external carotid restenosis in our patients, although this may overestimate its frequency.

THE SIZE OF THE PROBLEM

In 1997/98, about 3300 patients had primary carotid reconstruction in England, a figure that is increasing annually.[13] Following surgery, approximately 10% of patients develop a restenosis of greater than 50% diameter reduction, whereas severe restenosis (greater than 70%) may occur in a little over half this number.[14,15] Therefore, about 165 patients may develop severe restenosis each year, a population too small for meaningful study.

CAUSES OF RESTENOSIS

Restenosis within the first 2 years of surgery is predominantly caused by pseudointimal hyperplasia, whereas progression of atherosclerosis is more likely in late recurrence.[16] A carotid kink forming either initially or as scar tissue develops can cause turbulent flow and overestimation of stenosis.[17] Restenosis may therefore have several differing aetiologies and treatment need not be similar to that for primary carotid disease. Pseudointimal hyperplasia, kinking and atheroma may all be present although those experienced in duplex imaging may be able to estimate the approximate contribution of each.

Who requires intervention?

Degree of stenosis

It is almost certainly inappropriate to apply the standard indication of symptomatic, greater than 70% internal carotid artery stenosis to the treatment of restenosis. Several studies failed to show an increased stroke risk in restenosis.[14,18,19] However, we and others have experienced patients who suffered disabling stroke when their restenosis progressed to complete occlusion.

Symptoms of cerebral ischaemia

Patients with symptoms attributable to carotid restenosis may, like those with primary stenosis, be at higher risk of stroke.[20] Despite this, stroke appears to be infrequent in patients with less severe restenosis. In those with less than 80% restenosis suffering a single minor transient ischaemic attack or episode of amaurosis fugax, intensifying platelet inhibitory therapy with aspirin or the addition of clopidogrel may be all that is required.

In our view restenosis of less than 70% is of doubtful clinical significance; reoperation is only likely to be considered when the stenosis is progressive and greater than 80%. Without good evidence, our approach has been to treat, by surgery or angioplasty, restenoses that are i) associated with recurrent appropriate symptoms despite adequate antiplatelet therapy, ii) rapidly progressing beyond 80% or iii) associated with a severe contralateral carotid stenosis or occlusion.

FREQUENCY OF RESTENOSIS

We conducted a review of carotid surgery in this unit to investigate the frequency of carotid restenosis and the outcome of further procedures. Each patient undergoing carotid surgery between January 1993 and December 1998, under the care of one consultant (CNMcC) was prospectively followed with colour duplex imaging (5MHz probe, ATL Ultramark 9 HDI) at 6 weeks, 6 months and 1 year. Subsequent annual assessment was performed in those with a stenosis greater than 50%, progressive or symptomatic disease; asymptomatic patients with widely patent carotids were discharged. Internal and external carotid restenoses of greater than 70% were defined by the same criteria as the preoperative carotid stenosis. Complete occlusion was defined by an absent Doppler signal and reduced or reversed diastolic flow in the common carotid artery. Preoperative arch angiography was used only in very tight carotid stenosis, when there was doubt as to the patency of the internal carotid artery.[21] Restenoses and occlusions were counted separately.

Symptoms of cerebral ischaemia were recorded prospectively. In symptomatic patients with bilateral disease, the side with the more severe stenosis was operated on first. Length of follow-up was in months from surgery to the latest carotid duplex study before discharge, loss to follow-up, or reintervention.

Primary surgery

About 100 primary carotid procedures were carried out each year. Primary surgery was more frequently under general rather than local anaesthesia with 5000 units of heparin given intravenously before carotid clamping. Cerebral monitoring included cerebral oxygen saturation (CsO_2) measured by near-infrared spectroscopy (NIRS, INVOS 3100A, Somanetics) and transcranial Doppler sonography of middle cerebral artery blood flow velocity (TCD, Neuroguard). The indications for shunting were a fall in TCD mean velocity by more than 80% or a fall in CsO_2 of more than 12%. A routine carotid endarterectomy was performed in the 'pink plane' and intimal retention sutures were inserted when the intima was not firmly adherent. Dacron patch closure of the arteriotomy was used after 1995 if the distal internal carotid artery diameter was less than 6mm, previously patches were only used for arteries less than 5mm. When there was a risk of kinking due to an elongated and tortuous internal carotid artery, the proximal segment was excised and the internal carotid reimplanted.[22] Severe carotid dilating disease was excised and replaced with a 6mm Dacron interposition graft. External carotid endarterectomy was performed by initial dissection in the endarterectomy plane and the use of a haemostatic clamp to fracture the plaque. Then the plaque was removed en bloc by a combination of milking by external pressure and traction at the ostium of the vessel (Fig.1). Patients undergoing extra-anatomical procedures such as subclavian to carotid bypass were excluded.

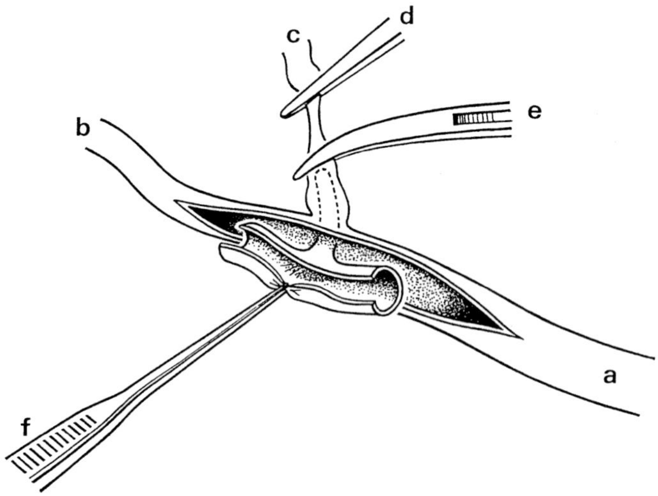

Fig. 1. External carotid endarterectomy. a: common carotid artery; b: internal carotid artery; c: external carotid artery; d: arterial clamp; e: small arterial clamp; f: forceps.

RESULTS

Over the 6 years from 1993 to 1998, 553 primary carotid procedures were performed on 509 patients. As patients with widely patent carotids were discharged at 12 months, follow-up was for a median of only 14 months (interquartile range 10–27).

Internal and common carotid procedures

Occlusion occurred in nine cases (1.5%) with restenosis occurring in 44 (8%) (Fig. 2). Only one of these was detected beyond 2 years following surgery.

Influence of operator and choice of procedure

There was a tendency for restenosis to occur a little more frequently following endarterectomy by a registrar compared with those by CNMcC but on review of the

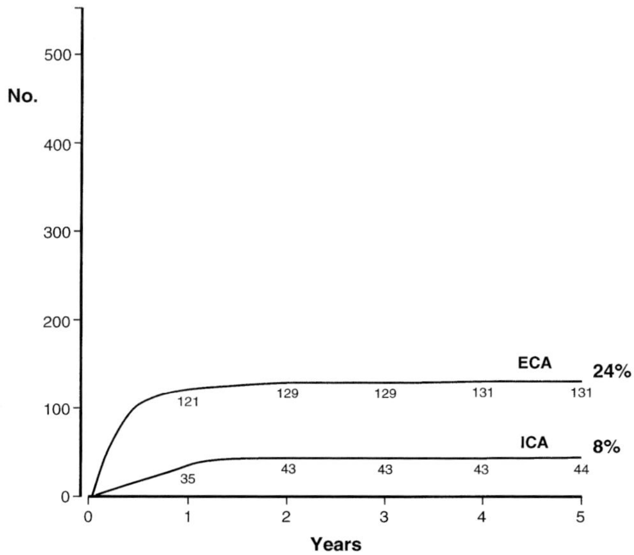

Fig. 2. Cumulative number of internal (ICA) and external (ECA) carotid restenoses in 553 primary operations.

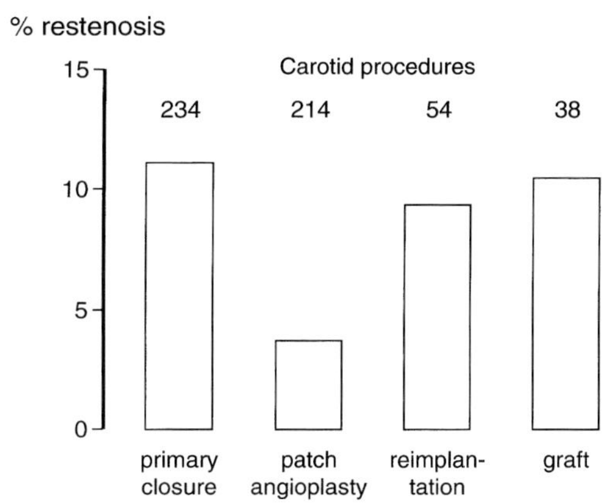

Fig. 3. Internal carotid restenosis rate for each of the four main carotid surgical procedures.

1993–1995 data, this possibly related to a reluctance to use patch closure. Prosthetic patch closure was associated with significantly fewer restenoses compared with the other procedures (Pearson's c^2=10.8, p=0.013, Fig. 3). Over the 6 years reviewed, the restenosis rate fell from 12% to 6% (Fig. 4) which may have been partly due to the increase in patch closure in this time, from 8% to over 70% of cases. The nine internal carotid occlusions all occurred by 15 months following surgery after primary closure in seven patients and after patch closure and graft replacement in one patient each.

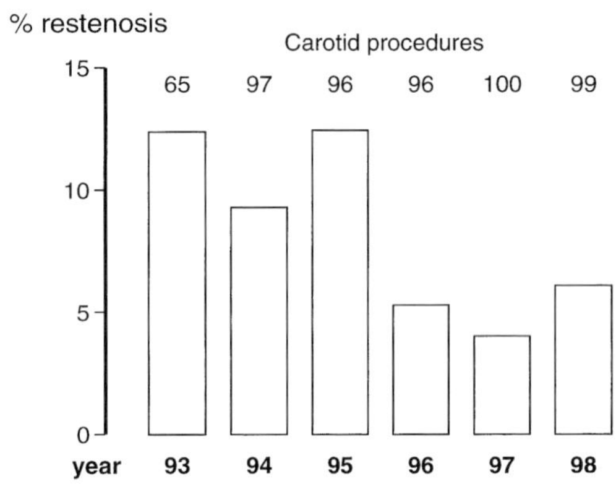

Fig. 4. Total number of primary internal carotid artery procedures and the restenosis rate by year.

External carotid artery

Postoperative occlusion occurred in ten of these, all but one within a year of surgery. Restenosis was found in 131 (24%, Fig. 2). Only two of these occurred after 2 years. The clinical relevance of external carotid restenosis is uncertain but this artery contributes substantially to the intracranial circulation in patients with severe internal carotid disease (Figs 5,6). External carotid stenosis is unlikely to be a problem when the internal carotid is widely patent but may become important if restenosis or occlusion of the internal carotid artery subsequently develops.

TREATMENT FOR RESTENOSIS

Twenty-six patients (4.7%) with internal carotid restenosis subsequently underwent re-intervention, 15 by open and 11 by endovascular procedures.

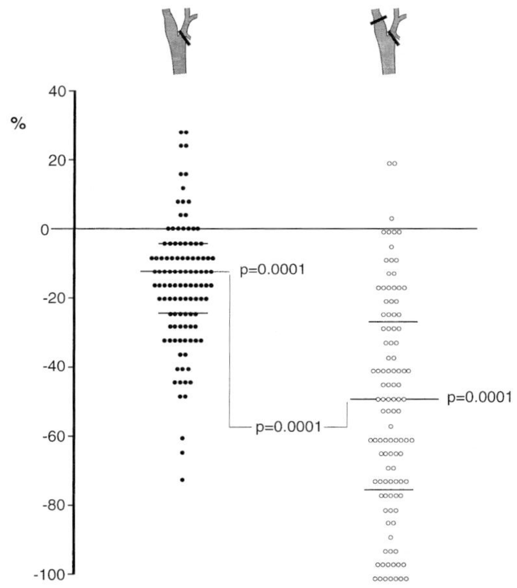

Fig. 5. Percentage fall in middle cerebral artery blood flow velocity by transcranial Doppler on clamping the external carotid and then the internal carotid in 108 patients undergoing carotid surgery. Results are expressed as median and interquartile ranges and demonstrate significant falls in middle cerebral blood flow on both external and internal clamping (Mann-Whitney U test).

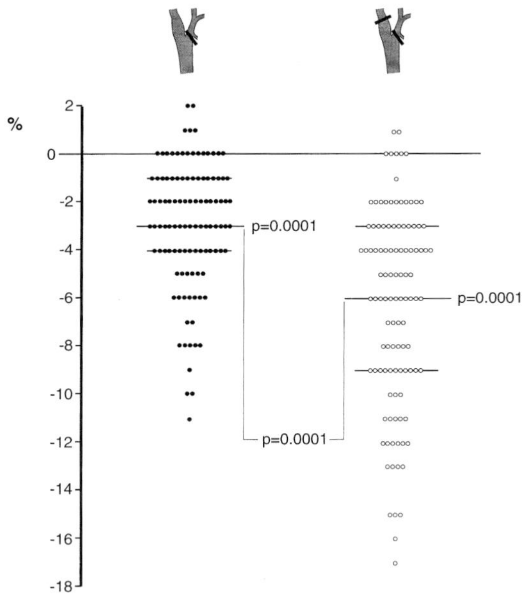

Fig. 6. Absolute fall in percentage cerebral oxygen saturation (CsO_2) on external carotid clamping and then clamping the internal carotid in 108 patients undergoing carotid surgery (Mann–Whitney U test). Results are expressed as median and interquartile ranges.

Surgery

Of the 15 patients requiring repeat surgery, ten were symptomatic. Interestingly, five patients developed 'global' symptoms of cerebral ischaemia suggesting a haemodynamic problem due to poor collaterals. Nine had contralateral internal carotid artery occlusions or tight stenoses. In two cases 'restenosis' was found at the first postoperative duplex image suggesting a residual problem following surgery.

In eleven patients with restenosis following primary closure, pseudointimal hyperplasia was removed in three and a kink was treated by patching in a further three cases; a formal endarterectomy was not required. All were closed using a patch angioplasty. Restenosis following graft replacement was treated by patch angioplasty (n=1) and partial graft excision and reanastomosis (n=2). None of the procedures required a shunt.

There were six complications following repeat surgery, comprising four nerve palsies (two transient and two permanent) and two haematomas requiring wound exploration. There were no perioperative strokes or deaths. Of the ten symptomatic patients, two had postoperative symptoms after repeat surgery, one with recurrent amaurosis fugax and another had a single episode of 'global' cerebral ischaemia. There were no late strokes during a mean follow-up of 20 months (range 0–50) months. There was one postoperative death due to cancer. Secondary restenosis was detected in two patients and one required a third operation.

Percutaneous angioplasty and stenting

Eleven patients underwent percutaneous transluminal angioplasty (PTA) for restenosis; two had symptoms of 'global' cerebral ischaemia and nine were asymptomatic. ECG and pulse oximetry were monitored continuously, and systemic blood pressure recorded at 5-minute intervals. Transcranial Doppler and near-infrared spectroscopy were used to monitor ipsilateral middle cerebral artery emboli and cerebral oxygen saturation, respectively. Once vascular access was achieved, 5000IU heparin was given intravenously, and prior to angioplasty 500mg atropine administered to prevent bradycardia or asystole on carotid sinus compression.

Our technique was to approach these lesions by femoral artery puncture to avoid dislodging common carotid atheroma during direct puncture, carotid dissection and thrombosis, neck haematoma, and post-procedure neck compression.[23] A 9F guiding catheter was used in case stent placement was necessary. The appropriate common carotid artery was accessed with a sidewinder II catheter (Cordis, UK) and the stenosis crossed using a Compass guidewire. A 6mm balloon (Courier, Boston Scientific or Cordis, Fig. 7) was used for dilatation in all but one case where a 5mm balloon was used.

The mean number of embolic events on TCD was 300 (range 176–400). These mainly occurred during contrast and saline injection and were likely to be due to air microbubbles or ultrasound reflections off the interface between blood and contrast. Protection balloons inflated in the distal cervical internal carotid artery have been used to reduce embolic events[24] but events are still recorded during the procedure either when the protection balloon is deflated or due to collateral flow through the external carotid artery.

We achieved our aim of residual stenosis no greater than 50% in all but one patient

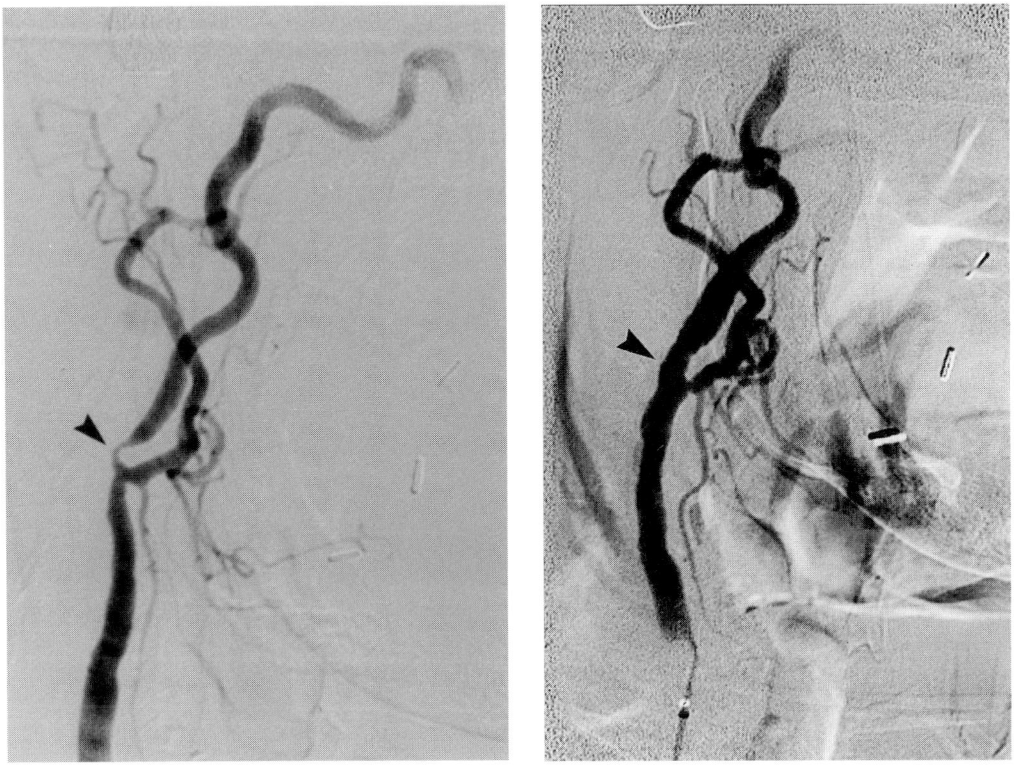

(a) (b)

Fig. 7. Digital subtraction angiography showing a tight stenosis at the origin of the internal carotid artery (a) successfully dilated by PTA (b).

in whom a 9mm Wallstent (Boston Scientific) was placed with a good result (Fig. 8). No complications occurred during the procedure but one patient developed a fatal haemorrhage into the contralateral hemisphere 8 hours later. This almost certainly was related to the procedure as the contralateral internal carotid artery had been occluded previously and contralateral middle cerebral artery filling was much improved following angioplasty.

During a mean follow-up of 17 months (range 1–36), there has been one death due to myocardial infarction, no strokes and a single episode of amaurosis fugax. One patient was found to have an asymptomatic occlusion of the relevant internal carotid artery at 3 months. The patient who underwent stent placement had a 70% asymptomatic restenosis at 3 months.

Endovascular or surgical treatment for restenosis?

In restenosis, where the complications of difficult repeat surgery may exceed potential benefits, PTA with or without stenting seems attractive. As a primary

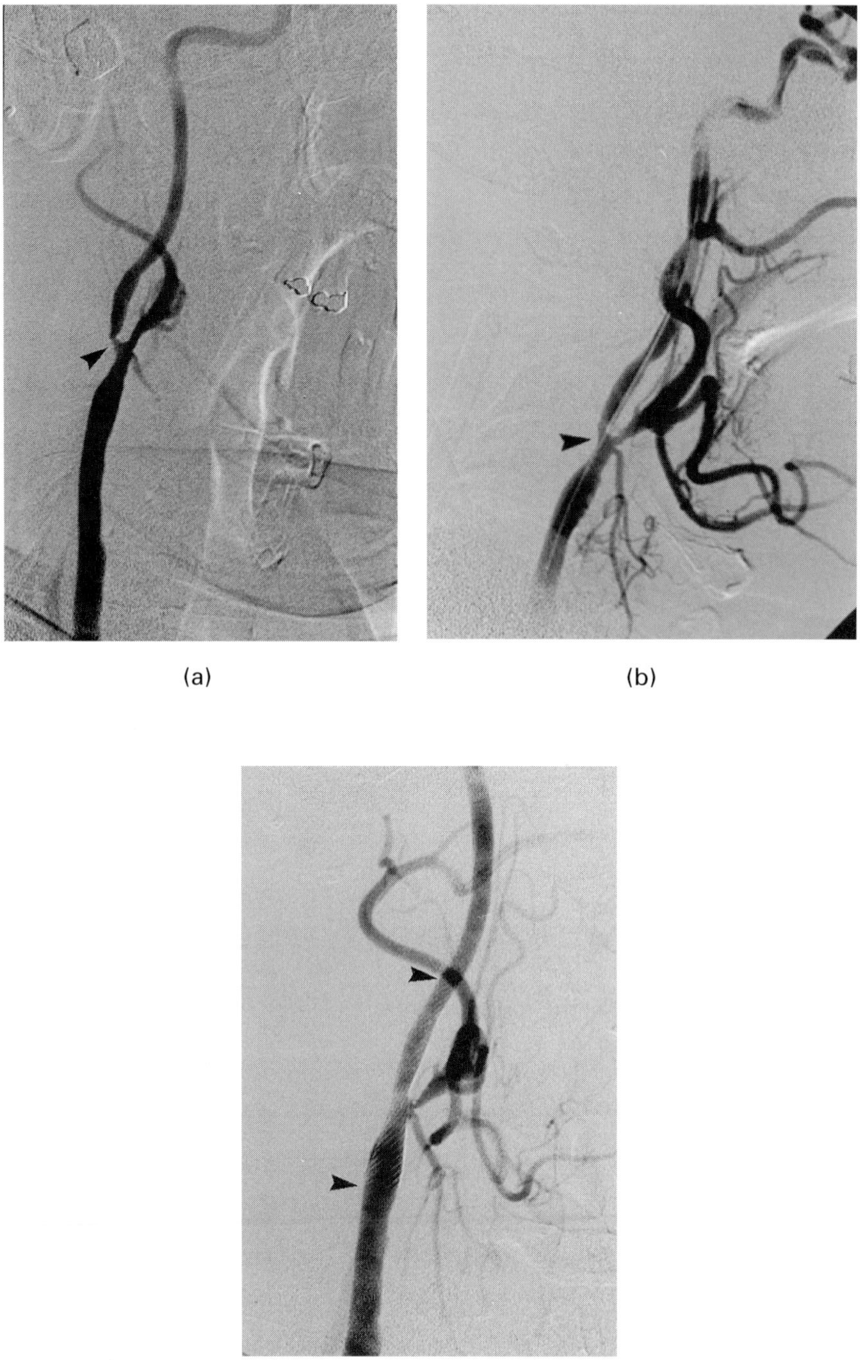

(a) (b)

(c)

Fig. 8. A tight internal carotid artery restenosis (a). Following angioplasty considerable recoil occurred (b) and a stent was placed (c).

procedure, the 30-day morbidity and mortality from the CAVATAS data were similar in surgical and PTA patients but there were more embolic events in PTA patients. In recurrent stenosis, involving intimal hyperplasia, PTA should carry a much lower risk of releasing emboli.

Theoretically, endoluminal therapy should carry a lower morbidity than repeat surgery as general anaesthesia and the complications associated with neck exploration are avoided. Neck haematoma is not a problem and the cranial nerves are not at risk. The endovascular technique is well tolerated and allows continuous communication with, and neurological assessment of, the patient. Balloon dilatation of the carotid may be painful[25] but not in our experience; we have found nitrous oxide and air inhalation provides effective pain relief during angioplasty procedures. Carotid occlusion times during PTA are also short (15–30 seconds) even for stent insertion. There remains the risk of atheroma embolism from the aorta or common carotid during catheterization and angioplasty which can be avoided in surgery by careful flushing. Post-angioplasty problems such as vessel wall dissection, spasm and localized thrombosis (rare) can also be treated endoluminally; dissection by immediate stent placement and thrombosis by aspiration thrombectomy and stenting.[26]

Whilst surgery of the external carotid artery attempts to improve its flow, PTA or stenting across its ostium may narrow or obstruct it. In our experience the external carotid remains patent, although its flow may be reduced. Recently, a double balloon technique has been described where a second balloon is placed in the external carotid artery and inflated simultaneously.[27] Long-term patency rates following PTA for restenosis are unknown, but PTA can be repeated if necessary. Stent deformation and detachment has been reported but should be infrequent.[28] Recurrent stenosis within a stent is usually due to further pseudointimal hyperplasia and although this has been reported to occur in 4% of patients at 12 months we suspect that it will occur more frequently.[29] Failure to access or to cross the lesion is seen in a small proportion of patients, particularly those with significant proximal disease or markedly angulated or kinked carotid vessels.

Primary stenting is now increasingly performed. This is of particular relevance in recurrent stenosis where scarring and fibrosis increase the likelihood of recoil following PTA. In most cases, pre-dilatation would be required with balloon moulding of the stent to the artery wall after deployment. Immediate patency rates using stents are higher than for PTA alone as the stent resists vessel wall recoil in these recurrent lesions.[30] Assessment during the procedure is by digital subtraction angiography but intravascular ultrasound can also be used.[31] Prior to placement, intravascular ultrasound may assist in deciding on the balloon diameter required, especially where stents are placed from common carotid artery to internal carotid artery where the failure of the stent to fully expand in the larger common carotid artery may lead to abnormal flow patterns and subsequent thrombosis or embolism.

Avoiding restenosis

Patch angioplasty reduced restenosis rates in two prospective and randomized trials.[32,33] Other studies that failed to identify a reduction in restenosis by patching were retrospective, where the choice of procedure may have been subject to selection bias, or included too few cases to make a comparison.[34–36] We found fewer restenoses with patch closure and a lower overall restenosis rate with selective prosthetic patch insertion for the small internal carotid artery.

Conservative treatment

The 18 patients with restenosis who did not undergo a second procedure were followed for a mean of 25 months (range 3–74). There were two cardiac deaths and three strokes, one in the ipsilateral and two in the contralateral hemisphere. Two patients recovered, but one suffered a dense hemiparesis and dysphasia from which recovery was poor. In all three, the carotid contralateral to the restenosis was previously occluded which raises the possibility that those with contralateral severe stenosis or occlusion may at higher risk of stroke.[37]

CONCLUSIONS

Few restenoses occurred after 18 months following carotid endarterectomy and routine carotid imaging is not justified beyond this time.[38,39] The number of patients suffering restenosis is too small to allow good evidence on indication for treatment. A prospective, multicentre randomized trial comparing surgery, endovascular and best medical treatments is clearly needed, but this may be impossible to arrange.

ACKNOWLEDGEMENTS

The authors would like to thank the following for their help in the preparation of this manuscript: Shirley Fearn for collecting many of the data and for Figs 1–3, Helen Carruthers for illustration, and Katharine Oakden for audit data.

REFERENCES

1. Piepgras DG, Sundt TM, Marsh WR *et al.*: Recurrent carotid stenosis. Results and complications of 57 operations. *Ann Surg* **203**: 205–213, 1986
2. Treiman GS, Jenkins JM, Edwards WH *et al.*: The evolving surgical management of recurrent carotid stenosis. *J Vasc Surg* **16**: 354–363, 1992
3. Hill BB, Olcott C, Dalman RL *et al.*: Reoperation for carotid stenosis is as safe as primary carotid endarterectomy. *J Vasc Surg* **30**: 26–35, 1999
4. Farrell B, Fraser A, Sandercock P *et al.*: Randomised trial of endarterectomy for recently symptomatic carotid stenosis: final results of the MRC European Carotid Surgery Trial (ECST). *Lancet* **351**: 1379–1387, 1998
5. Barnett HJM, Taylor DW, Haynes RB *et al.*: Beneficial effect of carotid endarterectomy in symptomatic patients with high grade carotid stenosis. *New Engl J Med* **325**: 446–453, 1991
6. Lattimer CR, Burnand KG: Recurrent carotid stenosis after carotid endarterectomy. *Br J Surg* **84**: 1206–1219, 1997
7. Steinke W, Kloetzsch C, Hennerici M: Carotid artery disease assessed by colour Doppler

flow imaging: Correlation with standard Doppler sonography and angiography. *Am J Neuroradiol* **154**: 1061–1068, 1990

8. Chang YJ, Golby AJ, Albers GW: Detection of carotid stenosis: From NASCET results to clinical practice. *Stroke* **26**: 1325–1328, 1995
9. Pan XM, Saloner D, Reilly LM *et al.*: Assessment of carotid artery stenosis by ultrasonography, conventional angiography and magnetic resonance angiography: Correlation with *ex vivo* measurement of plaque stenosis. *J Vasc Surg* **21**: 82–89, 1995
10. Alexandrov AV, Bladin CF, Maggisano R *et al.*: Measuring carotid stenosis. Time for a reappraisal. *Stroke* **24**: 1292–1296, 1993
11. AbuRahma AF, Robinson PA, Stickler DL: Analysis of regression of postoperative carotid stenosis from prospective randomised trial of carotid endarterectomy comparing primary closure versus patching. *Ann Surg* **229**: 767–773, 1999
12. Samson RH, Showalter DP, Yunis JP *et al.*: Hemodynamically significant early recurrent carotid stenosis: An often self limiting self-reversing condition. *J Vasc Surg* **30**: 446–452, 1999
13. Department of Health: *Hospital Episode Statistics (HES)* 1993–1998
14. Frericks H, Kievit J, Baalen JM *et al.*: Carotid recurrent stenosis and risk of ipsilateral stroke. *Stroke* **29**: 244–250, 1998
15. Baker WH, Koustas G, Burke K *et al.*: Intraoperative duplex scanning and late carotid artery stenosis. *J Vasc Surg* **19**: 829–833, 1994
16. Stoney RJ, String ST: Recurrent carotid stenosis. *Surgery* **80**: 705–710, 1972
17. Verlato F, Camporese G, Rocco S *et al.*: Carotid kinks – relationship to atherosclerosis and cerebral ischaemia. *J Vasc Invest* **2**: 65–69, 1996
18. Ganesan R, Cole R, Mackey A: Significance of carotid restenosis following endarterectomy. *Cerebrovasc Dis* **8**: 338–344, 1997
19. Bernstein EF, Torem S, Dilley RB: Does carotid restenosis predict an increased risk of late symptoms, stroke, or death? *Ann Surg* **212**: 629–636, 1990
20. Rothwell PM, Slattery J, Warlow CP: A systematic comparison of the risks of stroke and death due to carotid endarterectomy for symptomatic and asymptomatic stenosis. *Stroke* **27**: 266–269, 1996
21. Kirsch JD, Wagner LR, James EL *et al.*: Carotid artery occlusion: Positive predictive value of duplex sonography compared with arteriography. *J Vasc Surg* **19**: 642–649, 1994
22. Fearn SJ, McCollum CN: Shortening and re-implantation for tortuous internal carotid arteries. *J Vasc Surg* **27**: 936–939, 1998
23. Pratesi C, Credi G, Pulli R *et al.*: The role of endovascular surgery in carotid restenosis. *J Endovasc Surg* **2**: 36–41,1995
24. Theron J, Courtheaux P, Alachkar F *et al.*: New triple-coaxial catheter system for carotid angioplasty with cerebral protection. *Am J Neuroradiol* **11**: 869–874, 1990
25. Mounari LM, Belloni G, Moschini L *et al.*: Carotid pain during percutaneous angioplasty (PTA). Pathophysiology and clinical features. *Cephalalgia* **14**: 127–131, 1994
26. Lanzino G, Mericle RA, Lopes DK *et al.*: Percutaneous transluminal angioplasty and stent placement for recurrent carotid artery stenosis. *J Neurosurg* **90**: 688–694, 1999
27. Bergeron P, Chambron P, Hartungo I *et al*: Cervical carotid artery stenosis: which technique, balloon angioplasty or surgery? *J Cardiovasc Surg* **37** (Suppl 1): 73–75, 1996
28. Wholey MH, Wholey M, Bergeron P *et al.*: Current global status of carotid artery stent placement. *Cath Cardiovasc Diag* **44**: 1–6, 1998
29. Theron JG, Payell GG, Coskum O *et al.*: Carotid artery stenosis: Treatment with protected balloon angioplasty and stent placement. *Radiology* **201**: 627–636, 1996
30. Wholey M, Eles G, Jarmolowski CR *et al.*: Percutaneous transluminal angioplasty and stents in the treatment of extracranial circulation. *J Intervent Cardiol* **9**: 225–231, 1996
31. Diethrich EB, Ndiaye M, Reid D *et al.*: Stenting in the carotid artery: initial experience in 110 patients. *J Endovasc Surg* **3**: 42–62, 1996
32. AbuRahma AF, Robinson PA, Saiedy S *et al.*: Prospective randomized trial of bilateral carotid endarterectomies. *Stroke* **30**: 1185–1189, 1999
33. Ranaboldo CJ, Barros D'Sa AAB, Bell PRF *et al.*: Randomized controlled trial of patch angioplasty for carotid endarterectomy. *Br J Surg* **80**: 1528–1530, 1993

34. Nene S, Moore W: The role of patch angioplasty in prevention of early recurrent carotid stenosis. *Ann Vasc Surg* **13**: 169–173, 1999
35. Gelabert HA, El-Massry S, Moore WS: Carotid endarterectomy with primary closure does not adversely affect the rate of recurrent stenosis. *Arch Surg* **129**: 648–654, 1994
36. Rosenthal D, Archie JP, Garcia-Rinaldi R *et al.*: Carotid patch angioplasty: immediate and long term results. *J Vasc Surg* **12**: 326–333, 1990
37. Golledge J, Cuming R, Ellis M *et al.*: Clinical follow-up rather than duplex surveillance after carotid endarterectomy. *J Vasc Surg* **25**: 55–63, 1997
38. Johnson CA, Tollefson DFJ, Olsen SB *et al.*: The natural history of early recurrent carotid artery stenosis. *Am J Surg* **177**: 433–436, 1999
39. Fiorani P, Sbarigia E, Giannoni MF *et al.*: For how long should carotid endarterectomy surveillance be continued? *Int Angiol* **13**: 190–195, 1994

Endovascular interventions in the supra-aortic vessels

Tony Nicholson

INTRODUCTION

This chapter aims to describe the indications, technique and results of endovascular interventions in the supra-aortic vessels other than the internal carotid artery. Percutaneous transluminal angioplasty (PTA) of the subclavian arteries was first reported in 1980.[1]

There are now over 1000 cases of endovascular treatment in brachiocephalic arteries reported. An analysis of all these studies reveals an initial success rate varying from 90 to 100%, with an incidence of significant complications from 1 to 4%. The combined risk of death from stroke following supra-aortic intervention is less than 1%. Follow-up studies to 5 years have indicated patency rates of 90%.

Occlusions of the brachiocephalic arteries had a poor initial and late success rate before the development of intra-arterial stents. The use of stents has increased the initial success rate to 85% and the long-term success rate to 80% at 3 years. At present the results of thrombolysis for brachiocephalic occlusions is not clear. A limited personal experience indicates that occlusions treated within 6 weeks can be successfully recanalized with a low complication rate.

INDICATIONS FOR INTERVENTION IN THE SUPRA-AORTIC ARTERIES

Procedures in the brachiocephalic vessels should be limited to lesions that are clearly symptomatic. Close co-operation between vascular radiologist, surgeon and neurologist, where indicated, is mandatory. A uniform opinion should be sought prior to treatment and the patient should be warned of the potential risks and complications of the treatment, as indicated in the literature cited above. In addition, the patient should be counselled about therapeutic alternatives. An analysis of our own indications for intervention in the supra-aortic arteries since 1990 reveals that the majority of patients have been treated for vertebrobasilar insufficiency (VBI) ± subclavian steal (51%), followed by arm ischaemia or embolus (22%), global cerebral ischaemia (8%), transient ischaemic attacks (9%) and to improve inflow prior to vascular or neurosurgery (9%).

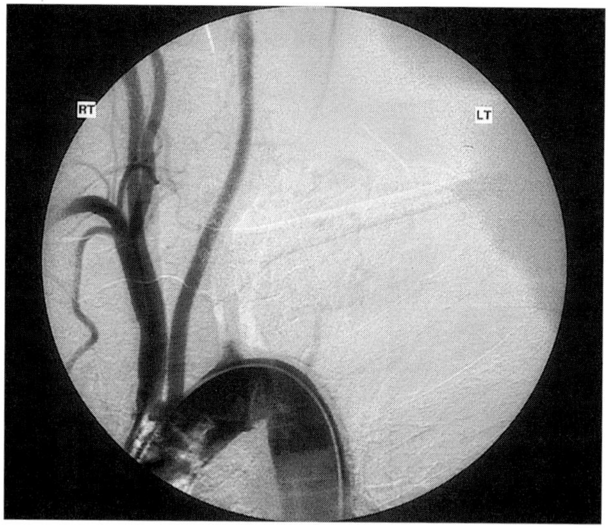

(a)

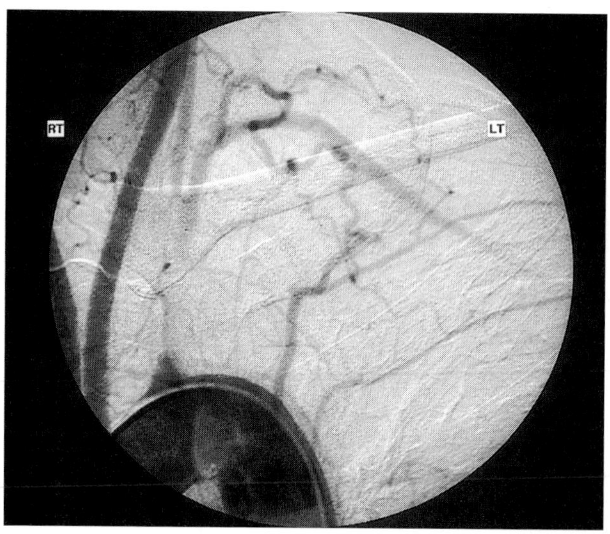

(b)

Fig. 1. Arch aortography in a patient with dizziness and arm ischaemia. (a) The left subclavian artery is occluded. (b) Late phase aortography. The distal left subclavian artery fills via retrograde flow down the left vertebral artery indicating vertebral steal syndrome.

PTA OF THE SUBCLAVIAN ARTERY

The subclavian steal syndrome was initially described in 1971[2] (Fig. 1a,b). A diagnosis of subclavian steal syndrome should only be made after arch aortography, as selective injections into the subclavian vessels can produce artificial steal. However, in a study of 1114 patients with extracranial occlusions of the innominate and subclavian arteries, only 168 demonstrated signs and symptoms of subclavian steal.[3] Stenosis of the left subclavian artery at its origin occurs more often than on the right side. Physical examination reveals reduction in blood pressure in one arm and often a supraclavicular bruit. A recently described phenomenon is the coronary subclavian steal syndrome, where a critical stenosis of the left subclavian artery leads to flow reversal through a patent LIMA graft, causing coronary hypoperfusion and angina[4] (Fig. 2a–d).

Method

Most subclavian stenoses can be approached from the transfemoral route (Fig. 3a,b). Our own practice is to use a 65cm long flexible 7F sheath so that we can monitor pressure and perform angiograms during and after the procedure. Left or right-sided stenoses can be approached and crossed using Sidewinder, Mani or Headhunter catheters, and curved hydrophilic wires. Once the lesion is crossed it is our practice to exchange the hydrophilic wire for a 180 or 260cm Amplatz stiff wire. A single bolus dose of heparin (5000 IU) is then administered. If any spasm is encountered in the subclavian or axillary arteries, it can be relieved with an intra-arterial injection of nitroglycerine (100μg). The subclavian artery varies in size considerably and it is our practice to always measure the size of the artery above and below the stenosis, and occasionally the size of the contralateral artery. Balloon sizes from 6 to 10mm in diameter are then used to dilate the stenoses, the balloon being inflated until the waist is abolished and inflation maintained for 2 minutes. The result is assessed by either arch aortography or by an injection through the sheath. If the result looks suboptimal, further balloon dilatation is carried out. Following this, if the result is still angiographically suboptimal or if there is a gradient of greater than 10mm across the lesion, it is our practice to deploy a stent in order to achieve the best possible result.

Most subclavian occlusions are proximal (Fig. 4a,b). It is usually not possible to approach them from the groin as it is not possible to gain firm catheter support to cross the occlusion. Such lesions have to be approached from the ipsilateral brachial or axillary artery. The brachial artery is preferred as it can often be easily punctured with a hand-held Doppler for percutaneous access but is also easier to cut down on to. At present, stents are being developed that can be delivered on 5F balloons through 6F sheaths and this will make percutaneous puncture more acceptable. If the percutaneous endovascular approach is made, the straight floppy end of a guidewire is passed through the puncture needle and into the axillary artery. A 6-8F sheath is then inserted and 5000 units of heparin are given immediately, along with 100μg of nitroglycerine, to avoid distal spasm. A high brachial puncture is safer than a low puncture. The subclavian occlusion is crossed with a combination of curved

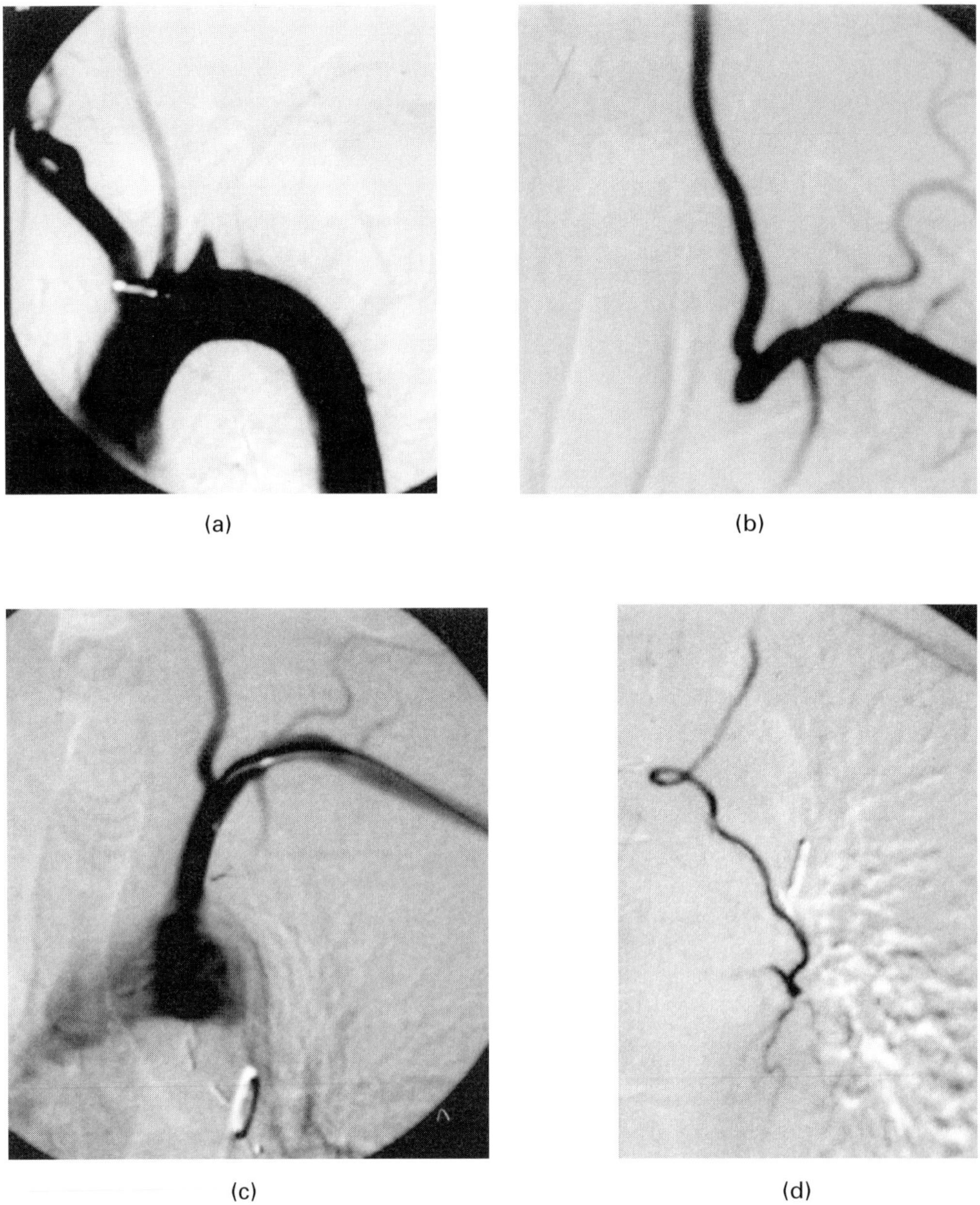

Fig. 2. Arch aortogram in a 50-year-old man, with angina on exertion and arm ischaemia (a), reveals an occluded subclavian artery with reversed flow in the vertebral and left internal mammary artery (b). He had undergone coronary bypass surgery 3 years earlier with a LIMA graft to his left anterior descending artery (LAD). The occlusion was crossed and stented from a left brachial cut down, with restoration of normal flow in both the vertebral artery and internal mammary graft (c) though clearly there is a stenosis in the LAD beyond the graft anastomosis (d) which was dealt with by angioplasty via the LIMA graft. (Courtesy of Dr Simon McPherson)

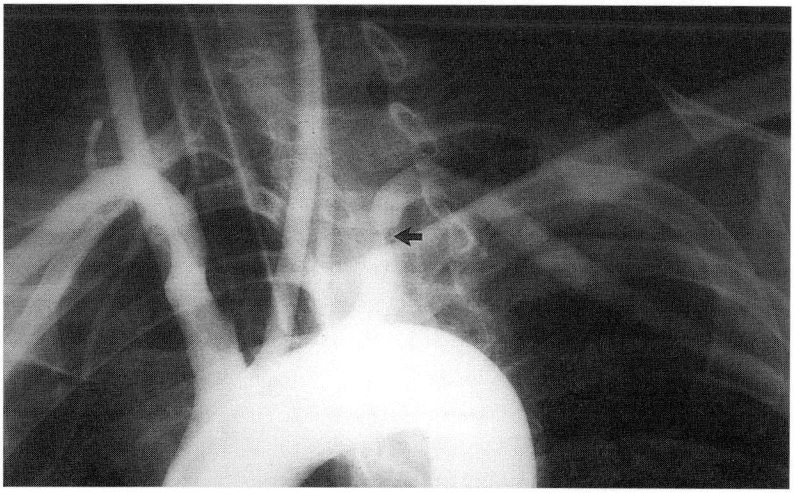

(a)

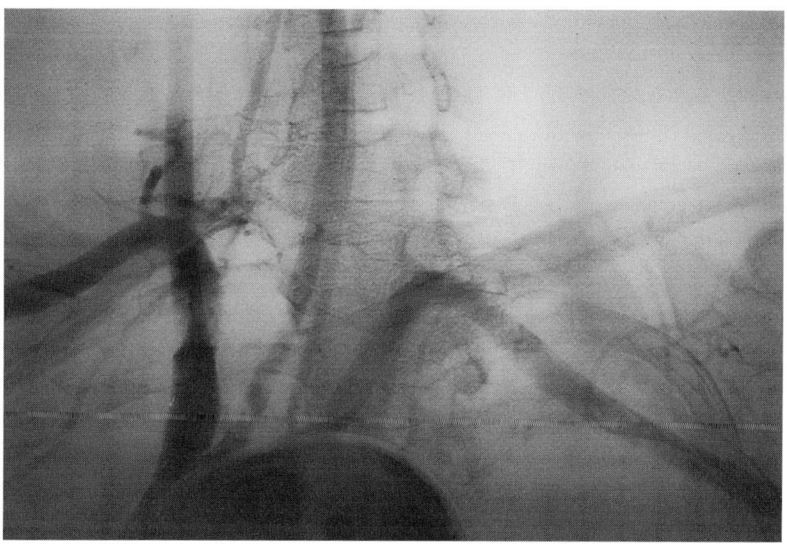

(b)

Fig. 3. Arch aortography in a patient following an acute embolic episode to the left fingers. The left radial pulse was impalpable and there was a 70mmHg difference in arm blood pressures. (a) Stenosis of the left subclavian artery distal to the left vertebral artery origin. (b) Simple 7 mm angioplasty from the right common femoral artery results in restoration of pulse and blood pressure and no further embolic episodes over a 12-month follow-up.

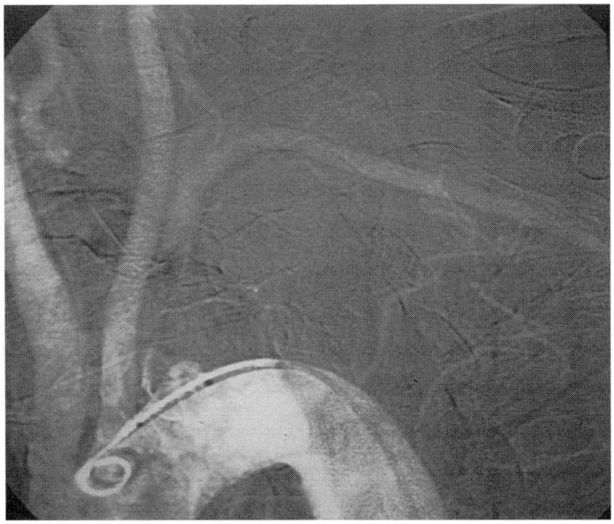

(a)

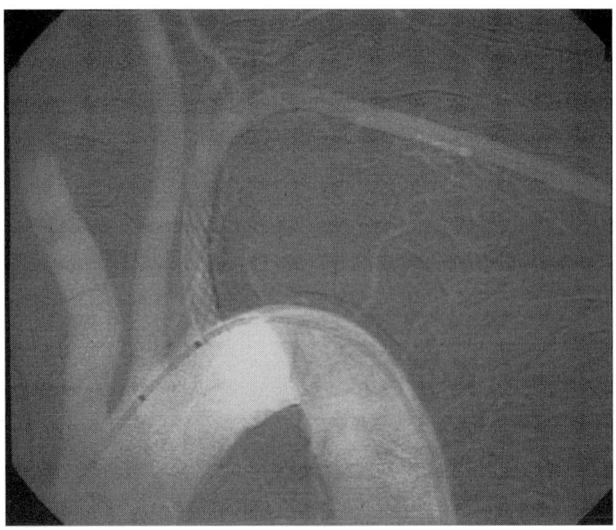

(b)

Fig. 4. Arch aortography in a patient with a pulseless left arm with symptoms of arm ischaemia. (a) The left subclavian artery is occluded from its origin to the origin of the left vertebral artery. (b) The occlusion was crossed from a left brachial arterial puncture and a 7mm x 3.9cm self-expanding stent inserted. The stent was then post-dilated to 7mm with restoration of arm pulses. The patient remains symptom free at 4 years.

glidewire and femorovisceral curved catheter. Occlusions at this site are often old and hard, and it is often necessary (intentionally or unintentionally) to recanalize them subintimally. Great care should be taken if the wire does not immediately re-enter the aorta, as it is possible to cause quite extensive dissections in the aortic arch. The subintimal approach can occasionally cause delayed pseudoaneurysms (Fig. 5). These can be successfully treated with stent-grafts (Fig. 6a,b). Sometimes it is not possible to cross such occlusions and as long as the patient has been fully informed and counselled beforehand, surgery becomes the only viable option. However, since 1990 we have managed to cross 85% of such proximal occlusions. It is my own practice to place short, self-expanding stents through such occlusions and then post-dilate them to an appropriate size. However, it is perfectly acceptable to pre-dilate such lesions and place balloon-mounted stents. Where occlusions extend up to the vertebral origin it is probably wise to deploy a stent with a large mesh size, as the origin may have to be crossed.

The potential for vertebral artery embolization during subclavian angioplasty is minimal, as the direction of blood flow within the vertebral artery is not supposed to change immediately but does so some 20 seconds to several minutes after the procedure.[5] This was based on duplex and Doppler findings. I have checked this on several occasions during subclavian angioplasty for subclavian steal, and have been unable to recreate these results (unpublished). Nevertheless, the incidence of significant vertebral artery embolus remains at less than 1%. It has also been reported that occlusion of the vertebral artery by adjacent stenotic plaque during angioplasty does not necessarily aggravate the symptoms and sometimes ablates them.[6]

Proximal right subclavian artery stenoses and occlusions can present special difficulties (Fig. 7a,b). Balloon inflation can compromise the ipsilateral carotid circulation. However, the carotid artery circulation can be protected by placing a wire in the carotid artery from the contralateral groin. Occlusions present a more difficult problem. It is often possible to accurately place a balloon-mounted stent exactly at the bifurcation of the common carotid and subclavian artery. However, there is always the risk of embolic material being squeezed into the carotid artery. In future it will be possible to protect the carotid artery from this occurrence but it is not possible at the present time to know the incidence of this complication. However, patients should be informed that it is a possibility and counselled as to the therapeutic alternatives. An analysis of the literature between 1980 and 1995 would suggest that the stroke rate is slightly higher for surgery at the present time (surgery 2.8% vs PTA ± stent 0.4%).

PTA OF THE VERTEBRAL ARTERY

Symptomatology of vertebral artery lesions is non-specific and therefore the indications for angioplasty are not well-defined. Symptoms such as dizziness, diplopia, nystagmus, ataxia, cortical blindness, weakness and memory disturbance, are so non-specific that it is often difficult to know the significance of the proven stenosis of the proximal vertebral artery. However, angioplasty can be performed under local anaesthetic, is of low cost, with a short hospital stay. Osteal stenoses of the vertebral artery are generally smooth lesions, unlike those of the carotid artery,

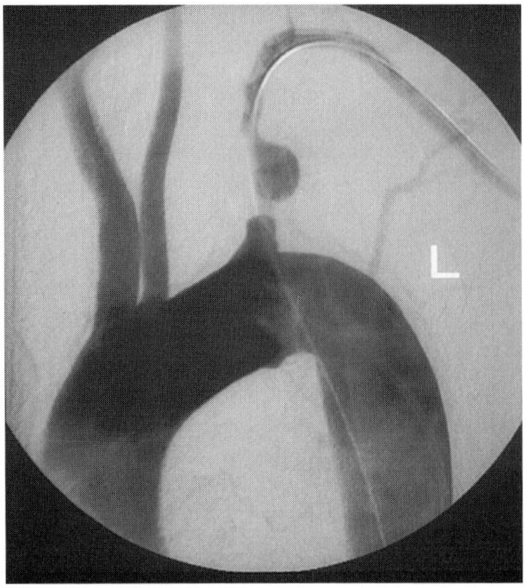

Fig. 5. Following percutaneous angioplasty of this left subclavian artery subintimal occlusion the pulse was briefly palpable and arm pressures normal with no gradient across the lesion. One week later the pulse was no longer palpable and the arm was ischaemic again. Arch aortography revealed restenosis with a pseudoaneurysm. Computed tomography follow-up a week later revealed that this was increasing in size.

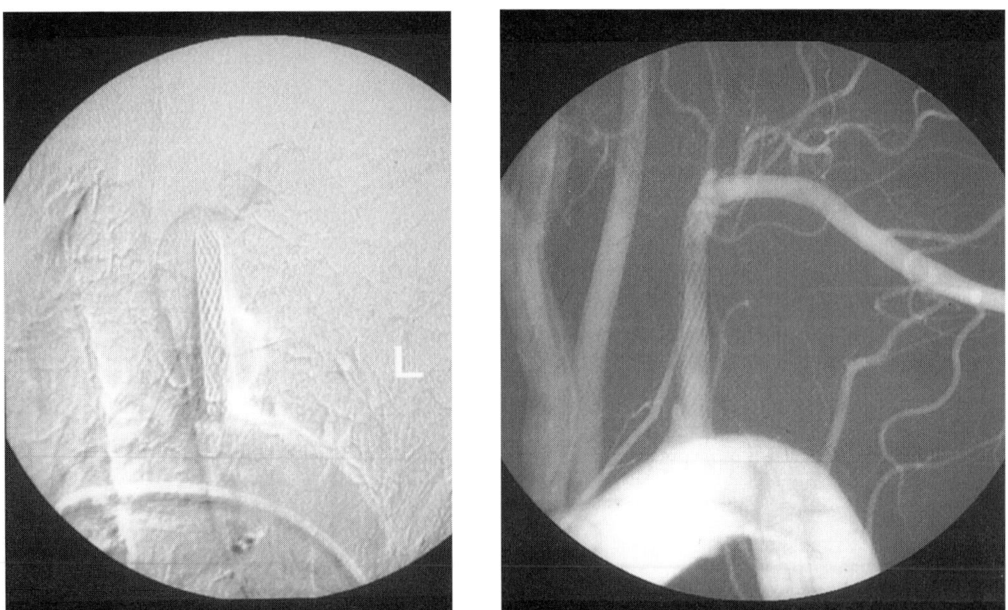

(a) (b)

Fig. 6. The pseudoaneurysm in Fig. 5 was treated from the right common femoral artery by the insertion of an 8mm x 3.6cm stent-graft (a) with restoration of flow and occlusion of the pseudoaneurysm (b). Flow in the left vertebral artery was preserved. The stent-graft was still patent at 1 year.

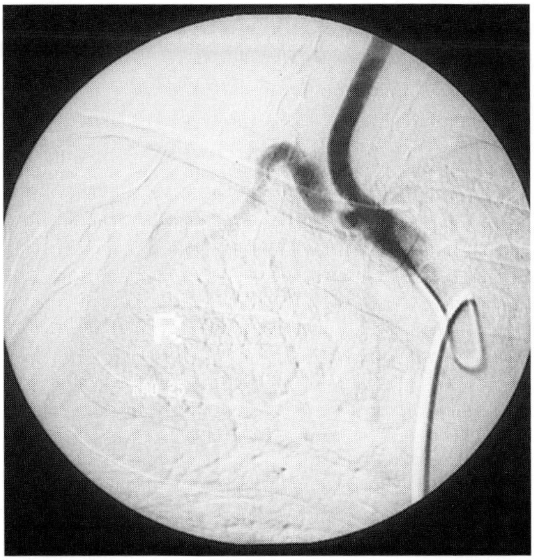

(a)

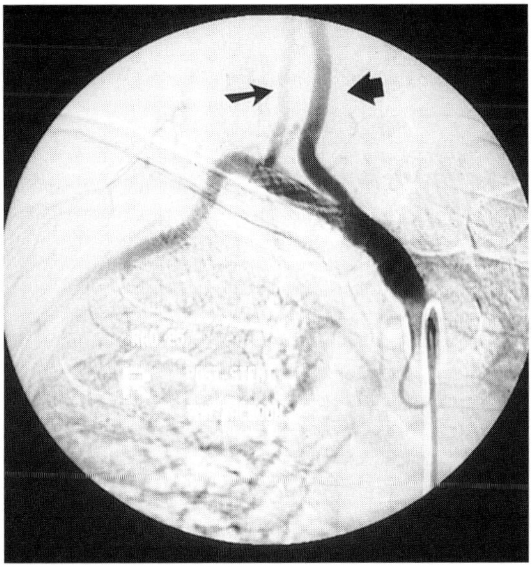

(b)

Fig. 7. Selective innominate angiography in the right anterior oblique position demonstrates a right subclavian origin stenosis (a) in a patient with right arm embolic disease. A short 7mm x 4cm balloon mounted stent has been placed with extreme accuracy at the junction of the right common carotid and subclavian arteries following a poor result from PTA alone (large arrow: right common carotid artery; small arrow: right vertebral artery). There were no further embolic episodes.

and reports suggest that there are few complications of angioplasty at this site.[7] Angioplasty of the vertebral artery can therefore be performed as a therapeutic trial, especially as 90% of vertebral artery lesions are osteal lesions accounting for 40% of all vertebrobasilar insufficiency cases.[8] The natural history of VBI indicates that 30% of patients remain asymptomatic after the initial episode, 50% have continued symptoms and 20% suffer a stroke.[9]

If significant carotid lesions are present then these should be corrected first. If the patient remains symptomatic after carotid endarterectomy then vertebral PTA can be performed as an adjunct.

Method

Vertebral artery angioplasty can be performed from a femoral approach. In elderly patients, where tortuosity and ectasia hinder this approach, the axillary or brachial artery can be used; 5000 units of intra-arterial heparin are administered prior to vertebral artery catheterization and a 4–6mm angioplasty balloon is used following measurement of the normal vessel adjacent to the stenosis. We usually use two inflations of 30 seconds. Though vertebral artery occlusion following angioplasty has been reported, it is not always symptomatic and often symptoms are cured.[6]

Of 125 patients reported in the literature between 1989 and 1993 technical success was reported in 116(93%). However, there is a lack of long-term follow-up, only three patients being reported with follow-up beyond 1 year, one of these having restenosis. If patients' symptoms are cured then it is ethically difficult to repeat angiography. However, if patients' symptoms are not cured or they have recurrent symptoms, repeat arch aortography is recommended. Recurrent stenosis, especially where symptoms were initially improved following angioplasty, should be treated with a stent (Fig. 8a,b). If the vertebral artery is only 4–6mm and the osteal stenosis is short, then it can be treated with either a renal or a coronary stent.

INNOMINATE ARTERY ANGIOPLASTY

Indications for innominate artery angioplasty include transient ischaemic attacks, right arm ischaemia and concomitant coronary artery disease, which requires bypass surgery. In our practice these lesions are almost exclusively atherosclerotic but angioplasty of the innominate artery and left common carotid artery in Takayasu's arteritis has been described.[10] Atherosclerotic lesions in the innominate artery are often large and ulcerated. If they co-exist with significant internal carotid artery lesions requiring endarterectomy, then angioplasty and stenting can be performed relatively safely at surgery. This will be described in the surgical section of this chapter. Balloon occlusion of the common carotid artery prior to angioplasty of the innominate artery has been successfully performed, with no sequelae.[11] Innominate and common carotid artery angioplasty from the percutaneous femoral approach will, in future, almost certainly be performed with some form of cerebral protection device in place.

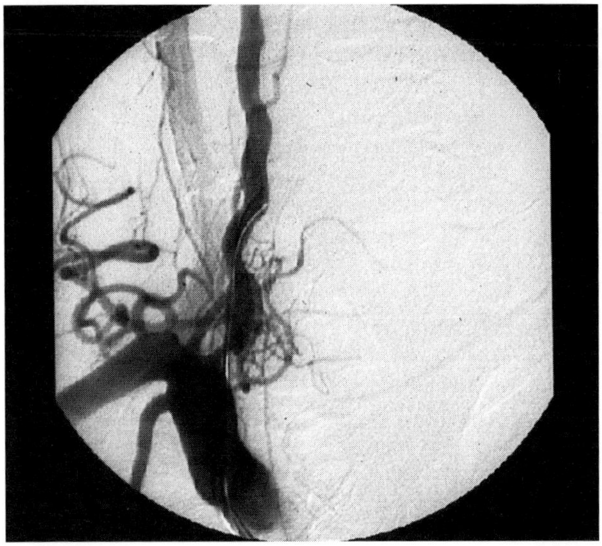

(a)

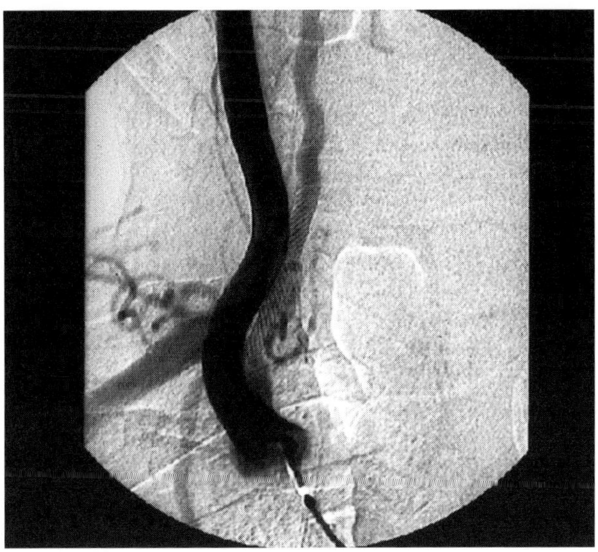

(b)

Fig. 8. Selective innominate angiography in a patient with dizziness and transient ischaemic attacks following left carotid endartrectomy reveals a right vertebral arterial stenosis (a). The left vertebral artery was hypoplastic and magnetic resonance angiography had not shown flow in the posterior communicating arteries. Previous PTA had failed and therefore a short self-expanding stent was inserted into the right vertebral artery origin with a good technical result (b). Clinically the patient was much improved but died of a myocardial infarction 7 months after the procedure.

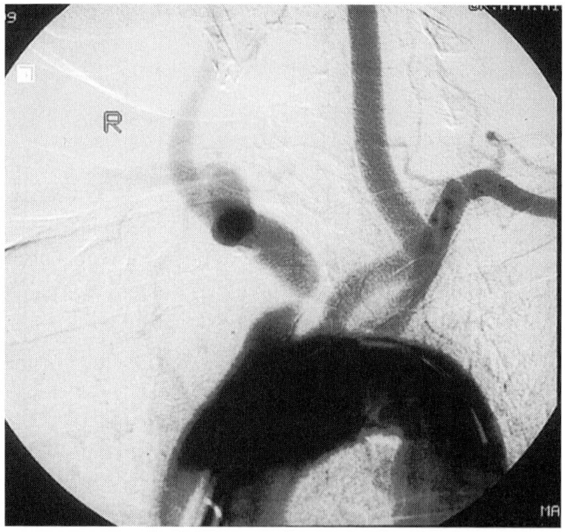

(a)

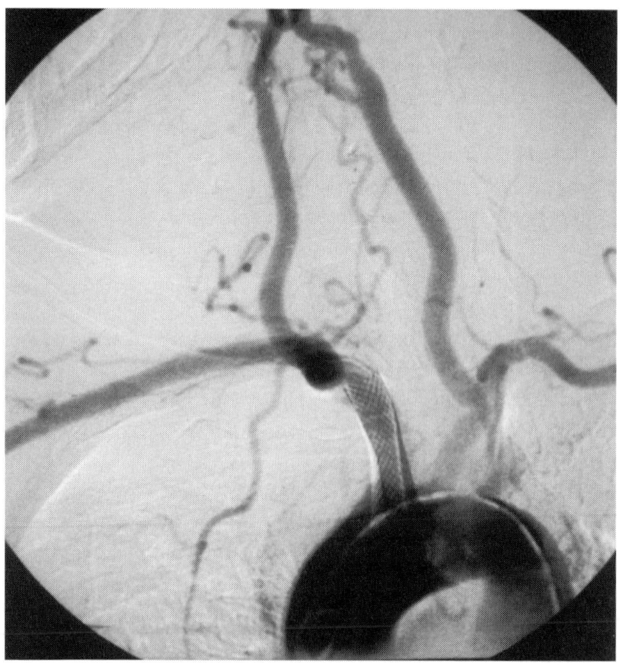

(b)

Fig. 9. Critical right innominate artery stenosis in a patient with crescendo transient ischaemic attacks and amaurosis fugax (a). The lesion was approached from the right brachiocephalic artery by cut-down and a 10mm x 3.9cm self-expanding stent deployed without predilatation. The deployed stent was then dilated to 10mm with a good angiographic result (b) and an excellent clinical response.

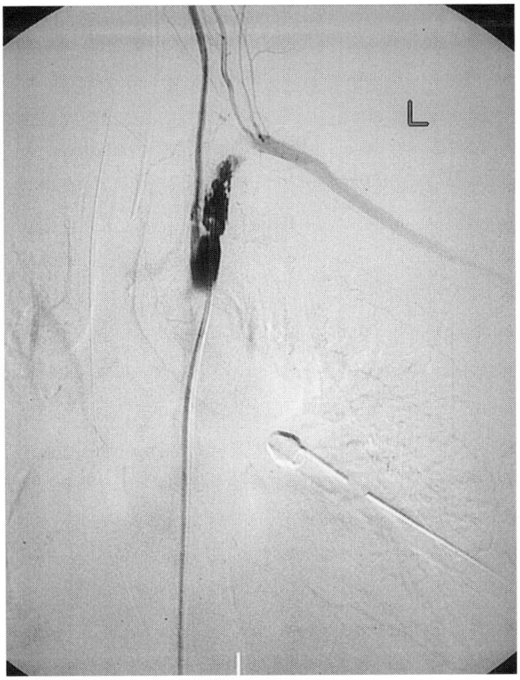

(a)

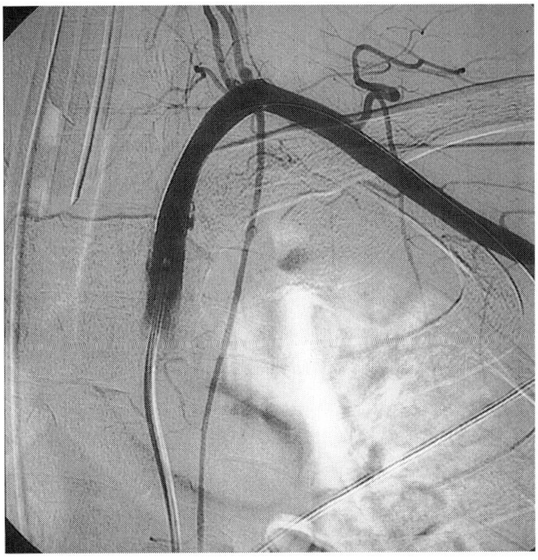

(b)

Fig. 10. Selective left subclavian angiography in a motorcyclist with an ischaemic left arm following an RTA reveals an almost occluded artery secondary to intimal disruption (a). This was simply treated by the insertion of a self-expanding uncovered stent from the right groin with restoration of left arm pulses (b).

Where stenotic lesions of the innominate or common carotid arteries are smooth and non-ulcerated, results have been good[12] (Fig. 9a,b). The results are certainly better than the surgical alternative, where a thoracotomy is required. Complication rates of surgery can be as high as 23% and include chylothorax, wound infection, phrenic nerve palsies and lymphatic fistulae.[13] However, careful analysis of the angiographic appearance of the lesion is recommended. Where the lesion is large, eccentric and ulcerated, angioplasty and stenting would best be performed with either percutaneous or surgical cerebral protection.

BRACHIOCEPHALIC TRAUMA

Traumatic lesions to the brachiocephalic arteries should be treated by embolization if they result in branch bleeding or stenting (covered or uncovered) for main arterial bleeding or arterial occlusion (Fig. 10a,b). Techniques are the same as already described.

SUMMARY

An analysis of the published literature suggests that the results of PTA, and more recently stenting, for lesions of the supra-aortic arteries are essentially the same as those achieved with modern surgical therapy. However, there appear to be fewer complications with endovascular therapy than are reported for surgical treatment. The initial technical results for patients with brachiocephalic occlusions were not quite so good but the introduction of stenting has improved the results considerably.

In view of the present experience with endovascular treatment for brachiocephalic lesions, PTA plus or minus a stent should be considered the treatment of choice for brachiocephalic stenoses, and primary stenting for occlusions.

REFERENCES

1. Bachman DM, Kim RM: Transluminal dilatation for subclavian steal syndrome. *Am J Roent* **135:** 995–996, 1980
2. Reivich M, Holling H, Roberts B *et al.*: Reversal of blood flow through vertebral artery and its effect on cerebral circulation. *New Engl J Med* **265:** 878–885, 1961
3. Burk DR, Gordon RL, Mishkin JD *et al.*: Percutaneous transluminal angioplasty of subclavian arteries. *Radiology* **164:** 699–704, 1987
4. Georges NP, Ferretti JA: Percutaneous transluminal angioplasty of subclavian artery occlusion for treatment of coronary subclavian steal. *Am J Roent* **161:** 399–400, 1993
5. Ringelstein EB, Szeumer H: Delayed reversal of vertebral artery blood flow following percutaneous transluminal angioplasty of the subclavian steal syndrome. *Neuroradiology* **26:** 189–198, 1984
6. Theron J: Angioplasty of supra-aortic arteries. *Semin Intervent Radiol* **4:** 331–342, 1987
7. Courtheaux P, Tounard EA, Theron J *et al.*: Transcutaneous angioplasty of vertebral artery atheromatous osteal stricture. *Neuroradiology* **27:** 259–264, 1985
8. Becker GJ: Non-coronary angioplasty. *Radiology* **170:** 921–940, 1989

9. Baker RN, Carroll RJ, Schwartz WS: Prognosis in patients with transient cerebral ischaemia attacks. *Neurology* **18:** 1157–1165, 1968
10. Hodgins GW, Dutton JW: Subclavian and carotid angioplasties for Takayasu's arteritis. *J Can Ass Radiol* **33:** 205–207, 1982
11. Vitek JJ, Raymon BC, Oh SJ: Innominate artery angioplasty. *Am J Neuroradiol* **5:** 113–114, 1984
12. Tsai FY, Matovich V, Hieschima G *et al.*: Percutaneous transluminal angioplasty of the carotid artery. *Am J Neuro Radiol* **7:** 349–358, 1986
13. De Bakey ME, Crawford ES, Cooley DA *et al.*: Cerebral arterial insufficiency. 1–11 year results following arterial reconstructive operation. *Am J Surg* **161:** 921–945, 1965

Surgical intervention for the supra-aortic vessels

MP Armon, J D Beard

INTRODUCTION

Endarterectomy of the common carotid artery, aortoinnominate bypass and subclavian–carotid artery bypass procedures were all first performed between 1950 and 1956. These operations and their variants have withstood the test of time for more than 40 years. However, endovascular procedures are now threatening to become the first-line option.[1]

The indications for intervention are well-established and apply equally to surgical and endovascular procedures. These are:

- *Subclavian steal syndrome*. During exercise, a stenosed or occluded subclavian artery 'steals' blood from the vertebral artery, distal to the occlusion. This may be seen on duplex ultrasonography or arteriography (Fig. 1), but usually only causes vertebrobasilar insufficiency (variable signs and symptoms which include: vertigo, ataxia, diplopia, visual field defects, dysphasia, dysarthria, and motor and/or sensory deficits) in the presence of concomitant occlusive lesions of the other extracranial vessels. In around 80% of cases, one or other carotid arteries or the contralateral vertebral artery is also diseased, interfering with the collateral supply to the posterior circulation. Treatment may therefore need to deal with multiple pathology and is only justified in the presence of definite disabling symptoms.
- *Upper limb ischaemia*. Brachiocephalic or subclavian occlusion rarely causes severe ischaemic symptoms due to the abundant collateral blood supply to the upper limb. However, disabling claudication, rest pain, digital ulceration or necrosis do occur in a minority of cases. Ulcerating plaques can cause digital ischaemia due to microembolization, ultimately leading to silting of the radial and ulnar arteries. Subclavian artery aneurysms often present with microembolization. Atherosclerotic degeneration is the usual cause of these and may be associated with an aberrant origin of the right subclavian artery (Kommerells' diverticulum). Aneurysms beyond the origin of the vertebral artery are usually due to post-stenotic dilatation caused by thoracic outlet compression (e.g. cervical rib). Non-traumatic common carotid aneurysms seem very rare.
- *Carotid territory symptoms*. Stenoses of the proximal common carotid and brachiocephalic arteries are potential sources of emboli, resulting in amaurosis fugax, transient ischaemic attacks and stroke. They are usually only identified during investigation of the carotid bifurcation. A combined approach to both lesions may therefore be required.

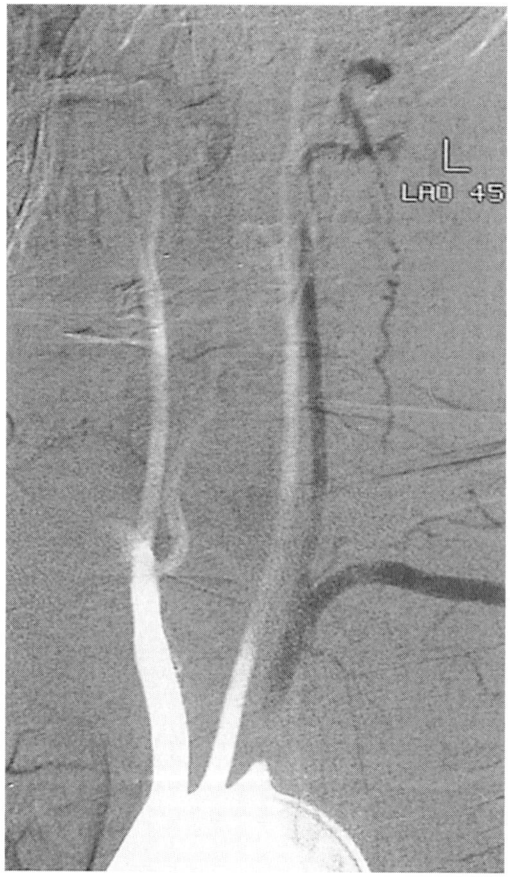

Fig. 1. Angiogram demonstrating a proximal subclavian artery occlusion and vertebral artery steal.

SUBCLAVIAN ARTERY

Subclavian artery lesions account for over 80% of great vessel surgery, with the left affected five times more commonly than the right. The majority of procedures are performed for subclavian steal syndrome. A number of procedures are available, the aims of which are:

- to restore antegrade flow to the vertebral artery,
- to remove any embolic source from the circulation,
- to restore flow to an ischaemic limb.

Extrathoracic procedures have come to be accepted as the best surgical treatment, except for proximal aneurysms (see section on brachiocephalic artery). The precise choice of procedure depends on the presence of disease in the other extracranial vessels. The most commonly used are outlined below:

Subclavian to carotid transposition

The subclavian disease must be confined to the proximal artery, terminating well short of the vertebral artery origin. The advantages of this technique are that it only requires one anastomosis, the diseased subclavian is excluded from the circulation and a bypass is avoided. The technique can also be used to avoid a thoracotomy or median sternotomy in cases of non-penetrating subclavian artery trauma.[2]

Technique

The patient is positioned with the neck hyper-extended and facing away, with the shoulder depressed to aid exposure of the subclavian artery behind the clavicle. A transverse incision is made 1–2 cm above the medial third of the clavicle, and deepened through platysma, the clavicular head of sternocleidomastoid and the inferior belly of omohyoid. The scalene fat pad is divided, as is scalenus anterior, taking care to preserve the phrenic nerve. The subclavian artery is identified deep to scalenus anterior, mobilized and controlled with silastic slings. The dissection is then continued medially to expose the proximal artery well beyond the vertebral origin and into the superior mediastinum. The vertebral artery must also be exposed over 1–2 cm to allow cranial rotation for the anastomosis.

The common carotid artery is exposed by medial retraction of the internal jugular vein and mobilized over a long length to avoid tension on the anastomosis. After heparinization, the proximal subclavian artery is divided and the proximal stump ligated with prolene sutures. An ellipse of common carotid artery is excised at the proposed anastomosis site. The subclavian artery is rotated through 90° and an end-to-side anastomosis performed with 5–0 or 6–0 prolene (Fig. 2). The distal common

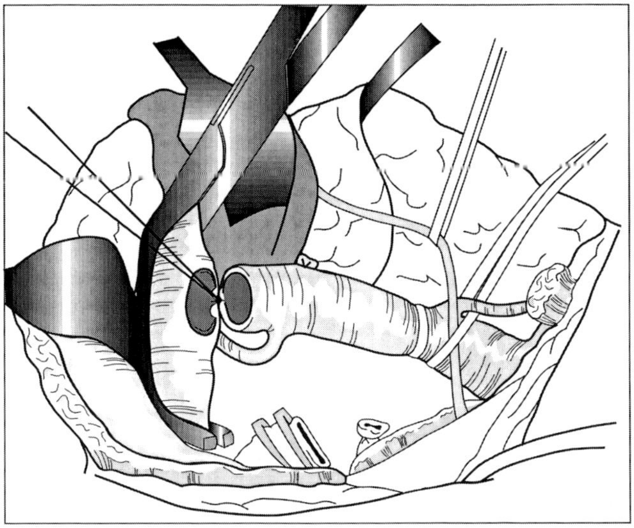

Fig. 2. Subclavian to carotid transposition.

carotid and vertebral clamps are removed last to minimize the risk of cranial embolization.

Carotid to subclavian transposition

This procedure is used for isolated proximal common carotid artery disease. The ipsilateral subclavian artery must be free of disease. The technique is virtually identical to the previously described operation, except that a longer length of common carotid artery must be mobilized (into the superior mediastinum) in order to swing it across to the proximal subclavian artery.

Carotid to subclavian bypass

This procedure can be used for either isolated proximal subclavian disease or for proximal common carotid artery disease (Fig. 3). In both scenarios, the vessel that is being used to provide inflow must itself be free of disease. If performed because of embolization, it must be combined with proximal ligation to exclude the embolic source. Vein or reinforced polytetrafluoroethylene (PTFE) may be used; PTFE is said to have a higher patency rate,[3] though a controlled comparative trial has not been performed. A Miller vein cuff can be used with any transposition or bypass to facilitate the anastomoses and reduce tension[4] (Fig. 4).

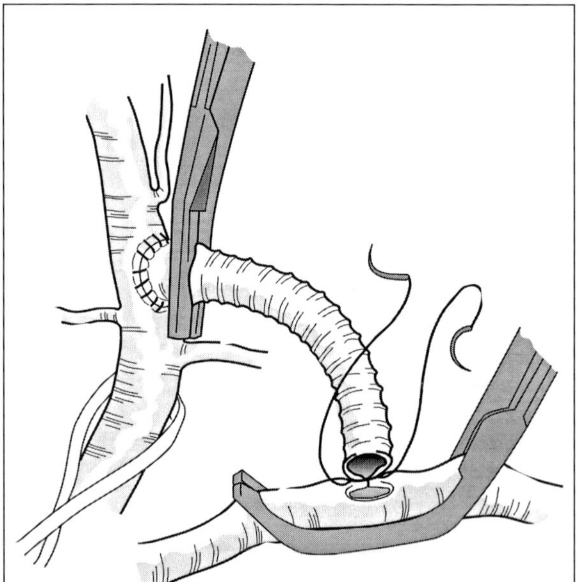

Fig. 3. Carotid to subclavian bypass using a PTFE graft.

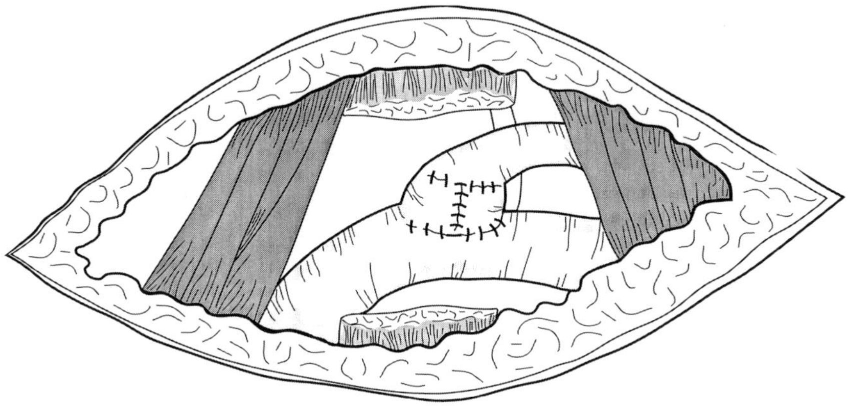

Fig. 4. A Miller vein cuff facilitating a subclavian to subclavian bypass with PTFE.

Carotid to carotid bypass

This uncommon procedure can be used for proximal common carotid disease when the ipsilateral subclavian artery is also diseased and cannot be used as a source of inflow.

Subclavian to subclavian bypass

This is an alternative approach for the patient with an isolated subclavian artery lesion in whom the proximal common carotid artery is also diseased and cannot be used as a source of inflow. However, an extra-anatomical bypass crossing the trachea or sternum can make subsequent procedures (tracheostomy, CABG, arch reconstruction) problematical.

Axillary to axillary bypass

A similar procedure to the above using a longer graft probably with a lower long-term patency rate but avoiding the deeper dissection required for subclavian exposure. In addition to the drawbacks mentioned above, it is at greater risk of skin erosion and infection.

Results

Due to the comparative rarity of these conditions, reported results are based on case series performed usually by enthusiasts in large centres. Kretschmer reported a 100% 10-year patency rate for 33 transpositions, compared with 74% for carotid–subclavian bypass in a retrospective review.[5] Criado's review of seven series endorsed the view that unilateral cervical operations produced excellent results with the transposition procedures giving the best outcome. There was no mortality or neurological complications in 112 transpositions and no late restenosis in the two largest series (accounting for 99 of the 112 patients).[6]

BRACIOCEPHALIC ARTERY

Brachiocephalic artery disease is uncommon, accounting for only 3% of all the procedures in Criado's review. The majority of patients have neurological symptoms, frequently in combination with upper limb ischaemia. Surgery involves either a direct approach (arch reconstruction, innominate endarterectomy) or an indirect, extra-anatomical procedure (subclavian–subclavian artery bypass, axillo–axillary artery bypass, carotid–carotid or carotid–subclavian artery bypass). The latter are easier to perform and can be done without a median sternotomy. However, advocates of a direct approach argue that the aorta provides a better source of inflow, particularly in the (frequent) presence of multiple vessel disease, and that median sternotomy itself has become a safe procedure with low inherent morbidity and mortality. In enthusiasts hands, the results are good with long-term relief of symptoms in 87–90% of patients. Perioperative stroke rates range from 0 to 7.6% and mortality rates from 0 to 15%.[7]

COMMON CAROTID ARTERY

Fewer than 2% of patients with carotid territory symptoms have common carotid lesions. When they do occur, the indications for surgery are identical to those for carotid bifurcation disease. Not infrequently, these lesions are identified during investigation of patients with symptomatic bifurcation stenoses. It appears impossible to determine which stenosis is the source of the symptoms and therefore both require treatment. A combined surgical–endovascular approach seems best as surgical repair would require extensive dissection and a purely endovascular approach risks cerebral embolization (Fig. 5).

Combined carotid endarterectomy and proximal stenting for multi-level disease

The carotid bifurcation is exposed as for a standard carotid endarterectomy. We prefer general anaesthesia with transcranial Doppler monitoring or awake monitoring under regional cervical blockade. Stenting of the proximal lesion can take place either before or after the carotid endarterectomy is completed. We have generally proceeded with stenting first. A test clamp is placed on the internal carotid artery and if there is no fall in middle cerebral artery velocity on transcranial Doppler or no neurological deficit, the clamp can remain in place during stenting to reduce the risk of atheroembolism. However, it is possible to proceed without a clamp via a direct common carotid artery puncture if necessary. Otherwise, a longitudinal arteriotomy is performed and following predilatation of the common carotid artery stenosis, a Palmaz stent is deployed retrogradely under fluoroscopic control. Any debris can then be flushed out through the arteriotomy. A completion angiogram is performed before proceeding to the bifurcation endarterectomy. Alternatively, the endarterectomy can be carried out first and a sheath placed into the common carotid

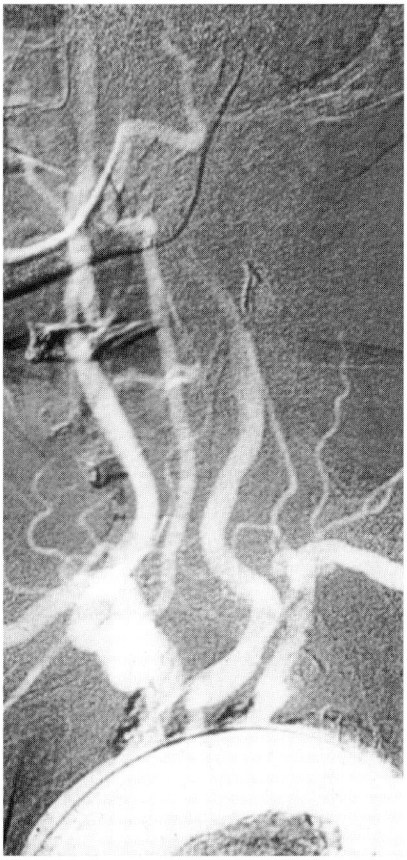

Fig. 5. Arteriogram showing combined proximal and distal carotid stenoses and marked tortuosity.

artery for stenting before placing the final sutures in the patch repair. After completion angiography and flushing the vessels, the patch is closed in the usual fashion.

This technique has been used in eight patients in Sheffield with excellent results to date. All eight had symptomatic, greater than 70% stenoses of the internal carotid artery. Seven had additional proximal common carotid artery disease and one had a brachiocephalic artery stenosis. Six patients were operated on under general anaesthetic and two under a regional cervical block. One stent was placed by direct puncture of the common carotid artery before endarterectomy, six were placed via the arteriotomy before endarterectomy, and one was placed after completion of the endarterectomy. The diameter of the stent varied from 7 to 9 mm and the length from 2 to 3 cm. There were no postoperative deaths or strokes. Two wound haematomas occurred, probably due to aggressive antiplatelet therapy and one of these required surgical drainage. One transient hypoglossal nerve palsy was also noted. No recurrence of symptoms has occurred in the follow-up period (median 20 months, range 3 to 31 months), but one patient developed a restenosis of the common carotid artery at 15 months. This patient had severe hyperlipidaemia and an abnormal common carotid artery arising from the brachiocephalic trunk.

Other authors have described similarly good results with combined angioplasty[8] and stenting.[9]

CONCLUSIONS

There seems little doubt that simple stenoses of the supra-aortic arteries are now best treated by angioplasty or stenting. The same is probably true for short occlusions, with surgery being reserved for failed endovascular treatment and longer occlusions. The traditional transfemoral approach to endovascular stenting is not ideal for these lesions. Percutaneous transfemoral arteriography combined with deployment of the stent via a brachial arteriotomy obviates these problems.[10] However, there are no prospective comparative series of endovascular versus surgical treatment. Randomized trials are unlikely to be performed because of the small numbers of such lesions.

REFERENCES

1. Harris NJ, Cameron I, Beard JD, Gaines P: Percutaneous stenting of proximal subclavian artery occlusion. *Eur J Vasc Endovasc Surg* **9:** 479–480, 1995
2. Mason PF, Beard JD: Chest and subclavian artery trauma: avoiding thoracotomy. *Eur J Vasc Surg* **7:** 90–91, 1993
3. Ziomek S, Quinones-Baldrich WJ, Busuttil RW *et al.*: The superiority of synthetic arterial grafts over autologous veins in carotid subclavian bypass. *J Vasc Surg* **3:** 140–145, 1986
4. Thompson MM, Beard JD, Bell PRF: Subclavian-to-subclavian bypass facilitated by the use of an interposition vein cuff. *Br J Surg* **78:** 630–631, 1991
5. Kretschmer G, Teleky B, Marosi L *et al.*: Obliterations of the proximal subclavian artery: to bypass or to anastomose. *J Cardiovasc Surg* **32:** 334–339, 1991
6. Criado FJ: Extrathoracic management of aortic arch syndrome. *Br J Surg* **69:** S45–S51, 1982
7. Cherry KJ: Arteriosclerotic occlusive disease of brachiocephalic arteries. In: Rutherford RB (Ed), *Vascular Surgery* pp. 935–953. London, Philadelphia: WB Saunders, 1995
8. Levien L *et al.*: Retrograde balloon angioplasty of brachiocephalic or common carotid artery stenoses at the time of carotid endarterectomy. *Eur J Vasc Endovasc Surg* **15:** 521–527, 1998
9. Queral LA, Criado FJ: The treatment of focal aortic arch branch lesions with Palmaz Stents. *J Vasc Surg* **23:** 368–375, 1996
10. Whitbread T, Cleveland TJ, Beard JD, Gaines PA: A combined approach to the treatment of proximal arterial occlusions of the upper limb with endovascular stents. *Eur J Vasc Endovasc Surg* **15:** 29–35, 1998

AORTIC ANEURYSM OPPORTUNITIES

The control of matrix metalloproteinases: a potential therapeutic option for aneurysmal disease?

Adriano M Henney

INTRODUCTION

Abdominal aortic aneurysms are a potentially fatal disorder affecting up to 9% of the population over the age of 65. With the increase in this population in the United States of America and Europe projected to be in excess of 60% between now and the year 2050, the treatment of abdominal aortic aneurysms is an escalating problem, and one which continues to present very real therapeutic challenges as we enter the new Millennium. It is well-known that, apart from their frequent appearance in the ageing population, abdominal aortic aneurysms are associated with atherosclerosis, male gender, cigarette smoking, pulmonary emphysema, and high blood pressure. It is also well-documented that the occurrence of aneurysms has a familial tendency, suggesting a genetically inherited component, although this is incompletely defined. In a nutshell, abdominal aortic aneurysm is an example of a complex trait. That is, a disease which arises from the modification by common genetic variation in a number of genes of the responses within an individual to a variety of environmental stimuli. Whatever the specific aetiology, ultimately the defect arises from inflammatory destruction of the vascular connective tissue, resulting in the irreversible degeneration of the elastic component of the aortic media. A number of studies have implicated the release of proteases by infiltrating macrophages in this process. Recent investigations have focused attention on one enzyme family in particular, the matrix metalloproteinases (MMPs), although it is far from clear that these are indeed the only culprits. More likely, matrix destruction in the aneurysmal aorta arises from a burden of proteolytic activity to which matrix metalloproteinases will contribute their own effects. This chapter will focus on MMPs, the role they play in matrix remodelling, how this is controlled naturally and what opportunities may exist for pharmacological intervention to control activity.

MATRIX REMODELLING

Extracellular matrix remodelling, involves both the synthesis and degradation of matrix components. This is a normal phenomenon associated with, for example, angiogenesis, tissue morphogenesis, growth and wound healing. This process is tightly controlled, through complex cell–cell and cell–matrix interactions involving the production of resident connective tissues, enzymes, activators, inhibitors and regulatory agents such as growth factors and cytokines.[1] Disruption of these regulatory processes is likely to contribute to a variety of pathological states. For instance, unregulated expression of matrix-degrading enzymes is partially the cause of the accelerated breakdown of extracellular matrix in arthritic disease, tumour invasion and metastasis while, on the other hand, inadequate production of these enzymes is associated with the excessive accumulation of connective tissue in systemic sclerosis.[1,2]

In the cardiovascular system, the connective tissue matrix provides blood vessels not only with structural support, but it also has multiple biological functions. For example, it is an important medium through which essential nutrients are transported across the vessel wall, and it acts as a site for the accumulation of secreted products and cell debris. It also plays a role in regulating cell migration and proliferation, and the engagement of cell-surface integrins with specific matrix components is known to influence gene expression.

Vascular matrix is predominantly composed of proteoglycans, collagen and elastin, as well as smaller amounts of fibronectin, laminin and various plasma components. These components interact to form a complex network which confers on blood vessels their elastic physical characteristics. Blood vessels are subjected to perpetual mechanical stress, and there is a need for regular remodelling to repair and replace proteins that have become worn if proper function is to be maintained. Connective tissue remodelling is, therefore, an essential physiological process associated with the maintenance of blood vessel integrity.

MATRIX REMODELLING IN VASCULAR DISEASE

The reshaping and reconstitution of the vascular connective tissue matrix is a phenomenon which underlies many vascular diseases. In atherosclerosis, the wide spectrum of plaque architecture which develops from the normal, regular patent vessel clearly involves extensive matrix remodelling.[3–5] These plaques evolve through a process of vascular reconstruction which results in the creation of a lesion in which up to 60% of the intimal volume is connective tissue. Similarly, the appearance of neointimal hyperplasia in response to injury of the vessel during angioplasty involves the deposition of new matrix as part of the repair process, occupying up to 80% of the lesion volume. Remodelling of ventricular tissue after an ischaemic event is another repair mechanism which results in the formation of scar tissue and altered ventricular function.

In the case of abdominal aortic aneurysms, the reshaping of the matrix as part of the underlying atherosclerotic process is taken a stage further, with the irreversible destruction of the aortic media associated with chronic transmural inflammation.[6] The consequent loss of medial elastin and the accompanying reduction in smooth muscle cell density are thought fundamentally to contribute to alterations in the biophysical properties of the infrarenal aorta, resulting in dilatation.

All of these examples include a number of common processes which contribute to the alterations in vascular architecture characteristic of the pathological state. For example, the infiltration of circulating monocytes into the vessel wall, the migration and proliferation of smooth muscle cells and the movement of endothelial cells during neovascularization requires that the cells traverse major extracellular barriers, including the basal lamina and a dense mesh of interstitial proteoglycans and collagen, before they can migrate and multiply. But, irrespective of the cell involved, a fundamental prerequisite for these activities is the degradation of the pericellular matrix to permit movement and/or division. Once at the site of the insult, cells will contribute to matrix remodelling either through the synthesis of new matrix components, for example by smooth muscle cells and fibroblasts, and/or degradation of existing connective tissue, principally by macrophages or neutrophils, but in some cases by mesenchymal cells too. As mentioned above, the net outcome in the vessel wall or myocardium reflects the balance struck between the concomitant synthesis and degradation of matrix components.

PROTEASES AND MATRIX REMODELLING

The key enzymes contributing to extracellular matrix turnover are endopeptidases from three major classes: the metalloproteinases, the serine proteinases and the lysosomal proteinases.[1,7,8] Matrix degradation initially takes place extracellularly. Except in special circumstances such as bone resorption, extracellular matrix degradation is thought to occur at neutral pH values, and is catalysed primarily by the metallo- and serine proteinase families, both of which have neutral pH optima.

The metallo- and serine proteinase classes are linked in an activation cascade, with the metalloproteinases being downstream of the serine proteinases.[1] In general, the serine enzymes have broader substrate specificities than the metalloproteinases which tend to be more specialized. The major serine proteinase, namely plasmin, is also responsible for the dissolution of fibrin clots, thus making a connection with another process relevant in atherosclerotic disease: fibrinolysis. Under normal conditions, the lytic potential of these enzymes is held in check by their specific activators and inhibitors.[9]

MATRIX METALLOPROTEINASES: A BRIEF OVERVIEW

The MMPs are a family of at least 20 zinc-containing endopeptidases which are structurally related, and which were originally defined by their ability to mediate the degradation of extracellular matrix macromolecules such as collagen, elastin and proteoglycans. These enzymes are generally expressed at low levels in normal adult tissue. They are upregulated during matrix remodelling not only in degenerative disease pathology, but also during normal growth and repair. All MMPs are classified as a family on the basis that: (i) they are secreted as latent zymogens requiring activation for proteolytic activity; (ii) they degrade extracellular matrix components; (iii) they function at neutral pH; (iv) they contain Zn^{2+} at their active sites and require Ca^{2+} for stability; and (v) they are inhibited by specific tissue inhibitors of metalloproteinases (TIMPs).

The MMP family was originally divided into three main subgroups, based mainly on their substrate preferences and domain structure: the interstitial collagenases, the type IV collagenases and the stromelysins. The family has expanded recently to include membrane-bound MMPs which now constitute a fourth group. Two MMPs, matrilysin (MMP-7, degrading non-fibrillar collagens) and macrophage metalloelastase (MMP-12, relatively non-specific but very active against elastin), are anomalous in that they do not appear to fit into any of the subgroups described so far. Each subgroup consists of two or more enzymes with similar substrate specificity. The collagenases (MMP-1, interstitial, MMP-8, neutrophil and MMP-13, collagenase-3) are relatively specific, mainly degrading the fibrillar interstitial collagens at a single locus within the native helical structure at about three-quarters of the distance from the N-terminus. The type IV collagenases (MMP-2 and MMP-9) are so named because they were originally described as enzymes active against type IV collagen, a major component of basement membrane. In addition they also degrade non-helical collagens and other basement membrane proteins such as fibronectin. These enzymes also have high affinity for elastin and gelatins (denatured collagen that has lost the typical triple helix), the latter suggesting a role in the further extracellular degradation of denatured collagen. The stromelysins (MMP-3 and MMP-10) degrade a broad range of substrates and are capable of activating other members of the MMP family from their latent state. Even though it is included in this grouping, stromelysin-3 (MMP-11) is not as closely related to the other two structurally and has very limited activity on matrix components, but is very active in degrading α-$_1$ antitrypsin. There are currently four membrane type MMPs (MT-MMPs, MMP-14 through MMP-17) whose substrate preferences remain to be defined. It is known that MMP-14 degrades a variety of matrix components, and both this and MMP-16 act as activators of latent MMP-2. Five new candidate MMPs (MMP-19 through MMP-23) have recently been described and their function is currently under investigation.

THE CONTROL OF MATRIX METALLOPROTEINASE ACTIVITY

The activity of MMPs is controlled at three levels: expression of the respective genes is under tight transcriptional control, the secreted latent proteins need to be activated before they can degrade matrix and, finally, active enzymes are inhibited by specific tissue inhibitors (TIMPs) or non-specific inhibitors such as α_2-macroglobulin (Fig. 1).

As connective tissue turnover in healthy adult tissues is normally very low, MMP expression will also be low. However, substantial evidence now exists to indicate that both MMPs and their inhibitors are inducible through the action of cytokines (e.g. IL-1, IL-6), growth factors (e.g. PDGF, TGFβ, FGF) and hormones (retinoids and glucocorticoids) operating at the transcriptional level.[1,7,8] This is the mechanism through which cells will respond to signals inducing synthesis during growth and repair, as well as those associated with complex inflammatory and other disease associated pathways. Genetic studies have shown that common variation in the promoters of MMPs does affect the transcription of these genes.[10,11] In tissues, this may cause inter-individual differences in levels of expression which, at a local cellular level, may affect the extent to which the pericellular matrix is remodelled and may thus have an impact on disease progression.[11,12]

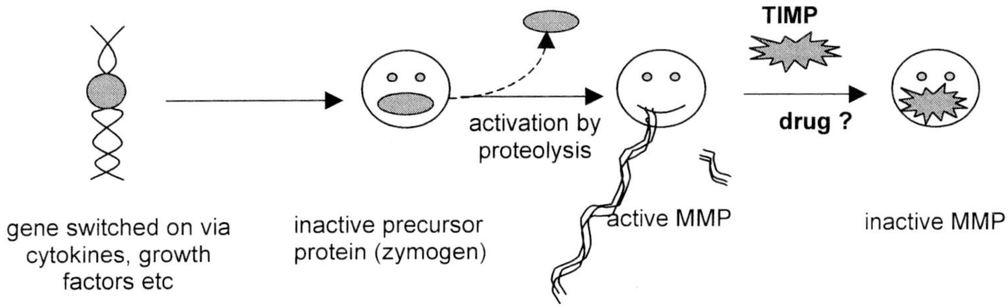

Fig. 1. Control of matrix metalloproteinases.

The majority of MMPs are secreted as inactive zymogens which are subsequently activated in the pericellular and extracellular environment. Although the precise mechanism for MMP activation *in vivo* has been the subject of debate for a number of years, plasmin has been implicated as the principal physiological activator of MMPs. This view has been strengthened recently by elegant experiments using gene knockout technology targeting the plasminogen activation system.[13] The involvement of plasmin as an activator offers a further, more complex level of regulation, in that activation of plasmin itself is the subject of a complex cascade. Again through the use of knockout technology, it appears that the latent MMP activation mechanism is mediated by urokinase bound to its receptor, rather than tissue plaminogen activator. This effectively focuses activation close to the cell surface and may limit the extent to which active enzymes are present in the wider matrix.

One member of the family, MMP-2, is not activated by plasmin, but, as mentioned above, it has been shown that it can be activated on the cell surface through the assembly of a ternary complex consisting of the zymogen, TIMP-2 and MMP-14. It is unclear whether other MMPs are activated at the surface of the cell by similar, MT-MMP-dependent mechanisms.

Once secreted, the activity of the MMPs is counteracted by the presence of their specific natural inhibitors, TIMPs. In addition, the potent destructive potential of these enzymes is held further in check by non-specific protease inhibitors such as α_2-macroglobulin. Whilst TIMPs require no further post-translational processing to exhibit their activity, they appear in many cases to be co-regulated with MMPs at the transcriptional level. To date, four TIMPs have been identified, which are encoded by four separate genes: TIMPs 1, 2 and 4 are secreted in a soluble form, whilst TIMP-3 is found bound to the extracellular matrix. With the exception of TIMP-4 which is more selective, the remainder of the TIMPs act effectively against all MMPs by forming inhibited, non-covalent, 1:1 stoichiometric complexes with MMPs and blocking access to their substrate. It has been suggested that gelatinases A and B can form complexes with TIMPs in their zymogen forms as well as active forms, whereas collagenase-type and stromelysin-type MMPs only form complexes after exposure of the active site.

MATRIX METALLOPROTEINASES AND VASCULAR DISEASE

Since the first demonstration of MMP expression in atherosclerotic lesions some 10 years ago, interest in this enzyme family and its role in the mechanisms underlying cardiovascular disease has expanded considerably.[4,14]

Initial work with MMPs in atherosclerosis was prompted by the knowledge that plaque disruption frequently occurs in the 'shoulder' regions where there is significant macrophage accumulation.[15] As macrophages produce a number of proteases capable of degrading matrix, including MMPs, it was reasoned that their presence in large numbers may contribute to excess degradation and consequent destabilization of the supporting connective tissue matrix, weakening the plaque and leading to lesion disruption. Analysis of human coronary artery sections by *in situ* hybridization identified stromelysin-1 (MMP-3) transcripts in atherosclerotic lesions.[16] Extensive expression of the stromelysin-1 gene was localized to large clusters of macrophages that contained intracellular lipid deposits, particularly in the regions considered prone to rupture, such as the plaque shoulders. These observations were supported and extended subsequently by other investigators.[17–21] Using immunocytochemistry, it was shown that non-atherosclerotic arteries contained ubiquitous immunoreactive MMP-2, TIMP-1 and TIMP-2, which were localized to smooth muscle cells in all layers of the arteries. These lesion-free arteries stained only weakly or not at all for three other MMPs: MMP-1, MMP-3 and MMP-9. In contrast to the normal arteries, atheromata stained for all MMPs and TIMPs tested. Increased immunoreactivity of MMP-1, MMP-3 and MMP-9 co-localized with macrophages, smooth muscle cells, lymphocytes and endothelium, particularly in the fibrous cap, the shoulders of the lesions, and the base of the lesions' lipid core. Due to the presence of natural inhibitors and as all MMPs are secreted as zymogens requiring activation, an increase in MMP immunoreactivity does not necessarily equate to raised enzymatic activity. For this reason, Galis and colleagues used a modified *in situ* zymography technique to investigate whether atherosclerotic plaques contained activated MMPs.[17,18] This method detected and localized MMP activity microscopically in tissue sections, showing both gelatinolytic and caseinolytic activity in regions of plaques where there was increased expression of immunoreactive interstitial MMP-1, MMP-3 and MMP-9. In contrast to the affected areas, non-atherosclerotic arteries and uninvolved regions of atherosclerotic specimens did not exhibit enzymatic activity determined by this method.

As described earlier in this article, extensive vascular connective tissue remodelling is fundamental to the development, progression and subsequent rupture of abdominal aortic aneurysms. Not surprisingly, much of the blame for the destructive tissue pathology is laid at the door of proteolytic enzymes. In recent years the MMPs have gained particular favour over other enzyme classes in this context, probably because of their specialized involvement in connective tissue metabolism. However, to exclude other classes at this stage would be premature, as there is no clear evidence favouring a particular culprit, if indeed there is only one. For example, very recent data on cystatin C implicates a role for cysteine proteases in abdominal aortic aneurysms, adding further to the complexity of aneurysmal disease.[22]

Focusing attention here on the MMPs, there are four members of the family which have the capacity to attack the vascular matrix components which are most severely affected in abdominal aortic aneurysms. Those able to degrade mature elastin under physiological conditions, as it is laid down in the vessel wall, are the two gelatinases MMP-2 and MMP-9, and the two unclassified enzymes (see above) MMP-7 and MMP-12. Of these, MMP-2 and MMP-9 have been shown often to be the most abundant both in explant organ culture experiments and by assessment of expression in human abdominal aortic aneurysms tissues. However, the picture describing cause and effect in abdominal aortic aneurysms is anything but clear. For example MMP-9 expression has been shown to be elevated in abdominal aortic aneurysms and also in aorto-occlusive disease, in some cases showing no differences between the two at the RNA level, whilst others using enzyme-linked immunosorbent assay (ELISA) suggested 10-fold and 6-fold increases respectively.[23,24] Additionally, a relationship has been described between MMP-9 RNA levels in diseased tissues and aortic diameter by computed tomographic scan.[25] Here it was observed that MMP-9 expression was significantly higher in moderate diameter (5–6.9cm), but not small (<4 cm) or large (>7 cm) aneurysms, so how is this phenomenon explained? The suggestion was that MMP-9 contributed to the propensity to expansion of moderate aneurysms, whereas other mechanisms, including wall stress, affected the rapid expansion and high rupture rates characteristic of large aneurysms.

Many of these reports are descriptive, taking snap shots of expression patterns in the end-stage of a chronic progressive disease. However, as stated elsewhere in this article, evidence supporting elevated expression of specific enzymes in diseased tissues reflects only the *potential* for increased activity in the tissue. As TIMP expression is also elevated in abdominal aortic aneurysms and as these inhibitors are abundant in aortic tissue, it will be the balance between these proteins and the amount of active enzyme that will dictate the net burden of MMP-mediated matrix degradation. This was investigated in a study comparing abdominal aortic aneurysm and aorto-occlusive disease, using *in situ* zymography.[26] Here it was confirmed that MMP expression was elevated in diseased aortas and that this translated into the appearance of active enzyme. No difference could be shown between the proteolytic patterns seen in abdominal aortic aneurysms and aorto-occlusive disease, from which the authors concluded that MMP imbalance was questionable as a primary cause of aneurysm formation versus occlusive disease. Thus, even though the enzymes are present in the diseased tissue, precisely how they contribute to the course of disease remains unclear.

New information has emerged in the last year from experiments using targeted inactivation of a variety of genes in mouse models of atherosclerosis, which may help us to unravel the complexities of the protease cascades which operate in the pathogenesis of abdominal aortic aneurysms. An elegant series of experiments studied mice deficient in apolipoprotein E (ApoE) alone or in combination with a deficiency in t-PA or of u-PA. Analysing the atherosclerotic aorta in these animals indicated that loss of u-PA activity protected them from medial destruction and aneurysm formation.[13] The suggestion was that this probably arose from a reduced plasmin-dependent activation of latent MMPs. Subsequent studies by this group and others have shown that MMP-12 may be a key enzyme in the macrophage-mediated proteolysis of the aorta.

Despite the amount of evidence implicating MMPs in the pathogenesis of cardiovascular and other diseases, much of this is 'guilt by association'. Very little offers a direct causal relationship, for example through the description of defects in MMP/TIMP genes and resulting disease phenotypes. This is perhaps surprising, given the tight, complex control of enzyme activity and the consequent opportunity for deficiencies in the cascade to cause an imbalance between synthesis and degradation of matrix. As an analogy, the clotting cascade is similarly complex, but in contrast it is littered with genetic defects affecting function. The discovery of mutations in the TIMP-3 gene in patients with the ocular condition Sorsby's fundus dystrophy was the first evidence linking a rare mutation in an MMP/TIMP gene to a disease caused by defective connective tissue remodelling.[27] We have speculated for some time that common genetic variants, which disrupt or modulate the cascade controlling MMP activity, may contribute to the pathogenesis of multifactorial diseases in which deficiencies in connective tissue remodelling is a feature. The TIMP-3 paper provided a 'proof of principle', albeit in a rare disorder rather than a common complex trait, that correct maintenance of the balance between active enzyme and inhibitor is critical to preserving the function of the extracellular matrix.

In the last 10 years, there has been an explosion of interest in the use of molecular genetic tools to study the impact of small effects of a variety of genes in multifactorial diseases, as opposed to large effects of single genes in rare disorders. Our own studies have focused on MMPs and atherosclerosis and provide further evidence in support of MMPs as important candidates in atherogenesis. Initially working with MMP-3, we described a common genetic variant in the promoter which affected transcription of the gene *in vitro* and which was associated with the progression of atherosclerosis.[10,12] Similar studies published very recently on MMP-9 described a number of variants both in the promoter and the coding region, some of which have a functional impact *in vitro*.[11] Again, associations with disease endpoints were described, and we also observed a trend between variation in the gene and circulating MMP-9 levels. Similar data emerging from studies on MMP-12 have been reported in abstract form and are due to be published in the near future. These studies suggest that other common genetic variants may exist in this family which *modify*, rather than drastically disrupt, the function of the proteins, and which may be important in determining the extent to which connective tissue is remodelled to establish and progress complex cardiovascular disease traits. In this way, subtle differences in the control of activity between individuals could contribute to variation not only in disease progression but also to the response to environmental challenge in its broadest sense.

Whilst it is well-known that abdominal aortic aneurysm has a familial tendency, suggesting a genetic component, specific gene defects have not been described. Genetic approaches, similar to those described above, using appropriately powered case-control studies may offer new insight into the pathogenesis of abdominal aortic aneurysms.

INHIBITION OF PROTEASE ACTIVITY IN VASCULAR DISEASE: AN OPPORTUNITY?

For a long time, MMPs have been considered tempting pharmacological targets, and substantial work has been done in pursuit of small molecule inhibitors for use in particular in the treatment of cancer and arthritis. A recent review documents the information currently available on aspects of the medicinal chemistry of the various classes of MMP inhibitors which have been tested, and also covers questions related to the feasibility of selective inhibition of specific members of the MMP family.[28]

Evidence does exist in the literature to suggest that blocking MMP activity will have a beneficial effect on aneurysm formation. Vascular overexpression of TIMP-1, or dosing with doxycyline or various hydroxamate-based inhibitors, such as British Biotech's BB94, reduced or abolished the progression of aneurysms in experimental models in rodents.[29–32] Interestingly, similar studies in ApoE-deficient mouse models of atherosclerosis also showed reduced lesion progression, reinforcing the role of MMPs in those models of atherosclerosis.[33]

Thus, it would appear that it is feasible to mount an MMP inhibitor drug discovery programme to find something suitable to use in abdominal aortic aneurysms. The questions we have to face in considering the development of such a compound are not trivial, whether it is for abdominal aortic aneurysms, another cardiovascular indication or, for that matter, any chronic disease. For example:

- *What other activities are MMPs involved in which inhibition would affect?* We know that these enzymes are critical to a range of normal physiological processes. How many of these are likely to cause problems if the drug is given for prolonged periods in an elderly population?
- *How would the drug be best administered and to whom?* Ideally the plan would be to find a drug with a profile suitable for once-daily oral dosing, but this is not always possible. Under these circumstances would alternative dosing schedules or parenteral administration be acceptable and/or attractive to this patient group? Given an effective drug, how would this be targeted? Would the only option be to offer it to an 'at risk' group with slightly enlarged aortic diameter, or are there alternatives?
- *What hurdles would we encounter in clinical development of drugs?* How would we go about designing a proof of concept study to evaluate the potential for this approach in man as opposed to animal models? If this proved encouraging, how would we design a dose-ranging trial, and what would be the end-points we could measure over how long to see an effect? As with all clinical trials, this information would be needed to assess the feasibility and cost of the development, and this would need to be considered alongside the commercial estimates of the market potential.

These questions are not intended to deter or diminish interest, but more to act as a stimulus for discussion in considering the best way to overcome the hurdles in pursuit of MMP inhibition as a therapeutic option.

CONCLUSION

Substantial evidence is available indicating that MMPs are major players in the remodelling of vascular connective tissue in cardiovascular diseases. The precise contribution made by individual members of the family to the pathophysiology remains unclear, but emerging technologies, in particular in genetics, may offer the possibility of unravelling the complexities of these processes and point the way to the best therapeutic targets. The available evidence suggests that inhibition of MMP activity may indeed be an option for the treatment of abdominal aortic aneurysms. But although this includes the use of synthetic 'drug-like' compounds, the evidence is based mainly on animal models, which may or may not be appropriate or accurate parallels to the human disease. The only real way to evaluate the potential of this approach will be to take a safe and potent inhibitor into a human proof of concept study, the design of which is likely to be difficult, but perhaps not impossible.

ACKNOWLEDGEMENT

Work on the molecular genetics of MMPs in the author's former laboratory was generously funded by the British Heart Foundation.

REFERENCES

1. Murphy G, Reynolds J: Extracellular matrix degradation. In: Royce PM, Steinman B (Eds), *Connective Tissue and its Heritable Disorders*, pp. 287–316. New York: Wiley-Liss Inc., 1993
2. Birkedal-Hansen H, Moore WGI, Bodden MK *et al.*: Matrix metalloproteinases: a review. *Crit Rev Oral Biol Med* **4:** 197–250, 1993
3. Stary HC, Blankenhorn DH, Chandler B *et al.*: A definition of the intima of human arteries and of its atherosclerosis-prone regions. *Arterioscler Thromb* **12:** 120–134, 1992
4. Libby P: Molecular bases of the acute coronary syndromes. *Circulation* **91:** 2844–2850, 1995
5. Davies MJ: Stability and Instability: two faces of coronary atherosclerosis. The Paul Dudley White Lecture 1995. *Circulation* **94:** 2013–2020, 1996
6. Halloran BG, Baxter BT: Pathogenesis of aneurysms. *Semin Vasc Surg* **8:** 85–92, 1995
7. Matrisian LM, Hogan BLM: Growth factor-regulated proteases and extracellular matrix remodelling during mammalian development. *Curr Topics Development Biol* **24:** 219–259, 1990
8. Alexander Werb Z: Extracellular matrix degradation. In: Hay ED (Ed), *Cell Biology of Extracellular Matrix* 2nd edn, pp. 255–302. New York: Plenum Press, 1991
9. Birkedal-Hansen H: Proteolytic remodelling of extracellular matrix. *Curr Opin Cell Biol* **7:** 728–735, 1995
10. Ye S, Eriksson P, Hamsten A. *et al.*: Progression of coronary atherosclerosis is associated with a common genetic variant of the human stromelysin-1 promoter which results in reduced gene expression. *J Biol Chem* **271:** 13055–13060, 1996
11. Zhang BP, Ye S, Hermann SM *et al.*: Functional polymorphism in the regulatory region of the gelatinase B gene in relation to severity of coronary atherosclerosis. *Circulation* **99:** 1788–1794, 1999
12. Ye S, Watts GF, Mandalia S: Genetic variation in the human stromelysin promoter is associated with progression of coronary atherosclerosis. *Br Heart J* **73:** 209–215, 1995

13. Carmeliet PL, Moons R, Lijnen M *et al.*: Urokinase-generated plasmin activates matrix metalloproteinases during aneurysm formation. *Nature Genet* **17:** 439–444, 1997
14. Dollery CM, McEwan JR, Henney AM: Matrix metalloproteinases and cardiovascular disease. *Circulat Res* **77:** 863–868, 1995
15. Richardson PD, Davies MJ, Born GVR: Influence of plaque configuration and stress distribution of fissuring of coronary atherosclerotic plaques. *Lancet* **ii:** 941–944, 1989
16. Henney AM, Wakeley PR, Davies MJ *et al.*: Localization of stromelysin gene expression in atherosclerotic plaques by *in situ* hybridization. *Proc Nat Acad Sci USA* **88:** 8154–8158, 1991
17. Galis ZS, Sukhova GK, Lark MW, Libby P: Increased expression of matrix metalloproteinases and matrix degrading activity in vulnerable regions of human atherosclerotic plaques. *J Clin Invest* **94:** 2493–2503, 1994
18. Galis ZS, Muszynski M, Sukhova GK *et al.*: Enhanced expression of vascular matrix metalloproteinases induced *in vitro* by cytokines and in regions of human atherosclerotic lesions. *Ann N Y Acad Sci* **748:** 501–507, 1995
19. Galis ZS, Sukhova GK, Kranzhofer R, *et al.*: Macrophage foam cells from experimental atheroma constitutively produce matrix-degrading proteinase. *Proc Nat Acad Sci USA* **92:** 402–406, 1995
20. Brown DL, Hibbs MS, Kearney M *et al.*: Identification of 92-kD gelatinase in human coronary atherosclerotic lesions. Association of active enzyme synthesis with unstable angina. *Circulation* **91:** 2125–2131, 1995
21. Nikkari ST, O'Brien KD, Furguson M, *et al.*: Interstitial collagenase (MMP-1) expression in human carotid atherosclerosis. *Circulation* **92:** 1393–1398, 1995
22. Shi G-P, Sukhova GK, Grubb A. *et al.*: Cystatin C deficiency in human atherosclerosis and aortic aneurysms. *J Clin Invest* **104:** 1191–1197, 1999
23. McMillan WD, Patterson BK, Keen RR *et al.*: In situ localisation and quantification of mRNA for 92 kD type-IV collagenase and its inhibitor in aneurysmal, occlusive and normal aorta. *Arterioscer Thromb Vasc Biol* **15:** 1139–1144, 1995
24. Thompson RW, Holmes DR, Mertens RA *et al.*: Production and localisation of 92-kilodalton gelatinase in abdominal aortic aneurysms. *J Clin Invest* **96:** 318–326, 1995
25. McMillan WD, Tamarina NA, Cipollone M *et al.*: Size matters: The relationship between MMP-9 expression and aortic diameter. *Circulation* **96:** 2228–2232, 1997
26. Knox JB, Sukhova GK, Whittemore AD, *et al.*: Evidence for altered balance between matrix metalloproteinases and their inhibitors in human aortic diseases. *Circulation* **95:** 205–212, 1997
27. Weber BH, Vogt G, Pruett RC *et al.*: Mutation in the tissue inhibitor of metalloproteinases-3 (TIMP3) in patients with Sorsby's fundus dystrophy. *Nature Genet* **8:** 352–356, 1994
28. Whittaker M, Floyd CD, Brown P *et al.*: Design and therapeutic application of matrix metalloproteinase inhibitors. *Chem Rev* **99:** 2735–2776, 1999
29. Allaire E, Forough R, Clowes M *et al.*: Local over-expression of TIMP-1 prevents aortic aneurysm degeneration and rupture in a rat model. *J Clin Invest* **102:** 1413–1420, 1998
30. Curci JA, Petrinec D, Liao S *et al.*: Pharmacologic suppression of experimental abdominal aortic aneurysms. a comparison of doxycycline and four chemically modified tetracyclines. *J Vasc Surg* **28:** 1082–1083, 1998
31. Bigatel DA: The matrix metalloproteinase inhibitor BB-94 limits expansion of experimental abdominal aortic aneurysms. *J Vasc Surg* **29:** 130–138, 1999
32. Moore G *et al.*: Suppression of experimental abdominal aortic aneurysms by systemic treatment with a hydroxamate-based matrix metalloproteinase inhibitor (RS 132908). *J Vasc Surg* **29:** 522–532, 1999
33. Rouis M, Adamy C, Duverger N *et al.*: Adenovirus-mediated over-expression of tissue inhibitor of metallopro-teinase-1 reduces atherosclerotic lesions in apolipoprotein E-deficient mice. *Circulation* **100:** 533–540, 1999

Non-steroidal anti-inflammatory drugs and abdominal aortic aneurysms

Ian J Franklin, Lesley Walton, Trevor Bayston, Louise C Brown, Roger M Greenhalgh, Janet T Powell

INTRODUCTION

Three crucial pathophysiological features seem to be central to the formation of abdominal aortic aneurysms. These are inflammation, excessive proteolysis with loss of elastic tissue and loss of vascular smooth muscle. The result is a thickening but weakening of the aortic wall, which dilates under the haemodynamic load until rupture occurs. The triggers that start the whole process are far from clear, and there is uncertainty of a chicken and egg nature over which of the three critical processes drives the others. However, evidence is accumulating, and it is indeed plausible, that chronic inflammation in the aneurysm wall promotes excessive destruction of elastin and collagen. Associated with this is the characteristic loss of vascular smooth muscle. A better understanding of these events is allowing the development of drug therapies to limit aneurysm growth. One approach is to depress excessive matrix metalloproteinase (MMP) activity with selective inhibitors, thus preventing elastin and collagen destruction. An alternative approach is to dampen the chronic inflammatory processes in the aneurysm wall. If the hypothesis is correct, that an unknown trigger precipitates a chronic inflammatory response which results in excessive connective tissue destruction leading to arterial dilatation, then reducing the inflammatory drive should result in a slower rate of expansion. This chapter examines the evidence to support this strategy, focusing on non-steroidal anti-inflammatory drugs as agents to limit aneurysm growth.

INFLAMMATION IN THE ANEURYSM WALL

Two kinds of aortic aneurysm are readily recognizable at operation; 'ordinary' or 'atherosclerotic' aneurysms and the so-called 'inflammatory' aneurysm. Inflammatory aneurysms are characterized by a thick, white wall densely adherent to surrounding structures and surgical reconstruction is technically much more demanding. However, the majority of aneurysms are of the 'ordinary' variety, considered until relatively recently to be a complication of atherosclerosis and referred to as atherosclerotic aneurysms.

The clear distinction observed macroscopically between inflammatory and ordinary aneurysms is not apparent under the microscope. Histological analysis

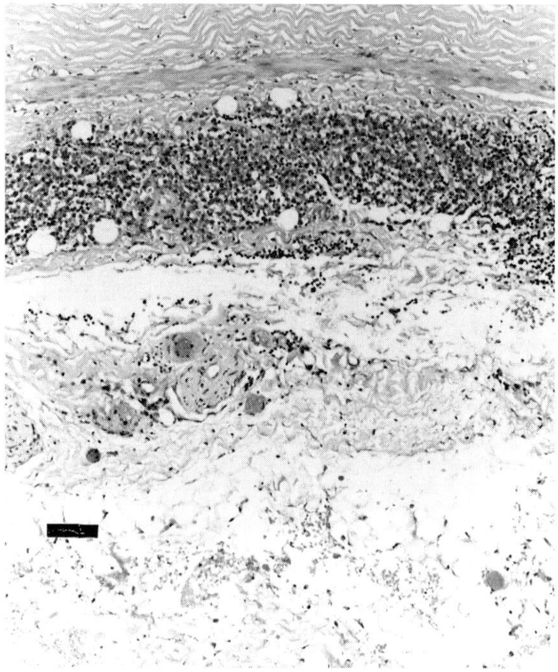

(a)

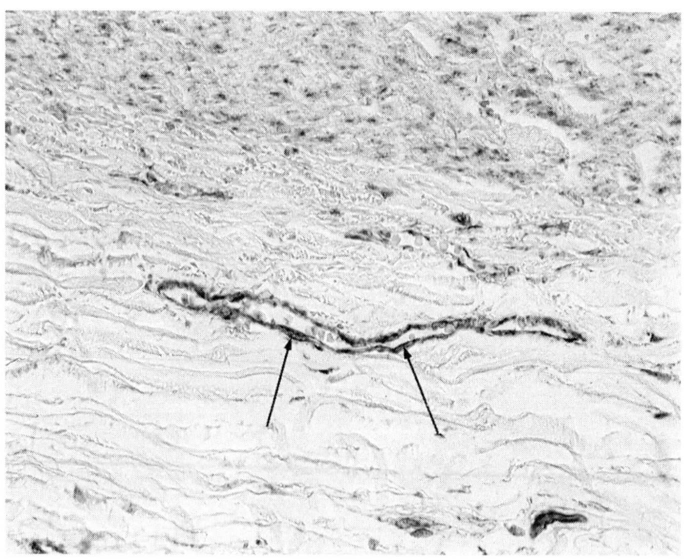

(b)

Fig. 1. (a) Section through an abdominal aortic aneurysm, showing the striking number of inflammatory cells present in the adventitia and at the adventitia/medial junction. At the top acellular, collagen-rich media can be seen. The scale bar shows 100μm. (b) Endothelial cells (arrowed) of the vasa vasorum in the adventitia stain positively for the cytokine TNF-α, a characteristic of activated endothelium.

reveals that over 80% of aneurysm walls exhibit features of inflammation, but the degree of inflammation is highly variable.[1] Heavily inflamed aneurysms are more likely to be symptomatic[2] and there is a positive correlation between degree of inflammation and aneurysm diameter.[3]

The nature of the inflammatory infiltrate seen in aortic aneurysms is different from that seen in stenosing atherosclerotic disease.[4] The appearances are those of a chronic inflammatory response with a high proportion of lymphocytes and macrophages but few neutrophils. In contrast to stenosing atherosclerotic disease, in aneurysms the infiltrate is concentrated in the outer layers of the vessel wall, in the adventitia and media (Fig. 1a). The infiltrate frequently surrounds vasa vasorum, which are increased in number. These vasa vasorum have the characteristics of activated endothelium, secreting the inflammatory cytokines tumour necrosis factor alpha (TNF-α) and monocyte chemoattractant protein-1 (MCP-1) (Fig. 1b).

Many studies have confirmed high levels of cytokine production in the aneurysm wall. TNF-α, IL-1β, IL-6, IL-8, MCP-1 and IFN-γ have all been detected in elevated amounts compared with occlusive or normal aorta.[5–7] These cytokines have multiple actions including attraction and activation of monocytes and potentiation and perpetuation of the inflammatory response.[8] In particular, they have the ability to promote production of proteolytic enzymes by macrophages,[9] increase the degradation of collagen and other components of the extracellular matrix and to induce apoptosis in vascular smooth muscle,[10] processes strongly implicated in aneurysm development.

THE SIGNIFICANCE OF PROSTAGLANDIN E2 IN ANEURYSM DEVELOPMENT

Of all the inflammatory mediators present in aneurysm wall, prostaglandin E2 (PGE2) is emerging as among the most significant. Aneurysm biopsies in explant culture produce very large quantities of PGE2 compared with normal aorta, which produces very little.[11] PGE2 is synthesized by cyclo-oxygenase (COX) of which there are two isoenzymes, COX1 and COX2. COX1 is constitutively expressed in a large number of healthy tissues including gastric mucosa and vascular endothelium. COX2 expression is low in normal tissues but appears in response to inflammatory stimuli (Fig. 2). Neither COX1 or COX2 is detectable in normal aorta but COX2 has been localized by immunohistochemistry and *in situ* hybridization to macrophages in the inflammatory infiltrate in abdominal aortic aneurysm wall.[11] Since the action of MMPs has been shown to be PGE2-dependent,[12] these findings raise the possibility that PGE2 is an important mediator of aneurysm formation and that its synthesis results from COX2 expression in adventitial macrophages and other cells.

THE EFFECT OF PROSTAGLANDIN E2 ON AORTIC SMOOTH MUSCLE

In the normal aorta, the predominant cell type is the vascular smooth muscle cell, arranged in concentric elastic lamellae in the tunica media. The smooth muscle cells contribute both to the tone of the vessel wall and synthesize the bulk of the matrix

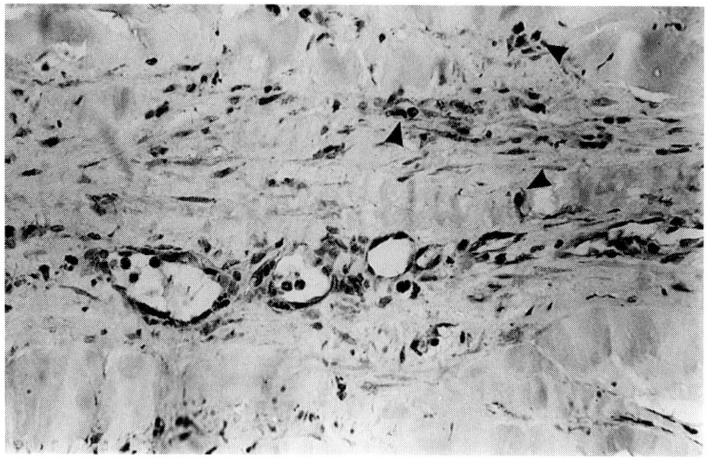

Fig. 2. Macrophages (arrowed) and vasa vasorum in the aneurysm wall stain strongly for cyclo-oxygenase 2.

proteins and are therefore important in maintaining structural integrity. In addition, smooth muscle cells influence extracellular matrix turnover by expression of MMPs and MMP inhibitors. In the aneurysm wall therefore there is an apparent conflict between synthesis of connective tissue proteins by aortic smooth muscle cells, and matrix degradation by infiltrating inflammatory cells. This suggests that smooth muscle cell function might be a pivotal factor in the formation of aortic aneurysms. Any diminution in smooth muscle cell numbers would deplete a population of cells capable of maintaining vessel tone and synthesizing components of the extracellular matrix and could contribute a to weakening and dilatation of the aorta.

A consistent and striking histological feature of abdominal aortic aneurysm is the marked reduction in the number of smooth muscle cells in the media of aortic aneurysms relative to normal and atherosclerotic aortas. The decrease in the smooth muscle cell population of aneurysm wall coincides with chemical and ultrastructural evidence of smooth muscle cell apoptosis.[13]

Intact smooth muscle cells remaining within the aneurysm wall display loss of cell volume, cytoplasmic contracture , dissolution of cytoskeletal actin fragments and distortion of intracellular organelles. The nuclei show clumping and fragmentation of chromatin, changes consistent with apoptosis. Physiological cell death is frequently characterized by fragmentation of genomic DNA producing the so-called DNA laddering seen on gel electrophoresis. *In situ* end-labelling, a technique used to localize fragmented DNA, has shown that such DNA is not present in normal aorta and is confined to intimal atherosclerotic plaque in atherosclerotic occlusive disease. In contrast, large numbers of vascular smooth muscle cells in aneurysm wall contain fragmented DNA in the nuclei, providing further evidence for vascular smooth muscle cell apoptosis in aortic aneurysms.

These morphological and histochemical findings are supported by molecular studies. The protein p53 has been implicated in the induction of physiological cell death in a range of tissues including vascular smooth muscle cells[14] and is used as a marker for apoptosis. Using a combination of immunohistochemistry and reverse transcriptase polymerase chain reaction, p53 and p53 mRNA was localized to the cytoplasm and nuclei of smooth muscle cells and detected in greater quantities in aneurysm tissue (by nearly 4-fold) compared with normal and atherosclerotic occlusive aorta.[15]

These findings taken together suggest that the smooth muscle cell population in aortic aneurysms is depleted by apoptosis and that this process may occur, at least in part, through mechanisms involving increased expression of p53. The stimuli leading to induction of physiological cell death remain to be defined though a number of different mechanisms have been proposed.

High concentrations of oxidants produced by atheroma[10] and hypoxia due to occluded vasa vasorum[16] have both been proposed as mechanisms which might deplete smooth muscle cell population in aneurysm wall. The chronic inflammation seen in the media and adventitia of aneurysms may have deleterious effects on smooth muscle cells. Many of the cytokines produced by inflammatory cells, for example IL-1β, TNF-α and IFN-γ, are known to induce apoptosis in vascular smooth muscle cells *in vitro*,[17] and these mediators are present in high concentrations in aneurysmal wall.

Aortic tissue cultured in the laboratory shows outgrowth and proliferation of aortic smooth muscle; smooth muscle cell cultures are derived from such techniques. A key observation was that cultures containing large numbers of mononuclear cells

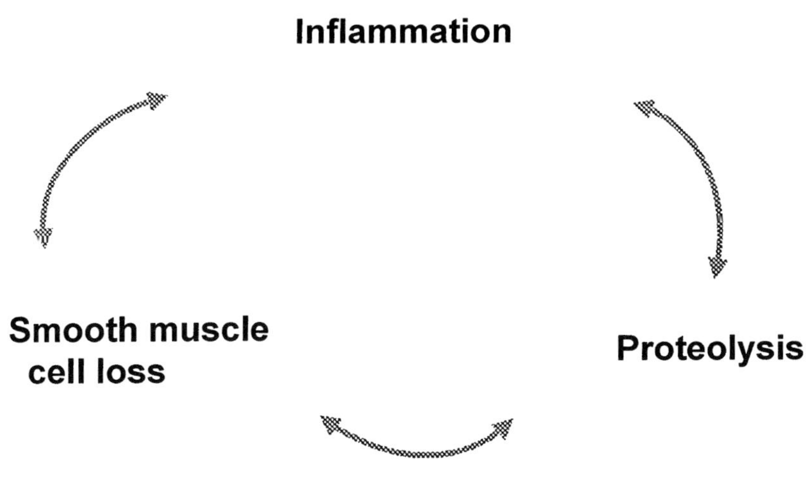

Fig. 3. The three corner stones of aneurysm pathogenesis. All aortic aneurysms to a varying degree exhibit features of chronic inflammation, excessive proteolysis and depletion of aortic smooth muscle. The primary stimulus triggering the dilating process is unclear but attempting to modify these key processes with drugs is a logical approach to limit aneurysm growth.

appeared to show poorer growth of smooth muscle cells than biopsies containing fewer inflammatory cells. This lead to the hypothesis that macrophages were producing a compound that was depressing the population of aortic smooth muscle. Further studies were directed by the observation that the toxic effects of a compound to reduce smooth muscle cell proliferation could be abolished when indomethacin was added to the cultures: a range of other drugs including those inhibiting nitric oxide synthase were ineffective.[18] This suggested that the toxic compound was a prostanoid or prostanoid metabolite. The number of smooth muscle cells present in aortic wall depends on the balance between the rates of proliferation and cell death. We sought to characterize the prostanoid metabolite capable of inhibiting aortic smooth muscle cell proliferation.

High-performance liquid chromatography of conditioned media from abdominal aortic aneurysm explant cultures demonstrated that the compound was indeed a prostanoid metabolite, and co-eluted with PGE2.[18] When macrophages were isolated from the aneurysm wall they secreted large amounts of PGE2 and macrophages in the aneurysm wall stained strongly for cyclo-oxygenase 2. Therefore, the principal cellular source of the PGE2 in the aneurysm wall appeared to be macrophages.

These observations prompted a detailed study in our laboratory of the effect of PGE2 on the rate of growth of aortic smooth muscle cells. Smooth muscle cell cultures isolated from normal and aneurysmal aortas were incubated in the presence of different concentrations of PGE2. The rates of proliferation were assessed by measuring uptake of bromodeoxyuridine, a reflection of DNA synthesis. Cell death rates were measured by oligonucleosome assay, a measure of apoptosis.

The results were clear-cut and striking. PGE2 caused a concentration dependent inhibition of the rate of proliferation of smooth muscle cells isolated from both normal and aneurysmal aortas (Fig. 4). The IC50 was in the region of 23 ng/ml for

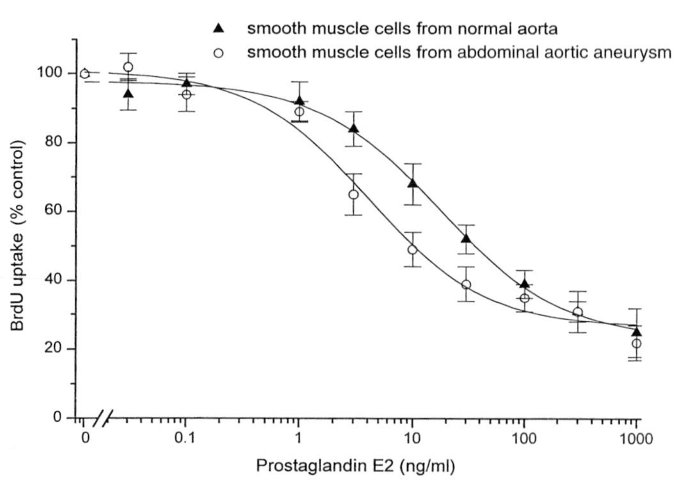

Fig. 4. Prostaglandin E2 inhibits DNA synthesis in cultured aortic smooth muscle cells.

cells derived form normal aorta and 6 ng/ml for those isolated from aneurysmal aorta.

A reverse effect was observed for rates of apoptosis of abdominal aortic aneurysm derived smooth muscle cells cultured in the presence of PGE2. PGE2 seemed to enhance the rate of apoptosis as estimated by oligonucleosome assay (Fig. 5).

These data therefore indicated that PGE2 had detrimental effects on aortic smooth muscle cells. It depressed the rate of proliferation and appeared to increase levels of apoptosis of aneurysm smooth muscle cells. Elevated concentrations of PGE2 in aneurysm wall therefore might account for the smooth muscle cell loss seen in the walls of abdominal aortic aneurysms. The corollary of this would be that agents reducing the excessive COX2 activity in aneurysm wall might have potential to limit aneurysm expansion.

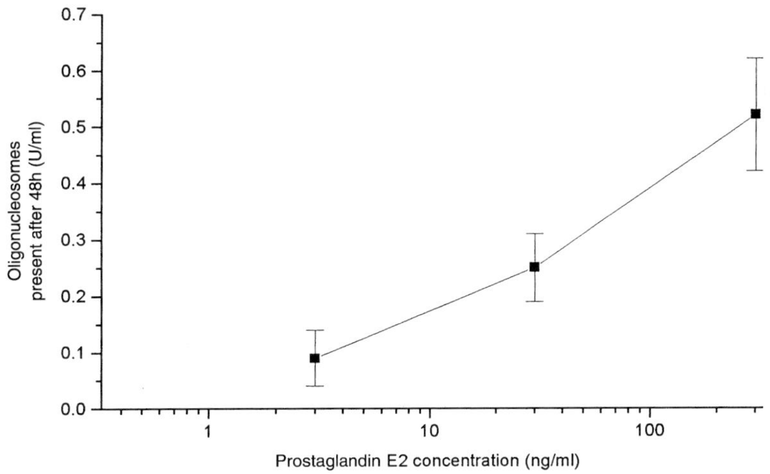

Fig. 5. Prostaglandin E2 increases oligonucleosome formation in smooth muscle cells cultured from aneurysm biopsies.

THE INFLUENCE OF NON-STEROIDAL INFLAMMATORY DRUGS ON ANEURYSM TISSUE

Aneurysm biopsies retrieved at open surgical abdominal aortic aneurysm repair are viable in tissue culture for 6 or more days.[19] Such explant cultures of aneurysm tissue are a useful way of assessing the effect of candidate drugs to limit aneurysm expansion on the behaviour of the target tissue. Aortic explants produce very high concentrations of PGE2, far in excess of the levels found to depress aortic smooth muscle cell proliferation and augment apoptosis. When abdominal aortic aneurysm explants were cultured in the presence of therapeutic concentrations of indomethacin, PGE2 production was almost completely abolished. Since indomethacin is an effective inhibitor of COX2, this result might be expected. More surprising was the finding that production of the cytokines IL-1β and IL-6, both implicated in aneurysm development, was also significantly reduced.[19] These studies demonstrated that COX2 inhibition had the potential to interrupt inflammatory cascades in aneurysm tissue. In particular, the excessive production of PGE2, demonstrated to be detrimental to aortic smooth muscle, could be abrogated by a non-steroidal anti-inflammatory drug (NSAID). These *in vitro* experiments suggested it would be worthwhile examining whether NSAIDs have an effect on aneurysm growth rates in patients.

DO NON-STEROIDAL ANTI-INFLAMMATORY DRUGS ALTER ANEURYSM GROWTH RATES?

In an observational case-controlled study, patients taking NSAIDs with abdominal aortic aneurysms 4.0–5.5 cm in diameter at presentation, entered locally into the UK Small Aneurysm Study and followed up for aneurysm growth for more than 12 months were identified.[18] These patients included 12 men and three women who were mainly taking the drugs (NSAIDs) for joint problems. Sixty-three other patients matched for age, sex, smoking and initial aneurysm diameter were selected as control subjects. Systolic blood pressures were slightly higher in the group taking NSAIDs and plasma cholesterol levels were slightly higher in the controls but these differences were far from significant. The usage of other drugs was not different between the two groups. Low dose aspirin (75 mg/day) was taken by three of the 15 NSAID takers and 21 of the 63 non-takers. Aneurysm diameters were measured by ultrasound every 3–6 months. Growth rates were calculated by linear regression analysis from a minimum of three separate scans over a median follow-up period of 24 months. The repeatability of diameter measurement was within 2 mm.

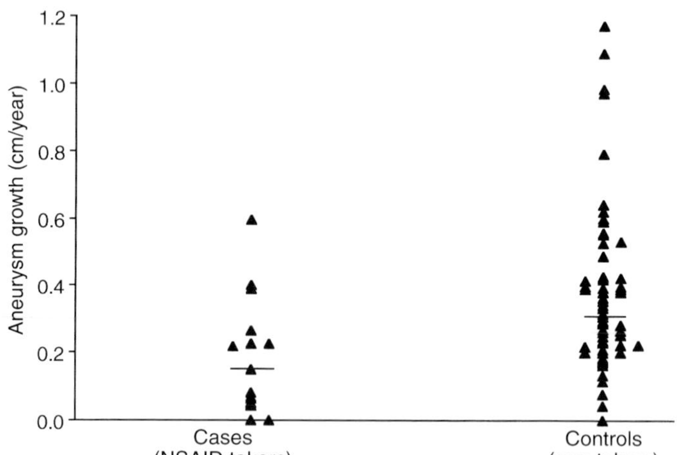

Fig. 6. Effect of NSAIDs in abdominal aortic aneurysm growth rates. Abdominal aortic aneurysm diameters were measured by ultrasound on a minimum of four occasions over a median follow-up interval of 2 years to derive growth rates for each aneurysm. The range of expansion rates was wide for both groups but the aneurysms seemed to grow more slowly in the patients taking NSAIDs than in the non-takers.

The median aneurysm growth rate in the NSAID takers was 1.5 mm/year compared with 3.2 mm/year for the controls (p=0.001, Mann-Whitney U test, Fig. 6).

CYCLO-OXYGENASE 2 INHIBITORS

The main adverse effects of NSAIDs are those of peptic ulceration. PGE2 is produced in gastric mucosa by COX1 and modulates gastric acid secretion and stimulates release of bicarbonate.[20] Inhibition of COX1 by NSAIDs therefore leads to reduced PGE2 production and a decrease in gastric pH. Specific COX2 inhibitors are becoming available which should have the beneficial effects of COX2 inhibition in aneurysm wall while avoiding the gastroduodenal complications caused by inhibition of COX1. Prospective randomized controlled trials are needed to determine whether the promising effects of COX2 inhibition in aneurysm tissue *in vitro* and the apparent effect of halving abdominal aortic aneurysms expansion rates in patients are borne out in clinical practice.

REFERENCES

1. Rose AG, Dent DM: Inflammatory variant of abdominal atherosclerotic aneurysm. *Arch Path Lab Med* **105:** 409–413, 1981
2. Rijbroek A, Moll FL, von Dijk HA *et al.*: Inflammation of the abdominal aortic aneurysm wall. *Eur J Vasc Surg* **8:** 41–46, 1994
3. Freestone T, Turner RJ, Coady A *et al.*: Inflammation and matrix metalloproteinases in the enlarging abdominal aortic aneurysm. *Arterioscler Thromb Vasc Biol* **15:** 1145–1151, 1995
4. Koch AE, Haines GK, Rizzo RJ *et al.*: Human abdominal aortic aneurysms. Immunophenotypic analysis suggesting an immune-mediated response. *Am J Pathol* **137:** 1199–1213, 1990
5. Newman KM, Jean-Claude J, Li H *et al.*: Cytokines that activate proteolysis are increased in abdominal aortic aneurysms. *Circulation* **90:** II224–II227, 1994
6. Szekanecz Z, Shah MR, Pearce WH, Koch AE: Human atherosclerotic abdominal aortic aneurysms produce interleukin (IL)-6 and interferon-gamma but not IL-2 and IL-4: the possible role for IL-6 and interferon-gamma in vascular inflammation. *Agents Actions* **42:** 159–162, 1994
7. Koch AE, Kunkel SL, Pearce WH *et al.*: Enhanced production of the chemotactic cytokines interleukin-8 and monocyte chemoattractant protein 1 in human abdominal aortic aneurysms. *Am J Pathol* **142:** 1423–1431, 1993
8. Libby P, Geng YJ, Aikawa M *et al.*: Macrophages and atherosclerotic plaque stability. *Curr Opin Lipidol* **7:** 330–335, 1996
9. Page RC: The role of inflammatory mediators in the pathogenesis of periodontal disease. *J Period Res* **26:** 230–242, 1991
10. Pollman MJ, Yamada T, Horiuchi M, Gibbons GH: Vasoactive substances regulate vascular smooth muscle cell apoptosis. Countervailing influences of nitric oxide and angiotensin II. *Circulat Res* **79:** 748–756, 1996
11. Holmes DR, Wester W, Thompson RW, Reilly JM: Prostaglandin E2 synthesis and cyclooxygenase expression in abdominal aortic aneurysms. *J Vasc Surg* **25:** 810–815, 1997
12. Corcoran ML, Stetler-Stevenson WG, Brown PD, Wahl LM: Interleukin 4 inhibition of prostaglandin E2 synthesis blocks interstitial collagenase and 92-kDa type IV collagenase/gelatinase production by human monocytes. *J Biol Chem* **267:** 515–519, 1992
13. Thompson RW, Liao S, Curci JA: Vascular smooth muscle cell apoptosis in abdominal aortic aneurysms. *Coronary Artery Dis* **8:** 623–631, 1997

14. Bennett MR, Evan GI, Schwartz SM: Apoptosis of rat vascular smooth muscle cells is regulated by p53-dependent and -independent pathways. *Circulat Res* **77:** 266–273, 1995
15. Lopez-Candales A, Holmes DR, Liao S *et al.*: Decreased vascular smooth muscle cell density in medial degeneration of human abdominal aortic aneurysms. *Am J Pathol* **150:** 993–1007, 1997
16. Zatina MA, Zarins CK, Gewertz BL, Glagov S: Role of medial lamellar architecture in the pathogenesis of aortic aneurysms. *J Vasc Surg* **1:** 442–448, 1984
17. Geng YJ, Wu Q, Muszynski M *et al.*: Apoptosis of vascular smooth muscle cells induced by in vitro stimulation with interferon-gamma, tumor necrosis factor-alpha, and interleukin-1 beta. *Arterioscler Thromb Vasc Biol* **16:** 19–27, 1996
18. Walton LJ, Franklin IJ, Bayston T *et al.*: Inhibition of prostaglandin E2 synthesis in abdominal aortic aneurysms: implications for smooth muscle cell viability, inflammatory processes, and the expansion of abdominal aortic aneurysms. *Circulation* **100:** 48–54, 1999
19. Franklin IJ, Walton LJ, Greenhalgh RM, Powell JT: The influence of indomethacin on the metabolism and cytokine secretion of human aneurysmal aorta. *Eur J Vasc Endovasc Surg* **18:** 35–42, 1999
20. Hojgaard L, Mertz NA, Rune SJ. Peptic ulcer pathophysiology: acid, bicarbonate, and mucosal function. *Scand J Gastroenterol* (Suppl) **216:** 10–15, 1996

The potential benefit of improving lung and renal function before elective aortic procedures

Janet T Powell, Anthony R Brady, Roger M Greenhalgh
for The UK Small Aneurysm Trial Participants

The modern era of aortic aneurysm repair started almost 50 years ago when Dubost and colleagues in Paris resected an abdominal aortic aneurysm using a homograft replacement for the abdominal aorta. The use of homografts was short-lived being rapidly replaced by prosthetic grafts of man-made fibres. Open elective repair of an abdominal aortic aneurysm with a Dacron inlay graft is now a standard procedure performed by all vascular surgeons and has been considered one of the safest and most durable operations performed.

A SUCCESSFUL OPERATION?

The safety of open elective surgical repair of abdominal aortic aneurysms may be a myth. Through the 1970s and 1980s, vascular surgeons have been impressed by the reports from single surgical centres showing a 30-day operative mortality of less than 2% associated with elective aneurysm repair. All these personal series are small, the number of patients rarely exceeding 300. In addition, the series may be started and stopped at convenient points to display results to best advantage. During the 1990s, several studies have reported the 30-day mortality associated with open elective surgical repair of abdominal aortic aneurysms in population series.[1–6] These population studies provide a different perspective to indicate that the 30-day operative mortality for this operation lies between 4.4% and 7.6%. Three large studies have reported from North America. In the Canadian Aneurysm Study, the 30-day mortality was 5.4%.[1] The experience from the Mayo Clinic records a 30-day mortality of 5.5%[2] whilst a State-wide study in Michigan reports a 30-day mortality of 5.6%.[3] In Europe, there have been two studies, one reporting from the northern region of England where the operative mortality in patients under 80 years of age was 7.6%,[4] and in the Netherlands where the 30-day operative mortality was 6.8%.[5] A more recent study from Western Australia shows the best results with a 30-day operative mortality of 4.4% for men.[6] These figures would suggest that elective surgical repair of an aneurysm kills somewhere between 1 in 15 and 1 in 21 patients, Table 1. This is not a safe operation. In this context, it becomes particularly important to identify the factors which predict 30-day operative mortality, especially if some of those factors may be correctable prior to surgery.

Some vascular surgeons reading the paragraph above may be full of dismay. However, they should not be. The results quoted above exemplify the performance of qualified vascular surgeons across the world. It would not appear as though

Table 1. Mortality within 30 days of elective aneurysm repair

Study region	*Year reported*	*30-Day mortality (%)*	*No. of patients*	*Ref.*
Canada	1994	5.4	680	1
Minnesota	1993	5.5	243	2
Michigan	1994	5.6	8185	3
Northern England	1995	7.6	662	4
Netherlands	1994	6.8	1289	5
Western Australia	1998	4.4	1257	6
UK Small Aneurysm Trial	2000	5.6	820	8

surgeons in the North Atlantic are better than their colleagues in Europe or Australia. Moreover, the national figures for England and Wales, collected from Hospital Episode Statistics, which include aneurysm repairs performed by general surgeons who may undertake just one or two repairs a year, would indicate that the 30-day operative mortality reaches 10% or more.[7] These figures would imply that the operative mortality for elective aneurysm repair by the non-specialist could be in excess of 15%. This is clearly unacceptable and such surgeons should be discouraged from performing this operation.

The UK trial participants have used the opportunities presented by the UK Small Aneurysm Trial to identify the prognostic risk factors associated with 30-day operative mortality in patients undergoing elective surgical repair of small aneurysms. During the course of this trial, in which 1090 patients participated, a total of 820 patients underwent open elective surgical repair of their aneurysm. Amongst these, 46 died within the first 30 days to give an operative mortality of 5.6%,[8] in line with the studies quoted above. However, with only 46 deaths, the statistical approach to the identification of prognostic risk factors was limited to the investigation of just 13 variables. To have included further patient and policy variables would have greatly increased the chance of random associations being found. With this limitation of being able to investigate only 13 prognostic risk factors, return to reading the literature was necessary, to ensure that we could make the appropriate selection.

Most of the deaths following elective aneurysm repair have been attributed to cardiac causes and there has been much discussion of how cardiac function influences postoperative outcome.[9] In some centres, coronary artery bypass surgery has been recommended before aneurysm repair.[10] Therefore it was clear that we had to include a measure of cardiac function. Only two such measures were available to us, the resting electrocardiogram (ECG) and the cardiothoracic ratio. During the UK Small Aneurysm Trial, the assessment of fitness for surgery had been left to local decisions and the procedures for investigating cardiac fitness varied from centre to centre. However, the ECGs and the cardiothoracic ratio had been collected by the dedicated trial co-ordinators and the ECGs read and coded by two independent observers. For this reason, we chose to use the resting ECG as our parameter of cardiac function. Other important causes of postoperative mortality include renal failure, multi-organ failure, and various forms of pulmonary dysfunction. For these reasons, we chose serum creatinine and the forced expiratory volume, FEV_1, as factors to put into our model. Previously there has also been considerable discussion as to whether elective surgery should be offered to smokers since smoking impacts on the pulmonary status: We used self-reported patient smoking status as another variable. We also had to include age, sex, the randomized group of the patient, and the aneurysm diameter at the time of surgery as variables for consideration. For some people, tenderness of the aneurysm to palpation has been associated with impending rupture and the use of a bifurcated graft rather than a tube graft which requires an additional anastomosis and implies more extensive disease which may prolong the cross clamping time. Therefore both tenderness and whether a tube or bifurcated graft was placed were used as other important variables. In addition, it was necessary to include policy variables. These included the type of hospital, whether it was a teaching hospital or a district general hospital, whether the operation was performed by a fully qualified surgeon or by a senior trainee, and how frequently the surgeon performed this operation. All these variables were identified in the predetermined statistical plan.

SUBJECTS, METHODS AND CAUSES OF DEATH

Of the 1090 patients in the UK Small Aneurysm Trial, 841 underwent aneurysm repair between September 1991 and June 1998 when the trial closed. Eight emergency operations and 13 endovascular repairs were excluded leaving a group of 820 patients undergoing elective open surgical repair. This included 516/563 patients randomized to early elective surgery where the median time between randomization and surgery was 1.8 months, and 304/527 patients randomized to ultrasound surveillance where the median time between randomization and surgery was 35 months.[11] Therefore the patients undergoing surgery in the group initially randomized to ultrasound surveillance were both older and had larger aneurysms at the time of surgery, the largest aneurysm having reached 7cm in diameter. All the patients had been flagged at the Office of National Statistics which provided us with a copy of the death certificate when the patient died. The immediate causes of death in the 46 patients who died within the first 30 days of their surgery are shown in Table 1. As had been anticipated, nearly half of the patients died from a cardiac problem. The univariate associations between 30-day mortality and the chosen 13 prognostic variables were first investigated using χ^2 tests for categorical variables and T tests for continuous variables. Following this, multiple logistic regression was performed to adjust the potential confounding effects between variables. These variables divided naturally into three groups: primary, biological and policy variables. And the results of these are listed in Table 2.

EXPECTED AND UNEXPECTED RESULTS

With 46/820 patients dying within 30 days, the operative mortality was 5.6%, (95% confidence interval, 4.1–7.4%).[8] Most of these deaths occurred within the first 20 days (Fig. 1) and the immediate causes of death are listed in Table 2. The in-hospital

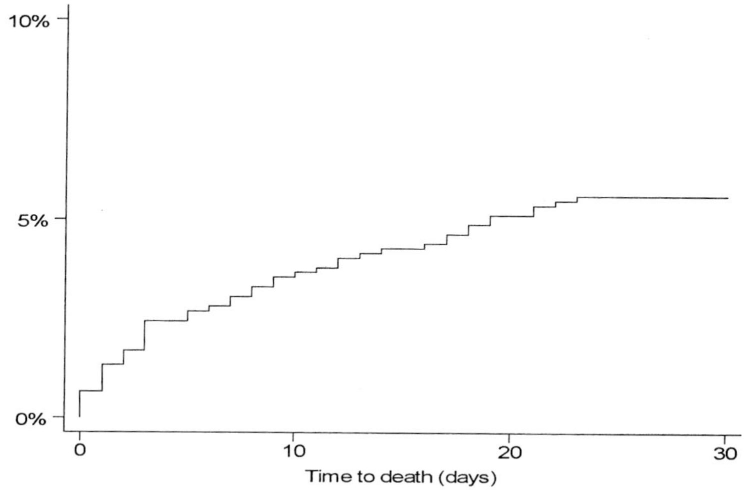

Fig. 1. Postoperative mortality for 820 patients undergoing elective aneurysm repair. Cumulative percentage according to time after surgery.

Table 2. Immediate cause of death[a] for 46 post-operative deaths

Cause of death	*No. %*
Cardiac	19 (41)
Pulmonary problems[b]	7 (15)
Renal failure	5 (11)
Sepsis	4 (9)
Multiorgan failure	3 (6)
Pulmonary embolism	3 (6)
Haemorrhage	3 (6)
Stroke	1 (2)
Bowel infarction	1 (2)

[a]Evaluated from death certificates. [b]Two chronic obstructive airways disease; five bronchopneumonia.

mortality was very similar with 47 of 820 deaths (5.7%) and all these in-hospital deaths occurred within 40 days of surgery. The univariate analyses (Table 3) indicated that patients who died within 30 days of their operation were slightly older than those who survived ($p = 0.03$). Other studies also have reported that older patients may do less well and this finding might have been anticipated.

Others have reported that women fare worse after elective aneurysm surgery but our results provided no evidence for this. Equally, there was no evidence that any of the variables associated with the aneurysm itself, whether the aneurysm was tender, the diameter at the time of surgery and whether a tube or bifurcation graft was used, appeared to significantly influence postoperative mortality. It was perhaps unexpected that neither ECG evidence of cardiac ischaemia nor smoking status were associated with 30-day mortality. Interestingly, none of the policy variables,

Table 3. Relation between preoperative prognostic factors and 30-day postoperative mortality: univariate analyses

Variable[a]	*Survived (n=774)*	*Died (n=46)*	*Significance test p-value*[b]
Primary variables			
Mean (SD) age at operation (years)	69.9 (4.4)	71.3 (4.2)	0.03
Sex			
Male	647 (84%)	37 (80%)	
Female	127 (16%)	9 (20%)	0.58
Mean (SD) FEV_1 ([litre] 18)	2.22 (0.74)	1.87 (0.62)	0.003
Mean (SD) creatinine ([μmol/litre] 27)	107.4 (30.3)	122.2 (44.6)	0.002
Evidence of ischaemia on ECG (10)	292 (38%)	20 (43%)	
Possible/Probable	472 (62%)	26 (57%)	0.48
Unlikely			
Smoking status (2)			
Current	289 (37%)	19 (41%)	
Ex/Never	483 (63%)	27 (59%)	0.60
Randomized group			
Surveillance	284 (37%)	20 (43%)	
Early surgery	490 (63%)	26 (57%)	0.36
Aneurysm variables			
Mean (SD) aneurysm diameter at operation (cm)	4.94 (0.55)	5.03 (0.56)	0.31
Tender aneurysm at operation	63 (8%)	5 (11%)	0.51
Graft type (13)			
Straight	588 (77%)	32 (76%)	
Bifurcated	177 (23%)	10 (24%)	0.92
Policy variables			
Type of hospital			
Teaching	284 (37%)	12 (26%)	
District General	490 (63%)	34 (74%)	0.15
Mean (SD) volume of surgery[c] (17)	20.8 (17.2)	20.0 (17.1)	0.76
Surgeon rank (18)			
Consultant	620 (82%)	37 (84%)	
Registrar/Senior Registrar	138 (18%)	7 (16%)	0.70

ECG: electrocardiography. [a]Numbers in ( ): number missing for 820 patients. [b]t-test for continuous variables, χ^2 test for categorical variables. [c]Number of abdominal aortic aneurysms operations surgeon performed during the trial period.

including the type of hospital, the volume of surgery performed and the operating surgeon's rank, had important influence on postoperative mortality. Of these, the one that came closest to significance was whether the surgery was performed in a district general or teaching hospital. In teaching hospitals, there were 12 of 284 deaths to give a 30-day operative mortality of 4.2% whilst in district general hospitals, there were 34 of 490 deaths giving a postoperative mortality of 6.9%. The senior trainees may have operated under the eagle eyes of their more senior supervisors and their results compared more than favourably with the results of their peers.

The two most significant factors associated with an increase 30-day mortality were lung function and renal function as assessed by FEV_1 and serum creatinine respectively.[8] The relationship between postoperative risk and both FEV_1 and creatinine appeared to be approximately linear (Fig. 2). Both FEV_1 and creatinine remain significantly associated with postoperative mortality after adjustment for other prognostic variables even though the level of significance fell to 1%. This reduction in statistical significance was largely due to these variables being correlated with age since both lung function and renal function were worse in older patients. The statistical significance of age effect was lost after adjustment for FEV_1 and creatinine ($p = 0.08$). From Fig. 2, it is clear that a decrease in FEV_1 of 1 litre approximately doubles the 30-day mortality risk and that each increase in creatinine of 40 μmole/litre increases the risk at approximately 40%.

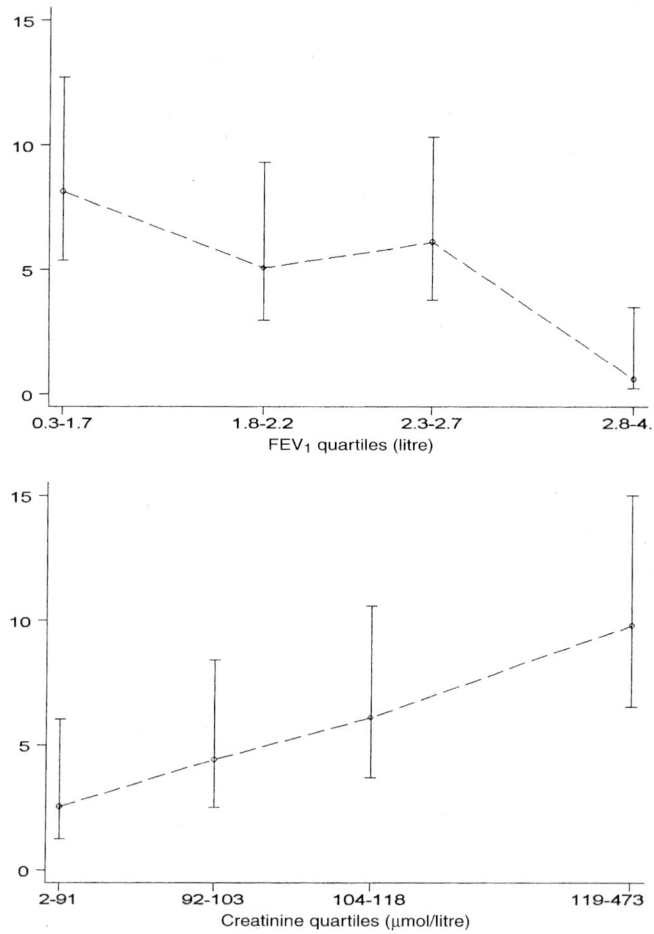

Fig. 2. 30-Day postoperative mortality risk by quartiles of FEV_1 and creatinine (estimate and 95% confidence interval).

VIGILANCE AND PRECAUTIONS WHICH MIGHT INCREASE SURVIVAL AFTER OPEN ELECTIVE SURGICAL REPAIR OF AN ABDOMINAL AORTIC ANEURYSM

The UK Small Aneurysm Trial was established in 1991 and power calculations were based upon data from single-centre studies which had suggested that the 30-day mortality following elective aneurysm repair was 2% or less. This had allowed the calculation that with 500 patients randomized into each arm of the trial, there should have been sufficient power to detect a significant improvement in long-term survival for those patients undergoing early elective surgery. The trial was started before most of the population-based studies and large cohorts investigations were published. The disagreement between reported mortality rates from hospital-based and population-based studies of elective surgery have been highlighted recently, with the comment that prospective studies provide the best documentation of postoperative morbidity and mortality.[12] UK Small Aneurysm Trial results are in keeping with all the other large studies published from Europe, across the North Atlantic in North America, and as far away as Western Australia.[1–7] In the UK trial, the 30-day postoperative mortality was 5.6%. One in 18 patients undergoing this supposedly safe procedure did not survive for 1 month beyond the operation.

In terms of identifying the important preoperative risk factors which may allow us to reduce this postoperative mortality in the future, the most surprising finding was that evidence of myocardial ischaemia in the resting ECG did not predict postoperative outcome. There are those who may criticise the trial for not having included other assessments of cardiac function, such as cardiac ejection faction, thallium scanning or exercise testing. Not each of these investigations would have been performed in every centre and the difficulties of standardizing reporting and data emanating from such testing would have been overwhelming. However, it is certain that the resting ECG does not provide a useful guide when assessing the risk of a major operative procedure such abdominal aortic aneurysm repair.

Nineteen of the 46 deaths were attributed to cardiac causes, with insufficient oxygen delivery to the rest of the body. Impaired lung function also leads to impaired oxygen delivery. Two recent publications suggest that surgeons could do much to increase oxygen delivery following elective surgery.[13,14] A randomized study showed that preoperative chest physiotherapy reduced pulmonary complications after major abdominal surgery and a separate trial showed the importance of optimizing preoperative oxygen delivery. These are measures, which could be implemented in all centres performing elective aneurysm repair. Not only was lung function, as measured by FEV_1, such an important prognostic indicator of postoperative mortality, it was also one of the most important prognostic factors of long-term mortality. Poor lung function also had a major impact on the cost of aneurysm repair with patients with poor lung function having an increased length of postoperative stay in the hospital.[15] Although previous studies have pointed to the problems of performing aneurysm repair for patients with poor lung function, the UK study is perhaps the first study that has used such high quality data with few missing values. Moreover the clinical measurements were taken by five specially trained regional co-ordinators to reduce measurement error. In addition, lung function was reported numerically as both FEV_1 and FVC and this allowed analyses which could be adjusted for other risk factors. Most previous studies have identified poor lung function on the basis of a single threshold value. Both FEV_1 and creatinine have been modelled as continuous variables to allow the production of the data shown in Fig. 2.

The other important risk factor identified in the UK study elevated serum creatinine concentration as an index for poor renal function has also been in previous studies as a possible factor relating to increased postoperative mortality. This is particularly true in recent studies of endovascular stenting of abdominal aortic aneurysms.[16] The options for treating poor renal function may be fewer than options for treating poor lung function. However, a recent case report has suggested that renal stenting might reduce the postoperative risk following aneurysm repair.[17] In addition, it would be particularly important to avoid therapeutic agents, which might further impair renal function.

The role of age in determining surgical policy has been controversial. Most previous studies have found a univariate association between older age and higher postoperative risk. However, the two other very important risk factors, which we have identified as being associated with postoperative mortality, poor lung function and poor renal function, increase with age. Age was no longer a significant factor after it had been adjusted for creatinine and FEV_1 in the UK data, which provided no indication that elective surgical repair should be denied to patients on the grounds of age alone.

As a population study, the UK study drew attention to the risk of death of 1 in 8 from operation[8] and it is therefore pertinent to provide practical suggestions to improve operative results. These suggestions are likely to have implications for those patients undergoing open surgical procedures for aortic occlusive disease, as well as those undergoing endovascular aneurysm repair. These new approaches should ensure optimization of oxygen delivery and judicious use of preoperative chest physiotherapy.

ACKNOWLEDGEMENTS

The UK Small Aneurysm Trial was supported by grants from the Medical Research Council and the British Heart Foundation to the University of Edinburgh and Imperial College at Charing Cross. The analysis of postoperative mortality was performed by Anthony R Brady, who is supported by a grant from the BUPA Foundation to Imperial College at Hammersmith and Charing Cross campuses. The trial would not have been possible without the participation of all the vascular surgeons and trial co-ordinators listed on page 209, the Regional Trial Directors, Professors PRF Bell, RM Greenhalgh, M Horrocks, CN McCollum and CV Ruckley.

UK SMALL ANEURYSM TRIAL

Steering committee

Professor RM Greenhalgh (***Chairman***)
Professor JT Powell (Imperial College at Charing Cross), Professor FGR Fowkes, Dr JF Forbes, Professor CV Ruckley (University of Edinburgh)

Writing committee

Professor JT Powell ***(Chair)***
L Brown, Professor RM Greenhalgh, Professor FGR Fowkes, Professor CV Ruckley

Monitoring committee

Professor PA Poole-Wilson (***Chair***)
Sir N Browse, Professor CJ Bulpitt, Professor K Burnand, Dr EC Coles, Dr A Fletcher

Trial co-ordinators

Sue Blair, Rebecca Clark, Carol Devine, Karen Ferguson, Sheila Hearn, Eileen Kerracher, Sarah Logan, Anna McCabe, Razia Meer-Baloch, Michelle Mossa, Anna Rattray, Katie Wilson

ECG coding

Mrs N Keen, Mrs C Rose

Blood analysis

R Mir Hassaine

TRIAL PARTICIPANTS (number of randomized patients recruited in brackets)

SW ENGLAND AND SOUTH WALES

Regional Trial Director:	**Professor M Horrocks**
Royal United Hospital:	Mr J Budd (6)
	Professor M Horrocks (23)
Bristol Royal Infirmary:	Mr RN Baird (12)
	Mr P Lamont (10)
Derriford Hospital:	Mr DC Wilkins (6)
	Mr S Ashley (3)
Dorset County Hospital:	Mr K Flowerdew (9)
Frenchay Hospital:	Mr A Baker (7)
Gloucester Royal Infirmary:	Mr J Earnshaw (1)
	Mr B Heather (3)
Morrison Hospital:	Mr C Gibbons (14)
Neville Hall Hospital:	Mr RL Blackett (8)
New Royal Bournemouth General Hospital:	Mr SD Parvin (30)
North Devon District General Hospital:	Mr DR Harvey (1)
Princess of Wales Hospital:	Mr R Hedges (1)
Princess Margaret Hospital:	Mr D Finch (6)
	Mr DB Hocken (2)
Southampton General Hospital:	Mr GE Morris (1)
	Mr CP Shearman (4)
Southmead Hospital:	Mr P Lear (4)
Torbay Hospital:	Mr P Lewis (5)
Yeovil District General Hospital:	Mr RJ Clarke (5)

SCOTLAND AND NE ENGLAND

Regional Trial Director:	**Professor CV Ruckley**
Edinburgh Royal Infirmary:	Mr AM Jenkins (1)
	Professor CV Ruckley (28)
Aberdeen Royal Infirmary:	Mr GG Cooper (18)
	Mr J Engeset (38)
	Mr R Naylor (1)
Ayr Hospital:	Mr G Stewart (16)
Dryburn Hospital, Durham:	Mr JCumming (10)
Dumfries and Galloway Royal Infirmary:	Mr J McCormick (8)
Dunfermline and West Fife Hospital:	Miss A Howd (9)
	Mr A Turner (6)
Falkirk and District Infirmary:	Mr DR Harper (5)
	Mr RC Smith (6)
Freeman Hospital:	Mr J Chamberlain (10)
	Mr AG Jones (12)
	Mr MG Wyatt (2)
Gartnavel General Hospital:	Mr AJ McKay (13)
Ninewells Hospital:	Mr JC Forrester (3)
	Mr P McCollum (30)
	Mr PA Stonebridge (3)
Perth Royal Infirmary:	Mr AIG Davidson (2)
Queen Elizabeth Hospital:	Mr R Baker (4)
Royal Victoria Infirmary:	Mr JLR Forsythe (1)
	Mr D Lambert (8)
Royal Northern Infirmary:	Mr JL Duncan (11)

THE MIDLANDS

Regional Trial Director:	**Professor PRF Bell**
Leicester Royal Infirmary:	Professor PRF Bell (25)
	Mr D Ratliff (1)
Derbyshire Royal Infirmary:	Mr KG Callum (16)
	Mr KG Nash (17)
Glenfield General Hospital:	Mr DS McPherson (7)
Kettering and General District Hospital:	Mr RE Jenner (4)
	Mr R Stewart (5)
Kidderminster General Hospital:	Mr PR Armitstead (8)
Leicester General Hospital:	Mr WW Barrie (5)
Northampton General Hospital:	Mr DB Hamer (6)
	Mr S Powis (5)
Northern General Hospital:	Mr LD Coen (2)
	Mr J Michaels (4)
	Mr CL Welsh (3)
Nottingham Queen's Medical Centre:	Mr BR Hopkinson (5)
	Mr PW Wenham (14)
Royal Hallamshire Hospital:	Mr J Beard (25)
Sandwell District General Hospital:	Mr A Auckland (3)
Worcester Royal Infirmary:	Mr J Black (7)
	Mr R Downing (6)
Worcester Royal Infirmary:	Mr NC Hickey (3)

LONDON AND SE ENGLAND	
Regional Trial Director:	**Professor RM Greenhalgh**
Charing Cross Hospital:	Mr AH Davies (2)
	Professor RM Greenhalgh (39)
	Mr D Nott (5)
Colchester General Hospital:	Mr ARL May (33)
Epsom District Hospital:	Mr R McFarland (11)
Guy's Hospital:	Mr P Taylor (15)
Hillingdon Hospital:	Mr JWP Bradley (3)
	Mr T Paes (9)
Ipswich Hospital:	Mr AEP Cameron (7)
Joyce Green Hospital:	Mr A McIrvine (18)
Lewisham Hospital:	Mr D Negus (4)
	Mr PR Taylor (10)
Medway Hospital:	Mr CM Butler (2)
	Mr RW Hoile (1)
Newham General Hospital:	Mr B Pardy (11)
Princess Alexandra Hospital:	Miss J Ackroyd (9)
Royal Free Hospital:	Mr G Hamilton (4)
Royal Hampshire County Hospital:	Mr R Lane (1)
Royal Surrey County Hospital:	Mr AEB Giddings (21)
St Georges's Hospital:	Mr J Dormandy (5)
	Mr R Taylor (9)
St Peter's Hospital:	Mr M Thomas (18)
St Thomas' Hospital:	Mr KJ Burnand (7)
University College Hospital:	Mr M Adiseshiah (3)
West Middlesex Hospital:	Mr P Pattison (1)
West Norwich Hospital:	Mr J Clarke (8)
	Mr J Colin (9)
Wexham Park Hospital:	Mr P Rutter (4)
Whipps Cross Hospital:	Mr S Brearley (14)
	Mr M Pietroni (1)

N ENGLAND AND NORTH WALES	
Regional Trial Director:	**Professor CN Mc Collum**
University Hospital South Manchester:	Professor CN McCollum (12)
Arrowe Park Hospital:	Mr MG Greaney (2)
	Mr D Reilly (7)
Blackburn Royal Infirmary:	Mr WG Paley (1)
Blackpool, Victoria Hospital:	Mr M Lambert (16)
Burney General Hospital:	Mr R Hughes (16)
Clatterbridge Hospital:	Mr S Blair (2)
Cumberland Infirmary:	Mr JEG Shand (1)
Grimsby District General Hospital:	Mr LA Donaldson (1)
Hull Royal Infirmary:	Mr JMD Galloway (2)
	Mr AR Wilkinson (21)
Leeds District General Hospital:	Mr M Gough (16)
Leigh Infirmary:	Mr J Mosley (1)
Macclesfield General Hospital:	Mr DM Matheson (19)
Manchester Royal Infirmary:	Mr M Walker (4)
Oldham Royal Hospital:	Mr N Hulton (4)

Pontefract General Infirmary:	Mr MI Aldoori (4)
	Mr CK Yeung (1)
Royal Preston Hospital:	Mr AR Hearn (6)
Royal Lancaster Infirmary:	Mr J Kelly (18)
Stafford General Hospital:	Mr D Durrans (2)
	Mr B Gwynn (3)
Stoke City General Hospital:	Mr GB Hopkinson (13)
Telford General Hospital:	Mr RGM Duffield (18)
The Infirmary Rochdale:	Mr IG Schraibman (3)
York District Hospital:	Mr R Hall (3)
	Mr SH Leveson (4)
Glan Clwyd Hospital, Rhyl:	Mr J Clark (3)
	Mr O Klimach (23)

REFERENCES

1. Johnston KW: Nonruptured abdominal aortic aneurysm: Six-year follow-up results from the multicenter prospective Canadian aneurysm study. *J Vasc Surg* **20:** 163–170 1994
2. Hallet JW, Naessens JM, Ballard DJ: Early and late outcome of surgical repair for small abdominal aortic aneurysms: A population-based analysis. *J Vasc Surg* **18:** 684–691, 1993
3. Katz DJ, Stanley JC, Zelenock GB: Operative mortality rates for intact and ruptured abdominal aortic aneurysms in Michigan: An eleven-year statewide experience. *J Vasc Surg* **19:** 804–817, 1994
4. Berridge DC, Chamberlain J, Guy AJ, Lambert D: Prospective audit of abdominal aortic aneurysm surgery in the northern region from 1988 to 1992. *Br J Surg* **82:** 1066–1070, 1995
5. Akkersdijk GJ, van der Graaf Y, van Bockel JH *et al.*: Mortality rates associated with operative treatment of infrarenal abdominal aortic aneurysm in the Netherlands. *Br J Surg* **81:** 706–709, 1994
6. Norman PE, Semmens JB, Lawrence-Brown MMD, Holman CDJ: Long-term relative survival after surgery for abdominal aortic aneurysm in Western Australia:population-based study. *Br Med J* **317:** 852–856, 1998
7. Department of Health. *Hospital Episode Statistics 1989–1996*. London: Department of Health, 1997
8. UK Small Aneurysm Trial Participants: Risk factors for post-operative mortality following elective surgical repair of abdominal aortic aneurysm: results from the UK Small Aneurysm Trial. *Br J Surg* 2000 (in press)
9. D'Angelo AJ, Puppala D, Farber A *et al.*: Is preoperative cardiac evaluation for abdominal aortic aneurysm repair necessary? *J Vasc Surg*. **25:** 152–156, 1997
10. Golden MA, Whittemore AD, Donaldson MC, Mannick JA: Selective evaluation and management of coronary artery disease in patients undergoing repair of abdominal aortic aneurysms. A 16-year experience. *Ann Surg* **212:** 415–420, 1990
11. The UK Small Aneurysm Trial Participants: Mortality results for randomised controlled trial of early elective surgery or ultrasonographic surveillance for small abdominal aortic aneurysms. *Lancet* **352:** 1649–1655, 1998
12. Blankensteijn JD, Lindenburg FP, Van der Graaf Y, Eikelboom BC: Influence of study design on reported mortality and morbidity rates after abdominal aortic aneurysm repair. *Br J Surg* **85:** 1624–1630, 1998
13. Fagevik OM, Hahn I, Nordgren S *et al.*: Randomised controlled trial of prophylactic chest physiotherapy in major abdominal surgery. *Br J Surg* **84:** 1535–1538, 1997
14. Wilson J, Woods I, Fawcett J *et al.*: Reducing the risk of major elective surgery: randomised controlled trial of preoperative optimisation of oxygen delivery. *Br Med J* **318:** 1099–1103, 1999

15. UK Small Aneurysm Trial Participants: Length of stay following elective abdominal aortic aneurysm repair. *Eur J Vasc Endovasc Surg* **6:** 185–191, 1998
16. Walker SR, Yusuf SW, Wenham PW, Hopkinson BR: Renal complications following endovascular repair of abdominal aortic aneurysms. *J Endovasc Surg* **5:** 318–322, 1998
17. Sullivan TM, Hertzer NR: Stenting of the renal artery to improve renal function prior to thoracoabdominal aneurysm repair. *J Endovasc Surg* **5:** 56–59, 1998

The UK EndoVascular Aneurysm Repair (EVAR) trials: background and methodology

Roger M Greenhalgh, Louise C Brown, Janet T Powell
for The UK EVAR Trial Participants

SUMMARY

The EndoVascular Aneurysm Repair (EVAR) Trials began recruitment on 1 September 1999 and are funded initially for 4 years by a National Health Service Health Technology Assessment Programme grant. Since 1996 training centres for the use of endovascular stent-grafts for abdominal aortic aneurysm repair have been established and progress audited in the National Registry of Endovascular Treatment of Aneurysms (RETA). At the start of the Trials 13 national centres identified themselves as eligible and trained in the use of endovascular aneurysm repair. Trial co-ordinators at these 13 UK centres have been trained at Charing Cross Hospital in correct protocol procedures and collection of Health Related Quality of Life (HRQL). Trained operators enter patients undergoing aortic aneurysm repair into randomized trials of (1) EVAR compared with Open repair (OR) in fit patients and (2) EVAR and best medical treatment against best medical treatment in patients unfit for open repair. Each trial will compare EVAR against current best alternative in terms of mortality, costs and graft durability as well as generic and patient specific health related quality of life; 1080 patients will be entered over 4 years, 800 in Trial 1 and 280 in Trial 2.

BACKGROUND TO THE PROJECT

The incidence of abdominal aortic aneurysm in England and Wales has been increasing. From 1950 to 1984 age standardized mortality rose 20-fold in men to 47.1 per 100000 population and 11-fold in women to 22.2 per 100000.[1] The authors concluded that the trends were not wholly compatible with increases in diagnosis and surgery because there were inconsistencies by age and sex and increases had occurred in the number of complicated as well as uncomplicated cases. Similarities to the trends were noted in North America, elsewhere in Europe and Australasia and so the authors concluded that there was a true increase in the incidence of abdominal aortic aneurysms. At the beginning of this decade Parodi *et al.* in Argentina[2] and Volodos in the Ukraine introduced EVAR in sicker patients with shorter hospital stay. These pioneers used hand-made stent-graft systems beginning with a repair to lie entirely within the abdominal aorta (aorto–aortic graft). Subsequently it has been shown that the aorto–aortic EVAR can be used in less than 10% of patients and bifurcation systems have been developed which enable approximately 25% of aneurysms to be managed by an EVAR method.[3] 'Home-made systems' have been introduced in this country in Nottingham[4] and Leicester.[5] These systems have employed an aortouni–iliac EVAR system. The second side is occluded using a Dacron sac and stent and the procedure completed with a femorofemoral crossover graft just leaving the patient with two small incisions in the groins and minimum pain. The Nottingham group[4] have shown that using their system, 75% of all abdominal aortic aneurysms could be managed by EVAR.

The Registry for Endovascular Treatment of Aneurysms (RETA)

The National RETA registry was initiated in January 1996 to audit 'home-made' and commercially available EVAR systems deployed within the UK. Annual audits have been conducted and reports are available to the EVAR Trial Management Committee, principally to be advised when centres are trained.

According to the 1998 data, patients have been classified as either fit or unfit for open repair (OR). The proportions of each are given in Fig.1 and represent the distribution of patients that would enter EVAR Trial 1 (fit for OR) or EVAR Trial 2 (unfit for OR). It is clear that the operative mortality at 30 days is significantly worse for unfit patients ($\chi^2 = 23.4$, $p < 0.001$).

In patients suitable for open repair the data for 1996, 1997 and 1998 (Fig. 2) show decreasing 30-day mortality. It must be remembered that not all EVAR procedures in the UK are recorded in these data.

EVAR is currently being used both for fit for OR patients (75%) and unfit for OR patients (25%). Consequently it is appropriate to pose the question of the original National Health Service Research and Development Health Technology Assessment commissioning brief **what is the cost-effectiveness of aortic stenting versus other**

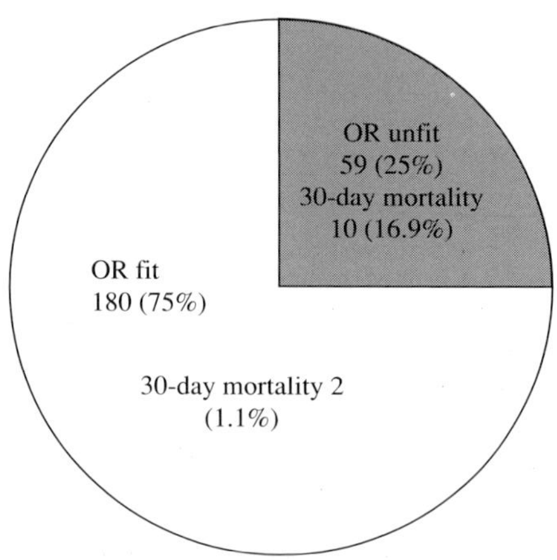

Fig. 1. RETA data for 30-day EVAR mortality (1998) according to fitness for Open Repair (OR), (n=239).

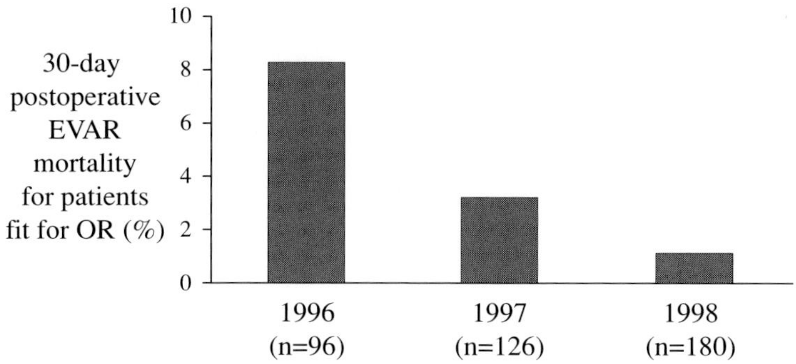

Fig. 2. Data for 30-day postoperative mortality for patients classified as fit for open repair (OR). Taken from RETA annual reports from 1996 to 1998 (n=number of EVARS performed in that year).

innovative methods versus open repair for elective abdominal aortic aneurysms? Currently the accepted alternative to EVAR is open repair (OR) in patients who are fit enough for the procedure. For those that are not fit for open repair, EVAR is currently being used as an adjunct to best medical treatment. Should it be? Can best medical treatment be 'innovative'? We have shown that smoking increases the growth rate of small abdominal aortic aneurysms[6] and so after EVAR one can no longer expect the aortic dimensions proximal and distal to the stents to remain constant if a patient continues to smoke. Consequently innovative best medical treatment could involve the setting up of smoking advice clinics using nicotine replacement therapy in the trial centres with measurement of smoking markers for compliance. Careful control of blood pressure including reduction in pulse pressure should be advocated. EVAR procedures are being performed in the UK on patients less than fit for OR and this is a potentially expensive exercise for the NHS and the appropriate trial would be to assess any adjuvant benefit of EVAR beyond current best medical practice, particularly any treatment which can slow the expansion of the aortic aneurysm.

In considering a random allocation trial of EVAR versus OR, it is argued that the operative mortality for the commercially available stent grafts is very low. Blum *et al.* in Freiburg, Germany using the Mintek System in 140 patients, reported a 0.7% 30-day mortality.[7] Moore *et al.*[8] in North America reported a 33% 30-day mortality in 30 patients using another commercially available device. The Eurostar Audit of Systems in Europe has data on 400 procedures with a 30-day mortality of 4% for mainly commercially available systems.[9] At present, commercially available systems can only be used in up to 25% of aneurysms and generally in the less diseased or extensive abdominal aortic aneurysms with suitable anatomical dimensions. We had no alternative but to base our calculations on the pilot data of RETA which included aortouni–iliac data of 'home-made systems' which brings to 75% the proportion of patients correctable by EVAR.[10]

THE UK SMALL ANEURYSM TRIAL

The results of The UK Small Aneurysm Trial were reported in two back-to-back papers published in *The Lancet* on 21 November 1998.[11] During the 4 years of recruitment from August 1991 to 1995, 1090 patients aged 60–76 presenting with asymptomatic, infrarenal aortic aneurysm sized between 4.0 and 5.5cm were randomized either to regular ultrasound surveillance or elective open repair. Patients were followed for a further 3 years in terms of mortality, cost-effectiveness and health-related quality of life. Kaplan–Meier survival analysis indicated that surgical intervention for abdominal aortic aneurysm was not justified in terms of all-cause mortality, cost-effectiveness or health related quality of life. Survival was similar in both groups and regular surveillance was found to be a safe and reliable mode of treatment to monitor the aneurysm until it grew to 5.5cm, became tender, grew fast (>1.0cm/year) or ruptured. The 30-day operative mortality for patients randomized to elective surgery in the UK Small Aneurysm Trial was 5.8% and an annual rupture rate of 1% was found. Accordingly, no benefit was found for early surgical intervention (within 3 months of randomization for sizes of 4.0–5.5cm). Instead, surveillance to 5.5cm was seen to be better. We see no reason to modify these findings for EVAR at this stage and aortas > 5.5cm will be considered for surgery.

From the Freeman Hospital, Newcastle, Berridge *et al.* reported a 5 year prospective audit on 1131 patients undergoing surgery for abdominal aortic aneurysms from 1988 to 1992.[12] The Teaching Hospital 30-day mortality was 3.9% and District General Hospital mortality 12.0%. The audit showed a far greater mortality for over 80-year-olds (23.8%), than under 80-year-olds (7.6%). Hopkinson in Nottingham has also found higher mortality in patients older than 85 years undergoing EVAR.[10]

ELIGIBILITY OF REGIONAL CENTRES

The training of surgeons and radiologists (operators)

The success of the new technique is thought to be highly device-, operator- and centre-dependant and therefore hospitals need to demonstrate competence at performing the new procedure before it can realistically compete with current alternative best medical or surgical practice. Eligible centres need to meet the learning curve requirements of the Joint Working Party for The Vascular Surgical Society of Great Britain and Ireland (VSSGBI) and The British Society of Interventional Radiology (BSIR). These requirements specify that any centre must have performed at least 20 endovascular procedures, at least 10 by the eligible operator and at least 5 per device. Trial co-ordinators at centres entering patients are trained before the first patient is entered and skills will be checked during the trial and compared between centres.

Role of associated hospitals

It is important that patient recruitment is as high as possible. Each trained regional centre will also act as a specialist centre in its own area. It may be possible for surrounding non-vascular specialist hospitals to support recruitment by referring vascular patients believed to be suitable for the EVAR Trials to that regional centre. If anatomically suitable for EVAR and agreeable to randomization the patient would receive treatment at the regional centre. Thus *all* EVAR, OR, best medical treatment and follow-up would be performed at the regional centre and or patients unsuitable for EVAR are returned.

GENERALIZABILITY AND THE EVAR STUDY

It will be of particular importance that patients found to be unsuitable for an EVAR device are recorded at initial consultation. Numbers of unsuitable patients and reasons for this will determine what proportion of patients with abdominal aortic aneurysm are anatomically suitable for an EVAR device at the national level. Thus, all patients registered for anatomical suitability assessment for an EVAR device will form the 'EVAR Study' and Trial patients will be drawn from this pool of patients with abdominal aortic aneurysm. Figure 3 demonstrates the relationship between the Study and Trials. Some of the eligible centres act as both the District General Hospital and Regional Centre for their area. These centres will provide reliable population information about the proportion of patients throughout the country who could be treated by EVAR.

ENTRY CRITERIA

Age at least 60 years

A minimum age of 60 years is chosen as surgeons may wish to manage patients under 60 years in a different way because frequently there is an associated genetic cause where expansion rates and extent of aortic aneurysm may be extreme, such as Marfan syndrome. No upper age limit is thought necessary as very elderly patients

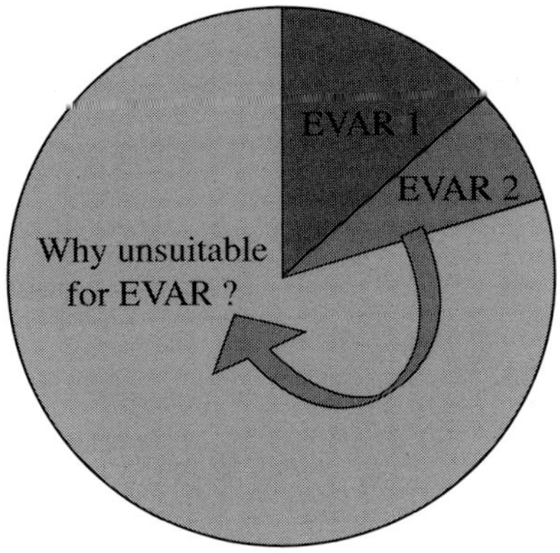

Fig. 3. Generalizability relationship between EVAR Study and Trials.

may benefit from the use of an EVAR device and their recruitment will be important for achieving the numbers required.

Size of abdominal aortic aneurysm

The criterion for entry into both trials will be an aneurysm diameter measuring ≥ 5.5cm according to a computed tomographic (CT) scan. The UK Small Aneurysm Trial has shown that it is safe to leave abdominal aortic aneurysms until they reach this size. However, reproducibility differences between duplex ultrasound and CT scanners can lead to significant variation in abdominal aortic aneurysms diameters. Duplex scanning tends to produce diameters smaller than CT scanning and therefore we recommend that patients presenting with a ≥ 5.0cm aneurysm on duplex should be sent for a CT scan to determine whether the aneurysm is ≥5.5cm in any diameter on CT scan and thus suitable for EVAR Trial entry. Tender aortic aneurysms and contained ruptures may be included provided the aneurysm measures at least 5.5cm on a CT scan and suitable EVAR equipment is available at such short notice. Tender aneurysms < 5.5cm requiring surgery will only have the options of open repair or surveillance.

Anatomical suitability for EVAR

This is assessed by spiral CT or conventional CT combined with conventional angiography with a marked catheter to enable the calculation of length. The trial co-ordinator needs to work closely with the local radiologist and appropriate training centre and document how the aneurysm was assessed and how the size and type of EVAR device was selected. Patients found to be unsuitable for an EVAR device will not be flagged for mortality at The Office of National Statistics but reasons for unsuitability will be collected. Patients referred from associated hospitals will be returned there for treatment if an EVAR device is found to be unsuitable.

Fitness for surgery

This is determined locally by the surgeon, radiologist, anaesthetist and cardiologist. It was originally thought that ASA grades I, II and III would indicate entry to EVAR Trial 1 and ASA IV patients would permit entry into EVAR Trial 2. However, despite the simplicity of ASA grade it can be open to different interpretation at each centre and has proved too difficult to use as a classification system for EVAR Trials 1 or 2. Recently, more sophisticated tests have not been good predictors of outcome in vascular surgery.[13,14] It has been appreciated during the UK Small Aneurysm Trial that fitness 'inflation' has emerged with respect to the size of aneurysm. Patients who were earlier described as 'unfit for OR' and later developed a larger aneurysm were suddenly deemed 'fit for the procedure'. This could equally happen for these current trials. For the purposes of pragmatism, fitness is determined at the local level for these trials. Recommended cardiac, respiratory and renal guidelines have been provided as outlined in Fig. 4 and baseline data will be used to assess fitness of randomized patients at the final analysis. These guidelines may help provide some conformity of fitness classification for EVAR Trials 1 or 2.

Recommended guidelines for assessment of patient fitness for open repair and suitability for EVAR Trial 1 or 2

Patient fitness for open repair is decided at the local level, however, these guidelines may provide some assistance.

Cardiac status

Normally, patients presenting with the following cardiac symptoms would not be recommended for any surgical intervention:

- Myocardial infarction within last 3 months
- Onset of angina within the last 3 months
- Unstable angina at night or at rest

Normally, patients presenting with the following symptoms would be unsuitable for open repair (EVAR Trial 1) but may be suitable for EVAR Trial 2:

- Severe valve disease
- Significant arrhythmia
- Uncontrolled congestive cardiac failure

Respiratory status (no constraints for EVAR Trial 2)

Open repair (EVAR Trial 1) would not be recommended for patients presenting with the following respiratory symptoms:

- Unable to walk up a flight of stairs without shortness of breath (even if there is some angina on effort).
- $FEV_1 < 1.0$ litre
- $PO_2 < 8.0$ kPa
- $PCO_2 > 6.5$ kPa

Renal status (no constraints for EVAR Trial 2)

Open repair might not be recommended for patients presenting with serum creatinine levels greater than 200mmol/litre. These patients may be suitable for EVAR Trial 2.

Fig. 4.

Randomization

Randomization is performed for each trial using 50:50 ratio randomization tables constructed by the STATA package. Randomization is stratified by centre and is only performed when all data have been received at Charing Cross. This enables patients to be randomized into the relevant trial and simultaneously flagged for mortality at The Office of National Statistics.

Figure 5 demonstrates the entry protocol for patients into both trials.

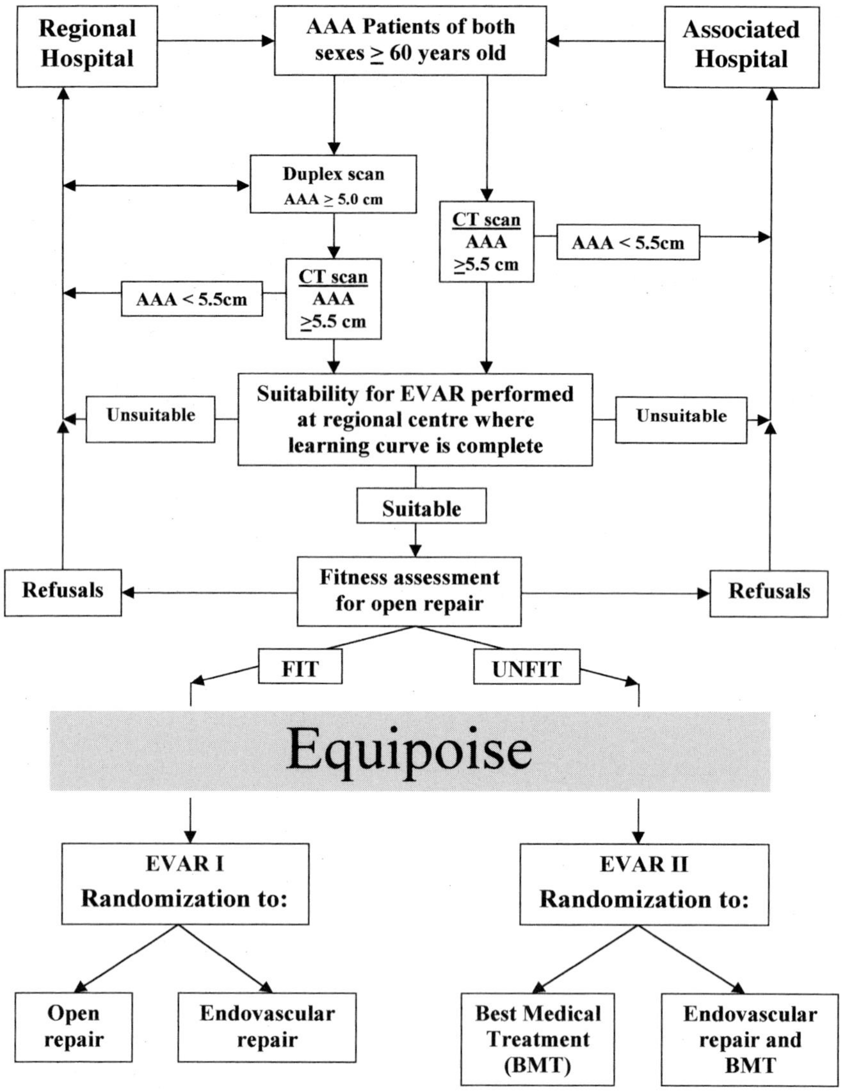

Fig. 5. Summary of recruitment procedure for EVAR Trials. (AAA: abdominal aortic aneurysm.)

OUTCOME MEASURES

Mortality for EVAR Trial 1

From The UK Small Aneurysm Trial data, 30-day operative mortality was calculated for patients who were randomized to observation but whose aortic aneurysms subsequently grew to larger than 5.5cm when surgery was performed (n=191). Eleven patients were dead at 30 days leading to a 30-day operative mortality of

5.76%. Sample size calculations were performed using 5.76% for open repair 30-day mortality and the RETA 30 day mortality figures for 1996–1998. Figure 6 shows how the annual fall in EVAR 30-day mortality has reduced the numbers required to show a difference between OR and EVAR should there be one. Thus, we may need to randomize as few as 361 patients in each arm.

Sample size calculations are calculated to provide 90% power at the 5% significance level

	Open repair [UK Aneurysm Trial]	EVAR [RETA 1996 data]	EVAR [RETA 1997 data]	EVAR [RETA 1998 data]
Number dead at 30 days / Total operated	11/191	8/96	4/126	2/180
30-day operative mortality	5.76 %	8.3 %	3.2 %	1.1 %
Numbers required per group (total recruitment) to detect difference between EVAR and OR		2205 (4410)	1448 (1896)	361 (722)

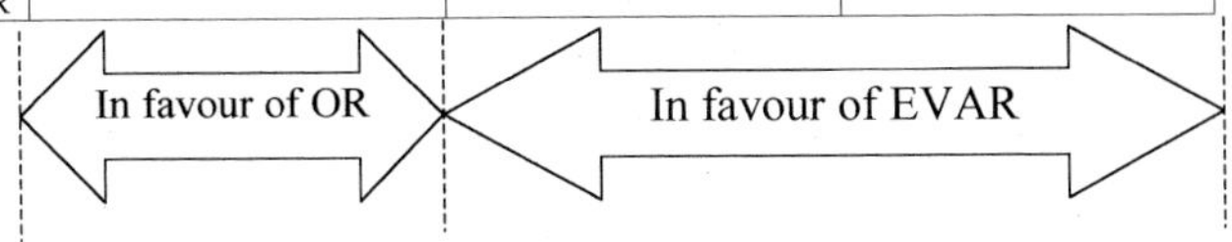

Fig. 6. Numbers of patients required for EVAR Trial 1 to detect a difference in 30-day postoperative mortality.

Mortality for EVAR Trial 2

From the UK Small Aneurysm data, we know that unfit for OR patients with best medical treatment have a mortality at 10 months of 22% and 50% at 2 years. The Nottingham 30-day EVAR mortality at 10 months for patients unsuitable for open repair is 40%. Therefore, mortality is likely to be high for EVAR Trial 2 patients and we expect to see a difference between the two arms early on during recruitment. Stopping rules are currently being decided by the DMEC who will regularly be checking (1) patient recruitment (2) deaths.

The incidence of endoleaks from EVAR (durability of procedure)

Endoleaks will be classified in the manner suggested by Geoffrey White of Sydney, Australia:[15]

Endoleak type I	Perigraft leak at proximal or distal end
Endoleak type II	Retrograde endoleak from patent lumber artery
Endoleak type III	Fabric tear
Endoleak type IV	Graft porosity
Endoleak type V	Endopressure

Health-related quality of life (HRQL)

In measuring HRQL a combination of specific and generic instruments was recommended e.g.[16] Specific instruments are useful for clinical evaluation; their narrow focus makes them more responsive to small but clinically important changes in health. Generic instruments are useful for economic evaluation and for comparisons across groups of patients; their comprehensive nature also enables them to detect unforeseen effects of treatment. There are two main types of generic instrument – health profiles and utility measures. Health profiles measure HRQL across a number of distinct dimensions and thus assess the effect of health care on different aspects of HRQL. Utility measures incorporate the values that individuals attach to HRQL and thus produce a single index of HRQL suitable for economic evaluation. The portfolio of instruments to measure HRQL in the proposed trials was designed to be comprehensive yet brief. It is completed by patients in the form of a questionnaire – at recruitment and subsequently 1, 3 and 12 months after surgery or the beginning of medical treatment as appropriate. The questionnaire includes three generic instruments – the Short-Form 36-item (SF-36) Health Survey, EuroQol and the Spielberger questionnaire assesses patient anxiety. The SF-36 is a health profile comprising eight distinct scales including physical and social functioning, role limitation, mental health, vitality, pain and general health.[17] It has been shown to be valid, reliable and responsive to changes in health in British patients.[18–20] The EuroQol is a validated utility measure comprising five items covering mobility, self-care, usual activities, pain, anxiety and depression.[21] The HRQL states defined by the various combinations of responses to these items have been valued by the general public for use in cost-utility analysis. Unfortunately we know of no specific instrument designed to measure HRQL in patients suffering from abdominal aortic aneurysms; this has been confirmed by a recent systematic search of Medline. One likely reason for this lack is the wide range of effects that this condition has on patients. In these circumstances we have proposed to use one specific instrument, the Patient Generated Index (PGI). This is a quasi-specific HRQL instrument that focuses on the concerns of the *individual* patient with a given condition rather than concerns derived by the investigator for the *typical* patient with that condition.[22] Patients nominate and rate on a scale the five most important aspects of their lives affected by their condition. The final score represents the gap between their current health status and their expectations in those areas of their lives in which they would most value an improvement. Thus the PGI measures the effect of the condition on quality of life as defined by the patient. There is good evidence for the acceptability, validity, reliability and responsiveness of this instrument.

Economic evaluation

Within each of the two subtrials the type and extent of economic evaluation will depend crucially upon the clinical outcome of that trial:

1. If one technology produces a clinically better outcome than another at significantly lower cost, then clinical and financial criteria both lead to the same conclusion.
2. If there is no clinically significant difference in outcome between two

technologies under comparison, then the least cost option is preferable (cost minimization analysis[23]).

3. If one technology produces a clinically better outcome than another at higher cost, then we shall undertake marginal cost-utility analysis[23] (based on mortality and the EuroQol[21]) and, if appropriate, marginal cost-effectiveness analysis[23] (based on the PGI[22]).

NHS costs will be collected. These will include the length of time in hospital (subdivided into intensive care, high dependency care, acute care and convalescent care), and theatre costs (subdivided into the length of operation and the use of staff, tests and drugs).

Under scenario 3 we shall use the EuroQol to estimate changes in health utility. One advantage of using the EuroQol is that it expresses changes in HRQL on a ratio scale. Thus cost-utility ratios in the form of cost per quality-adjusted life year (QALY) can be constructed from changes in mortality (if any) and in HRQL. Comparisons can then be made with other health care interventions. If there is no significant change in mortality, however, care will be needed because the EuroQol is less responsive to change than most condition-specific measures. To reduce the possibility of a Type II error, we shall also undertake a cost-effectiveness analysis based on the PGI.

We shall subject our results to extensive sensitivity analysis. First we shall identify the critical components of the cost and outcome by varying all estimated parameters in the analysis individually, to see how the economic findings are affected. Those parameters which lead to substantial changes in these findings will be varied over plausible ranges in combination to see whether the main conclusions are altered.[24]

As this economic evaluation is being undertaken alongside a randomized trial, both cost and outcome data will be subject to random variation. Therefore we shall estimate confidence intervals for costs, outcomes, cost-utility ratios and cost-effectiveness ratios. The last two will use the resampling technique known as bootstrapping.[25]

FOLLOW-UP

All trial patients are flagged for mortality at The Office of National Statistics. HRQL data are collected at 1, 3 and 12 months following treatment and cost-evaluation data have been based on operation costs and graft durability issues during the course of follow-up. Any adverse events are also to be collected, e.g. tender or ruptured abdominal aortic aneurysm, conversion to open repair, myocardial infarction, stroke, renal failure and amputation. CT scan is used for assessment of growth rates, persistent endoleaks and durability which could vary with stent-graft type. CT scan follow-up is at 1 and 3 months, 1 year, 2 years, 3 years and 4 years for EVAR patients in Trials 1 or 2. CT scan follow-up is performed annually for patients randomized to open repair in EVAR Trial 1. CT scan follow-up is collected at 6 monthly intervals for best medical treatment patients in EVAR Trial 2.

THE UK EVAR TRIAL PARTICIPANTS

Trial Steering Committee

Professor RJ Lilford (*Chairman*)

Professor RM Greenhalgh, Professor PRF Bell 1999–2000, Dr SC Whittaker 1999–2000

Data Monitoring and Ethical Committee

Professor P Poole-Wilson (*Chairman*)

Dr EC Coles, Professor CV Ruckley, Mr WB Campbell, Dr MRE Dean, Dr MST Ruttley

Trial Management Committee

Professor RM Greenhalgh (*Chairman*)

Professor DJ Allison, Professor MJ Buxton, Professor JT Powell, Professor IT Russell
Professor SG Thompson, Mr JD Beard, Mr PL Harris 1999–2000, Dr JDG Rose 1999–2000

Regional Trial Participants Committee

Mr SD Parvin, Dr DFC Shepherd, *Bournemouth General Hospital*
Professor RM Greenhalgh, Dr AWM Mitchell, *Charing Cross Hospital, London*
Mr MG Wyatt, Dr JDG Rose, *Freeman Hospital, Newcastle*
Mr PR Taylor, Dr JF Reidy, *Guy's Hospital, London*
Mr AR Wilkinson, Dr DF Ettles, *Hull Royal Infirmary*
Mr M Gough, Dr S McPherson, *Leeds General Infirmary*
Professor PRF Bell, Dr NG Fishwick, *Leicester Royal Infirmary*
Mr PL Harris, Dr DA Gould, *Liverpool Royal Hospital*
Professor M Walker, Dr NC Chalmers, *Manchester Royal Infirmary*
Mr JD Beard, Dr PA Gaines, *Northern General Hospital, Sheffield*
Professor BR Hopkinson, Dr SC Whittaker, *Queen's Medical Centre, Nottingham*
Mr M Adiseshiah, Dr MJ Raphael, *University College Hospital, London*
Professor CN McCollum, Dr R Ashleigh, *University Hospital of South Manchester*

Data and Trial Management

Miss LC Brown, Mr GR Barton

Trial Co-ordinators

Sara Baker, Lesley Wilson, Marion Aukett, Jennie Bryce, Rona Hooper, Bet Hughes, Janis Martin, Paul Fulford, Marilyn Ireland, Sarah Spencer, Cindy Tomlinson, Carol Devine

REFERENCES

1. Fowkes FGR, MacIntyre CCA, Ruckley CV: Increasing incidence of aortic aneurysms in England and Wales. *Br Med J* **298:** 33–35, 1989
2. Parodi JC, Palma JC, Barone HD: Transfermoral intraluminal graft implantation for abdominal aortic aneurysm. *Ann Vasc Surg* **5:** 491–497, 1991
3. Andrews SM, Cuming R, MacSweeney ST *et al.*: Assessment of feasibility for endovascular prosthetic tube correction of aortic aneurysm. *Br J Surg* **7:** 917, 1995
4. Yusef SW, Baker DM, Hind RE *et al.*: Endoluminal transfemoral abdominal aortic aneurysm repair with aorto-uni-iliac graft and femorofemoral bypass. *Br J Surg* **82:** 916, 1995
5. Nasim A, Thompson MM, Sayers RD *et al.*: Endovascular repair of abdominal aortic aneurysm: an initial experience. *Br J Surg* **83:** 516–519, 1996

6. MacSweeney STR, Ellis M, Worrell PC *et al.*: Smoking and growth rate of small abdominal aortic aneurysms. *Lancet* **344:** 651–652, 1994
7. Blum U, Voshage G, Lammer J *et al.*: Endoluminal stent grafts for infra-renal abdominal aortic aneurysms. *New Engl J Med* **336:** 13–20, 1997
8. Moore WS, Rutherford RB for the EVT investigators: Transfemoral endovascular repair of abdominal aortic aneurysms. Results of the North American EVT phase 1 Trial. *J Vasc Surg* **23:** 543–553, 1996
9. Harris P: The need for clinical trials of endovascular abdominal aortic aneurysms stent/graft repair: The Eurostar Project. *J Endovasc Surg* **4:** 72–77, 1997
10. Yusef SW, Whitaker SC, Chuter TAM *et al.*: Early results of endovascular abdominal aortic aneurysm repair with aorto uni iliac graft and femoro femoral bypass. *J Vasc Surg* **25:** 165–172, 1997
11. The UK Small Aneurysm Trial Participants. Results for randomised controlled trial of early elective surgery or ultrasonographic surveillance for small abdominal aortic aneurysms. *Lancet* **352:** 1649–1660, 1998
12. Berridge DC, Chamberlain J, Guy AJ, Lambert D on behalf of the Northern Vascular Surgeons Group: Prospective audit of abdominal aortic aneurysm surgery in the northern region from 1988 to 1992. *Br J Surg* **82:** 906–910, 1995
13. D'Angelo J, Pappalo D, Farber A *et al.*: Is preoperative cardiac evaluation for abdominal aortic aneurysm repair necessary? *J Vasc Surg* **25:** 152–156, 1997
14. Höltzenbein J, Kretschmer G, Glanzl R *et al.*: Endovascular abdominal aortic aneurysm treatment: Expensive prestige or economic alternative? *Eur J Vasc Endovasc Surg* **14:** 265–272, 1997
15. White GH, May J: Failure of endovascular repair of abdominal aortic aneurysms: endoleak, adverse events and grading of technical difficulty. In: Greenhalgh RM (Ed), *The Durability of Vascular and Endovascular Surgery*. London: WB Saunders, 1999
16. Streiner DL, Norman GR: *Health Measurement Scales: A Practical Guide to Their Development and Use*. Oxford: Oxford University Press, 1989
17. Ware JE, Sherbourne CD: The MOS 36-item short-form health survery (SF-36): conceptual framework and item selection. *Med Care* **30:** 473–483, 1992
18. Garratt AM, Ruta DA, Abdalla MI *et al.*: The SF-36 health survey questionnaire: an outcome measure suitable for routine use within the NHS? *Br Med J* **306:** 1440–1444, 1993
19. Ruta DA, Abdalla MI, Garratt AM, Russell IT: The SF-36 health survey questionnaire: reliability in patient populations. *Qual Hlth Care* **3:** 180–185, 1994
20. Garratt AM, Russell IT, Abdalla MI: The SF-36 health survery questionnaire: responsiveness to changes in health status in four common clinical conditions. *Qual Hlth Care* **3:** 186–192, 1994
21. The EuroQol Group. EuroQol – a new facility for the measurement of health-related quality of life. *Hlth Policy* **16:** 199–208, 1990
22. Ruta DA, Garratt AM, Leng M *et al.*: A new approach to the measurement of quality of life – the patient-generated index. *Med Care* **11:** 1109–1126, 1991
23. Drummond MF: *Economic Analysis Alongside Clinical Trials*. London: Department of Health, 1994
24. Torgerson DJ, Spencer A: Marginal costs and benefits. *Br Med J* **312:** 35–36, 1996
25. Campbell MK, Torgerson DJ: Confidence intervals for cost-effectiveness ratios: the use of bootstrapping. *J Hlth Serv Res Pol* **2:** 1997

The Dutch Randomized Endovascular Aneurysm Management (DREAM) Trial

Jan D Blankensteijn

GRANT GIVING BODY

The Dutch Fund for Investigative Medicine is the grant giving body of the Dutch Health Insurance Council. It is the largest sponsor of clinical research in the Netherlands. The Health Insurance Council uses this fund to obtain cost-effectiveness data from randomized trials evaluating new therapies in medicine.

APPLICATION HISTORY

In 1995, the first application for the Dutch Randomized Endovascular Aneurysm Management (DREAM) trial was submitted. At this time, only one endovascular (tube) device was commercially available (EVT, Endovascular Technologies, Menlo Park, Calif. USA). The primary endpoint was operative mortality and endovascular surgery was expected to bring it down from 7% to 0.5%. The application was rejected, as the device was considered too experimental. Indeed, the initial EVT device ran into hook break issues in January 1995. In addition, the inclusion rate was considered too low to run a randomized trial with tube grafts only.

In the following years, three more applications were rejected for reasons related to the experimental nature of the procedure. In January 1998, the fifth application was submitted. This time the trial would include any commercially available device, which was both CE-marked (for European Union approval) and Food and Drug Administration – Investigational Device Exemption (FDA-IDE) labelled. Now, the primary endpoint was a combined operative mortality and morbidity, to be reduced from 20% in open surgery to 10% in conventional surgery. The trial was again rejected because the Health Insurance Council believed that too many devices in the trial would dilute the data. It took another three submissions of the trial to get the Council to approve more than two devices to be included. This January 1999 application has now been granted 1.9 million Euro.

THE DREAM TRIAL

The DREAM trial is a randomized multicentre study of elective treatment of an infrarenal abdominal aortic aneurysm. In this study, the cost-effectiveness of endovascular abdominal aortic aneurysm repair is compared with that of conventional, transabdominal surgery, in patients considered suitable for both types of treatment (ASA I-III). The primary endpoint is combined operative mortality and morbidity. Secondary endpoints and additional assessments include quality of life, length of hospital stay, and costs. A total of 400 patients will be randomized over a 1.5- to 2-year period.

REQUIREMENTS FOR PARTICIPATION

Requirements for devices to be included in the trial consist of the European CE-mark and Preliminary Market Approval (PMA) or IDE of the FDA.

The participating physicians and centres are required to comply with the guidelines for endovascular abdominal aortic aneurysm repair of the Endovascular Safety Committee of the Dutch Society for Vascular Surgery and the Dutch Society for Radiology. Specifically, surgeons and radiologists are required to co-operate in the trial. They must have passed their learning curve in endovascular abdominal aortic aneurysm repair (more than 20 procedures) and have their scrub nurses and radiology technicians specifically trained for the endovascular procedure. Furthermore, the participating centres are required to have a yearly volume of at least 30 conventional abdominal aortic aneurysm repairs, 10 endovascular abdominal aortic aneurysm repairs, and 50 endovascular procedures (i.e. PTA, stent placement).

Any configuration of endovascular abdominal aortic aneurysm treatment is allowed including tube, bifurcated, and mono-iliac devices, extension cuffs, and suprarenal fixation according to the preference of the investigator.

TRIAL EXECUTION

Pending approval of the budget, the steering committee is currently setting up the organizational structure of the trial. A device and centre selection committee will be installed. The trial is anticipated to start mid-2000.

After a 5-year struggle to get the necessary funds, it has come to the attention of the primary investigator that many co-applicants have lost their initial enthusiasm for a randomized trial. Nevertheless, the need for a randomized trial is still there. In addition, the Health Authority of the Dutch Government is now seeking to enforce the self-regulating ability of the Vascular Surgery and Interventional Radiology profession in the Netherlands. It has categorized endovascular abdominal aortic aneurysm repair an experimental treatment modality that should only be applied in centres of excellence, in the context of a carefully controlled, clinical investigation. The DREAM trial is a prototype for such a study. Although the Dutch Department of Health has the ability legally to restrict new treatment modalities to certain centres, it is hoped that vascular surgeons and interventional radiologists will self-regulate and prevent unlimited expansion of endovascular abdominal aortic aneurysm repair at this stage.

CONCLUSION

The DREAM trial will provide patients with safe and controlled introduction of a new technology, the medical community with valid scientific knowledge on the merits of endovascular abdominal aortic aneurysm repair, the government with a blueprint for centralized health care in vascular surgery, and the Health Insurance Council with cost-effectiveness data on this new therapy for Dutch health care.

Abdominal aortic aneurysms – surgical versus endoluminal repair: the French prospective randomized (ACE) trial

Jean-Pierre Becquemin, Alexandre D'audiffret, for the ACE Trialists

INTRODUCTION

Currently, a randomized trial (TEAM) is underway in France to compare the endovascular approach with conventional surgery in high risk patients; whatever the results, this study will not provide evidence of the superiority of one approach versus the other in patients with abdominal aortic aneurysms and acceptable surgical risks. Thus it was decided to conduct a randomized prospective trial to establish the potential benefit and long-term results of this approach. The study was designed by a group of vascular surgeons, interventional radiologists, methologists and specialists in health economics and will be supported financially by the PHRC (Programme Hôpitalier de Recherche Clinique, section of the Ministry of Health).

STUDY DESIGN

The ACE project (**A**neurysme de l'aorte abdominal: **C**hirurgie versus **E**ndoprothèse) is a French multicentre prospective randomized trial designed to compare the 30-day mortality, the 2-year mortality, the postoperative, and follow-up morbidity between conventional surgical and endoluminal repair. A total of 1120 patients will be enrolled over a 3-year period and followed for 2 years. The figure has been determined by statistical analysis based on an overall surgical mortality of 5.8%, and a mortality of 1.5% in the endovascular group.

Centres selection

Each participating team will consist of at least one vascular surgeon and one interventional radiologist with experience of various endovascular techniques and having participated in at least ten endoprostheses deployments (five as a first assistant and five as the principal surgeon). Furthermore, the selected centre should guarantee a recruitment of at least 15 aneurysms a year and benefit from a surgical mortality inferior to 7% for conventional non-emergent surgical repair.

Patient selection

Patients between 50 and 90 years old with a non-ruptured abdominal aortic aneurysm greater or equal to 50 mm and belonging to class 1 or 2 of the SVS/ISCVS[1] operative risk classification meeting the following anatomical criteria:

- healthy upper aneurysmal neck equal or greater to 1.5 cm;
- end of the aneurysmal process at least 1.5 cm proximal to one of the common iliac bifurcation;
- no significant superior mesenteric artery stenosis;
- an angle less or equal to 80% of the iliac arteries and aneurysmal neck;
- external iliac arteries greater than 6 mm in diameter.

Patients with severely angulated, heavy calcified, thrombotic or aneurysmal upper neck and with aneurysms involving both hypogastric arteries will be excluded.

Preoperative evaluation
Patients will be selected following:

- clinical examination with assessment of the surgical risks according to the SVS/ISCVS;
- assessment of the anatomical features by arteriography with a graduated catheter and abdominal CT scan;
- informed consent signed.

The completed patient's file will then be submitted to the core lab for the final approval.

Choice of endoprostheses

Graft deterioration has been reported with some early endoprosthesis, although there is no evidence that the current type of endoprosthesis may influence results. Thus, the choice of endoprosthesis will be left to the preference of the involved team according to availability and experience. However, only commercially available grafts with the CE (European Union approval) mark will be permitted, and implanted grafts will be scrutinized by a safety committee. The grant from the Ministry of Health will not cover the purchase of the devices. Currently, devices are brought by each hospital, within a global budget. In private centres grafts are not reimbursed, and negotiations with the Social Security Department are going on to obtain funds.

Follow-up

Follow-up visits will be scheduled at 1, 6, 12, and 24 months and consist of a clinical examination and a duplex-scan study. In addition patients randomized in the endovascular arm of the study will undergo a computed tomography (CT) scan with contrast. If an endoleak is detected, a CT scan will be performed 3 months later in order to assess the need for further intervention. A plain abdominal X-ray will also be performed at the same interval to assess the metallic structure of the prosthesis.

Clinical and imaging data will be compiled and sent to a committee consisting of independent experts responsible for the proper conduct of the trial and analysis of critical events.

Endpoints

The primary endpoint is the 30-day mortality. Secondary endpoints are 30-day morbidity and 2-year mortality. As well, all complications, re-intervention, and conversion during the follow-up will be computed. In patients treated by endovascular techniques, the evolution of the aneurysmal sac and of the prosthesis will be followed. Finally, total costs and quality of life will be compared in both groups.

RANDOMIZATION PROCESS AND GENERAL ORGANIZATION

Patient inclusion will be determined in each investigation centre by the vascular surgeon, the interventional radiologist, and the anaesthesia team. The patient's chart, CT-scan and angiogram will be subsequently transmitted to the co-ordination centre for final approval and randomization. To avoid selection bias, any good risk patient treated for abdominal aortic aneurysm and not included in the study will be recorded in a separate register.

In order to guarantee the quality of this study, a number of committees will be created:

- Scientific committee: function as the co-ordination nucleus.
- Centre selection committee (lists of centres already approved).
- Committee responsible for endpoints validation (consisting of independent experts).
- Committee for adverse events.
- Committee for the imaging studies.
- Committee responsible for the proper progress of the study.

STATISTICS AND DATABASE MANAGEMENT

All data will be gathered and verified by the co-ordination centre (University of Creteil, Paris Val de Marne). Results will be analysed on an 'intent to treat' basis. Primary and secondary endpoints will be compared by χ^2 for qualitative variables and *t*-tests or ANOVA tests for quantitative variables. Survival curves will be compared using Log–Rank tests. Additional logistic regression will be performed in order to assess the influence of prognostic factors on the type of intervention.

PLANNING OF STUDY

Final approvement of grant application should be released by the end of November 1999. Randomization should start somewhere between June and September 2000.

REFERENCE

1. Hollier LH, Taylor LM, Oschner J: Recommended indications for operative treatment of abdominal aortic aneurysms. Report of subcommittee of the joint council of the Society for Vascular Surgery and the North American chapter of the International Society for Cardiovascular Surgery. *J Vasc Surg* **15**; 1046–1056, 1992

Eurostar: the need to audit new generations of devices separately

Peter L Harris

INTRODUCTION: THE EUROSTAR REGISTRY

The Eurostar Project was launched in 1996 with the objective of collating information on the results of endovascular treatment of abdominal aortic aneurysms. Because the efficacy of the new technology of intra-aortic stent-grafting was, and remains, unproven, it was considered essential to recruit as many patients as possible, as quickly as possible in order to develop a database large enough to allow conclusions to be drawn within the shortest possible time. Achievement of this objective necessitated a large scale multicentred international study. In most European countries access to endovascular devices has been less restricted than in other parts of the world, most notably the United States of America, and for this reason Europe represented a very suitable setting for such a study.

By August 1990 a total of 1930 patients had been registered by 73 physicians in 14 European countries. An analysis of the aggregated database is published twice yearly and is available without restriction to all interested parties. The analysis includes the following:

1. preoperative details of the patients and the anatomical characteristics of their aneurysms;
2. the types of devices used;
3. complications encountered intraoperatively;
4. outcome of the procedure as judged by angiography on completion;
5. 30-day mortality and complication rates;
6. long-term results as determined by examination clinically and by contrast enhanced tomography at 1, 3, 6, 9, and 12 months after operation and at yearly intervals thereafter.

The follow-up information includes all adverse events and the frequency and indications for secondary intervention.

PROBLEMS OF COMPARATIVE ANALYSIS: TECHNICAL EVOLUTION/CLINICAL EVALUATION 'LAG-TIME'

The registry provides very reliable information about procedural complication rates, the relative performance of different devices in terms of complications encountered during deployment including intraoperative endoleaks and conversion rates.

However, comparison between first, second and subsequent generations of endovascular devices in terms of their longer term performance poses considerable problems due to the short duration of follow-up of the newer devices. Inevitably the analysis of the aggregated database is influenced by the results associated with early generations of devices of which there are larger numbers followed up for longer periods of time. It is unavoidable that scientific analysis of results will lag behind the 'cutting edge' of the new technology because of the time necessary for clinical evaluation.

THE NEED FOR COMPARATIVE STUDIES

There are important differences between devices, in terms of their structure and their mode of deployment, that make it essential to evaluate them individually and to compare their performance in clinical practice. This process is integral to progressive evolution of design and technology as applied to aortic endografts. Validation in the clinical setting of the responses of device manufacturers to any observed shortcomings of earlier generations of endograft is similarly important.

The number of different types of devices and their diversity of structure and design are increasing progressively making the task of comparative analysis ever more difficult.

TYPES OF DEVICE INCLUDED IN THE EUROSTAR STUDY

The Eurostar Registry was established to monitor the results of commercially manufactured endografts with a CE mark indicating that they had been approved for clinical application in the European Union. Registration of patients treated with homemade devices constructed on site was discouraged and these will not be considered in this analysis.

Devices can be ordered arbitrarily into four different generations according to the time of their introduction into the market or their present status in preparation for marketing as shown in Table 1. In August 1999 there were seven different devices that had been deployed in more than 50 patients registered on the Eurostar database as shown in Table 2. This table also shows the mean duration of follow-up of the patients with these different devices. At this time Stentor and Vanguard devices accounted for 62% of the total and more than 90% of those with a follow-up of more than 1 year. Stentor and Vanguard devices therefore, predominantly influence analysis of the aggregated database for outcomes at 1 year and beyond.

A classification of devices in terms of their structure (modular or one-piece), type of stent (balloon or self-expanding, fully or partially stented), mechanism of fixation, the materials from which they are constructed, and introducer-systems is highly relevant in the context of comparative analysis. Evaluation of these specific design features may be as informative as that of individual devices.

Of the devices included on the Eurostar database all except the Ancure (Endovascular Technologies) are modular in construction. Ancure is a one-piece

Table 1. Commercially manufactured devices for endovascular aortic aneurysm repair

1st Generation
Stentor (Mintec)
2nd Generation
Vanguard (Boston Scientific Corp.)
Ancure (Endovascular Technologies)
AneuRx (Medtronic)
Talent (World Medical)
Stentford (Stentford)
3rd Generation
Zenith (Cook)
LIFEPATH (Baxter)
4th Generation
Excluder (Gore)
Endologics (Bard)
Cordis (Cordis)
Anaconda (Sulzer/Vascutec)

Table 2. The number of different endovascular devices for aortic aneurysm repair included in the Eurostar database and their mean duration of follow-up

	No. of patients	*Mean follow-up (months)*
Stentor	333	11.15
Vanguard	826	7.16
AneuRx	285	4.3
Talent	228	4.2
Zenith	69	2.0
Ancure	55	6.1
Excluder	51	1.6
Other	24	4.2

bifurcated graft that has been constructed to mimic, as closely as possible, a conventionally sutured aortic graft. Standard gauge Dacron material is used whereas ultrathin fabrics are employed in other devices.

Metallic components

There is considerable variation in the structure of the metallic framework of the different devices. Stentor, Vanguard, AneuRx and Excluder endografts are all fully stented. This provides good column strength that is said to improve the stability of the device and reduce the risk of stent migration. In Stentor and Vanguard endografts the metallic frame is on the inside whereas in the AneuRx and Excluder devices the metallic frame is external. Talent and Zenith endografts are supported by interrupted circumferential stents. These provide hoop strength but very little columnar strength. In the Talent endograft thin longitudinal metallic strips have been incorporated to provide column strength. The Ancure graft is completely devoid of stents apart from those at the proximal and distal fixation sites. The stents in all of the devices that have been included in the Eurostar database to date are self-expanding, although a balloon is used in the Ancure system to help the fixation hooks penetrate the aortic wall, and soft latex balloons are used in the other devices for 'moulding' purposes. The LIFEPATH endograft (Baxter) employs balloon-expanded stents. This device has become available in Europe only recently and the number included in the Eurostar registry, to date, is small.

Mechanism of fixation

The Ancure endograft, which has no intrinsic columnar strength, relies on hooks at both proximal and distal fixation sites to maintain stability of the device. Stentor, Vanguard, Zenith and Excluder endografts all have small barbs to assist their fixation. The AneuRx and Talent devices rely on column strength, alone, to prevent migration.

Materials used for construction

With the exception of the Ancure endograft specially adapted thin-wall fabrics are used for the construction of aortic endografts in order to minimize their bulk and the diameter of the introducer-system. The Excluder and Endologic devices are constructed from polytetrafluoroethylene (PTFE) whereas Dacron is the fabric component of all other devices. In currently available endografts the metal frame is constructed either from nitinol or stainless steel.

Introducer-systems

The technique for the deployment of most modular grafts is very similar. There are, however, some minor variations. The AneuRx system incorporates a 'fishing reel' gadget that facilitates smooth and controlled deployment of the endograft. The Excluder device utilizes a unique 'jacket' constructed from PTFE to reduce the bulk and increase the flexibility of the system. Once in position the device itself deploys very rapidly when the cord lacing the 'jacket' is withdrawn.

AGGREGATED EUROSTAR RESULTS

Operative procedure and results to 30 days[1]

The endovascular device was deployed successfully in 1886 (97.7%) of the 1930 procedures registered with Eurostar. Risk factors for failure to complete the procedure included an aneurysm diameter in excess of 60 mm and the need for adjuvant procedures.

The 30-day mortality was 2.1%. Significant risk factors for perioperative death were ASA (American Society of Anesthesiologists) grade III and IV, patients considered to be unfit for open repair and a requirement for adjuvant procedures.

Systemic complications occurred within the first 30 days of operation in 126 patients (8.6%). Complications of this type occurred significantly more frequently in patients aged over 75 years, in those with impaired cardiac function and in those who were considered to be unfit for conventional surgery.

The incidence of endoleak on the completion angiogram was found in 16.7%. However, computed tomographic imaging at 1 month identified an endoleak in only 10% and it is assumed that the remainder closed spontaneously. Independent risk factors for intraoperative endoleaks were female gender, age over 75 years, and an aneurysm diameter in excess of 60 mm.

The overall technical success rate as defined by the Ad Hoc Committee of the Society for Vascular Surgery and the International Society for Cardiovascular Surgery[2] was 72%. Minor additional endovascular procedures to facilitate access and to correct intraoperative endoleaks accounted for most of the 'failures'.

Intermediate and long-term results

The cumulative survival rate following operation for the total population of patients is shown in Fig. 1. At 3 years it was 82.6%.

To date rupture of the aneurysm following endovascular repair has been reported in 14 Eurostar patients with a fatal outcome in nine (85.6%). In addition another 31 patients have required late conversion to open repair, and in these patients the mortality rate was 19%. The rate of rupture approximates to 1.5% per annum and the conversion rate to twice this figure. These are incontrovertibly 'hard endpoints' that signify that there is a small, but significant risk of treatment failure following endovascular aneurysm repair.

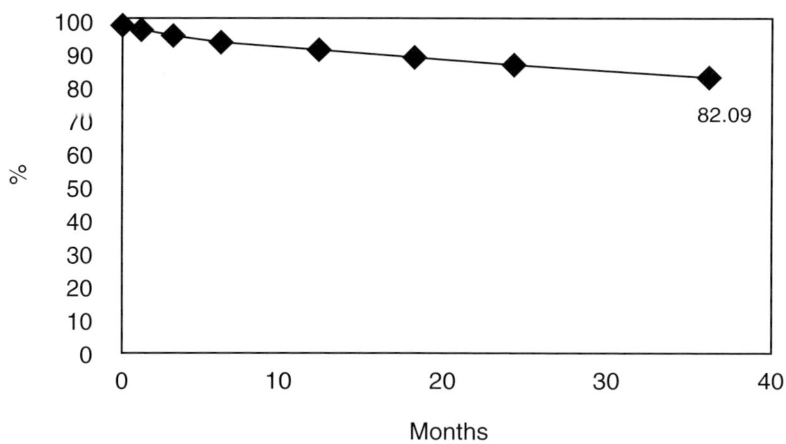

Fig. 1. Eurostar Registry: Cumulative survival of the total patient population for endovascular repair of abdominal aortic aneurysms.

The cumulative rate of freedom from endoleak is shown in Fig. 2. It can be seen that new endoleaks are detected at a steady rate of approximately 20% per year, at least for the first 3 years. However, the cumulative proportion of patients free from persistent endoleak at 3 years is 88%. This would suggest that most late endoleaks are resolved satisfactorily by secondary intervention. It is of interest to note that secondary endoleaks arise primarily from either the distal fixation site or from the body of the device. Studies carried out in Liverpool and elsewhere have shown that changes in stent-graft and vessel morphology are important factors in the causation of late endoleaks[3] (Fig. 4).

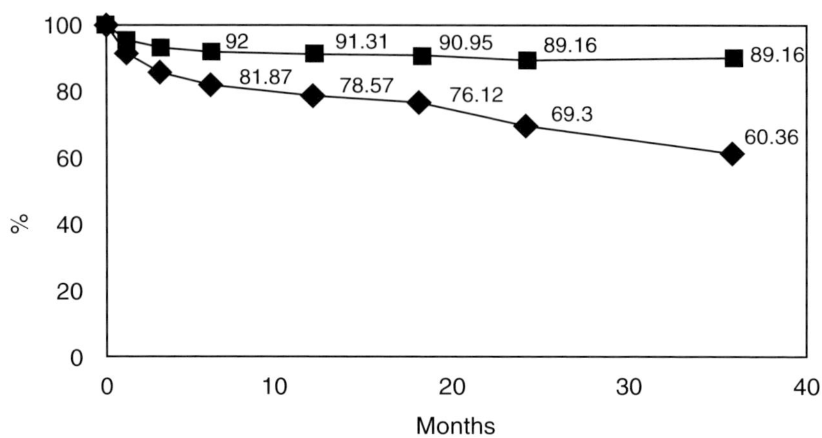

Fig. 2. Eurostar Registry. Cumulative rates of endoleak (lower curve) and persistent endoleak (upper curve).

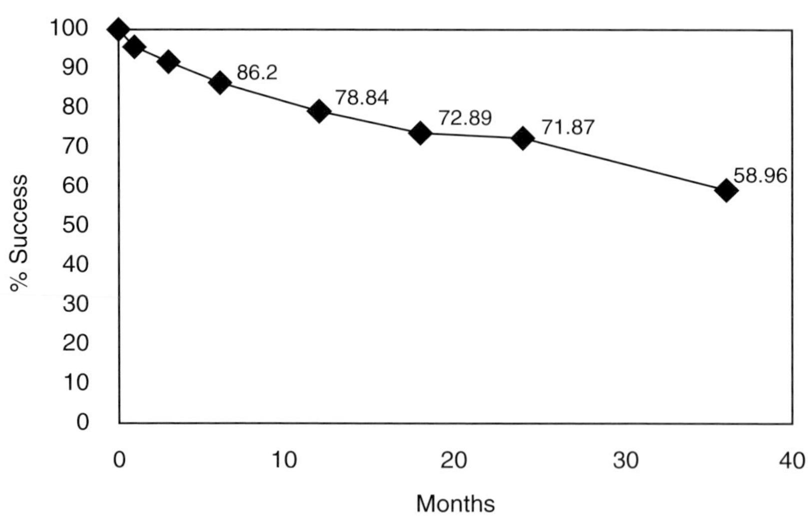

Fig. 3. Eurostar Registry. Cumulative rate of survival and freedom from secondary intervention combined.

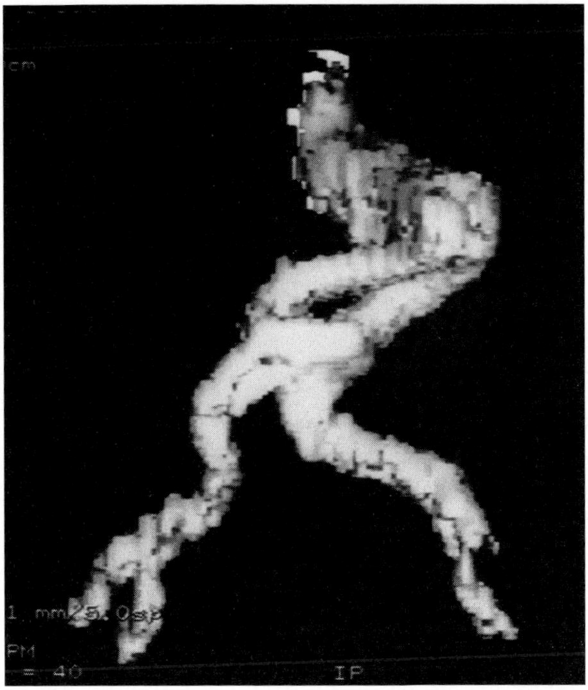

Fig. 4. Three-dimensional reconstruction from helical computed tomography scan of aortic endograft (Vanguard, Boston Scientific Corporation) showing distortion and secondary distal type I endoleak.

Although it has been established that there is a relationship between the presence or absence of an endoleak and continuing expansion or contraction of the aneurysm sac, it is also becoming apparent that this relationship is inconstant. Analysis of Eurostar data shows that the aneurysm sac continued to expand in 36% of patients in whom no endoleak had been detected. Conversely the aneurysm sac was seen to contract in 18% of patients in whom an endoleak had been detected. The significance of this finding is that reliance upon the detection of an endoleak as a guide to the eventual outcome of the operation is unsafe. In other words the absence of an endoleak does not equal treatment success.[4] It is pressure or endotension within the aneurysm sac that causes it to expand, and it is now very clear that endotension may exist in the absence of a detectable endoleak. Until techniques are evolved to measure endotension within the sac non-invasively, morphological changes in the aneurysm itself represent the only reliable means for predicting failure of treatment. One-third of all patients registered with Eurostar required some form of secondary intervention within 3 years. The combined figure for cumulative rate of survival and freedom from secondary intervention was 59% at 3 years (Fig. 3). The majority of secondary interventions were relatively minor endovascular procedures. However, 31 patients required late conversion to open repair (see above).

DEVICE SPECIFIC COMPLICATIONS

Failure to complete the procedure

Failure to complete the endovascular procedure was reported in 2.3% of Eurostar patients necessitating conversion to an open operation. Multivariant analysis showed that the diameter of the aneurysm was the only anatomical variable that had an adverse independent correlation with this complication. However, two specific devices had a significant negative influence. There were 9.6% failures to complete the procedure in patients receiving Ancure (EVT) endografts and 7.5% in those receiving Talent endografts as opposed to 1.6% with all other devices combined and these differences were statistically significant.[1] Deployment of the Ancure device is considered by many to be more complicated that that of most other devices and this may be a factor. However, many of the Ancure devices in the Eurostar Registry were implanted between 1994 and 1996 and these constitute a relatively early experience of the endovascular approach to aortic aneurysm repair. Latest modifications to the introducer-system for the Ancure device make them easier to use than earlier models and lower complication rates have been reported. Analysis of the patient population shows that Talent endografts have tended to be deployed in patients with difficult vascular anatomy. Specifically they have been used to treat aneurysms with shorter and wider necks. This is because Talent endografts were originally offered in larger sizes than other types of device. A patient population at higher risk may explain the higher primary conversion rate associated with a Talent endograft rather than any deficiencies within the graft itself.

Changes in aneurysm and device morphology

Buckling and kinking of the endograft postoperatively has been observed most frequently in Stentor and Vanguard devices. However, these changes tend to develop 12 months or more after the operation, and, at present, there are far more Stentor and Vanguard endografts that have been exposed to this risk than any other device. Distortion of other types of endograft has certainly been observed, but it will be some time before it can be determined whether the incidence is similar to that seen with the earlier generations of device. In the meantime new prototypes of the Vanguard device that have been modified to make them resistant to deformation are under evaluation.

It is becoming apparent that aneurysms that have been effectively excluded from endotension diminish in size after operation. This contraction involves not only the transverse dimension, but also the length of the aneurysm. Studies in Liverpool have shown that postoperative distortion of endografts and complications arising as a result of this distortion are related to reduction in the longitudinal dimension of the aneurysm.[3] These studies were carried out upon patients who had received Stentor and Vanguard devices. However, it was recently reported that in patients who had received other types of device that no reduction occurred in the length of the aneurysm. This raises the possibility that the rate of contraction of an aneurysm postoperatively and, therefore, the effectiveness with which it has been excluded from endotension may be dependent upon the type of device used. If true this could have important implications for the future construction and design of endografts.

There is no evidence to suggest that intraoperative endoleaks occur more frequently with some devices than others. At present it is too soon to draw conclusions about later complications including new endoleak, stent-graft migration, device limb thrombosis and delayed rupture and conversion, because of the disparity in the duration of follow-up of the different devices. However, it will be of great practical interest to see whether any correlation between these complications and the type of device used becomes apparent as the Eurostar database matures.

CONCLUSIONS

Endovascular repair is a relatively new technique, for the treatment of aortic aneurysms, that is still undergoing a process of technological evolution and clinical evaluation. The first of these is very heavily dependent upon the second. Comparative evaluation of the performance of the different types of device available is essential to guide future advances in basic endovascular technologies and their appropriate application in clinical practice .

The Eurostar database confirms that endovascular aneurysm repair is a very successful strategy for the majority of the patients treated in the short and medium term. However, the data generated by Eurostar shows also that there is a small, but significant risk of failure with potentially disastrous consequences for the individuals concerned. Future evolution of stent-graft design and their clinical application should be directed towards reducing, if not eliminating, this risk.

Because there is an unavoidable time lag between the cutting edge of the technology and proper clinical evaluation, this process inevitably is slower than most physicians would like. Studies on a large scale, of which the Eurostar Registry is a good example, offer the best opportunity to provide the necessary information in the shortest possible time. As new endografts become available it is essential to maintain a high level of recruitment into these studies, in order that the relative merits and disadvantages of each can be evaluated.

EUROSTAR COLLABORATORS

Executive team

P L Harris, *Liverpool, UK*: **Chairman and Project Director**
V Riambau i Alonso, *Barcelona, Spain*: **Secretary and Southern European Coordinator**
J Buth, Eindhoven, *The Netherlands*: **Executive Director of the Data Registry Centre and Northern European Coordinator**
C Mialhe, *Draguignan, France*: **Membership Director**
J-P Becquemin, *Paris, France*: **Sponsorship Director**
L Norgren, *Lund, Sweden*: **Publications Director**
R Laheij, *Eindhoven, The Netherlands*: **Data Manager**

International Advisory Steering Committee

R Baird, *Bristol, UK*
J Blankensteijn, *Utrecht, The Netherlands*
U Blum, *Freiberg, Germany*
P Cao, *Perugia, Italy*
R Edwards, *Glasgow, UK*
G Kretschmer, *Vienna, Austria*

A Nevelstein, *Leuven, Belgium*
F Moll, *Nieuwegein, The Netherlands*
H Myhre, *Trondheim, Norway*
W Stelter, *Frankfurt, Germany*

Collaborators
H R Dopp, *Groningen, The Netherlands*
Dr van Dijk, Heiloo, *The Netherlands*
Dr Chalabli, *Aachen, Germany*
Prof. Michalak, *Lublin, Poland*
Dr Moll van Otterlo, *Den Haag, The Netherlands*
Dr Sambeek, *Rotterdam, The Netherlands*
Prof. Shanik, *Dublin, Ireland*
Dr Uberoi, *Gateshead, UK*
Dr Schroe, *Genk, Belgium*
Dr Barendrecht, *Nijmegen, The Netherlands*
Dr van Overhagen, *Den Haag, The Netherlands*
Dr van Elst, *St Truiden, Belgium*
Dr de Vries, *Arnheim, The Netherlands*
Prof. van der Ham, *Rotterdam, The Netherlands*
Dr Abbott, *Chester, UK*
Dr Massin, *Gilly, Belgium*
Dr Odink, *Heerlen , The Netherlands*
Dr Verhelst, *Brussels, Belgium*
Dr Voshage, *Hanover, Germany*
Dr de Smet, *Rotterdam, The Netherlands*
Dr Berg, *Luxembourg, Luxembourg*
Prof. Maurer, *Munich, Germany*
Prof. Dondelinger, *Liege, Belgium*
Dr Johnsen, *Hamburg, Germany*
Prof. Eikelboom, *Utrecht, The Netherlands*
Dr van Iersel, *Doetinchem, The Netherlands*
Mr. Darke, *Bournemouth, UK*
Prof. Klempa, *Bremen, Germany*
Dr Stabel, *Turnhout, Belgium*
Dr Wisselink, *Amsterdam, The Netherlands*
Dr Vermassen, *Gent, Belgium*
Dr Kasper, *Cologne, Germany*
Dr Pamler, *Ulm, Germany*
Prof. Sievert, *Frankfurt, Germany*
Dr Swedenborg, *Stockholm, Sweden*
Prof. Van Bockel, *Leiden, The Netherlands*
Dr Kasprzak, *Regensburg, Germany*
Dr Kolvenbach, *Dusseldorf, Germany*
Prof. Loeprecht, *Augsberg, Germany*
Dr Bender, *Veldhoven, The Netherlands*
Prof. Kvernebo, *Oslo, Norway*
Dr Geelkerken, *Enschede, The Netherlands*
Dr Veihofer, *Bonn, Germany*
Mr Scott, *Leeds, UK*
Dr Ettler, *Hull, UK*
Dr Jivegard, *Gothenberg, Sweden*
Dr Bleyn, *Antwerp, Belgium*
Dr Kranendonk, *Tilberg, The Netherlands*
Dr Possiers, *Bonheiden, Belgium*
Dr Ashleigh, *Manchester, UK*

Mr R Taylor, *London , UK*
Mr P Taylor, *London, UK*
Dr Tordoir, *Maastricht, The Netherlands*
Dr Enzler, *Zurich, Switzerland*
Dr Balm, *Amsterdam, The Netherlands*
Mr Wyatt, *Newcastle, UK*
Mr Wolfe, *London, UK*
Prof. Kroeze, *Oslo, Norway*
Prof. Betzler, *Essen-Ruttenscheid, Germany*
Dr Hamming, *Tilberg, The Netherlands*
Prof. Allenberg, *Heidelberg, Germany*
Dr von Duber, *Mainz, Germany*
Prof. van Vliet, *Nijmegen, The Netherlands*
Dr Cairols, *Barcelona, Spain*
Prof. Fernandes e Fernandes, *Lisbon, Portugal*
Dr Scoccianti, *Rome, Italy*
Dr Meaulle, *Grenoble, France*
Dr Vasseur, *Lille, France*
Prof. Favre, *St Etienne, France*
Prof. Rousseau, *Toulouse, France*
Prof. Kreitmann, *St Laurent du Var, France*
Dr Marzella, *Nanterre, France*
Dr Age, *Lyon, France*
Dr Giraud, *Toulouse, France*
Prof. Gaux, *Paris, France*
Dr Magne, *Grenoble, France*
Prof. Marty-Ane, *Montpellier, France*
Prof. Cossio, *Madrid, Spain*
Prof. Balas, *Athens, Greece*
Dr Criado, *Madrid, Spain*
Dr Orron, *Tel Aviv, Israel*
Dr Cardon, *Nimes, France*
Dr Tagarro, *Madrid, Spain*
Dr Sanchez-Coll, *Madrid, Spain*
Prof. Morach, *Tel Aviv, Israel*
Dr Amicabile, *Nancy, France*
Dr de Blas, *Tenerife, Spain*
Dr Coppi, *Modena, Italy*

REFERENCES

1. Buth J, Laheij RJF on behalf of the Eurostar collaborators: Early complications and endoleaks after endovascular abdominal aortic aneurysm repair. Report of a multicentre study. *J Vasc Surg* **31**: 134–146, 2000
2. Ahn SS, Rutherford RB, Johnston KW *et al.*: Reporting standards for infrarenal endovascular abdominal aortic aneurysm repair. *J Vasc Surg* **25**: 405–410, 1997
3. Harris PL, Brennan J, Martin J *et al.*: Longitudinal shrinkage following endovascular aneurysm repair: a source of intermediate and late complications. *J Endovasc Surg* **6**: 11–16, 1999
4. Gilling-Smith GL, Martin J, Sudhindran S *et al.*: Freedom from endoleak after endovascular aneurysm repair does not equal treatment success. *Eur J Vasc Endovasc Surg* (in press)
5. Singh-Ranger R, McArthur T, Lees W, Adiseshiah M: Abdominal aortic aneurysms: Sac diameters shrink but their lengths increase after endovascular repair (abstract). Presentation to the European Society for Vascular Surgery. Copenhagen 1999.

Endoluminal building of the aortic grafts for abdominal aortic aneurysm disease

Michael MD Lawrence-Brown, James B Semmens, Brendan M Stanley, Kurt Liffman, Ahn Bui, Murray Rudman, David E Hartley

INTRODUCTION

Age is the greatest risk factor for aortic aneurysmal disease. The aging, healthier population presents a different spectrum of diseases. Education, communication and technology changes bring with them an increasing demand on an expectation of health services. Higher quality, durable, minimally invasive and pain-free interventions are now becoming the norm. These are the factors that have driven endoluminal grafting for abdominal aortic aneurysm.[1] The highly invasive, painful open surgery for abdominal aortic aneurysms, accompanied by its long recovery period will be avoided where possible by those undergoing prophylactic repair of aneurysms which are or will be posing a threat to life or limb.[2]

There has been a progressive evolution of devices and endoluminal grafts for aortic and iliac aneurysmal disease through the 1990s. Initially, straight tube grafts were used in the aorta (Fig. 1a).[3] Grafts of varying diameter were then used through the aorta and into the iliac vessels to accommodate for length assessment problems which are exaggerated by the tortuosity resulting from the lengthening of the arteries when they become aneurysmal (Fig. 1b). The aortouni-iliac grafts were soon replaced by aortobi-iliac (bifurcated) grafts because of the desire to preserve normal anatomy; with the added bonus of eliminating a substantial open procedure (Fig. 1c).[1,4–6]

Two-piece aorto-iliac grafts formed the basic unit for endoluminal repair. Extension pieces were added,to the iliac limbs to treat short-falls in the design or accompanying iliac aneurysmal disease. Extension pieces have also been added to the proximal end of endoluminal grafts, usually for the purpose of correcting a deployment error, or bolstering the support to counter an endoleak. Standard three-piece units are replacing the two piece modules because they better lend themselves to addressing length assessment problems, and for storing 'off the shelf' modules (Fig. 1d). The development and use of fenestrated grafts (Fig. 1e) paves the way for major vessel preservation.

THORACIC ABDOMINAL ANEURYSMS

When the lower end of the thoracic abdominal aorta involves, or is close to, the coeliac axis, it presents a problem of fixation and seal. Initially it was feared that migration would be downward and essential visceral vessels would be occluded by

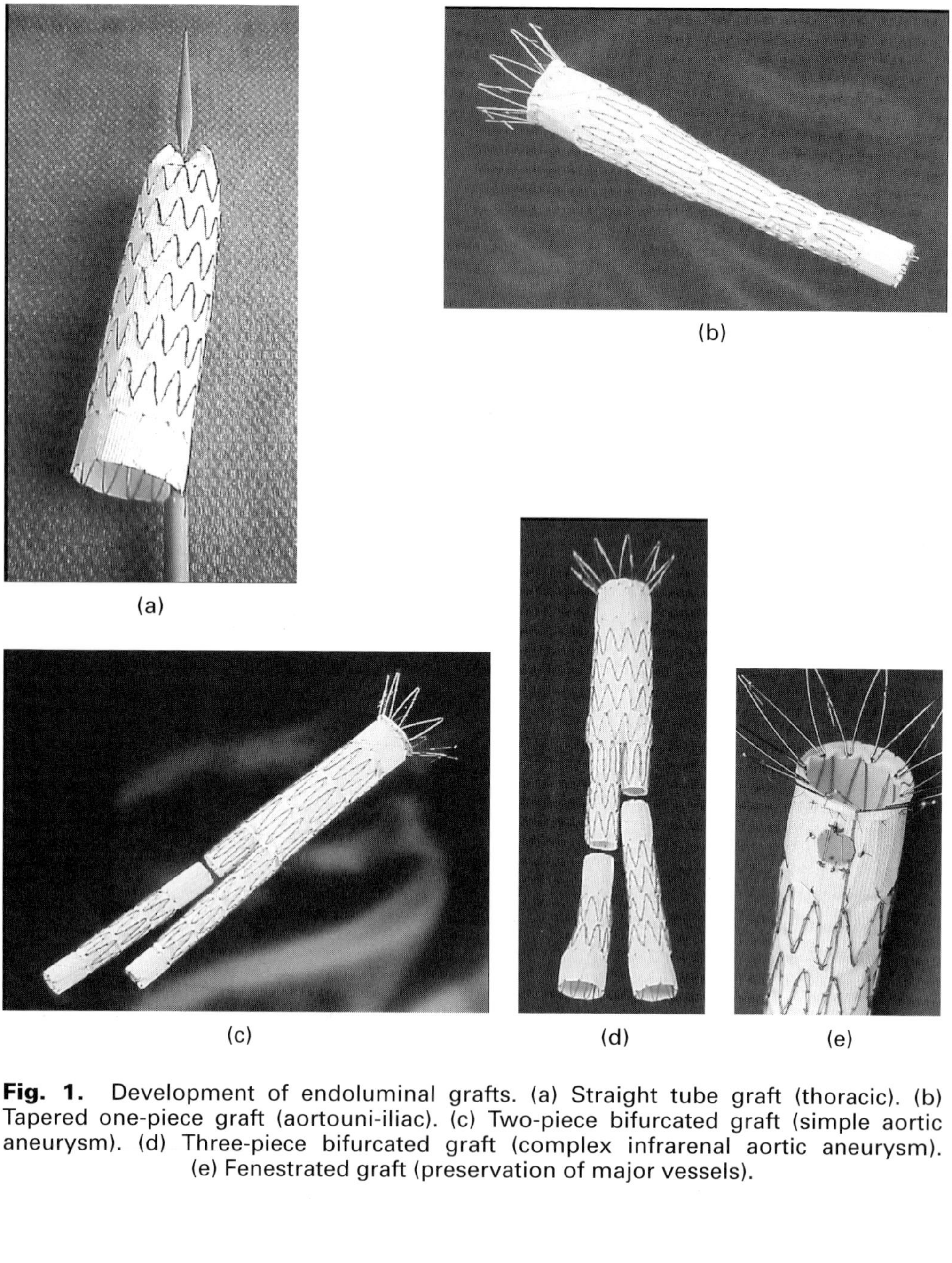

Fig. 1. Development of endoluminal grafts. (a) Straight tube graft (thoracic). (b) Tapered one-piece graft (aortouni-iliac). (c) Two-piece bifurcated graft (simple aortic aneurysm). (d) Three-piece bifurcated graft (complex infrarenal aortic aneurysm). (e) Fenestrated graft (preservation of major vessels).

the migrating graft. Further knowledge of how the forces work[7] suggests that the graft will lift out of the coeliac area with a resulting distal endoleak, repressurising the aneurysm. Initially this problem was addressed by a laparotomy, ligation and division of the coeliac axis at the origin, transaortic suture fixation of the graft and a re-inforced circumferential Dacron band (Fig. 2). Fenestration and stent fixation was

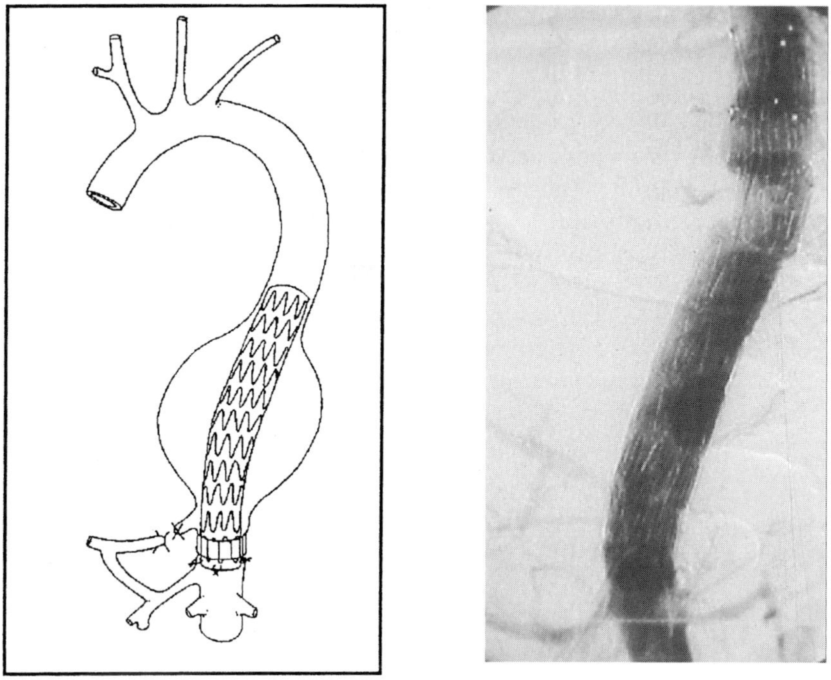

(a) (b)

Fig. 2. Endoluminal repair of thoracic aorta aneurysm including transaortic suture (five sutures) fixation of the graft and re-enforced circumferential Dacron band: (a) is a cartoon of the plane X-ray presented in (b).

the step required to eliminate the open part of the procedure and to achieve secure attachment. The combined open and endoluminal technique is shown in Fig. 2. Fixation of the thoracic graft with a fenestration and stent is discussed below (see Fig 6).

The two-piece and the three-piece systems are the start of the endoluminal building process. While much work is progressing towards treating infrarenal abdominal aortic aneurysms, work has also progressed to treat thoracic aortic aneurysmal disease. Initially single straight tubes were again used for the straightforward descending thoracic aneursym. Often the thoracic aortic aneurysm extends proximally and distally so that the normal aorta above and below the dilated portion is relatively short. Length assessment may be even more difficult in a thoracic aortic aneursym where the chamber is larger and the curve of the lie of the graft unpredictable. These length assessment difficulties are further complicated by complex curvatures in the dilated thoracic aorta.[7] Two-piece trombone grafts for thoracic aortic aneursyms are routinely used now, especially when careful placement of the distal end is required so as not to encroach upon the visceral or vessels.

ILIAC ARTERY INVOLVEMENT

At the lower end of the abdominal aorta, aneurysmal disease may extend along the common iliac artery and occasionally into the internal iliac artery. In our experience, the external iliac artery has never been involved in aneurysmal disease. The problem at this end is to endeavour to preserve the internal iliac artery, at least on one side, to preserve pelvic blood flow, and to make sure that the internal iliac artery does not retrograde fill an aneurysm cavity of the common iliac artery so as to constitute a risk of further iliac expansion, or flow back into a dominating aortic aneurysm. In the absence of mural thrombus in the common iliac artery, we routinely preserve the internal iliac artery if the diameter of the common artery is less than 25 mm, by constructing, or adding, a cuff to the base of the graft. The three-piece design enables close proximation of the graft to the internal iliac origin by the use of the trombone technique. Length assessment and accurate deployment in the iliac vessels requires

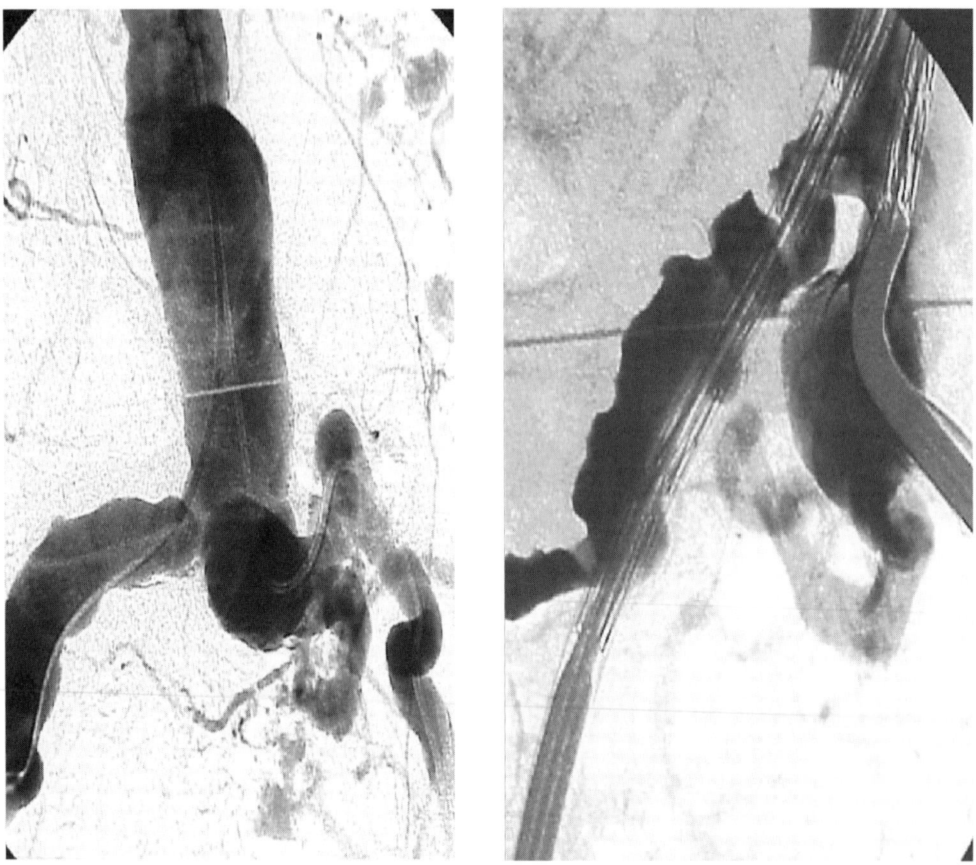

(a) (b)

Fig. 3. Tortuousity of the iliac arteries (a) with concertining of iliac vessels on the delivery device (b).

both care and skill. This is because of the tortuousity and actual length changes of the iliac vessels on the relatively stiff delivery system. Bunching of the vessel on the delivery device may occur, similar to knitting on a knitting needle. Herein is the requirement of skilful deployment by adjusting to the changing length. Special imaging techniques and contrast delivery is usually necessary (Figs 3a,b).

ADVENT OF THE FENESTRATED GRAFT

The routine treatment of the thoracic aorta, the infrarenal aorta and the iliac vessels with endoluminal grafting means that only the area across the visceral and renal vessels and across the arch of the aorta remain to be included. The advent of fenestrated grafts with preservation of flow into the orifices of essential vessels heralds the possibility of stent-grafting the whole of the aorta and the iliac systems.

Moving from a straight tube to a two-piece bifurcated system integrates from two dimensions to three dimensions. The need for control and accuracy of deployment of one module in order to accept the second becomes important. For aorto-iliac aneurysmal disease the necessity for accurate rotational deployment is not so critical and errors may be salvaged with good catheter skills and adjuvant interventional devices. For the preservation of the orifice of an essential vessel by the placement of fenestration in a covered graft over this orifice – the rotational accuracy is of paramount importance. The degree of accuracy demanded increases for every additional vessel preserved, both for the construction of the graft and its deployment.

The success of endoluminal grafting for infrarenal aneurysms relies on a complete durable seal in the neck of the aneurysm. When the walls of the neck are approximately parallel, the present recommendation is for a 20-mm long neck: this strict criteria, however, excludes many aneurysms from endoluminal repair. Even if the operator does not adhere to the criteria there comes a point at which no further compromise can be made. Asymmetry of the renal arteries or a significant lower pole vessel are ready examples of limited available neck which may otherwise be suitable. To overcome these problems, and increase the area of the attachment zone and seal, fenestrated grafts were developed. This has opened the door to link the thoracic and infrarenal domains.

The principles of fenestrating a graft to preserve renal or visceral vessels are based upon accurate planning and construction of the graft.[8] It also requires control and accuracy of deployment especially rotational manoeuvrability to allow exact positioning of the fenestration over the intended orifice. Accurate planning and construction requires high quality three-dimensional computerized tomography imaging and good angiography. Controlled and accurate positioning of the fenestrated system is based on partial deployment of the graft to allow rotational as well as caudal and cephalic movement to position the fenestration over the orifice of the target vessel. Once positioned and still partially deployed the vessel is cannulated from inside the graft through the fenestration into the vessel with a guidewire. The guidewire is then given added support with either a guide catheter or inflated rigid balloon; this then acts to track the fenestration down to its orifice on completing deployment of the graft. Further fixation of the orifice through the fenestration with a stent (covered or uncovered) prevents a change in the position of the main graft from the orifice or causes the orifice to move with the graft and parent artery as a unit.

The two systems, which allow partial deployment, will be described. The first method employs a fenestration in the body of the usual suprarenal fixation graft. Once the sheath has been retracted to open the short limb but prior to releasing the top cap containing the uncovered suprarenal fixation stents, the body is cannulated with a guidewire, which is then manipulated out through the fenestration into the target vessel. The top cap is then released to complete deployment (Fig. 4).

This group following bench modelling and animal experimentation reported the second method.[9] A posterior longitudinal column brings about this partial deployment where the graft has been infolded. The loose fold of Dacron is gathered and held together by a trigger wire threaded through the material in a lace fashion.

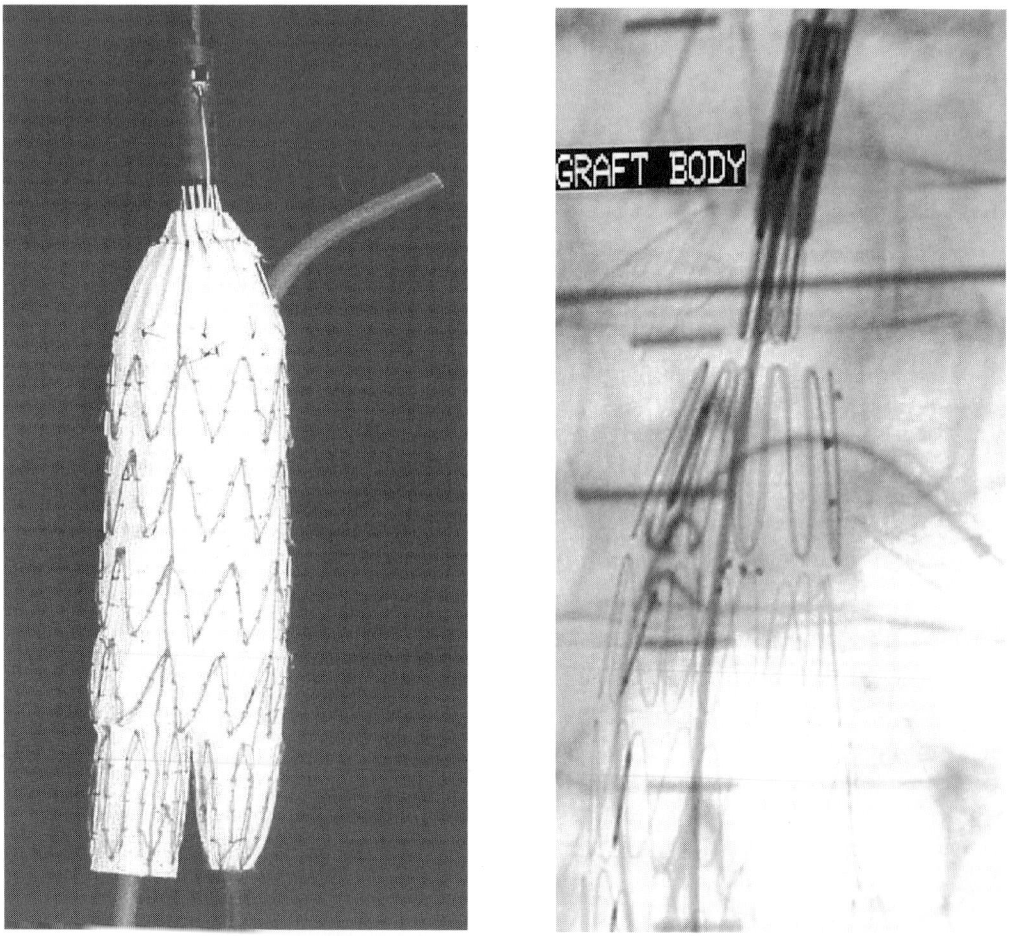

(a) (b)

Fig. 4. Aligning and deploying the fenestrated graft: fenestrated graft (a); plane X-ray of graft deployment (b).

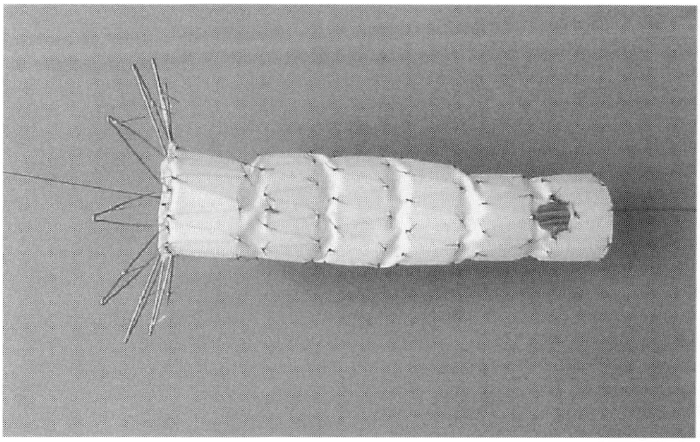

Fig. 5. The use of fenestration to preserve orifices of major vessels.

Once the sheath is removed the graft is partially deployed once positioning etc is complete; the coaxial trigger wire is removed to complete deployment of the system.

This second system is useful for preservation of orifices away from the leading end and also allows building of a graft via the use of extension pieces (Fig. 5). The extension can occur proximally or distally depending on the aneurysm being treated i.e. infrarenal with renal preservation or thoracic with preservation of the coeliac axis.

The feasibility of treating a thoracic aneurysm and an infrarenal aortic aneurysm with preservation of a vessel has now been demonstrated (Fig. 6). Combining these together such as the following example shows the treatment of a thoracoabdominal dumbbell aneurysm with preservation of the coeliac vessel.

As elegant as these examples may appear they are undoubtedly crude by comparison with what is likely to be developed with imaging technology. The ability to visualize the vessels from within and to reconstruct the image promises much with the advances with computerized tomography scanning and magnetic resonance angiography. Improved imaging for vascular surgeons, in the theatre setting must be part of the modern vascular theatre and will be essential for the accuracy required. Preparedness and special training must be addressed if vascular surgeons wish to be involved with the treatment of vascular disease in the future.

FORCES ACTING ON AN ENDOLUMINAL GRAFT

The design and use of an endoluminal graft requires an understanding of the expected forces which the graft will encounter once it is placed within an abdominal aortic aneurysm (Fig. 7).[7] Three approaches can be used to evaluate the forces. The first is experimental, where an experimental rig is built to measures the forces on the graft. Many investigators would be satisfied with obtaining such measurements.

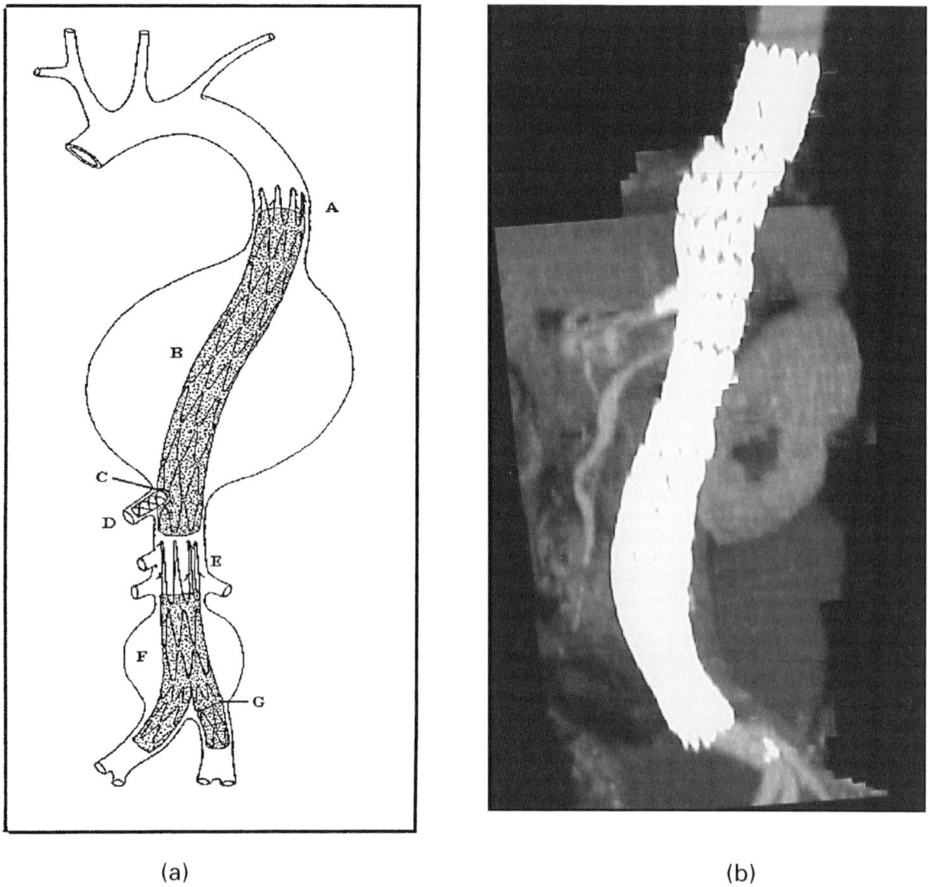

Fig. 6. Treatment of a thoracoabdominal dumbbell aneurysm with preservation of the coeliac vessels: (a) is a cartoon of the plane X-ray presented in (b). (A uncovered anchor stent of thoracic graft, B covered stent. C fenestration, D palmaz stent, E open anchor stent of abdominal graft, F covered stent, G join).

However, there will be circumstances encountered by the surgeon, which are not covered by a certain set of experiments, e.g. the convoluted blood vessel geometries of elderly patients often require the use of individually tailored grafts. To do an individual experiment for each patient may not be practical. To accommodate such cases it is desirable to obtain a general physical understanding of the system, and, possibly, a set of mathematical equations that can be used to obtain a moderately accurate estimate of the forces on the graft. This is known as 'force balance analysis', and is a standard engineering way of solving such problems.

A third approach is to use computational fluid dynamics (CFD). This involves modelling the flow of blood in the graft by solving the equations of fluid flow via numerical methods. The increasing processing speed of computers is making CFD a relatively practical and inexpensive option. The following discussion reports on CFD

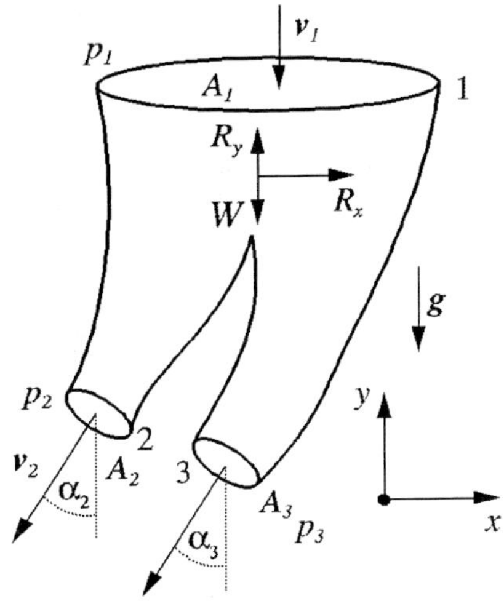

Fig. 7. The characteristic velocity, pressure, area and force vectors required to compute the restraining forces on a bifurcated, bent pipe of varying cross-sectional area. The gravitational force is assumed to act in the negative *y* direction.

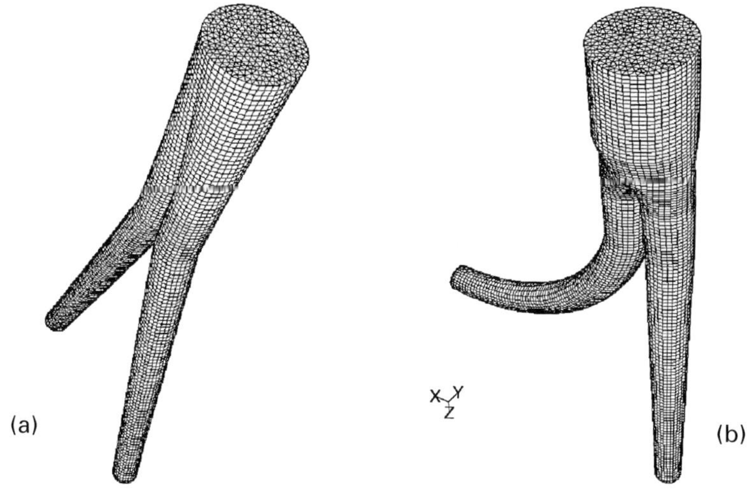

Fig. 8. Computational domains for CFD calculations. (a) The flat or in-plane domain. (b) The bent leg domain.

and force balance analysis methods to estimate the forces on the Zenith bifurcated endoluminal graft.

The Zenith endoluminal graft is a flexible bifurcated pipe of varying cross-section. We schematically depict this device in Fig. 8. Blood enters the proximal end of the graft, which we label by the number 1, and exits via the distal ends 2 and 3. The velocities, v, and pressures, p, of the blood are shown, as are the areas, A, of the different ends of the pipe. The proximal end of the graft is aligned so that the direction of the inlet blood flow is in the negative y direction. The two outlet legs of the graft are at angles α_1 and α_2 to the vertical, and gravity, g, acts in the negative y direction. R_x and R_y are the restraint forces required to keep the graft in position, while W is the weight of the graft.

From conservation of mass[10] one can show that:

$$A_1 v_1 = A_2 v_2 + A_3 v_3 \tag{1}$$

or

$$Q_1 = Q_2 + Q_3 \tag{2}$$

where $Q_i = A_i v_i$ is the volume flow rate through the ith opening of the graft.

Equations (1) and (2) simply say, in mathematical terms, that the volume flow rate of blood entering the graft, Q_1 $(=A_1 v_1)$ is equal to the sum of the volume flow rates of blood leaving the graft, $Q_2 + Q_3$ $(=A_2 v_2 + A_3 v_3)$. If we assume that

$$Q_2 = f Q_1 , \tag{3}$$

where f is a constant ≤ 1, then Eqn (2) implies that:

$$Q_3 = (1-f)\, Q_1. \tag{4}$$

In turn, Eqns (3) and (4) give:

$$v_2 = f\,(A_1/\,A_2)\,v_1 \tag{5}$$

and

$$v_3 = (1-f)(\,A_1/\,A_3)\,v_1\,. \tag{6}$$

In non-mathematical terms Eqns (5) and (6) demonstrate that if the area of a pipe becomes smaller as the liquid flows along the pipe then the speed of the flow will increase. Similarly, if the area of the pipe increases then the speed of the flow will decrease.

To compute the restraining forces for the graft, we require the momentum conservation equation.[10] Standard engineering analysis using the momentum equation allows us to derive expressions for the restraint forces, R_x and R_y:

$$R_x = -p_2 A_2 \sin\alpha_2 - p_3 A_3 \sin\alpha_3 - \rho\, v_2^2 A_2 \sin\alpha_2 - \rho\, v_3^2 A_3 \sin\alpha_3 \tag{7}$$

and

$$\begin{aligned} R_y = {} & p_1 A_1 - p_2 A_2 \cos\alpha_2 - p_3 A_3 \cos\alpha_3 + \\ & \rho\, v_1^2\, A_1 - \rho\, v_2^2\, A_2 \cos\alpha_2 - \rho\, v_3^2\, A_3 \cos\alpha_3 + \rho V g + m g \,, \end{aligned} \tag{8}$$

where ρ is the mass density of blood, V is the volume of the graft, g the acceleration due to gravity and m the mass of the graft. If we know the values for the pressure and velocities of the blood on both ends of the graft then Eqns (7) and (8) can be used to calculate the forces required to keep the graft in place. Sometimes, however, it is difficult to determine the pressures at the distal ends of the graft and so we can use the conservation of energy[10] to derive expressions to compute these values:

$$p_1/\gamma + v_1^2/2g + y_1 = p_i/(+v_i^2/2g + y_i + h_L\,, \tag{9}$$

where $\gamma = \rho g$ is the weight density of blood, y_1 is the height of the inlet, h_L is the energy loss due to friction, i refers to the ith outlet, i.e., i refers to outlets 2 or 3, and y_i is the height of the ith outlet.

Equations (1), (7), (8) and (9) provide the basis for understanding the flow in a graft via analytic equations. However, due to the complex flow structures that may develop in a graft, such equations should be treated with caution.

A more detailed treatment of the problem can be done by using computational fluid dynamics to solve the equations of fluid motion on a mathematical grid that typically takes the shape of the object of interest. As an example of this gridding process, the CFD grids used to compute the forces on the Zenith graft are shown in Fig. 8. In the present CFD study, the influence of gravity was ignored (which is equivalent to assuming that the patient is in a horizontal position) and a peak inlet flow speed of approximately 60 cm/s and a peak pressure of 100 mm Hg (13.2 kPa) was used to approximate blood flow. The assumption that blood behaves as a 'Newtonian fluid' was also made: that is, the friction between separate, but adjacent, 'fluid packets' is proportional to how fast those fluid packets are moving relative to each other. This is a good approximation for blood flowing through the aorta, where the relatively high flow speed also ensures that the rheological properties of blood are fairly constant, with a dynamic viscosity $\mu = 0.0036\ \mathrm{Ns/m^2}$ and blood density $\rho = 1060\ \mathrm{kg/m^3}$.[11]

In this study, it was assumed that the blood flow was steady and turbulent. The former assumption was made for computational convenience and should give a moderately accurate value for the peak forces on the graft if peak flow rates are used. The latter assumption was necessary, because the high flow speeds in the aorta nearly guarantee that the blood is turbulent or partially turbulent in that region.

Turbulence in fluid dynamics refers to the propensity of fluids to form a cascade of eddies (whirlpools of fluid) of all different sizes. The number of eddies is, usually, inversely proportional to the size of the eddy. So there are only a few, very large eddies and a large number of small eddies. The intriguing and, from the engineer's point of view, frustrating aspect of turbulence is that the smallest eddies can dramatically affect the large scale motion of the flow, a bit like the 'tail waving the dog', so to speak. The size of these 'tail' eddies is usually much smaller than the smallest grid volume that can be created with current computer technology. So, it is necessary to model this 'subgrid' turbulence with a specifically designed turbulence model. In this simulation we used the 'RNG k-ε' model, which is a moderately robust turbulence model that has been developed by engineers and scientists over the last 30 years or so.[12,13]

For the symmetrical, flat graft, the blood flow produced a downward force of around 3.1 Newton and symmetrical side forces that cancelled out to give no resultant side force. The curved geometry produced a side force, acting to the left, of around 1.5 Newton and a downward force of 4.4 Newton. By placing the appropriate values into Eqns (7) and (8), it was found that the analytic formulae gave similar values for the restraint forces required to keep the graft in place.

In addition to these calculations, we also calculated the forces on grafts with a proximal inlet diameter of 3 cm and a distal outlet diameter of 1 cm. For these cases, the flat geometry produced a downward force of 7.12 Newton and the curved geometry produced downward and side forces of 8.24 Newton and 1.3 Newton, respectively. The side force may act to displace the distal legs of the graft from their initial positions in the iliac vessels.

CONCLUSION

Major advances in the design and patency of endoluminal grafts have occurred during the 1990s such that the endoluminal procedure now offers a real alternative to open repair in the treatment of aneursym disease. Its feasibility has eased the restrictions of its use and increased the scope of treatment of aneurysms with more complex morphology. Modular building and the ability to preserve blood flow into the orifices of essential vessels with the use of fenestrated grafts has opened the door for treatment of the whole aorta and iliac systems. However, while early results of this technology have been encouraging, the issue of long-term durability is still of central importance in ultimate success.

Understanding the forces acting within the pressurized aorta, and upon the stent-graft, and how they may affect the ongoing performance of the stent graft is important for lasting effective exclusion of the aneurysm. The preliminary data presented here indicate that the blood flow forces upon the stent-graft may be close to the force threshold required to dislodge the stent-graft when relying on radical attachment alone.

ACKNOWLEDGEMENTS

We would like to thank Ms Christine McComb for the graphic design illustrations of the endoluminal grafts.

REFERENCES

1. Lawrence-Brown MMD, Hartley D, MacSweeny S *et al.*: The Perth endoluminal bifurcated graft system – development and early experience. *J Cardiovasc Surg* **4**: 706–712, 1996
2. Harris PL, Buth J, Mialhe C *et al.*: The need for clinical trials of endovascular abdominal aortic aneurysm stent-graft repair: The EUROSTAR Project. *J Vasc Surg* **4**: 72–77, 1997
3. Parodi JC, Palmaz JC, Barone HD: Transfemoral infraluminal graft implantation for abdominal aortic aneurysms. *Ann Vasc Surg* **5**: 491–499, 1991
4. Gordon M, Lawrence-Brown MMD, Hartley D *et al.*: A self-expanding endoluminal graft for treatment of aneurysms: results through the development phase. *Aust NZ J Surg* **66**: 621–625, 1996
5. Van Schie G, Sieunarine K, Lawrence-Brown MMD, Hartley D: The Perth bifurcated endovascular graft for infrarenal aortic aneurysms. *Semin Intervent Radiol* **15**: 63–69, 1996

6. Lawrence-Brown M, Sieunarine K, Hartley D *et al.*: The Perth HL-B bifurcated endoluminal graft: a review of the experience and intermediate results. *J Cardiovasc Surg* **6**: 220–225, 1998
7. Lawrence-Brown MMD, Semmens JB, Hartley DE *et al.*: How is durability related to patient selection and graft design with endoluminal grafting for abdominal aortic aneurysm? In: Greenhalgh RM (Ed), *Durability of Vascular and Endovascular Surgery*, pp. 375–385. London: WB Saunders, 1999.
8. Lawrence-Brown M M D, Sieunarine K, Hartley D *et al.*: Should an anchor stent cross the renal artery orifices when placing an endoluminal graft for abdominal aortic aneurysm? In: Greenhalgh RM (Ed), *Indications in Vascular and Endovascular Surgery*, p. 261. London: WB Saunders, 1998.
9. Browne TF, Hartley D, Purchas S *et al.* A fenestrated covered suprarenal aortic stent. *Eur J Vasc Endovasc Surg* **18**: 449, 1999
10. Gerhart PM, Gross RJ, Hochstein JI: *Fundamentals of Fluid Mechanics* 2nd edn. Reading, Mass: Addison Wesley, 1992
11. Skovberg F: Blood viscosity in normal and diabetic subjects: a clinical-hemorheological study. Kobenhavn, FADL, 1974
12. Launder BE, Spalding DB: The numerical computation of turbulent flows. *Comput Meth Appl Mech Eng* **3**: 269–289, 1974
13. Chodbury D: *Introduction to the renormalization group method and turbulence modelling.* Fluent Inc. Technical Memorandum p.107, 1993

The Ancure endovascular graft: development, design, and FDA trial results in the USA

David H Deaton

INTRODUCTION

The Ancure graft was the brainchild of Harrison Lazarus, a vascular surgeon in Utah. Designs, patents and a company to pursue animal and clinical testing were in place in the late 1980s well before the first reports of clinical endovascular grafting. A start-up company, EndoVascular Technologies (EVT), was incorporated in 1989 and became a public company in 1996 with an initial public stock offering. Guidant Corporation acquired EVT in 1997. EVT began operations in Menlo Park, California and their operations as Guidant/CVS continue there. Ten years of experimental and clinical work culminated in the first approval of an endovascular graft in the USA by the US Food and Drug Administration (FDA). The Ancure tube and bifurcated endovascular grafts for patients with abdominal aortic aneurysm were approved on 29 September 1999.

HISTORY OF THE ANCURE GRAFT

The original EVT endovascular graft, known as EGS (Endovascular Grafting System) was a tube graft. After extensive *in vitro* and *in vivo* animal testing[1] an FDA Phase I trial was begun in humans in February 1993. Dr Wesley Moore performed the first human graft at the University of California, Los Angeles.[2] That case was successful and all subsequent clinical research was done under FDA approved protocols. *The FDA protocols were designed to compare endovascular abdominal aortic aneurysm repair with conventional repair in patients that were elective candidates for conventional open surgical abdominal aortic aneurysm repair*. Unlike most early work with endovascular grafts, compassionate and emergent indications were not addressed and the basic design of the graft was kept constant. Phase I trials were designed to assure the technical ability of the graft delivery system to perform in a manner consistent with its design and make sure there were no major unexpected technical problems with the implantation. Phase I trials for the tube and bifurcated configurations of the Ancure graft were done between 1993 and 1995 and were the first clinical trials of an endovascular graft in the USA.

Phase II trials were designed to compare the endovascular repair with conventional repair with respect to safety and efficacy. Phase II trials for the tube,[3] bifurcated and aorto-iliac Ancure grafts were completed between 1995 and 1998. Twenty concurrent centres were allowed by the FDA to participate in the Phase II trials. The trials were strictly controlled and all follow-up radiological interpretation was subjected to multiple reviews by a panel at a Core Laboratory facility in the Cleveland Clinic. The Core Lab reading was recorded as the final reading for all radiological follow-up. Clinical data at all investigative centres were audited by clinical specialists from Guidant (formerly EVT), by independent clinical trial auditors, and by FDA auditors at selected centres.

The only dysfunction related to graft integrity was hook breaks identified in the original design of tube and bifurcated grafts in 1994. This defect was not recognized by the investigative centres but was first noted by EVT engineering staff. EVT immediately stopped all trials and informed the FDA of the finding. The clinical trials were never officially stopped by the FDA in recognition of EVT's proactive approach to recognition and address of the defect.

Hook breaks in the original graft design (i.e. pre-1995) occurred in approximately 10–20% of grafts at 12 months. Some grafts with multiple hook breaks experienced graft migration and conversion to open repair was performed in a small minority of cases. This development was significant for both the design of the Ancure graft and the entire field of endovascular aortic grafting for it documented the significant forces placed on these grafts *in vivo*. It also showed that *despite a stationary location for 1 year, grafts migrated without intact mechanical fixation*. This suggests that 'healing', or biologic incorporation, is not an effective method of chronic fixation for endovascular grafts and that competent mechanical attachment is necessary for the life of the graft. Engineering calculations allowed the documentation of the forces on the proximal attachment and a simple reconfiguration of the hooks allowed a many-fold increase in strength. The hooks have no mechanical junctions or welds and are independent of the radial component responsible for initial deployment. *No hook on an EGS/Ancure graft has broken since the new attachment system was introduced in 1995*. There have not been any defects in graft integrity noted since the introduction of the current graft in 1995.

A major change in the delivery system of the Ancure graft was introduced in the Autumn of 1998. While the graft remained essentially identical to previous iterations, the delivery system was simplified and made more intuitive. The graft is now available in the USA, Europe and Australia.

ANCURE GRAFT DESIGN

The original graft was designed to imitate, as closely as possible, the result of open surgical replacement of the aorta. The inventors reasoned that if a graft that adhered to the principles of open surgical repair could be implanted via femoral access the long-term performance would likely mimic the remarkably durable nature of conventional surgical aortic prostheses. This heightened the challenge of acute implantation but lessened the uncertainties of chronic graft performance.

To that end a single piece (i.e. non-modular) woven polyester fabric identical to that used in conventional vascular grafts was utilized. A proximal and distal attachment system was fashioned to allow self-expanding initial deployment at a desired location followed by balloon driven implantation of a series of eight hooks through all layers of the aortic wall. The body and limbs of the Ancure graft are essentially identical to conventional grafts without any mechanical reinforcement or support. Radio-opaque markers are aligned in characteristic orientations (i.e. longitudinal on the body and radial on the limbs) on different locations of the graft to allow fluoroscopic identification of the orientation and position of the graft. The delivery system allows the graft to be controlled with respect to both rotation and longitudinal location at three separate attachment sites. The inability to reconstrain or adjust the attachment system after deployment required delivery catheter engineering that guaranteed precision deployment and avoidance of premature release.

The basic design concepts (e.g. compliant and unsupported graft with positive transmural fixation) of the Ancure graft are identical to the precepts of conventional aortic prostheses. These characteristics made delivery system design more challenging but avoided the larger risks of chronic performance related to changes in the basic characteristics of graft composition, biomechanical characteristics, and method of graft fixation.

GRAFT ATTACHMENT

The method of graft attachment to the vasculature is unique to the Ancure graft. The radial force of each attachment system is minimal and, unlike many endovascular grafts, is not designed to play a major role in fixation. Rather, fixation is primarily dependent on metal hooks penetrating the vessel wall and seated in the load bearing portion of the vessel wall, the adventitia. There are four pairs of hooks that are each separately attached to the graft material independent of each other and of the radial deployment framework. This gives the attachment a discrete longitudinal location rather than attachment distributed over a length of vessel. Proximal attachment in the perirenal aorta devotes 100% of the proximal attachment integrity to the portion of the infrarenal aorta least likely to dilate and least likely to be involved with pathologic changes.

The attachment system also has a high degree of radial compliance allowing it to achieve a seal when the vessel is irregular and non-circular. Its low force self-expanding nature allows it to respond to small diameter changes characteristic of radial compliance in the aorta during the cardiac cycle. The proximal neck of the graft is typically oversized to the native perirenal aortic diameter by 1–3 mm. If the neck expands over time the graft will follow the neck expansion up to the original size of the graft. The hooks impart purchase to the aortic wall to a diameter as large as 4 mm greater than the graft size (i.e. the hooks extend 2 mm past the graft border on each side).

Longitudinal compliance and the absence of columnar strength is another distinguishing feature of the Ancure graft. This characteristic prevents mechanical coupling of the proximal attachment site (i.e. perirenal aorta) and the aortic bifurcation and allows the maintenance of native aortic elasticity during the cardiac cycle and prevention of longitudinal motion or stress of the proximal attachment relative to the vessel. Longitudinal compliance also allows the graft to adapt to the

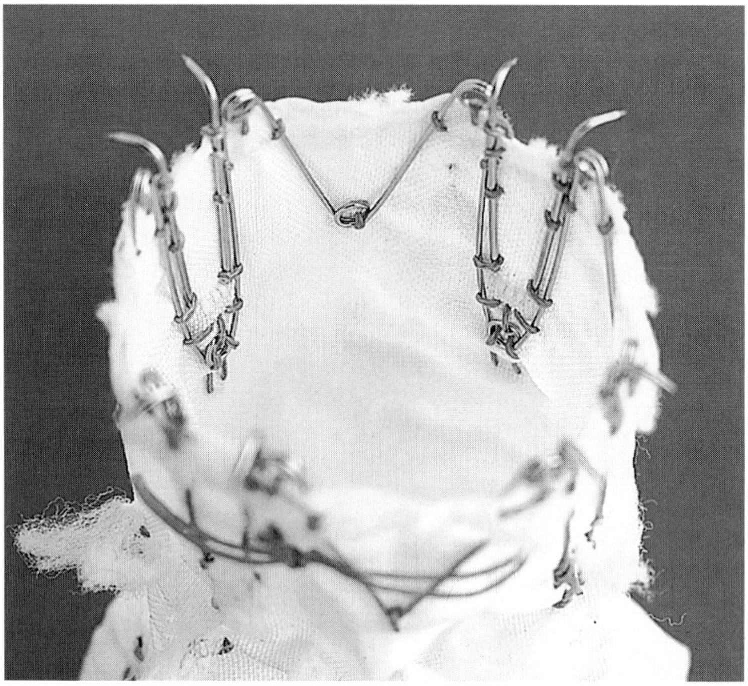

Fig. 1. Proximal attachment of the ANCURE™ Endograft®. Radial deployment framework separate from hook attachments

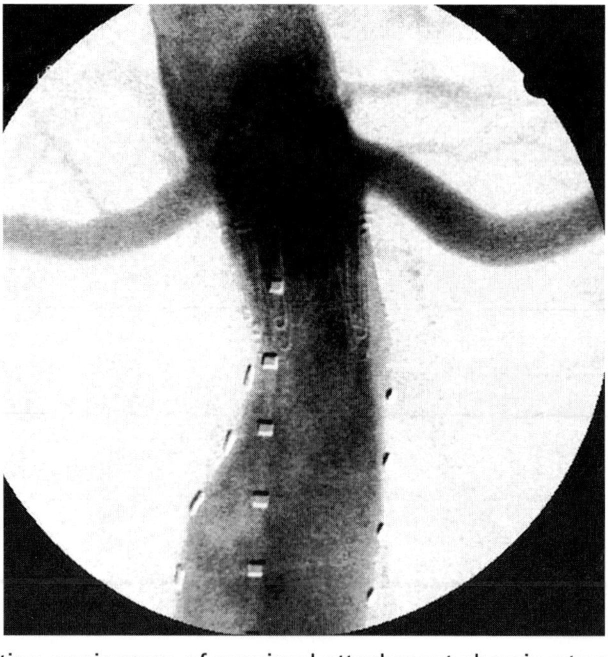

Fig. 2. Completion angiogram of proximal attachment showing transmural purchase of hooks in juxtarenal position.

normal tortuosity of native anatomy rather than trying to force the arterial anatomy to adapt to a straight graft. This allows the proximal attachment to orient to the local axis of the proximal aortic neck irrespective of angulation to the axis of the aneurysm and lower aorta. Chronic changes in aortic length and configuration as a result of aortic remodelling are also accommodated by the unsupported nature of the graft.

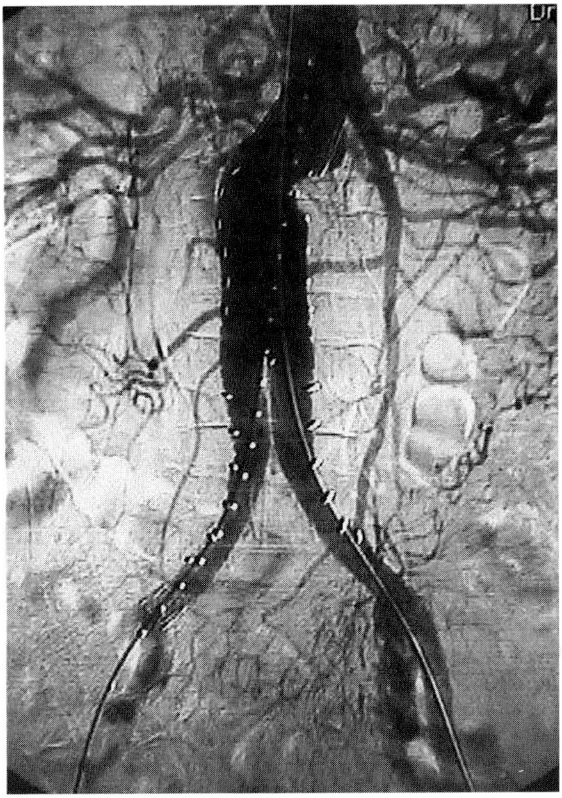

Fig. 3. Completion angiogram of a bifurcated graft in a 7-cm aneurysm. Note adaptation of graft to significant proximal neck turtuosity relative to aortic axis.

PATIENT SELECTION

Patient selection is one of the most important factors in achieving technical success in endovascular grafting. The majority of problems that prevent technical success involve access issues in the iliac vasculature. Lack of adequate external iliac diameter, tortuosity, and vessel calcification are the leading factors affecting access and can act synergistically to prevent graft delivery.

The proximal neck of the aorta must be 26 mm in diameter or less for currently available graft dimensions. A proximal neck length of 15 mm or greater has been used as an inclusion criteria for all of the US trials. Distally, a 25 mm or greater length segment of normal iliac must be present for implantation and seal of the iliac limbs. The iliac limbs are one half the diameter of the body of the graft and this characteristic has significant implications for implantation as discussed later.

RESULTS OF THE BIFURCATED GRAFT IN US PHASE II TRIALS

The results of the Phase II trial in the USA for the bifurcated graft are continuously updated as data on follow-up are returned and validated.[4] The results that were presented to the Advisory Panel for the Center for Device and Radiologic Health of the FDA are summarized in this section. In general these results are the 1-year follow-up of patients with tube and bifurcated grafts presented to the FDA in June of 1999; 5-year follow-up of all patients enrolled in the Phase II trials was mandated by the FDA at the time of approval.

Trial design

The trials for tube and bifurcated grafts were concurrently controlled, non-randomized trials for patients with abdominal aortic aneurysms who were candidates for conventional repair. Originally the trial was designed to be randomized but this quickly proved futile during the tube trial. Very few patients were candidates for an endovascular tube graft and to assign half to surgical therapy would have made accrual nearly impossible. The phenomenon of 'trial shopping' also began to occur with patients assigned surgical therapy withdrawing and going to another clinical site to be randomized again with the belief that their luck, as they perceived it, would be better. Controls were identical to treated patients with respect to nearly all patient demographics and medical history. They were significantly different only in specific vascular dimensions related to candidacy for endovascular grafting: proximal neck length and iliac diameter. Patients still had to be amenable to infrarenal clamping and have no evidence of clinically significant iliac occlusive disease (i.e. normal femoral pulses and normal ankle brachial indices) to participate in the control arm of the study.

Technical success

Most centres experienced a technical success rate of ≈90% in the early phases of the trial and/or learning curve of a particular centre. It should be remembered that these trials represented the initial experience with any endovascular technique for most centres and was the first endovascular aortic trial in the USA. Centres and surgeons with experience now have current technical success rates over 95%. The single largest impediment to technical success is iliac access making patient selection an important determinant of graft deployment.

Operative parameters

A variety of operative parameters were tabulated during the trials. All data analysis was done on an 'intent to treat' basis so that any complications occurring in a patient originally assigned to endovascular therapy accrued to endovascular irrespective of actual treatment.

Operative time was similar between all groups ranging from 130 to 167 minutes. *Blood loss* was reduced significantly from 800 cc in control patients to 200cc and 300cc in tube and bifurcated endovascular patients respectively. *Hospital stay* was also reduced from an average of 6 days for open surgical patients versus 2–3 days for endovascular patients. *Mortality* was 2.7% in controls compared with 0% and 2.5% in tube and bifurcated endovascular patients respectively.

A composite index (i.e.the IDE (Investigational Device Exemption) Composite Safety Measure) of expected complications following aortic surgery was used to track and characterize the general morbidity of the procedures. The index included death, bleeding, renal, respiratory, wound, cardiac, bowel, vascular and ischaemic complications and rated the severity according to a scale of mild, moderate, and severe where appropriate. If a patient experienced either a moderate or severe manifestation of any complication they were counted as positive with respect to the index. Control patients had an index of 44% while tube and bifurcated endovascular patients had rates of 20% and 29% respectively.

Of particular interest were cardiac, renal, and respiratory complications. Cardiac complications occurred in 21% of controls versus 10% and 13% of tube and bifurcated endovascular patients. *Renal* complications occurred in 3% of controls versus 8% and 2% of tube and bifurcated endovascular patients. Renal complications include all

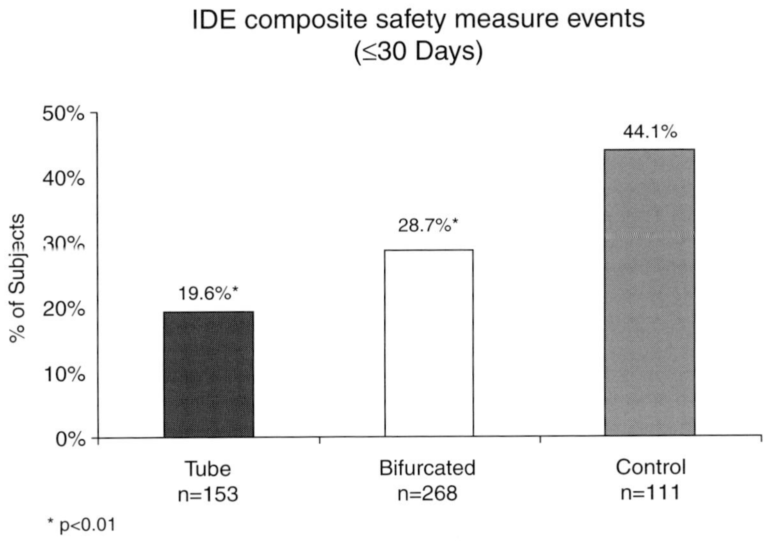

Fig. 4. The IDE composite index representing whether or not a patient experienced moderate or severe complications in the categories represented by the composite for surgical controls and tube and bifurcated endovascular grafts.

patients with a rise in creatinine of 30% for any period of time. Fewer than 1% of patients required any dialysis. There were no renal artery occlusions, early or late, during the study. Of note, in the more recent experience with the Ancure bifurcated graft in 89 patients presented to the FDA, renal insufficiency has been reduced from 8% to 2%. *Respiratory* complications occurred in 22% of controls versus 7% and 10% of tube and bifurcated endovascular patients. In general, marked improvements in complication rates were achieved in the primary areas of morbidity surrounding conventional aneurysm repair.

Perigraft flow/endoleaks

The subject of perigraft flow, or endoleaks as they are more commonly known, has fuelled much debate in endovascular grafting literature. Endovascular grafting has no surgical precedent or analogue with respect to the placement of a graft inside an intact blood vessel. For this reason there is no antecedent experience or theory in the appreciation and evaluation of the presence of liquid blood in the aneurysm sac outside the graft after endovascular exclusion. It should be remembered that 'endoleak' is an image, not a diagnosis, and the challenge of its appreciation lies in correlating the image with a diagnosis and outcome. The most popular classification system[5,6,7] applied to this image is one based on the presumed source of the endoleak. Roughly speaking, this system relates the source of the liquid blood to a failure of the graft to prevent direct communication to aortic pressure (Types 1, 3, and 4 endoleak) or a failure of the technique of endovascular grafting to prevent transaneurysmal tributary-to-tributary flow (Type 2 endoleak). The former category represents failure modes specific to the graft itself while the latter represents a failure mode generalized to the technique rather than the graft.

Type 3 and Type 4 endoleaks are associated with failure modes related to features not found in the Ancure graft. No Type 3 or 4 endoleaks were detected during these studies. At 1 year, tube graft patients had an overall perigraft flow rate 27.1% with 6% in the Type 1/Indeterminate category and the remainder in the Type 2 category. At 1 year, bifurcated graft patients had an overall perigraft flow rate of 30% with 4% in the Type 1/Indeterminate category and the remainder in the Type 2 category. Of the 4% of bifurcated patients with 'Type 1/Inderterminate' endoleak, half were identified as 'Type 1' and half as 'indeterminate'.

The incidence of perigraft flow with the Ancure graft related to aneurysm tributaries is higher than most reports of aortic stent-grafts at about 30%. This may be a result of the compliant nature of the graft which does not induce the degree of stasis in the aneurysm sac that a rigid graft does. It may also have a relationship to the fact that this study was the only one that employed a stringent core radiologic reading facility independent of all clinical sites in a prospective fashion. Certainly the readings done by both radiologists and surgeons at investigative sites were often different from the readings rendered by the core laboratory. Much of this was due to the inherent subjective nature of radiologic image interpretation but also to the very conservative interpretation that was the core laboratory's mandate.

In any case the finding of perigraft flow, or endoleak, while initially presumed to be negative, has not had a significant impact on the effectiveness of aneurysm exclusion as measured by aneurysm growth or rupture. Very few patients with Type

2 perigraft flow have had aneurysm growth. None have been converted for this finding. *No aneurysm in the US Phase II bifurcated graft trial has ruptured since the inception of the trial in 1995.* While careful follow-up of all patients in the trial continues the initial concerns about perigraft flow resulting from aneurysm tributaries seems unwarranted. Indeed patients without perigraft flow have had aneurysm growth in this and other studies making the diagnosis of ineffective aneurysm exclusion difficult. The relationship between the presence of perigraft flow and the potential for aneurysm growth, and presumably risk of rupture, will be an ongoing subject of interest for vascular surgeons as we define the limits of expected outcomes after endovascular grafting.

Aneurysm growth

The harder endpoint of *aneurysm growth* was also examined with a change of 5 mm, considered significant for change. At 1 year, 94% of tube graft patients had either an unchanged (51%) or decreasing aneurysm (43%). At 1 year, 98% of bifurcated graft patients had either an unchanged (50%) or decreasing aneurysm (48%). Of patients with an increase in aneurysm size (n=9), eight had perigraft flow while one did not. Type 2 perigraft flow would theoretically be a very small threat to continued aneurysm expansion since it represents collateral bed physiology with a marked reduction in mean pressure and pulse pressure. Perigraft flow is clearly associated with a higher risk of future aneurysm growth but the majority of patients with this finding had unchanged or decreasing aneurysm diameter. Dynamic angiography lends the most accurate information on the source and dynamics of perigraft flow and future analysis promises better diagnosis of persistent aneurysm pressurization, with or without endoleak. The correlation of perigraft flow and the diagnosis of continued aneurysm pressure and growth will be one of the most important areas of future research and characterization.

Graft patency

The body of the Ancure graft did not experience any stenoses or thromboses during the trials. The unsupported iliac limbs were susceptible to a number of hazards that lead to limb stenosis and rarely thrombosis. Fortunately, no patient with limb stenosis or thrombosis experienced limb-threatening ischaemia or tissue loss.

As a result of being constrained to the native vasculature the unsupported limbs of the Ancure graft are susceptible to severe tortuosity and native stenoses. They can also be twisted on implantation. The ratio of proximal diameter to iliac limb diameter is 2:1 raising the potential for the iliac limbs to be significantly larger than the native iliac diameters (e.g. 13 mm limb in a 9 mm iliac). When these problems were encountered, radial support in the form of a stent was often used in the portion of the limb constrained to the diseased native iliac vasculature. As the trial progressed a sensitivity for these problems developed and intervention migrated almost entirely to the operative setting rather than postoperative.

A total of 38% of patients received some form of adjunctive therapy to maintain or restore patency in a limb. Some of these interventions were made on based on the perception of threat to limb contour in the operating suite while others were directed at documented defects. The majority of interventions, 34% (i.e. 89% of interventions), were in the form of balloon angioplasty or stent placement, primarily done at the time of implantation. In patients that had these procedures there were no recurrences of limb stenosis or need for reintervention. There were no other problems related to stent placement in terms of operative complication profiles, blood loss, operative time, or late complications. No patient with limb stenosis or thrombosis experienced limb threatening ischaemia or tissue loss.

Identification of poor iliac limb configuration has become an essential part of the Ancure implantation and experienced users employ a variety of techniques to identify these problems including multiplanar angiography, pressures and intravascular ultrasound. Angioplasty and stent placement has become a common and easy adjunctive procedure at the time of implantation. The addition of radial support in the limbs after implantation of the graft allows for selective and targeted use of the most appropriate stent design and length for the offending anatomy without introducing rigid elements into the dynamic portion of the graft in the aorta.

OTHER GRAFT PERFORMANCE PARAMETERS

A variety of complications related to endovascular grafts and covered stents has been reported in the literature. These include erosion of grafts through the aortic wall, aortoduodenal fistulas, migration of grafts covering renal arteries, migration distally, modular disjunction, and mid-graft perforation from metallic erosion. Since the inception of these trials in 1995, the durability of a successfully placed Ancure graft has been remarkable with no reports of graft perforation, graft extrusion/erosion, attachment system fracture or graft dilatation or rupture. Migration has been limited to unusual circumstances of massive proximal neck dilatation (i.e. more than 6 mm dilatation, n=1) or an improperly placed graft (n=1). Overall, migration has occurred in fewer than 0.5% of cases.

CONSIDERATION OF SPECIFIC GRAFT COMPONENTS

Proximal attachment

Proximal fixation is an important issue for any graft employing a transmural fixation technique. The same properties that make the graft resistant to migration and secure in its location prevent movement or adjustment of its location after deployment. This makes accurate proximal deployment crucial. Theoretic concerns regarding lack of column strength and the potential for the graft to be pushed beyond its intended attachment site by blood flow ('blow back') also exist.

To date, the proximal aortic attachment of the Ancure graft has been very precise allowing reliable implantation of the proximal hooks within 1–2 mm of the intended site in the majority of cases. Refinements in deployment technique including angulation of the C-arm and magnification have also made accurate graft placement easier. None of the grafts were placed over a renal orifice in the US Phase II study and there were no reports of late renal occlusion. Perigraft flow related to the proximal attachment is rare (less than 2%) and is essentially non-existent at 1 year. No late conversions as a result of proximal perigraft flow have been recorded. No perigraft flow related to the proximal attachment has been recorded as a late occurrence.

Body of the graft

The body of the graft is identical to woven polyester grafts used in open surgical procedures. There have been no incidences of occlusion, leak, tear, or any other dysfunction of the body of the graft since the inception of its use in 1993.

Iliac limbs

The iliac limbs of the bifurcated graft are by definition one-half the diameter of the trunk portion of the graft. The susceptibility of the unsupported limbs within disease iliac vasculature to become stenotic as a result of redundant graft material has been described. This occurs about one-third of the time. Generally it is easily relieved by adding radial support in the form of a stent that serves to flatten out any redundant graft material and to distribute any acute angulation from tortuosity over a longer length of the vessel. The size, length, and type of stent used is tailored to the particular situation. The addition of radial support to the limb of the graft results in very little additional operative time. Care must be taken to recognize the potential for iliac obstruction since its presence as assessed by angiography is sometimes occult. Intravascular ultrasound is a valuable diagnostic adjunct when limb obstruction is suspected but is not detected by angiography.

Iliac limb attachment

The iliac attachment also uses hooks to fix it to the arterial wall. When perigraft flow related to iliac attachment is detected it is almost always (more than 90%) correctable with the addition of an endovascular manipulation, usually radial support with a stent. Perigraft flow from an iliac attachment (Type 1) or from aneurysm tributaries (Type 2) can be difficult to distinguish on duplex ultrasound or computed tomography scans. If an aneurysm continues to grow, further investigation with angiography or other techniques is warranted. In our series of over 60 cases at East Carolina University, two of three aneurysms that had grown at 2 years were found to have iliac attachment incompetence easily remedied by stent placement. Both of these patients were thought to have Type 2 perigraft flow prior to investigation with angiography. Migration of the iliac attachment site has not been recorded in the US series.

ANEURYSM OUTCOME

No aneurysm in the US bifurcated graft trial has ruptured since the inception of the trial in 1995. Late conversions were performed for some of the early grafts that experienced hook breaks and migration but none of the current grafts used since 1995 have experienced that problem. The chronic performance of the Ancure bifurcated graft has been excellent to date without any report of graft perforation or graft extrusion/erosion through the vascular wall.

SUMMARY

The integrity and chronic performance of the proximal attachment to isolate the aneurysm sac adequately to prevent further growth is probably the single most important determinant of successful endovascular aneurysm exclusion. To date, the performance of a transmural attachment that addresses the inherent inability of endovascular grafts to 'heal', or become biomechanically incorporated, has been excellent. The unibody compliant design has allowed the graft to adapt to native anatomy both acutely and chronically as aortic remodelling occurs in the face of physiologic alteration. The fate of perigraft flow and its management remain significant questions that will demand further research and follow-up. It is likely that a more aggressive approach to perigraft flow diagnosis will be pursued in the future since it is often amenable to simple endovascular therapy.

The original premise, that achieving implantation of a graft adherent to the principles of conventional repair would mimic the long-term success of open repair, has been realized to date. The utility and potential failure modes for grafts that employ novel techniques of fixation (e.g. radial force, column strength, suprarenal stents) and novel graft characteristics (e.g. metal/fabric interaction in the aneurysm cavity, modularity) are still under evaluation with respect to durability.[8,9] They will need to surpass the standards set by more conventional grafts to justify the inherent uncertainty of their chronic performance. It is equally important to evaluate the presentation mode of failure. If graft failure can be detected on an elective basis and intervention, either endovascular or open, pursued in an elective and controlled setting the tolerance for these defects might be considerable. On the other hand, if failure presents as a catastrophic and unheralded event the tolerance for such possibilities is likely to be low. The amenability of each graft type to future modification (i.e. open surgical conversion/modification) in the face of failure is another important consideration when committing patients to novel technology.

The Ancure graft has demonstrated a very high degree of implantation reliability, reproducibility and accuracy. Its unibody design avoids the pitfalls of modular junctions but also confers upon it lessened applicability with respect to pathological anatomy (e.g. large common iliac diameters, variant iliac lengths, larger aortic necks). These principles of design and their engineering implications have made adoption of this graft delivery system slower as a result of a longer learning curve and the attraction of stent-graft systems with a large degree of similarity to bare stent deployment techniques. With this in mind it is important to remember that the goal of endovascular grafting is to provide aneurysm therapy that is equivalent and without compromise relative to open surgical aneurysm therapy. The benefits of early reductions in morbidity and faster recovery do not outweigh the commitment to aneurysm repair integrity. If we are to maintain the validity of endovascular procedures it is important to proceed diligently towards broadening the applicability of endovascular aortic grafting within the constraints of procedural integrity rather than modifying the integrity of the procedure to enhance applicability.

REFERENCES

1. Quinones-Baldrich WJ, Deaton DH, Mitchell RS *et al.*: Preliminary experience with the EndoVascular Technologies bifurcated endovascular aortic prosthesis in a calf model. *J Vasc Surg* **22**: 370–381, 1995
2. Moore WS, Rutherford RB: Transfemoral endovascular repair of abdominal aortic aneurysm: results of the North American EVT phase 1 trial. EVT Investigators. *J Vasc Surg* **23**: 543–553, 1996
3. Edwards WH, Jr., Naslund TC, Edwards WH Sr *et al.*: Endovascular grafting of abdominal aortic aneurysms. A preliminary study. *Ann Surg* **223**: 568–575, 1996
4. Deaton DH, Bogey WM, Chiang K *et al.*: Bifurcated endovascular grafting for abdominal aortic aneurysm. *Ann Vasc Surg* **13**: 23–31, 1999
5. White GH, Yu W, May J: Endoleak – a proposed new terminology to describe incomplete aneurysm exclusion by an endoluminal graft [letter]. *J Endovasc Surg* **3**: 124–125, 1996
6. White GH, Yu W, May J *et al.*: Endoleak as a complication of endoluminal grafting of abdominal aortic aneurysms: classification, incidence, diagnosis, and management. *J Endovasc Surg* **4**: 152–168, 1997
7. White GH, May J, Waugh RC, Yu W: Type I and Type II endoleaks: a more useful classification for reporting results of endoluminal abdominal aortic aneurysms repair [letter]. *J Endovasc Surg* **5**: 189–191, 1998
8. Riepe G, Heilberger P, Umscheid T *et al.*: Frame dislocation of body middle rings in endovascular stent tube grafts. *Eur J Vasc Endovasc Surg* **17**: 28–34, 1999
9. Norgren L, Jernby B, Engellau L. Aortoenteric fistula caused by a ruptured stent-graft: a case report. *J Endovasc Surg* **5**: 269–272, 1998

AneuRx outcomes 2000

Rodney A White

INTRODUCTION

The recent Food and Drug Administration (FDA) approval of the first endovascular prostheses to treat abdominal aortic aneurysms in the USA and the increasing use of several types of endovascular grafts in many European countries establishes important benchmarks in the rapid evolution of this technology. The concept that arterial aneurysms can be excluded by endovascular devices was reduced to practice less than 10 years ago with the first several years of important clinical observations being made following implantation of 'hand-made' devices. The early successes that have been observed with the first commercially available prostheses have been duplicated with remarkable consistency worldwide. The early clinical success has stimulated the development of many new prototype prostheses with new devices being rapidly acquired by large medical companies once feasibility is established. The early consolidation of this technology to large corporations with significant resources for further research and development signals an ever increasing refinement of the technology as new solutions to address current limitations and future challenges are identified.

New clinical studies are being initiated with devices that offer novel delivery mechanisms and lower profile catheter components. These include one- to three-piece modular systems that can be used to exclude an abdominal aortic aneurysm with a bifurcated prosthesis. The modular concept has been adapted to many devices and enhances the number of patients that can be treated by adding extension cuffs of various configurations. These can be used to extend the length of the device, to secure fixation in ectatic vessels using a bell-bottom configuration, and to obtain suprarenal fixation using uncovered stent designs. The Medtronic AneuRx bifurcated device for treating abdominal aortic aneurysm is the first modular device approved by the US FDA for commercial sale and has been used in many countries around the world with similar success.

THE ANEURX MODULAR BIFURCATED ENDOVASCULAR GRAFT

The Medtronic AneuRx (Medtronic AneuRx, Inc., Santa Rosa, California) modular bifurcated endovascular prosthesis incorporates multiple component parts that can be used in various ways to treat each patient's unique pathology (Fig. 1). Versatility is a key characteristic of the system. The modular components allow varying diameters and linear lengths to be tailored to the patient's pathology and anatomy

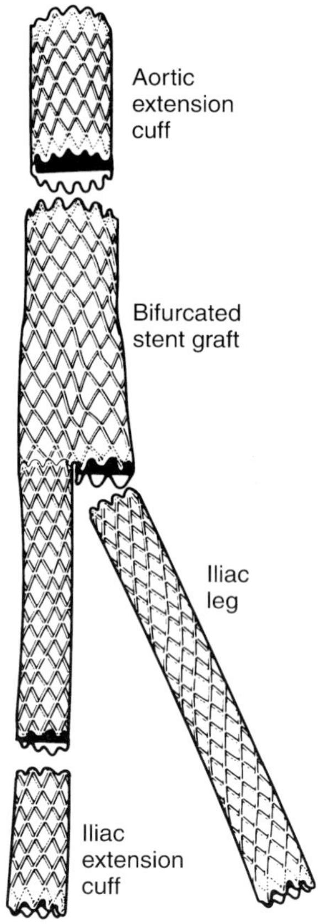

Fig. 1. The AneuRx modular bifurcated device has multiple components in various diameters and lengths so that the device can be deployed to accommodate various aneurysm and attachment vessel morphologies.

without compromising fixation points. These characteristics give the modular bifurcation prosthesis a degree of conformability that increases the number of patients that can be treated. The AneuRx device is composed of a thin-walled polyester vascular prosthesis lining the flow surface and a series of nitinol stents sutured end-to-end along the external surface of the fabric.

A key device component is nitinol, a self-expanding nickel-titanium alloy that serves as a strong yet flexible exoskeleton resistant to compression and kinking. Nitinol is radiopaque, and the device is distinctly marked at the critical endpoints to promote clear visualization during implantation. The self-expanding nitinol stent–polyester graft combination optimizes sealing at the proximal and distal attachment sites, while the full-length exoskelton provides column strength and stable fixation.

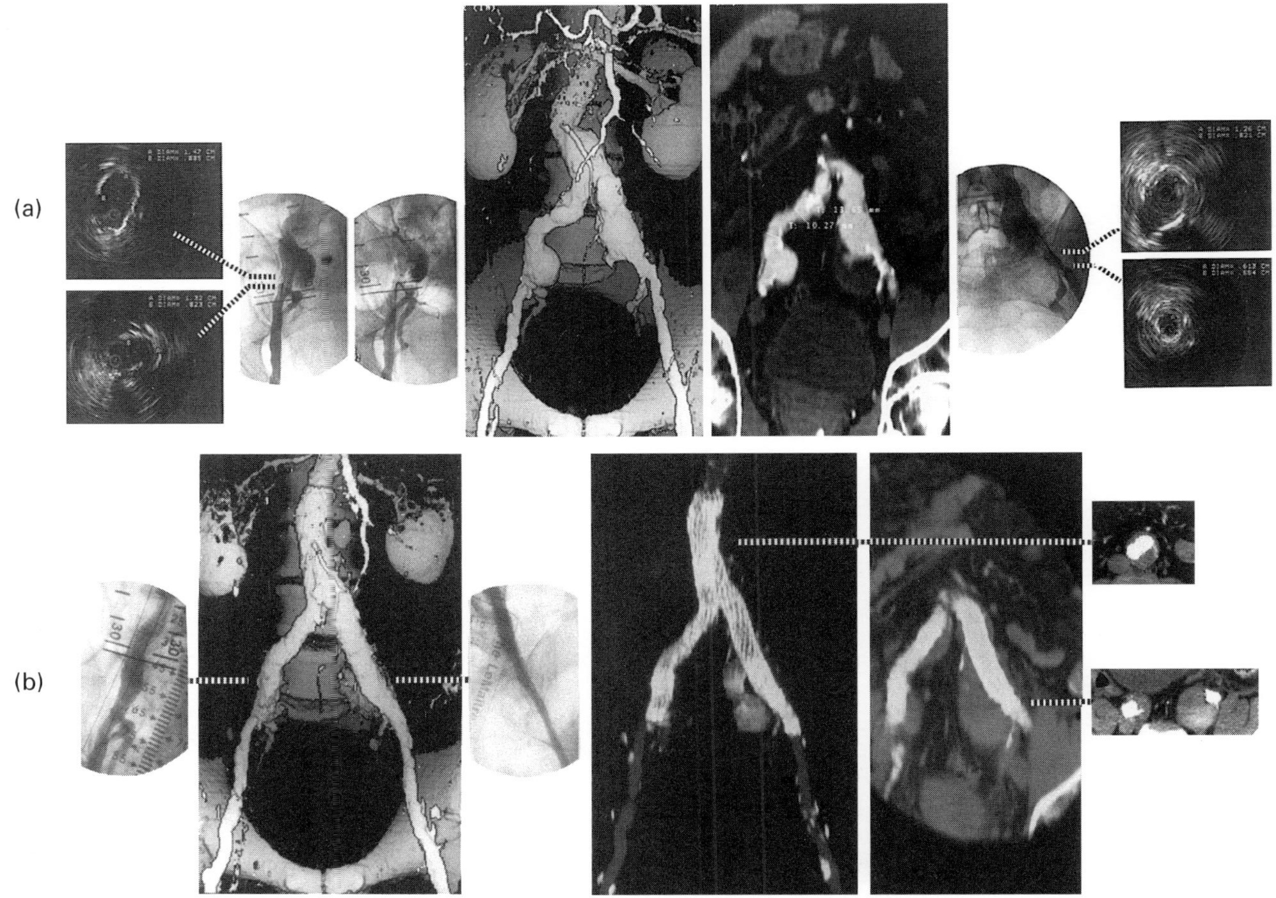

Fig. 2. (a) A patient with complex aorto-iliac aneurysms including a 5cm abdominal aortic aneurysm and 6cm left and 4cm right common iliac artery aneurysms. The patient was evaluated pre-intervention with spiral CT (centre panels), angiography, and intravascular ultrasound (right and left images) to assess candidacy for endovascular intervention. Using these images and the potential for customizing both length and diameter of the device using the AneuRx device, the patient was successfully treated with exclusion of all aneurysms and preservation of hypogastric artery flow. (b) Comparison of the spiral CT images acquired at 48 hours post-deployment with the angiographic images obtained after placement of the device showing the alignment of the component pieces.

Dimensional adaptability is an additional appealing feature of the AneuRx device. Dimensional variability includes adaption of the device to both length and diameter characteristics of the aneurysm and attachment vessels. Proximal length adjustment is facilitated by the proximal sealing cuffs. Distal extender cuffs allow distal length and diameter adjustments enabling deployment in more complex iliac anatomy (Fig. 2).

CLINICAL UTILITY

The ultimate test of any device is the success when introduced to clinical practice. There have been several published studies addressing the safety and utility of the AneuRx bifurcated device for treatment of abdominal aortic aneurysms.[1–4] These include concurrent studies that occurred in various European countries during the same interval while controlled clinical Investigational Device Exemption (IDE) studies were performed in the USA under FDA approved protocols. The European studies have been used to support introduction of this technology in many countries, while the US data recently presented to the FDA Circulatory Advisory Panel on 23 June 1999, and received conditional approval.[5] Following satisfactory compliance of the manufacturer regarding the outlined conditions, unrestricted clinical sale of the AneuRx device for aorto-iliac aneurysmal disease was granted in October 1999 in the USA. Although the European data will not be reviewed in detail in this discussion, the papers are recommended for those seeking further information related to utility of this device.[2–3] An important observation is that the initial clinical results related to success rates and low incidence of significant complications have been reproduced by many investigators in both the European and US studies.

The major discussion in this manuscript will be to briefly outline the results of Phase II data that were reported in the USA to the FDA panel, with the complete FDA submission being available as part of the official federal records containing the information that was reported at the 23 June 1999, Panel Meeting. Additional reports summarizing these data have been published or have been submitted for peer review publication and will form the basis for the official references regarding these studies.[4,6,7]

The FDA study in the USA was performed to evaluate the safety, efficacy and clinical utility for endovascular repair of abdominal aortic aneurysms using the AneuRx endoluminal graft compared with an open surgery control group. The inclusion criteria for this study were that patients had an aneurysm greater than 5cm diameter, or greater than 4cm with an increase of more than 0.5cm in the past 6 months. A minimum of 1cm of non-aneurysmal aortic neck distal to the most inferior major renal artery between 18 and 26mm diameter was required. Common iliac arteries were less than 16mm in diameter and access vessels were patent enabling delivery of the device via the ileofemoral arteries. Patients were entered into the study after extensive discussion with the patient and interested family members and having the patient sign consents for both conventional surgery and the endoluminal bypass procedure on a form approved by the Institutional Review Board of each hospital. Patients were excluded if their aneurysm was acutely rupturing, if the aneurysm had thoracic, suprarenal or ileofemoral components that would require exclusion of both hypogastric arteries, or if the aneurysm was inflammatory or due to vascular trauma. The exclusion criteria including morbid obesity or other clinical conditions that inhibit X-ray visualization of the aorta, connective tissue disease or hypercoagulability, acute renal failure, acute systemic infection, or life expectancy or inability of the patient to be available for 1-year follow-up.

A concurrent controlled surgical group was enrolled and included 66 patients from the investigational sites conducting the study. Each investigational centre was required to enter five patients with abdominal aortic aneurysms meeting inclusion criteria for the endovascular procedure. These five patients were enrolled prior to any investigational centre beginning implantation of the AneuRx endovascular devices. A total of 416 patients with attempted placement of endovascular prostheses were enrolled, with 415 patients being treated. One patient had a myocardial infarction just prior to treatment and was not considered further in the endoluminal group. The study consisted of 89% male and 11% female patients with an average age of 73.8 years. American Society of Anesthesia grade of patient morbidity was 1–4.

During the study, the patients were evaluated for both primary and secondary trial endpoints. The primary endpoints were used to determine eventual safety and efficacy of the device. The secondary endpoints were factors that were compared with the operative surgical group during the hospitalization.

Primary end-points

The primary endpoints evaluated in this study were technical success, mortality and major morbidity, aneurysm rupture, aneurysm diameter, conversion to open surgery repair, patency, stent fracture, device migration, additional procedures, and the incidence of endoleaks.

Technical success was determined for both the endovascular surgery procedure and conventional surgical controls on an intention to treat basis. All 66 surgery controls were successfully implanted with a 100% technical success. Of the 415 patients with attempted endovascular prosthesis deployment 405 were successfully treated for a 97.6% technical success. There was no statistical difference between the conventional surgical and endovascular prosthesis technical success. Of the ten patients who were not treated successfully with endovascular prostheses, seven were not implanted due to vessel access difficulty. Three patients had surgical repair due to device malposition. These ten patients will be considered in further discussions of the results.

The second primary end-point was a comparison of mortality and major morbidity. Seven of the 415 endovascular graft patients died (2%) compared with none in the surgery control group (0%), with no statistical difference. In the follow-up of both groups to 1-year post-procedure, six patients died in the surgery control group (9%) compared with 26 in the endoluminal group (6%), no statistical difference. Major perioperative morbidity was statistically different between the two groups with there being 30 events in the endoluminal graft group (7%) and 10 events in the surgery controls (15%). The 50% reduction in perioperative major morbidity in the endoluminal graft group combined with no difference in mortality accentuates comparability of the endovascular treatment with a conventional surgical procedure in the perioperative interval.

There were two aneurysm ruptures in the 405 patients during the study. One occurred at 18 hours after the procedure in an elderly female who experienced chest and abdominal pain that could not be differentiated from an acute myocardial infarction. A computed tomography (CT) angiogram demonstrated minimal extravasation of contrast through the fabric of the device with a retroperitoneal haematoma. For this reason, the patient was converted to an open surgical repair. A second rupture occurred in a patient 14 months post-procedure following treatment with an endoluminal graft. Review of the case demonstrated that the device had a marginal seal in a short angled neck throughout the interval of the implantation, and that the rupture was due to the development of a proximal endoleak. The patient was successfully converted to an open surgical repair. Aneurysm ruptures have been reported in other series.[7–10] The 0.05% aneurysm rupture in this study is comparable with the frequency that is being reported worldwide with other devices. Comparison with the surgical literature where aneurysms in the 5–6cm range would normally increase by approximately 4mm diameter per year, with a 10% rupture rate per year offers a comparison of the rupture rate in untreated aneurysms to the 0.5% rupture rate reported in this study. Although the rate of rupture is dramatically decreased by endovascular exclusion with a concomitant decrease in aneurysm size in the endoluminal graft treatment group compared with the conventional surgical patients, these patients should be informed that there is a less than 1% rupture risk associated with endovascular repair and that this remains as a challenge for future evolution of the technology.

In this study, aneurysm diameter increased by more than 5mm diameter in fewer than 4% of patients at any follow-up interval. In contrast, aneurysm diameter approximately decreased in 10% of patients at each 6-month follow-up interval. At 1 year, nearly 20% of patients demonstrated a decrease.

An important endpoint in any endovascular graft study is conversion to open surgical repair. In this study, 2% of the total population (8 of 415) underwent surgical conversion. Three were for device malposition and were mentioned earlier in this report. Two additional patients were those described presenting with aneurysm rupture. One patient had an elective conversion at 6 months for an endoleak and two patients underwent endovascular conversion at the time of the procedure when access through the ileofemoral vessels was inadequate. Both of these patients had consented prior to the procedure for the conversion.

Patency of the conventional surgical and endoluminal grafts were both 98% in each group. One patient with conventional surgery underwent an iliac limb thrombosis that was cleared with thrombolysis. Eight patients in the endovascular group had limb thrombosis with four being restored by extra-anatomic bypasses, and four were restored to patency using catheter techniques. The secondary patency in both the surgical and endovascular graft patients was 100%.

Throughout the study, there was no evidence of stent fracture. Migration, defined as any movement of the device by CT or flat plate examination occurred in less than 2% of the patients at any interval. Two patients that had displacement, had endoleaks that were repaired with addition of a cuff. This finding emphasizes, the importance of monitoring device position related to fixed anatomic landmarks as an indicator of potential problems.

An additional important endpoint in this study is additional procedures required during the time of follow-up in order to maintain function of the device. These included 19 patients who had cuff placements for endoleaks (4.7%). Of the 19 patients with endoleaks, 16 received corrections with an additional modular component. The remaining secondary interventions were in the nine patients who had limb thrombosis discussed in the proceeding section.

Detection and treatment of endoleaks is an extremely important component in the follow-up of endovascular graft patients. Endoleaks in this modular device can occur at various sites as depicted in Fig. 3. These include proximal, distal, junctional, transgraft, branch flow or indeterminate origin. As the device consists of a porous polyester fabric, flow across the device can be documented for 24–48 hours following the procedure by contrast CT in 20–30% of patients. Transgraft flow was found to have no consequence and usually stopped within 48 hours. Throughout the study, any endoleak associated with aneurysm enlargement was investigated and considered for treatment. Proximal, distal or junction leaks were considered to be pressurized leaks and treatment was recommended. The modular design of the prosthesis expedited successful treatment in most patients, as discussed. At 1-year, the incidence of proximal distal and junctional leaks was in six patients or 1.75%. The branch flow leaks constituted 9.5% and indeterminate leaks were 4.7%.

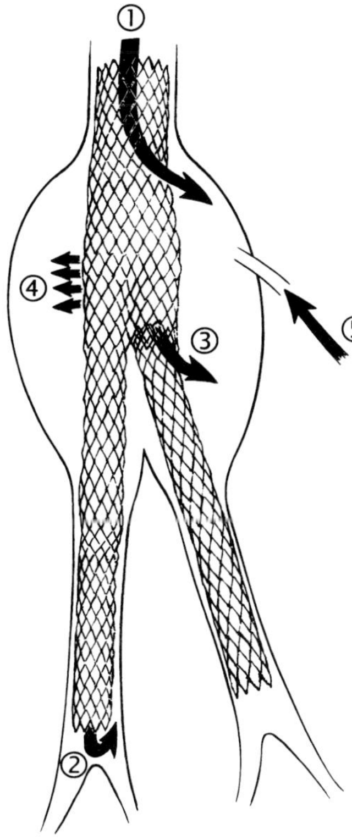

Fig. 3. Potential sources of endoleaks in the modular AneuRx device: 1) proximal, 2) distal, 3) junctional, 4) transgraft, and 5) branch flow.

Secondary endpoints

Secondary endpoints assessing clinical utility including procedure time, blood loss, transfusions, time to extubation, time to ambulation and normal diet, time in the intensive care unit, and hospital stay were also compared between the surgery control and endovascular patients. The analysis demonstrated that the endovascular graft group had significantly reduced secondary clinical endpoints with all variables being reduced by nearly two-thirds compared with the conventional surgery group.

Risk-benefit analysis

Following completion of this study, a risk-benefit analysis of the data demonstrated that there was no difference in mortality with the 50% reduction in major morbidity. The technical success rate of 98% at discharge and surgical conversion rate of 2% combined with the major benefit of secondary endpoints led to the recommendation for approval of this device.

Based on potential risks including perioperative mortality, aneurysm rupture, aneurysm expansion, surgical conversion, and thrombosis of the device, a primary success rate at 1 year was determined to be 89.6%. When considering the secondary patencies that occurred in patients with successful secondary procedures, the secondary success rate at 1 year increased to 92%. Further analysis of these parameters has demonstrated that the primary and secondary success rate at 18 months is 92 and 88%.[6]

DISCUSSION

The AneuRx bifurcated endoluminal graft is exemplary of the advances that have been made in endovascular therapy, and of the potential for further development in this field. The AneuRx device was developed and tested in the experimental laboratory over approximately 2 years,[11] and was then investigated in patients for an additional 3.5 years which demonstrates the significant effort that is required for new devices to reach a clinical setting. In one regard, the developmental phase before use in clinical practice appears to be quite long. From a broader perspective, the rapid development of endovascular graft technologies has been quite short and successful compared with many other biomedical development projects. The widespread interest and application of these devices and the ability to select patients and provide successful treatment in the majority of patients represents an optimistic perspective regarding the eventual potential for continued rapid development of endovascular technologies to treat many vascular disorders.

The AneuRx bifurcated endoluminal graft offers an innovative means to treat abdominal aortic aneurysms and now has clinical applicability for many patients. The obvious candidates for repair are those with aneurysms that have significant co-morbid conditions that would make conventional repair either prohibitively high-risk or not possible. This patient group also has the highest risk for morbid complications using the technology, so that patient selection and endovascular skill are paramount issues in treating these patients. Since the devices have been approved by many regulatory agencies for widespread use in all patients who would normally be treated with conventional surgery, a well informed presentation of the benefits and potential risk of this technology compared with conventional surgical repair is required. Although this paper provides a brief and preliminary report of data regarding the AneuRx device that will be expanded in subsequent peer review publications, it contains important information that can be made available to better inform patients. When one reviews the current knowledge related to conventional vascular procedures, the long-term durability is a major advantage, even though associated problems requiring either reintervention by endovascular or conventional surgical repair are significant over time. With regard to the endovascular technologies, the long-term perspective for comparability with conventional surgical repair and any statement regarding more or less potential for complications remains speculation. Although those who are skeptical about endovascular technology would say that durability will be compromised, they are overlooking the fact that rapid evolution has occurred in all perspectives related to endovascular prosthesis development and use, and that new methods to treat potential complications and eliminate them with enhancements to current devices will most certainly reduce the risk of complications and make it applicable to a much broader group of patients. Although the current AneuRx endoluminal technologies may only be applicable to 50% or more of current patients receiving treatment for abdominal aortic aneurysms, the early success and rapid evolution highlights the potential for broader utilization of these devices in the future.

REFERENCES

1. White RA, Donayre CE, Walot I *et al.*: Modular bifurcation endoprosthesis for treatment of abdominal aortic aneurysms. *Ann Surg* **226**: 381–391, 1997
2. Biasi GM, Piglionica MR, Meregaglia D *et al.*: European multicenter experience with modular device (Medtronic AneuRx) for the endoluminal repair of infrarenal abdominal aortic aneurysms. *J Maladies Vasculaires* **5**: 374–380, 1998
3. Nolthenius PPT, Berg JD, Biasi GM *et al.*: Endoluminal repair of infrarenal abdominal aortic aneurysms using a modular stent-graft: One-year clinical results from a European multicenter trial. *Cardiovasc Surg* **5**: 503–507, 1999
4. Zarins CK, White RA, Schwarten D *et al.*: For the investigators of the Medtronic AneuRx clinical trial: AneuRx stent-graft versus open surgical repair for abdominal aortic aneurysms: Multicenter perspective clinical trial. *J Vasc Surg* **29**: 292–303, 1999
5. FDA Circulatory Advisory Panel, Gaithersberg, MD, 23 June 1999
6. Zarins CK, White RA, Hodgson KJ *et al.*: Endoleak as a predictor of outcome following endovascular aneurysm repair: AneuRx multicenter clinical trial. *J Vasc Surg* (in press)
7. Zarins CK, White RA, Fogarty TJ, Nolan S: Aneurysm rupture following endovascular repair: AneuRx multicenter clinical trial using the AneuRx stent-graft. *J Vas Surg* (in press)
8. May J, White GH, Waugh R *et al.*: Rupture of abdominal aortic aneurysms: A concurrent comparison of outcome of those occurring after endoluminal repair versus those occurring *de novo*. *Eur J Vasc Endovasc Surg* **18**: 344–348, 1999

9. Alimi YS, Chakfe N, Rivoal E *et al.*: Rupture of abdominal aortic aneurysm after endovascular graft placement and aneurysm size reduction. *J Vasc Surg* **28**: 178–183, 1998
10. Krohg-Sorensen K, Brekke M, Drolsum A *et al.*: Periprosthetic leak and rupture after endovascular repair of abdominal aortic aneurysm: The significance of device design and long-term result. *J Vasc Surg* **29**: 1151–1158, 1999
11. White RA, Fogarty TJ, Kopchok GE *et al.*: Evaluation of a modular endovascular prosthesis in a canine aortic aneurysm model. *J Vasc Surg* **24**: 1034–1042, 1996

Custom manufacturing of aortic stent-grafts to expand applicability of endovascular repair

Frank J Criado, Eric P Wilson, Jennifer A Martin, Snehal C Patel, Scott A Bovard

INTRODUCTION

The development of stent-graft technology for repair of aortic aneurysms represents nothing short of a revolution in our specialty. The initial 10-year evolutionary phase of this new era in vascular intervention began with the pioneering work of Parodi *et al.* in Buenos Aires,[1] and culminated with the approval of two abdominal aortic aneurysm devices by the Food and Drug Administation (FDA) in the USA in 1999. Currently available stent-grafts (Table 1) reflect the state of the art in the year 2000. With few exceptions, these endografts are modular in design and contain a metal frame that provides column strength and kink/compression resistance. Nitinol and Dacron are the two most common components; stainless steel and PTFE are used less frequently. Self-expansion is the preferred mode of deployment.

The notion of 'anatomical suitability' describes morphological characteristics that relate to technological limitations in design and manufacturing. Minimum proximal aortic neck dimensions of 26 mm diameter and 15 mm length are required in most cases. Similarly, iliac artery diameter must be 14–16 mm. These limitations can seriously handicap applicability of stent-graft repair[2] and exclude many high-risk patients who tend to have large, complex aneurysms – the precise clinical subset where a less-invasive approach can be of most benefit (Fig.1).

Table 1. Abdominal aortic aneurysm stent-graft devices

Ancure (Guidant)
AneuRx (Medtronic AVE)
Talent (Medtronic AVE)
Vanguard (Boston Scientific Vascular)
Excluder (W L Gore)
Zenith (Cook)
LifePath (Baxter)
Endologix (Bard)
Cordis bilateral aortoiliac (Cordis Endovascular)
Anaconda (Sulzer Vascutek)

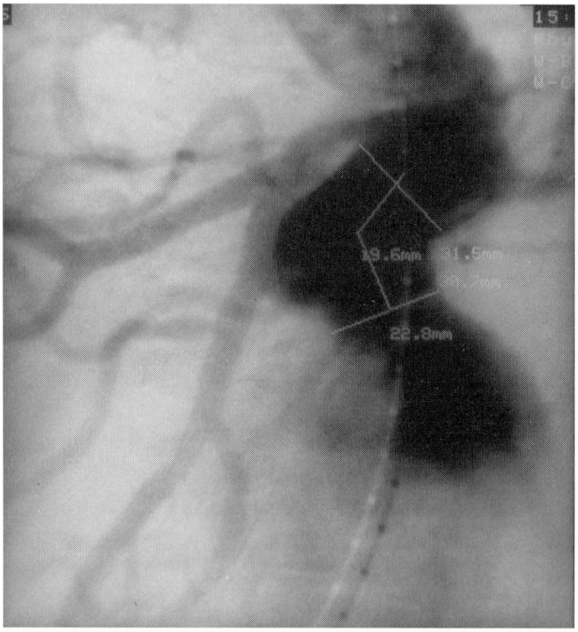

(a)

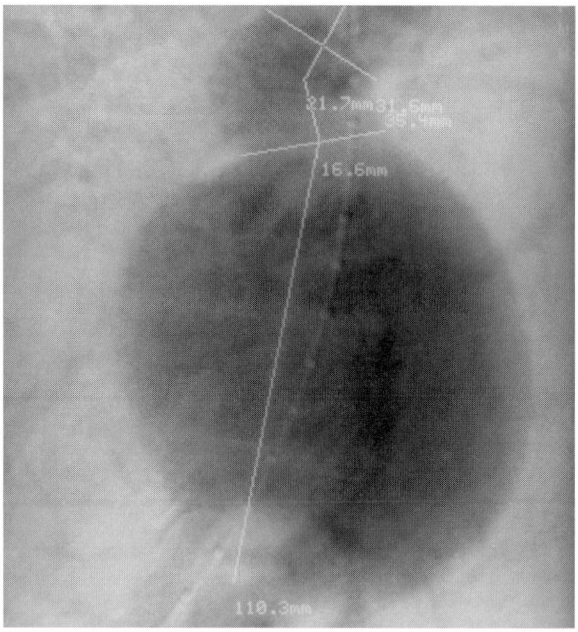

(b)

Fig. 1. Abdominal aortic aneurysm of 10 cm with challenging neck anatomy and large diameter. Patient was treated successfully with a customized Talent stent-graft.

Table 2. Talent stent-graft (dimensional possibilities)

	Diameter	*Length*
Bifurcated devices		
Aortic	16–36 mm	35–75 cm
Iliac	8–20 mm	5–20 cm
Straight-tube devices		
Abdominal, iliac, thoracic	8–46 mm	5–20 cm

Commercially produced stent-graft devices are manufactured in various sizes and lengths, but choices are limited to a number of 'standard' configurations. Exceptionally, World Medical/Medtronic AVE (maker of the Talent stent-graft system) offers unique customization possibilities.[3] These involve dimensional (Table 2) as well as configurational options. The following Talent customization features have been found valuable in dealing with the anatomical challenge of many large, complex abdominal aortic aneurysms.

- *Proximal neck diameter* – 36 mm grafts allow placement in aortic necks up to 32 mm in diameter. We have successfully treated more than ten patients with necks greater than 30 mm in diameter. It must be emphasized, however, that large necks show a tendency for progressive dilatation over time that may lead to secondary endoleak and aneurysm rupture (Fig. 2a,b).
- *Neck length* of at least 10 mm is required to achieve proper anchoring and sealing with all stent-graft devices – Talent included. We have had a chance to do implants on a handful of patients with neck lengths of 5–10 mm. Trans/suprarenal fixation is quite important in such cases, made possible by the 'bare spring' design at the top end of the Talent endograft (Fig. 3), but it should be made clear that proper fixation and sealing in such a short length can only be achieved when the neck is not angulated or funnel-shaped. The combination of short length (less than 15 mm), trapezoidal configuration, and angulation (Fig. 4) increase the risk of failure exponentially, and should be looked upon as anatomical contraindications to endovascular repair.
- *Short distance* (less than 90 mm) between renal arteries and bifurcation may dictate design of a short aortic section to avoid possible deployment of both limbs into the (same) ipsilateral iliac artery. The dictum 'when in doubt, make it shorter' describes a useful principle: modular endografts can always be extended distally, but cannot be shortened after deployment.
- *Narrow aortic bifurcation*, especially when associated with circumferential calcification (on computed tomography) can preclude safe deployment of a standard bifurcated stent-graft. Custom designs with narrow reverse-taper limbs (Fig. 5a–c) allow placement and aneurysm exclusion on patients who may not be candidates for conventional surgery.
- *Iliac artery diameter* can be a limiting factor on patients with large vessels. The Talent iliac limbs can be manufactured with a maximum diameter of 20 mm, permitting placement in arteries that are up to that calibre. The risk of progressive

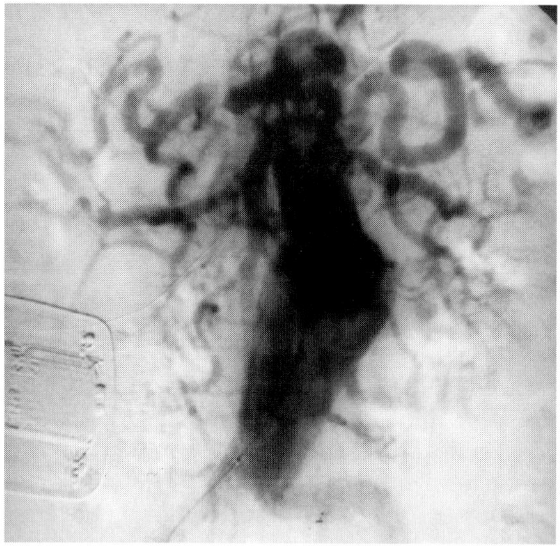

(a)

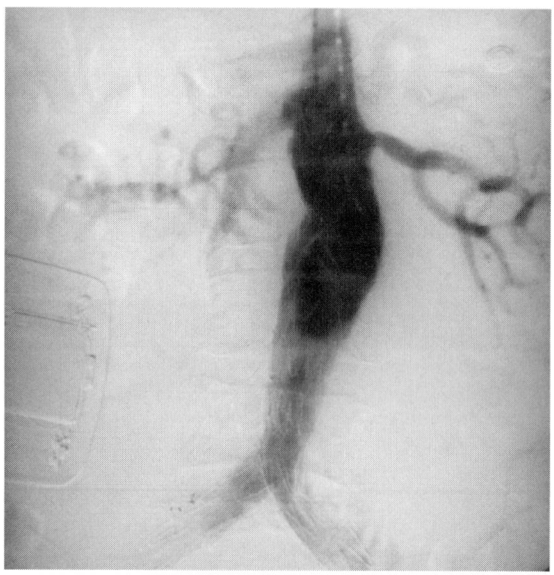

(b)

Fig. 2. Aortogram of large abdominal aortic aneurysm with a 32-mm diameter infrarenal neck (a). Aneurysm exclusion was achieved with an oversized Talent endograft + proximal extension cuff (b). Patient did well for 18 months, but experienced aneurysm rupture at 18 months from secondary endoleak at proximal attachment site.

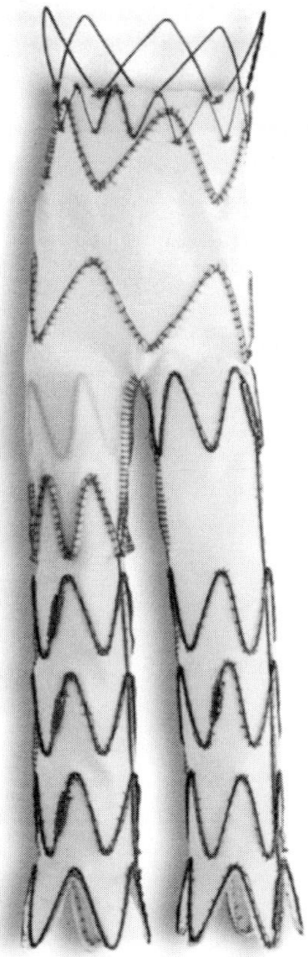

Fig. 3. Uncovered bare spring at top end of Talent stent-graft.

iliac enlargement is quite small in that size range, and rupture has not been reported in iliac arteries less than 20 mm in diameter.[4]

- *Aortouni-iliac configurations* are useful alternatives for patients with associated iliac artery disease, applicable in 10–15% of abdominal aortic aneurysm implants in our experience (Fig. 6). It is also of interest that a 'bifurcated' main section can be converted into a uni-iliac design by placing an occluding oversized aortic cuff or a custom 'converter endograft' (Fig. 7). This is occasionally necessary in case of access failure across the short contralateral leg.

STENT-GRAFT CUSTOMIZATION FOR THE THORACIC AORTA

The thoracic aorta presents both unique challenges and an excellent opportunity for stent-graft technology. Early results with endoluminal treatment of thoracic aortic aneurysms and Type B aortic dissection are encouraging.[5,6]

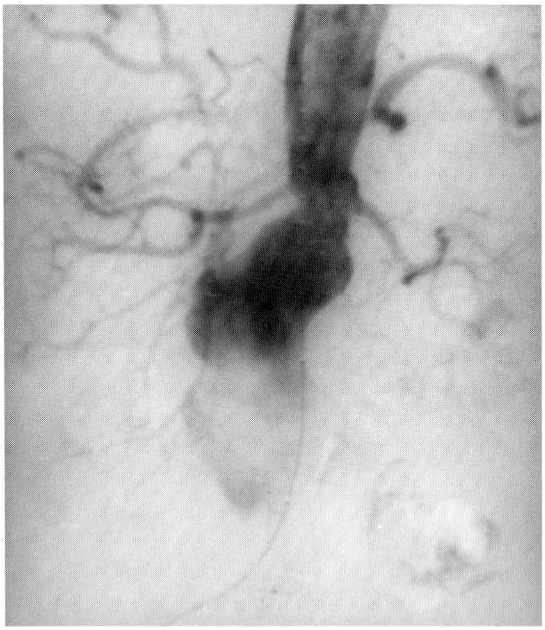

Fig. 4. Example of unsuitable neck anatomy.

- Some of the most vexing anatomical difficulties occur in the *parasubclavian aorta* involving that segment from the distal aortic arch to the proximal portion of the descending thoracic aorta (Fig. 8). Flexibility and conformability are important endograft characteristics for deployment in this area. Management of the left subclavian artery itself can be a significant issue. At times, graft coverage of the vessel origin may be necessary to gain additional critical length to achieve apposition and sealing distal to the left common carotid artery (Fig. 9). Preliminary revascularization of the subclavian artery, (i.e. carotid–subclavian bypass) is largely unnecessary, and can always be done after the fact if indicated, but possible reflux back into the aorta may be an issue when treating a large proximal descending aneurysm, and dictate preliminary vessel occlusion (or ligation) in preparation for endovascular grafting.

It is important to emphasize that the term *customization* (as used in this chapter) is meant to describe design/dimensional possibilities that can be translated into a commercial device manufactured by a major company in the endovascular industry. Such custom stent-grafts are made with the same rigorous standards and quality controls as those adhered to in the fabrication of 'off-the-shelf' devices. 'Homemade' endografts, on the other hand, are assembled on site by surgeons and other physicians following their own conceptions and guidelines. The materials and techniques are not standardized or subjected to systematic quality control testing.

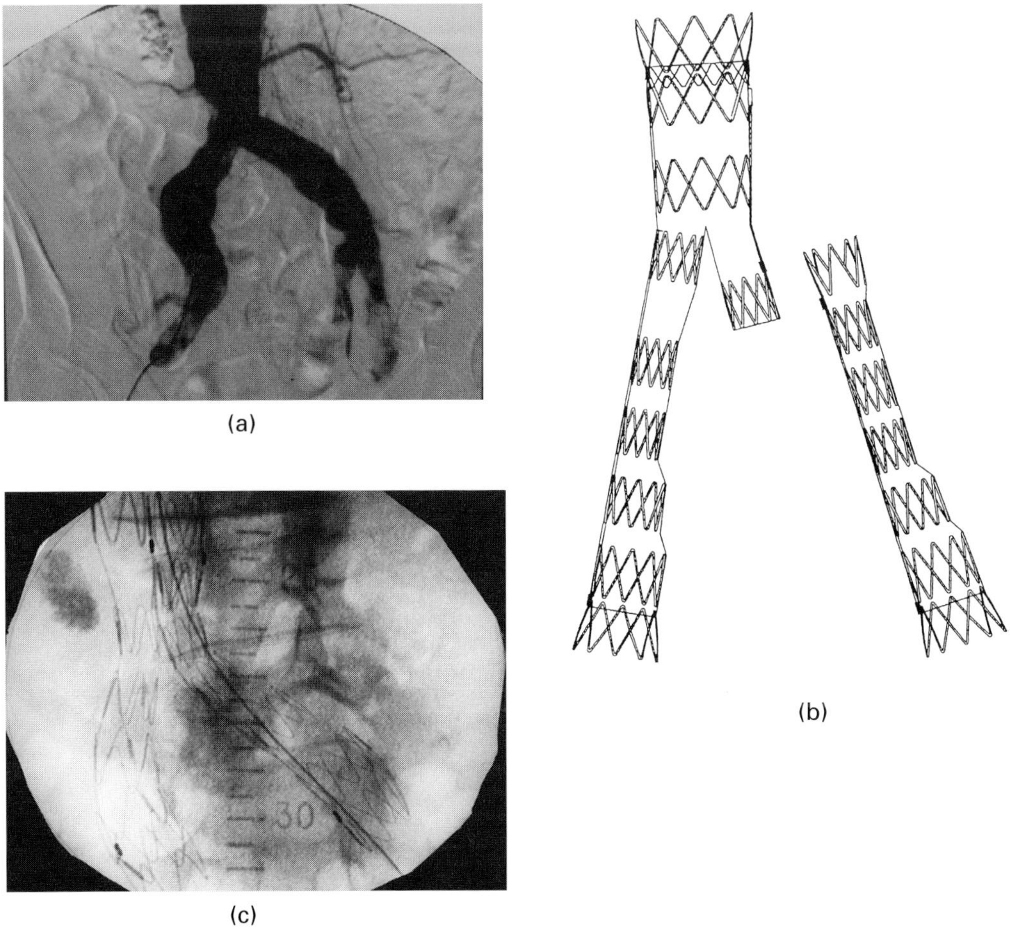

Fig. 5. Combination of narrow/hardened aortic bifurcation with large iliac arteries (a). Custom design (b) allowed endovascular treatment (c).

The authors do not endorse the teaching or 'showcasing' of such homemade devices, for wider application would undoubtedly lead to increased risks of technical and device failures.

A final word of caution is in order: custom manufacturing of devices to expand clinical use of stent-graft repair may be recommended for carefully selected cases only. Such aggressive endovascular approach can be justified on some abdominal aortic aneurysm patients who are unfit for major surgery, or those with thoracic aortic lesions where surgical treatment carries considerable risks of serious morbidity and mortality. Currently available evidence does not support undertaking endovascular repair in situations of borderline morphology when patients are suitable candidates for conventional surgical treatment.

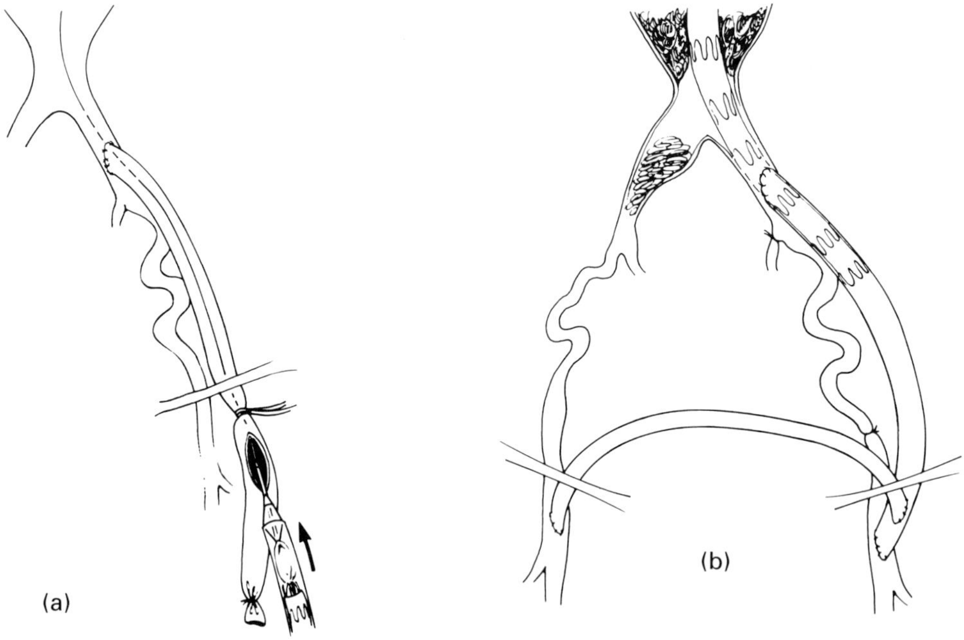

Fig. 6. Diagrammatic illustration of aortouni-iliac/iliac-conduit technique.

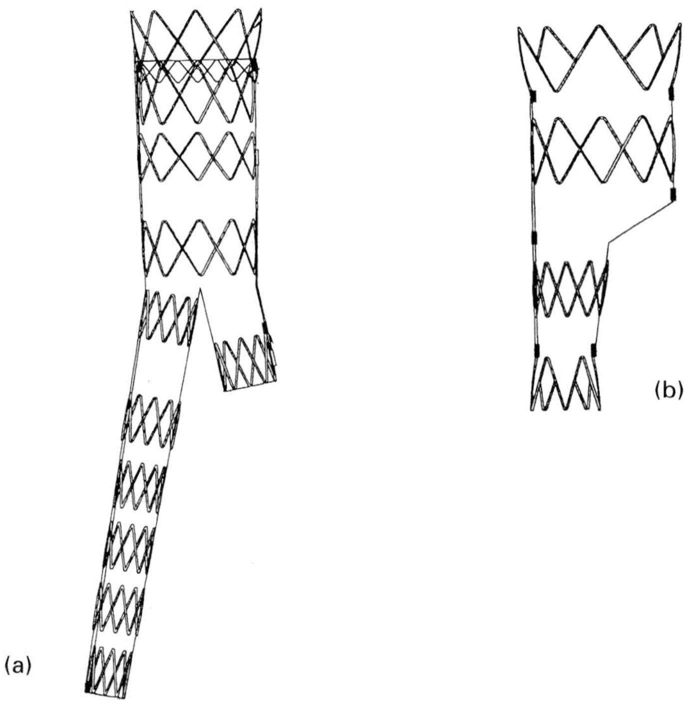

Fig. 7. Main section of Talent system (a) was implanted, but access-related failure precluded deployment of contralateral limb. Custom-design ‘converter’ endograft (b) can be used to make it into an aortouni-iliac design.

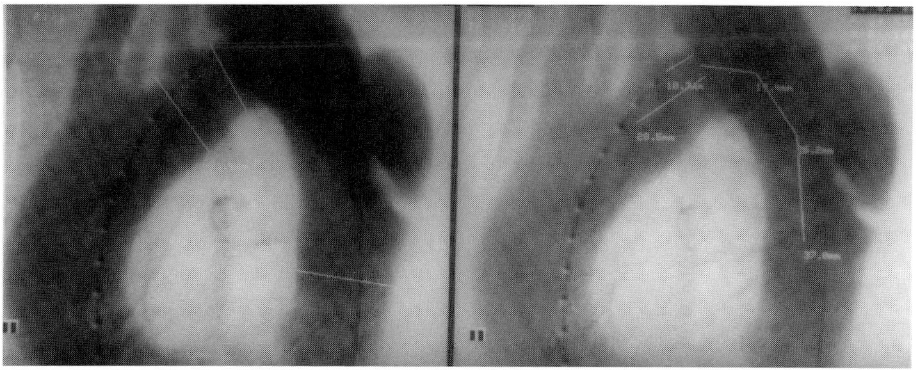

Fig. 8. Saccular aneurysmal dilatation of dissected proximal descending thoracic aorta. Note proximity to origin of left subclavian artery.

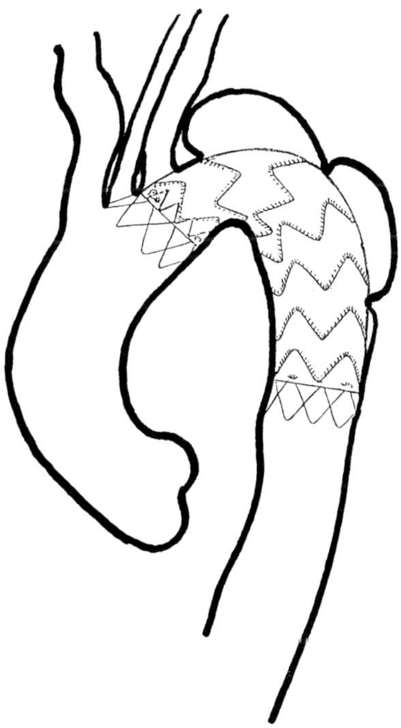

Fig. 9. Proposed endovascular repair, with coverage of subclavian artery and bare-spring fixation across left common carotid.

REFERENCES

1. Parodi JC, Palmaz JC, Barone HD: Transfemoral intraluminal graft implantation for abdominal aortic aneurysms. *Ann Vasc Surg* **5**: 491–499, 1991
2. Armon MP, Hopkinson BR: How much does an aortouni-iliac stent-graft increase the endovascular options for abdominal aortic aneurysm repair? In: Greenhalgh RM (Ed), *Indications In Vascular And Endovascular Surgery*, pp. 221–227. London: WB Saunders, 1998

3. Criado FJ, Abul-Khoudoud O, Wellons E *et al.*: The Talent abdominal aortic aneurysm stent graft: technical approaches and results of aneurysm exclusion. In: Greenhalgh RM (Ed), *The Durability Of Vascular And Endovascular Surgery*, pp. 433–448. London: WB Saunders, 1999
4. Criado FJ, Fairman R, Greenberg RK: Endovascular exclusion of abdominal aortic aneurysms with the Talent stent-graft system: Problem solving and alternative techniques. *Talent Technical Guidebook*. World Medical, Medtronic AVE, 1999
5. Mitchell RS, Miller DC, Dake MD. Stent-graft repair of thoracic aortic aneurysms. *Semin Vasc Surg* **10**: 257–271, 1997
6. Nienaber CA, Fattori R, Lund G *et al.*: Nonsurgical reconstruction of thoracic aortic dissection by stent-graft placement. *New Engl J Med* **340**: 1545–1559, 1999

Recent Vanguard experience and the introduction of Vanguard III

Svante Horsch, Kiriakos Ktenidis, Georg-Wilhelm Albrecht-Früh

HISTORY

The development of operative measures employing minimal access is developing rapidly particularly in the treatment of vascular disease. Of special mention is the abdominal aortic aneurysm, which is treated by a large transperitoneal incision. Moore attempted the thrombosis by wire of syphilitic aneurysms in the seventeenth century.

Endovascular treatment of abdominal aortic aneurysms has been in use since 1990, when Juan Parodi performed these procedures in the human.[1] In the early years self-constructed stent-graft combinations were implanted. However, in 1992 specially manufactured devices came into use, first with an uni-piece design, and more recently with a modular modification. This latter version, which is now used on a large scale, has a metal stent frame along its entire length. The Boston Scientific Company manufacture the Vanguard device, which, like its predecessor the Mintec produced Stentor, incorporates zig-zag shaped nitinol stent rows on the inside of the Dacron graft. The apices of the different zig rows are connected by polypropylene sutures.

METHODS

From January 1997 to August 1999 100 patients (12 women and 88 men with an average age of 69.6 years, range 48–87 years) were selected for endovascular treatment of an infrarenal abdominal aortic aneurysm with a Vanguard prosthesis. The patients were classified according to the American Society of Anesthesiologists (ASA) Physical Status as class II (n=56), class III (n=52) or class IV (n=2); 24 suffered from a compensative renal insufficiency, of which four patients had a preoperative creatinine value of more than 2 mg/dl. In addition to cardiac, pulmonary and renal risk factors 34% of patients were distinctly overweight (more than 120% of their normal weight/height value) and 24 patients had undergone multiple previous laparatomies. Of these patients one had a bladder resection with implantation of a neobladder using a part of the jejunum and three had a colostomy. In one patient the conventional aneurysm resection had to be abandoned due to inflammatory adhesions 8 months previously. The indication for the treatment of the aneurysms was confirmed if the diameter of the aneurysm exceeded 4.5 cm, if the aneurysmal sac was more than double than the lumen of the aorta, if a growth tendency had been documented or if the morphology of the aneurysm implied therapy. Important criteria for inclusion was a segment of thrombus-free aorta between the lower renal artery and the commencement of the aneurysm of at least 1.5 cm or more and the iliac arteries needed to allow access to aorta via the groin. The aneurysms were classified according to the Heidelberg classification.[2] The distribution and the implanted prothesis are demonstrated in Fig. 1.

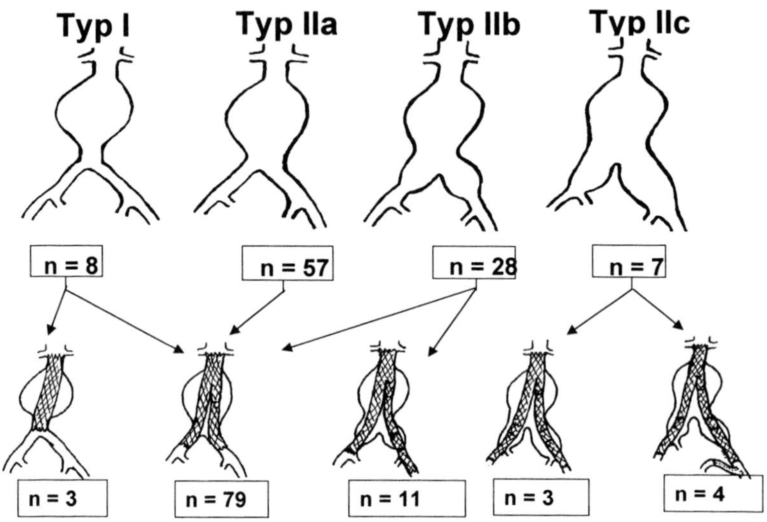

Fig. 1. Heidelberg classification of 100 abdominal aortic aneurysms and implanted prostheses.

Eight patients had an aneurysm which was limited to the aorta and with a proximal and distal neck and could be classified as Type I. In 57 cases the aneurysm ended at the aortic bifurcation (Type IIA) and 28 times the aneurysm was classified as Type II B due to aneurysmic dilatation of the iliac arteries. In seven patients with partially major co-morbidities endoluminal therapy was planned despite a Type IIC aneurysm, which applied iliac aneurysms bilaterally. The average aneurysm diameter was 4.8 cm (maximum 7.5, minimum 3.7 cm). Five aneurysms were classified as sacciform, and three aneurysms presented an inflammatory component.

Despite a distal aneurysm neck of more than 1.5 cm, only three sacciform aneurysms were treated by means of a tubular prosthesis. In 97% of patients a bifurcational prosthesis was considered necessary. The most frequently implanted prosthesis had a proximal diameter of 24 mm (35%) and 26 mm (29%). Other prosthesis diameters of 28 mm (14%) and 30 mm (15%) were only available from the beginning of 1998.

RESULTS

All implantations were done in an operating theatre with patients under general anaesthesia with the possibility for an immediate conversion to open surgery. Generally the femoral artery was dissected and the main part of the prosthesis implanted via an arteriotomy in the femoral artery. A purely percutaneous implantation of the contralateral wire graft leg was successful in 72% of patients; in all others the groin artery on the left-hand side was additionally dissected in order to achieve an additional local disobliteration, or to exclude difficult arterial punctures and thereby avoid a postoperative bleeding. In three patients an aneurysm spurium had to be excluded after arterial puncture.

A total of 27 patients required additional vascular procedures (four cubital access routes, two percutaneous transluminal angioplasties (PTA) of the renal artery, eight PTA of the iliac arteries, two retrograde iliac disobliteration, two iliac-femoral bypass grafts, four internal iliac artery bypass grafts and 14 femoral desobliteration, usually bilaterally).

We placed our grafts as proximal as possible, so that in more than 40% of the cases the open wire covered at least one renal artery. Fortunately an aneurysmal inclusion of this proximal piece of aorta within the region of the renal arteries is seen rather seldomly. Placement of the short leg of the wire graft was possible in a free-style manoeuvre from the puncture side in most cases. In five cases an additional crossover manoeuvre and in four cases the additional cubital access had to be chosen in order to successfully place the leg of the stent graft.

A correct placement of the prosthesis was possible in 97% of cases; however, an additional five proximal cuffs in three patients and 40 distal extensions in 23 patients were required. In eleven patients a patent but partially stenotic or aneurysmatic internal iliac artery was overstented unilaterally, in 7% bilaterally. Four of these patients received a bypass on to the internal iliac artery unilaterally. Two of these bypasses occluded asymptomatically in the follow-up period.

The average operative time, inclusive of all additional procedures was 124 minutes, with a dramatic time difference noted once the first learning problems were overcome (105 minutes for the last 50 procedures). Average radiation time was 22.8 minutes (6–128 minutes) and 102 ml of contrast medium (45–270 ml) were used. In the early postoperative phase 59% of patients were monitored in the intensive care unit for roughly 17 hours. The other patients were transferred to the ward after brief monitoring in the intensive care unit. The average hospital stay (inclusive of the patients who had to be converted to open surgery) were 7.3 days.

An emergency operation of a 76-year-old patient suffering from numerous other illnesses was successfully performed on a contained rupture of a 1.8 cm abdominal aortic aneurysm. The entire aneurysm was included by means of a bifurcated prosthesis within 1.5 hours. The operative mortality was 2% in the series and was not influenced by concomitant disease, but cases of conversion.

Conversions

Three patients were converted to the conventional open repair after an initial endoluminal treatment was partially attempted. A 78-year-old patient with a heavily calcified and stenosed and kinked iliac artery was perforated after attempted PTA. He was converted to an extraperitoneal conventional repair on an emergency basis. Due to further complications and the linked extended intensive care period, the patient developed a severe pneumonia and died. Due to an accidential misplacement of the graft suprarenally, an 82-year-old patient developed a mesenterial and renal ischaemia which ended in a fatality despite conversion. A conversion due to unpassable iliac stensosis bilaterally, which was performed under the same anaesthesia but not under emergency conditions was well tolerated by an 86-year-old patient.

Follow-up observations

Follow-up has included clinical and laboratory examination, biplanar non-contrast radiography, duplex scanning and contrast-enhanced computed tomography (CT). Over the mean 15-month follow-up (range 3–32) nine patients were reoperated, predominantly for endoleaks in five patients, but no aneurysm showed an increase in diameter.

A reperfusion of the aneurysm sac is not always identifiable on the intraoperative angiography, and for this reason a postoperative CT-scan is obligatory to recognize early leakages. According to the classification by White *et al.*[3,4] reperfusions can be classified in our patients as Types I, III and IV. In our patient group a total of 10% primary endoleaks, one proximal and three distal leakages were identified, some of them nearly retrospectively. Out of three secondary endoleaks one was classified as distal and two as collateral reperfusion. After diagnosis proximal or distal leakages (Type I A or B) secondary endovascular repair was performed. Three reperfusions, where the primary leakage site could not be identified, closed spontaneously and in five patients lumbar artery or inferior mesenteric artery leaks are under close observation.

Thromboses

Three graft thromboses were diagnosed in the follow-up period. In two cases a thrombectomy was no longer possible. One of these patients was treated 6 months ago with a bifurcated graft and an extension passanger graft on each side. An increased angulation at the connecting area of the left limb was found as an incidental finding. A few days later, while planning to implant an addional stent, thrombosis probabely due to disconnection took place and was corrected by a crossover bypass graft. The process is illustrated in Fig. 2. Two higher grade stenoses were treated by PTA or a local desobliteration. The development of stenoses in the left iliac artery and the simultaneous increase of a distal leak is shown in Fig. 3.

Aortoduodenal fistula

To date only one late conversion has been necessary. A 57-year-old patient with a Type II B aneurysm was treated in January 1999 by stent-graft combination. He suffered from other major concomitant illnesses and adiposity. A biiliac prosthesis was implanted endoluminally. After an initial uncomplicated procedure the patient suffered increasing peripheral ischaemia. Within the following 6 months three further operations were performed in an attempt to improve the peripheral perfusion (retrograde iliac desobliteration, femoropopliteal bypass bilaterally). A secondary endoleak, which was retrogradly perfused via the inferior mesenteric artery, was closely monitored over the next 6 months. Before the planned operative exclusion of this reperfusion the patient developed an aortoduodenal fistula with or caused by a proximal infection of the prosthesis. The patient was lost despite an emergency operative intervention.

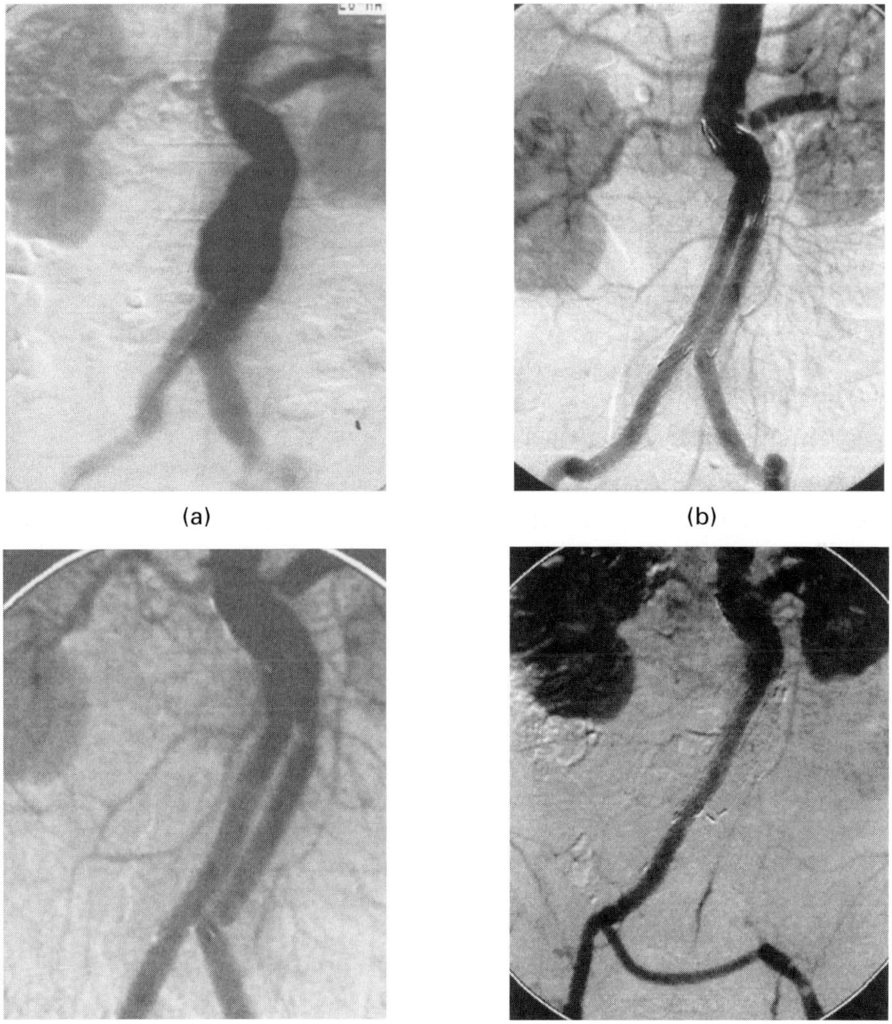

Fig. 2. Limb disconnection after 6 months: (a) preoperative; (b) postoperative; (c) 6 months control; (d) 2 weeks later after thromboses and crossover.

Deformation of prostheses

Knots and wire breakages were followed by plane X-rays. Particularly in cases of more distinct kinkings in the aortal prosthetic segment knot breakages (more than 20%) were noticed in at least one position by a widening of the middle stents. A leakage caused by the mentioned deformation has not, however, to date been documented. A proximal dislocation has so far not occurred, but at least two distal migrations of the prosthetic limb led to thromboses or leakages. Distinct proof of stent breakages and this leading to complications have to date not been unequivocally proven.

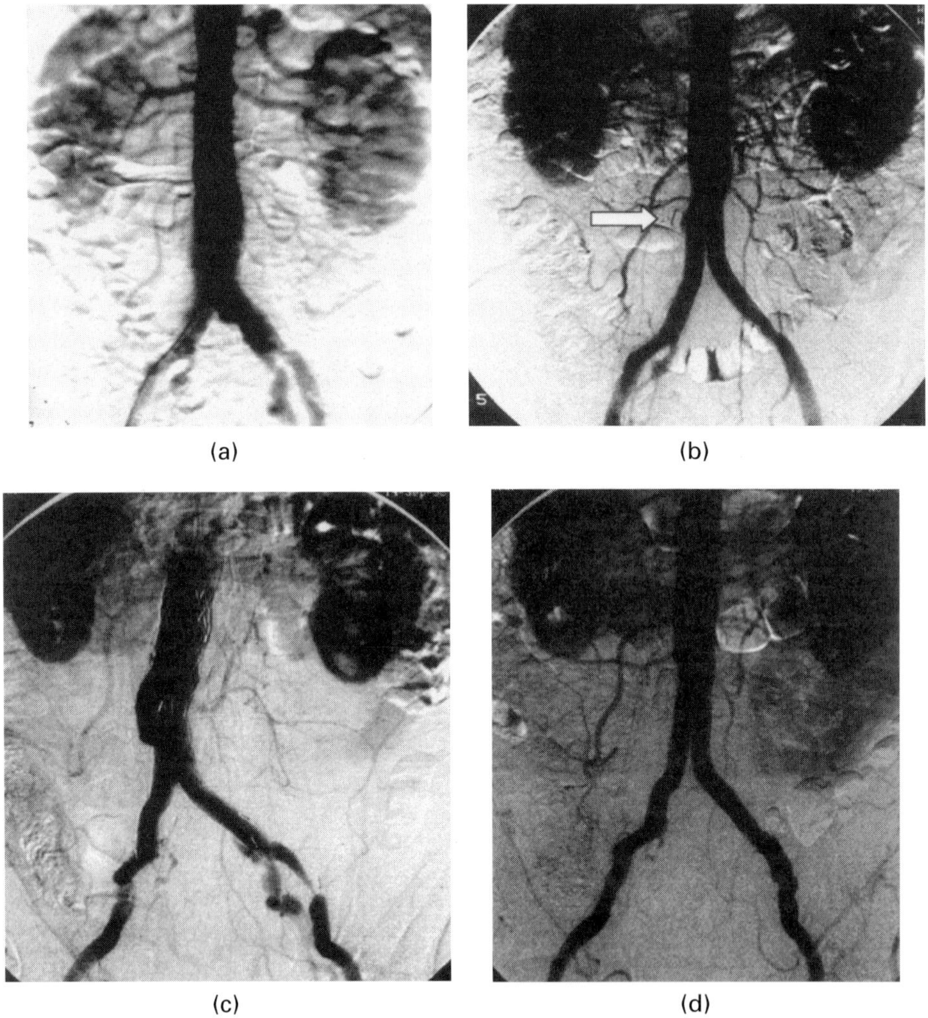

Fig. 3. Movement of the limb of the prosthesis with stenosis and leakage: (a) preoperative; (b) postoperative – small leakage; (c) 6 months postoperative; (d) post-desobliteration and ligation.

DISCUSSION

In comparison with other patient groups that have been reported, a high degree of covering of the internal iliac artery is noticeable. However, only one gluteal ischaemia and one colonic ischaemia were noticed. In both of these patients a unilateral overstenting of the internal iliac artery had been performed. Both were treated expectantly and did not require further surgery. Three of the seven patients where the internal iliac arteries were occluded developed gluteal claudication, which, however, showed an improvement after 6–12 months.

The cause of the aortoduodenal fistula has never been clearly defined. Compared with other reports[5,6] the relatively numerous vascular procedures after implantation of an endoluminal aortic stent and following prosthetic infections with cutaneous bacteria is noticeable.

The changes in the prosthetic materials and shape caused by knot breakages and curvages, which has been noticed in the close follow-up examinations have been frequently discussed.[7] A link between suture breakages and leakages has not been found so far.[8] Also an expected dilatation of the aneurysm neck or the proximal dislocation of the graft have not been noticed. Also Umscheid[9] reported, that he found no neck dilatation, proximal stent moving, or late caudal dislocation. Indeed three of his explanted stent grafts demonstrated that the uncovered proximal stent had completely healed into the aortic wall and was covered by an intimal layer.

It is, however, definite, that the deformation of the prosthesis, particularly the proximal kinking of the wire legs in a large aneurysm can lead to dislocation and thrombosis years later. Tortuosity of the native vessels is thus a source of complication in the long-term follow-up, just as it is during implantation.[9]

Long-term follow-up and comparisons will show, whether the Vanguard system will develop more frequent problems of this nature as the Vanguard design has a flexible stent frame and the nitinol wires are relatively thin. The prosthesis can be easily compressed circumferentially and it is not as rigid at other systems. We have preferred using more flexible systems for the treatment of aneurysms with severely kinked vessels, as we believe, that eventually every graft will in the long-term adapt to the longitudinal and radial forces of the vessel into which it was implanted.

THE VANGUARD III SYSTEM

The Vanguard aortic endograft was derived from the MinTec endovascular prosthesis that had been used in Europe since 1994. Whereas the MinTec system was excessively permeable and liable to late failure due to a structural design feature resulting in a full-length manually sewn fabric seam, the Vanguard system is manufactured out of a substantially modified fabric, stent and delivery system which has been newly developed. This has already led to much improved early results and leads one to hope for a decreased late complication rate. The most obvious and long-expected change lies in the now-available increased iliac diameter of a graft up to 16 mm diameter. Initially a definite standard combination, where the iliac leg of the graft measures half the aortal diameter was offered. Additionally a further standard (153 mm and 165 mm) length of 180 mm was introduced. The adapted prosthesis design is demonstrated in the Fig. 4. and shows the tighter stent configuration in the main part of the prosthesis and the hourglass-shaped lengthened docking limb. The nitinol wire has been strengthened and the contralateral iliac limb was fitted with an uncovered stent row at the proximal end. With this system the holding capacity as well as the sealing of the two components to each other is definitively improved without doubt.

In conclusion it can be said, that the endovascular exclusion of abdominal aortic aneurysm has proved to be successful and the minimal operative stress for the patient is a great improvement to the therapeutic options. Particularly kinkings as well as large aneurysms present a distinct stress for the prosthetic material, which needs to be improved judging by the found complications. The further development in form of the Vanguard system to the Vanguard III prosthesis seems to be a marked improvement in to this direction.

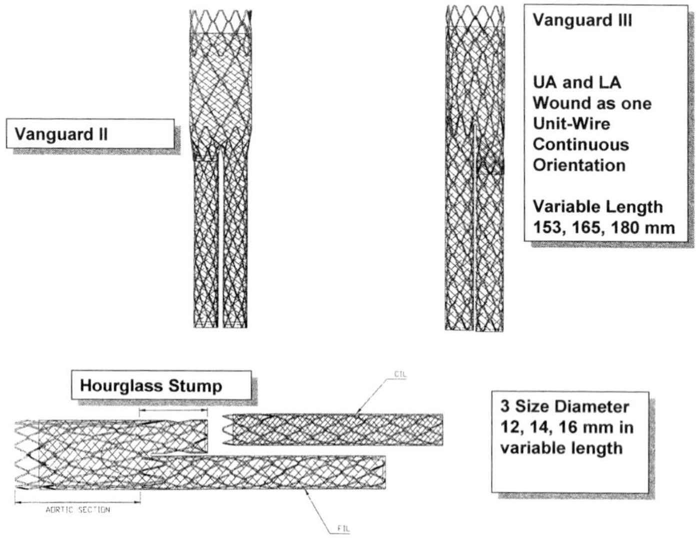

Fig. 4. The adapted prosthesis design.

REFERENCES

1. Parodi JC, Palmaz JC, Barone HD: Transfemoral intraluminal graft implantation for abdominal aortic aneurysms. *Ann Vasc Surg* **5**: 491–499, 1991
2. Allenberg JR, Schumacher H, Eckstein HH, Kallinowski F: Das infrarenale abdominelle Aortenaneurysma (AAA): Morphologische Klassifikation als Entscheidungshilfe für das Therapieverfahren. *Zentralbl Chir* **121**: 721, 1996
3. White GH, May J, Waugh RC *et al.*: Type III and Type IV endoleak: Toward a complete definition of blood flow in the sac after endoluminal AAA repair. *J Endovasc Surg* **5**: 305–309, 1998
4. White GH, Yu W, May J *et al.*: Endoleak as a complication of endoluminal grafting of abdominal aortic aneurysms: Classification, incidence, diagnosis and management. *J Endovasc Surg* **4**: 152–168, 1997
5. Tiesenhausen K, Hausegger KA, Amann W, Koch G: Aortoduodenale Fistel nach endovaskulärer Rekonstruktion eines abdominellen infrarenalen Aortenaneurysma. *Gefässchir* **4**: 101–104, 1999
6. Norgren L, Jernby B, Engellau L:Aortoenteric fistula caused by ruptured stent-graft. *J Endovasc Surg* **5**: 269–272, 1998
7. Boyle JR, Thompson MM, Code-Baker EG *et al.*: Torsion and kinking of unsupported aortic endografts: Treatment by endovascular intervention. *J Endovasc Surg* **5**: 216–221, 1998
8. Brennan J, Harris P, Tielbeek A, Buth J *et al.*: The significance of suture breakage in stent-graft used for abdominal aortic aneurysm. *Eurostar ESVS Abstact* 1998
9. Umscheid Th, Stelter WJ: Time-related alteration in shape, position, and stucture of self-expanding, modular aortic stent-grafts: A 4-year single-center follow up. *J Endovasc Surg* **6**: 17–32, 1999

The Baxter system

Hardy Schumacher, Jens-Rainer Allenberg

INTRODUCTION AND BACKGROUND

Due to progress in endovascular surgery, it is now possible to treat aneurysms without an abdominal surgical procedure.[1] This new therapeutic approach consists of transfemoral introduction of a metallic scaffold coupled with a vascular graft.[2] When the endovascular graft device is deployed and expanded within the aneurysmal blood vessel, it creates a new aortic lumen for blood flow effectively excluding the aneurysm sac from the flow while maintaining perfusion to the lower limbs. Several preliminary studies have demonstrated the feasibility[3] and a number of endoluminal graft designs are currently marketed outside the USA or are under clinical investigation in Europe. Some device systems consist of novel combinations of off-the-shelf marketed products for general vascular use; others are specifically designed for use in abdominal aortic aneurysm repair but are manufactured from biomaterials with little or no implant history.[4] None of the currently available endovascular graft systems have been specifically designed to meet the intrinsic requirements of abdominal aortic aneurysm morphology (e.g. tortuosity) while taking advantage of proven clinical history of the device materials.[5]

The Vascular Systems Division of Baxter Healthcare Corporation (Baxter) has developed an endovascular graft system for the treatment of abdominal aortic aneurysm. Development of prototype versions of the Baxter Lifepath abdominal aortic aneurysm graft commenced in 1991 and the first clinical case was in 1993. The bifurcated graft design is a direct adaptation of the SYDNEY™ device developed by Geoffrey H White and Weiyun Yu and described in the literature.[6] The first-generation system was a straight aorto-aortic tube graft and a delivery system for endoluminal placement and balloon deployment. The second-generation system is a bifurcated graft which is intended to be delivered to the lesion site via the femoral arteries following surgical cut-down. The generic name of the Baxter device is Baxter Endovascular Graft System, the proprietary name is Baxter LIFEPATH™ abdominal aortic aneurysm straight tube and bifurcated endovascular graft system. Based on clinical data from a pilot study, it is approved as a class IIb medical device in the European Community and bears the CE mark. An international feasibility study (prospective, multicentre, controlled, non-randomized) to support the US submission to the Food and Drug Administration (FDA) is conducted in up to 15 clinical sites in the USA, Australia and Europe.

PRIOR CLINICAL INVESTIGATIONS OF THE WHITE–YU GRAFT

As of June 1997, a total of 112 procedures have been performed with endovascular grafts (straight, double-straight overlap (Trombone™), aortoiliac, bifurcated, and more complex graft designs) that have been modified for each patient by the investigators Geoffrey H White MD and Weiyun Yu MD, in Sydney, Australia. The experience has shown promise in the treatment of aortic aneurysms in the infrarenal abdominal position as well as thoracic and iliac aneurysms.[7,8] Of the 112 procedures, 27 used bifurcated graft designs on 26 patients in the treatment of abdominal aortic aneurysms; 22 of the 26 patients were classified as high risk for open repair of abdominal aortic aneurysms. A preliminary graft design was unsuccessfully used for the first three patients who were converted to open surgical repair. The final 23 patients received bifurcated grafts which resemble the Baxter clinical device.

The graft materials used by GH White *et al.* were Vascutek woven polyester PET (base material of Gelweave®, vascular graft prosthesis) or BARD woven polyester (Softwoven®, vascular graft prosthesis), and stainless steel (316 L) or Elgiloy® wireforms. Endoluminal delivery has been successful via femoral or retroperitoneal iliac artery approaches. Patients have been followed for up to 3 years postoperatively.

In the 23 bifurcated patients to date who received a graft similar to the current Baxter LIFEPATH device, perioperative (i.e. within 30 days of surgery) mortality for elective endoluminal repair of abdominal aortic aneurysm was 4% (one of 23 cases), long-term mortality was 0%, and complications encountered to date have been acceptable when compared with open repair or with other available systems.[9,10] Treatment success was 91% (21 of 23 cases). Of the two unsuccessful cases: one patient had a failed implant when the balloon became entrapped within the graft and the graft was displaced requiring open repair to seal the aneurysm; the second patient developed graft thrombosis. Since the aneurysm was effectively sealed by the thrombosed graft, the patient was revascularized by axillofemoral bypass. This high risk patient subsequently died following myocardial infarction on the third postoperative day.

Endoleak, defined as blood flow outside the endoluminal graft but contained within the native aneurysm sac, was 0 of 21 (0%) early term and three of 21 (14%) late term cases. This compares favourably with the 21% unresolved endoleak rate reported by Moore *et al.* for the Endovascular Technologies, Inc. (EVT) Endovascular grafting system.[11] Two of Dr White's patients had endoleak due to leak from the iliac limbs and were repaired by secondary endoluminal graft implantation. One of these patients subsequently underwent conversion to open surgical repair because of continued perfusion of the abdominal aortic aneurysm sac by backflow from patent lumbar arteries. The third patient underwent open surgical repair for management of proximal graft endoleak. Endoleak in two of the three patients was a result of the iliac limb grafts overlapping 1 cm or less. The case of proximal endoleak was a result of the proximal graft placed too distally within the neck of the abdominal aortic aneurysm.

There were no other device complications observed in these patients. Local and vascular complications were as follows: retroperitoneal access to iliac artery required on one side (four patients), patch or graft repair of femoral artery sheath access site (two patients), and wound infection (one patient). Most of these complications and the graft thrombosis were felt to be associated with the relatively large diameter (29 Fr external), non-flexible delivery sheath. The Baxter LIFEPATH system has now incorporated a 19–20 Fr, flexible delivery system to reduce these complications.

The medical complications observed during the prototype clinical trial were:

myocardial infarction (two patients), angina pectoris (three patients), respiratory (two patients) and fever (eight patients). All patients have been followed up by contrast-enhanced computed tomographic (CT) scans with no evidence of other graft thrombosis or stenosis to date (100% patency). There has been no observed incidence of graft migration. Diminishment in aneurysm size has been consistently observed in successfully treated cases.[7]

THE BAXTER LIFEPATH™ SYSTEM: DEVICE DESIGN AND CHARACTERISTICS [Figs 1–4]

The LIFEPATH abdominal aortic aneurysms bifurcated graft is intended for treatment of infrarenal abdominal aortic aneurysms which have at least a 15 mm proximal neck length and do not involve the renal arteries; and have at least a 15 mm non-aneurysmal attachment zone in each iliac artery. The first-generation Baxter endovascular graft system includes a straight aorto–aortic tube graft and delivery system for endoluminal placement and balloon deployment. It has been specifically designed for flexibility, thus allowing conformation of the wireform-supported graft to the aneurysm morphology. It is made of one or more tubes depending on the aneurysm morphology. The system is modular. The grafts fit together in an overlap area using the Trombone technique, which allows virtual customization of the graft length intraoperatively. The prosthetic device portion is composed of a woven polyester graft of standard thickness (0.03 mm) with independent balloon expandable annealed Elgiloy wireforms providing secure attachment between graft and wireform. The wireforms are interwoven into and fully integrated throughout the length of the graft for optimal radial strength. Sutures are not required to hold wires in place. The graft is fully supported yet wireforms are independent (not linked together), to minimize concern of graft twisting or kinking. At the end sections of the graft, the wireforms are more dense to ensure the proper fixation adjacent to the device in the aneurysm necks. The LIFEPATH abdominal aortic aneurysm straight tube graft is available in five different diameters of 19 mm to 27 mm (in 2 mm increments) each of them delivered in two different lengths of 60 mm and 90 mm.

The Baxter LIFEPATH bifurcated endovascular graft is second-generation and is made up of three individual units: a bifurcated graft trunk with two iliac extension grafts (three piece modular design) and delivery systems for endoluminal placement. The bifurcated system employs both balloon-expanded and self-expanding Elgiloy wire. The woven polyester graft material is identical in composition and strength to material used in grafts that are commercially available for open repair.

The bifurcated trunk has a straight proximal section approximately 5 cm in length and two limbs that extend approximately 2.5 and 3.7 cm below the bifurcation. The overall length of graft is 9.2 cm. One leg is shorter than the other contralateral for easier identification under fluoroscopy. The top or proximal portion of this trunk contains four independent wireforms of annealed Elgiloy® with a fifth wireform composed of heat-treated spring-tempered Elgiloy. Elgiloy is a lightweight wire made from corrosion-resistant alloy that has excellent

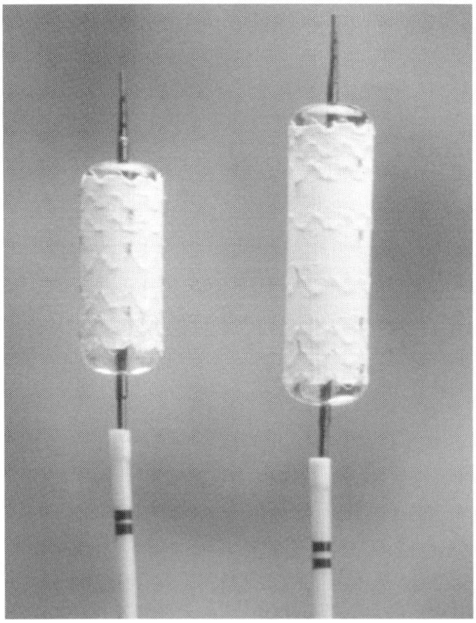

Fig. 1. LIFEPATH abdominal aortic aneurysm straight graft expanded with balloon inflation.

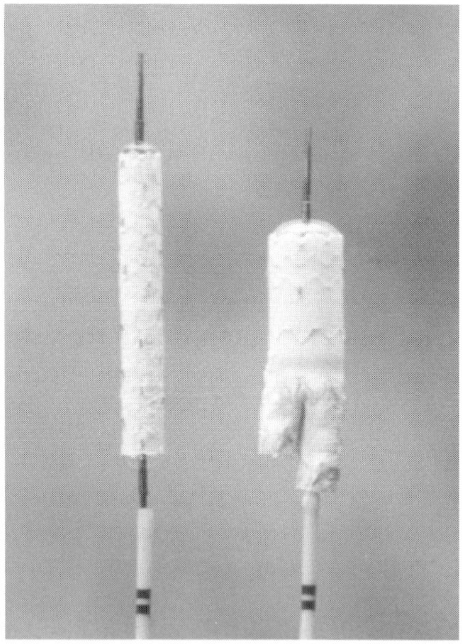

Fig. 2. LIFEPATH abdominal aortic aneurysm bifurcated graft (modular design) components: main trunk/ one iliac limb.

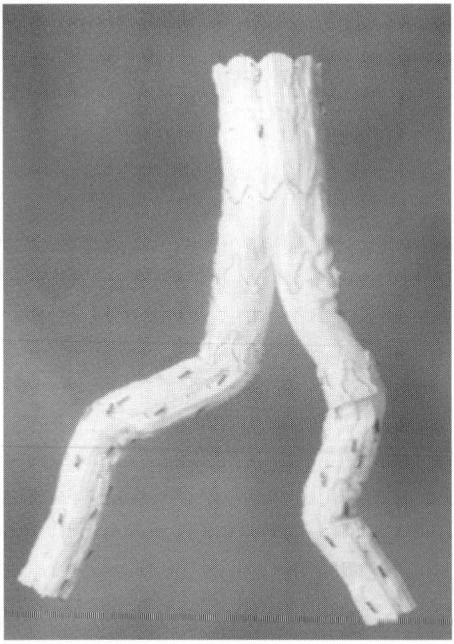

Fig. 3. LIFEPATH abdominal aortic aneurysm bifurcated graft three-piece design: final configuration.

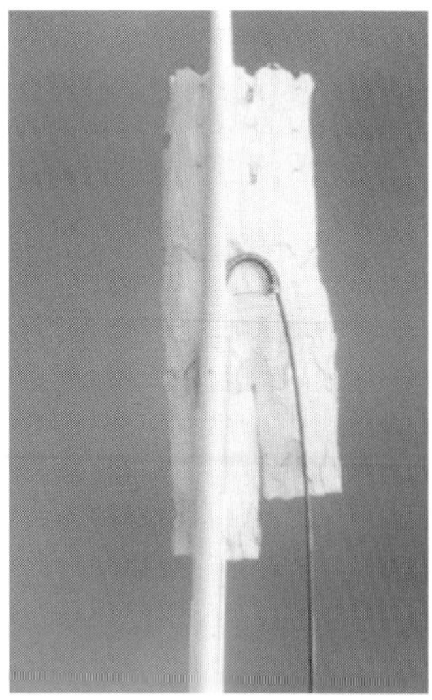

Fig. 4. Deflected directional catheter with terumo glidewire for crossover edure.

fatigue-resistant characteristics. It has an extensive clinical history over 20 years as a long-term implantable material, including use in heart valve bioprotheses (Carpentier-Edwards). These wireforms are more radiolucent and interwoven into the polyester graft matrix and provide attachment of the bifurcated trunk to the proximal aorta following deployment via balloon expansion. The two limbs contain wireform components made of spring Elgiloy®. These self-expanding leg portions of graft are incorporated to assure that the balloon can be removed without pulling the graft out of position. The proximal portion of the iliac extension grafts are anchored within the limbs of the bifurcated graft trunk (a minimum of 2 cm overlap is required). The distal portions are anchored into their respective iliac arteries. The iliac grafts are made of independent wireforms to make it virtually impossible to kink, twist or occlude. The flexibility designed in the iliac graft system allows movement to mirror aneurysm morphology changes over time. The iliac graft system will 'accordion' to accept potential shortening of the aneurysm, virtually eliminating concern that the graft will shift in the aneurysm. The iliac graft is tromboned into the bifurcated graft leg. Currently, the bifurcated trunk is available in four diameters at the proximal neck: 21, 23, 25 and 27 mm. The iliac extension grafts are available in four diameters at the distal neck: 10, 12, 14 and 16 mm; and three lengths: 43, 80 and 110 mm. The overlap zone does not vary regardless of the proximal trunk diameter or the distal diameters of the extension grafts. The proximal diameter of the iliac extension grafts is fixed at 14 mm wide, while the distal leg portion of the bifurcated graft is 13 mm; the oversize creates a tight seal, and would require over 2.72 kg (6 lb) of force to pull apart. Different distal diameters are accommodated by tapering the extension graft and the balloon used to deploy it.

The delivery system includes five components: two introducer sheaths, the bifurcated graft and two iliac graft delivery catheters. The introducer sheaths contain an introducer with a very flexible tip and lubricious hydrophilic coating for initial placement and passive haemostatic valve system (three valves) located in the sheath head. The prosthetic device is mounted over a deployment balloon and housed within a loader. The balloon is non-compliant with a unique square shoulder ensuring full opening at proximal and distal ends of graft. The balloon fills from the centre to eliminate the potential of the graft sliding off during expansion. The loader fits within the introducer sheath unit, facilitating easy transfer of the device into the introducer sheaths for deployment into the aorta. An optional component of the system is the directional catheter to help establish the contralateral guidewire position. This is a dual lumen catheter designed to assist the surgeon gain access to the 'contralateral' leg. It is introduced over a 0.035 'superstiff' guidewire and positioned on the fourth wireform counting from the top. This procedure eliminates concern about passing the terumo glidewire behind wireforms inside the graft. Once positioned, the cover sheath is pulled back and the channel directed by a thumb actuator in the same direction as the thumb tab is pointing.

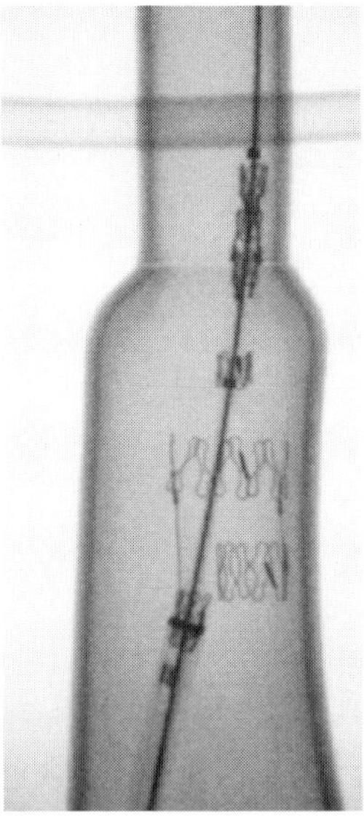

Fig. 5.

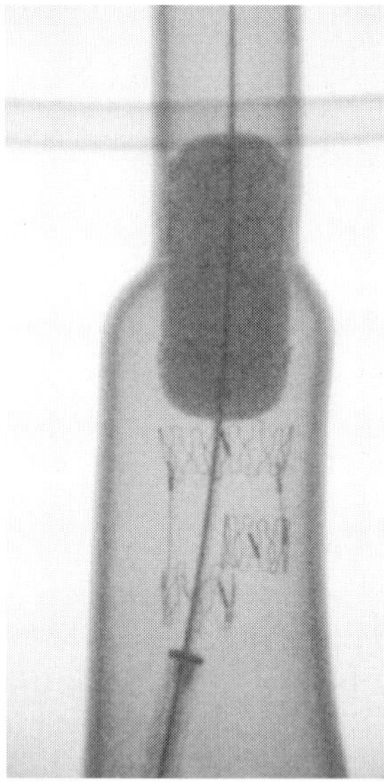

Fig. 6.

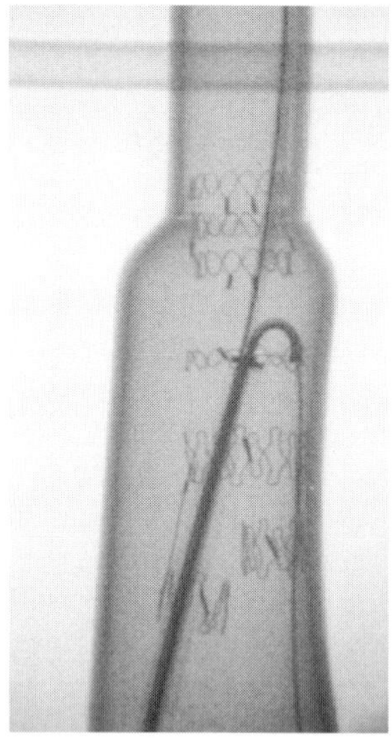

Fig. 7.

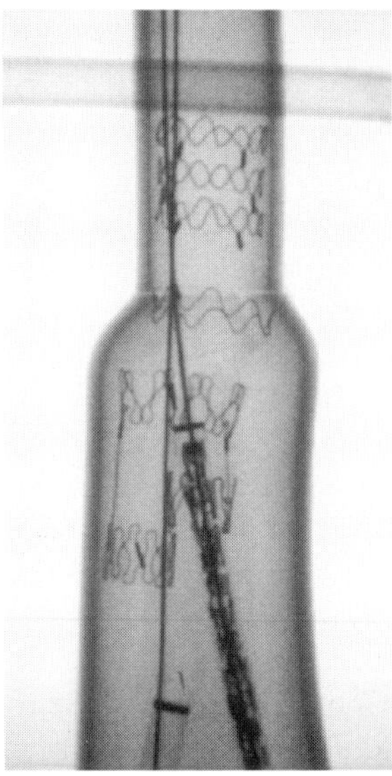

Fig. 8.

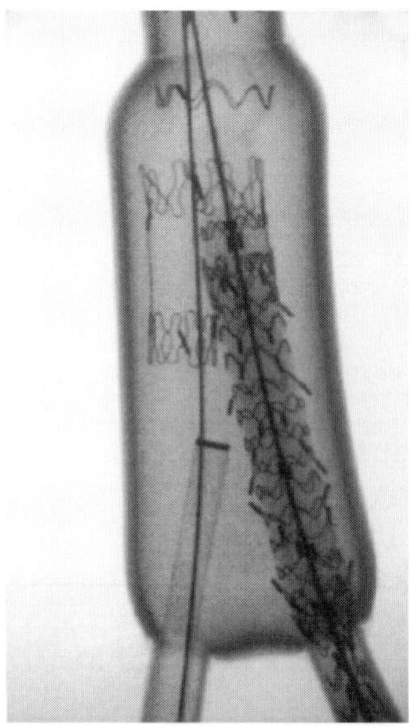

Fig. 9.

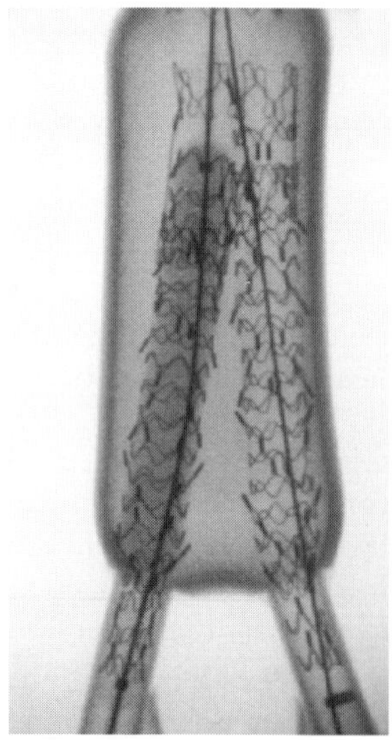

Fig. 10.

Figs 5–10. Implantation procedure LIFEPATH abdominal aortic aneurysm bifurcated graft (fluoroscopic view). **Fig. 5.** Main graft in infrarenal position, sheath pulled back, contralateral self-expanding iliac limb opened, balloon-expandable main trunk ready for deployment. **Fig. 6.** Main trunk deployment with balloon inflation to 2 atm for 30 seconds. **Fig. 7.** Deflecting catheter in place for Terumo glidewire crossover. **Fig. 8.** Contralateral iliac graft through 16 Fr introducer sheath in position (bridging 2cm). **Fig. 9.** Deployment of contralateral iliac limb. **Fig. 10.** Deployment of ipsilateral iliac limb.

PATIENT SELECTION: OPTIMAL IMAGING TECHNIQUE, MORPHOLOGICAL CLASSIFICATION AND GRAFT SIZING

[Figs 11–15]

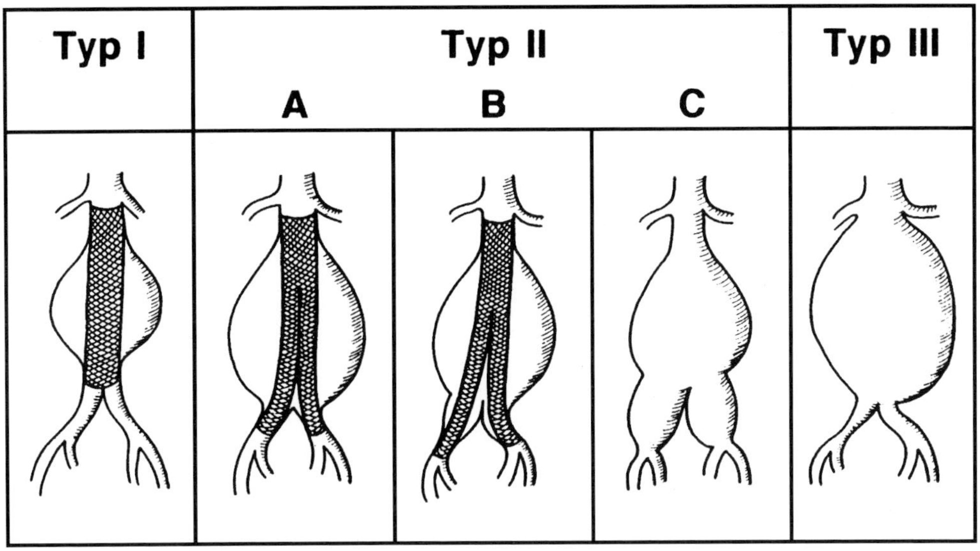

Fig. 11. Heidelberg abdominal aortic aneurysm classification.

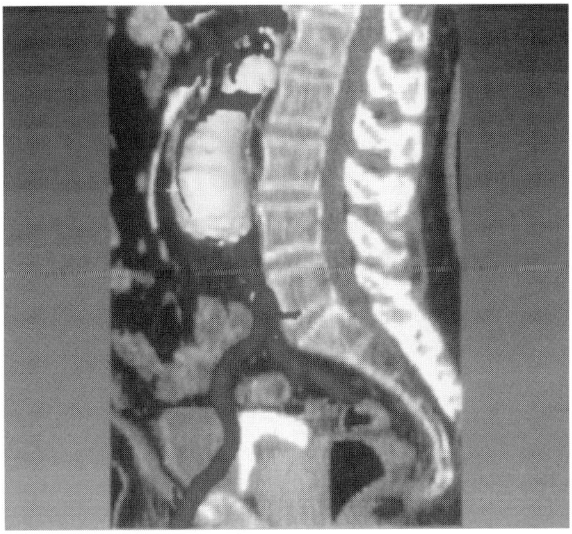

Fig. 12.

Figs 12–15 (pp. 311–313). Patient evaluation and procedure planning with PREVIEW.
Fig. 12. Infrarenal aortic aneurysm 3D reconstruction CTA scan.

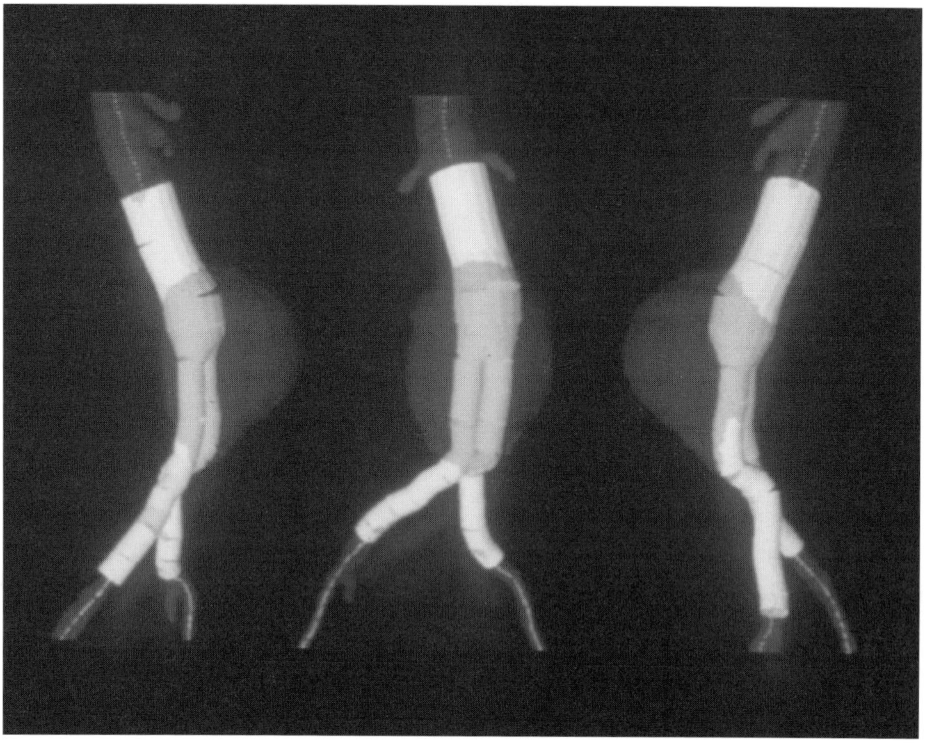

Fig. 13. Virtual grafting.

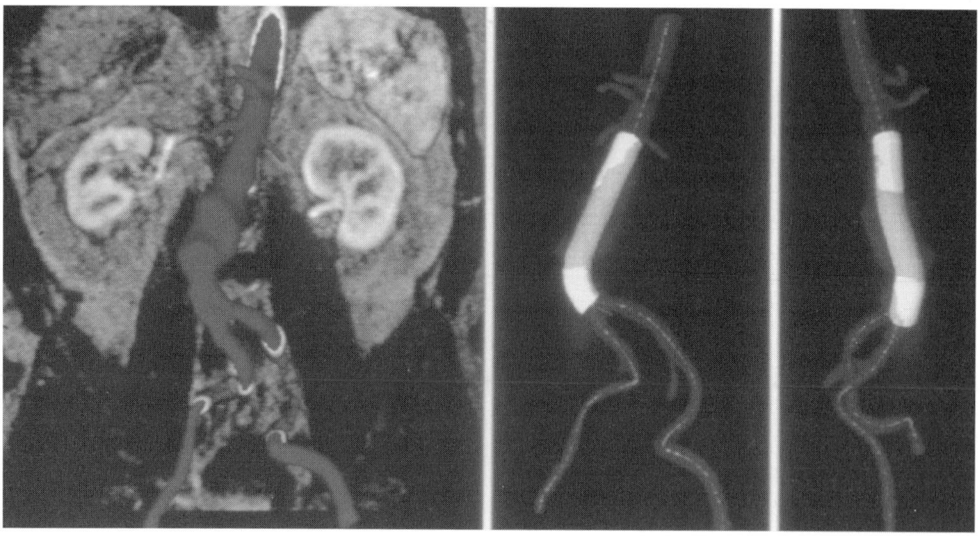

Fig. 14. Infrarenal aortic aneurysm 3D reconstruction MRA and virtual grafting.

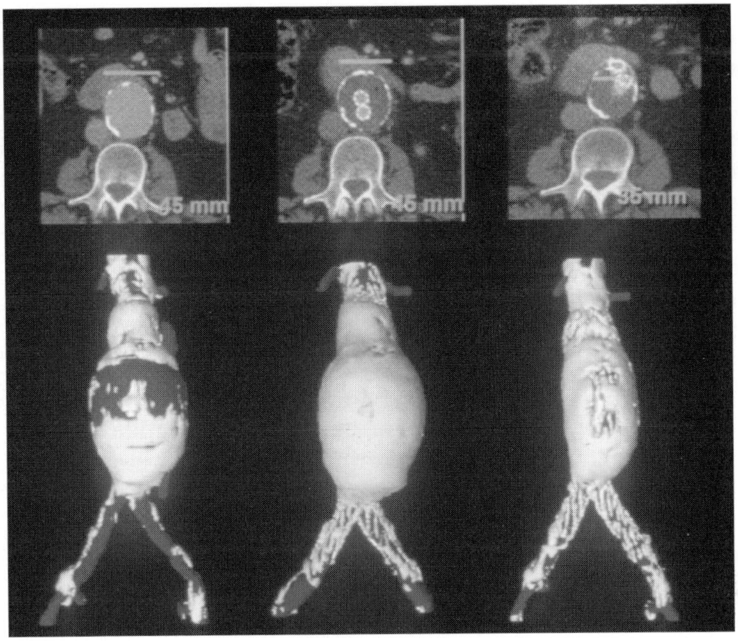

Fig. 15. Follow-up analysis with volume measurements.

Anatomical definition and accurate measurements are critical elements for successful endovascular aortic grafts for abdominal aortic aneurysm. Evaluation of the aorto-iliac segment depends on conventional imaging methods, usually axial CT and arteriography at many institutions, increasingly supplemented by computerized image processing. For a typical bifurcated graft, many measurements are necessary, including the length and diameter of the proximal neck, the distal cuff, and the dimensions of the iliac arteries. Measurements for an endovascular tube graft are only slightly less complex. Undersizing endograft diameter can contribute to inadequate sealing around the stents leading to endoleak or graft migration. Conversely, oversizing endograft diameter may lead to crimping or folding of the graft material leading to occlusion or aortic enlargement. Grafts which are too short or too long may similarly have attachment problems, endoleak, kinking, or occlusion of important branches. Thus, appropriate sizing and placement of endografts requires a preprocedure imaging system which can determine the lengths and diameters of tortuous vessels with a high degree of accuracy.

While diameter measurements with CT scan can be difficult, using CT to determine the length for a proposed endograft is even more difficult even with spiral CT; the current standard is to perform angiography for length measurements and evaluation of occlusive disease prior to endovascular repair. All the currently used methods have limitations, but spiral CT angiography (CTA) with three-dimensional (3D) reconstruction offers unique benefits.

We have participated in the testing of a system which stores CTA data, 1-2 mm axial reconstructions, multiplanar reconstructions, and an interactive 3D model of the data on a CD-ROM disk (PREVIEW™, Medical Media Systems). The images are stored on the CD-ROM disk along with software which allows image display and measurements to be performed on a personal computer. The system can also be used with MRA data. This specialized measurement software and unique aspects of the 3D reconstructions are the key to eliminating the problems associated with conventional preoperative measurement techniques. A novel software algorithm is used to display the centreline of the blood flow channel in the infrarenal aorta and iliac arteries, which allows length measurements along the vessel centreline, even in tortuous iliac segments. Graft paths along a line other than the centreline can also be chosen and modified in real time on the PC ('virtual graft'). Spiral CT with 3D reconstruction and specialized software will soon become the gold standard for the preoperative evaluation of patients prior to endovascular abdominal aortic aneurysm repair due to its unique imaging capabilities, superior measurement accuracy, lower cost, lower radiation dose and lower patient morbidity.[12]

Computer-aided surgery-planning software for abdominal aortic aneurysm is a industry-standard software development for viewing patient-specific data on a personal computer through a unique approach, which improves visualization, navigation, and decision support capabilities for both open and endovascular surgery. Raw scan data are extracted from CT scans and rendered into a 3D format. This 3D modelling technology and user interface provides a patient-specific model with a rapid visual access to the full range of information, including accurate 3D assessment of abdominal aortic aneurysm morphology and pathology, interactive multiplanar reconstructions, measurements, and views to assist the surgeon in understanding of complex 3D relationships. It provides an optimal system for patient evaluation and selection for endovascular repair of abdominal aortic aneurysm and in the postoperative evaluation of stent deployment and/or complications, such as endoleaks.[12,13]

Classification of abdominal aortic aneurysm is described by Schumacher *et al.*[14,15] illustrating the locations for the various parameters taken from CT and/or angiographic images. Neck and cuff are defined as the segments of non-dilated, thrombus-free vessels necessary for the attachment of the endovascular grafts. Based on these definitions abdominal aortic aneurysms are classified according to the anatomic variations illustrated in Fig. 11.

According to these anatomic criteria the appropriate endovascular graft can be selected. Repair of aneurysms with a good non-aneurysmal proximal neck of ≥ 15 mm length below the renal arteries, as well as a distal neck of ≥ 20 mm above the aortic bifurcation allow fixation or attachment of a straight tube endoluminal graft. Patients with abdominal aortic aneurysms having these criteria are estimated to be less than 5% of all abdominal aortic aneurysm endovascular patients. There is a trend towards fewer cases eligible for straight tube graft repair.[10]

Critical elements of the endovascular grafting system are graft selection and sizing in accordance with the abdominal aortic aneurysm morphology. This is the key factor to ensure accurate and secure endoluminal graft deployment.[15]

THE PROPRIETARY DEPLOYMENT PROCEDURE: PRINCIPAL STEPS OF OPERATION

[Figs 5–10]

While the patient is appropriately anaesthetized (general or peridural anaesthesia) and lying supine, the operative fields are prepared per routine protocol. Bilateral groin incisions are performed to expose the common femoral arteries. The patient is then anticoagulated with intravenous heparin. An 8 Fr sheath is inserted into the ipsilateral common femoral artery using the Seldinger needle technique. A guidewire and angiographic catheter is advanced to the level of the renal arteries in the abdominal aorta. An aortogram is then performed. An Amplatz superstiff guidewire is exchanged and the angiographic catheter and the 8 Fr introducer sheath are removed.

The 19 Fr main introducer sheath assembly is inserted over the guidewire from the ipsilateral side and the tip of the sheath is advanced until it is above the proximal neck of the aneurysm, just above the renal arteries. The introducer is removed while leaving the main sheath and guidewire *in situ*. The bifurcated graft delivery assembly is then connected to the sheath head over the guidewire. The graft is delivered by advancing the pusher. The sheath may be rotated to allow for the correct orientation of the bifurcated graft. Once the graft has reached the planned level of deployment, the main introducer sheath is retracted until the bifurcated graft is fully exposed to the circulation.

Final adjustments are made to the bifurcated graft position before deployment of the graft. The graft is deployed by inflating the main balloon to maximum inflation. The balloon is then deflated and the balloon catheter is removed through the introducer sheath while leaving the sheath and guidewire *in situ*.

The Baxter directional catheter is inserted over the wire through the haemostatic valve of the main introducer sheath. The directional catheter is advanced to the level of the bifurcated graft septum and the tip is manually deflected over the septum. A 0.035 inches guidewire is inserted through a second guidewire channel in the directional catheter. This wire is advanced over the graft septum to cannulate the contralateral limb of the bifurcated graft and continue into the contralateral common iliac artery until it reaches the femoral artery. The guidewire is then retrieved by a transverse arteriotomy of the contralateral common femoral artery.

A contralateral exchange catheter is advanced over the contralateral guidewire until it is well inside the bifurcated graft. The deflection of the directional catheter tip is released and the catheter withdrawn through the main introducer sheath. Care should be taken during this step to check that both iliac extensions are selectively cannulated with one guidewire (fluoroscopy in oblique position).

The contralateral 16 Fr introducer sheath assembly is advanced over the superstiff guidewire until it is well within the contralateral limb of the main graft. The contralateral iliac extension graft delivery assembly is then connected to the sheath head over the guidewire. The iliac extension graft is delivered by advancing the pusher. The iliac extension is positioned to provide for a minimum of 2 cm overlap with the contralateral limb and is deployed by inflating the iliac extension balloon. After deflating the balloon, the balloon catheter is left in position. The 19 Fr introducer is reinserted into the main introducer sheath and the entire assembly is advanced until the tip of the sheath reaches above the main graft septum. After positioning, the ipsilateral iliac extension graft is deployed by inflating the iliac extension ballooon. Simultaneously, the contralateral iliac extension balloon is also reinflated (Kissing Balloon). Both iliac balloon extensions are then simultaneously deflated and removed. A completion angiogram is then performed and both sheaths are removed.

CLINICAL SUCCESS: THE HEIDELBERG EXPERIENCE

[Figs 16–24]

Prior to market release both the straight tube graft and bifurcated device were subject to clinical investigations in Australia, Europe and the USA. The study protocol is a multicentre, prospective, controlled, non-randomized clinical study.

Due to the regularities, a subset of test group data (first 16 patients) were summarized. These data were gathered on patients treated at the Department of Vascular Surgery, Ruprecht-Karls University of Heidelberg. The patient were treated by the investigator Professor Allenberg or his co-investigator Dr Schumacher.

All of the 16 patients were male and Caucasian. The mean age of patients at treatment was 66.9 years (50–78 years). The first two patients with saccular abdominal aortic aneurysms were treated with the Baxter endovascular straight tube

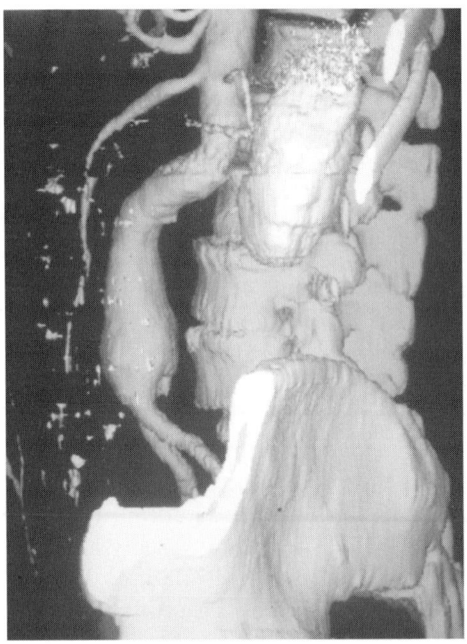

Fig. 16.

Figs 16–19 (pp. 316–318). Abdominal aortic aneurysm with kinking proximal neck and iliac arteries: preoperative CTA; postoperative CTA; 2D reconstruction with graft in place; plain X-ray.

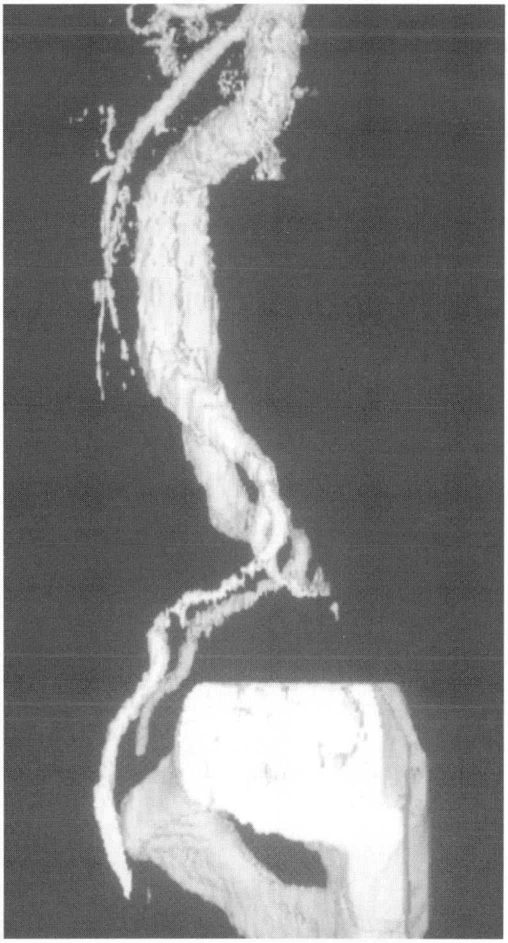

Fig. 17.

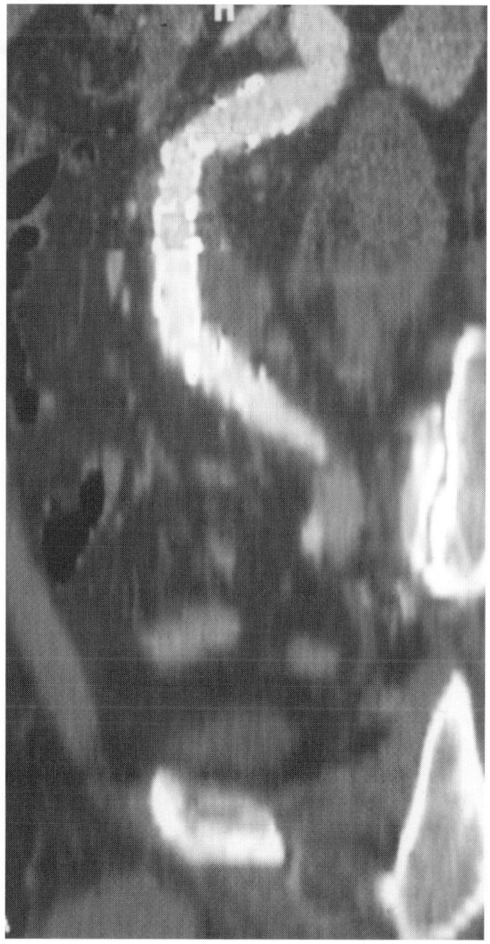

Fig. 18.

graft (April and September 1997) and 14 patients with the bifurcated graft by elective repair enrolled in the study between March and September 1999. The sac diameter of the aneurysm treated was on average 51.5 mm (40–61 mm).

Both tube graft implants required two overlapping grafts. One case was resolved with modification of the procedure to reverse the trombone technique due to tightness of the distal aortic cuff. Both interventions were successfully completed with no further reintervention.

For both patients 2-year follow-up data are available. Both are alive with the graft in place. The diameter of the abdominal aortic aneurysm shows complete shrinkage in one case and a significant reduction in the other.

Among the 14 patients with the Lifepath abdominal aortic aneurysm bifurcated graft system 12 implantations (85.7%) were totally uneventful and required no further intervention. In two cases (14.3%) displacement either of the trunk or the iliac limb was observed intraoperatively. In one case an additional intraoperative

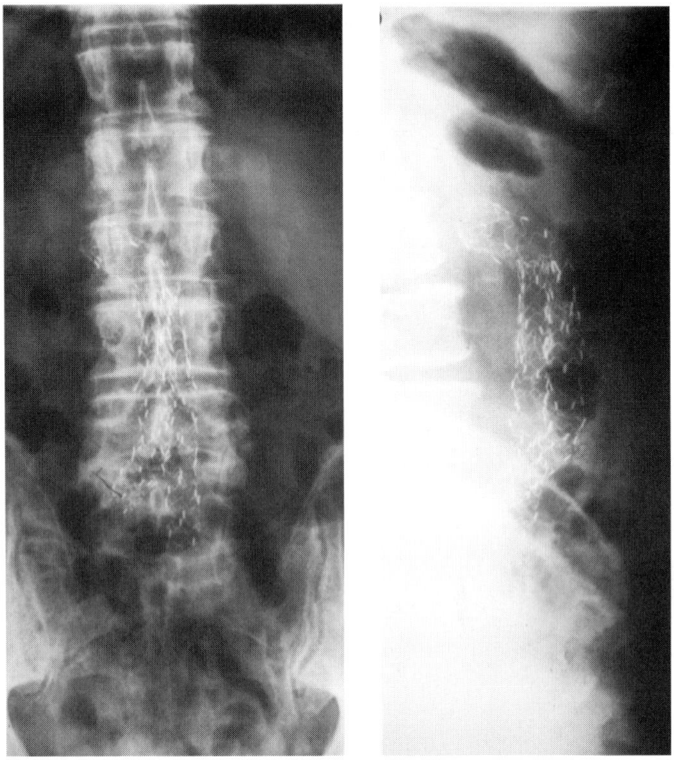

Fig. 19.

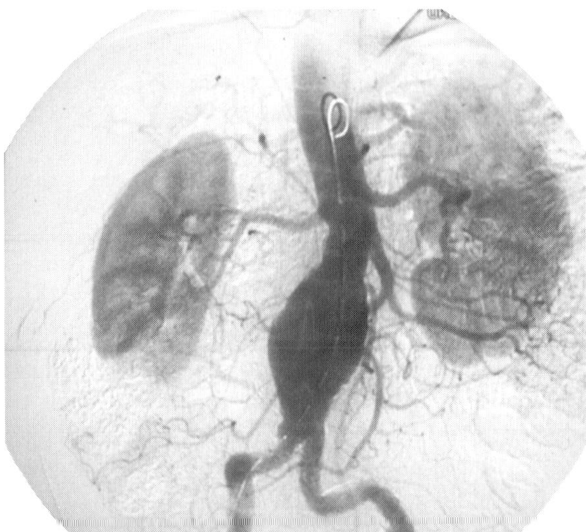

Fig. 20.

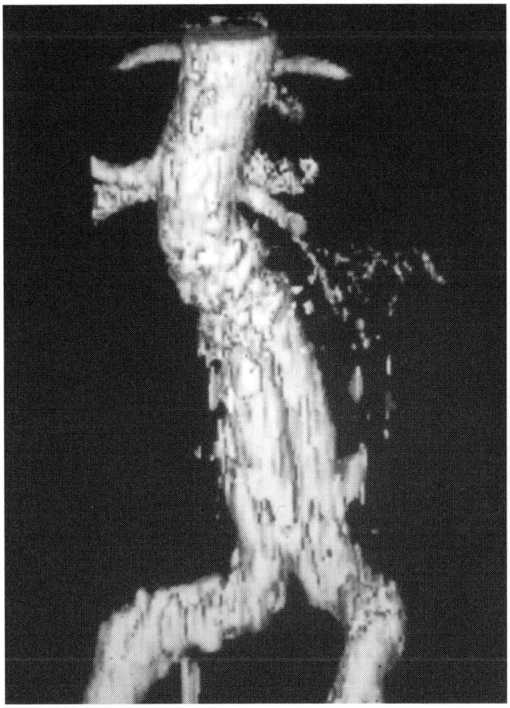

Fig. 21.

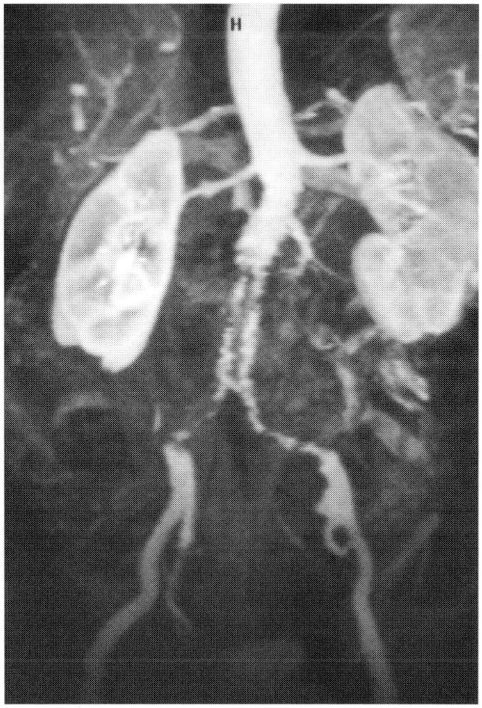

Fig. 22.

Figs 20–24 (pp. 318–320). Abdominal aortic aneurysm with iliac tortuosity left side and 90-degree kinking right side: preoperative angiography, postoperative CTA with graft in place.

procedure (proximal extension with an aortic cuff, custom-made by cutting a 6 cm trunk down to 4 cm) was required to ensure correct placement of the graft. The other case could only be resolved successfully with conversion to open surgery. All these reinterventions were successfully completed. Overall procedure duration to implant the Lifepath bifurcation (skin incision to skin closure) averaged 2.2 hours (1.13–3 h). The two cases with reintervention/conversion lasted 4 and 5 hours.

Perioperative endoleak was seen in one (tube graft) of these 16 cases being a persistent lumbar branch artery flow which sealed spontaneously and was no longer present in the follow-up after 3 months.

With the device misplacement being corrected during the surgical procedure the overall operative success rate (technical success) was 93.7%.

The patient with the unsuccessful deployment (malpositioning) of the bifurcated main trunk followed by incomplete exclusion of abdominal aortic aneurysm and conversion to open repair, developed a severe cholesterol embolism resulting in gluteal, bowel and limb ischaemia. Surgical reintervention on postoperative days 1 and 2 was necessary with placement of a transperitoneal internal iliac artery bypass and resection of the colon sigmoideum due to occlusion of the patent inferior mesenteric artery and internal iliac artery embolization.

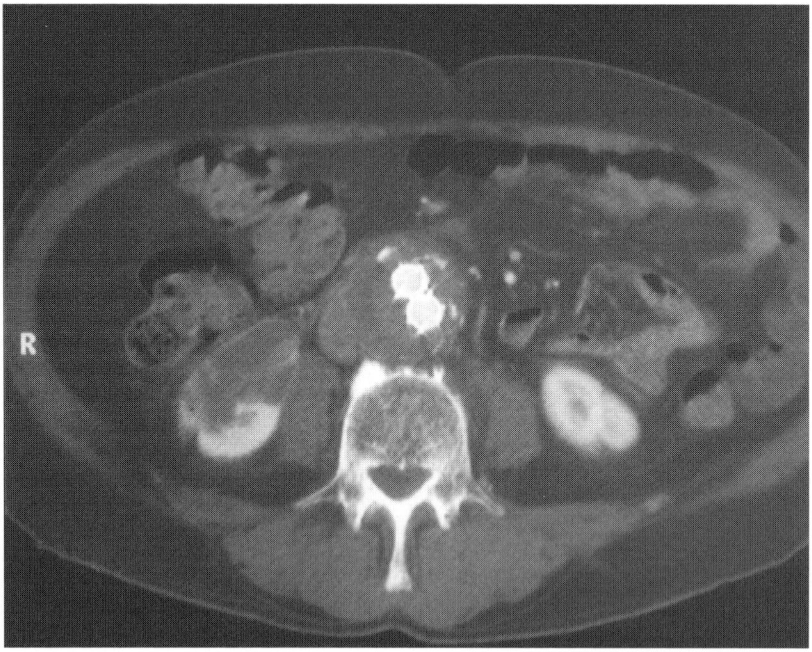

Fig. 23.

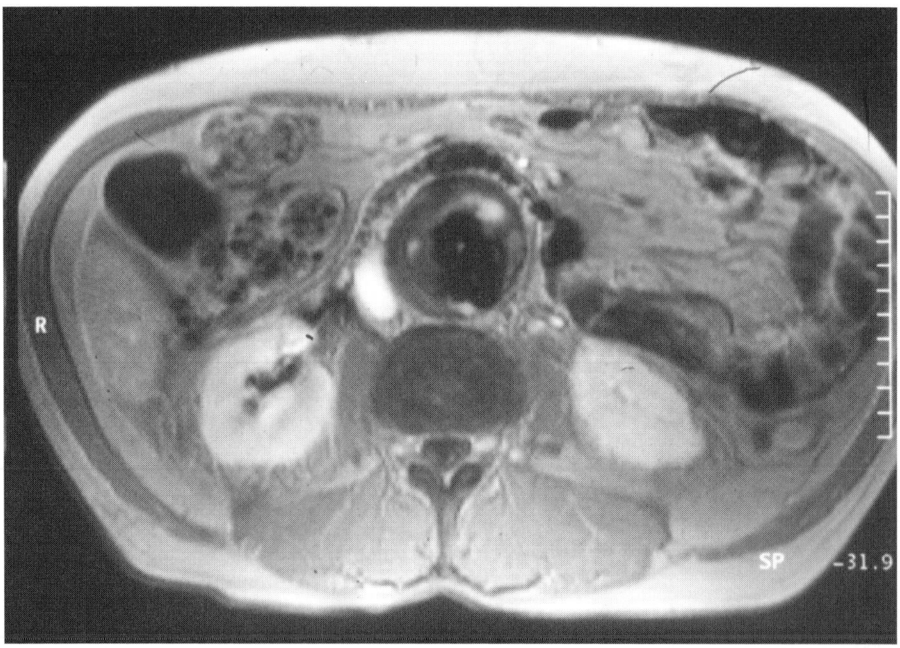

Fig. 24.

Figs 23, 24. MRT and MRA at follow-up; metal artefacts with false positive results: endoleakage and occlusion.

Hospital discharge was on average on postoperative day 5. For all 16 patients 30-day and 3-month postoperative follow-up data are available, at which point no technical or severe clinical complications were observed. Follow-up data at 6 months are available for nine of a possible nine patients. All patients were alive with the graft in place (except the patient with the conventional aortobiiliac bypass). In the CT scans, the diameter of the abdominal aortic aneurysm sac shows a reduction and no signs of growth nor any endoleaks.

Mid-term success at 2-year follow-up is likely for both possible patients with tube endografts. Both patients are alive with the graft in place. The CT scan shows no sign of endoleak and a significant reduction of sac diameter; in one patient the aneurysm no longer exists as complete shrinkage was achieved.

CONCLUSIONS AND OUTLOOK

The Baxter LIFEPATH abdominal aortic aneurysm endovascular graft system has excellent results at short-term follow-up. Proper patient selection and accurate measurements and graft sizing are critical elements for successful endovascular aortic grafting. The handling of the delivery system is very comfortable especially in difficult iliac anatomy with kinking, tortuosity or calcification due to the very flexible tip which gradually stiffens.

Of course, long-term results have to be awaited before this system fully earns its adequate place among the other different endovascular systems in the treatment of aneurysmatic disease.

REFERENCES

1. Allenberg JR, Schumacher H: Endovasculäre Rekonstruktion des infrarenalen abdominellen Aortenaneurysmas (AAA). *Chirurg* **66**: 870–877, 1995
2. Parodi JC, Palmaz J, Barone H: Transfemoral intraluminal graft implantation for abdominal aortic aneurysms. *Ann Vasc Surg* **5**: 491–499, 1991
3. Schumacher H, Eckstein HH, Allenberg JR: (Endovascular prosthesis: evolution, state-of-the-art and perspectives of a new technology). *Chirurg* **70**: 858–867, 1999
4. Mialhe C, Amicabile C: Traitement endovasculaire des aneurisme de l'aorte sous-renale par l'endoprothese Stentor. Serie preliminaire. *J Mal Vasc* **20**: 290–295, 1995
5. Parodi JC, Barone H, Piraino R *et al.*: Endovascular treatment of abdominal aortic aneurysms: lessons learned. *J Endovasc Surg* **4**: 102–110, 1997
6. White GH, Yu W, May J *et al.*: A new non-stented balloon-expandable graft for straight or bifurcated endoluminal bypass. *J Endovasc Surg* **1**: 16–24, 1994
7. White GH, Yu W, May J *et al.*: Three years experience with the White-Yu endovascular GAD graft for transluminal repair of aortic and iliac aneurysms. *J Endovasc Surg* **4**: 124–136, 1997
8. White GH, Yu W, May J *et al.*: Design developments and long-term results of a balloon-deployed endovascular graft for the repair of abdominal aortic aneurysms. *J Endovasc Surg* **3**: 28–83, 1996
9. Cuypers Ph, Buth J, Harris PL *et al.*: Realistic expectations for patients with stent-graft treatment of abdominal aortic aneurysms. Results of a European Multicentre Registry. *Eur J Vasc Endovasc Surg* **17**: 507–516, 1999

10. May J, White GH, Yu W *et al.*: Concurrent comparison of endoluminal versus open repair in the treatment of abdominal aortic aneurysms: analysis of 303 patients by life table method. *J Vasc Surg* **27**: 213–221, 1998
11. Moore WS, Rutherford RB: Transfemoral endovascular repair of abdominal aortic aneurysm: results of the North American EVT phase 1 trial. *J Vasc Surg* **23**: 543–553, 1996
12. Allenberg JR, Schumacher H, Robbie P: (Computer-assisted evaluation of aortic aneurysm morphology for choosing the method of therapy). *Langenbecks Arch Chir Suppl* **115**: 105–107, 1998
13. White GH, Yu W, May J *et al.*: Endoleak as a complications of endoluminal grafting of abdominal aortic aneurysms: classification, incidence, diagnosis, and management. *J Endovasc Surg* **4**: 152–168, 1997
14. Schumacher H, Allenberg JR, Eckstein HH: Morphological classification of abdominal aortic aneurysm in selection of patients for endovascular grafting. *Br J Surg* **83**: 949–950, 1996
15. Schumacher H, Eckstein HH, Kallinowski F *et al.*: Morphometry and classification in abdomi-nal aortic aneurysms: patient selection for endovascular and open surgery. *J Endovasc Surg* **4**: 39–44, 1997

The team approach to EVAR complications I: Device-related problems

John DG Rose, Ralph Jackson, Tim A Lees, Michael G Wyatt

INTRODUCTION

The last decade of the twentieth century was marked by expanding investment in the opportunities provided by minimally invasive procedures and the endovascular repair of aortic aneurysms has been a prime example of this phenomenon. The application of transluminal catheter and guidewire-based techniques to the treatment of aortic aneurysms has highlighted the potential benefits of a combined surgical and radiological team. There are now a large number of published non-randomized case series showing the feasibility of endovascular aneurysm repair and suggesting early morbidity and mortality at least equivalent to open surgery.[1] However, there does appear to be a significant incidence of device- (and non-device)-related problems[1,2] which can conveniently be divided into early (primary) and late (secondary) complications.

The main focus of this part of the chapter will be on the device-related problems that arise after the endovascular repair of abdominal aortic aneurysms (EVAR). As an illustration of what can be achieved by the 'Team' approach, we will draw on the experience of the first 100 aortic stent grafts implanted at the Freeman Hospital (Table 1) and followed up according to the Eurostar protocol.

EVAR COMPLICATIONS

The device-related complications of EVAR include:
- Endoleak formation
- Limb occlusion
- Graft migration
- Rupture

Although most of these problems can be treated using endovascular techniques, surgery may be required either in the urgent situation or following radiological failure. The surgical techniques available for the treatment of EVAR complications include:

- Proximal banding (laparoscopic / laparotomy)
- Extra-anatomical bypass
- Open conversion

Endoleak

Endoleak is defined by the presence of blood flow outside the endograft and within the aneurysm sac after completion of the primary procedure,[3] either at the time of the completion angiogram or at subsequent computed tomography (CT) follow-up. There are several causes of such leaks and these have been classified[4] into primary and secondary, types I-IV. The management of endoleaks depends primarily on the suspected site of the leak.

Proximal endoleak

A short or otherwise suboptimal proximal neck precludes the use of endovascular repair in between 30 and 50% of patients with abdominal aortic aneurysms.[5] If stent grafts are deployed in patients with unsuitable necks, there is a high risk of technical failure including stent graft migration and the development of immediate or late proximal leaks.

Immediate stent graft migration usually requires conversion to open repair (see below).

A proximal leak may be evident at the end of the primary procedure, usually when much time has been exhausted trying to abolish such a leak (Fig. 1 a,b). This appears to carry the greatest potential for early rupture (Fig. 1c), especially if there is no outflow for the endoleak.[6] The major causes of this situation include underestimation of the diameter of the proximal aortic neck, misplacement of the device and unfavourable proximal neck anatomy. The first two causes can usually be dealt with quite simply by deploying a proximal cuff of adequate diameter in the immediate infrarenal neck.

If the proximal neck is very angulated or has concave margins (Fig. 1a) it may prove impossible to achieve a satisfactory seal, even with an additional large proximal cuff. For this reason most commercial devices are issued on the assumption that proximal neck angulation is less than 60° and that the profile of the implantation site is smooth and straight.

The endoleak that results from proximal neck angulation or irregularity may be fixed by endovascular means through the deployment of a large (uncovered) Palmaz stent, stretching out the proximal margin of the stent graft and forcing contact with the aortic wall. However, where endovascular techniques fail, surgical banding of the proximal aortic neck may prevent the need for open repair.

Open banding. Surgical banding involves the placement of a nylon tape around the neck of the aortic aneurysm, below the renal arteries but above the aneurysm sac. This results in tightening of the aortic tissue around the contained stent resulting in cessation of the proximal endoleak and depressurization of the aneurysm sac. Surgical banding can be performed via a mini-laparotomy or laparoscopically (trans- or retro-peritoneal).

Reports of this technique are generally anecdotal and we have experience of two cases. The first involved a Vanguard graft placed into a *severely* tortuous aortic neck. This resulted in a large proximal leak that was successfully treated, using a mini-laparotomy technique, with two nylon tapes around the aortic neck. The second case involved a large proximal leak around a Zenith endograft via an irregular and

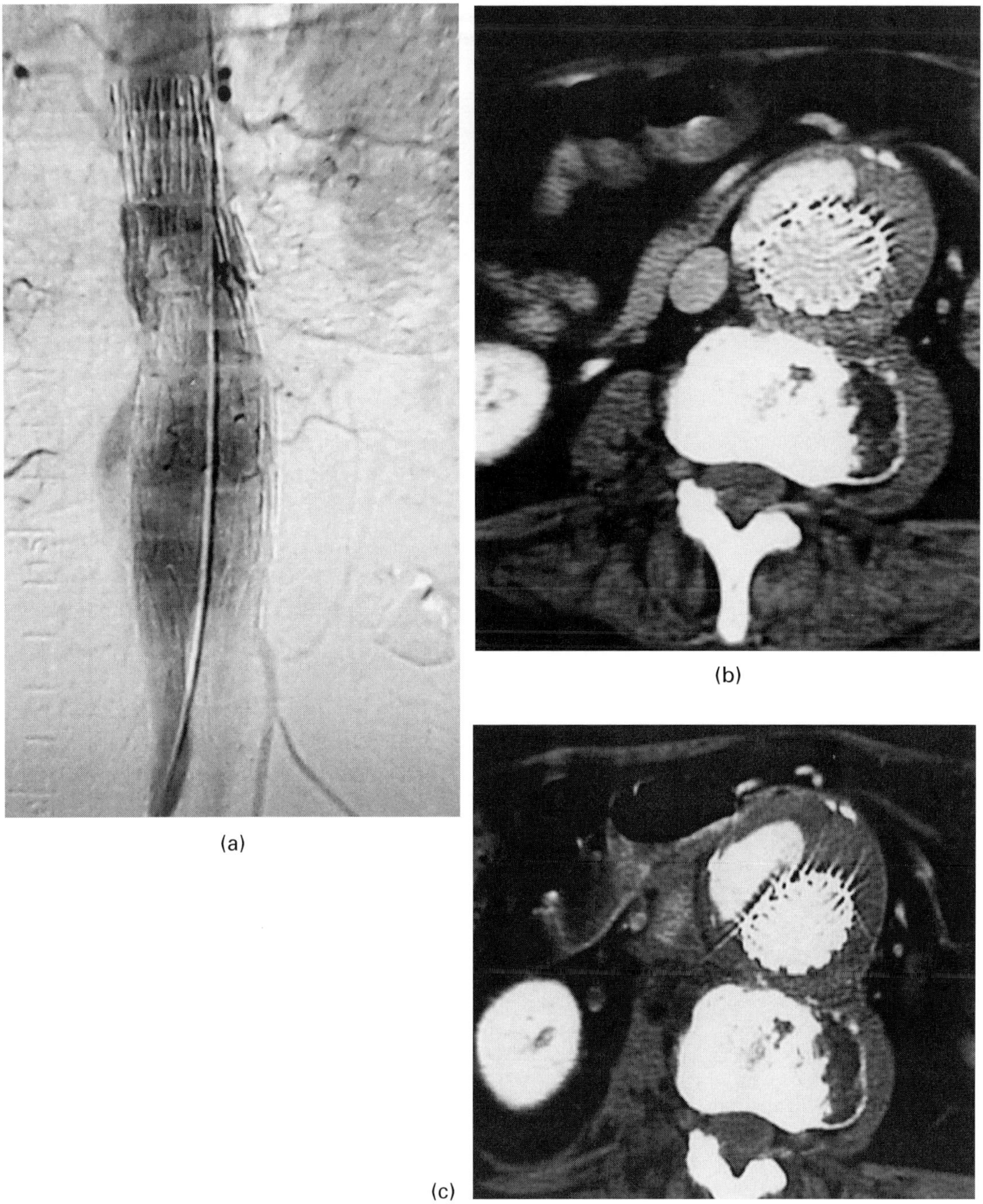

Fig. 1. (a) Post-procedure angiogram (Zenith endograft) showing persistent perigraft contrast flow despite prolonged balloon dilation of proximal stent mechanism. Note the concave internal profile of the proximal aortic neck around the endograft. (b) CT scan at 24 hours confirming large proximal endoleak. (c) CT scan through same area at 10 days, showing continued endoleak but now with contained rupture.

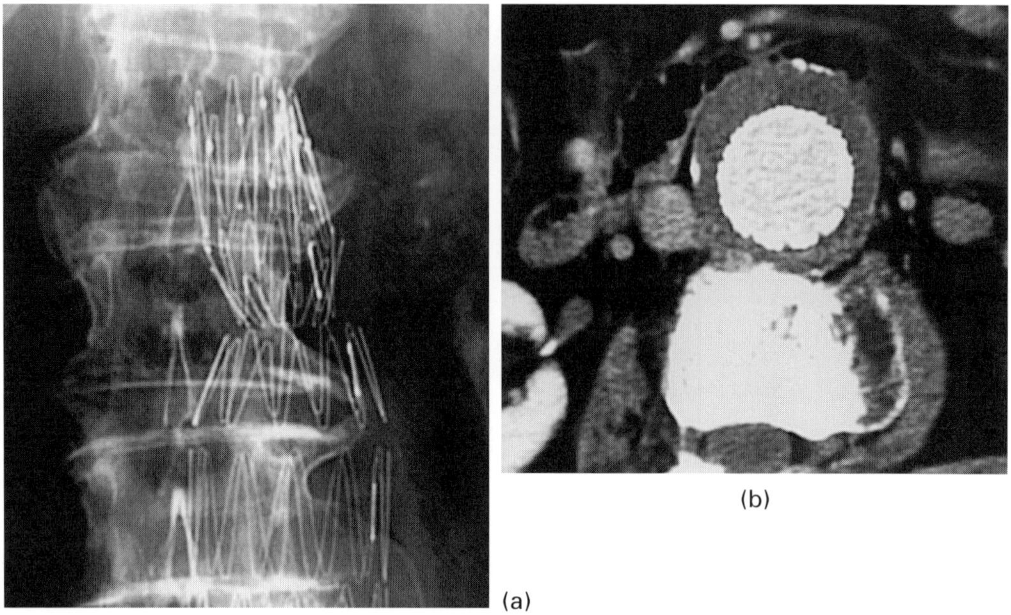

(a) (b)

Fig. 2. (a) Plain radiograph, showing annular constriction between 2nd and 3rd stents of the Zenith graft, due to the (surgically placed) external band. (b) CT scan at 3 months. No sign of previous endoleak.

concave aortic neck. This was successfully treated using the same technique (Fig. 2). In both instances the profile of the proximal aortic neck suggested that a rigid stent would not exclude the persistent endoleak around the outside of the stent-graft and external banding of the aorta seemed the more appropriate option.

Late proximal endoleaks will no doubt occur, but not in our experience to date. Providing that the leak is detected prior to rupture there should be no reason why this complication could not be treated in the same manner as an early proximal endoleak.

Distal endoleaks

There are two distal implantation sites for bifurcate systems, and in the case of modular devices at least one junctional site, at which the potential for endoleak exists. Providing that the correct preoperative calibrations have been made and that a satisfactory junctional overlap is achieved during endograft deployment, then early endoleaks from these sites are unusual.

Late or secondary endoleaks from the junctional areas and distal implantation sites are the most frequent late device complication after EVAR. The causes are probably multifactorial,[7,8] but factors such as severe angulation of the proximal neck, aneurysm sac or iliac vessels, poor junctional overlap of modular devices and inherent stent-graft defects have to be considered. The Freeman Hospital experience of distal endoleak is exhibited in Table 1. Note that all the secondary endoleaks have been

Table 1. Device-related complications: 100 cases EVAR, 1995–1999

Males : Females		91 : 9	
Age: median (range)			72 (45–89)
Abdominal aortic aneurysm diameter: median (range)		5.9 (4.2–9.2)	
Bifurcated grafts : aortomonoiliac		91 : 9	
Endoleak		*11*	
	Primary:	5 on postop CT	2 proximal, banded 3 distal: 2 sealed < 3 months 1 persisted*
	Secondary:	6:	endovascular:
		3 late limb disconnections (or dislocations)	re-stenting
		3 sac reperfusion*	embolization
Limb occlusion		*10 (5 within 30 days)*	
		2 intraoperative	femorofemoral crossover grafts
		1 embolus	embolectomy(combined)
		3 outflow disease	endovascular (2), crossover graft (1)
		4 graft distortion	crossover grafts (3)
Graft migration		*3*	
	Primary:	1 Palmaz-PTFE	open conversion
	Secondary:	2 Stentor (33 months)	proximal cuff
		Talent (18 months)	proximal cuff
Abdominal aortic aneurysm rupture		*1*	
		1 Vanguard (15 months)	died during surgery

successfully treated by endovascular means. The leak site is identified at angiography, crossed with a guidewire and then bridged by an additional section of stent-graft (Figs 3, 4).

Distal endoleaks due to holes in the graft material have been demonstrated in surgical explants and at post-mortem studies but are thought to be rare – six in more than 3000 Vanguard implants worldwide.[9] However, we have come across one such case and this is demonstrated in Fig. 5.

Re-perfusion of the aneurysm sac by collateral vessels

These endoleaks (type II) usually appear insignificant, are often apparent on the first postoperative CT scan and provide a constant aggravating reminder that the

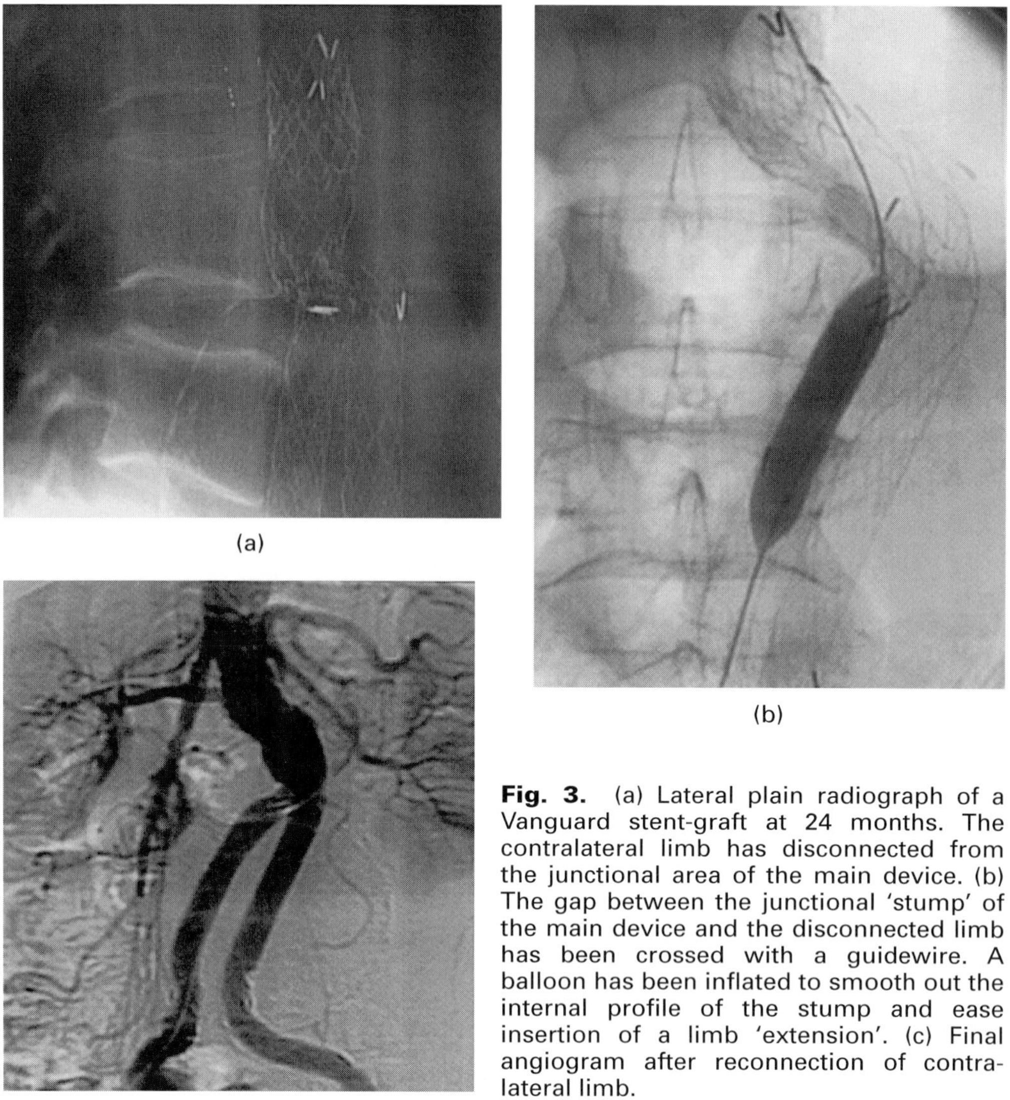

(a) (b) (c)

Fig. 3. (a) Lateral plain radiograph of a Vanguard stent-graft at 24 months. The contralateral limb has disconnected from the junctional area of the main device. (b) The gap between the junctional 'stump' of the main device and the disconnected limb has been crossed with a guidewire. A balloon has been inflated to smooth out the internal profile of the stump and ease insertion of a limb 'extension'. (c) Final angiogram after reconnection of contralateral limb.

endovascular repair of aneurysms does not entirely remove the sac from the general circulation in all cases. There is an argument for attempting to occlude all patent lumbar and inferior mesenteric arteries prior to the deployment of aortic endografts. However, this would add a vast amount of interventional time to the patient's preoperative management, not to mention the radiation and contrast doses, the risks of embolizing gut or spinal arteries and the extra costs involved. There is also evidence to suggest that ignoring the patent lumbar and inferior mesenteric vessels, seen on many pre-EVAR assessments, does not lead to a greater incidence of type II endoleaks.[10,11] Our experience thus far mirrors that of others, whereby the persistent

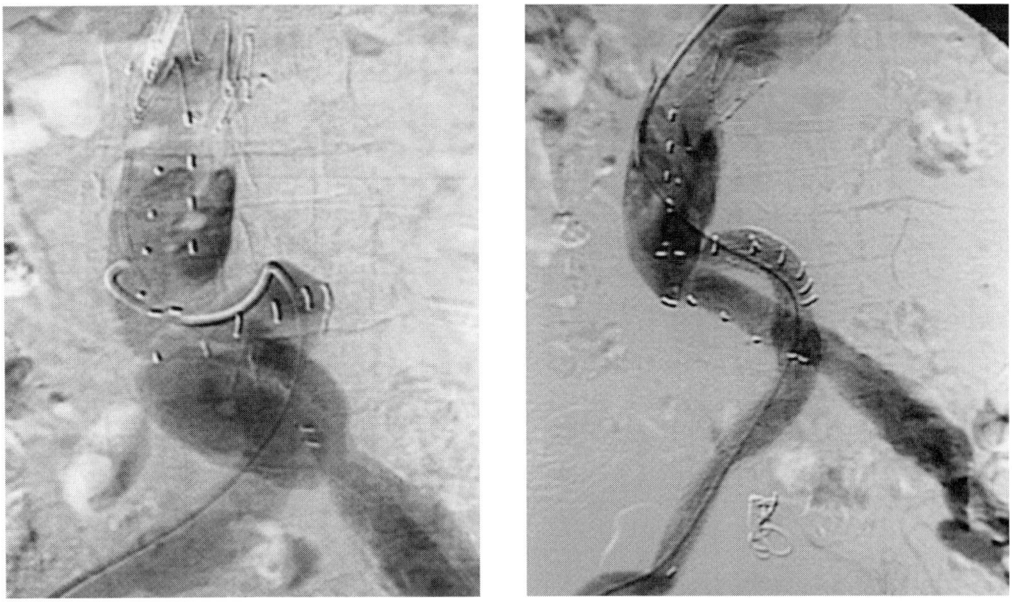

(a) (b)

Fig. 4. (a) Angiogram demonstrating a large distal endoleak through the dislocated right limb of an EVT graft. The distal crown of the right limb has migrated upwards into the aneurysm sac. (b) The right limb of the EVT graft has been reconnected to the right common iliac artery with a Gore extension.

endoleak related to reperfusion can be treated by embolization via the internal iliac artery and the ilio-lumbar collaterals.[12,13] This is often a time consuming procedure utilizing microcatheters and is not lightly embarked upon as several procedures may be required (Fig. 6). The direct transcutaneous injection of embolic material into the aneurysm sac has been discussed as a possible method of managing the reperfusion endoleak, but there is no reported experience of this technique.

Graft occlusion

There is a significant incidence of endograft limb occlusion,[14,15] particularly evident amongst the first generation of bifurcated devices, where 10% occlusion rates have been noted.[16] This concurs with our own experience (Table 1). The incidence of endograft occlusion is low in the immediate postoperative phase, but occasional problems arise where the outflow through the external iliac is compromised. This may be due to inadequately treated pre-existing stenotic disease, or to endothelial shearing and dissection during device insertion. Prompt intervention by a 'combined' procedure, with Fogarty thrombectomy and placement of an uncovered metal stent may be all that is required.

However, our first two such cases were not amenable to endovascular salvage and proceeded to extra-anatomical bypass grafts. Two further graft limb occlusions arose as a direct result of intra-procedural manipulations during the primary operation and one of these underwent immediate femorofemoral crossover grafting.

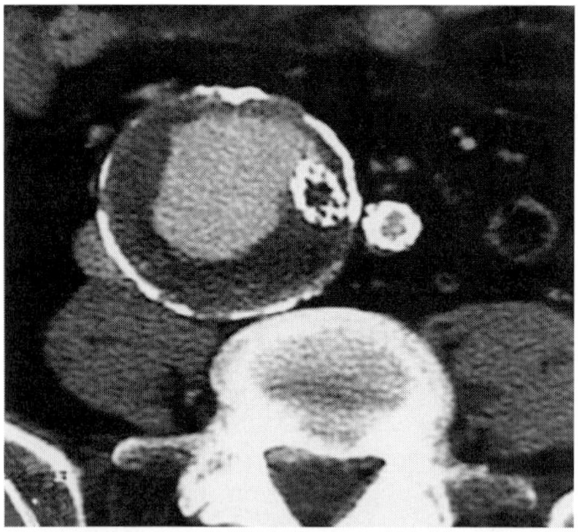

(a)

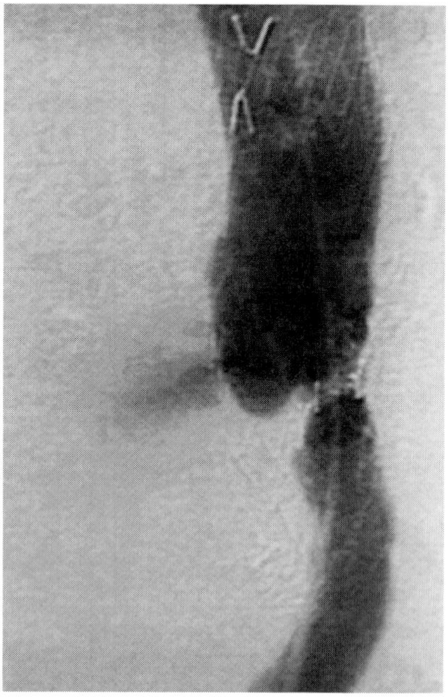

(b)

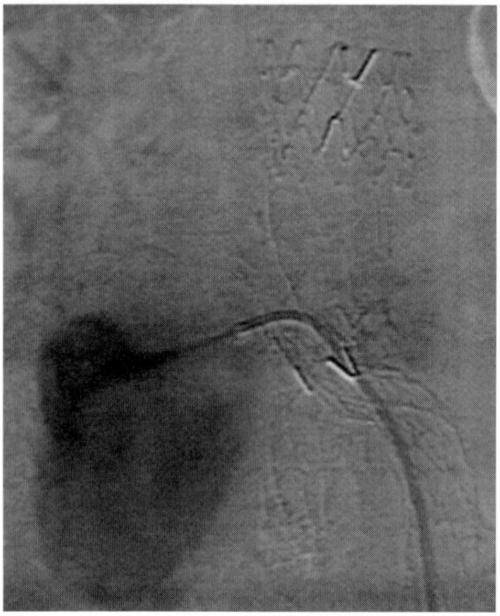

(c)

Fig. 5. (a) Bifurcated Stentor device. Endoleak in right common iliac aneurysm. Right limb had previously occluded. (b) Angiogram showing contrast exit through a perforation in the right side of the distal body of the Stentor graft. Related to the apex of an adjacent stent 'zig'. (c) Catheter tip projects through hole in graft. Repaired by insertion of a Talent aorto-mono-iliac endograft.

Our series also includes one patient with recurrent emboli from an atheromatous thoracic aorta and limb occlusion at 3 weeks. He required a 'combined' procedure via a small femoral cut-down with initial negotiation of the occluded segment by catheter and subsequent Fogarty embolectomy.

Late endograft occlusion

In one of five occlusions after 30 days, there was disease in an adjacent vascular segment rather than a primary stent-related problem and this was treated by endovascular means with combined thrombectomy and stenting (Fig. 7).

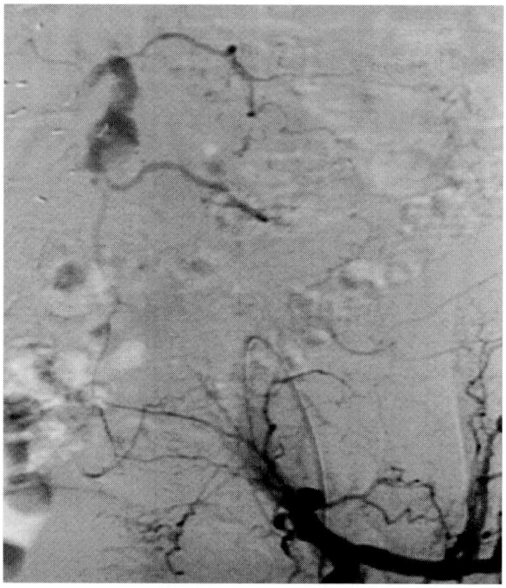

Fig. 6. Selective angiogram of left internal iliac artery. There are several tiny ascending branches producing a type II endoleak into the aneurysm sac with outflow into lumbar arteries.

Extra-anatomic bypass. The four remaining cases were related to secondary stent-graft limb distortion and kinking with or without dislocation (Fig. 8). These patients, and one of the peroperative occlusions, had chronic occlusions with continued exclusion of the aneurysm. So far, four of the five have been managed by surgical crossover grafts when symptoms of claudication have become problematic and further intervention deemed to be justified. Treatment was with femorofemoral crossover grafts, essentially converting bifurcated endografts to aortouni-iliac grafts with crossovers.

Migration (with or without endoleak)

Migration of the aortic endograft from the proximal neck down into the aneurysm sac during the primary procedure, unless correctable, will obviously lead to immediate technical failure and open conversion (see below).

The incidence of secondary device migration seems gratifyingly low.[17] The downward migration of the proximal fixation mechanism should be identified on the follow up plain radiographs (Fig. 9) and ideally will be noticed prior to the formation of a significant proximal endoleak. The prompt insertion of an appropriate proximal cuff (Fig. 9e) will then be required, usually via a femoral cutdown. It is mandatory for all companies producing aortic endografts to have an easily available proximal cuff (Fig. 10) for such occasions.

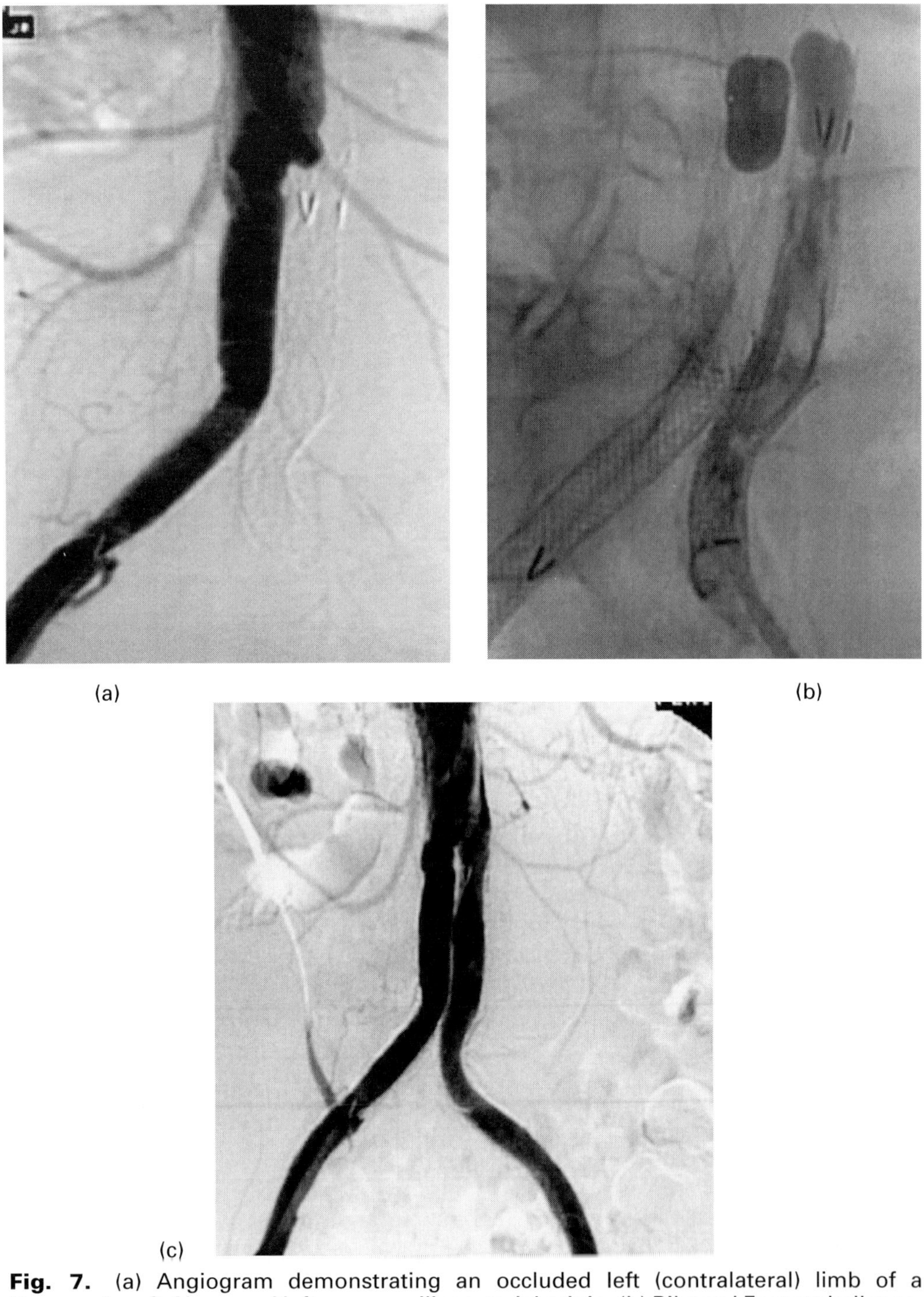

Fig. 7. (a) Angiogram demonstrating an occluded left (contralateral) limb of a Vanguard graft. Narrowed left common iliac arterial origin. (b) Bilateral Fogarty balloons. The right-sided balloon to prevent thrombus entering the origin of the right common iliac. Left balloon pulled through the blocked limb. (c) Angiogram after recanalization of the occluded left limb.

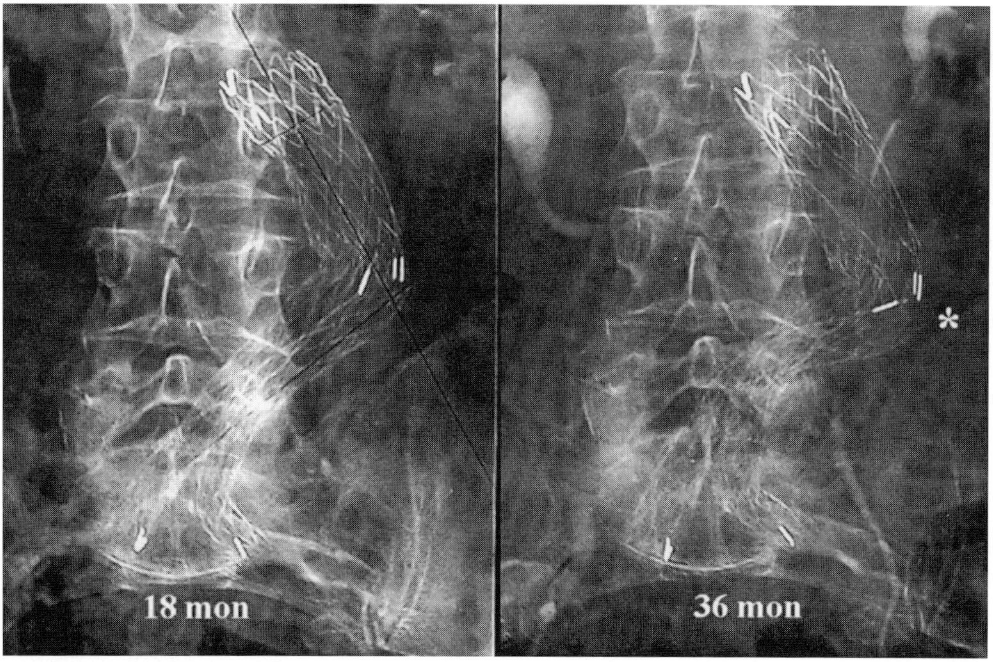

(a) (b)

Fig. 8. (a, left side of image) Radiograph at 18 months post-EVAR. Vanguard stent graft is buckling towards left side. (b, right side of image) Radiograph at 36 months shows further kinking of the graft associated with left limb disconnection at the junctional site (markers separated). This limb had recently occluded.

Open conversion

Conversion to open repair following EVAR may be primary or secondary. The mortality associated with primary conversion was initially reported as 43%.[18] More recently, this mortality has improved as the incidence and indications for conversion to open repair have changed.[19] The largest series of aortic stent-graft conversion to open repair has recently been reported from the Royal Prince Alfred Hospital in Sydney, Australia.[17] Over a period of 6 years, endoluminal methods were used to repair 204 aortic aneurysms. Conversion to open repair was required in 34 patients (17 primary and 17 secondary repairs). In the first 3-year period 17% of patients required primary conversion. This dropped to 3% in the later 3-year period, suggesting better patient selection and the use of more robust devices. The mortality following primary conversion to open repair was 18%.

Other centres report similar results[20–22] with the incidence of conversion to open repair ranging from 2% to 25%.

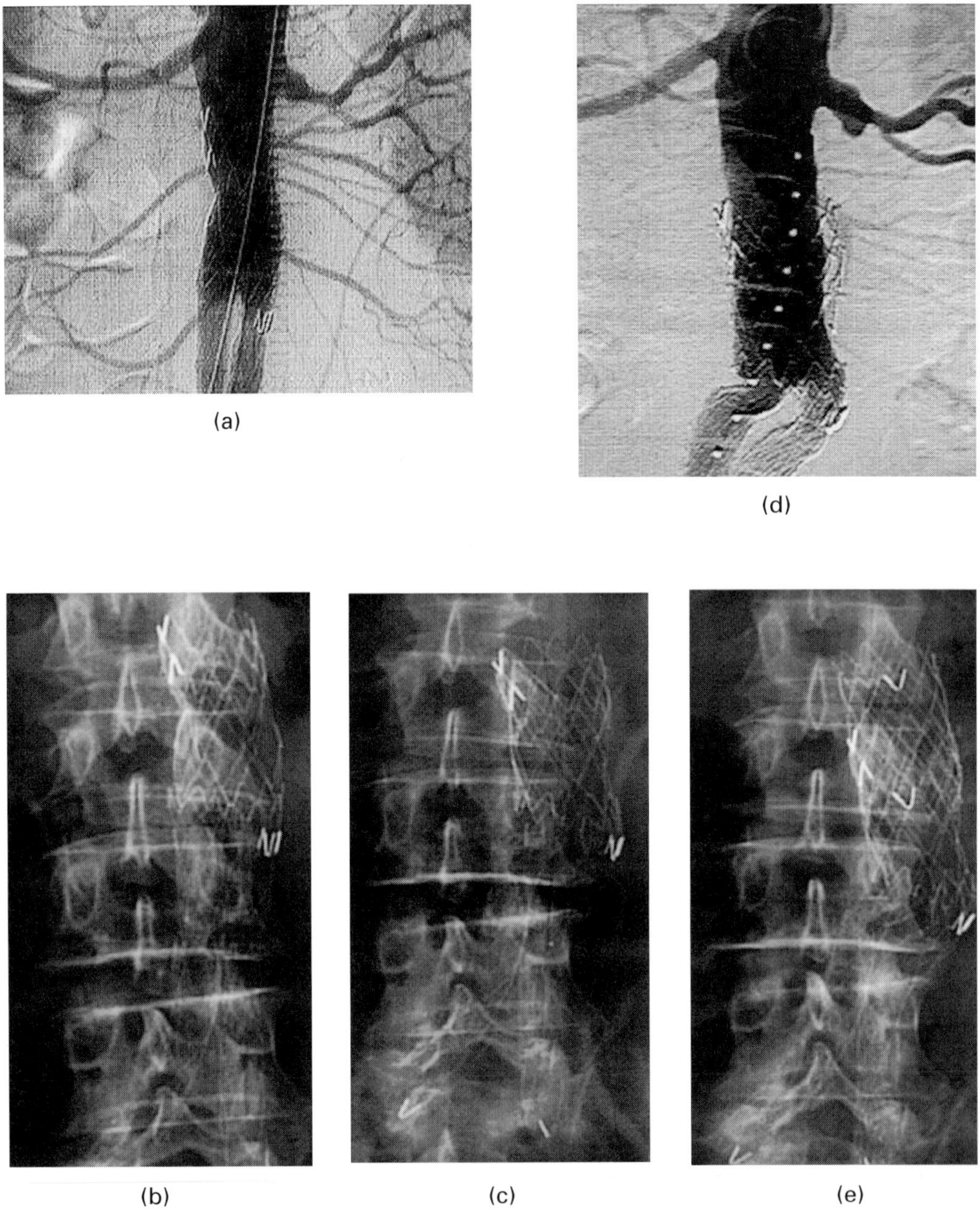

Fig. 9. (a) Post-procedural angiogram after primary Vanguard procedure. Note top stent marker within a few millimetres of left renal artery. (b) Baseline plain radiograph pre-discharge. (c) Plain radiograph at 33 months. Stent-graft buckling at bifurcation with evidence of distal migration. (d) Angiogram at 33 months. Confirmed downward migration of proximal end of Vanguard in relation to left renal artery. (e) Plain radiograph demonstrating the proximal Vanguard 'cuff' within and overlapping the upper end of the primary stent-graft.

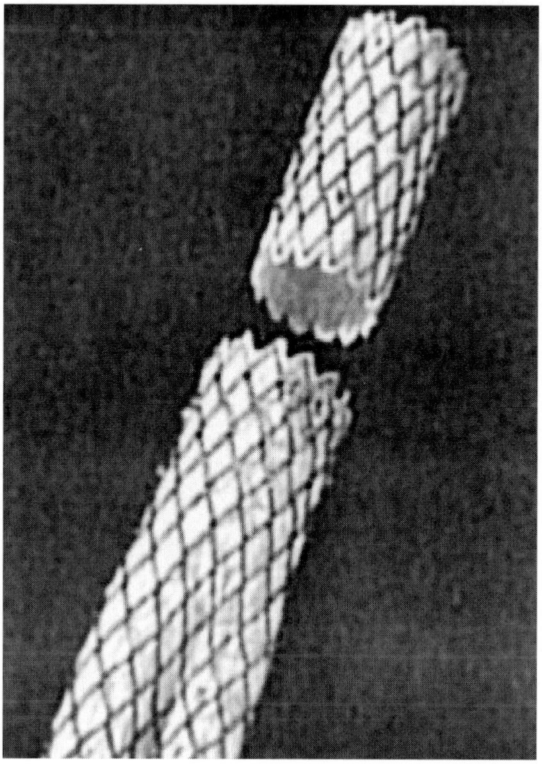

Fig. 10. Proximal cuff for the AneuRx device.

Surgical conversion – operative techniques

The techniques described[17] for surgical conversion are:

- Conventional open abdominal aortic aneurysm repair
- Modified conventional open abdominal aortic aneurysm repair
- Supracoeliac aortic control
- Amputation of infrarenal endoprosthesis from suprarenal component.

Conventional open repair is used in patients in whom attempted endoluminal repair has to be abandoned due to access problems or immediate proximal migration of the device. No stent graft is present within the aortic neck or iliac segments and a standard open repair is possible.

Modified conventional open repair is required in the presence of stent graft material within the aortic neck and iliac arteries. Here clamps are applied to the appropriate vessels but are opened and closed in sequence to allow removal of the underlying endograft.

Supracoeliac control of the abdominal aorta is required when endografts have been inadvertently deployed above the renal arteries, or in patients with rupture of the proximal neck or suprarenal retainment of the introduction device (both deployment related). In addition, a temporary suprarenal clamp may be required for patients with known proximal endoleaks, presenting as rupture and following the removal of an infected prosthesis to enable oversewing of the infrarenal aorta.

Occasionally, grafts with suprarenal bare stent elements (Figs 1,2) become incorporated into the aortic wall and cannot safely be removed in their entirety. In this instance, cutting of the metal frame or fabric has been described with incorporation of the proximal amputated prosthesis into the suture line.[23] In summary, conversion to open repair following EVAR is uncommon, with most series reporting incidences of approximately 2–7%. Although initial mortality rates were high, with increasing experience, careful case selection and accurate planning, these rates are dropping to acceptable levels. In our own series of 100 stent-graft deployments, only one patient has required open conversion. This was a primary conversion following immediate proximal migration of a Leicester aortouni-iliac device. No commercial devices have required primary or secondary conversion.

Rupture

In the absence of long-term follow-up of second-generation aortic stent-grafts, it is difficult to be certain of the efficacy of the endovascular technique with regard to the prevention of aneurysm rupture. As with device migration, rupture of an aortic aneurysm following EVAR is unusual in the early- and medium-term. The national database[24] quotes a 1.3% incidence of rupture and we have had one such event in our first 100 cases.

The management of aneurysm rupture post-EVAR should be according to conventional surgical principles, but obviously the exact approach to open repair would be dictated by the type of stent-graft *in situ* (see above). It is interesting to note a recent comparison of mortality as a result of secondary aneurysm rupture (following EVAR) with the mortality of a concurrent series of primary ruptures,[25] which seemed to indicate that EVAR might have a beneficial effect.

CONCLUSION

The complementary skills of the vascular surgeon and the interventional radiologist lend themselves ideally to the opportunity provided by the management of EVAR complications. Catheter and guide wire expertise is required to recanalize disconnected or blocked endograft limbs. Surgical attention to the careful control of the access site is needed to minimize blood loss or distal embolization during such 'endovascular' procedures. Conventional surgical skills are necessary to insert extra-anatomical grafts, to fix the more problematic proximal endoleaks and to cope with the (rare) open conversions. The formation of a surgical and radiological vascular team probably represents 'best practice' in these circumstances.

REFERENCES

1. Woodburn KR, May J, White GH: Endoluminal abdominal aortic aneurysm surgery. *Br J Surg* **85**: 435–443, 1998
2. Harris PL: The highs and lows of endovascular aneurysm repair: the first two years of the Eurostar Registry. *Ann R Coll Surg Engl* **81**: 161–165, 1999
3. White GH, Yu W, May J: 'Endoleak' – a proposed new terminology to describe incomplete aneurysm exclusion by an endoluminal graft. *J Endovasc Surg* **3**: 124–125, 1996
4. White GH, May J, Waugh RC *et al.*: Type III and Type IV Endoleak : towards a complete definition of blood flow in the sac after endoluminal AAA repair. *J Endovasc Surg* **5**: 305–309, 1998
5. Malina M, Brunkwall J, Lindblad B *et al.*: Endovascular management of the juxtarenal aortic aneurysm: can uncovered stents safely cross the renal arteries? *Semin Vasc Surg* **12**: 182–191, 1999
6. Gordon MK, Lawrence-Brown MMD, Hartley D *et al.*: A self-expanding endoluminal graft for treatment of aneurysms: Results through the development phase. *Aust NZJ Surg* **66**: 621–625, 1996
7. Schurink GWH, Aarts NJM, van Bockel JH : Endoleak after stent-graft treatment of abdominal aortic aneurysm: a meta-analysis of clinical studies. *Br J Surg* **86**: 581–587, 1999
8. Harris P, Brennan J, Martin J *et al.*: Longitudinal aneurysm shrinkage following endovascular aortic aneurysm repair: a source of intermediate and late complications. *J Endovasc Surg* **6**: 11–16, 1999
9. Nielsen M : Boston Scientific EAG Physician Advisory Board Recommendations (personal communication): May 14, 1999
10. Walker SR, Halliday K, Yusuf SW *et al.*: A study on the patency of the inferior mesenteric and lumbar arteries in the incidence of endoleak following endovascular repair of infra-renal aortic aneurysms. *Clin Radiol* **53**: 593–595, 1998
11. Broeders IA, Blankensteijn JD, Eikelboom BC: The role of infrarenal aortic side branches in the pathogenesis of endoleaks after endovascular aneurysm repair. *Eur J Vasc Endovasc Surg* **16**: 419–426, 1998
12. Golzarian J, Struyven J, Abada HT *et al.*: Endovascular aortic stent-grafts: transcatheter embolization of persistent perigraft leaks. *Radiology* **202**: 731–734, 1997
13. Kato N, Semba CP, Dake MD: Embolization of perigraft leaks after endovascular stent-graft treatment of aortic aneurysms. *J Vasc Int Radiol* **7**: 805–811, 1996
14. Lawrence-Brown M, Hartley D, MacSweeney S *et al.*: The Perth Endoluminal Bifurcated Graft System – Development and Early Experience. *J Cardiovasc Surg* **4**: 706–712, 1996
15. Umscheid T, Stelter WJ: Time-related alterations in shape, position and structure of self-expanding, modular aortic stent-grafts: a 4 year single-center follow-up. *J Endovasc Surg* **6**: 17–32, 1999
16. Chuter TA, Risberg B, Hopkinson BR *et al.*: Clinical experience with a bifurcated endovascular graft for abdominal aortic aneurysm repair. *J Vasc Surg* **24**: 655–666, 1996
17. May J, White GH, Harris JP: Techniques for surgical conversion of aortic endoprosthesis. *Eur J Vasc Surg* **18**: 284–289, 1999
18. May J, White GH, Yu W *et al.*: Conversion from endoluminal to open repair of abdominal aortic aneurysms: a hazardous procedure. *Eur J Vasc Endovasc Surg* **14**: 4–11, 1997
19. May J, White GH, Yu W *et al.*: Endovascular grafting for abdominal aortic aneurysms: changing incidence and indications for conversion to open operation. *Cardiovasc Surg* **6**: 194–197, 1998
20. Blum U, Voshage G, Lammer J *et al.*: Endoluminal stent grafts for infrarenal abdominal aortic aneurysms. *New Engl J Med* **336**: 13–20, 1997
21. Parodi JC, Barone A, Piraino R, Schonholz C: Endovascular treatment of abdominal aortic aneurysms: lessons learned. *J Endovasc Surg* **4**: 102–110, 1997
22. Thompson MM, Sayers RD, Nasim A *et al.*: Aorto-mono-iliac endovascular grafting: difficult solutions to difficult aneurysms. *J Endovasc Surg* **4**: 174–181, 1997
23. Lawrence-Brown M: (personal communication) 1999

24. Joint Working Party, Vascular Surgical Society of Great Britain and Ireland and the British Society of Interventional Radiologists, *Third Report on the Registry for Endovascular Treatment of Aneurysms (RETA)*. 1999
25. May J, White GH, Waugh R *et al.*: Rupture of abdominal aortic aneurysms: A concurrent comparison of outcome of those occurring after endoluminal repair versus those occurring *de novo*. *Eur J Vasc Endovasc Surg* **18**: 344–348, 1999

The team approach to EVAR complications II: Laparoscopic vascular surgery – current state and application

A Darzi, N Cheshire

INTRODUCTION

There is currently growing interest in the application of minimally invasive surgical techniques for reconstruction of the aorta. At the present time, worldwide, experience of laparoscopic aortic surgery is limited and there are few data to confirm the potential advantages of the technique. The new skills being learned from our laparoscopic colleagues, however, may help in the management of other retroperitoneal problems such as the insertion of stents for complex aortic disease and the management of complications of endovascular surgery – the minimally invasive advantages of endovascular repair of abdominal aortic aneurysms (EVAR) are lost if complications require major surgical intervention for correction. The application of laparoscopy and other minimally invasive techniques may enable EVAR complications such as types I and II endoleak to be managed surgically without major trauma or the use of large abdominal incisions.

It is valuable to review the current state of the art in laparoscopic aortic surgery before looking forward to how further refinement of the techniques may be applied to management of EVAR complications in the future.

USE OF LAPAROSCOPY IN VASCULAR SURGERY

Laparoscopic abdominal aortic aneurysm repair

The introduction and wide acceptance of laparoscopy have revolutionized general surgery. Laparoscopic surgery is now preferred by both patients and surgeons because of reduced postoperative complications and shorter hospital stays. Laparoscopic applications in vascular surgery have focused on aortic surgery in an attempt to provide similar benefits.

Adequate exposure of an infrarenal abdominal aortic aneurysm for open surgery typically requires a midline incision extending from the xyphoid to the pubis and is associated with considerable postoperative pain. Retroperitoneal dissection and bowel manipulation during the procedure contribute significantly to postoperative ileus and fluid shifts. Traditionally, patients stay in an intensive care or high dependency environment for 1–3 days, followed by 5–10 more days in the hospital. Many patients require 6 weeks for convalescence before resuming normal activities.

Because trocars or small incisions are used in laparoscopic surgery, postoperative pain is reduced, which in turn diminishes the potential for cardiovascular and pulmonary complications. Relief of pain after standard abdominal procedures, (including the use of epidural anaesthesia) is associated with limited improvement in postoperative vital capacity and functional residual capacity. Better pulmonary function has been found after laparoscopic than after open surgery; First-day postoperative open cholecystectomy patients have pulmonary function decreased by 50%, as measured by forced vital capacity, 1-second forced expiratory volume, and 25–75% forced expiratory flow, whereas laparoscopic patients have function decreased by approximately 25%. This can be explained by decreased trauma to the abdominal wall, decreased changes in pulmonary volume, and decreased levels of pain. Laparoscopic surgery also causes less tissue damage and trauma than do corresponding open procedures. Recent studies have investigated whether the decreased physical trauma and faster recovery times associated with laparoscopic procedures can be linked to lower levels of stress hormones.[1] During laparoscopic procedures, increases in serum metabolites and hormones, including glucose, cortisol, prolactin, b-endorphin, epinephrine, norepinephrine, dopamine, and interleukin-6, are related to operative stress, but compared with equivalent open procedures, the magnitude of the biologic response is decreased, reflecting a perceived minimization of stress.

With any laparotomy, the patient's core body temperature decreases with time because of patient exposure to a cool environment. Patients undergoing aortic reconstruction are prone to hypothermia (< 35.7ºC).[2] Significant coagulopathy is associated with intraoperative hypothermia,[3] and avoidance of hypothermia in laparoscopic procedures by the use of smaller incisions and the lack of intestinal evisceration is expected to result in less operative blood loss.

EARLY CLINICAL EXPERIENCE

The application of laparoscopic techniques to intra-abdominal vascular procedures is not new: laparoscopic exposure of the aorta during para-aortic lymph node dissection, and laparoscopically assisted aortic reconstruction procedures have all been performed previously in human beings.

Retroperitoneoscopy

In 1993, Dion and colleagues[4] reported on the first laparoscopically assisted aortobifemoral bypass. Balloon dissection was used to create a retroperitoneal cavity, similar to the technique used in laparoscopic preperitoneal hernia repair, which then allowed dissection of the distal aorta and proximal iliac arteries. The aortic anastomosis was performed through a midline minilaparotomy without laparoscopic assistance. Standard groin incisions were then made, the limbs of the graft were brought down, and end-to-side anastomoses were hand-sewn.

The relatively simple approach of balloon dissection and retroperitoneoscopy may be valuable for vascular surgeons in the management of EVAR complications. It can be used to expose the infrarenal aorta, inferior mesenteric artery, common iliac arteries and the lumbar sympathetic trunks. The technique requires only three port site incisions in the flank and can be used for sympathectomy[5] and ligation of lumbar arteries and the inferior mesenteric artery for endoleak control. In addition, the exposure obtained theoretically allows laparoscopic placement of external bands around the aortic neck or common iliac arteries. This has been advocated by some authors to seal proximal or distal landing site endoleak and to minimize or control graft migration.

Transperitoneal aortic approaches

Continued modifications of laparoscopy, including use of a transperitoneal approach, gasless abdominal wall suspension, and the development of bowel retractors, led to the first completely laparoscopic procedure involving a vascular anastomosis. By using a mechanical lift device (thus avoiding the need for pneumoperitoneum), Berens and Herde[6] were able to use conventional vascular instruments for vessel clamping and suturing to perform two iliofemoral bypasses, one aortobifemoral bypass, and one aortoiliac endarterectomy. In this series, all patients tolerated regular diet by postoperative day 2, and all were discharged on postoperative days 2 or 3.

Techniques developed in the animal laboratory have been brought into the human arena for laparoscopically assisted abdominal aortic aneurysm repair.[7] Under institutional review board approval, patients with infrarenal abdominal aortic aneurysms requiring tube grafts and with no contraindications to laparoscopy were carefully selected. The operative goals were to laparoscopically dissect the neck of the aneurysm and both iliac arteries and then, through a minilaparotomy, to cross-clamp the aorta and repair the aneurysm using a conventional open Creech technique. A preliminary study of 20 patients has been completed. In 18 patients, the dissection was successfully completed. In one patient, conversion to a standard open incision was necessary because of inadequate port placement. One patient was converted because of multiple adhesions caused by a previous hysterectomy.In the animal studies, the dissection ports were placed in the lower abdomen. Although these port positions were ideal for the iliac dissection, they were too low to get over the hump of the aneurysm and reach the neck. Modifications in the trocar location resulted in successful laparoscopic dissection of the neck of the aorta and the iliac vessels.

In the immediate postoperative period, three patients experienced minor complications, all unrelated to laparoscopy. One patient developed a superficial wound infection requiring 2 additional days of intravenous antibiotics. Another patient developed a mild case of rhabdomyolysis following the release of plaque emboli from an iliac cross-clamp; this condition was successfully treated by intravenous hydration. In one patient who had undergone an uncomplicated laparoscopically assisted abdominal aortic aneurysm repair 8 days after undergoing combined coronary artery bypass grafting and aortic and mitral valve replacements, a pericardial effusion developed that necessitated a pericardial window.

One major complication, postoperative left colon ischaemia, occurred. This patient underwent Hartmann's procedure and subsequently became ventilator dependent. Operative times averaged 4.09 ± 0.92 hours, longer than the standard times of 3.0–3.5

hours for open approaches. Laparoscopic time, which accounted for approximately 40% of the total operative time, was 1.40 ± 0.45 hours. With increased experience, this operative time decreased to less than 1 hour. Most patients were extubated within hours of the completion of the procedure. The mean duration of nasogastric tube suction was 1.3 ± 0.7 days, and 14 of 18 patients tolerated a clear liquid diet by postoperative da 2y. The mean intensive care unit stay was 2.2 ± 0.9 days, and the mean length of hospitalization was 5.8 ± 1.6 days. Within 2 or 3 weeks after surgery, patients returned to their preoperative levels of energy, activity, and appetite. No deaths occurred in this study.

The application of transperitoneal techniques to the management of EVAR complications may not confer significant advantages over retroperitoneoscopy unless access to more difficult areas such as the internal iliac arteries are required.[8] The approaches described above allow access to the aortic neck, the aneurysm sac and inferior mesenteric artery and the iliacs but usually require more port sites than a flank approach in order to contain the small bowel out of the operative site. In addition, this approach is associated with the risk of inadvertant bowel injury that is not a feature of retroperitoneal miminally invasive surgery.

FUTURE DEVELOPMENTS

At present, laparoscopically assisted abdominal aortic aneurysm repair has been performed principally on aneurysms that can be treated using tube grafts, but as Dion,[4] Ahn,[3] Gough[8] and others[9] have demonstrated, the iliac arteries can be managed through port site incisions. Refinement of iliac approaches is important for laparoscopic surgical management of EVAR and its complications. Furthermore, the use of laparoscopy in placing a bifurcated graft for an abdominal aortic aneurysm is a natural progressive step in the marriage of our current skills and those demonstrated for aortoiliac disease.

Another problem that must be tackled before laparoscopic aortic surgery becomes commonplace is control of lumbar artery backbleeding into the operative field. Aortic mobilization and clipping of lumbar vessels from outside the aorta is feasible although carries some risk of damage to the retroaortic venous plexus and embolization from atherosclerotic aortic plaques. Currently available laparoscopic stapling devices frequently cannot occlude patent vessels from within the lumen of atherosclerotic aorta. As instrumentation is developed, however, newer ways of controlling the significant bleeding which can be seen from patent lumbar vessels will be developed and may also be useful for the control of endoleak. Likewise, as secure laparoscopic vascular clamps are developed, the need for minilaparotomy should be obviated, and a totally laparoscopic aortic reconstruction and EVAR complication management procedure should evolve.

Currently, the minimal size limit for aneurysm repair in most series is approximately 5.0 cm. Investigators generally believe that open surgery for aneurysms of less than 5.0 cm is not beneficial because of an adverse risk-benefit ratio considering current mortality rates.[10] If total laparoscopic abdominal aortic aneurysm repair can be performed with minimal morbidity and mortality, operations on smaller aneurysms may well be considered appropriate, particularly because of improved anatomic exposure for laparoscopy.

SUMMARY

Since the first description of abdominal aortic aneurysms by sixteenth-century anatomist Vesalius, the history of this disease has reflected the remarkable progress of vascular surgery.[11,12] From initial attempts of ligation and sclerosis to the recent advances of endovascular and laparoscopic repair, present-day vascular surgeons are supplied with a technically evolving choice of therapeutics. None of these procedures is mutually exclusive; currently, great interest lies in the use of laparoscopy to provide extraluminal control at the neck of aneurysms, to work with endoluminal grafts, and to control collateral vessel endoleaks.

Laparoscopic vascular surgery must not be introduced into the clinical arena based only on the assumption that it is feasible. Clearly, it is a technically challenging procedure with a steep learning curve that requires specialized instrumentation and sophisticated laparoscopic suturing capability; however, with continued investigation, including prospective randomized trials, laparoscopic treatment of aortic aneurysms may become a standard option for high-risk patients.

REFERENCES

1. Lefebvre G, Thirion AV, Vauthier-Brouzes D *et al.*: Laparoscopic surgery versus laparotomy: Comparative analysis of stress markers. *J Gynecol Obstet Biol Reprod* **21**: 507–511, 1992
2. Cambria RP, Brewster DC, Abbott WM *et al.*: Transperitoneal versus retroperitoneal approach for aortic reconstruction: A randomized prospective study. *J Vasc Surg* **11**: 314–325, 1990
3. Ahn SS, Clem MF, Braithwaite BD *et al.*: Laparoscopic aortofemoral bypass. *Ann Surg* **222**: 677–683, 1995
4. Dion YM, Katkhouda N, Rouleau C *et al.*: Laparoscopy-assisted aortobifemoral bypass. *Surg Laparosc Endosc* **3**: 425–429, 1993
5. Cheshire NJ Darzi AW: Retroperitoneoscopic lumbar sympathectomy *Br J Surg* **84**: 1094–1095 1997
6. Berens ES, Herde JR: Laparoscopic vascular surgery. Four case reports. *J Vasc Surg* **22**: 73–79, 1995
7. Kline RG, D'Angelo AJ, Chen MHM *et al.*: Laparoscopically assisted abdominal aortic aneurysm repair: First 20 cases. *J Vasc Surg* **27**: 81–88, 1998
8. Gough MJ MacMahon M: A minimally invasive technique allowing ligation of the internal iliac artery during endovascular repair of aortic aneurysms with a aorto-uni-iliac device. *Eur J Vasc Endovas Surg* **16**: 535–536, 1998
9. Chen MHM, Murphy EA, Halpern V *et al.*: Laparoscopic-assisted abdominal aortic aneurysm repair. *Surg Endosc* **9**: 905–907, 1995
10. Nevitt MP, Ballard DJ, Hallett JW: Prognosis of abdominal aortic aneurysms: A population-based study. *N Engl J Med* **321**: 1009–1014, 1989
11. Parodi JC, Palmaz JC, Barone HD: Transfemoral intraluminal graft implantation for abdominal aortic aneurysms. *Ann Vasc Surg* **5**: 491–499, 1991
12. Resnikoff M, Darling RC, Chang BB *et al.*: Fate of the excluded abdominal aortic aneurysm sac: Long-term follow-up of 831 patients. *J Vasc Surg* **24**: 851–855, 1996

PERIPHERAL ARTERIAL OPPORTUNITIES

Intermittent claudication issues

Exercise programmes in intermittent claudication

Patrick Chong, Jon Golledge, Roger M Greenhalgh,
Alun Davies

INTERMITTENT CLAUDICATION – BACKGROUND AND TREATMENT OPTIONS

It is estimated that 5% of males and 2.5% of females at or over the age of 60 have symptoms of intermittent claudication.[1–2] The natural history of intermittent claudication is considered 'benign', as 70% of patients will have stable or improved symptoms at 5 years and only 1% require amputation.[3–4] Claudicants may suffer severe limitation in their daily activities due to mobility impairment.

Non-interventional or medical therapy consists of risk factor modification for tobacco, hypertension, diabetes and lipids together with advice on exercise.[5–6] There is no consensus on the exact role of pharmacotherapy in intermittent claudication. Naftidrofuryl,[7–8] pentoxifylline[9–15] and cilostazol[16] have all been advocated but have presently not gained widespread acceptance. However, aspirin is commonly prescribed with the rationale of preventing secondary cardiovascular events. The large Antiplatelet Trialists meta-analysis showed that long-term aspirin therapy contributed to a reduction in overall non-fatal and fatal cardiovascular events.[17]

Angioplasty (PTA) or surgical revascularization is usually considered for claudicants with symptoms affecting their work or lifestyle after failing an adequate trial of conservative medical therapy. Since interventional therapy carries some risk, its use in patients with intermittent claudication has been questioned.[18–20]

Exercise therapy has been advocated as first-line treatment for intermittent claudication. It is well tolerated by the majority of claudicants with the exception of those with limiting cardiopulmonary or musculoskeletal conditions[21] and it does not subject claudicants, who may have a high prevalence of concomitant cardiac and cerebrovascular disease, to the adherent risks of PTA or surgery. The evidence for exercise therapy is considered.

MEASURING THE BENEFIT DERIVED FROM EXERCISE PROGRAMMES

An important factor in the determination of the effectiveness of exercise programmes for intermittent claudication is the choice of a suitable outcome measure for the condition. Due to the unreliability of walking distance estimation in clinic,[22] researchers have tried to quantify the severity of claudication symptoms by measuring endpoints based around treadmill testing. Treadmill protocols can be either fixed load with no increase in walking speed or gradient throughout the test or graded load with gradual increments in either speed or gradient. During exercise on a treadmill, the start of claudication pain (Initial Claudication Distance or ICD) and subsequent point of maximum claudication pain (Absolute Claudication Distance or ACD) are recorded. Reproducibility is a problem with treadmill testing.[23] Patient motivation may also introduce an unpredictable bias into results. A single treadmill test has a high coefficient of variation (30–45%)[24] and endpoints based on ICD[25] or fixed load treadmill tests[26] are less accurate. Although not perfect, the ACD measured on a graded load treadmill protocol has the best reproducibility and should be utilized if treadmill testing is considered.[27–28]

The impact of treatment on the quality of life in intermittent claudication is an increasingly important issue. Researchers have utilized generic tools such as the SF-36, the EuroQol (European Quality of Life Scale) and the NHP (Nottingham Health Profile) in an attempt to quantify the impact of intermittent claudication on a patient's daily living activity.[28] Some disease-specific questionnaires have been developed for use in claudicants such as the Walking Impairment Questionnaire (WIQ)[29–30] and the Claudication Scale (CLAU-S).[31] The criticism of generic tools is that they are intended to be used with any disease state and thus are not sensitive enough to detect small but important changes in a patient's health status as a result of treatment. Although the WIQ has been designed as an intended disease-specific instrument for intermittent claudication, it relies largely on the patient's estimation of walking and stair-climbing ability which is inaccurate[22] and does not adequately assess the full impact of intermittent claudication upon a patient's daily quality of life. The CLAU-S is a long 80-item questionnaire that has been validated against the NHP. It consists of nine sections, four of which correspond to a well-described instrument for measuring mood states, the Profile of Mood States (POMS).[32] CLAU-S requires 14 minutes on average to complete and the English translation of the questionnaire has not yet been validated.

THE EVIDENCE FOR EXERCISE

Foley first described the benefit of exercise therapy in patients with peripheral arterial occlusive disease in the form of daily walks in 1957.[33] Almost a decade later in 1966, this observation was followed up by Larssen and Lassen[34] in a study of 14 claudicants randomly allocated between a control group with placebo tablets and a group asked to take a daily 1 hour walk with instructions to rest only at the point of maximum claudication. The outcome measures were maximum anterior tibial muscle blood flow and treadmill walking distance. At 6 months, no significant differences were noted in maximum blood flow measurements between the two groups but there was a significant increase in ICD ($p<0.001$) and ACD ($p<0.025$) on treadmill testing.

Over the subsequent 30 years, exercise therapy in patients with intermittent claudication has been studied extensively. Brandsma's meta-analysis in 1998 identified 82 studies of exercise therapy for intermittent claudication.[35] Strict inclusion criteria that required study randomization and the reporting of either walking distance or treadmill time as outcome measures meant that only ten studies involving 124 patients undergoing exercise were left for the meta-analysis[20,34, 36–43] (Table 1). The mean improvement in walking distance or time was 105% at the end of training.

A Cochrane Library review in 1998[44] identified nine randomized controlled trials of sufficient quality involving just over 200 patients undergoing exercise therapy for intermittent claudication[20,34,36,38,40–42,45–46] (Table 1). Results showed that exercise therapy significantly improved ACD with a mean overall improvement of 150%.

A meta-analysis of 21 randomized and non-randomized studies by Gardner and Poelhman[47] involving exercise therapy for intermittent claudication attempted to highlight some important recommendations. Mean improvement following exercise therapy was 179% for ICD and 122% for ACD. The most effective mode of exercise was walking ($p<0.001$) and programmes advocating a target of walking to near maximal pain as an endpoint produced greater symptomatic improvement than those that advised resting at the initial onset of pain ($p<0.001$). The frequency of exercise advised was more than three times a week for at least 30 minutes on each occasion and the duration of the rehabilitation programme required to be at least 6 months or longer ($p<0.001$). Older patients (>65 years) were more likely to derive benefit from an exercise programme and surprisingly outcome was not significantly different between supervised and non-supervised programmes.

Existing limitations with exercise therapy studies

The weaknesses of studies involving exercise therapy for intermittent claudication are that most are non-randomized and the numbers studied have been small. In Brandsma's meta-analysis, only one study out of ten had more than 25 subjects.[20] The mean walking distance improvement of 105% stated by Brandsma is invalid as the meta-analysis has confused studies using the pain-free walking distance or ICD with those using the maximum walking distance or ACD as the main endpoint.

There has been an overdependence on the use of treadmill walking distances as an outcome measure in the majority of exercise studies. Most have opted for the more variable fixed load protocol instead of the graded load protocol that has better reproducibility.[40,42,43] Two studies have used treadmill walking both as a means of exercise training as well as outcome testing thus introducing the possibility of error due to a 'learning effect' bias.[40,42]

The correlation between a patient's daily functional ability and treadmill walking is unclear and the evaluation of the impact of exercise therapy on quality of life has

Table 1. Randomized controlled trials of exercise therapy for intermittent claudication

Name	*Subjects in exercise programme (total no. in study)*	*Control group*	*Training mode and supervision*	*Duration (weeks) Frequency (days per week) Length (min)*	*Treadmill testing protocol and endpoint*	*% Increase in endpoints at the end of study (control)*	*p-Value difference between control and study group*
Studies in Leng's Cochrane Library Review and Brandsma's meta-analysis							
Larsen *et al.* 1966[34]	7(14)	N / P	W None	24w / daily / 60min	Fixed MWT	106 (-10)	Not significant
Dahlloff *et al.* 1974[36]	10(18)	N / P	DLE yes	12w / 3dpw / 30min	Fixed	100 MWD	p<0.001 (0)
Lundgren *et al.* 1989[20] [a]	25(50)	S S/DLE/W	DLE+W yes	24w / 3dpw / 30min	Fixed MWD	51 (163)	Not significant
Creasy *et al.* 1990[38]	16(36)	PTA	DLE+W combination	24w / 2dpw / 30min	Graded MWD	210 (70)	Not significant
Hiatt *et al.* 1990[40]	10(19)	N / P	TM yes	12w / 3dpw / 30min	Graded MWT	165 (20)	p<0.05
Mannarino *et al.* 1991[41] [b]	10(30)	D1 D1/W	W no	24w / 2dpw / 60min	Fixed ICT	86 (38)	p<0.06
Hiatt *et al.* 1994[42]	10(29)	N / P	TM yes	24w / 2dpw / 60min	Graded MWT	74 (36)	p<0.05

Studies included in Brandsma's meta-analysis							
Ernst *et al.* 1987[37]	22(42)	N / P	TM+W combination	8w / 5dpw / NS	Fixed MWD	122 (16)	Not stated but significant
Kiesewetter *et al.* 1987[39]	15(30)	D2	DLE yes	6w / 5dpw / 60min	Fixed ICD	28 (40)	Not available
Regensteiner et al. 1996[43]	10(29) St	N / P	TM yes	12w / 3dpw / 60min	Graded	74 MWT	p<0.05 (36)
Studies included in Leng's Cochrane Library Review							
Holm *et al.* 1993[45]	6(12)	N / P	DLE yes	16w / 3dpw / 30min	NS MWD	122 (0)	Not stated but significant
Ciufetti *et al.* 1994[46]	NS(30)	D3	W combination	12w / 2dpw / 60min	Fixed MWD	62 (88)	p<0.001

N/P Nothing or placebo
DLE Dynamic leg exercises
PTA Angioplasty
S Surgery
St Strength training
D1 Dipyridimole + aspirin
D2 Drug therapy
D3 Pentoxifylline

MWD Maximum walking distance
MWT Maximum walking time
IWD Initial walking distance
ICD Initial walking time
NS Not stated
W Walking
TM Treadmill

[a]Three-arm study with surgery only and surgery plus exercise in the other two groups.
[b]Three-arm study with antiplatelet only and antiplatelet plus exercise in the other two groups.

not been adequately addressed. In the last 10 years, researchers have begun to acknowledge the importance of quality of life assessment in exercise therapy studies.[40,42,43,48,49] Instruments used in exercise therapy studies have been mainly generic quality of life assessment tools such as the Medical Outcomes Study SF-36[48] and the Nottingham Health Profile (NHP)[49] with the exception of the Walking Impairment Questionnaire (WIQ).[21] As previously discussed, these questionnaires may not be an accurate reflection of the full impact of intermittent claudication on patient quality of life.

Another reservation with exercise therapy for intermittent claudication is the suggestion that training in claudicants may trigger a series of ischaemic reperfusion episodes leading to oxygen-derived free radical generation, neutrophil activation and a generalized increase in vascular permeability. This systemic endothelial inflammatory response may potentially be harmful and has been postulated as a cause for the two- to three-fold increased mortality rate observed in the claudicant population due to stroke or myocardial infarction not simply explained by the progression of atherosclerosis.[50–53] However, a study by Tisi has shown that the biological markers of this exercise-induced inflammatory response can be attenuated through regular exercise training over 3–6 months and thus the concern over adverse systemic effects may be unjustified.[54]

The mechanism for improvement in exercise therapy

Various explanations have been forwarded for the benefits seen in claudicants following an exercise programme.[55] They include adaptations in skeletal muscle enzyme activity,[36] more efficient clearance of ischaemic metabolic byproducts,[40] decreases in blood viscosity and changes in erythrocyte filterability,[37] improved blood flow through collateral vessels,[37] inhibition of progression of atherosclerotic disease,[56] changes in pain perception[57] and other factors such as improved walking economy.[58]

Although exercise has been postulated to increase the efficiency of oxidative metabolism of skeletal muscle, studies evaluating the activity of oxidative or glycolytic enzymes in skeletal muscle have failed to demonstrate any increase in activity with training.[59–61] In chronic ischaemia and exercise to claudication pain, skeletal muscle concentrations of acylcarnitines, a byproduct of abnormal metabolism, increase mitochondrial. Although a reduction in the plasma concentration of acylcarnitine has been observed in subjects with the best response to exercise training,[40] research is still in progress to determine the exact role of muscle carnitine metabolism in the treatment of intermittent claudication.

Improvements seen following an exercise programme may be in part due to a 'learning' effect as some trials have utilized the treadmill both as a training tool and as a means of testing for outcome.[40,42] Altered walking technique, improved gait and walking efficiency due to training have also been cited as explanations for the benefit seen with exercise.[42]

In general, haemodynamic studies have shown no correlation between improved exercise performance and changes in ankle brachial pressure index or calf muscle blood flow.[44,61] Despite the many investigations into the mechanisms for benefit in exercise therapy for intermittent claudication, the precise reason for the improvement seen in pain-free walking ability remains to be elucidated.[55]

Comparison between exercise and other options

A comparison of exercise therapy for intermittent claudication with other treatment options in the Cochrane Library review[44] explored the effectiveness of exercise against placebo tablets,[34,36,45] the normal level of physical activity[40,42,] pharmacotherapy[41,46] and endovascular or surgical intervention.[20,38] Outcome measures analysed were walking distances, ankle brachial pressure index, calf blood flow, subjective symptomatic measures, adverse events and mortality.

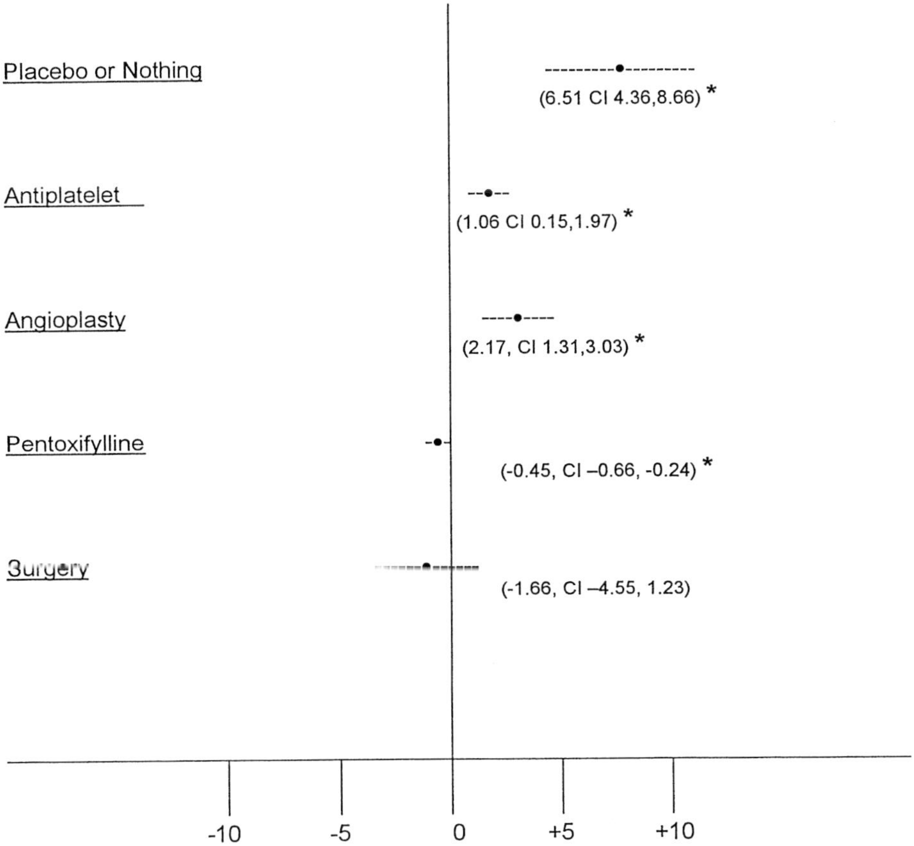

Fig. 1. Odds ratios for maximum walking distance improvements in comparisons between exercise therapy and other treatment options for intermittent claudication. *Denotes a significant difference between exercise therapy and controls. (Adapted from Ref. 44.)

The meta-analysis showed that exercise therapy produced significantly improved walking distances to controls when compared against placebo or nothing, antiplatelet therapy and PTA. Meanwhile, walking distances were not significantly longer in the surgical controls and significantly better in the pentoxifylline treated controls (Fig. 1).

In general, haemodynamic differences in ankle brachial pressure index changes or maximum calf blood flow were unremarkable between exercise therapy and controls except when compared with surgery which produced significant improvements in ankle brachial pressure index and maximum calf blood flow postoperatively. However, two patients in the exercise group developed critical ischaemia requiring surgery whereas several patients in the surgical group had major complications necessitating further procedures (three requiring thrombectomy and three requiring re-reconstructive surgery) with two deaths reported (Fig. 1).

EXERCISE THERAPY VERSUS ANGIOPLASTY: A COMPARISON OF SYMPTOMATIC BENEFIT

So far, two small, randomized controlled trials from Oxford and Edinburgh comparing exercise therapy and PTA have suggested that PTA may not have any additional benefit over exercise therapy in intermittent claudication.[38,62] Although initial mean walking distance for the PTA group at 6 months was non-significantly higher than the exercise therapy group, thereafter between 6 and 12 months, there was a gradual decline in the walking time for the PTA group while there was a steady increase in the exercise therapy group, so that walking time was significantly longer in the exercise therapy group by 12 months.[38] Follow-up at 6 years showed no significant differences between both groups in median walking distance (exercise therapy 150m versus PTA 180m, $p>0.05$) or median ankle brachial pressure index.[63]

A summation analysis was performed to compare the symptomatic benefit of exercise therapy versus PTA in intermittent claudication. Symptomatic success for the PTA studies is defined as an improvement up at least one category according to the subjective clinical criteria suggested by the joint council of the Society for Vascular Surgery (SVS) and the North American Chapter of the International Society for Cardiovascular Surgery (ISCVS) reporting guidelines[64] and symptomatic success for the exercise therapy studies is stated as the doubling of the ACD on treadmill testing (≥100% improvement) at 6 months. Studies were only included when results were available for patients with intermittent claudication alone and excluded if the proportion of patients with symptomatic success at a minimum of 6 months was not documented. A computer search for English language abstracts published between 1966 and April 1999 yielded nine exercise therapy[20,24,26,28,52,57,65–67] and 12 PTA[38,62,68–77] studies for analysis. Results are summarized in Table 2.

Although data from the summation suggests that PTA provides better results at 6 months, the analysis is more important in demonstrating the difficulties that exist

Table 2. Summation analysis of exercise therapy versus angioplasty for intermittent claudication

Exercise studies				*Angioplasty studies*			
Author	*Patients (n)*	*Patients with symptomatic success at 6 months*	*Percentage of patients with symptomatic success at 6 months*	*Author*	*Patients (n)*	*Patients with symptomatic success at 6 months*	*Percentage of patients with symptomatic success at 6 months*
Larsen *et al.* 1966[34]	7	5	71	Mortajeme *et al* 1980[74].	45	33	73
Alpert *et al.* 1969[57]	19	7	37	Krepel *et al.* 1985[70]	138	94	81
Dahlloff *et al.* 1974[36]	18	7	40	Blankensteijn *et al.* 1986[68]	31	26	81
Ekroth *et al.* 1978[66]	148	61	41	Morin *et al.* 1986[76]	681	531	78
Clifford *et al.* 1980[65]	21	0	0	Johnston *et al.* 1987[71]	667	567	85
Lundgren *et al.* 1989[20]	25	9	35	Creasy *et al.* 1990[38]	20	5	25
Mannarino *et al.* 1989[67]	8	1	13	Johnston *et al.* 1992[72]	236	189	80
Creasy *et al.* 1990[38]	16	12	75	Matsi *et al.* 1995[75]	106	69	65
Whyman *et al.* 1996[62]	32	11	35	Whyman *et al.* 1996[62]	30	21	69
				Katzenschlager *et al.* 1996[73]	24	17	71
				Nyamekye *et al.* 1996[77]	50	33	66
				Golledge *et al.* 1999[69]	43	27	63
Total	294	113	Mean 38	Total	2071	1612	Mean 77

when comparing exercise therapy with PTA given the present available published data. Exercise therapy studies were small and only one programme lasted longer than 6 months. Eleven of 12 exercise therapy studies utilized the more variable fixed-load treadmill test as an endpoint. There was a lack of a uniform outcome endpoint for exercise therapy and PTA studies. For a valid comparison of these therapies in a large randomized trial, a validated endpoint for the assessment of symptomatic benefit in intermittent claudication is required and the most effective and feasible exercise programme needs to be defined.

FUTURE OPPORTUNITIES IN EXERCISE THERAPY FOR INTERMITTENT CLAUDICATION

While there is some evidence to support the use of exercise therapy in intermittent claudication, the prime role of exercise therapy is unclear due to the lack of clear outcome assessment. The optimal exercise programme, patient compliance and cost-effectiveness are also unclear.

It will be difficult to draw any meaningful conclusions from any future trial comparing the efficacy of exercise therapy to other options like angioplasty or surgery for intermittent claudication unless a validated disease-specific health related quality of life measurement for claudicants is available.

Future trials of exercise programmes for intermittent claudication should also include an assessment of subsequent secondary cardiovascular events and all-cause mortality as outcome measures in order to explore the usefulness of exercise therapy in the overall reduction of the costs of managing the claudicant population.[28]

REFERENCES

1. Jelnes R, Gaardsting O, Hougaard Jensen K *et al.*: Fate in intermittent claudication: outcome and risk factors. *Br Med J (Clin Res Ed)* **293**: 1137–1140, 1986
2. Reunanen A, Takkunen H, Aromaa A: Prevalence of intermittent claudication and its effect on mortality. *Acta Med Scand* **211**: 249–256, 1982
3. Imparato AM, Kim GE, Davidson T, Crowley JG: Intermittent claudication: Its natural course. *Surgery* **78**: 795–799, 1975
4. Kannel WB, Shurtleff D: The natural history of arteriosclerosis obliterans. *Cardiovasc Clin* **3**: 37–52, 1971
5. Golledge J: Lower limb arterial disease. *Lancet* **350**: 1459–1465, 1997
6. Regensteiner JG, Hiatt WR: Medical management of peripheral arterial disease. *J Vasc Intervent Radiol* **5**: 669–677, 1994
7. Scottish Intercollegiate Guidelines Network 1998. SIGN Secretariat, Royal College of Physicians, 9 Queen Street, Edinburgh EH2 1JQ.
8. Girolami B, Bernardi E, Prins MH *et al.*: Treatment of intermittent claudication with physical training, smoking cessation, pentoxyfilline, or nafronyl. *Arch Int Med* **159**: 337–345, 1999
9. Di Perri T, Guerrini M: Placebo controlled double blind study with pentoxifylline of

walking performance in patients with intermittent claudication. *Angiology* **34**: 40–45, 1983

10. Strano A, Davi G, Avellone G *et al.*: Double-blind, crossover study of the clinical efficacy and the haemorheological effects of pentoxyfilline in patients with occlusive arterial disease of the lower limbs. *Angiology* **35**: 459–466, 1984
11. Lindgarde F, Jelnes R, Bjorkman H *et al.*: Conservative drug treatment in patients with moderately severe chronic occlusive peripheral arterial disease: Scandinavian Study Group. *Circulation* **80**: 1549–1556, 1989
12. Ernst E, Kollar L, Resch KL: Does pentoxyfilline prolong the walking distance in exercised claudicants? A placebo-controlled double blind trial. *Angiology* **43**: 121–125, 1992
13. Porter JM, Cutler BS, Lee BY *et al.*: Pentoxyfilline efficacy in the treatment of intermittent claudication: multicentre controlled double-blind trial with objective assessment of chronic occlusive arterial disease patients. *Am Heart J* **104**: 66–72, 1982
14. Reilly DT, Quinton DN, Barrie WW: A controlled trial of pentoxyfilline (Trental 400) in intermittent claudication: clinical, haemostatic and rheological effects. *NZ Med J* **100**: 445–447, 1987
15. Dettori AG, Pini M, Morrati A *et al.*: Acenocoumarol and pentoxyfilline in intermittent claudication: a controlled clinical study: the APIC study group. *Angiology* **40**: 237–248, 1989
16. Beebe HG, Dawson DL, Cutler BS *et al.*: A new pharmacological treatment for intermittent claudication: results of a randomized, multicentre trial. *Arch Int Med* **159**: 2041–2050, 1999
17. Antiplatelet Trialists Collaboration: Secondary prevention of vascular disease by prolonged antiplatelet treatment. *Br Med J (Clin Res Ed)* **296**: 320–331, 1988
18. Belli AM, Cumberland DC, Knox AM: The complication rate of percutaneous peripheral balloon angioplasty. *Clin Radiol* **41**: 380–383, 1990
19. Capek P, McLean GK, Berkowitz HD. Femoropopliteal angioplasty: factors influencing long-term success. *Circulation* **83** (Suppl I): I-70–I-80, 1991
20. Lundgren F, Dahllof AG, Lundholm K *et al.*: Intermittent claudication: surgical reconstruction or physical training? A prospective randomized trial of treatment efficiency. *Annl Surg* **209**: 346–355, 1989
21. Regensteiner JG, Steiner JF, Hiatt WR: Exercise training improves functional status in patients with peripheral arterial disease. *J Vasc Surg* **23**: 104–115, 1996
22. Watson CJE, Collin J: Estimates of distance by claudicants and vascular surgeons are inherently unreliable. *Eur J Endovasc Vasc Surg* **16**: 429–430, 1998
23. Perakyla T, Tikannen H, Von Knorring J, Lepantalo M: Poor reproducibility of the exercise test in assessment of claudication. *Clin Physiol* **18**: 187–193, 1998
24. Harris KA, Meads GE: A single treadmill test does not accurately quantitate claudication. *Can J Surg* **30**: 446–448, 1987
25. Chaudry H, Holland A, Dormandy J: Comparison of graded versus constant treadmill test protocols for quantifying intermittent claudication. *Vasc Med* **2**: 93–97, 1997
26. Cachovan M, Rogatti W, Creutzig A *et al.*: Treadmill testing for evaluation of claudication: comparison of constant-load and graded exercise tests. *Eur J Endovasc Vasc Surg* **14**: 238–243, 1997
27. Hiatt WR, Hirsch AT, Regensteiner JG, Brass EP: Clinical trials for claudication. Assessment of exercise performance, functional status and clinical endpoints. Vascular clinical trialists. *Circulation* **92**: 614–618, 1995
28. Labs KH, Dormandy JA, Jaeger KA *et al.*: On behalf of the Basel PAOD Clinical Trial Methodology Group. Trans-Atlantic Conference on Clinical Trial Guidelines in Peripheral Arterial Obstructive Disease Clinical Trial Methodology. *Eur J Endovasc Vasc Surg* **18**: 253–265, 1999
29. Regensteiner JG, Steiner JF, Panzer RJ, Hiatt WR: Evaluation of walking impairment by questionnaire in peripheral arterial disease. *J Vasc Med Biol* **2**: 142–152, 1990
30. McDermott MM, Kiang L, Guralnik JM *et al.*: Measurement of walking endurance and walking velocity with questionnaire: validation of the walking impairment

questionnaire in men and women with peripheral arterial disease. *J Vasc Surg* **28**: 1072–1081, 1998

31. Spengel FA, Brown TM, Dietze S *et al.*: The Claudication Scale (CLAU-S): A new disease-specific quality of life instrument in intermittent claudication. *Dis Manage Hlth Outcomes* **2** (s1): 65–70, 1997
32. McNair D, Lorr M, Droppleman LF: *EITS Manual for the Profile of Mood States*. San Diego: Educational and Industrial Testing Services, 1971
33. Foley WT: Treatment of gangrene of the feet and legs by walking. *Circulation* **15**: 689–700, 1957
34. Larssen OA, Lassen NA: Effect of daily muscular exercise in patients with intermittent claudication. *Lancet* **ii**: 1093–1095, 1966
35. Brandsma JW, Robeer BG, van den Heuvel S *et al.*: The effect of exercises on walking distance of patients with intermittent claudication: A study of randomized clinical trials. *Phys Ther* **78**: 278–288, 1998
36. Dahllof AG, Bjorntorp P, Holm J, Schersten T: Metabolic activity of skeletal muscle in patients with peripheral arterial insufficiency: Effect of physical training. *Eur J Clin Invest* **4**: 9–15, 1974
37. Ernst EEW, Matrai A: Intermittent Claudication, exercise and blood rheology. *Circulation* **76**: 1110–1114, 1987
38. Creasy TS, McMillan PJ, Fletcher EWL *et al.*: Is percutaneous transluminal angioplasty better than exercise for claudication? – Preliminary results from a prospective randomised trial. *Eur J Vasc Endovasc Surg* **4**: 135–140, 1990
39. Kiesewetter H, Blume J, Gerhards M, Leipnitz G: Gehtraining und medikamentose therapie bei der peripheren arteriellen verschlusskrankheit. *Vasa* (Suppl.) **20**: 384–388, 1987
40. Hiatt WR, Regensteiner JG, Hargarten MS *et al.*: Benefit of Exercise conditioning for Patients with peripheral arterial disease. *Circulation* **81**: 602–609, 1990
41. Mannarino E, Pasqualini L, Innocente S *et al.*: Physical training and antiplatelet treatment in Stage II peripheral arterial occlusive disease: Alone or combined? *Angiology* **42**: 513–521, 1991
42. Hiatt WR, Wolfel EE, Meier RH, Regensteiner JG: Superiority of treadmill walking exercise versus strength training for patients with peripheral arterial disease. *Circulation* **90**: 1866–1874, 1994
43. Regensteiner JG, Steiner JF, Hiatt WR: Exercise training improves functional status in patients with peripheral arterial disease. *J Vasc Surg* **23**: 104–115, 1996
44. Leng GC, Fowler B, Ernst E: Exercise for intermittent claudication. The Cochrane Library. 9 April 1998.
45. Holm J, Dahllof AG, Bjorntorp P, Schersten T: Enzyme studies in muscles of patients with intermittent claudication.: effect of training. *J Clin Lab Invest* **128**: 201–205, 1993
46. Ciufetti, Paltriccia R, Lombardini R *et al.*: Treating peripheral arterial occlusive disease: pentoxyfilline versus exercise. *Int Angiol* **13**: 33–39, 1994
47. Gardner AW, Poelhman ET: Exercise rehabilitation programs for the treatment of claudication pain. *J Am Med Assoc* **274**: 975–980, 1995
48. Patterson RB, Pinto B, Marcus M *et al.*: Value of a supervised exercise programme for the therapy of arterial claudication. *J Vasc Surg* **25**: 312–329, 1997
49. Tisi P, Shearman C: The impact of treatment of intermittent claudication on subjective health of the patient. *Hlth Trends* **30**: 109–113, 1998/99
50. Tisi PV, Shearman CP: Biochemical and inflammatory changes in the exercising claudicant. *Vasc Med* **3**: 189–198, 1998
51. Tisi PV, Shearman CP: The evidence for exercise-induced inflammation in intermittent claudication: should we encourage patients to stop walking? *Eur J Vasc Endovasc Surg* **15**: 7–17, 1998
52. Leng GC, Lee AJ, Fowkes FG *et al.*: Incidence, natural history and cardiovascular events in symptomatic and asymptomatic peripheral arterial disease in the general population. *Int J Epidemiol* **25**: 1172–1181, 1996

53. Criqui MH, Langer RD, Fronek A *et al.*: Mortality over a period of 10 years in patients with peripheral arterial disease. *New Engl J Med* **326**: 381–386, 1992
54. Tisi PV, Hulse M, Chulakadabba A *et al.*: Exercise training for intermittent claudication: does it adversely affect biochemical markers of the exercise-induced inflammatory response? *Eur J Vasc Endovasc Surg* **14**: 344–350, 1997
55. Remijnse-Tamerius HCM, Duprez D, De Buyzere M *et al.*: Why is training effective in the treatment of patients with intermittent claudication? *Int Angiol* **18**: 103–112, 1999
56. Pancera P, Prior M, Zannoni M *et al.*: Micro- and macrocirculatory, and biohumeral changes after a month of physical exercise in patients with intermittent claudication. *Scand J Rehabil Med* **27**: 73–76, 1995
57. Alpert JS, Larsen OA, Lassen NA: Exercise and intermittent claudication: Blood flow in the calf muscle during walking studied by the Xenon-133 clearance method. *Circulation* **34**: 353–359, 1969
58. Schoop W: Mechanism of beneficial action of daily walking training of patients with intermittent claudication. *Scand J Clin Lab Invest* **31**(s128): 197–199, 1973
59. Henrikkson J, Nygaard E, Andersson J, Eklof B: Enzyme activities, fibre types and capillarization in calf muscles of patients with intermittent claudication. *Scand J Clin Lab Invest* **40**: 361–369, 1980
60. Regensteiner JG, Wolfel EE, Brass EP *et al.*: Chronic changes in skeletal muscle histology and function in peripheral arterial disease. *Circulation* **87**: 413–421, 1993
61. Radack K, Wyderski RJ: Conservative management of intermittent claudication. *Ann Int Med* **113**: 135–146, 1990
62. Whyman MR, Fowkes FGR, Kerracher EMG *et al.*: Randomised controlled trial of percutaneous transluminal angioplasty for intermittent claudication. *Eur J Vasc Endovasc Surg* **12**: 167–172, 1996
63. Perkins JM, Collin J, Creasy TS *et al.*: Exercise training versus angioplasty for stable claudication. Long and medium results of a prospective randomised trial. *Eur J Endovasc Vasc Surg* **11**: 409–413, 1996
64. Rutherford D *et al.*: Recommended standards for reports dealing with lower extremity ischaemia: Revised version. *J Vasc Surg* **26**: 517–538, 1997
65. Clifford PC, Davies PW, Hayne JA, Baird RN: Intermittent claudication: Is a supervised exercise class worth while? *Br Med J* 1503–1505, 1980
66. Ekroth R, Dahllof AG, Gundevall B *et al.*: Physical training of patients with intermittent claudication. *Surgery* **84**: 640–643, 1978
67. Mannarino E, Pasqualini L, Menna M *et al.*: Effects of physical training on peripheral vascular disease: A controlled study. *Angiology* 5–10, 1989
68. Blankensteijn JD, Van Vroonhoven TJ, Lampmann L: Role of percutaneous transluminal angioplasty in aorto-iliac reconstruction. *J Cardiovasc Surg* **27**: 466–468, 1986
69. Golledge J, Ferguson K, Ellis M, *et al.*: Outcome of femoropopliteal angioplasty. *Ann Surg* **229**: 146–153, 1999
70. Krepel VM, Van Andel GJ, Van Erp WFM, Breslau PJ: Percutaneous transluminal angioplasty of the Femoropopliteal artery: Initial and long-term results. *Radiology* **156**: 325–328, 1985
71. Johnston KW, Rae M, Hogg-Johnston SA *et al.*: 5-Year results of a prospective study of percutaneous transluminal angioplasty. *Ann Surg* **206**: 403–413, 1987
72. Johnston KW. Femoral and popliteal arteries: Reanalysis of results of balloon angioplasty. *Radiology* **183**: 767–771, 1992
73. Katzenschlager R, Ahmadi A, Minar E *et al.*: Femoropopliteal artery: Initial and 6-month results of color duplex-guided percutaneous transluminal angioplasty. *Radiology* **199**: 31–334, 1996
74. Mortajeme A, Keifer JW, Zuska AJ: Percutaneous transluminal angioplasty of the Iliac Arteries. *Am J Roentgenol* **135**: 937–944, 1980
75. Matsi PJ, Manninen HI: Impact of different patency criteria on long term results of femoropopliteal angioplasty: Analysis of 106 consecutive patients with claudication. *J Vasc Intervent Radiol* **6**: 159–163, 1995

76. Morin JF, Johnston KW: Improvement after successful percutaneous transluminal dilatation treatment of occlusive peripheral arterial disease. *Surg Gyn Obs* **163**: 453–457, 1986
77. Nyamekye I, Sommerville K, Raphael M: Non-invasive assessment of arterial stenoses in angioplasty surveillance: A comparison with angiography. *Eur J Vasc Endovasc Surg* **12**: 471–481, 1996

Medical management of intermittent claudication

Jill JF Belch

INTRODUCTION

The medical management of intermittent claudication is a complex area which includes strategies for vascular risk reduction, lifestyle advice and direct pharmacotherapy for the vascular disease. Although this chapter describes medical management, the implementation of such management and its follow-up requires a multidisciplinary team which includes not only vascular physicians, vascular surgeons and interventional radiologists but many of the professions allied to medicine and, importantly, our primary care colleagues. This chapter will concentrate on the medical management of intermittent claudication. The issue which will be addressed in this chapter requires a shared care approach. Such a management plan should be established for each individual unit and Fig. 1 shows that in use by Tayside Vascular Services.

INTERMITTENT CLAUDICATION

Intermittent claudication is a marker for multisystem vascular disease. Clinicians have long recognized that intermittent claudication of the lower limb is associated with potentially lethal coronary atherosclerosis. Brodie, in 1841[1] recorded the following:

> *I say, that this (angina pectoris) exactly corresponds to the sense of weakness and want of muscular power which exists in persons who have the arteries of the legs obstructed or ossified.*

These words spoken nearly 150 years ago were the first record of the clinicians' appreciation of multisystem vascular disease. Subsequent workers[2] have validated this but the strength of the link between peripheral arterial occlusive disease (PAOD) of the lower limb and coronary artherosclerosis has only recently been appreciated. We now recognize that the main risk for the patient with intermittent claudication is not lower limb amputation but myocardial infarction or stroke. Intermittent claudication is the prime symptom of lower limb ischaemia and the natural history of leg disease in claudicating patients is usually benign. We know that fewer than 5% of patients require amputation and indeed spontaneous remission of symptoms occurs frequently. Despite the benign nature of the claudication, patient mortality,

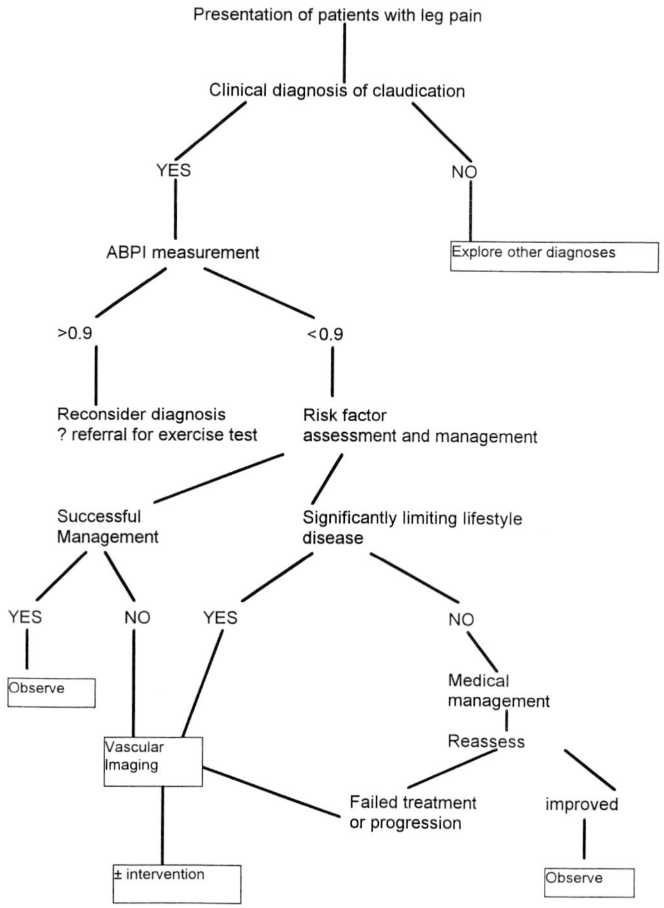

Fig. 1. Suggested shared care management plan for East of Scotland/Tayside vascular unit.

however, is three to four times higher than in non-claudicating patients of a similar age.[3] This increase in mortality is brought about by an increased prevalence of cardiovascular disease at other sites. Approximately 50% of patients die from ischaemic heart disease, 15% from cerebral vascular events, 10% from abdominal vascular pathology and only 25% of patients die from non-vascular events. The strength of association between PAOD and cardiac mortality is such that even in asymptomatic disease (detected by a decreased lower limb blood pressure) the relative risk of a cardiac event is very much increased (Table 1). Currently therefore the main thrust for the vascular physician in these patients is directed at reducing the risk of thrombotic stroke and ischaemic heart disease, in addition to reducing or preventing progression of leg ischaemia.

Table 1. The ankle brachial pressure index (ABPI) as a marker for increased cardiovascular risk[77]

Subjects	*ABPI*	*Event*	*Relative risk (95% CI)*
Population study	<0.40	Total mortality	4.49 (3.52–5.64)
Population study	<0.85	Total mortality	2.36 (1.60–3.48)
Elderly men (≥50 years)	<0.90	IHD mortality	2.0 (1.4–2.9)
Elderly women	<0.90	IHD mortality	2.1 (1.4–3.1)
Hypertensive patients	<0.90	Total mortality	4.1 (2.0–8.3)

Major targets have been set by our cardiological colleagues to be achieved by the year 2000. These relate to vascular event reduction and coronary disease, making modification of risk factors a major remit for these physicians. *The Health of The Nation* is a British Government white paper whose targets include a reduction in death rate from stroke and ischaemic heart disease by at least 40% in people under 65 years of age and 30% in those aged between 65 and 74 years. Similar strategies are in place in North America with the Healthly People 2000 Objectives. Until fairly recently, however, despite major public health campaigns and doctor education programmes, combined with government directives described above, physicians have failed to significantly increase risk factor modification after myocardial infarction. Action on Secondary Prevention through Intervention to Reduce Events study (ASPIRE, 1996)[4] showed that approximately 50% of subjects diagnosed as glucose intolerant at the time of their vascular event had received no treatment by 6 months, over 75% of the population had a blood cholesterol above the recommended level, and 25% remained hypertensive. As it can be difficult for the patient presenting with leg symptoms to appreciate that this is a symptom for more generalized vascular risk it is possible that the rate of take-up of risk factor modification is even lower in the patient with intermittent claudication. Apart from cigarette smoking, the importance of vascular risk factors is not yet widely recognized and historically, in Britain at least, vascular physicians who would manage these are in short supply. In most of Europe and in a limited fashion in the USA, vascular physicians work with the vascular surgeons and radiologists as part of a multidisciplinary team. This situation is now undergoing a change with most vascular surgeons and radiologists working closely with their physician colleagues to decrease vascular risk.

RISK FACTORS FOR INTERMITTENT CLAUDICATION

Although there have been relatively few cohort studies in PAOD, there have been numerous cross-sectional studies which have demonstrated the risk factors associated with the development of intermittent claudication (Table 2). Available evidence suggests that cigarette smoking[5], hypertension[6], diabetes mellitus[7] and

Table 2. Risk factors for intermittent claudication

Risk	*Management*
1. Other cardiovascular events e.g. myocardial infarction stroke	• Antiplatelet agent aspirin/dipyridamole clopidogrel for aspirin 'failures'
2. Smoking	• Cessation programme counselling nicotine replacement e.g. patch gum spray
3. Dyslipidaemia	• Lipid lowering therapy diet ± drug target = cholesterol <5.0mmol/litre high density lipoprotein ≥20% triglycerides <1.8mmol/litre
4. Hypertension	• Antihypertensive therapy Select ACE inhibitor calcium channel blockade diuretic Avoid β blockade (unless vasodilatory) Target blood pressure <140/85 (in diabetes <140/80) (NB 25% will have renal artery stenosis. Watch renal function)
5. Diabetes	• Check for hyperglycaemia Fasting glucose ≥7.8mmol/litre If borderline glucose (random or fasting) glucose tolerance test with fasting and 2h sample 2h sample <7.8mmol/litre normal ≥7.8–11.0 impaired ≥11.1 diabetic
6. Obesity	• Check for obesity BMI ≥30 Low fat, high fibre diet, healthy eating Calorie control
7. Thrombophilia	• Consider referral for thrombophilia screen (inherited or acquired) Suspect if: young (<50 years of age) connective tissue disease, e.g. SLE additional history of unexplained venous thrombosis previous failed vascular reconstruction strong family history of thrombosis

SLE: Systemic lupus erythematosus
BMI: Body Mass Index

dyslipidaemia[8] are key factors in the development of claudication and each will be addressed in turn. Thrombotic and haemorrheological abnormalities are also known to be involved in risk for PAOD. One of the best recognized is increased platelet aggregation[9] and also increased plasma fibrinogen[10] and decreased fibrinolysis.[11] More recently interest has focused on the white blood cell as a risk factor in PAOD[12] and on increased oxidative stress/free radical generation.[13] Of these, platelet activation has been best studied and the use of antiplatelet agents in intermittent claudication should by now be established clinical practice.

Platelet aggregation

Platelet aggregation is increased in intermittent claudication and the role of such aggregates in arterial thrombosis has been well documented. Other relevant aspects of platelet behaviour include the involvement of platelet released products. Beta thromboglobulin (βTG) is a marker of platelet activation *in vivo*. Levels of βTG had been shown to be increased in the plasma of patients with intermittent claudication.[14] The biological actions of βTG are not fully understood. However, they include a contribution to neutrophil activation through the formation of neutrophil activating peptide. Platelet factor 4 (PF4) which neutralizes the bodies natural anticoagulant, heparin, and platelet derived growth factor (PDGF) which stimulates proliferation of vascular smooth muscle cells, are also released from activated platelets and may play a role in atherosclerosis. Platelet release of plasminogen activator inhibitor-1 (PAI-1), which decreases fibrinolysis by inhibiting the activation plasminogen activator, may also contribute to this process. Other potentially relevant platelet released products which may be important in intermittent claudication include thromboxane A_2 (TXA_2) and serotonin (5HT). Both cause vasoconstriction, and increased levels of TXB_2, the stable metabolites for TXA_2 have been reported in intermittent claudication.[15] Aspirin inhibits TXA_2 formation which may be one mechanism of action for its beneficial effects in intermittent claudication.[16] Although a weaker vasocontrictor, serotonin still induces platelet aggregation. Patients with intermittent claudication have lower platelet 5HT levels than matched controls suggesting increased release into the plasma,[17] and thus increased platelet activation. In the claudicating patient therefore there are multiple reports of both increased platelet aggregation, which may occlude the microcirculation, and of increased platelet release. The release products may have a secondary potentiating effect for the development of continuing vessel damage/ atherosclerosis.

Antiplatelet agents

The study of pharmacotherapy for PAOD in general has been difficult, because of this disorder's variable natural history. The evaluation of antiplatelet therapy as a treatment for claudication symptoms has been attempted but the studies are small and there have been very few randomized trials of sufficient size to clearly define the efficacy of such drug therapy.[18] The current interest in agents relates to their use as

Table 3. Antiplatelet agents and intermittent claudication (IC) (Ticlopidine not licensed for IC in the UK)

Clinical situation	*Antiplatelet agents providing benefit*
1. Primary prevention of IC	Not yet studied Study in diabetic patients[20] with asymptomatic disease (POPADAD) is under way
2. Primary prevention of PAOD surgery	Aspirin[21]
3. Secondary prevention of IC progression (angiographic)	Aspirin and dipyridamole,[22] ticlopidine[39,40]
4. Prevention of re-occlusion after re-vascularization	Aspirin,[19] aspirin and dipyridamole[30], ticlopidine[37]
5. Prevention of coronary and cerebrovascular events in PAOD	Aspirin,[23] clopidogrel,[32] ticlopidine[37]

PAOD: Peripheral arterial occlusive disease

prophylactic treatments against other arterial events and disease progression, as we now realize that the platelet may be involved in the other manifestations of arterial disease in a claudicating patient such as thrombotic stroke, angina and myocardial infarction. The antiplatelet strategies in claudication which have been evaluated are summarized in Table 3.

Aspirin in intermittent claudication

Of all the antiplatelet agents aspirin is the most commonly used. This probably reflects the fact that aspirin is the best studied agent in clinical trials and currently is the cheapest agent available. Its action includes irreversible inhibition of the cyclo-oxygenase enzyme through acetylation of the serine residue number 529 near the active site of the enzyme.[19] Platelet aggregation is therefore decreased and the synthesis, and thus release, of TXA_2 is attenuated. As the platelets are unable to synthesize new enzyme, they are therefore inactive for their 8–10 day lifetime.

Primary prevention of intermittent claudication. No published study has yet proven that aspirin will prevent the primary development of intermittent claudication in a normal population. Very large numbers would be required for such a study. One method of decreasing population numbers is to increase the risk in the population to be enrolled. Two such studies are currently underway, where aspirin is being evaluated in patients with decreased ankle brachial blood pressure index (ABPI) (Table 1) but who are currently asymptomatic in terms of intermittent claudication symptoms. One of the studies is a population study, and the second is a study in patients with diabetes.[20] This second study, Prevention Of Progression of Arterial Disease And Diabetes (POPADAD), is recruiting 1600 patients with ABPI measurement less than 0.99 and randomizing them to either aspirin plus placebo, antioxidant plus placebo, aspirin and antioxidant or double placebo. The study is double-blind, randomized and of 5 years duration. The endpoint is a composite one of vascular events and vascular mortality. This is a Scotland-wide study with patients being recruited from the majority of regions within Scotland. Results should be available in 2005.

Primary prevention of vascular surgery. Aspirin has been used in subjects to decrease the occurrence of stroke and myocardial infarction. In the USA the Physicians Health Study[21] evaluated the primary prevention of requirement of peripheral vascular surgery using aspirin treatment. Every other day 325mg of aspirin were given to healthy doctors; the study was double-blind and placebo controlled. The risk of undergoing surgery for PAOD in the aspirin group was decreased by 46% (p=0.03) when compared with the control population. Interestingly a subgroup analysis suggested that those doctors already suffering from claudication were found to require less vascular surgery than the controls with claudication who took placebo therapy. Aspirin did not, however, affect the likelihood of developing claudication *de novo* in the study period.

Prevention of intermittent claudication progression. The studies which have examined the ability of aspirin to prevent intermittent claudication progression have been small. Hess *et al.*[22] evaluated 240 patients and showed that aspirin and dipyridamole inhibited progression of intermittent claudication as measured by angiography. They also indicated that the combination of aspirin and dipyridamole was superior to aspirin alone. This latter result, however, may have been obtained because the pre-study occurrence of vascular stenosis occurred more frequently in the aspirin group. This may explain the failure to obtain a statistically significant difference from placebo with aspirin alone.

Aspirin in the prevention of coronary and cerebral vascular events in intermittent claudication. The most convincing data in support of the use of aspirin in intermittent claudication comes from the antiplatelet trialists collaboration. In this meta-analysis of 174 randomized trials of various antiplatelet drugs (mainly aspirin) the data showed a decrease in non-fatal myocardial infarction, non-fatal stroke and vascular death in patients with cardiovascular disease treated by antiplatelet therapy.[23] Interestingly in a subgroup analysis of high-risk patients, which included those with a history of vascular surgery, peripheral angioplasty or intermittent claudication, the percentage of risk reduction versus placebo were as follows; 32% for the risk of vascular disease, myocardial infarction or stroke; 32% also for non-fatal myocardial infarction; 46% for non-fatal stroke and 20% for death from vascular causes. The dosage of aspirin most frequently used was between 75 and 325mg per day. There is no evidence that the higher doses were more effective than the lower ones.

Antiplatelet therapy and prevention of re-occlusion after revascularization. There is a significant failure rate following arterial surgery.[24] Vein grafts have a failure rate of

12% compared with approximately 49% for artificial materials over 5 years. The underlying mechanisms of occlusion are likely to be due in part to platelet behaviour. Early thrombosis can occur due to activation of platelets on the exposed artificial surface. Stenosis at surgical anastomosis may take place because of smooth muscle cell proliferation which may in part be related to PDGF release.[25] The first randomized control studies evaluated either aspirin alone or in combination with dipyridamole, another antiplatelet agent Both agents decreased reocclusion rates.[26–28] These early studies are supported by the antiplatelet trialists collaboration meta-analysis.[29] In this meta-analysis 3000 PAOD patients were enrolled with anti-platelet agents being given for a mean duration of 19 months. Results showed that the risk of occlusion was decreased by 25% among the control patients, to 16% in those patients receiving antiplatelet therapy. Translated to patient numbers, the addition of aspirin to the therapeutic regime will prevent nine out of every 100 patients experiencing a vascular graft occlusion ($p<0.0001$).[30] Again, a variety of aspirin doses were used and the higher doses were not significantly more effective than the lowest dose of 75mg per day.

It is of interest that although aspirin does appear to prevent secondary vascular events in patients receiving vein grafts, it does not increase vein graft patency rates. In one of the largest studies to date,[31] 549 patients were studied following vein graft surgery. No statistically significant differences in the occlusion rates were detected between the (active) aspirin- or placebo-treated groups. Nevertheless, because of the proven benefits of antiplatelet therapy in secondary prevention of vascular events elsewhere, aspirin or other alternative agent should still be given to these patients. A compound affecting other mechanisms of the coagulation cascade may be of use in improving vein graft patency and warfarin has been evaluated in this respect.[33]

Precautions with aspirin. Aspirin is contraindicated in patients with active peptic ulceration and gastrointestinal haemorrhage. It should be remembered that previous peptic ulceration is not a contraindication if ulcer prophylaxis e.g. H2 receptor antagonists, proton pump inhibitors are given concurrently. If aspirin intolerance is mainly due to gastrointestinal side-effects these may be minimized by alternate day dosing. Efficacy does not appear to be lost with this regime.[21] On the rare occasions when true aspirin intolerance can occur, alternative drug therapies are dipyridamole, clopidogrel or ticlopidine (not currently licensed for this indication in the UK). The recent CAPRIE study makes clopidogrel an attractive alternative for the aspirin intolerant patient.[32]

Clopidogrel

Clopidogrel blocks the activation of platelets by adenosine diphosphate (ADP), by selectively and irreversibly blocking the binding of this agonist to its receptor on platelets. It therefore affects the ADP-dependent activation of the group IIb-IIIa complex.[33] Clopidogrel is chemically related to ticlopidine, but with a potentially greater antithrombotic effect[36] and without the same degree of leucopenia occurrence.[34] Clopidogrel, 75mg per day, appears to be equipotent to ticlopidine 250mg twice per day. The Clopidogrel versus Aspirin in Patients at Risk of Ischaemic

Events (CAPRIE) study[32] investigated potential benefits of clopidogrel versus aspirin in reducing the risk of vascular death, myocardial infarction and stroke in patients with vascular disease; 19 185 patients were evaluated and over 1960 first vascular events. Clopidogrel reduced the event rate by 5.32% per annum versus 5.83% with aspirin (p=0.043). These reflect a relative rate reduction of 8.7% in favour of clopidogrel. There were no major differences in safety issues between the two compounds, with neutropenia occurring in 0.1% of clopidogrel patients and 0.17% of those in the aspirin group. An *ad hoc* subgroup analysis demonstrated that patients with intermittent claudication appeared to benefit to a greater extent with clopidogrel than other patient populations, with an event rate per annum of 3.1 compared with 4.86 in the aspirin group of patients, a relative risk reduction of 23.8% (95% CI 8.9–36.2) in favour of clopidogrel (p=0.0028). As approximately 30% of all patients given aspirin develop gastrointestinal side-effects, a reasonable strategy is first to combine the aspirin with a gastric protectant, and if this fails change to clopidogrel. The advent of this drug is a significant improvement to our therapeutic armamentarium in terms of tolerated antiplatelet drugs.

Dipyridamole

Dipyridamole is another antiplatelet agent that has been available for many years. There are three potential mechanisms of action of this drug in terms of antiplatelet effect. First it may increase or potentiate the effects of prostacyclin (PGI_2). Second it may inhibit cellular uptake of adenosine, thereby increasing the plasma concentration of this antiplatelet vasodilator agent,[35] and finally, it inhibits the platelet phosphodiesterase, the enzyme which breaks down cyclic-AMP. Clinical studies of dipyridamole have used doses ranging from 75 to 400mg/day, usually in three divided doses. The drug, however, is now available in a slow-release preparation which appears to encourage compliance, particularly within the elderly population. There has been much controversy over the use of dipyridamole in combination with aspirin. In the 1970s, there was excitement about the potential benefits of the combination of aspirin and dipyridamole but by the 1980s aspirin alone was the favoured choice. More recently the large stroke studies have convincingly demonstrated benefits of the combination treatment and certainly Hess, Mietaschk and Deichsel[22] did find the combination more effective in the prevention of peripheral graft failure. It is our current practice to use both aspirin and a slow-release preparation of dipyridamole in patients with stroke or transient ischaemic attack but to use aspirin or clopidogrel alone in patients with intermittent claudication unless symptoms appear to be progressing when dipyridamole is added to the regime. In stable intermittent claudication we usually reserve dipyridamole for the aspirin intolerant with clopidogrel becoming our first choice as there is more evidence base for this latter.

Ticlopidine

Although not licensed for intermittent claudication within the UK, ticlopidine is a potent antiplatelet agent with results in European studies which merit its inclusion in this text. It mediates its antiplatelet effect by interfering with the binding of macromolecules such as fibrinogen to the group IIb IIIa complex.[36] Given in a dose of 250mg twice a day, it can cause leucopenia in 1–2% of patients given the drug. Despite this profile of side-effects, it has been shown to be efficacious, although clopidogrel availability has attenuated the use of ticlopidine with its use now being limited to patients requiring stents. Ticlopidine decreases cardiac events as shown by a meta-analysis of a number of intermittent claudication studies where a statistically significant reduction in the rate of fatal and non-fatal cardiovascular events occurred following ticlopidine treatment: 3% in the group receiving ticlopidine compared with 9% of the controls. Furthermore, the Swedish TIclopidine Multicentre Study (STIMS)[37,38] showed a reduction in events such as transient ischaemic attack, strokes and myocardial infarction in patients with intermittent claudication. Mortality was also decreased when analysis was carried out on an intention to treat basis. Further analysis of the STIMS data[41] also showed a reduction in requirement for leg vascular surgery following treatment with ticlopidine. These data support the earlier work by the EMATAP group[39] where ticlopidine was shown to significantly reduce the need for vascular surgery.

Ketanserin

Ketanserin is an antiplatelet agent that produces its effect through selective $5HT_2$ receptor antagonism. This results in inhibition of serotonin-induced platelet aggregation. The Prevention of Atherosclerotic Complications with Ketanserin (PACK)[40] trial evaluated the effect of ketanserin on vascular events and/or vascular death. In contrast to the data for aspirin, clopidogrel and ticlopidine, ketanserin did not attenuate these endpoints. In view of these results, ketanserin can not be recommended as a prophylaxis for vascular events in intermittent claudication.

Intravenous perioperative atenolol

The recent work by Mangano *et al.* is of interest.[41] In this study atenolol is given intravenously immediately pre- and post-operatively to patients undergoing surgery. Follow-up was with oral medication and the regime was compared with placebo. The patient population were patients undergoing surgery and at risk of cardiovascular events. All operations were non-cardiac, but included 81 patients out of a total of 200 undergoing major peripheral vascular surgery. It was suggested that atenolol might have a number of beneficial effects such as modifying perioperative arrhythmia but also including antiplatelet effects. At 6 months, all-cause mortality was significantly decreased in the atenolol group compared with the control population (0% versus 8%, $p<0.001$), at 1 year (3% versus 14%, $p=0.05$) and at 2 years (10% versus 21%, $p=0.019$). The principal cause for reduction in death was attenuation of cardiac related deaths. Further work in this area is needed, and a study with the newer non-vasoconstrictor betablockers is planned.

Conclusion

There is convincing evidence that antiplatelet agents such as aspirin and clopidogrel are effective in preventing cardiac and stroke events in patients with intermittent claudication. Additionally they will decrease occlusion rate following synthetic vascular graft insertion. It is therefore recommended that antiplatelet drug prescription for these patients should be made unless there is a clear contraindication to such therapy for that individual patient.

Smoking habit

The smoking of tobacco has long been known to increase the risk of intermittent claudication and to contribute to its progression.[42] Cigarette smokers have a significantly higher prevalence of atherosclerosis and of another tobacco-related peripheral vascular disease, thromboangiitis obliterans (Buerger's disease).[43] Of all the risk factors, the use of tobacco correlates most strongly with the development of intermittent claudication. There are multifactorial reasons why cigarette smoking produces its vascular morbidity and mortality. The smoke from burning tobacco contains over 3000 components, of which nicotine and carbon monoxide have been the best studied.[44] Carbon monoxide directly reduces oxygen availability and is atherogenic. Nicotine raises the systolic blood pressure and increases heart rate. Tobacco smoking induces platelet aggregation and decreases fibrinolysis[45] and also damages the vascular endothelium. Smoking also appears to adversely effect the lipid profile,[44] with serum cholesterol levels averaging 3% higher in the smoking population than in non-smoking controls. The Framingham study[46] convincingly demonstrated the link between tobacco smoking and intermittent claudication. The smokers were twice as likely to develop intermittent claudication, and indeed 70–90% of patients with intermittent claudication smoke or are ex-smokers.

Intermittent claudication is more likely to progress to critical limb ischaemia in subjects who smoke and amputation occurs less frequently in non-smokers.[47] Vascular grafts are more likely to fail if smoking continues. In one study the 1-year cumulative patency rate for femoropopiteal vein bypass grafts was 63% in smokers and 84% in non-smokers.[48] Prioritizing smoking cessation is an important part of the medical management of intermittent claudication and must be given a firm priority not only by the clinician but also by their Trusts and Health Boards.

To stop smoking is difficult. Although the majority of smokers would like to cease, and at least 75% have tried to stop smoking more than once,[49] 90% are physically addicted to nicotine.[50] Disappointingly 75% of those who give up smoking restart within 3 months.[51] There are two aspects to nicotine dependence; the psychological dependence and the physiological dependence. Thus when smokers try to quit smoking they experience both behavioural and physical withdrawal symptoms. It is important to reassure the patient that these withdrawal symptoms are short-lived, as they can exert a strong influence on the smoker's will to stop. It also underlines the need for support to be offered in overcoming both aspects of the addiction. Only 5% of patients with intermittent claudication successfully give up smoking after receiving only medical advice.[52] However, provision of increasing support through counselling or a clinic improves cessation rates.[53] The medical management of intermittent claudication includes giving the patient the opportunity to be referred to the area smoking cessation clinic, which may be either in primary care or a hospital based facility. It should, however, exist, and Health Boards and Trusts should be pressurized to develop these facilities. Judicious nicotine replacement therapy is effective as an aid to smoking cessation[54] by overcoming the physical addiction in the initial phases. The first type of nicotine replacement therapy to become widely available was nicotine chewing gum.[55] Other forms of nicotine replacement therapy are transdermal patches, intranasal sprays and inhalers. These later forms of therapy may attenuate some problems seen with the gum such as the transfer of dependency to the gum.[56] A meta-analysis of 53 trials of nicotine replacement therapy (42 chewing gum, nine patch, one spray and one inhaler) evaluated data on 17703 subjects.[57] Nicotine replacement therapy increased the odds ratio for abstinence as follows; 1.61 for gum, 2.07 for patch, 2.92 for nasal spray and 3.05 for inhaled nicotine. The authors concluded that the currently available forms of nicotine replacement therapy are effective aids to smoking cessation. It should be remembered that nicotine replacement therapy, however, is contraindicated in acute myocardial infarction, unstable angina and in patients with cardiac arrhythmias.

Hypertension

The development of PAOD has been associated with elevation in blood pressure. Some workers favour a raised systolic blood pressure as being the most important component[58] with some favouring an association with both diastolic and systolic increases.[59] The results from prospective studies, however, are less convincing.[46,60] Nevertheless, the general cardiovascular effects of hypertension are undisputed and it is well recognized that an elevation in blood pressure contributes to aneurysm formation. Patients with substantial hypertension, particularly with higher nocturnal pressures, show a higher mortality, an increased preponderance of left ventricular hypertrophy and more cerebral lacunar infarcts.[61] Epidemiological studies show cardiovascular events often occur in the early hours of the morning and a rapid increase in blood pressure is evident in these early hours. In combination with other factors, such as platelet aggregation and white blood cell activation that also peak at this crucial time[62] hypertension may have a role in both the acute and chronic presentation of PAOD. The management of elevated blood pressure has recently been simplified with the issuing of the Scottish Intercollegiate Guidelines Network (SIGN) guideline on the management of hypertension[63] and the publication of the British Hypertension Society Guidelines in 1999.[64] Of relevance to medical management of intermittent claudication are two particular recommendations. The first of these is that therapy should be started in all patients with sustained systolic blood pressure ≥160mmHg or sustained diastolic blood pressures ≥100mmHg despite non-pharmacological measures such as diet, exercise etc. The second is that drug treatments is indicated in patients with sustained systolic blood pressures between 140 and 159mmHg or diastolic blood pressures between 90 and 99mmHg if there is evidence of established cardiovascular disease. This obviously includes intermittent claudication. The optimum target range is a systolic blood pressure of ≥140mmHg and a diastolic of ≥85mmHg. The target is even tougher for those patients with diabetes and this should be remembered, as many of our intermittent claudication patients have this disorder. A target of ≥140/80mmHg is recommended for these patients. Three long-term double-blind studies have compared all the major classes of antihypertensive drug therapy in patients with hypertension; thiazides; beta blockers; calcium antagonists; ACE inhibitors, and alpha blockers[65–67] and overall showed no consistent or important differences as regards anti-hypertensive efficacy, side-effects or quality of life. However, in general, hypertensive patients whose blood pressure is controlled by thiazides or beta blockers have a persistent excess risk of coronary/death.[68,69] These drug classes change glucose intolerance and lipid profiles in a dose-dependent fashion. In a patient population suffering from dyslipidaemia and who have a tendency towards diabetes mellitus, these compounds may be best avoided. It is of interest that the new vasodilating beta blockers may not be contraindicated in intermittent claudication. In general, however, ACE inhibition or calcium channel blockade is preferred (Table 2).

A note of caution must be introduced for patients with borderline intermittent claudication and critical limb ischaemia. It may be that perfusion to the limbs is only maintained via the elevated blood pressure. Too rapid a fall in blood pressure may significantly worsen the symptoms and particular care must be taken with these patients, in the same way that patients with severe carotid disease should be treated cautiously.

Dyslipidaemia

The characteristic lesion in patients with intermittent claudication is atherosclerosis, the fat-rich fibrous plaque, composed of a central cholesterol core with an overlying cap of smooth muscle cells and collagen covered by endothelium. This composition varies widely from solid hard plaques of mainly smooth muscle cells to those containing large pools of cholesterol covered only by a thin fibrous cap. These latter are the dangerous plaques which tend to fissure and ulcerate.

Dyslipidaemia contributes in three ways to intermittent claudication. First elevated levels of lipids are available for the early vascular damage i.e. fatty streaks. Second, the cholesterol rich plaques are occlusive narrowing the vessel. Furthermore they may be unstable and may rupture stimulating *in situ* thrombosis formation. This increases the risk of thrombus-cholesterol emboli formation. Finally endothelial function is perturbed affecting flow in the microcirculation. Patients with intermittent claudication and dyslipidaemia have decreased endothelial vasodilatory responses which can be normalized by lipid lowering therapy.[70] The relationship between cholesterol level and ischaemic heart disease risk is continuous with no obvious cut-off point being 'safe'. It is likely to be the same for patients with intermittent claudication. In general, increased lipid levels occur most commonly in the elderly intermittent claudication patient, and intermittent claudication patients with diabetes[71] and in obese intermittent claudication subjects.[72] The Framington study, after 26 years, found cholesterol to be a weak but significant risk factor for claudication.[46] A Danish study running for 10 years found cholesterol levels at the age of 50 years to correlate with ABPI. This finding was independent to other risk factors.[73] Reduced high density lipoprotein has been detected in intermittent claudication[74] and is associated with an increased disease severity.[75] In the Edinburgh Artery Study there are strong inverse relationships between high density lipoprotein cholesterol and intermittent claudication which persisted after adjustment for other lipids, obesity and diabetes.[76] Elevated serum triglyceride levels have been found in a majority of the studies of intermittent claudication.[77] Longitudinal studies[73,78] have been carried out. Of the 2759 men in the Basel study,[79] 174 developed disease during 5 study years and of these almost 60% had increased triglyceride levels in their blood. Interestingly, the strong apparent relationship between intermittent claudication and an increased triglyceride level may be explained by the increase in low density lipoprotein which provides the vascular risk.[77]

Clinical studies

There have been no clinical studies targeting patients with intermittent claudication with the occurrence of vascular events as an end-point. The attempts to establish such a study have met with lack of enthusiasm by the pharmaceutical industry who perceive the coronary arena as the larger market. The situation has now been overtaken by events with recommendations for lipid lowering therapy if there is a >3% chance of a vascular event per annum, such a risk occurring in patients with intermittent claudication. Some early studies of intermittent claudication looked at progression of disease rather than vascular risk and although some regression with lipid lowering therapy has been seen, many investigators remain unconvinced due in part to the short-term follow-up of these studies.[77]

There have been a number of major clinical studies in the field of lipid lowering in recent years. These include the Scandinavian Simvastatin Survival Study (4S),[80] the West of Scotland Coronary Prevention Study (WOSCOPS)[81] and the Cholesterol and Recurrent Events (CARE) trials.[82] The 4S evaluated 4444 subjects with a past history of myocardial infarction or angina with cholesterol levels between 5.5–8.0mmol/litre and triglyceride ≥2.5mmol/litre. The median duration of treatment was 5.4 years at which point the study was terminated because of a 30% decrease is overall mortality with simvastatin treatment. This was caused by a 42% decrease in ischaemic heart disease mortality. Furthermore, major coronary events were reduced as was the need for coronary revascularization. Stroke was also less frequently seen in the treated group. These data suggest that four out of nine deaths occuring in a group of subjects with a cholesterol over 5.5mmol/litre will be prevented by treatment. The CARE trial was also a secondary prevention study with 4195 patients with a past history of myocardial infarction enrolled. After 5 years there were 24% fewer coronary deaths and non fatal myocardial infarctions in the prevastatin group. There was a 27% decrease in the need for coronary revascularization and angioplasty. The importance of this trial is that the statin appeared to be beneficial in secondary prevention even when cholesterol levels were at that time defined as 'normal'. WOSCOPS, a primary prevention trial, showed benefit from lipid lowering but is less relevant to the intermittent claudication patient. It is our current practice to intervene if total cholesterol is over 5.0mmol/litre or low density lipoprotein cholesterol is over 3.0mmol/litre.

Lipid lowering therapy

Adherence to a lipid lowering diet can reduce blood lipid values by a moderate 10–15%. Our own somewhat pragmatic regime is to concentrate the patient's mind on smoking cessation whilst we improve their lipid profile pharmacologically. There are many lipid lowering drugs that are effective but involvement of a dietitian at this point is useful. A number of drugs can be used for reducing low density lipoprotein cholesterol. The statins (HMG-CoA reductase inhibitors) are preferred for patients with multiple risk factors. This relates to the majority of intermittent claudication patients who do not exercise, who smoke and who may be obese. In patients with intermittent claudication who are diabetic, a mixed hyperlipidaemia may be found i.e. triglycerides are also increased. In this case fibrates may be selected because of their stronger effects on triglycerides and high density lipoprotein cholesterol. Nevertheless, statins are well tolerated alternatives in patients with diabetes and mixed hyperlipidaemia did well on statin therapy in the secondary prevention studies.[80]

Diabetes mellitus

Intermittent claudication and the presence of diabetes mellitus are events that frequently co-incide. It has been estimated that 50% of all diabetic patients have evidence of PAOD 10–15 years after diabetes disease onset.[83] Additionally the extent of the disease measured angiographically correlates with glucose intolerance.[84] Almost one-third of below-knee amputations are performed on diabetic patients. This figure rises to nearly half of all amputations when distal amputations are include in this figure. Some of the problems for the diabetic limb results from diabetic microvascular disease[85] and some from the macrovascular disease[86] which occurs at an earlier age probably with its roots in childhood.[87] Asymptomatic peripheral arterial disease as detected by a decrease in ABPI occurs in approximately 20% of all diabetic patients with no other evidence of vascular disease (POPADAD screening of 8000 patients, unpublished observations) and in 25% of all diabetic patients.[88] The aetiology of diabetic vascular disease is multifactorial and complex and includes contributions from hypertension, dyslipidaemia, oxidative stress and decreased free radical scavenging,[89,90] and abnormalities of haemostasis and fibrinolysis,[91] including abnormalities of platelet behaviour as described earlier.

The occurrence of overt diabetes and intermittent claudication is well recognized. What is less well appreciated is the occurrence of occult diabetes in patients with claudication. The familiar picture of distal disease on angiography (Fig. 2) or increased ABPI (due to vessel stiffening) can lead to the retrospective diagnosis of diabetes mellitus as a cause for the patient's intermittent claudication. Of 100 consecutive patients presenting to our vascular surgeons, 40% had abnormal glucose tolerance tests.[92] All these 40 patients had normal random or fasting blood sugar levels and were diagnosed only on the basis of a glucose tolerance test. The difficulty is knowing which patients require glucose tolerance tests in the presence of a normal fasting or random glucose levels. It is our current practice to administer such a test to the two groups of patients as described above. Firstly those in whom the distal distribution of peripheral arterial disease would clinically arouse the suspicion of diabetes, and secondly those with a raised ABPI in the presence of symptomatic intermittent claudication. Another clue to underlying diabetes is a 'diabetic' lipid profile where both total plasma cholesterol or fasting triglyceride levels are elevated and high density lipoprotein levels are lowered. Diabetes mellitus is consistently underdiagnosed in intermittent claudication[93] and this can have serious consequences. Detection of "asymptomatic" diabetes mellitus in the patient with intermittent claudication is a major contribution to the medical management of these patients. It should be remembered that all risk factors are synergistic in terms of vascular disease, not merely additive,[94] and the failure to diagnose underlying diabetes in a smoking claudicant will have serious consequences for that patient.

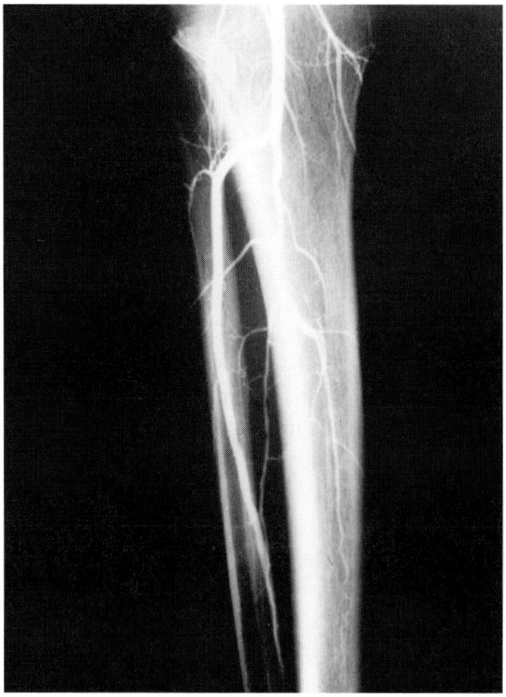

Fig. 2. Diabetic angiogram with disease.

Thrombophilia in a patient with intermittent claudication

The prothrombotic or hypercoagulable state can be classified into two broad categories, acquired and hereditary, the latter often referred to as an inherited thrombophilia disorder. Although some of the haemostatic risk factors mentioned above, such as increased platelet activity, may contribute an acquired hypercoaguable state, in PAOD, the term acquired thrombophilia is usually reserved for well defined syndromes such as the antiphospholipid syndrome. (This was previously called the lupus anticoagulant.) The name change was brought about for two good reasons. First although it can be associated with systemic lupus erythematosus, this is by no means necessary and second, anticoagulant refers to the behaviour of the blood *in vitro* not *in vivo*.

The inherited thrombophilia disorders are frequently characterized by venous thrombosis. More recently, however, we see that they may be relevant to patients with PAOD. There are a number of provisional reports of patients with inherited thrombophilias experiencing arterial thrombosis. In particular a significant incidence of these syndromes appears to occur in patients undergoing vascular surgery. In prospective studies, the overall incidence of hypercoagulability in general varies from 10 to 25% and increases to about 50% in the presence of clinical markers for thrombophilia.[95,96] It is important to identify these patients preoperatively because short- and medium-term failure rates of the vascular graft are reported to be approximately 50%.[95,97] If such patients are being considered for surgery, there is of course the additional risk of the development of deep vein thrombosis at the operative time point. As hereditary thrombophilia occurs only infrequently in this patient group, it is not possible to make a formal recommendation for screening of PAOD patients with intermittent claudication. Probably a selective approach, reserving screening to those patients with bypass failure, is appropriate[98] or if the patient has an additional history of unexplained venous thrombosis.

Protein C and Protein S deficiency

Protein C and its co-factor protein S are physiological inhibitors of coagulation. Protein S deficiency appears to be linked, in particular, with arterial thrombosis.[99] However there have also been reports of patients with protein C deficiency developing arterial thrombosis manifest clinically by an embolic phenomenon.[100,101] Recent studies have shown that an inherited defect, resistance to activated protein C, may be important also in arterial thrombus formation, however this factor V Leiden mutation[102] has not been evaluated in intermittent claudication.

Antithrombin III deficiency

As with protein C and S deficiencies, this abnormality is more commonly associated with venous thrombosis. It may however occur more frequently in subjects with arterial disease where, like protein C, it occurs in association with thromboembolism secondary to arterial clot formation.[103] These abnormalities can be detected if clinical suspicion has been aroused by asking the haematology colleagues for a thrombophilia check on a clotting screen blood sample (citrate anticoagulant).

Homocysteinaemia

The development of premature atherosclerosis, in combination with arterial and venous thrombosis, are clinical features of homocysteinaemia.[104] Homocysteinaemia causes endothelial cell dysfunction and damage and in particular decreased fibrinolysis.[105] Homozygous patients are diagnosed early because of disease severity but patients with heterozygous disease present merely with premature atherosclerosis. It has been estimated that between 20 and 40% of patients presenting with premature PAOD have heterozygous homocysteinaemia.[106] Pyridoxine supplementation may reduce thrombotic events in homozygous patients. However, it is not known whether this or other vitamins affect the course of the premature atherosclerosis in the heterozygous sufferers. Nevertheless, it is usual to supplement these patients with vitamin B6 and perhaps vitamin B12 even if they are heterozygous for the defect.

Antiphospholipid syndrome

Of all the hyperanticoaguable states that have been reported in PAOD patients, the APS is the most frequently detected.[107] The antiphospholipid syndrome as diagnosed by an increase in anticardiolipin antibody titres in the blood, and by the finding of a prolonged APTT, defines two distinct but related populations each associated with an increased risk of arterial and venous thrombus formation.[108] The antiphospholipid syndrome is associated with postoperative thrombosis of arterial reconstructions.[109] A serum sample sent to immunopathology will allow detection of this disorder by the measurement of anticardiolipin antibodies and will allow the diagnosis of antiphospholipid syndrome to be made. Treatment is with anticoagulants where there is evidence of thrombosis but this may not always protect against recurrent thrombus formation.[110] Aspirin is used if antiphospholipid syndrome is detected as an incidental finding in an otherwise normal individual or secondary to fetal loss.

Conclusion

When a patient presents with intermittent claudication an ideal opportunity presents itself for the critical assessment of vascular risk factors. Intervention at this time is likely not only to decrease the risk of coronary and cerebral events but to limit progression of the arterial disease in the periphery, although this latter is theoretical rather than proven. Modifying risk is important now and is likely to become even more important in the future when management strategies for the more recently described risk factors become available. The newer emphasis on the importance of oxidative stress[111] in intermittent claudication as a contributor to direct vascular damage and as a mechanism for oxidizing lipids[112] has opened up a number of potential therapeutic avenues. The recently begun POPADAD study (Prevention of Progression of Asymptomatic Diabetic Arterial Disease)[20] evaluates not only the effect of aspirin but also an antioxidant cocktail on cardiovascular mortality in asymptomatic patients with low ABPIs and diabetes mellitus. Another area of current interest is the role of endothelial activation, with expression of specific cell adhesion molecules and increased leukocyte adhesion. There is an association between restenosis following peripheral angioplasty and plasma E-selectin levels.[113] E-selectin is a cell adhesion molecule specific to activated endothelium. Antibodies for cell adhesion molecules are now being developed to provide us with interesting therapeutic and diagnostic interventions for the future.

DRUG TREATMENT OF INTERMITTENT CLAUDICATION

The drug treatment of intermittent claudication is a contentious area due to doubts over the effectiveness of this intervention and consequent concern over the use of Health Services resource. A number of guidelines have been developed to guide prescribing physicians in this area.[114] There are four oral drug therapies that have a licence for use as a treatment for intermittent claudication in the UK: naftidrofuryl (Praxilene®), oxpentifylline (Trental®), inositol nicotinate (Hexopal®) and cinnarizine (Stugeron Forte®). Various studies have evaluated these drugs for effectiveness in alleviating the leg pain associated with walking, delaying the progression of the disease and dealing with the associated mortality.

Naftidrofuryl

Naftidrofuryl is reported to have vasoactive effects. It is known to have a local anaesthetic action[115] and has been shown to act at tissue level in improving tissue oxygenation, increasing ADP levels and reducing lactic acid, thus potentially improving symptoms of claudication. The drug is mainly administered orally for the treatment of intermittent claudication and the recommended maximum dose is 200mg three times per day.

A number of double-blind placebo-controlled studies of naftidrofuryl as a treatment for intermittent claudication have been completed.[116–124] These studies show a placebo response which produces an average improvement in pain-free walking distance of approximately 25%. In general a further 30% improvement can be expected in patients taking naftidrofuryl with walking times being measured at 3 or 6 months post-treatment initiation. These estimates are supported by two major analysis of four and five of the studies respectively.[125,126]

Naftidrofuryl may lead to a slight improvement in symptoms of patients suffering moderate disease (claudicant distance less than 500 metres). It may therefore be considered for symptomatic benefit. However, if the decision is made to use naftidrofuryl, assessment of benefits should be undertaken at 3–6 months with the compound stopped if no benefit has been obtained.

Oxpentifylline (Trental®)

This was one of the first drugs approved for the treatment of intermittent claudication. Both the drug and its metabolites are vasodilators which may also improve the flow properties of blood. The mechanism whereby it produces this effect is thought to be related to an increase in blood cell deformability and a reduction in plasma fribrinogen levels. The main use of this drug, given orally, is for the treatment of intermittent claudication with a recommended dose of 400mg three times per day. There have been a number of double-blind, placebo-controlled studies of oxpentifylline which employed treadmill testing.[133] Only two of these studies were statistically significant in terms of a favourable outcome of oxpentifylline and one of these was a retrospective subanalysis of short distance claudicants[130] already included in another study.[127] A meta-analysis of ten randomized, double-blind, controlled studies[127–132,134,135] concluded that the limited amount and quality of reported data precluded an overall reliable estimate of efficacy of this drug.[136] Thus in the absence of consistent clinical trial evidence, it is not possible to make any recommendation on the use of oxpentifylline in this indication.

Inositol nicotinate (Hexopal®)

This drug is currently licensed in the UK for intermittent claudication (dose 3–4g daily). The reported mechanism of action includes a hypolipidaemic, fibrinolytic and vasodilatory action. It is also reported to inhibit oxidative metabolism in ischaemic tissue.

Four double-blind, randomized, placebo-controlled trials are presented in the literature.[137–139] Of these trials three were primary care based and used subjective or questionable objective criteria for assessment of intermittent claudication without treadmill use.[137,138,140] None of these trials showed clear evidence of benefit over placebo for this drug. This drug is therefore not recommended for use in the treatment of intermittent claudication.

Cinnarizine (Stugeron Forte®)

The drug is currently licensed in the UK for intermittent claudication at a dose of 75mg three times a day. Its action is reported to be via antagonism of vasoconstrictor substances.[141] Additional benefits on blood rheology have been reported.

Whilst there are a number of placebo-controlled, single-dose or short-term studies, the majority of these evaluate blood flow measuring techniques rather than treadmill walking distance. All these studies took place on the 7th day with the result that they cannot be used in support of this drug as a long-term treatment for intermittent claudication. Six controlled studies evaluated cinnarizine over a period ranging from 4 weeks to 6 months.[141–146] Standardized treadmill measured walking distances were not calculated in these although patient measured (subjective) walking times were recorded in three.[142,143,146] In two studies timed pacings using a metronome were evaluated[141,145] and in one, laboratory measures only were evaluated (Xenon clearance). Thus there are no studies of cinnarizine which meet currently accepted guidelines on the clinical investigation of drug therapy for intermittent claudication. It is therefore not possible to make a recommendation on the use of cinnarizine in the treatment of intermittent claudication.

Conclusion

If the patient's symptoms are sufficiently severe to merit drug treatment, it is reasonable to consider naftidrofuryl for the symptomatic relief of moderate disease. Reassessment of the requirement for the drug should be made after 3–6 months. Inositol nicotinate is not recommended for the treatment of intermittent claudication. There is insufficient evidence to make a recommendation on the use of cinnarizine or oxpentifylline in the drug treatment of this disorder.

SUMMARY

From the above it can be seen that the presentation of intermittent claudication to the vascular clinician can provide the ideal opportunity for medical intervention. Vascular risk modification, in particular, should be implemented with the introduction of antiplatelet therapy. Consideration of a vasculitic element to the disease can be given if acute phase responses are elevated or the clinical picture unusual.

REFERENCES

1. Brodie BC: Lectures on mortification delivered at the medical theatre of St George's Hospital. Lecture V. In: Gazette S (Ed), *New Series of London Med* **52**: 714, 1841
2. McKenna M, Wolfson S, Kuller L: The ratio of ankle and arm arterial pressure as an independent predictor of mortality. *Athersclerosis* **87**: 119–128, 1991
3. Leng GC, Fowkes FGR: The epidemiology of peripheral arterial disease. *Vasc Med Rev* **4**: 5–18, 1993
4. ASPIRE Steering Group: A British Cardiac Society survey of the potential for the secondary prevention of coronary disease: ASPIRE (Action on Secondary Prevention through Intervention to Reduce Events). *Heart* **75**: 334–342, 1996
5. Levy LA: Smoking and peripheral vascular disease. Epidemiology and podiatric perpective. *J Am Pediatr Med Assoc* **79**: 398–402, 1989
6. Strano A, Novo S, Avellone G *et al*.: Hypertension and other risk factors in peripheral arterial disease. *Clin Exp Hypertens* **15**: 71–89, 1993
7. Beks PJ, MacKaay AJ, de Neeling JN *et al*.: Peripheral arterial disease in relation to glycaemic level in an elderly Caucasian population: the Hoorn study. *Diabetologia* **38**: 86–96, 1995
8. Fowkes FG, Dunbar JT, Lee AJ: Risk factor profile of non-smokers with peripheral arterial disease. *Angiology* **46**: 657–662, 1995
9. Belch, JJF, McKay A, McArdle B *et al*.: A double blind study of the effect of prostacyclin infusion in severe peripheral vascular disease. *Lancet* **8320**: 315–317, 1983
10. Lowe GDO, Donnan PT, McColl P *et al*.: Blood viscosity, fibrinogen and activation of coagulation and leucocytes in peripheral arterial disease: the Edinburgh Artery Study. *Br J Haematol* **7**(Suppl 1): 12–17, 1991
11. Smith FB, Lowe GD, Fowkes FG *et al*.: Smoking, haemostatic factors and lipid peroxides in a population case control study of peripheral arterial disease. *Atherosclerosis* **102**: 155–162, 1993
12. Belch JJF, Sohngen M, Robb R *et al*.: Neutrophil count and amputation in critical limb ischaemia. *Int Angiol* **18**: 139–144, 1999
13. Belch JJF, Mackay IR, Hill A *et al*.: Oxidative stress is present in atherosclerotic peripheral arterial disease and further increased by diabetes mellitus. *Int Angiol* **14**: 385–388, 1996
14. Zahavi J, Zahavi M: Enhanced platelet release reaction, shortened platelet survival time and increased platelet aggregation and plasma thromboxane B_2 in chronic obstructive arterial disease. *Thromb Haemostas* **53**: 105–109, 1985
15. FitzGerald GA, Smith B, Pederson AK, Brash AR: Increased prostacyclin biosynthesis in patients with severe atherosclerosis and platelet activation. *New Engl J Med* **310**: 1065–1068, 1984
16. Lau CS, Scott N, Brown JE *et al*.: Increased activity of oxygen free radicals during reperfusion in patients undergoing percutaneous peripheral artery balloon angioplasty. *Int Angiol* **10**: 244–246, 1991a
17. Barradas MA, Gill DS, Fonseca VA *et al*.: Intra-platelet serotonin with diabetes mellitus and peripheral vascular disease. *Eur J Clin Invest* **18**: 399–404, 1988
18. Cameron HA, Waller PC, Ramsay LE: Drug treatment of intermittent claudication: a critical analysis of the methods and findings of published clinical trials, 1965–1985. *Br J Clin Pharmacol* **26**: 569–576, 1988
19. Patrono C: Aspirin as an antiplatelet drug. *New Engl J Med* **330**: 1287–1294,1994
20. The POPADAD Study Group: The Prevention of Progression of Arterial Disease and Diabetes (POPADAD) (Submitted)
21. Goldhaber SZ, Manson JE, Stampfer MJ *et al*.: Low-dose aspirin and subsequent peripheral arterial surgery in the Physicians' Health Study. *Lancet* **340**: 143–145, 1992
22. Hess H, Mietaschk A, Deichsel G: Drug-induced inhibition of platelet function delays progression of peripheral occlusive arterial disease: a prospective double-blind arteriographically controlled trial. *Lancet* **i**: 415–419, 1985
23. Antiplatelet Trialists' Collaboration: Collaborative overview of randomised trials of

antiplatelet therapy – I: Prevention of death, myocardial infarction, and stroke by prolonged antiplatelet therapy in various categories of patients. *Br Med J* **308**: 81–106, 1994

24. Taylor P, Wolfe J, Tyrell M *et al.*: Graft stenosis: justification for 1-year surveillance. *Br J Surg* **77**: 1125–1128, 1990
25. Reidy MA, Jackson C, Lindner V: Neointimal proliferation: control of vascular smooth muscle cell growth. *Vasc Med Rev* **3**: 156–167, 1992
26. Green RM, Roedersheimer LR, De Weese JA: Effects of aspirin and dipyridamole on expanded polytetrafluoroethylene graft patency. *Surgery* **92**: 1016–1026, 1982
27. Goldman M, Hall C, Dykes J *et al.*: Does indium-platelet deposition predict patency in prosthetic arterial grafts? *Br J Surg* **70**: 635–638, 1983
28. Clyne CAC, Archer TJ, Atuhaire LK *et al.*: Random control trial of a short course of aspirin and dipyridamole (persantin) for femorodistal grafts. *Br J Surg* **74**: 246–248, 1987
29. Antiplatelet Trialists' Collaboration: Collaborative overview of randomised trials of antiplatelet therapy – II: Maintenance of vascular graft or arterial patency by antiplatelet therapy. *Br Med J* **308**: 159–168, 1994
30. Lualdi J, Goldhaber SZ, Manson JE: The role of antiplatelet agents in patients with peripheral vascular disease. *Vasc Med Rev* **6**: 109–119, 1995
31. McCollum C, Alexander C, Kenchington G *et al.*: Antiplatelet drugs in femoropopliteal vein bypasses: a multicenter trial. *J Vasc Surg* **13**: 150–162, 1991
32. CAPRIE Steering Committee: A randomised, blinded, trial clopidogrel versus aspirin in patients at risk of ischaemic events (CAPRIE). *Lancet* **348**: 1329–1338, 1996
33. Herbert JM, Tissinier A, Defreyn G, Maffrand JP: Inhibitory effect of clopidogrel on platelet adhesion and intimal proliferation following arterial injury in rabbits. *Arterioscler Thromb* **13**: 1171–1179, 1993b
34. Herbert JM, Frechel D, Vallee E *et al.*: Clopidogrel, a novel antiplatelet and antithrombotic agent. *Cardiovasc Drug Rev* **11**: 180–188, 1993
35. Fitzgerald GA: Dipyridamole. *New Engl J Med* **316**: 1247–1257, 1987
36. McTavish D, Faulds D, Goa KL: Ticlopidine: an updated review of its pharmacology and therapeutic use in platelet-dependent disorders. *Drugs* **40**: 238–259, 1990
37. Janzon L, Bergquist D, Boberg J *et al.*: Prevention of myocardial infarction and stroke in patients with intermittent claudication: effects of ticlopidine. Results from STIMS, the Swedish Ticlopidine Multicenter Study. *J Intern Med* **227**: 301–308, 1990
38. Bergqvist D, Almgren B, Dickinson JP: Reduction of requirement for leg vascular surgery during long-term treatment of claudicant patients in Ticlodipine: Results from the Swedish Ticlodipine Multicentre Study (STIMS). *Eur J Vasc Endovasc Surg* **10**: 69–76, 1995
39. Blanchard J, Carreras LO, Kindermans M and the EMATAP Group: Results of EMATAP: a double-blind placebo-controlled multicentre trial of ticlodipine in patients with peripheral arterial disease. *Nouv Rev Fr Hematol* **35**: 523–528, 1993
40. Prevention of Atherosclerotic Complications with Keranserin Trial Group: Prevention of atherosclerotic complications: controlled trial of ketanserin. *Br Med J* **298**: 424–430, 1989
41. Mangano DT, Layug EL, Wallace A, Tateo I: Effect of Atenolol on mortality and cardiovascular morbidity after noncardiac surgery. *New Engl J Med* **335**: 1713–1720, 1996
42. Krupski WC: The peripheral vascular consequences of smoking. *Ann Vasc Surg* **5**: 291–304, 1991
43. Beurger L: Thrombo-angiitis obliterans: a study of the vascular lesions leading to presenile spontaneous gangrene. *Am J Med* **136**: 567–580, 1908
44. McGill HC: The cardiovascular pathology of smoking. *Am Heart J* **115**: 250–257, 1988
45. Belch JJF, McArdle B, Burns P *et al.*: The effects of acute smoking on platelet behaviour, fibrinolysis and haemorrheology in habitual smokers. *Thromb Res* **51**: 6–8, 1984
46. Kannel WB, McGee DL: Update on some epidemiological features of intermittent claudication: the Framingham Study. *J Am Ger Soc* **33**: 13–18, 1985
47. Hughson WG, Mann JI, Tibbs DJ *et al.*: Intermittent claudication: factors determining outcome. *Br Med J* **1**: 377–379, 1978
48. Wiseman SA, Kenchington GF, Dain R *et al.*: The influence of smoking and plasma factors on femoropopliteal vein graft patency. *Br Med J* **299**: 643–646, 1989

49. Russell MAH: The nicotine trap: a 40 year sentence for four cigarettes. *Br J Addiction* **85**: 293–300, 1990
50. Jarvis MJ, Russell MAH: Treatment for the cigarette smoker. *Int Rev Psychiat* **1**: 139–147, 1989
51. Benowitz NL: Pharmacologic aspects of cigarette smoking and nicotine addiction. *New Engl J Med* **319**: 1318–1330, 1988
52. Fiore MC *et al.*: Methods used to quit smoking in the United States. *J Am Med Assoc* **263**: 2760–2765, 1990
53. Abelin T *et al.*: Controlled trial of transdermal nicotine patch in tobacco withdrawal. *Lancet* **7**: 7–10, 1989
54. Silagy C, Mant D, Fowler G, Lodge M: Meta-analysis on efficacy of nicotine replacement therapies in smoking cessation. *Lancet* **343**: 139–142, 1994
55. Lam W, Sze PC, Sacks HS, Chalmers TC: Meta-analysis of randomised controlled trials of nicotine chewing-gum. *Lancet* **ii**: 27–30, 1987
56. Hughes JR, Hatsukami DK, Skoog KP: Physical dependence on nicotine in gum. *J Am Med Assoc* **255**: 3277–3279, 1986
57. Henningfield JE, Radzius A, Cooper TM, Clayton RR: Drinking coffee and carbonated beverages blocks absorption of nicotine from nicotine polacrilex gum. *J Am Med Assoc* **264**: 1560–1564, 1990
58. Schroll M, Munck O: Estimation of peripheral arteriosclerotic disease by ankle brachial pressure measurements in a population study of 60 year-old men and women. *J Chron Dis* **34**: 261–269, 1981
59. Reid DD, Holland WW, Hummerfelt S, Rose G: A cardiovascular survey of British postal workers. *Lancet* **i**: 614–618, 1966
60. Da Silva A, Widmer LK, Ziegler HW *et al.*: The Basle longitudinal study: report on the relation of initial glucose level to baseline ECG abnormalities, peripheral arterial disease and subsequent mortality. *J Chron Dis* **32**: 797–803, 1979
61. Shimada K, Kawamoto I, Matsubayashi K *et al.*: Diurnal blood pressure variations and silent cerebrovascular damage in elderly patients with hypertension. *J Hypertens* **10**: 875–878, 1992
62. Bridges AB, Fisher TC, Scott N *et al.*: Circadian rhythm of white blood cell aggregation and free radical status in healthy volunteers. *Free Radical Res Commun* **16**: 89–97, 1992
63. Scottish Intercollegiate Guidelines Network (SIGN): A National Clinical Guideline. *Drug therapy for peripheral vascular disease* 1998
64. Ramsay LE, Williams B, Johnston GD *et al.*: Guidelines for management of hypertension: report of the third working party of the British Hypertension Society. *J Human Hypertens* **13**: 569–592, 1999
65. Neaton JD *et al.* for the Treatment of Mild Hypertension Study Research Group. Treatment of Mild Hypertension Study. Final results. *J Am Med Assoc* **270**: 713–724, 1993
66. Materson BJ *et al.* for the Department of Veterans Affairs Cooperative Study Group on Antihypertensive Agents: Single-drug therapy for hypertension in men. A comparison of six antihypertensive agents with placebo. *New Engl J Med* **328**: 914–921, 1993
67. Philipp T *et al.* on behalf of the HANE Trial Research Group: Randomised, double blind, multicentre comparison of hydrochlorothiazide, atenolol, nitrendipine, and enalapril in antihypertensive treatment: results of the HANE study. *Br Med J* **315**: 154–159, 1997
68. Collins R *et al.*: Blood pressure, stroke and coronary heart disease. Part 2, short-term reductions in blood pressure: overview of randomised drug trials in their epidemiological context. *Lancet* **335**: 827–838, 1990
69. Clausen J, Jenson G. Blood pressure and mortality: an epidemiological survey with 10 years follow-up. *J Hum Hypertens* **6**: 53–59, 1992
70. Khan F, Belch JJF. Cholesterol-lowering and endothelial cell function in forearm skin of patients with hypercholesterolaemia with hypercholesterolaemia and peripheral vascular disease. *Internat Angiol* **14**(Suppl 1): 356, 1995
71. Laakso M, Ronnemaa T, Pyorala *et al.*: Atherosclerotic vascular disease and its risk factors in non-insulin dependent diabetics and non-diabetic subjects in Finland. *Diabetes Care* **11**: 449–463, 1988

72. Van Gaal L, Rillaerts E, Creten W, De Leeuw I: Relationship of body fat distribution pattern to atherogenic risk factors in non-insulin depdendent diabetes. Preliminary results. *Diabetes Care* **11**: 103–106, 1988
73. Cardia G, Grisorio D, Impedovo G *et al.*: Plasma lipids as a risk factor in peripheral vascular disease. *Angiology* **41**: 19–22, 1990
74. Angquist KA, Johnson O, Ericsson M, Tollin C: Serum lipoproteins and apoliproproteins A1 and A11 in male patients with peripheral arterial insufficiency. *Acta Chir Scand* **148**: 675–678, 1982
75. Jacobson UK, Dige-Pedersen H, Gyntelberg F, Svendsen UG: 'Risk factors' and manifestiations of arteriosclerosis in patients with intermittent claudication compared to normal persons. *Dan Med Bull* **31**: 145–148, 1984
76. Fowkes FGR, Housley E, Riemersma RA *et al.*: Smoking, lipids, glucose intolerence and blood pressure at risk factors for peripheral atherosclerosis compared with ischaemic heart disease in the Edinburgh Artery Study. *Am J Epidemiol* **135**: 331–340, 1992
77. Fowkes FG, Allan PL, Tsampoulas C *et al.*: Validity of duplex scanning in the detection of peripheral arterial disease in the general population. *Eur J Vasc Surg* **6**: 31–35, 1992
78. Blankenhorn DH, Brooks SH, Selzer RH *et al.*: The rate of atherosclerosis change during treatment of hyperlipoproteinuria. *Circulation* **57**: 355, 1978
79. Zelis R, Manson DT, Braunwald E *et al.*: Effects of hyperlipoproteinemias and their treatment on the peripheral circulation. *J Clin Invest* **49**: 1007, 1970
80. Scandinavian Simvastatin Survival Study Group: Randomised trial of cholesterol lowering in 4444 patients with coronary heart disease: the Scandinavian Simvastatin Study (4S). *Lancet* **344**: 1383–1389, 1994
81. Shepherd J, Cobbe SM, Ford I *et al.*: Prevention of coronary heart disease with pravastatin in men with hypercholesterolaemia. *New Engl J Med* **333**: 1301–1307, 1995
82. Sacks FM, Pfeffer MA, Moye LA *et al.*: The effect of pravastatin on coronary events after myocardial infarction in patients with average cholesterol levels. *New Engl J Med* **335**: 1001–1009, 1996
83. Brandman O, Redisch W: Incidence of peripheral vascular changes in diabetes mellitus. *Diabetes* **2**: 194–198, 1953
84. Kingsbury KJ: The relation between glucose tolerance and atherosclerotic vascular disease. *Lancet* **2**: 1374–1379, 1996
85. Connor H: The economic impact of diabetic foot disease. In: Connor H, Boulton AJM, Ward JD (Eds), *The Foot in Diabetes* pp. 145–149. Chichester: John Wiley, 1987
86. Wilson S, Jennings PA, Belch, JJF: Detection of microvascular impairment in type 1 diabetes by laser Doppler flowmetry. *Clin Physiol* **12**: 197–210, 1992
87. Belch JJF, Greene SA, Litttleford R *et al.*: Impaired skin blood flow response to heat in children with insulin dependent diabetes. *Int J Angiol* **5**: 189–191, 1996
88. Elhadd TA, Robb R, Jung RT *et al.*: Pilot study of prevalence of asymptomatic peripheral arterial occlusive disease in patients with diabetes attending a hospital clinic. *Pract Diabetes Int* **16**: 163–166, 1999
89. Jennings PE, McLaren M, Scott N *et al.*: The relationship of oxidative stress to thrombotic tendency in type 1 diabetic patients with retinopathy. *Diabetic Med* **8**: 860–865, 1991
90. Belch JJF, Mackay IR, Hill A *et al.*: Oxidative stress is present in atherosclerotic peripheral arterial disease and further increased by diabetes mellitus. *Internat Angiol* **14**: 385–388, 1996
91. McLaren M, Jennings PE, Forbes CD, Belch JJF: Fibrinolytic response to venous occlusion in diabetic with and without micro-angiopathy compared to normal age and sex matched controls. *Fibrinolysis* **4**: 116–117, 1990
92. Green F, Stonebridge P, Levison R, Belch JJF: The prevalence of occult diabetes in patients with intermittent claudication (submitted)
93. Gerstein HC, Yusuf S: Dysglycaemia and risk of cardiovascular disease. *Lancet* **347**: 949–950, 1996
94. Mühlhauser I: Smoking and Diabetes. *Diabet Med* **7**: 10–15, 1990

95. Donaldson MC, Weinberg DS, Belkin M *et al.*: Screening for hypercoagulable states in vascular surgical practice: a preliminary study. *J Vasc Surg* **11**: 825–831, 1990
96. De Frang RD, Edwards JM, Moneta GL *et al.*: Repeat leg bypass after multiple prior bypass failures. *J Vasc Surg* **19**: 268–277, 1994
97. Ahn SS, Kalunian K, Rosove M *et al.*: Postoperative thrombotic complications in patients with the lupus anticoagulant; increased risk after vascular procedures. *J Vasc Surg* **7**: 749–756, 1988
98. Eldrup-Jorgensen J, Flanigan DP, Brace L *et al.*: Hypercoaguable states and lower limb ischaemia in young adults. *J Vasc Surg* **9**: 334–341, 1989
99. Schafer AI, Kroll MH: Nonatheromatous arterial thrombosis. *Ann Rev Med* **44**: 155–170, 1993
100. Coller BS, Owen J, Jesty J *et al.*: Deficiency of plasma protein S, protein C, or antithrombin III and arterial thrombosis. *Arteriosclerosis* **7**: 456–462, 1987
101. De Stafano V, Leone G, Micalizzi P *et al.*: Arterial thrombosis as a clinical manifestation of congenital protein C deficiency. *Ann Hematol* **62**: 180–183, 1991
102. Dahlback B, Hildebrand B: Inherited resistance to activated protein C is corrected by anticoagulant cofactor activity found to be a property of factor V. *Proc Natl Acad Sci USA* **91**: 1396–1400, 1994
103. Hirsh J, Piovella F, Pini M: Congenital antithrombin III deficiency. *Am J Med* **87**: 34S–38S, 1989
104. Rees MM, Rodgers GM: Homocysteinemia: association of a metabolic disorder with vascular disease and thrombosis. *Thromb Res* **71**: 337–359, 1993
105. Rodgers GM, Conn MT: Homocysteine, an atherogenic stimulus reduces protein C activation by arterial and venous endothelial cells. *Blood* **75**: 895–901, 1990
106. Taylor LM Jr, Porter JM: Elevated plasma homocysteine as a risk factor for atherosclerosis. *Semin Vasc Surg* **6**: 36–45, 1993
107. Eldrup-Jorgensen J, Brace L, Flanigan DP *et al.*: Lupus-like anticoagulants and lower extremity arterial occlusive disease. *Circulation* **80** (Suppl III): III-54–III-58, 1989
108. Bick RL, Baker WF: Anticardiolipin antibodies and thrombosis. *Hematol/Oncol Clin North Am* **6**: 1287–1299, 1992
109. Rosove MH, Brewer PMC: Antiphospholipid thrombosis: clinical course after the first thrombotic event in 70 patients. *Ann Intern Med* **117**: 303–308, 1992
110. Ginsburg KS, Liang MH, Newcomer L *et al.*: Anticardiolipin antibodies and the risk for ischemic stroke and venous thrombosis. *Ann Intern Med* **117**: 997–1102, 1992
111. Lau CS, Khan F, McLaren M *et al.*: The effects of thromboxane receptor blockade on platelet aggregation and digital skin blood flow in patients with secondary Raynaud's syndrome. *Rheumatol Int* **11**: 163–168, 1991
112. Hickman P, McCollum PT, Belch JJF: Neutrophils may contribute to the morbidity and mortality of claudicants. *Br J Surg* **81**: 790–798,1994
113. Belch JJF, Shaw JW, Kirk G *et al.*: The white blood cell adhesion molecule E-selectin predicts restenosis in patients with intermittent claudication undergoing percutaneous transluminal angioplasty. *Circulation* (in press)
114. Scottish Collegiate Guidelines Network: *Drug Therapy for Peripheral Vascular Disease*. Sign Publication No. 27, 1998
115. Waters KJ, Craxford AD, Chamberlain J: The effect of naftidrofuryl (Praxilene) on intermittent claudication. *Br J Surg* **67**: 249–251,1980
116. Adhoute G, Bacourt F, Barral M *et al.*: Naftidrofuryl in chronic arterial disease. Results of a six month controlled multicenter study using naftidrofuryl tablets 200mg. *Angiology* **37**: 160–167, 1986
117. Kriessmann A, Neiss A: Clinical effectiveness of naftidrofuryl in intermittent claudication. *Vasa Suppl* **24**: 27–32, 1988
118. Trubestein G, Böhme H, Heidrich H *et al.*: Naftidrofuryl in chronic arterial disease. Results of a controlled multicentre study. *Angiology* **35**: 701–708, 1984
119. Adhoute G, Andreassian B, Boccalon H *et al.*: Treatment of stage II chronic arterial disease of the lower limbs with the serotonergic antagonist naftidrofuryl: Results after 6 months of a controlled, multicentre study. *J Cardiovasc Pharmacol* **16**: S75–S80, 1990

120. Becker HM, Elert O, Haring R *et al.*: Effectiveness of Dusodril-P in arterial occlusive diseases. A multicentric double-blind study. *Med Welt* **30**: 1602–1606, 1979
121. Karnik R, Valentin A, Stollberger C *et al.*: Effects of naftidrofuryl in patients with intermittent claudication. *Angiology* 234–240, 1988
122. Moody MP, Al-Khaffaf HS, Lehert P *et al.*: An evaluation of patients with severe intermittent claudication and the effect of treatment with naftidrofuryl. *J Cardiovasc Pharmacol* **23**: S44–S47, 1994
123. Pohle W, Hirche P, Barnmeyer J *et al.*: Double-blind study of naftidrofuryl-hydrogen oxalate in patients suffering from occlusive peripheral arterial disease. *Med Welt* **30**: 269–272, 1979
124. Clyne CA, Galland RB, Fox MJ *et al.*: A controlled trial of naftidrofuryl (Praxilene) in the treatment of intermittent claudication. *Br J Surg* **67**: 347–348, 1980
125. Lehert P, Riphagen FE, Gamand S: The effect of naftidrofuryl of intermittent claudication: a meta analysis. *J Cardiovasc Pharmacol* **16**: 81–86, 1990
126. Lehert P, Comte S, Gamand S *et al.*: Naftidrofuryl in intermittent claudication. A retrospective analysis. *J Cardiovasc Pharmacol* **23**: S448–S452, 1994
127. Porter JM, Cutler BS, Lee BY *et al.*: Pentoxifylline efficacy in the treatment of intermittent claudication: Multicenter controlled double-blind trial with objective assessment of chronic occlusive arterial disease. *Am Heart J* **104**: 66–72, 1982
128. Perhoniemi V, Salmenkivi K, Sunberg S *et al.*: Effects of flunarizine and pentoxifylline on walking distance and blood rheology in claudication. *Angiology* **35**: 366–372, 35
129. Gallus AS, Gleadow F, Supont P *et al.*: Intermittent claudication: a double-blind crossover trial of pentoxifylline. *Aust NZ J Med* **15**: 402–409, 1985
130. Reich T, Gillings D: Effects of pentoxifylline on severe intermittent claudication. *Angiology* **38**: 651–656, 1987
131. Chopra HK, Chopra KL, Aggarwal KK *et al.*: Pentoxifylline (Trental) – a new drug for the treatment of peripheral chronic occlusive arterial disease. *J Med* **19**: 89–107, 1988
132. Lindgarde F, Jelnes R, Bjorkman H *et al.*: Conservative drug treatment in patients with moderately severe chronic peripheral arterial disease. *Circulation* **80**: 1549–1556, 1989
133. Dettori AD, Pini M, Moratti A: Acenocoumarol and pentoxifylline in intermittent claudication. A controlled clinical study. *Angiology* **40**: 237–248, 1989
134. Strano A, Davi G, Avellone G *et al.*: A double-blind, crossover study of the clinical efficacy and the haemorheological effects in patients with occlusive arterial disease of the lower limbs. *Angiology* **35**: 459–466, 1984
135. Acetto B: Beneficial hamorheologic therapy of chronic peripheral arterial disorders with pentoxifylline: results of double-blind study versus vasodilator-nylidrin. *Am Heart J* **103**: 864–869, 1982
136. Radack K, Wyderski RJ: Conservative management of intermittent claudication. *Ann Intern Med* **113**: 135–146, 1990
137. Tyson VC: Treatment of intermittent claudication. Practitioner 223: 121–126, 1979
138. Head A: Treatment of intermittent claudication with inositol nicotinate. *Practitioner* **230**: 49–54, 1986
139. Kiff RS, Quick CR: Does inositol nicotinate (Hexopal) influence intermittent claudication? A controlled trial. *Br J Clin Pract* **42**: 141–145, 1988
140. O'Hara J, Jolly PN, Nicol CG: The therapeutic efficacy of inositol nicotinate (Hexopal) in intermittent claudication: a controlled trial. *Br J Clin Pract* **42**: 377–383, 1988
141. Forconi S, Guerrini M, Pecchi S *et al.*: Haemorheological and peripheral haemodynamic action of flunarizine in patients suffering from peripheral obliterative arterial disease. An open controlled clinical pharmacological study. *Clin Terapia Cardiovascolare* **3**: 11–20, 1984.
142. Adrianensen H: A randomised double-blind trial of cinnarizine. *Clin Trials J* **6**: 191–193, 1969
143. Verhaegen H, Roels V, Adrriansen H *et al.*: The arteriolar affects of cinnarizine and flunarizine. *Angiology* 261–278, 1974
144. Staessen AJ: Treatment of circulatory disturbances with flunarizine and connarizine. *Curr Ther* **6**: 59–71, 1977
145. Mashiah A, Patel P, Schraibman IG *et al.*: Drug therapy in intermittent claudication: an objective assessment of the effects of three drugs on patients with intermittent claudication. *Br J Surg* **65**: 342–345, 1978

146. Barber JH, Reuter CA, Jageneau AH *et al.*: Intermittent claudication: a controlled study in parallel time of the short-term and long-term effect of cinnarizine. *Pharmatherapeutica* **2**: 401–407, 1980

The secondary use of antiplatelet and oral anticoagulant therapy in patients with peripheral arterial occlusive disease

Marco JD Tangelder, James A Lawson, Ale Algra,
Bert C Eikelboom

INTRODUCTION

The progress of medical technology in the twentieth century has been overwhelming. Medical knowledge and efficacy of treatment is now more and more promising. As a result, average survival has improved, and ageing has increased the prevalence of vascular diseases. At the very beginning of the twenty-first century, evidence-based medicine has become an established feature. Efficacy of treatment modalities are compared in randomized controlled trials, the gold standard. Data from randomized trials are pooled to understand precise effects of treatment. In this new era of high quality medicine we incline towards a broader view of vascular patients. Outcome of trials should not asses graft patency only but the spectrum of ischaemic events including mortality. Furthermore, quality of life, being the most important outcome from the patients' point of view, has become an established measure of effect. Fortunately, treatment of vascular patients is increasingly practised in a multidisciplinary setting, which gives a complete insight into patients with generalized disease. Despite all progress made, vascular patients are still at high risk for complications due to progression of atherosclerosis.[1–5] Intermittent claudication, for instance, is associated with a two- to five-fold increased relative risk of ischaemic cardiovascular disease.[6] It is therefore of major importance to offer vascular patients the optimal antithrombotic treatment known at the moment. Numerous clinical trials have been conducted to determine the efficacy of antithrombotic drugs in coronary artery and cerebrovascular diseases. However, there are few properly conducted randomized controlled trials in patients with intermittent claudication or critical ischaemia of the lower extremities, particularly trials investigating the efficacy of antithrombotic drugs in maintaining graft or angioplasty patency and preventing cardiovascular and cerebrovascular complications. In this chapter we will provide an overview of the actual evidence on clinical effects of antithrombotic therapy in patients with manifest peripheral arterial occlusive disease.

Table 1. Recommendations for antithrombotic therapy in patients with peripheral arterial occlusive disease

Patient category	*Recommendation*
Intermittent claudication	Low-dose aspirin
Peripheral angioplasty	Low-dose aspirin
Peripheral vascular surgery	
venous bypass	Oral anticoagulants, target range 3–4 INR
non-venous bypass	Low-dose aspirin
thrombendarterectomie	Low-dose aspirin

INR: International normalized ratio

ANTITHROMBOTIC THERAPY IN THE NON-OPERATIVE MANAGEMENT OF INTERMITTENT CLAUDICATION

Antiplatelet drugs

All unconfounded (i.e. where the allocated treatment in one group did not differ from that in the other, in any aspect other than antiplatelet therapy) randomized trials of antiplatelet therapy in various categories of patients, available before March 1990, in which vascular events were studied systematically, were included in an impressive meta-analysis by the Antiplatelet Trialists' Collaboration.[7] Subgroup analysis of 22 randomized controlled trials in patients with intermittent claudication only just failed to demonstrate a significant beneficial effect on vascular events, defined as non-fatal myocardial infarctions, non-fatal strokes, or vascular deaths, of antiplatelet therapy compared with placebo. The most evidence came from the 15 trials studying ticlopidine versus placebo. Only four trials in which aspirin was compared with placebo, showed no effect of aspirin on reduction of vascular events at all. The risk reduction in vascular events in all categories of patients was highly significant in favour of antiplatelet therapy compared with controls: 27% ($2p<0.00001$). The thrombosis prevention trial demonstrated a similar 20% reduction in ischaemic heart disease in high risk men treated with aspirin compared with placebo ($p=0.04$).[8]

Promising results were recently achieved with a new generation of platelet inhibitors. The efficacy in reducing the risk of ischaemic events of clopidogrel (chemically related to ticlopidine) was compared with that of aspirin in patients with ischaemic stroke, myocardial infarction or peripheral arterial occlusive disease in the CAPRIE study.[9] The relative risk reduction for the composite outcome of stroke, myocardial infarction or vascular death was highest in the subgroup of patients with peripheral arterial disease: 23.8% (95% confidence interval [CI] 8.9–36.2) in favour of clopidogrel. However, this group consisted of a repository of patients with intermittent claudication, or a history of claudication with previous amputation or vascular reconstruction or angioplasty. In contrary, there was no difference between both treatments in the other subgroups of patients with recent stroke (relative risk reduction 7.3%; 95% CI –5.7–18.7) and recent myocardial infarction (relative risk reduction –3.7%; 95% CI –22.9–12.0). The overall risk reduction was only just significant in favour of clopidogrel: 8.7% (95% CI 0.3–16.5).

Evidence of the efficacy of platelet inhibitors, especially aspirin, in patients with intermittent claudication is still insufficient. Supposed evidence is to a large extent an extrapolation of (positive) results of large trials or meta-analyses in various categories of high-risk patients. Given the divergent results in several categories of patients it is doubtful whether the lumping together of patients is justified. Irrespective of lack of evidence in patients with intermittent claudication, we feel that antiplatelet therapy is justified in these patients with a high cardiovascular and cerebrovascular risk profile, due to one underlying atherosclerotic disease. Convincing evidence of a superior platelet inhibitor is not available yet. For reasons of costs and convenience low-dose aspirin is recommended.

Oral anticoagulant therapy

A Dutch placebo-controlled trial, in which 300 patients with intermittent claudication, both conservatively and surgically treated, were randomized, demonstrated highly significant beneficial effects of long-term treatment with oral anticoagulants, target international normalized ratio (INR) range 2.8–4.8, during the 5-year follow-up.[10] The surgically treated group consisted of patients who had aortoiliac reconstructions only. Not only was the risk of progression of atherosclerotic lesions in peripheral vascular disease, as assessed by clinical description, ankle brachial index and treadmill exercise, reduced six-fold ($p<0.0001$) in patients treated with oral anticoagulants, but also progression of generalized vascular disease was delayed compared with the placebo-treated group. When the progression rates of cerebrovascular, cardiovascular and peripheral vascular disease were combined, the 5-year progression rate was reduced by factor 3, from 29% in the placebo group to 9% in patients treated with oral anticoagulants ($p<0.0001$). Although these results are convincing with regard to the occurrence of vascular events, they failed to demonstrate a significant beneficial effect of oral anticoagulant treatment in terms of reduction of total mortality compared with the placebo group. The frequency of bleeding complications appeared to be very moderate, although there were two fatal intracerebral haemorrhages in the treated group.

A randomized comparison between oral anticoagulants and aspirin in patients with intermittent claudication has not been performed yet. For reasons of costs, convenience and associated adverse effects, treatment with aspirin seems to be the most sensible choice for the present.

ANTITHROMBOTIC THERAPY AFTER PERIPHERAL ARTERIAL ANGIOPLASTY

Although there were no available data on the relative efficacy of antithrombotic therapy in patients after peripheral arterial angioplasty, the American College of Chest Physicians recommended in 1995 lifelong aspirin or other antiplatelet therapy.[11] These recommendations were based on extrapolations from data on coronary angioplasty. A Medline search in the period from 1994 until 1999 yielded no randomized controlled trials on the efficacy of antithrombotic drugs after angioplasty in peripheral arteries.

So far there is no evidence of efficacy of antithrombotic drugs for the prevention of occlusion of peripheral arteries treated by angioplasty. Given the fact that also these patients are at high risk for coronary and cerebrovascular events, prescription of low-dose aspirin seems to be justified.

ANTITHROMBOTIC THERAPY AFTER PERIPHERAL VASCULAR SURGERY

Antiplatelet therapy

In 1975 the first randomized controlled trial showed the protective action of aspirin on thromboembolic events in patients after infrainguinal bypass surgery.[12] Many randomized controlled trials studied the efficacy of antiplatelet therapy in maintaining vascular patency in various categories of patients; most of their results were pooled in the second part of the massive meta-analysis by the Antiplatelet Trialists' Collaboration.[13]

All unconfounded randomized trials of antiplatelet therapy in various vascular patients, available before March 1990, in which vascular graft or native arterial patency was studied systematically, were included. In a meta-analysis of the 11 studies concerning peripheral reconstructions in the lower extremities, they demonstrated a significant risk reduction of graft occlusion of 32% in patients who were given platelet inhibitors. The doses of aspirin used ranged from 600 to 1500 mg daily. In the first part of the Antiplatelet Trialists' Collaboration report, the effect of antiplatelet therapy on various vascular events, defined as non-fatal myocardial infarctions, non-fatal strokes, or vascular deaths were analysed.[7] Subgroup analysis of nine trials in patients with peripheral reconstructions failed to demonstrate beneficial effects of antiplatelet therapy compared with placebo. In the overview of all antiplatelet studies neither direct nor indirect comparisons of the effects of different regimens (aspirin, dipyridamole, sulphinpyrazone, ticlopidine and suloctidil) on vascular patency provided clear evidence that one antiplatelet regimen was more effective than an other, nor that the time at which treatment began made any difference to the results.

The composite outcome of ischaemic events is the most important outcome for patients with peripheral vascular disease. Therefore, we are interested in the long-term effects of antithrombotic therapy on graft occlusion, as well as on other vascular events. We recently undertook a meta-analysis of unconfounded trials to assess the impact of long-term treatment with aspirin, with or without other platelet inhibitors, and oral anticoagulants on occlusion of bypass grafts, and the occurrence of stroke, myocardial infarction, vascular and total mortality and the composite outcome of stroke, myocardial infarction or vascular mortality following infrainguinal bypass surgery.[14] Five randomized controlled trials comparing aspirin (with or without other antiplatelet therapy) with placebo after infrainguinal bypass surgery were included, resulting in a total of 816 patients (423 treated patients and 393 controls).[15–19] In 423 patients treated with antiplatelet drugs, 120 bypasses occluded (28,4%), compared with 144 occlusions in 393 randomized controls (36.6%). The relative risk is 0.78 (95% CI 0.64–0.95), meaning a proportional risk reduction of 22%. This corresponds with a significant absolute risk reduction of 8.2%.

Only three trials reported the number of strokes during follow-up. Among 351 patients treated there were 17 strokes, compared with 19 strokes among 312 controls resulting in a relative risk of 0.80 (95% CI 0.41–1.57). The same trials assessed the occurrence of myocardial infarction during follow-up. In the treated group fewer myocardial infarctions were reported: 25 among 351 patients, compared with 34 of 312 controls. The relative risk is 0.64 (95% CI 0.37–1.10). All trials reported both vascular and overall mortality at the end of the follow-up period. Among 423 patients allocated to antiplatelet treatment 33 died of a vascular cause compared with 43 among 393 controls (relative risk 0.71; 95% CI 0.47–1.09), the absolute risk reduction is 3.1%. The difference in total mortality is smaller: in both groups 50 patients died (relative risk 0.92; 95% CI 0.64–1.32) with an absolute risk reduction of 0.9%. Analysis of the composite outcome resulted in a total of 62 patients who suffered a vascular event among 423 treated patients compared with 65 patients with a vascular event among 393 control patients (relative risk 0.88; 95% CI 0.64–1.20). This corresponds with an absolute risk reduction of 2%. This meta-analysis demonstrated a reduction of the risk of graft occlusion by antiplatelet therapy. Unfortunately, the number of conducted randomized controlled trials is small, the number of patients in most of these trials is small and only a few trials studied cardiovascular and cerebrovascular events other than graft patency.

In all above mentioned trials a high dose of aspirin was administered, which is less effective and associated with more adverse effects than a low dose. High levels of aspirin cause besides inhibition of cyclo-oxygenase in platelets and thus thromboxane A_2 synthesis, which is responsible for platelet aggregation and vasoconstriction,[20–23] inhibition of cyclo-oxygenase in endothelial cells. This way endothelial prostacyclin production is diminished.[24,25] In contrast, prostacyclin is not only a powerful inhibitor of platelet adhesion and aggregation but also a vasodilator.[21,25,26]

A randomized controlled trial by Becquemin *et al.*[27] showed significant improvement of cumulative 2-year patency of infrainguinal vein bypasses in 243 patients treated with ticlopidine (82%) compared with placebo (63%), also if differences between treatment groups with regard to site of distal anastomosis were taken into account. Unfortunately, the study was too small to demonstrate a beneficial effect of ticlopidine on other ischaemic events studied.

Hitherto no difference in efficacy between various (combinations of) platelet inhibitors as well as various dosages have been proven. A low dose aspirin is, in theory, more effective than a high dose, and associated with fewer adverse effects. Besides, aspirin is available at a lower price than other platelet inhibitors. For these reasons, to-date, low-dose aspirin is the preferred antiplatelet therapy after peripheral bypass surgery.

Oral anticoagulants

Only two randomized controlled trials of oral anticoagulants versus no anticoagulation in patients after infrainguinal bypass surgery have been conducted. Kretschmer and colleagues studied the effect of long-term treatment with phenprocoumon, target INR 2.4–4.8, on vein graft patency, limb salvage and survival in patients operated for claudication or critical ischaemia.[28] Patency was determined by Doppler ultrasonography, when indicated followed by angiography. In 66 patients treated, 13 grafts occluded (19.7%), compared with 23 in 64 controls (35.9%), a relative risk of 0.55 (95% CI 0.30–0.99), meaning a proportional risk reduction of 45%. The corresponding absolute risk reduction is 16.2%. In the treated group there were four amputations (6.1%) compared with 13 (20.3%) in the control group (relative risk 0.30; 95% CI 0.10–0.87) with an absolute risk reduction of 14.2%. The number of strokes and myocardial infarctions were not reported in this trial. Therefore estimation of the effects of oral anticoagulants on the composite outcome was also not possible. Among the anticoagulated patients 27 (40.9%) died during 10 years of follow-up compared with 37 (57.8%) in the control group (relative risk 0.71; 95% CI 0.49–1.01), resulting in an absolute risk reduction of 16.9%.

The study reported one fatal gastrointestinal haemorrhage in the treated group. The second randomized controlled trial examined 116 patients after various operative reconstructions, i.e. vein bypass, polytetrafluoroethylene bypass and endarterectomy, because of severe intermittent claudication or critical ischaemia.[29] Intention to treat analysis showed no significant difference in patency rate, limb salvage and survival between the anticoagulated group and the control group. However, the level of anticoagulation of 1.8 to 2.8 INR was, in our view, inadequate.

Aspirin or oral anticoagulants after peripheral vascular surgery?

Although evidence on the efficacy of antiplatelet therapy and oral anticoagulants is weak in patients after peripheral bypass surgery, most of us consider it unethical not to prescribe antithrombotic medication. Up to now three randomized controlled trials comparing aspirin with oral anticoagulants in patients after infrainguinal bypass surgery or thrombendarterectomy have been accomplished. Already in the 1970s, Schneider *et al.* randomized 91 patients with a venous femoropopliteal bypass and 122 patients after thrombendarterectomy to treatment with either aspirin or aspirin plus dipyridamole or oral anticoagulant therapy. The overall 2-year patency rate did not differ significantly in the groups. However, subgroup analysis of patients after venous bypass surgery demonstrated a better patency rate in the group treated with oral anticoagulants than in both antiplatelet groups, which they did not distinguish: 87% versus 65%, $p<0.005$. In the group of patients after thrombendarterectomy, antiplatelet therapy proved to be favourable compared with oral anticoagulants: patency rates were 80% and 51% respectively, $p<0.002$.

In a recent trial 56 patients with vein bypasses who were at high risk for graft failure were randomized to a combination of warfarin and aspirin or aspirin only.[30] Aspirin (375mg daily) was started 1 day preoperatively and warfarin (target INR 2–3) 2 or 3 days; patients in the warfarin plus aspirin group received postoperative intravenous heparin. In 32 patients treated with warfarin plus aspirin, five (15.6%) grafts occluded compared with ten (41.7%) grafts in 24 patients treated with aspirin, with a corresponding relative risk of 0.38 (95% CI 0.15–0.95). This equals a proportional risk reduction of 62%. In the warfarin plus aspirin group five amputations were reported compared with nine in the aspirin group (relative risk 0.42, 95% CI 0.16–1.08). The number of myocardial infarctions and deaths were to small for reliable inferences on efficacy. In the warfarin plus aspirin group there were five bleedings reported compared with four bleeding complications in the aspirin group.

For lack of evidence from large trials of effects on all vascular events in patients after peripheral bypass surgery, members of the Dutch Society for Vascular Surgery decided in the early 1990s to conduct the Dutch BOA Study (Bypass, Oral anticoagulants or Aspirin Study).[31] Between 1 April 1995 and 1 March 1998 a total of 2650 patients from 80 centres were randomized to oral anticoagulant therapy (target INR 3–4.5) or 80mg aspirin daily. All patients who required an infrainguinal bypass graft for obstructive arterial disease were eligible for inclusion. The mean follow-up period was 21 months (median 20 months). The oral anticoagulants group (n=1326) had 308 graft occlusions compared with 322 in the aspirin group (n=1324) (hazard ratio 0.95; 95% CI 0.82–1.11), suggesting no overall benefit for either treatment. The hazard ratios of anticoagulants versus aspirin were essentially the same in patients with femoropopliteal (hazard ratio 0.97; 95% CI 0.81–1.16) and femorocrural bypass grafts (hazard ratio 0.95; 95% CI 0.70–1.30). Analysis stratified for graft material showed a lower risk of autologous vein graft occlusion in anticoagulated patients than in those on aspirin (hazard ratio 0.69; 95% CI 0.54–0.88), the number needed to treat to save one occlusion is 17. Conversely, the risk of non-venous graft occlusion was lower in patients treated with aspirin (hazard ratio 1.26; 95% CI 1.03–1.55), the number needed to treat is 15. The composite outcome event of vascular death, myocardial infarction, stroke or amputation occurred 248 times in the anticoagulant group and 275 times in the aspirin group (hazard ratio 0.89; 95% CI 0.75–1.06). Patients treated with oral anticoagulants suffered more major bleedings than patients treated with aspirin: 108 versus 56 (hazard ratio 1.96; 95% CI 1.42–2.71). The most adequate intensity of oral anticoagulation therapy, i.e. that intensity with the lowest incidence of both, ischaemic and haemorrhagic events, appeared to be between 3 and 4 INR. Given the results of this large trial we conclude that oral anticoagulation is the optimal treatment for preventing infrainguinal vein graft occlusion, and it also tends to be more effective in reducing ischaemic events, at an acceptable risk of haemorrhage. Aspirin is the first choice of treatment for preventing non-venous graft occlusion. Although it is associated with a somewhat higher risk of ischaemic stroke and myocardial infarction, the risk of haemorrhage is lower compared with that of oral anticoagulants.

REFERENCES

1. Criqui MH, Langer RD, Fronek A *et al.*: Mortality over a period of 10 years in patients with peripheral arterial disease. *New Engl J Med* **326**: 381–386, 1992
2. Jönssen B, Skau T: Outcome of symptomatic leg ischaemia: four year morbidity and mortality in Vadstena, Sweden. *Eur J Vasc Endovasc Surg* **11**: 315–323, 1996
3. Kannel WB, Skinner JJ Jr, Schwartz MJ, Shurtleff D: Intermittent claudication. Incidence in the Framingham Study. *Circulation* **41**: 875–883, 1970
4. Smith GD, Shipley MJ, Rose G: Intermittent claudication, heart disease risk factors, and mortality. The Whitehall Study. *Circulation* **82**: 1925–1931, 1990
5. Wolfe JHN: Defining the outcome of critical ischaemia: a one year prospective study. *Br J Surg* **73**: 321–321, 1986
6. Fowkes FG, Price JF, Leng GC: Targeting subclinical atherosclerosis. *Br Med J* **316**: 1764–1764, 1998
7. Antiplatelet Trialists' Collaboration: Collaborative overview of randomised trials of

antiplatelet therapy – I: Prevention of death, myocardial infarction, and stroke by prolonged antiplatelet therapy in various categories of patients. [published erratum appears in *Br Med J* 1994 Jun 11; **308**(6943): 1540]. *Br Med J* **308**: 81–106, 1994

8. The Medical Research Council's General Practice Research Framework: Thrombosis prevention trial: randomised trial of low-intensity oral anticoagulation with warfarin and low-dose aspirin in the primary prevention of ischaemic heart disease in men at increased risk. *Lancet* **351**: 233–247, 1998
9. CAPRIE Steering Committee: A randomised, blinded, trial of clopidogrel versus aspirin in patients at risk of ischaemic events (CAPRIE). *Lancet* **348**: 1329–1339, 1996
10. De Smit P, Van Urk H: The effect of long-term treatment with oral anticoagulants in patients with peripheral vascular disease. In: Tilsner V, Mathias FR (Eds), *Arterielle Verschlusskrankheit und Blutgerinnung* pp. 211–216. Basel: Roche, 1988
11. Clagett GP, Krupski WC: Antithrombotic therapy in peripheral arterial occlusive disease. *Chest* **4**(Suppl) 431–443, 1995
12. Zekert F: Klinische Anwendung von Aggregationshemmern bei arterieller Verschlusskrankheit. In: Zekert F (Ed), *Thrombosen, embolien und aggregationshemmer in der chirurgie*. pp. 68–72. Stuttgart: Schattauer, 1977
13. Antiplatelet Trialists' Collaboration: Collaborative overview of randomised trials of antiplatelet therapy – II: Maintenance of vascular graft or arterial patency by antiplatelet therapy. *Br Med J* **308**: 159–168, 1994
14. Tangelder MJD, Algra A, Lawson JA, Eikelboom BC: Systematic review of randomised controlled trials of aspirin and oral anticoagulants in the prevention of graft occlusion and ischaemic events after infrainguinal bypass surgery. *J Vasc Surg* **30**: 701–709, 1999
15. McCollum C, Alexander C, Kenchington G *et al.*: Antiplatelet drugs in femoropopliteal vein bypasses: a multicenter trial. *J Vasc Surg* **13**: 150–162, 1991
16. Donaldson DR, Salter MC, Kester RC *et al.*: The influence of platelet inhibition on the patency of femoro-popliteal dacron bypass grafts. *J Vasc Surg* **19**: 224–230, 1985
17. Goldman MD, McCollum CN: A prospective randomized study to examine the effect of aspirin plus dipyridamole on the patency of prosthetic femoro-popliteal grafts. *J Vasc Surg* **18**: 217–221, 1984
18. Green RM, Roedersheimer LR, DeWeese JA: Effects of aspirin and dipyridamole on expanded polytetrafluoroethylene graft patency. *Surgery* **92**: 1016–1026, 1982
19. Kohler TR, Kaufman JL, Kacoyanis GP *et al.*: Effect of aspirin and dipyridamole on the patency of lower extremity bypass grafts. *Surgery* **96**: 462–466, 1984
20. Hamberg M, Svensson J, Samuelssson B: A new group of biologically active compounds derived from prostaglandin endoperoxides. *Proc Natl Acad Sci* **72**: 2994–2998, 1975
21. Roth GJ, Stanford N, Majerus PW: Acetylation of prostaglandin synthase by aspirin. *Proc Natl Acad Sci* **72**: 3073–3076, 1975
22. Roth GJ, Majerus PW: The mechanism of the effect of aspirin on human platelets. I. Acetylation of a particulate fraction protein. *J Clin Invest* **56**: 624–632, 1975
23. Smith JB, Willis AL: Aspirin selectively inhibits prostaglandine production in human platelets. *Nature* **231**: 235–237, 1971
24. Burch JW, Baenziger NL, Stanford N, Majerus PW: Sensitivity of fatty acid cyclooxygenase from human aorta to acetylation of aspirin. *Proc Natl Acad Sci* **75**: 5181–5184, 1978
25. Moncada S, Higgs EA, Vane JR: Human arterial and venous tissue generates prostacyclin, a potent inhibitor of platelet aggregation. *Lancet* **i**: 18–21, 1977
26. Moncada S, Gryglewski RJ, Bunting S, Vane JR: An enzyme isolated from arteries transforms prostaglandin endoperoxides to an unstable substance that inhibits platelet aggregation. *Nature* **263**: 663–665, 1976
27. Becquemin JP: Effect of ticlopidine on the long-term patency of saphenous-vein bypass grafts in the legs. *New Engl J Med* **337**: 1726–1731, 1997
28. Kretschmer G, Herbst F, Prager M *et al.*: A decade of oral anticoagulant treatment to maintain autologous vein grafts for femoropopliteal atherosclerosis. *Arch Surg* **127**: 1112–1115, 1992
29. Arfvidsson B, Lundgren F, Drott C *et al.*: Influence on coumarin treatment on patency

and limb salvage after peripheral arterial reconstructive surgery. *Am J Surg* **159**: 556–560, 1990

30. Sarac TP, Huber TS, Back MR *et al.*: Warfarin improves the outcome of infrainguinal vein bypass grafting at high risk for failure. *J Vasc Surg* **28**: 446–457, 1998
31. The Dutch Bypass Oral Anticoagulant or Aspirin (BOA) Study Group. Efficacy of oral anticoagulants compared with aspirin after infrainguinal bypass surgery: a randomized trial. *Lancet* **355**: 346–351, 2000

PERIPHERAL ARTERIAL OPPORTUNITIES
Newer techniques

Is run-off percutaneous transluminal angioplasty worthwhile?

David Bergqvist, Duncan Ettles, Sadettin Karacagil,
Christer Ljungman, Anne-Marie Löfberg, A Tulga Ulus

INTRODUCTION

In recent years treatment of lower limb ischaemia has developed into a shared responsibility for surgeons and interventional radiologists in close cooperation. The surgical and endovascular procedures may be performed simultaneously or on different occasions. This clinical routine has developed gradually and is founded on experience, opinion or biased arguments from small case series, since solid scientific evidence is lacking. The clinician's dilemma is reflected in this chapter. He has to encounter the daily difficulties and challenges with clinical judgement and behaviour, which euphemistically is labelled clinical experience. On the other hand, solid scientific evidence, based on randomized studies, may be difficult to obtain for logistic reasons, e.g. when technical prerequisites for two available techniques such as balloon dilatation and open surgery differ considerably.

Although popliteal angioplasty was first undertaken in the 1960s , the results were disappointing, with frequent complications.[1,2] A major advance was heralded by the introduction of low profile percutaneous transluminal angioplasty (PTA) balloons and steerable hydrophilic guidewires which allow minimally traumatic access to the crural vessels. With these technical developments and accumulating experience, crural angioplasty has become more generally accepted and increasingly technically successful. However, the population treated by crural angioplasty differs significantly from those treated for iliac and femoral lesions. The majority of patients undergoing crural angioplasty are treated for rest pain or tissue loss. The objective of the procedure is preservation of a functioning pain-free limb. The cohort of patients tends to include more elderly patients with greater co-morbidity and a higher proportion of diabetes. Not surprisingly, a 5-year mortality of around 50% has been reported in this patient group.[3] While femorodistal bypass remains the gold standard of treatment for crural lesions, angioplasty is often the first step, also in case of these often complex lesions. Importantly, crural angioplasty rarely compromises the site of subsequent surgical reconstruction. The clinical indication of crural angioplasty is critical ischaemia and the use in severe claudicants remains controversial.

For the following discussion, the concept of run-off vessels depicts the arteries distal to the knee joint. The proximal vessels may be open, occluded or there may be a proximal reconstruction. In case of a bypass the distal anastomosis is included in the run-off. Only infrainguinal reconstructions are considered. From a prognostic point of view the quality of run-off arteries has an influence not only on the patency of a reconstruction but also on the long-term survival of the patient.[4] There are several situations where run-off PTA may be used.

- Isolated run-off PTA with patent proximal arteries. This means the presence of 'normal' flow to the diseased or distal popliteal artery with simultaneous lesions in the crural arteries. These patients have a high prevalence of diabetes mellitus. A prerequisite for success is the presence of a pedal outflow.[5] Published series with isolated run-off angioplasties are small.

- Distal PTA combined with a simultaneously performed femorodistal reconstruction (combined approach). The surgical reconstruction is most frequently a bypass but could also be an endarterectomy, or an endoluminal graft.[6–8] This combined approach is of practical importance but will not be further discussed because of the difficulty to evaluate each procedure separately.

- PTA in, or distal to, the distal anastomosis to prevent failure of a previous reconstruction, most frequently a bypass. The failing reconstruction is diagnosed either in a surveillance programme (asymptomatic) or because of the development of symptoms. PTA is then performed to obtain assisted primary patency.[9–11] Of 209 successfully performed below-knee bypasses 69 stenoses were detected at surveillance in 50 grafts.[12] Thirty stenoses were localized in the distal anastomosis and ten in run-off arteries; PTA was used as primary treatment, but the run-off angioplasties were not separately analysed. The 9-months assisted primary patency in the whole series was 72%.

- PTA in, or distal to, the distal anastomosis after emergent reopening (surgical or thrombolytic) of a failed reconstruction. PTA is performed to increase secondary patency. When the lesion is located to the distal anastomosis, it is most frequently due to pseudointimal hyperplasia. When the problem is located distal to the anastomosis, it is usually caused by progression of the arteriosclerotic process, which follows somewhat later compared with the development of pseudointimal hyperplasia. If thrombolysis is used to reopen an occluded reconstruction, the necessary intervention for the underlying lesion is often reduced to a limited or even elective procedure.[13–15] An underlying cause is detected in the majority of cases, in 81% in the STILE study[16] and in as many as 95% in the study by Hye *et al.*[17]

One of the problems with the literature dealing with run-off PTA is the rather great inhomogeneity in publications. This is seen both in inclusions, exclusions, report of the procedure and adjuvant pharmacotherapy and how various invasive combinations are handled. Obviously this makes analysis complicated, conclusions difficult to interpret and consequently recommendations may be flawed.

When reported series are evaluated for comparison of findings the following points need consideration:

- Indication for treatment. Various investigators differ considerably. The more distal the lesions the more strict should be the criteria for intervention.

- The exact technique for the distal angioplasty or open procedure may not be described.

- Handling of combined interventions, that is when different invasive methods have been used on different anatomical locations.
- The frequency and type of adjunctive measures. Various alternative treatments exist. Although important this chapter will not deal with problems related to cessation of smoking or pharmacological methods to increase patency.
- Diagnostic methodology used for follow-up as well as diagnostic criteria used for each method.
- Definition of success and failure. It is often difficult to realize if an intention-to-treat analysis has been performed or if various types of exclusions and drop-outs exist.
- Standards for reporting results may vary. The use of SVS/ISCVS standards are recommended and should be applied.[18,19]

TECHNIQUE

General considerations

A close co-operation between the referring vascular surgeon and the interventional radiologist is of utmost importance. All open and endovascular options must be discussed and a clear plan of treatment established prior to any intervention. Realistic objectives must be set. If the patient's general condition precludes surgical intervention, radiological intervention may offer the sole therapeutic option. This knowledge will considerably influence the approach and extent of any procedure. Where reconstructive surgery remains an alternative, the possible sites for anastomoses should be established. Clearly it is not in the patient's interest if a failed angioplasty compromises the site of distal graft insertion. The patient must be made aware of the aim of intervention, which is often healing of distal ulcers and relief of rest pain and long-term patency is less important. Crural angioplasty is rarely performed in isolation. Optimal inflow is necessary to ensure good distal flow and therefore proximal lesions should be treated prior to, or at the same time as the crural lesions.

Procedure

The optimal technique of crural angioplasty has never been clearly established and practice varies significantly between operators, institutions and countries. In most cases an antegrade approach is preferred by direct cannulation of the ipsilateral common femoral artery. A contralateral approach, however, is equally possible, especially with the advent of flexible support sheaths which can be passed across the aortic bifurcation. The contralateral approach may be of particular use in patients who have undergone thrombolytic therapy using the contralateral approach as this avoids a second puncture into the common femoral artery on the affected side. However, choice of approach is largely governed by the complexity and distribution of the crural lesions.

In general terms, the antegrade approach allows better directional control of guidewire and catheter postion and procedure times are reduced. A variety of catheter and guidewire systems are now available. Proximal crural lesions can be adequately dealt with using a 0.035 inch system and standard 5F PTA balloon catheters. More distal tibial lesions may be more appropriately managed using low profile 0.018 inch based systems with balloon diameters as small as 2mm, which are available in lengths of up to 8cm. After preliminary angiography, a bolus dose of 5000 units of heparin is administered. The choice and sequence of lesions to be angioplastied will vary widely between patients and clearly, where possible, maximum revascularization should be performed at each attendance. In the case of short and proximal focal stenoses, it may be possible to deal with each of the three crural vessels in turn. However, in more advanced cases the single vessel which provides remaining run-off may have to be recanalized over a considerable length. Balloon angioplasty of short focal stenoses in the crural vessels is rarely problematic. It is important to ensure that the guidewire remains within the main vessel and to avoid cannulation of the muscular branches as this can lead to spasm. Procedure times should be kept to a minimum and balloon inflation times rarely exceed 1 minute.

Recanalization of longer occlusions poses some additional technical problems. Where occlusions are longstanding, transluminal recanalization may be difficult and the technique of subintimal angioplasty, as described by Bolia,[20] may be employed (Fig. 1). The most important limitation of this technique, is in the presence of heavily

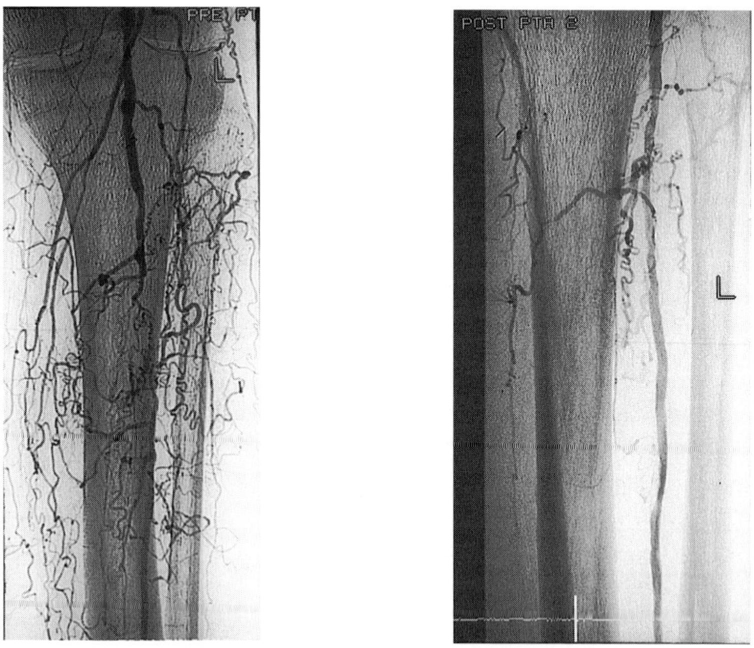

(a) (b)

Fig. 1a, b. Subintimal recanalization of long peroneal occlusion.

calcified vessels, where re-entry into the true lumen distally may be more challenging. When undertaking subintimal angioplasty, it is most important that the operator avoids crossing important collateral vessels by the subintimal channel and this requires both judgement and experience. After angioplasty repeat angiography is undertaken. The guidewire should never be withdrawn across the lesion before the angiography. In the majority of cases, a single balloon inflation will suffice to give a satisfactory angiographic result (Figs 2, 3). However, additional and longer inflations can sometimes be needed in the presence of extensive disease. Spasm may occur following balloon angioplasty and is often recognized by a varying but focal level of occlusion with a smooth appearance. Anti-spasmotic drugs are widely used, but there is little scientific support.

Where two or more crural vessels are selected for angioplasty and the lesions are complex or close to vessel bifurcations, it is sometimes useful to use additional guidewires to protect these vessels (Fig. 4). Generally, the most dominant is selected for angioplasty first of all, and subsequent angioplasties are performed after a satisfactory result at the initial site has been obtained.

It is common to continue heparinization (unfractionated or low molecular weight heparin) following crural angioplasties, particularly where complex or long lesions have been treated. In all cases, long-term aspirin therapy is prescribed unless contraindicated.

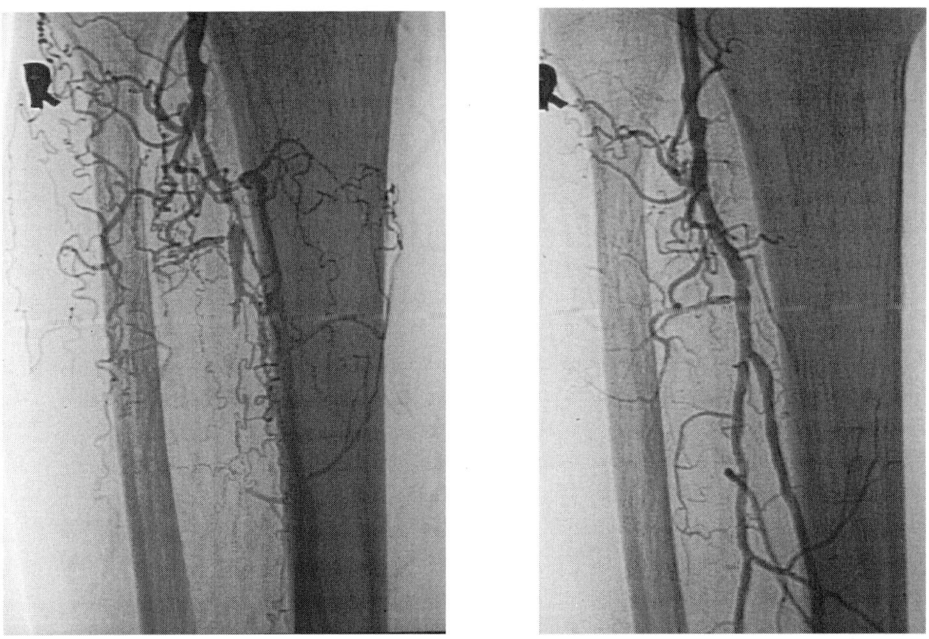

(a) (b)

Fig. 2a, b. Simple crural PTA.

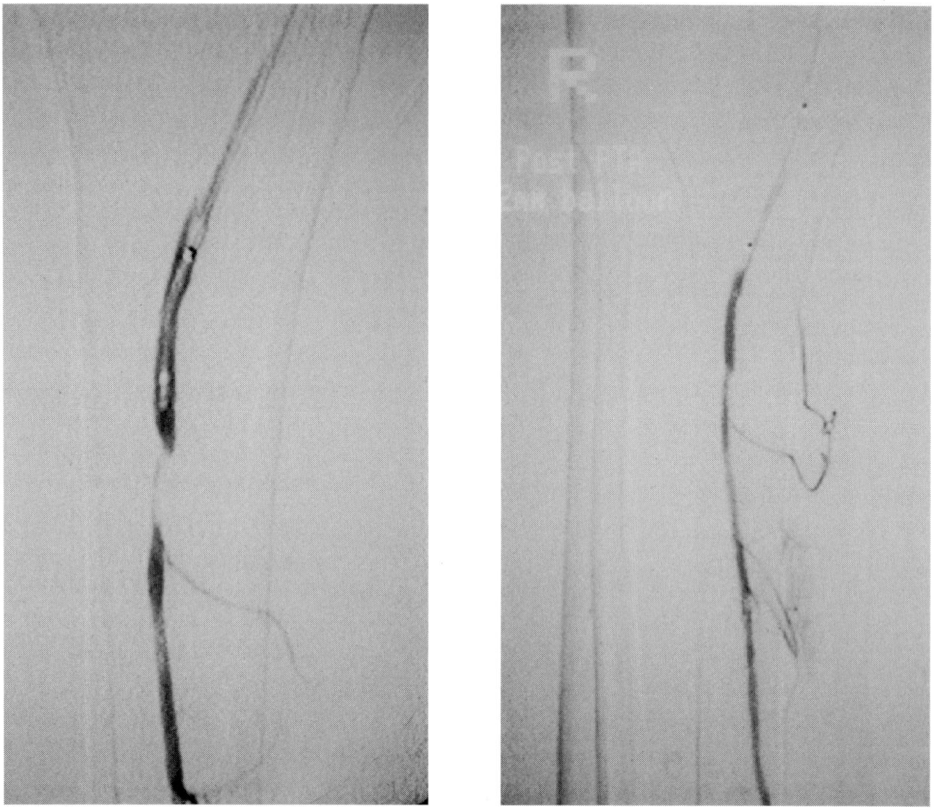

(a) (b)

Fig. 3a, b. PTA beyond femorodistal graft anastomosis.

Complications

PTA site thrombosis is rare but in some cases may require local installation of thrombolytic drugs. A bolus of 3-5mg rt-PA is often sufficient to disperse any acute thrombosis. If more extensive thrombotic occlusion is seen, low dose infusion of rt-PA (0.5mg/h) may be necessary. Dissection at the site of angioplasty is rare but may be catastrophic especially in the setting of single vessel run-off. In the first instance, more prolonged balloon inflations across the site of intimal disruption may be all that is needed to produce a satisfactory angiographic result. This may be unsuccessful and in rare instances the use of coronary stents will maintain patency at the angioplasty site. This is rarely, however, a long-term solution and early femorodistal bypass must be considered. In the case of attempted recanalization of long occlusions, vessel perforation or rupture may rarely occur. In these cases, there is no option but to discontinue the procedure.

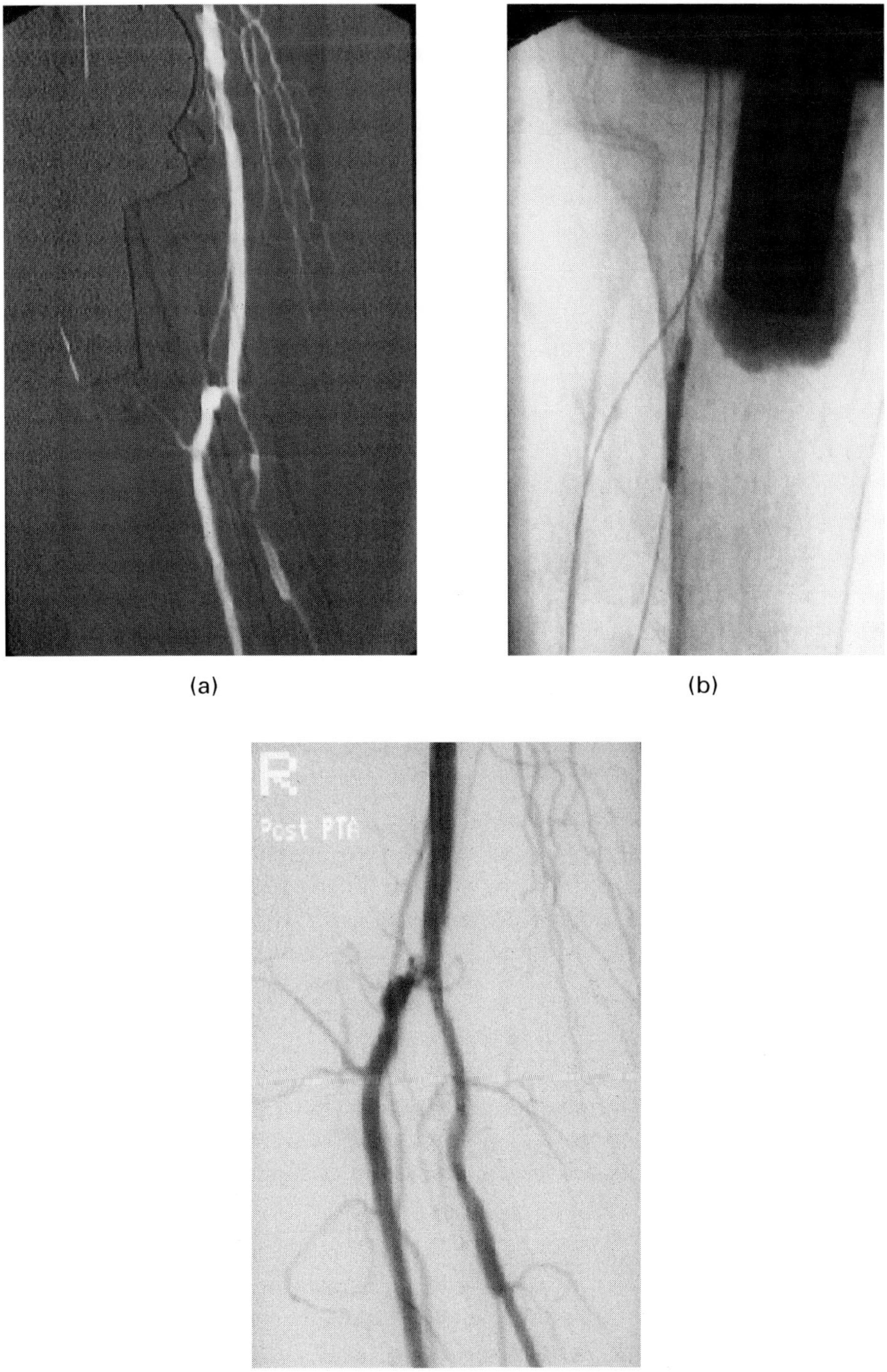

(a) (b) (c)

Fig. 4a, b, c. Complex crural PTA with double guidewires.

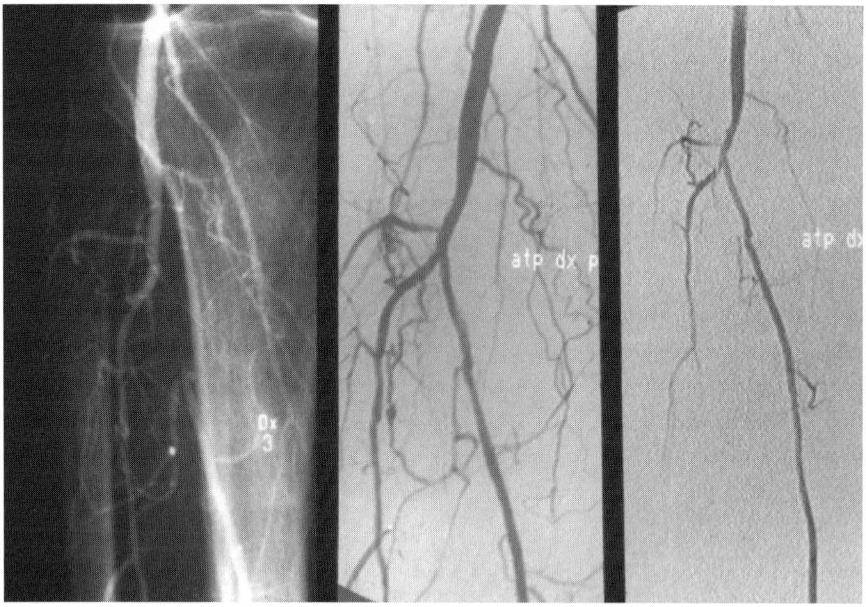

Fig. 5. PTA of posterior tibial artery occlusion with open artery at immediate control and at angiography after 2 years.

ISOLATED RUN-OFF PTA (FIG. 5)

Only few series analysed this treatment alone and in most publications it is presented in combination with a simultaneous proximal reconstruction.

In Table 1 reported publications are listed. The majority of series are small. The outcome after run-off PTA is poor in most publications but the results show wide variations. Parsons *et al.*[21] have published the largest series with a 1-year patency of only 13%. They concluded that 'PTA should not be considered as a primary treatment modality for patients with infrainguinal occlusive disease who also have limb threatening ischaemia, except in unusual circumstances'. The conclusion seems reasonable. On the other hand, in some patients with critical limb ischaemia the use of the simple therapeutic modality of crural artery PTA might be the primary choice of treatment in case of localized stenosis or segmental short occlusions.

SECONDARY RUN-OFF PTA THROUGH A PATENT PROXIMAL RECONSTRUCTION (FIGS 3, 6)

This approach is sometimes chosen to save a proximal reconstruction, when distal lesions are diagnosed at follow-up in a surveillance programme to detect asymptomatic stenoses.[10] It is not the aim of this chapter to deal with the value of graft surveillance. Different opinions exist, which has been discussed in previous Charing Cross symposia.[22,23]

Table 1. Studies on run-off PTA without combination with a simultaneous reconstruction

Author	*No of patients*	*No of lesions*	*Follow-up*	*Patency (%)*		*Limb-salvage*
				Primary	*Secondary*	
Criado *et al.*[5]	26	36	23 months			80
Löfberg *et al.*[32]	39		36 months (life table)	36		72
Durham *et al.*[33]	8	8	17 months			77
Favre *et al.*[34]	12		15 (3–61) months	46a(2 years)		
Callum *et al.*[35]	18		18 (1–48) months	38[a]	54	82
Wack *et al.*[36]	30	42	10.3 (1–35) months			82
Häuser *et al.*[37]	44	70	13.3 (1–50) months			77
Parsons *et al.*[21]	66	?	12 months	13 (1 year)		
Bolia *et al.*[20]	21	29	4 weeks			79
Brown *et al.*[38]	23	?	24 months (life table)			60

[a]In the patency calculation patients with a proximal reconstruction are also included

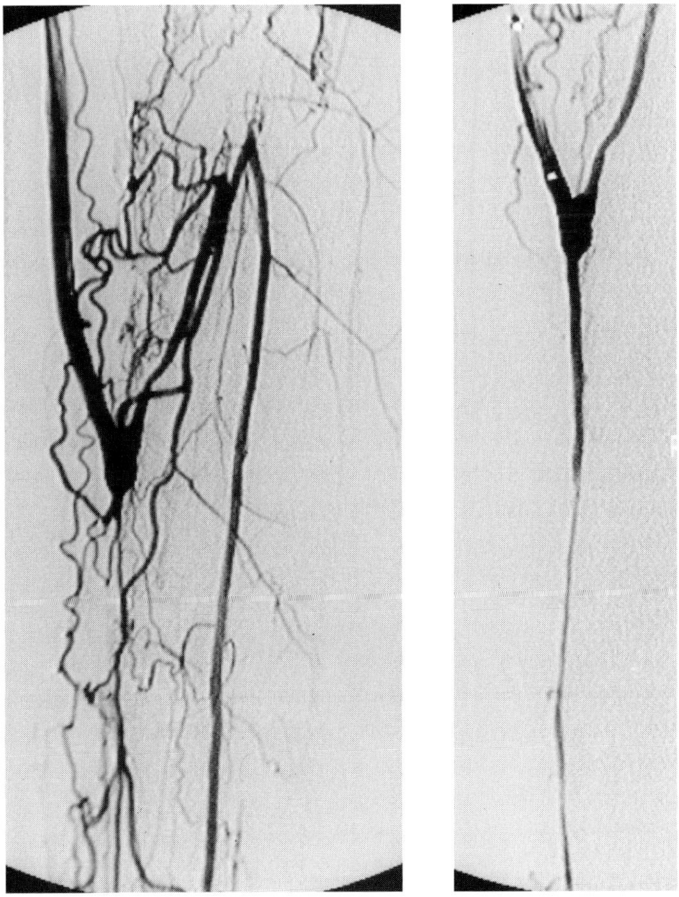

(a) (b)

Fig. 6a, b. PTA of an occluded posterior tibial artery distal to the distal anastomosis of a bypass.

The majority of the lesions detected during graft surveillance are localized within the vein graft itself but sometimes the pathological process is found in the distal anastomosis or distal to it, signifying progression of the arteriosclerotic disease.

In 40 patients (26 males, 21 diabetics, age 72:9 years) with a bypass to below-knee arteries we performed 50 PTA procedures at the distal anastomosis (n=23) or in crural arteries distal to the anastomosis (n=27). In 33 patients there was a more than 50% stenosis and in seven an occlusion. The original indication for surgery was critical limb ischaemia in 35 patients and severe claudication in five. The distal anastomosis was located to the below-knee popliteal artery in 15, anterior tibial artery in ten, posterior tibial artery in eight and peroneal in seven patients. There were 28 vein grafts, ten composite and two prosthetic grafts. The immediate success rate was 80% (n=32), four occluded and four had a remaining stenosis of more than 50%. The mean follow-up time was 14 months (1-72). Two patients died within 30 days and during follow-up a total of 13 died. The overall patency by Kaplan-Meier analysis was 55% at 1 year and 45% at 2 years. Patients with a vein graft reconstruction proximal to the PTA site had a significantly higher 2-year patency than those with a synthetic graft (69 versus 12%; p= 0.014). The run-off situation,[24] the indication for initial treatment, the site of the distal anastomosis, or the site of PTA (whether in the distal anastomosis or distal to it) did not influence patency results. In a Cox regression analysis only smoking negatively influenced the long-term patency. Two patients underwent amputation within 30 days and another two during the follow-up period.

RUN-OFF PTA AFTER REOPENING OF A FAILED BELOW-GROIN BYPASS

There are several mechanisms through which a bypass reconstruction in the below-groin position may fail ending with a thrombotic occlusion. Apart from graft thrombogenicity there may be a stenotic process in the graft or in the outflow tract. Reopening may be obtained by a surgical thrombectomy using a Fogarty catheter but the results are rather dismal.[25] An alternative, at least in recent occlusions (preferably less than 14 days), is thrombolysis. After successful thrombolysis a completion angiography will show a high incidence of lesions causing the occlusion. In these situations it seems reasonable to correct the lesion to avoid reocclusion. The longer the time since the primary arterial reconstruction the more probable that there will be progression of the arteriosclerotic process distally. A run-off PTA may therefore be worthwhile in these instances. Unfortunately, the case series reported below are very small and extremely heterogenous regarding reporting routines. In some publications native vessel and bypass graft occlusions are reported jointly. Consequently it is impossible to analyse the results for successfully lysed grafts with or without a run -off correction separately.

Gardiner *et al.*[26] used local thrombolysis in 72 grafts in 62 patients with an initial success rate of 69%, 84% if urokinase was used and 48% if streptokinase. The 1 year patency, using life table analysis, was 60%, the most important prognostic factor being the presence of a surgical (n=11) or endovascular (n=14) correctable lesion (86% versus 37%). Graft material, graft age and localization of anastomosis had no influence on patency after thrombolysis.

A similar initial success rate (33 of 45;77%) was reported by Rickard *et al.*[27] Of the 33 early successes 22 (67%) required further run-off PTA (in eight of which some form of surgical correction was made). The 1-year life table patency was around 8% for polytetrafluoroethylene (PTFE) grafts and around 45% for vein grafts. An even higher frequency of post-thrombolytic lesions causing occlusion was reported by Hye *et al.*,[17] 35 of 37 grafts or 95%. Anastomotic stenoses dominated and balloon angioplasty was used to correct the lesions in the majority. Although the number of procedures was small, the authors found support to speculate that grafts occluding within 1 year were likely to be suboptimal and should be replaced, whereas grafts occluding after more than 1 year should be treated with thrombolysis in combination with run-off or anastomosis reconstruction, most often PTA. This view has also gained support by other authors.[28–30] Vein grafts seem to fare worse than synthetic grafts after occlusion and local thrombolysis.[17,30] Thus, Hye *et al.*[17] found a mean secondary patency after thrombolysis of 24:6 months for PTFE grafts and 8:2 months for autologous vein grafts.

There is one prospective randomized study comparing thrombolysis and surgery of 124 occluded lower extremity bypass grafts.[16] Unfortunately, it is not possible to separately analyse the effect of run-off PTA on the outcome in this study.

Misra[31] combined graft thrombolysis with an endovascular thromboembolytic catheter endarterectomy for run-off correction in 15 occluded grafts (eight distal occlusions, seven distal stenoses of 90–99% and one anastomotic stenosis). All but one were open at 1-year follow-up.

CONCLUSION

Solid scientific evidence to allow conclusions whether run-off PTA is worthwhile is not available. Nonetheless, run-off PTA is used in various clinical situations. Proper randomized studies would be very difficult to perform. Notwithstanding the inherent difficulties with randomized studies, valuable experience could be gained in this field by adherence to proposed reporting standards. Such simple measures would allow for separate evaluation of the run-off PTA issue and for summarizing results from several smaller series. The available evidence lends some support for run-off PTA to prevent occlusion of femoropopliteal arteries and grafts. In addition it seems worthwhile to do run-off PTA after thrombolytic treatment for occlusion of synthetic below-groin grafts.

REFERENCES

1. Dotter CT, Judkins MP: Transluminal treatment of arteriosclerotic obstruction: Description of a new technique and a preliminary report on its application. *Circulation* **30:** 654–670, 1964
2. Sprayregen S, Snideraman KW, Sos TA: Popliteal artery branches: Percutaneous transluminal angioplasty. *Am J Roentgenol* **135:** 945–950 , 1980
3. Veith FJ, Gupta SK, Haidinger KR *et al.*: Changing arteriosclerotic disease patterns and management strategies in lower-limb threatening ischaemia. *Ann Surg* **212:** 402, 1990

4. Källerö S, Bergqvist D, Cederholm C *et al.*: Late mortality and morbidity after arterial reconstruction: The influence of arteriosclerosis in popliteal artery bifurcation. *J Vasc Surg* **2:** 541–546, 1985
5. Criado F, Twena M, Abdul-Khondoud O, Al-Soufi B: What are the indications for endovascular procedures below knee? In: Greenhalgh R (Ed), *Indications in Vascular and Endovascular Surgery* pp. 367–382. London: WB Saunders, 1998
6. Motarjeme A, Keifer JW, Zuska AJ: Percutaneous transluminal angioplasty as a complement to surgery. *Radiology* **141:** 341–346, 1981
7. Kugel R, Pereyra R: Combined femorotibial bypass and distal intraoperative transluminal angioplasty. *J Vasc Surg* **4:** 533–535, 1986
8. Lauber A, Marx A, John H *et al.*: Simultane chirurgische und katetertechnische Revascularisierung der unteren Extremität. *Helv Chir Acta* **60:** 739–741, 1993/94
9. Sanchez LA, Suggs WD, Marin ML *et al.*: Is percutaneous balloon angioplasty appropriate in the treatment of graft and anastomotic lesions responsible for failing vein bypasses? *Am J Surg* **168:** 97–101, 1994
10. Lundell A, Lindblad B, Bergqvist D, Hansen F: Femoropopliteal-crural graft patency is improved by an intensive surveillance program: A prospective randomized study. *J Vasc Surg* **21:** 26–34, 1995
11. Rutherford RB, Baker JD, Ernst C *et al.*: Recommended standards for reports dealing with lower extremity ischemia: revised version. *J Vasc Surg* **26:** 517–538, 1997
12. Tønnesen KH, Holstein P, Rordam L *et al.*: Early results of percutaneous transluminal angioplasty (PTA) of failing below-knee bypass grafts. *Eur J Vasc Endovasc Surg* **15:** 51–56, 1998
13. Gardiner GA Jr, Sullivan KL: Catheter-directed thrombolysis for the failed lower extremity bypass graft. *Semin Vasc Surg* **5:** 99–103, 1992
14. Nackman GB, Walsh DB, Fillinger MF *et al.*: Thrombolysis of occluded infra-inguinal vein grafts: Predictions of outcome. *J Vasc Surg* **25:** 1023–1032, 1992
15. Kroese A, Staxrud L, Sandbaeck G: When should we lyse an occluded femoropopliteal bypass? In: Greenhalgh RM (Ed), *Indications in Vascular and Endovascular Surgery* pp. 389–405. London: WB Saunders, 1998
16. Comerota AJ, Weaver FA, Hosking JD *et al.*: Results of a prospective, randomized trial of surgery versus thrombolysis for occluded lower extremity bypass grafts. *Am J Surg* **172:** 105–112, 1996
17. Hye JR, Turner C, Valji K *et al.*: Is thrombolysis of occluded popliteal and tibial bypass grafts worthwhile? *J Vasc Surg* **20:** 588–597, 1994
18. Rutherford R: Standards for evaluating results of interventional therapy for peripheral vascular disease. *Circulation* **83**(Suppl 1): 6–11, 1991
19. Ahn S, Rutherford R, Becker GJ *et al.*: Reporting standards for lower extremity arterial endovascular procedures. *J Vasc Surg* **9:** 1103–1107, 1993
20. Bolia A, Sayers RD, Thompson MM, Bell P: Subintimal and intraluminal recanalisation of occluded crural arteries by percutaneous balloon angioplasty. *Eur J Vasc Surg* **8:** 214–219, 1994
21. Parsons RE, Suggs WD, Lee, JJ *et al.*: Percutaneous transluminal angioplasty for the treatment of limb threatening ischemia: Do the results justify an attempt before bypass grafting? *J Vasc Surg* **28:** 1066–1071, 1998
22. Lennox AF, Wolfe J: Vein graft surveillance is worthwhile. In: Greenhalgh RM (Ed), *The Durability of Vascular and Endovascular Surgery* pp. 317–331. London: WB Saunders, 1999
23. Kirby PL, Davies A: Vein graft surveillance could be overrated. In: Greenhalgh RM (Ed), *The Durability of Vascular and Endovascular Surgery* pp. 333–341. London: WB Saunders, 1999
24. Karacagil S, Almgren B, Bowald S, Eriksson I: Angiographic criteria for prediction of early graft failure of secondary infrainguinal bypass surgery. *J Vasc Surg* **12:** 131–138, 1990
25. Graor RA, Risius B, Young JR *et al.*: Thrombolysis of peripheral arterial bypass grafts: Surgical thrombectomy compared with thrombolysis. *J Vasc Surg* **7:** 347–355, 1988
26. Gardiner GA, Harrington DP, Koltun W *et al.*: Salvage of occluded arterial bypass grafts by means of thrombolysis. *J Vasc Surg* **9:** 426–431, 1989

27. Rickard MJFX, Fisher CM, Soong CV *et al.*: Limitations of intra-arterial thrombolysis. *Cardiovasc Surg* **5:** 634–640, 1997
28. Durham JD, Geller SC, Abbott WM *et al.*: Regional infusion of urokinase into occluded lower-extremity bypass grafts: Long-term clinical results. *Radiology* **172:** 83–87, 1989
29. Ikeda Y, Rummel MC, Bhatnagar PK *et al.*: Thrombolysis therapy in patients with femoropopliteal synthetic graft occlusion. *Am J Surg* **171:** 251–254, 1996
30. Nackman GB, Walsh DB, Fillinger MF *et al.*: Thrombolysis of occluded infrainguinal vein grafts: Predictors of outcome. *J Vasc Surg* **25:** 1023–1032, 1997
31. Misra HP: Revascularization of the limbs with urokinase and TEC catheter endarterectomy for occluded bypass grafts. *Am J Surg* **166:** 756–759, 1993
32. Löfberg A-M, Lörelius L-E, Karacagil S *et al.*: The use of below-knee percutaneous transluminal angioplasty in arterial occlusive disease causing chronic limb ischaemia. *Cardiovasc Intervent Radiol* **19:** 317–322, 1996
33. Durham JR, Horowitz JD, Wright JG *et al.*: Percutaneous transluminal angioplasty of tibial arteries for limb salvage in the high-risk diabetic patient. *J Vasc Surg* **8:** 48–53, 1994
34. Favre JP, Do Carmo G, Adham M *et al.*: Results of transluminal angioplasty of infra-popliteal arteries. *J Cardiovasc Surg* **37:** 33–37, 1996
35. Callum K, Abdul-Hamid MA, Nash R *et al.*: Is popliteal and tibial angioplasty effective for critical ischaemia? In: Greenhalgh RM (Ed), *The Durability of Vascular and Endovascular Surgery* pp. 49–60. London, WB Saunders, 1999
36. Wack C, Wölfle KD, Loeprecht H *et al.*: Perkutane Ballondilatation bei isolierten Läsionen der Unterschenkelarterien mit kritischer Beinischämie. *VASA* **23:** 30–34, 1994
37. Häuser H, Bohndorf K, Wack CH *et al.*: Perkutane transluminale Angioplastie (PTA) isolierter Unterschenkelarterienstenosen bei kritischer arterieller Verschlusskrankheit. *Fortschr Röntgenstr* **164:** 238–243, 1996
38. Brown KT, Moore ED, Getrajdman GI, Saddekni S: Infrapopliteal angioplasty: Long-term follow-up. *J Vasc Intervent Radiol* **4:** 139–144, 1993

Endovascular correction of pseudoaneurysm

Hans O Myhre, Jan Lundbom, Jarlis Wesche, Staal Hatlinghus

INTRODUCTION

A pseudoaneurysm is a localized arterial dilatation caused by interruption of the elements forming the arterial wall. In some cases there may even be a pulsatile mass surrounded by fibrous, muscular or subcutaneous tissue only. Pseudoaneurysms can occur following traumatic arterial injuries, dissection, infection, or they can be located to the anastomosis of a previous vascular reconstruction (anastomotic false aneurysms).[1–3] Pseudoaneurysms occurring as a complication of dissection are often called false channel aneurysms.[4] Further, pseudoaneurysm formation is seen following thrombendarterectomy. The cause of anastomotic pseudoaneurysms is multifactorial and includes disintegration of the suture material, graft dilatation, stress at the anastomosis from compliance mismatch, degeneration of the host arterial wall and arterial hypertension. The incidence of this type varies between 2.8–6.7% in the literature depending upon the method of diagnosis.[1, 5–6]

Pseudoaneurysms of the aorta and iliac arteries are located in the retroperitoneal space, and can enlarge undetected in contrast to pseudoaneurysms with a more superficial location. Such factors may influence the indication for intervention. In general, conservative management should only be recommended when the pseudoaneurysm is accessible and when there is no evidence of aggressive enlargement. Recently, endovascular surgery has been introduced in the treatment of pseudoaneurysms and the purpose of this review is to evaluate this treatment modality based on our own experience and a review of the literature.

PREOPERATIVE EVALUATION

Prior to endovascular treatment the diameter and length of the lesion must be thoroughly evaluated. Neighbour arteries must be included in this investigation since a good proximal and distal point of fixation for the endograft is critical. Therefore the patient should undergo arteriography and computed tomography (CT) scans, while magnetic resonance imaging/angiography (MRI/MRA) and intravascular ultrasound are used on a selective basis. For pseudoaneurysms in superficial locations, colour-coded duplex scanning may be helpful. A careful preoperative evaluation of the arterial anatomy is essential for selection of a proper endograft, and for planning of the procedure.

The demand for an endoprosthesis of suitable size and design is perhaps even greater when used for pseudoaneurysm repair than for atherosclerotic aneurysmal disease. Improvization is often necessary, and the graft must be tailored according to the local anatomical conditions. For repair of small defects of the arterial wall, rather than larger lesions, flexible endografts can be accepted. Also the access must be planned and the vessel diameter measured. Consideration of arterial stenoses, tortuosity and kinking are important factors in the positioning and manipulation of the delivery system. Stenotic lesions can usually be dilated. Introducer systems up to 24 French (F) can usually be advanced via an arteriotomy of the common femoral artery. The different introducer systems must also be evaluated and various options are available. One can use introducer systems which can be placed in a proper position before the graft is inserted (Cook® Inc. Bloomington, IN, USA). They are flexible, but at the same time stiff enough in the longitudinal direction to avoid kinking. Furthermore, there are systems where the endoprosthesis is preloaded (Vanguard® Boston Scientific Corp. Natick, MA, USA. Talent®, World Medical Sunrise, FL, USA.) These systems are on the other hand somewhat stiffer. Finally, there are systems whereby the introducer is only inserted a short distance into the arterial tree and the endoprosthesis is introduced on a guidewire and advanced to cover the defect (Excluder® WL Gore & Associates, Flagstaff, AZ, USA). As in all preoperative evaluation, the patient's general medical condition should be taken into consideration before the indication for intervention is settled.

For practical purposes, mycotic aneurysms are included in this review. Although mycotic aneurysms in different arterial segments have been treated successfully by endovascular technique,[7,8] the possibility of infection must be thoroughly investigated.[9] Prior to selection of treatment modality, body temperature and erythrocyte sedimentation rate (ESR) as well as C-reactive protein (CRP) are recorded; CT scans and MRI could show a fluid collection or gas close to a previously inserted graft in case infection is present. Blood cultures should be taken when indicated. Some centres use neutrophil-specific white blood cell scans as the preferred method for diagnosing graft infection. Some cases of low grade infection hardly show any signs or symptoms at all. A disadvantage with the endovascular technique is that intraoperative microscopic evaluation as well as material for culture is difficult to obtain.

THORACIC AORTA

In this anatomic region pseudoaneurysms may occur following deceleration injuries usually affecting the descending thoracic aorta close to the orifice of the left subclavian artery. Furthermore, pseudoaneurysms may occur as a complication of aortic dissection (false channel aneurysm) and after previous operations for thoracic aortic aneurysms. Treatment by endovascular technique for such lesions has been reported,[10–16] even in mycotic aneurysms.[8]

The technique for treating pseudoaneurysms of the descending thoracic aorta is similar to that used for the management of atherosclerotic aneurysms in the same area. The procedure is carried out under general anaesthesia with fluoroscopic guidance in a fully equipped operating theatre; the patient should be prepared as for open surgery in case conversion becomes necessary. Our preference for repair of pseudoaneurysms of the descending thoracic aorta has been a 'home-made' endoprosthesis (Fig. 1) consisting of woven, uncrimped thin-walled polyester (Cooley Verisoft® Meadox Medicals Inc. Oakland NJ, USA) with Gianturco Z-stens® (Cook) sutured on the inside. The graft is tailored after careful preoperative measurement of the descending thoracic aorta. Usually, grafts of 15cm length are applied. For longer defects a second or third graft is applied with at least 3–4cm of overlapping. We prefer at least 2–3mm oversizing of the transverse diameter depending upon the type of endograft. Transoesophageal echocardiography is applied for accurate positioning of the stent-graft. Through a transverse arteriotomy of the common femoral artery, a 20–24 F Cook introducer is advanced into the artery, and pushed upwards into the thoracic aorta over a superstiff guidewire. A second guidewire or a catheter is also introduced from the brachial artery to define the exact position of the orifice of the subclavian artery, and make accurate deployment of the proximal part of the endograft easier.

During endovascular repair of the thoracic aorta, angulation of the aorta distal to the left subclavian artery must be taken into consideration when planning the procedure. This angulation seems to be more pronounced in elderly patients. At this stage, the inner dilator is removed from the introducer. The endograft is placed within the introducer and advanced to the proper position by a pushing mandril.

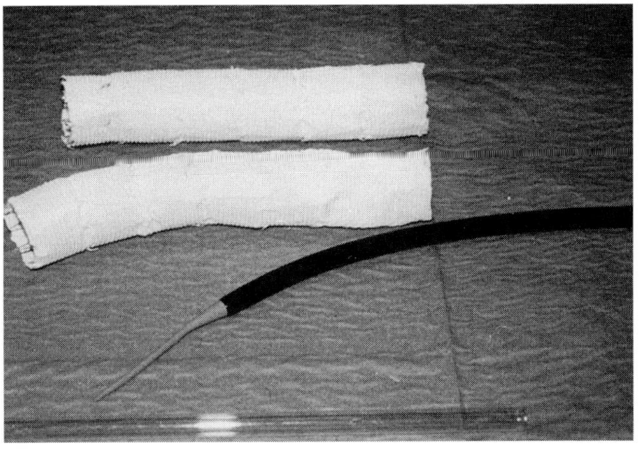

Fig. 1. Endoprosthesis made of polyester where Z-stents have been sutured on the inside. These endografts can be tailored according to the anatomy of the lesion. Also the introducer system is shown.

During deployment of the prosthesis the systolic blood pressure is decreased to about 60–80mm of mmHg by intravenous infusion of sodium nitroprusside. While the pusher is kept in place and the introducer removed, the endograft will expand. A post-deployment angiogram is obtained to control the position of the prosthesis. Both fluoroscopy and transoesophageal echocardiography are used to check for endoleaks. If present they should be repaired by an additional stent-graft during the same procedure. The orifice of the left common carotid artery should be identified and must not be covered by the endoprosthesis. However, the orifice of the left subclavian artery can be covered if the lesion is close to this artery. Revascularization of the subclavian artery for instance by a carotid–subclavian bypass may then be recommended. With this technique, the thoracic aorta can be excluded from the subclavian artery to the coeliac axis. It is likely that the rate of paraplegia and paraparesis is lower with this method than with open surgery.

In patients with false channel aneurysms as a complication of type B dissections, open surgery represents a major challenge with a relatively high morbidity and mortality rate.[4] In such cases, the entry of the dissection if patent, as well as the false aneurysm itself can usually be covered by an endoprosthesis.[13–15] (Figs 2, 3). In these patients we use the same technique as described for regular pseudoaneurysms.

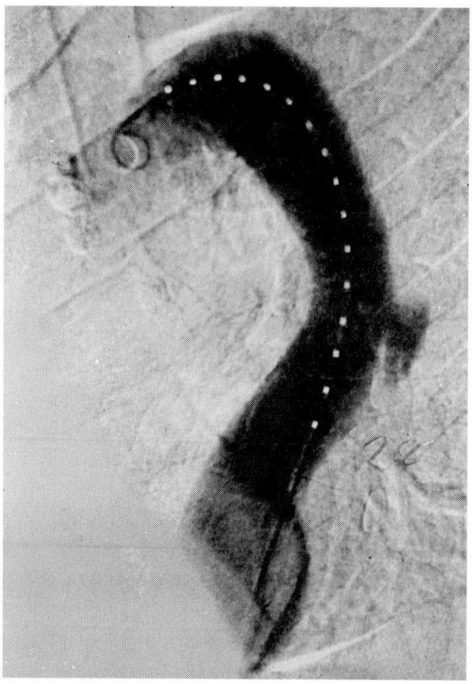

Fig. 2. Angiography of a patient with a false channel aneurysm occurring as a complication following a type B aortic dissection.

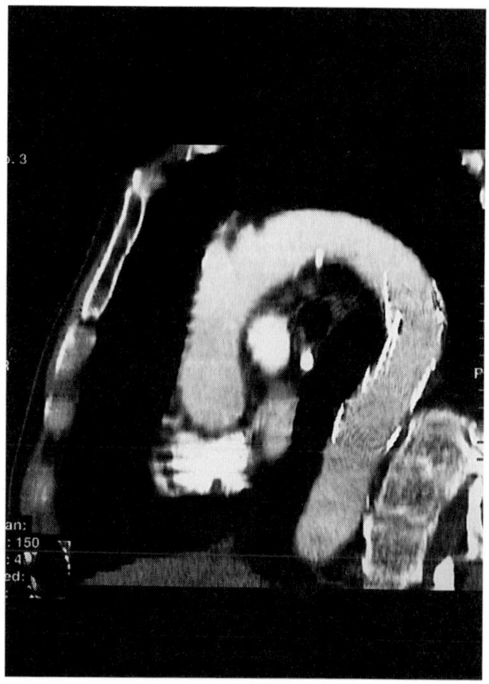

Fig. 3. CT scan from the patient described in Fig. 2. An endoprosthesis covers the orifice of the false channel aneurysm which has now been excluded from the circulation.

Post-traumatic pseudoaneurysms of the thoracic aorta are easily treated by the endovascular technique provided there is a neck of near-normal aorta of about 20mm from the left subclavian artery.[11,12,16] Traumatic lesions are usually of limited extent and are therefore ideal for endovascular repair from an anatomical point of view. Many of these patients are often young and we still do not know how these endoprostheses will perform in the long term. However, open surgery in these patients is often complicated, especially if there are multiple concomitant trauma. The application of extracorporeal circulation with heparinization may, in such cases, induce serious haemorrhage.

Even mycotic aneurysms of the thoracic aorta have been repaired by endovascular technique, and 24 months of observation time has been reported.[8] In spite of prolonged antibiotic therapy, one could suspect that the endoprosthesis might become infected in the long term. If, however, satisfactory long-term results can be obtained, endovascular technique offers definite advantages compared with open surgery in this group of patients.

CAROTID, INNOMINATE AND SUBCLAVIAN ARTERIES

Pseudoaneurysm formation of the carotid, the innominate and subclavian arteries is relatively rare. They can occur following closed trauma, percutaneous catheterization, and as a complication of previous vascular surgery. Pseudoaneurysms have also been observed following extensive surgery for malignancies of the neck, especially if irradiation therapy has been applied in the same area.[17] Several techniques have been applied in this region and even in cases of infection, endovascular treatment has been successfully applied. In those cases the defect has been bridged by a Palmaz® stent (Johnsen & Johnsen Co Warren NJ, USA) covered by autologous saphenous vein, and access can be obtained via the common femoral or the brachial arteries. Commercially available stent-grafts can be used for non-infected lesions. Perhaps endoprosthesis with the metal stents on the outside should be preferred in this region to minimize the risk of thromboembolic complications.[7, 18]

Post-traumatic pseudoaneurysms of the innominate artery are seen after deceleration injuries. Access to these lesions is obtained via the common carotid artery provided there is a neck of at least 1–1.5cm from the aortic arch. The common carotid artery may usually be clamped without the application of a shunt and a stentgraft or polytetrafluoroethylene prosthesis sutured to a Palmaz® stent[19] can be deployed at the proper position using an introducer on a guidewire. Should the orifice of the subclavian artery be covered by graft material, revascularization of the subclavian artery may be recommended.

For post-traumatic lesions of the subclavian artery, occluding transluminal balloons have been inserted via a remote artery e.g. the common femoral artery and advanced to the subclavian artery.[20] After inflation of the balloon the distal arterial blood pressure is decreased and open surgery then made possible. Coiling of false aneurysms has also been described,[21] but should only be applied as a last resort when

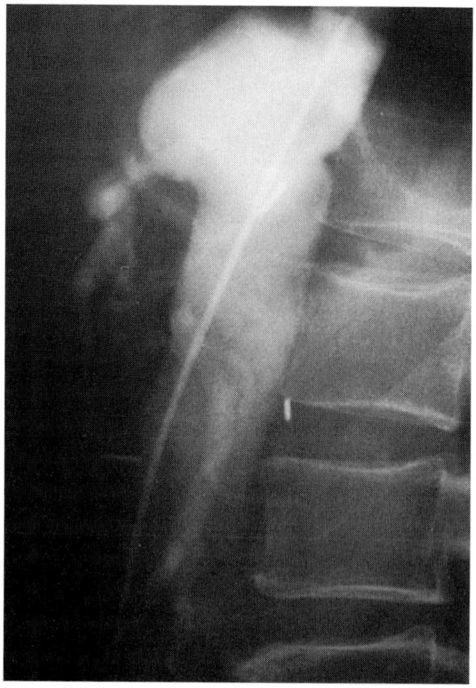

Fig. 4. Pseudoaneurysm formation of the cuff of aortic tissue including the coeliac, superior mesenteric and the renal arteries, in a patient who had been operated on for a type III thoracoabdominal aneurysm 10 years previously. Attempt of repair was made by excluding the diseased part of the aorta with an endoprosthesis applied within the old vascular graft, whereas extra-anatomic bypass was made to the patent visceral arteries.

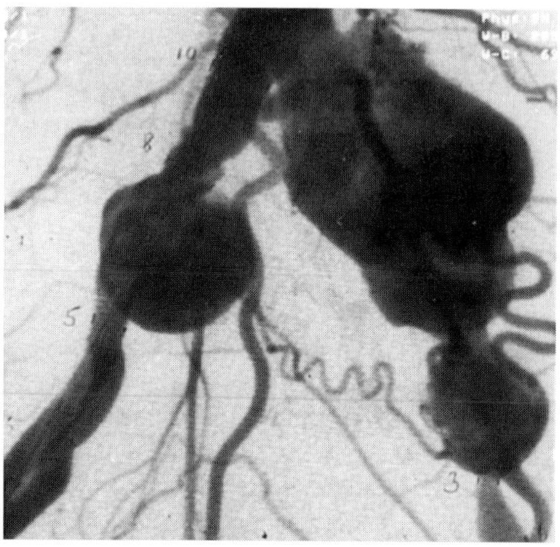

Fig. 5. Pseudoaneurysm formation after endarterectomy of the aorta and the iliac arteries 10 years previously. (From Ref. 25 with permission.)

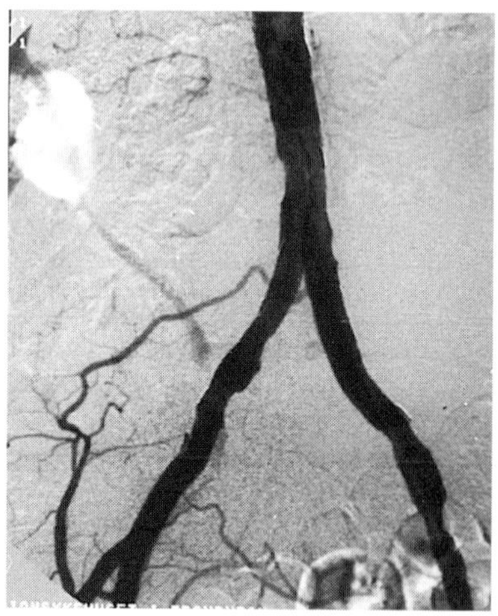

Fig. 6. Angiography from the patient in Fig. 5. Repair has been made by the application of a bifurcated modular endoprosthesis. (From Ref. 25 with permission.)

other possibilities are unavailable, due to the risk of further expansion and rupture of the aneurysmal sack. The most convenient access to lesions of the subclavian artery is usually obtained from the brachial artery. A guidewire is advanced into the proximal part of the subclavian artery and the orifice of the vertebral artery is identified. The endoprosthesis is delivered via a 7–10 F introducer into the brachial artery.[22–24]

PSEUDOANEURYSMS OF THE ABDOMINAL AORTA AND ILIAC ARTERIES

Pseudoaneurysms can occur following thoracoabdominal aneurysmal repair. We have observed this in one patient who was operated on for a type III aneurysm 10 years previously with resection and graft replacement (Fig. 4). The pseudoaneurysm included the cuff of abdominal aorta where the renal arteries, the superior mesenteric artery and the coeliac artery had been anastomosed to a side-hole in the vascular graft. Exclusion of the pseudoaneurysm was performed through an arteriotomy of the left femoral artery and with endovascular application of a 'home-made' stent-graft. In this particular case revascularization was only performed to the right renal artery, which was the only one patent. It is recommended that both renal arteries as well as the superior mesenteric artery and the coeliac axis are revascularized in these cases, this technique can be performed by the application of two bifurcated grafts anastomosed to the iliac arteries. The central part of the visceral arteries should be clip-ligated to avoid retrograde filling of the pseudoaneurysm.

Pseudoaneurysms may also occur following previous thrombendarterectomy of the aorta and the iliac arteries (Fig. 5). This is a rare condition, but is well suited for endovascular treatment.[25] Such repair is attractive since infection is unlikely to be a problem. For pseudoaneurysms of the aorta and the iliac arteries near the bifurcation, a modular bifurcated endoprosthesis is easily applied (Fig. 6).

Following previous aortoiliac graft implantation for aneurysmal or occlusive disease, pseudoaneurysms can occur both at the proximal and the distal anastomosis.[26] At the upper anastomosis, which usually has been performed end-to-end, an important question is whether there is a sufficient neck between the renal arteries and the suture line to allow for good fixation of an endoprosthesis.[27–30] In that case an endograft can be used to seal the leak following proper measurement of the lesion with arteriography and CT-scans. In case the upper anastomosis has previously been performed end-to-side there may be a problem with angulation of the endoprosthesis. If the anastomotic leak is located close to the renal arteries, it may be difficult to apply endoluminal technique. Provided the orifice of the pseudoaneurysm is located at the anterior or dorsal aspect of the anastomosis, one possibility is to bevel the implant so as not to cover the renal arteries, but a more proximal part of the aorta where the pseudoaneurysm is located.[25] Another option is to occlude the orifices of the renal

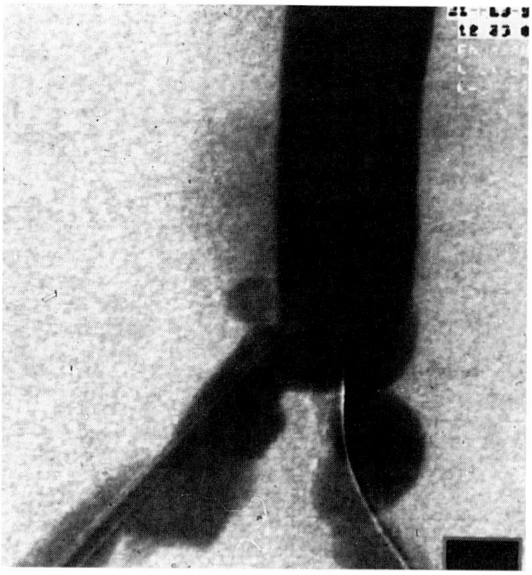

Fig. 7. False aneurysm at the distal anastomosis following insertion of a tube graft for infrarenal abdominal aortic aneurysm.

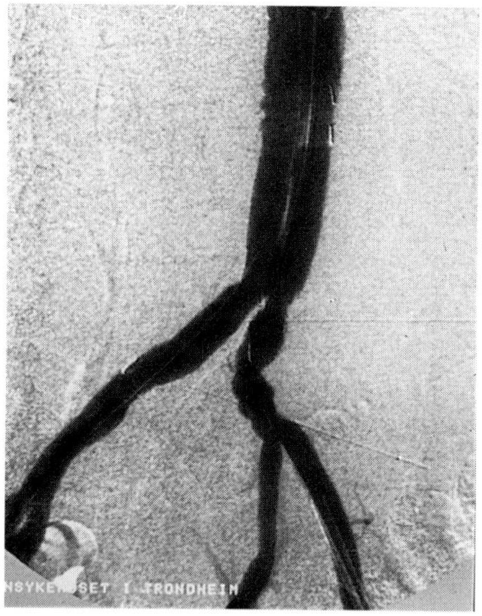

Fig. 8. The lesion described in Fig. 7 has been repaired by the application of a modular bifurcated endoprosthesis. (From ref. 25 with permission.)

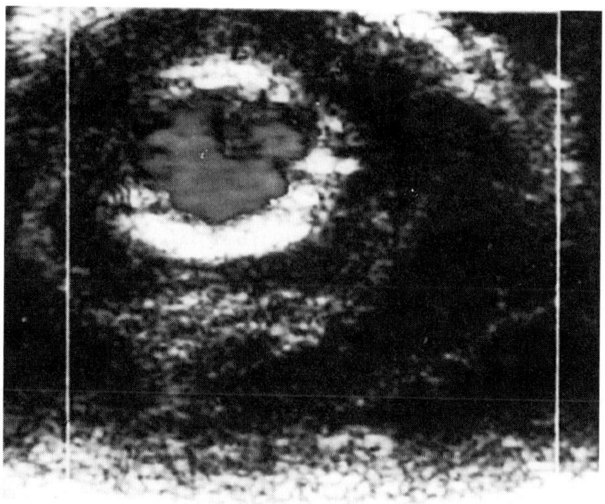

Fig. 9. Ultrasonography showing pseudoaneurysm in the iliofemoral region following insertion of an aortofemoral bypass graft 13 years previously. This pseudoaneurysm was repaired by endovascular technique using retrograde approach and stent-graft. Although a primary successful result was obtained, reocclusion occurred after 8 months necessitating a femorofemoral crossover bypass.

arteries with the endograft supplementing with extra-anatomic bypass. Finally, in selected cases there might be indication for aortouni-iliac tapered grafts to seal pseudoaneurysms of the abdominal aorta.[29] The contralateral common iliac artery is then occluded and a femorofemoral crossover bypass is performed. In the future, it is likely that endoprosthesis with side-arms will be available, in which case an endograft with two side-arms for the renal arteries can be applied for the treatment of pseudoaneurysms at this level.

For pseudoaneurysms at the distal anastomosis of a tube graft, the easiest method of repair is probably the application of a bifurcated modular endograft, which body is placed inside the previously inserted graft, excluding the pseudoaneurysm from the circulation (Figs 7, 8). Pseudoaneurysms at the distal anastomosis of an aortoiliac graft should be treated whenever its diameter is 50% wider than the native artery. Retrograde access through the common femoral artery is preferred for the repair of these lesions.[25,29,31] This method is particularly attractive whenever the primary anastomosis has been performed end-to-end, but it can also be used for end-to-side anastomosis. Provided preservation of blood flow to the internal iliac artery is desirable; a bifurcated graft can be applied, with one limb inserted into the old vascular graft limb, while the other is advanced into the common iliac artery which central part has been closed.

THE FEMOROPOPLITEAL ARTERIAL SEGMENT

One of the most common locations of anastomotic false aneurysms is the common femoral artery when it has been used as the recipient artery for an aortofemoral bypass procedure.[1,2,6] The occurrence is in the order of 3%.[2] There are flexible endografts which can be used for repair of such pseudoaneurysms using an approach from the contralateral femoral artery. However, the orifice of the profunda femoris artery should not be occluded. Provided there is sufficient distance between the lesion and the site of insertion of the introducer sheath, a stent-graft can be applied from the ipsilateral side using retrograde technique. We have repaired pseudoaneurysms at the distal anastomosis following aortofemoral bypass grafting using this technique (Fig. 9). However, this reconstruction occluded after 8 months, and it is our impression that the advantage of endovascular technique for repair of pseudoaneurysms in this region is limited. Usually an open operation for a pseudoaneurysm in the groin is straightforward and is in our opinion the currently preferred method.[3]

Iatrogenic pseudoaneurysms of the femoral artery are observed following various radiological procedures including cardiac catheterization. The incidence is in the order of 0.5%.[32] These patients are usually investigated because of cardiac disease and it is therefore advantageous to apply a method for repair where open operation is avoided. One method is to compress the defect with the probe of a duplex scanner whereby the blood flow into the pseudoaneurysm can be observed and abolished.[33,34] After a period of time, thrombosis of the pseudoaneurysm with subsequent shrinking is obtained. This method is easily applied in the groin and we have experience with successful outcome.

Anastomotic false aneurysms are rare following autologous saphenous vein bypass grafting, but the incidence is somewhat higher following the application of synthetic vascular grafts. Pseudoaneurysms may also occur at the anastomosis of composite grafts.[35] In this site pseudoaneurysms are also seen following trauma or as a complication after previous vascular surgery. The lesions can be repaired by transcutaneous technique using the antegrade route from the femoral artery. One can also expose the femoral artery and apply an endograft via an arteriotomy in the groin. Many of these lesions can be managed by the application of a flexible, commercially available stent graft.[36] In case infection is suspected,[37] repair can be obtained by the application of a Palmaz® stent which has been covered by autologous saphenous vein.[38]

COMPLICATIONS AND PROBLEMS

Following all types of endovascular repair, the patients must be followed with regular intervals since complications like endoleaks may occur. Small early endoleaks may be observed provided there is a good fixation of the endoprosthesis. Major early leaks and late endoleaks must be repaired as soon as they are detected. The patients must be followed by CT-scans and arteriography as necessary, especially if the site of repair is not easily controlled by clinical examination. Other possible complications are graft limb occlusion, a complication which hopefully will be minimized by recent modifications of the endoprosthesis. Migration and kinking of the endoprosthesis are seen, but perhaps to a lesser extent following pseudoaneurysm repair, since the endograft is then not placed within a large aneurysmal sack. The literature on endovascular repair of pseudoaneurysms usually consists of case reports or small series of patients with a maximum observation in the order of 5–7 years. Therefore, we still do not have enough long-term results to draw conclusions about the durability of the implants.

Patients who have been treated for pseudoaneurysms, and where infection may be suspected, should be followed thoroughly. In case of low-grade infection, which is often caused by *Staphylococcus albus*, a considerable time interval can be expected before the infection becomes manifest with clinical signs or symptoms. Patients who are treated for mycotic aneurysms should be followed with shorter intervals, and the duration of antibiotic therapy needs to be defined.

FUTURE ASPECTS

For patients with pseudoaneurysms we still do not know which graft is most suitable for endovascular treatment. A graft that is resistant to infection would be advantageous and perhaps antibiotic-bonded endografts will be available. It is also controversial whether the cover of the stent-graft should be on the inside or on the outside, or whether the stents should be incorporated in the prosthetic wall. The introducers should be flexible, but have enough axial strength to avoid kinking. It is likely that commercial endografts with side-arms will be available in the near future.[39] Such endografts would be useful for repair of pseudoaneurysms close to the renal arteries or to the left subclavian artery. Fenestration technique with the application of covered stents into the main prosthesis should be developed for the connection of side-branches to the main prosthesis. It should be stressed that many of these operations require excellent fluoroscopy equipment that must be available in the operating theatre since the patient should be prepared as for open surgery. Furthermore, complex lesions may require combined procedures including conventional surgery as well as endovascular technique.

REFERENCES

1. Earnshaw J: Anastomotic/false aneurysms. In: Horrocks M (Ed), *Arterial Aneurysms. Diagnosis and Management* pp. 209–220. Oxford: Butterworth–Heineman, 1995
2. Szilagyi DE, Smith RE, Elliott JP *et al.*: Anastomotic aneurysms after vascular reconstruction: Problems of incidence, etiology, and treatment. *Surgery* **78:** 800–816, 1975
3. Ernst CB: The surgical correction of arteriosclerotic femoral aneurysm and anastomotic aneurysm. In: Greenhalgh RM, Mannick JA (Eds), *The Cause and Management of Aneurysms* pp. 245–265. London, Philadelphia: WB Saunders Co., 1990
4. Borst HG, Heinemann MK, Stone CD: *Surgical Management of Aortic Dissection* Edinburgh: Churchill Livingston, 1996
5. Wandschneider W, Bull Ph., Denck H: Anastomotic aneurysms – an unsolvable problem. *Eur J Vasc Surg* **2:** 115–119, 1988
6. Nichols WK, Stanton M, Silver D, Keitzer WF: Anastomotic aneurysms following lower extremity revascularisation. *Surgery* **88:** 366–372, 1980
7. Parodi JC: Endovascular repair of abdominal aortic aneurysms and other arterial lesions. *J Vasc Surg* **21:** 549–557, 1995
8. Semba CP, Sakai T, Slonim SM *et al.*: Mycotic aneurysms of the thoracic aorta: Repair with use of endovascular stent-grafts. *J Vasc Intervent Radiol* **9:** 33–40, 1998
9. Rutter P, Wolfe J: Infected or mycotic aneurysms. In: Horrocks M (Ed), *Arterial Aneurysms Diagnosis and Management* pp. 221–230. Oxford: Butterworth–Heineman, 1995
10. May J, White G, Yu W *et al.*: Endoluminal repair of the atypical dissecting aneurysm of the descending thoracic aorta and fusiform aneurysm of the abdominal aorta. *J Vasc Surg* **22:** 167–172, 1995
11. Vlahakes GJ, Warren RL: Traumatic rupture of the aorta. *New Engl J Med* **332:** 389–390, 1995
12. Lagatolla N, Matson M, Self G *et al.*: Traumatic rupture of the aortic arch treated by stent grafting. *Eur J Vasc Endovasc Surg* **17:** 84–86, 1999
13. Slonim SM, Nyman U, Semba CP *et al.*: Aortic dissection: Percutaneous management of ischemic complications with endovascular stents and balloon fenestration. *J Vasc Surg* **23:** 241–253, 1996
14. Mitchell RS, Dake MD, Semba CP *et al.*: Endovascular stent-graft repair of thoracic aortic aneurysms. *Thorac Cardiovasc Surg* **111:** 1054–1062, 1996

15. Nienaber CH, Fattori R, Lund G *et.al.*: Nonsurgical reconstruction of thoracic aortic dissection by stent-graft placement. *New Engl J Med* **340:** 1539–1545, 1999
16. Deasphande A, Mossop P, Gurry J, Frydman G, Matalanis G, Walker P *et al.*: Treatment of traumatic false aneurysms of the thoracic aorta with endoluminal grafts. *J Endovasc Surg* **5:** 120–125, 1998
17. Myhre HO, Haaverstad R, Dahl T: Irradiation-induced carotid lesions. In: Greenhalgh RM, Hollier LH (Eds), *Surgery for Stroke* pp. 37–43. London: WB Saunders Co., 1993
18. May J, White GH, Waugh R, Brennan J: Endoluminal repair of internal carotid artery aneurysm: A feasible but hazardous procedure. *J Vasc Surg* **26:** 1055–1060, 1997
19. Chandler TA, Fishwick G, Bell PRF: Endovascular repair of a traumatic innominate artery aneurysm. *Eur J Vasc Endovasc Surg* **18:** 80–82, 1999
20. Nemes A, Pintér L, Hüttel K, Biró G, Acsády G: Proximal bleeding control obtained by a balloon catheter in the surgical repair of a left supraclavicular traumatic arteriovenous fistula. *J Vasc Surg* **25:** 587–590, 1997
21. Todd GJ: Complimentary surgical/interventional techniques for non-resective management of "inoperable" aneurysms: A second look. *Ann Vasc Surg* **12:** 248–254, 1998
22. May J, White GH, Waugh R *et al.*: Transluminal placement of a prosthetic graft-stent device for treatment of subclavian aneurysm. *J Vasc Surg* **18:** 1056–59, 1993
23. Marston WA, Criado E, Mauro, M Keagy BA: Transbrachial repair of an axillary artery pseudoaneurysm using a PTFE covered stent. *J Endovasc Surg* **2:** 172–176, 1995
24. May J, White GH, Yu W *et al.*: Endoluminal repair: A better option for the treatment of complex false aneurysms. *Aust NZJ Surg* **68:** 29–34, 1998
25. Lundbom J, Hatlinghus S, Aadahl P, Myhre HO: Endovascular treatment of vascular emergencies and complications following previous vascular surgery. *Eur J Vasc Endovasc Surg* (in press)
26. Treiman GS, Weaver FA Cossman DV *et al.*: Anastomotic false aneurysms of the abdominal aorta and the iliac arteries. *J Vasc Surg* **88:** 268–273, 1988
27. Lindblad B, Ivancev K, Chuter TAM *et al.*: Endovascular exclusion of juxtarenal anastomotic pseudoaneurysm. *Eur J Vasc Endovasc Surg* **12:** 116–118, 1996
28. Ohki T, Veith FJ: Five-year experience with endovascular grafts for the treatment of aneurysmal, occlusive and traumatic arterial lesions. *J Cardiovasc Surg* **6:** 552–565, 1998
29. White RA, Donayre CE, Walot I *et al.*: Endoluminal graft exclusion of a proximal para-anastomotic pseudoaneurysm following aortobifemoral bypass. *J Endovasc Surg* **4:** 88–94, 1997
30. Schönholz C, Donnini F, Naselli G *et al.*: Acute rupture of an aortic false aneurysm treated with a stent-graft. *J Endovasc Surg* **6:** 293–296, 1999
31. Weinberg DJ, Cronin DW, Baker AG: Infected iliac pseudoaneurysm after uncomplicated percutaneous balloon angioplasty and (Palmaz) stent insertion: A case report and literature review. *J Vasc Surg* **23:** 162–166, 1996
32. Roberts SR, Main D, Pinkerton J: Surgical therapy of femoral artery pseudoaneurysm after angiography. *Am J Surg* **154:** 676–680, 1987
33. Dorfman GS, Cronan JJ: Postcatheterization femoral artery injuries: Is there a role for nonsurgical treatment? *Radiology* **178:** 629–630, 1991
34. Fellmeth BD, Roberts AC, Bookstein JJ *et al.*: Postangiographic femoral artery injuries: Nonsurgical repair with US-guided compression. *Radiology* **178:** 671–675, 1991
35. Dorros G, Bates M, Kumar K: Percutaneous deployment of a polytetrafluoroethylene (PTFE) graft to repair a pseudoaneurysm produced by a graft to graft anastomotic dehiscence. *Catheterization Cardiovasc Diag* **32:** 372–375, 1994
36. Criado E, Marston WA, Ligush J *et al.*: Endovascular repair of peripheral aneurysms, pseudoaneurysms, and arteriovenous fistulas. *Ann Vasc Surg* **11:** 256–263, 1997
37. Seabrook GR, Schmitt DD, Bandyk DF *et al.*: Anastomotic femoral pseudoaneurysm: An investigation of occult infection as an etiologic factor. *J Vasc Surg* **11:** 629–634, 1990

38. Schneider PA, Abcarian PW, Leduc JR, Ogawa DY: Stent-graft repair of mycotic superficial femoral artery aneurysm using a Palmaz stent and autologous saphenous vein. *Ann Vasc Surg* **12:** 282–285, 1998
39. Inoue K, Sato M, Iwase T *et al.*: Clinical endovascular placement of branched graft for type B aortic dissection. *J Thorac Cardiovasc Surg* **112:** 1111–1113, 1996

Endoluminal treatment of peripheral aneurysms

Matthew B Matson, Anna-Maria Belli

INTRODUCTION

The traditional treatment for aneurysmal arterial disease has been open surgery in those patients with symptoms or significant clinical risk of complications such as rupture. The most common site for aneurysmal disease is the abdominal aorta, where endovascular treatment has recently emerged as an alternative to open surgery in some patients. Technological advances have made feasible the endovascular treatment of aneurysms at other sites. In some cases this may be achieved percutaneously, while other procedures require surgical cutdown for access, allowing collaboration between surgeon and interventional radiologist in the procedure. The results of endovascular therapy need to be evaluated and compared with those of traditional therapy.

ILIAC ANEURYSMS

Although the second most common site of intra-abdominal aneurysms after the aorta, isolated aneurysms of the iliac arteries are uncommon. A study of 35 265 autopsies in Malmö, Sweden discovered seven iliac artery aneurysms, giving a prevalence of 0.03%, of which one (14%) was ruptured.[1] The relative frequency of isolated iliac artery aneurysms compared with abdominal aortic aneurysms is 0.9–1.9%. They are found more commonly in men (5:1) with advancing age. Multiple aneurysms are reported in 33–66% of patients. In addition to isolated atherosclerotic aneurysms, iliac artery aneurysms are seen at the distal anastomoses of aortoiliac grafts inserted for treatment of abdominal aortic aneurysms, as well as pseudoaneurysms secondary to trauma.

The most important clinical consequence of iliac aneurysms is rupture, the risk of which is related to their size. In one set of authors' patients, the mean aneurysm size was 8.5 cm and rupture occurred in 51% of patients.[2] A later study reported on a group of asymptomatic patients with a mean aneurysm size of 3.4cm, in whom there was a rupture rate of 5.3% after a mean of 4.9 years.[3] The smallest reported ruptured aneurysm in the literature was 3cm.[1]

The operative mortality for treatment of ruptured iliac artery aneurysms is approximately 33%, whereas the mortality of elective operation is reported as 7–11%.[1,4] For this reason, elective treatment is currently recommended for iliac aneurysms when they reach 3cm. Endovascular treatment of iliac artery aneurysms can avoid the morbidity and mortality related to open repair, and has the advantage of being able to be performed under local anaesthetic.

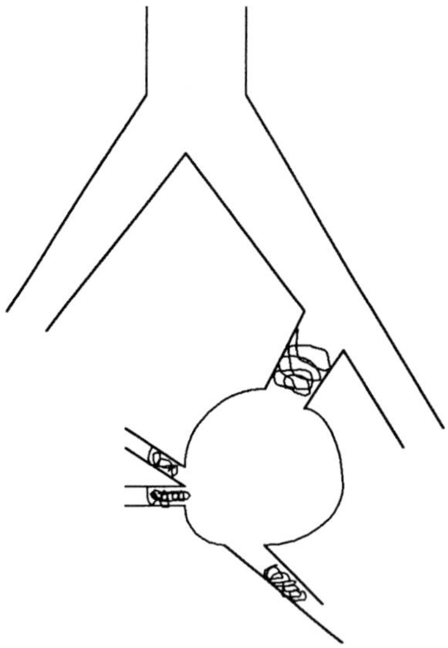

Fig. 1. Treatment of an internal iliac artery (IIA) aneurysm is achieved with coils alone when it is possible to occlude the entry and exit sites without causing limb ischaemia.

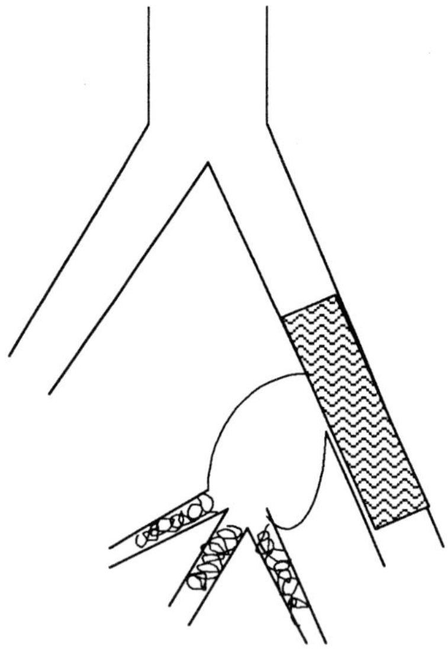

Fig. 2. Where there is no proximal neck to the IIA aneurysm, a stent-graft can be placed across the origin. Backfilling is prevented by placement of coils at the exit sites.

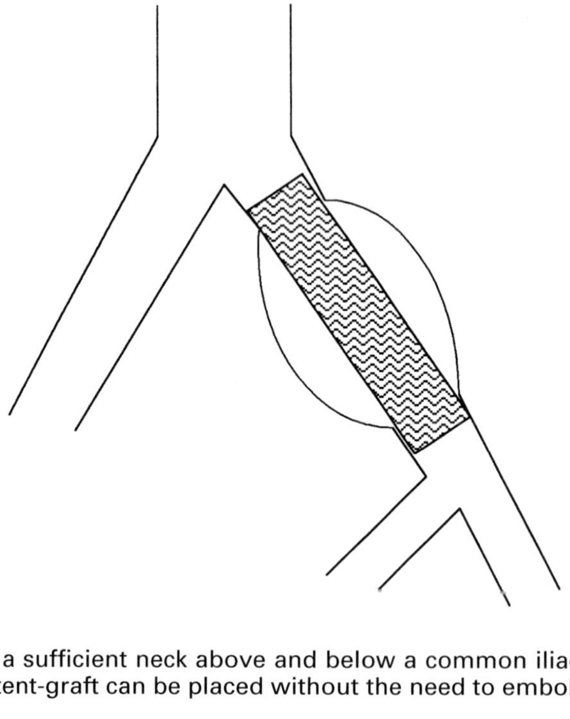

Fig. 3. Where there is a sufficient neck above and below a common iliac artery (CIA) aneurysm, a tubular stent-graft can be placed without the need to embolize the IIA.

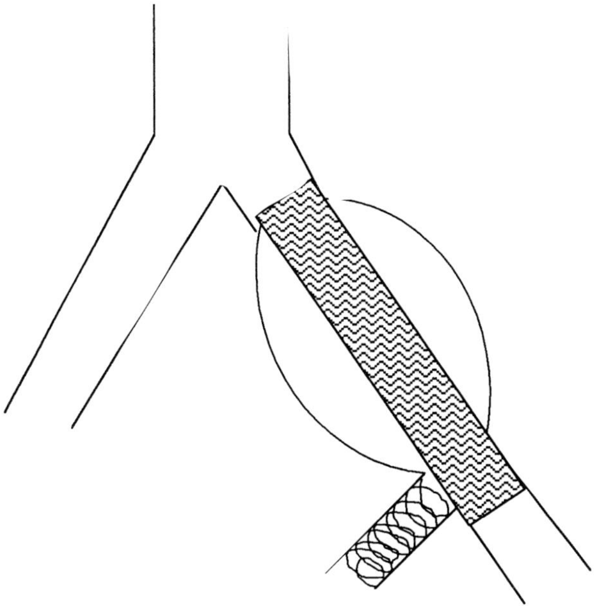

Fig. 4. When the CIA aneurysm extends to the origin of the IIA, a stent-graft can be placed across the origin, but the IIA must be coil embolized to prevent backfilling of the aneurysm sac.

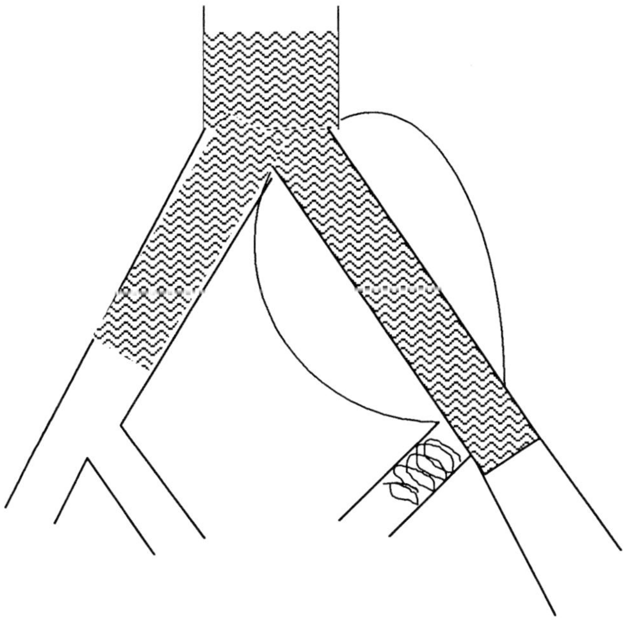

Fig. 5. For a CIA aneurysm extending proximally to the aortic bifurcation, a bifurcated aortic stent-graft can be employed to exclude the aneurysm.

There are various different approaches to the endovascular treatment of iliac aneurysms, dependent upon the site and morphology of the aneurysm. These are illustrated in Figs 1–5, and the underlying principles hold true for endovascular treatment of aneurysms at other sites.

In those situations where it is possible to occlude the entry and exit sites of an aneurysm safely without causing limb ischaemia, direct endovascular coil embolization is the simplest effective option. For example, aneurysms involving only the internal iliac artery can be managed by coil embolization, so long as there is a sufficient neck of normal artery proximal to the aneurysm and the distal artery or branches can be accessed to avoid backfilling. Coil embolization of the proximal internal iliac artery is also required as an adjunct to stent-graft treatment of common or external iliac artery aneurysms, when the stent-graft covers the origin of the internal iliac artery, in order to prevent backfilling. Common and external iliac artery aneurysms clearly cannot be treated by coil embolization without occluding flow to the limb, but have been treated in this way in combination with femorofemoral crossover bypass grafting.

Uncovered stents have been used to treat ulcerated plaques and focal aneurysms of the iliac arteries. The rationale is that the stent compresses the lesion, encourages thrombosis and allows smooth flow within the new lumen with subsequent endothelialization. Vorwerk used uncovered Wallstents to treat 13 ulcerated plaques and five focal aneurysms with a 4-year patency of 82%.[5] However, thrombosis of the sac is not guaranteed with uncovered stents. Furthermore, it is not known whether the sac, despite being thrombosed, remains under endotension and liable to expand when an uncovered stent is used.

Placement of a stent-graft allows exclusion of the aneurysm whilst maintaining flow to the limb. Ipsilateral percutaneous placement is possible with existing devices through 9 or 10F sheaths and technology continues to evolve. Assessment of the aneurysm with thin-section contrast-enhanced computed tomography (CT) scanning allows planning of the procedure. Angiography with a calibrated pigtail catheter is also useful for planning the necessary length of stent-graft required, particularly when the iliac arteries are tortuous. Embolization of the internal iliac artery with coils is necessary before stent-graft placement if the aneurysm involves the origin of the internal iliac artery and the stent-graft is to be placed across the origin. Coil placement within the proximal internal iliac artery, avoiding extension into its branches, is recommended to allow filling of pelvic branches via collaterals. This minimizes the risk of pelvic ischaemia and attempts to avoid painful buttock claudication.

Following stent graft placement, continued follow-up with CT and/or duplex is necessary to detect late complications such as leaks, occlusions or stenoses and to monitor the size of the aneurysm sac following exclusion.

Reported results of endovascular treatment of iliac artery aneurysms have been good, with initial technical success rates of 100% being the rule and patency rates of 90–100% after mean follow-up of 5.5–22 months.[6–9] No aneurysm ruptures have been reported in treated cases, but long-term results of effect on aneurysm sac size are awaited. The most commonly reported complications are late endoleaks, which can often be treated with further stent-graft placement, and late thrombosis. One group successfully lysed a fresh occlusion and placed a further stent successfully. One case of ipsilateral iliac venous thrombosis has been reported as a complication.

FEMOROPOPLITEAL ANEURYSMS

Atheromatous aneurysms of the common femoral artery and proximal superficial femoral arteries are rare. Iatrogenic pseudoaneurysms are far more common following percutaneous puncture. Recently, good results have been obtained for these by percutaneous injection of thrombin or fibrin glue directly into the pseudoaneurysm sac.[10–12] The common femoral artery is a difficult area to treat with stent-grafts as it is difficult to access and is a site of continuous flexion and extension, which leads to kinking of the stent-graft and increases the risk of neointimal hyperplasia and occlusion. Furthermore, placement of a stent-graft means that the femoral artery can no longer be used as a puncture site for access. Conversely, open surgical access is usually straightforward. Beregi treated two iatrogenic common femoral artery aneurysms with stent-grafts deployed via ipsilateral surgical cutdown onto the superficial femoral artery.[8] One case showed persistent leak into the aneurysmal sac and in the other the stent migrated and was removed at 3 days from what was subsequently demonstrated to be an infected aneurysm.

Popliteal artery aneurysms carry a low risk of rupture. The most common clinical presentation is with occlusion or distal embolization into the crural circulation, resulting in amputation in 20–50% of cases. Thrombolysis can be used to open up the distal vessels in acute occlusions. The aim of therapy is to recanalize the crural vessels, not the popliteal artery, and the catheter should be placed appropriately within the infrapopliteal vessels where possible. If patency of the run-off vessels can be restored, the surgical procedure is converted from a high-risk emergency operation to an elective operation with improved clinical outcome. With this approach, the limb salvage rate is approximately 80%, against which endovascular treatment must be judged.

Compared with results in iliac arteries, stents and stent-grafts placed in the superficial femoral and popliteal arteries have lower patency rates owing to smaller vessel size, slower flow and inadequate runoff. Stents within the popliteal artery at the knee joint are also prone to kinking. Nevertheless, in a report of two patients who declined surgery for their popliteal artery aneurysms, both were treated percutaneously from an ipsilateral antegrade puncture with uncovered Wallstents following thrombolysis of the run-off vessels. One required a further stent for a late leak, but both arteries remained patent with exclusion of the aneurysms at 25 and 47 months.[13] Using stent-grafts to treat popliteal aneurysms has obtained excellent short-term results,[8] but other groups have reported significant thrombosis rates in the medium-term, with primary and secondary patency rates of 30% and 43% respectively after 31 months.[14] Anticoagulation is not generally given nor currently recommended by the manufacturers for routine use after stent-graft placement.

INFRAPOPLITEAL ANEURYSMS

Reported cases of infrapopliteal aneurysms are very rare. Coil embolization and temporary balloon occlusion has been described to treat a peroneal artery aneurysm in a patient with Behçet's syndrome.[15] Current commercially available stent-grafts are too large for use in the infrapopliteal vessels.

ANEURYSMS OF THE GREAT VESSELS

Subclavian aneurysms are more often false aneurysms related to trauma than true isolated aneurysms. If a suitable neck is present, endovascular treatment can be with insertion of coils to thrombose and exclude the aneurysm while maintaining patency of the subclavian artery.

If it is not possible to embolize the aneurysm without occluding the vessel, the endovascular options are either to place coils anyway and occlude the subclavian artery or to place a stent-graft. While the former option seems less favourable, it should be remembered that this option will successfully exclude the aneurysm, that collateral formation in this area is good and that stents and stent-grafts in this location are associated with complications. Most experience has been gained with placement of uncovered stents in the subclavian arteries and veins for stenotic disease. Higher blood flow in the subclavian artery compared with the subclavian vein may protect against thrombosis, but both vessels are mobile and compressible between the clavicle and first rib upon arm abduction. This mechanical stress can lead to disruption and breakage of both stents and stent-grafts in the subclavian vein or artery.[16] Surgical resection of the first rib helps prevent this problem, but the vessel mobility remains.[17] Beregi treated five patients with covered stents for subclavian artery aneurysms.[8] Three of these were false aneurysms following trauma and the other two occurred following radiotherapy. Two (40%) remained patent at 22 and 42 months while the remainder thrombosed at 6 months. Other authors have reported single cases of successful treatment of subclavian aneurysms with stent-grafts with good medium-term patency.[18,19]

RENAL ARTERY ANEURYSMS

Renal artery aneurysms are being discovered more often because of modern imaging techniques such as CT. Nevertheless they are rare, with a prevalence of 0.1–0.3% based on studies of angiograms. They are strongly associated with fibromuscular dysplasia and hypertension and less so with atherosclerotic aneurysms at other sites.

The natural history of renal artery aneurysms has been controversial. Early reports suggested a high rate of rupture,[20] but a study of 36 656 autopsies, again from Malmö, found no cases of renal artery rupture and five studies of patients treated conservatively and followed for a mean of 3–10 years revealed no deaths attributable to the aneurysms.[21] Hence there is justification for some restraint when considering treatment of renal artery aneurysms, by endovascular or open technique. Rupture carries a mortality of around 10%; emergency nephrectomy is the life-saving treatment. Risk of rupture is increased in pregnancy and carries a mortality of around 50% for the mother and 80% for the fetus. Recommendations for treatment include dissection causing renovascular hypertension, local symptoms such as flank pain or haematuria, occurrence in pregnant women or women with a potential for pregnancy, thrombus in the sac with distal embolization or an aneurysm shown to be enlarging on serial imaging.[22] Asymptomatic aneurysms smaller than 2cm should be managed conservatively and followed. The management of asymptomatic aneurysms over 2cm is controversial; larger aneurysms and those with no calcification are at a greater risk of rupture.

For proximal aneurysms of the main renal artery, the open surgical technique of choice is *in situ* reconstruction with vein grafts. For focal aneurysms in this location, stent-grafting offers an alternative to open surgical reconstruction, so long as there is enough normal renal artery proximal and distal to the aneurysm. A case report documenting this technique reported aneurysm exclusion at 1 year.[23] For more distal aneurysms affecting the hilum and distal branches, if the neck of the aneurysm is sufficiently small, coil embolization can be performed and for intraparenchymal aneurysms, coil embolization is the treatment of choice. A superselective technique, using small co-axial catheters if necessary, allows treatment of the aneurysm while minimizing loss of functioning renal tissue.

ANEURYSMS OF VISCERAL ARTERIES

The most common site of visceral aneurysms is the splenic artery, accounting for about 60%. They are more common in women, occur most commonly in the distal third of the artery, are generally asymptomatic and carry a risk of rupture of about 2%, increased during pregnancy. Treatment is recommended for symtomatic aneurysms, aneurysms greater than 2cm and those in pregnant women or women with a potential for pregnancy.[24] Coil embolization of the aneurysm and proximal artery has been proposed as a preferred technique to surgery, since it allows preservation of the spleen, which acquires flow distally from collaterals.[25,26] Others recommend endovascular treatment only for older or high-risk patients unsuitable for surgery because of the risk of late rupture or abscess formation.[27]

Other visceral aneurysms arise from the hepatic artery, the superior mesenteric artery and the coeliac artery and its branches. Causes include infection, pancreatitis, vasculitis and trauma. Most will be asymptomatic, but rupture may occur into the gut, biliary tree or peritoneal cavity. In this instance, emergency transcatheter embolization may be life-saving. Possible agents are coils, polyvinyl alcohol or absorbable gelatin sponge. When using coils, it is important to occlude exit and entry sites. Good results can be achieved using embolization as the initial treatment of choice. Major high-risk surgery can be avoided or, if necessary, definitive surgery can be performed electively when the patient is stable.[28]

INFECTED ANEURYSMS AND ANTIBIOTIC PROPHYLAXIS

No data are available upon which to make an evidence-based decision regarding antibiotic prophylaxis. The risk of introducing infection during insertion of coils or stent-grafts percutaneously or through a small arteriotomy is probably very low.

However, the potential consequences are severe. Our practice is to give antibiotic prophylaxis for stent-graft insertion but not for coil insertion alone.

Infected aneurysms have generally been regarded as a contraindication to endovascular treatment, since the introduction of foreign material into an infected system acts as a focus for continued infection. Endovascular treatment of infected thoracic aneurysms in association with antibiotic treatment has been described in three patients.[29] One died of cardiac arrest but the other two remained well without septicaemic complications. However, these patients were unfit for major cardiothoracic surgery, which was the only alternative treatment. In peripheral aneurysms, surgery remains the first-line treatment for infected aneurysms.

SUMMARY

Improvements in catheter design have allowed the interventional radiologist selective access to all major arteries and this, along with advances in stent-graft technology have allowed the endovascular treatment of peripheral artery aneurysms at multiple sites. However, most series concentrate on feasibility and there are still few data on long-term outcomes. Technology continues to improve and the true place of these techniques is yet to be established.

REFERENCES

1. Brunkwall J, Haukusson H, Bengtsson H *et al.*: Solitary aneurysms of the iliac arterial system: an estimate of their frequency of occurrence. *J Vasc Surg* **12:** 219–220, 1990
2. Schuler JJ, Flanigan DP: Iliac artery aneurysms. In: Bergan J, Yao JST (Eds), *Aneurysms: Diagnosis and Treatment* pp. 469–485. New York: Grune & Stratton, 1982
3. McCready RA, Pairolero PC, Gilmore JC *et al.*: Isolated iliac artery aneurysms. *Surgery* **93:** 688–693, 1983
4. Richardson JW, Greenfield LJ: Natural history and management of iliac aneurysms. *J Vasc Surg* **8:** 165–171, 1988
5. Vorwerk D, Günther RW, Wendt G, Schürmann K: Ulcerated plaques and focal aneurysms of iliac arteries: Treatment with noncovered self-expanding stents. *Am J Roent* **162:** 1421–1424, 1994
6. Ruebben A, Tettoni S, Muratore P *et al.*: Percutaneous endoluminal bypass of iliac aneurysms with a covered stent. *Cardiovasc Interven Radiol* **22:** 339–342, 1998
7. Razavi MK, Dake MD, Semba CP *et al.*: *Radiology* **197:** 801–804, 1995
8. Beregi J-P, Prat A, Willoteaux S *et al.*: Covered stents in the treatment of peripheral arterial aneurysms: procedural results and midterm follow-up. *Cardiovasc Intervent Radiol* **22:** 13–19, 1999
9. Lacey NA, Matson MB, Taylor P *et al.*: Management of iliac aneurysms with covered stents: immediate and medium-term outcome. *Cardiovasc Intervent Radiol* **22**(Suppl 2): S114, 1999
10. Kang SS, Labropoulos N, Mansour A, Baker WH: Percutaneous ultrasound guided thrombin injection: a new method for treating post catheterization femoral pseudoaneurysms. *J Vasc Surg* **27:** 1032–1038, 1998
11. Loose HW, Haslam PJ: The management of peripheral artery aneurysms using percutaneous injection of fibrin adhesive. *Br J Radiol* **71:** 1255–1259, 1998

12. Matson MB, Morgan RA, Belli A-M: Percutaneous treatment of pseudoaneurysms using fibrin adhesive. Presented at BSIR, 1999
13. De Blas M, Merino S, Ortiz F *et al.*: Treatment of popliteal artery aneurysms with uncovered wallstents. *Cardiovasc Intervent Radiol* **22:** 336–339, 1999
14. Müller-Hülsbeck S, Link J, Schwarzenberg H *et al.*: Percutaneous endoluminal stent and stent-graft placement for the treatment of femoropopliteal aneurysms: early experience. *Cardiovasc Intervent Radiol* **22:** 96–102, 1999
15. Toyota N, Kimura F, Yoshida S *et al.*: Peroneal artery aneurysm treated by transcatheter coil embolization and temporary balloon occlusion in Behçet's disease. *Cardiovasc Intervent Radiol* **22:** 257–259, 1999
16. Rhodes AI, Gibson M, Al-Katoubi M: Mechanical Disruption of a Wallstent in the subclavian vein between clavicle and first rib. *J Intervent Radiol* **12:** 151–153, 1997
17. Kessel D, Robertson I, Scott J, Phipp L: Re: successful exclusion of subclavian aneurysm with covered nitinol stents (letter; comment). *Cardiovasc Intervent Radiol* **22:** 86–87, 1999
18. Patel AV, Marin ML, Veith FJ *et al.*: Endovascular graft repair of penetrating subclavian artery injuries. *J Endovasc Surg* **3:** 382–388, 1996
19. Szeimes U, Keuffer G, Stoeckelhuber B, Steckmeier B: *Cardiovasc Intervent Radiol* **21:** 246–249, 1998
20. Cerny JC, Chang C, Fry WJ: Renal artery aneurysms. *Arch Surg* **96:** 653-663, 1968
21. Tham G, Ekelund L, Herrlin K *et al.*: Renal artery aneurysms: natural history and prognosis. *Ann Surg* **197:** 348–352, 1983
22. Seki T, Koyangi T, Togashi M *et al.*: Experience with revascularizing renal artery aneurysms: is it feasible, safe and worth attempting? *J Urol* **158:** 357–362, 1997
23. Bui BT, Oliva VL, Leclerc G *et al.*: Renal artery aneurysm: treatment with percutaneous placement of a stent graft. *Radiology* **195:** 181–182, 1995
24. Babb R. Aneurysm of the splenic artery. *Arch Surg* **111:** 924–925, 1976
25. Reidy JF, Rowe PH, Ellis FG. Technical report: splenic artery aneurysm embolisation- the preferred technique to surgery. *Clin Radiol* **41:** 281–282, 1990
26. McDermott VG, Shlansky-Goldberg R, Cope C: Endovascular management of splenic artery aneurysms and pseudoaneurysms. *Cardiovasc Intervent Radiol* **17:** 179–184, 1994
27. Panayiotopoulos YP, Assadourian R, Taylor PR: Aneurysms of the visceral and renal arteries. *Ann R Coll Surg Engl* **78:** 412–419, 1996
28. Baker KS, Tisnado J, Cho S-R, Beachley MC: Splanchnic artery aneurysms and pseudoaneurysms: transcatheter embolization. *Radiology* **163:** 135–139, 1987
29. Semba SP, Sakai T, Slonim SM *et al.*: Mycotic aneurysms of the thoracic aorta: repair with the use of endovascular stent-grafts. *J Vasc Intervent Radiol* **9**: 33–40, 1998

Infrainguinal technical improvements? Subintimal angioplasty

A Bolia, PRF Bell, NJM London

INTRODUCTION

Severe claudication and critical limb ischaemia may result from occlusive disease of the superficial femoral and popliteal arteries but more commonly the disease may be in tandem with the distal vessel disease. Whilst treatment directed at the femoropopliteal segment may be sufficient for claudicants, any attempt at treating critical limb ischaemia by minimally invasive means has to be directed towards treating stenotic or occlusive lesions of the femoropopliteal segment and crural arteries.

Since the first description of percutaneous endoluminal treatment by Dotter in 1964[1] and subsequent development of the balloon catheter and its application by Gruntzig in 1974,[2] the treatment of peripheral vascular disease has been transformed.

Percutaneous transluminal angioplasty (PTA) has become an accepted and successful method of treatment for chronic atherosclerotic occlusive disease in the iliac and femoropopliteal segments.[3–10] As radiological techniques have advanced, attention has turned to lesions in the arterial tree which in the past were thought to be technically impossible. With the availability of low profile balloon angioplasty catheters and hydrophylic guidewires, attention has focused on lesions situated in the distal lower limb arteries. Recannalization of femoropopliteal occlusive disease and crural artery occlusions by subintimal angioplasty has been a standard practice in this unit for over 10 years. Subintimal angioplasty of long occlusions of the crural arteries is safe and effective and is an excellent alternative to reconstructive surgery in patients who are frequently elderly and frail. The good primary success rate, low complication rate and good limb salvage rates are comparable with reconstructive surgery and a relatively inexpensive strategy of management of critical limb ischaemia makes it an excellent alternative to reconstructive surgery.[11–22]

INDICATIONS

Subintimal angioplasty has an application in flush occlusions of the superficial femoral artery. Calcified and long occlusions may also be attempted. However, when an occlusion is 'fresh', less than 3 months old, then the procedure is not attempted. Recannalization is ineffective in such situations, the thrombus being too soft to be displaced by the balloon. In addition, there is a risk of embolism from the soft thrombus. More recently, diffuse long stenotic lesions of the superficial femoral

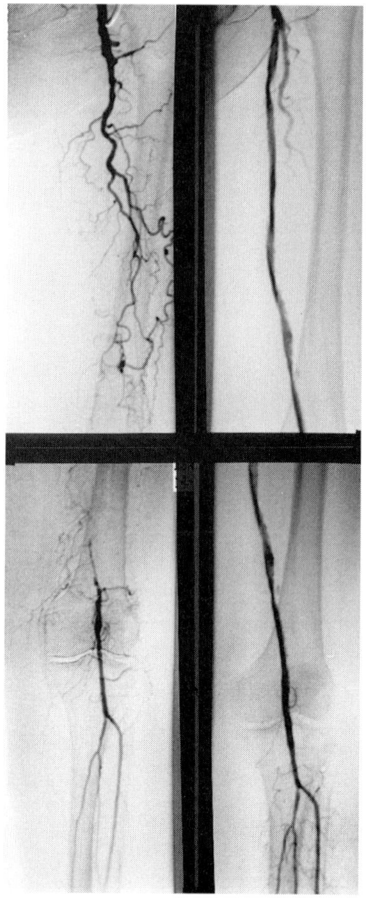

Fig. 1. There is a full length flush occlusion of the left superficial artery with reconstitution of the popliteal artery at mid level via collaterals. Subintimal angioplasty of the occlusion was carried out successfully. Note the typical spiral ribbon appearance of the dissection.

artery are also being treated with subintimal angioplasty, in the hope of improving long-term patency. Intraluminal angioplasty of diffuse long stenoses produce poor patencies.

The technique of subintimal angioplasty in the crural arteries is only applicable to occlusions of these vessels.[6,20] Whilst many occlusions of less than 3 months duration have been treated successfully, we generally prefer to recannalize mature occlusions, older than 3 months to prevent embolism from soft thrombus.

Suitable lesions may include occlusions of any of the three crural vessels. Lesions up to 3cm in length can usually be managed by an intraluminal crossing with a guidewire but longer lesions invariably demand the technique of subintimal angioplasty, hence any lesion between 3 and 30cm can be included. For the technique to be successful, the distal portion of the artery must be reasonably healthy. The presence of a relatively disease-free distal segment allows re-entry to be achieved and, more important, once an occlusion has been recannalized, the distal segment of the artery will be sufficiently accommodating to the improved flow that the recannalized segment will allow. Very diseased and poor distal segment beyond an occlusion is a relative contraindication for the subintimal technique, the reason being that re-entry in a diseased vessel is difficult to achieve. Moreover, despite a successful re-entry, the improved flow from the recannalized segment may not have anywhere to go, when the distal segment is severely diseased.

Occlusions extending from popliteal artery into the trifurcation is also a useful indication for the technique of subintimal angioplasty.[19] Recannalization of the popliteal artery may be carried out into one or more of the run-off vessels depending

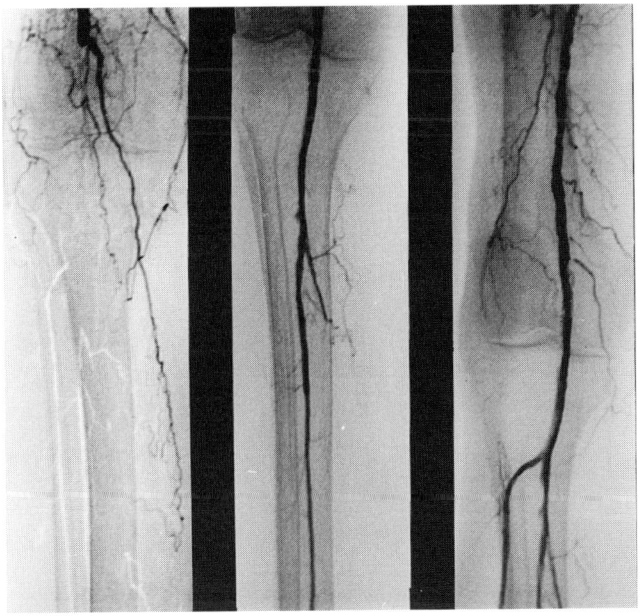

Fig. 2. There is an occlusion from the mid-popliteal artery extending into the anterior tibial and peroneal arteries. Subintimal angioplasty was first carried out into the peroneal artery. Once flow has been successfully established, an attempt is made to look for the origin of the anterior tibial artery with the help of a curved hydrophylic wire. A 'catch' is usually felt at the origin of the anterior tibial artery and when this happens, the tip of the wire is persued into the anterior tibial artery. Successful recanalization was finally achieved into both, the anterior tibial and the peroneal arteries.

on what vessels are patent distally.

PATIENTS AND METHODS

All patients presenting with severe and limiting claudication and critical ischaemia are initially investigated with colour duplex scan to characterize the arterial lesions. Diagnostic angiography is only performed as part of an intervention. The decision to intervene is based solely on the colour duplex scan.

One must make sure that there is adequate inflow before undertaking femoropopliteal and tibial recannalization. Therefore any proximal stenoses or occlusions in the aortoiliac segment are treated first before treating any infrainguinal lesions.

DESCRIPTION OF THE TECHNIQUE

The technique of recannalization of femoropopliteal occlusions has been extensively described.[11,12,23,24] Briefly, a Van Andel 5F catheter is introduced antegradely up to the level of the occlusion. A curved tipped hydrophylic guidewire (angled Terumo wire, 0.035, 180cm long, Terumo UK Ltd) introduced through the Van Andel catheter is directed towards the wall of the artery, at the level of the occlusion, and away from any important proximal collaterals. Advancing this wire usually causes a dissection. The catheter is then advanced into the occlusion. The wire is manipulated into a loop, which is then used to dissect the whole length of the occlusion. It is this loop in the wire, which allows re-entry back into the lumen distally.

Once the lesion has been crossed, the entire length of the dissection is dilated with an appropriate sized balloon at 10–12 atmospheres of pressure for 5-10 seconds at a time. All patients receive 300mg of aspirin (unless contraindicated) 1 day prior to the procedure, then 150mg of aspirin daily for 3 months following a successful procedure. Intra-arterial heparin is given at the start of the procedure up to a dose of 5000 units.

Access to crural arteries is achieved via an ipsilateral antegrade puncture of the common femoral artery, or more commonly, selectively the superficial femoral artery. Prior to crossing the crural occlusion, all patients receive 12.5mg of intra-arterial tolazoline (a vasodilator) to dilate distal arteries and to prevent spasm during the procedure. Despite this if spasm develops during the procedure, 100μg boluses of intra-arterial nitroglycerine are administered (up to a maximum of 500μg).

Short occlusions are recannalized intraluminally. If, however, dissection ensues during an attempted recannalization then subintimal angioplasty is carried out. For long occlusions subintimal angioplasty is attempted from the beginning of the procedure.[18,25]

The system employed for recannalizing crural arteries is based on a 5 French catheter and an 0.035 guidewire. The 5 F catheter/0.035 guidewire system is inherently stronger and therefore allows any forward force to be directed more effectively, thus allowing long occlusions to be crossed. The fine balloon catheters

(3.5 F) and wires (0.018) are avoided due to the lack of strength in the system that they offer. One added advantage of the former system is that the overall costs of the procedure are minimized.

Prior to an attempted recannalization, a diagnostic arteriogram is made through a simple catheter placed in the popliteal artery. The aim of this study is to get good assessment of the proximal vasculature, around the trifurcation, and more important, the quality of the distal vessels in the foot, particularly the anterior and posterior tibial arteries at the ankle and its branches leading into the foot. The better the quality of the vessels distally, the greater the chances of a successful recannalization.

The catheter is then substituted for a balloon catheter of the appropriate size (usually 3mm diameter and 2cm long balloon, 120cm long catheter). An angled hydrophylic guidewire (180cm long, 0.035inch diameter, Terumo UK Ltd) is used to make an initial entry into the occlusion. The same wire is used for crossing the lesion via a dissection and making a re-entry into the distal vessels. However, in view of the length of the occlusion and possible areas of calcification, the wire may not be strong enough to allow the passage through the full length of an occlusion. In such cases a stiff hydrophylic guidewire may become necessary.

Initial entry into the occlusion is made by using forward pressure on the tip of the angled hydrophylic guidewire. Dissection occurs easily with this manoeuvre. Once the tip of the wire has entered the occlusion, the balloon catheter is advanced over the wire into the occlusion. A small amount of dilute contrast medium may be used to confirm the position of the tip of the catheter and also, to check that a perforation has not occurred, this being a possible risk of the procedure. Once the tip of the catheter is within the occluded segment, the hydrophilic guidewire is manipulated in order to form a loop in the wire. This can be a difficult manoeuvre but as the guidewire is advanced forward, sooner or later, it comes across sufficient resistance for the tip not to advance forward and the wire will then begin to loop. As the loop begins to form, the balloon catheter may be advanced in order to enhance the formation of the loop.

Tibial vessels are delicate and the tip of the hydrophylic guidewire is liable to cause perforation relatively easily. In order to avoid this, undue force must not be used on the wire when the tip is its leading edge. However, once the loop has formed it is quite safe to advance the wire forward with minimal risk of perforation. To avoid perforation, it is preferable to form a loop in the guidewire 'above' the origin of the occlusion so that entry into the occlusion is made with the loop and not the tip of the guidewire. Formation of such a loop in a patent part of the artery proximally can be achieved by persuading the tip of the wire to enter a collateral. Once the tip is engaged into a collateral, forward pressure on the wire particularly with the help of the advancing balloon catheter may persuade the wire to form the appropriate loop.

Having formed a loop in the guidewire it is usually easy to advance the loop forward, causing a dissection through the wall of the crural artery. Any resistance to progression of the loop can be overcome by advancing the balloon catheter over the wire up to the level of the leading edge of the loop. This will strengthen one side of the loop with the balloon catheter and therefore any force applied on the wire will be directed onto the loop which can then be advanced forward. The dissection progresses forward with the help of the loop and the back up of the balloon catheter behind the loop. Having crossed most of the length of the occlusion, the loop is advanced into the patent part of the artery distally, there being a natural tendency for this to happen, depending on how disease free the distal segment is.

Once re-entry has been achieved, the entire length of the dissection is dilated using multiple sequential inflations at 8–10 atmospheres of pressure, with 5–10 second inflations at a time. The procedure is concluded with a further dose of tolazoline (12.5mg) in order to enhance the flow through the newly recannalized segment. In all cases of critical limb ischaemia, an attempt is made to recannalize as many vessels as are suitable for the procedure.

RESULTS

The impact of subintimal angioplasty on the treatment of critical limb ischaemia, and peripheral vascular disease generally, has been published elsewhere.[11–25]

In the femoropopliteal segment, an experience of the first 200 procedures has been published.[12] Of these 200 femoropopliteal occlusions 159 (80%) were successfully

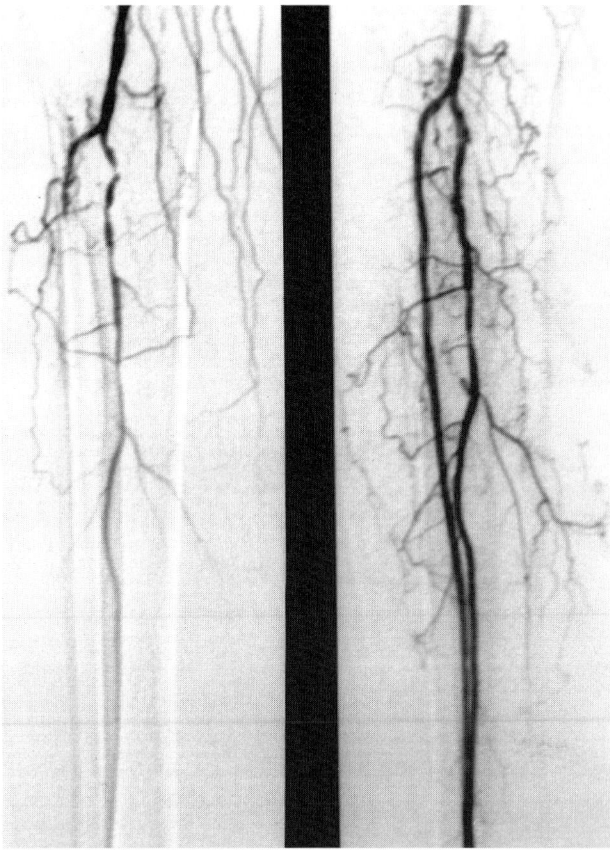

Fig. 3. This patient with critical ischaemia has one vessel run off but severe narrowing in the tibioperoneal trunk. This was successfully angioplastied intraluminally. Subsequently, a long occlusion of the anterior tibia artery was recannalized by subintimal angioplasty.

recanalized, the mean length of the occlusion being 11cm. The haemodynamic and symptomatic patencies of all successfully treated limbs at 36 months were 46% and 48% respectively.

Subsequent analysis of a further 275 procedures showed a primary success rate of 89% for a mean length of occlusion of 15cm. To date, over a thousand procedures carried out in the femoropopliteal segment proves that, for a mean length of occlusion of 15cm, over 85% can be recanalized primarily.

The impact on the treatment of critical limb ischaemia is evident from a study reporting a total of 222 separate referrals in 188 patients during a 12-month period in 1994.[21] A total of 94 (42%) limbs could be treated by balloon angioplasty, 14 (6%) by surgery and angioplasty and 54 (24%) by reconstructive surgery. This indicates a higher proportion of patients who could be treated by angioplasty than the national average of 24%.[26] This larger percentage of patients with critical limb ischaemia being treated by angioplasty is possible because of the ability of the technique of subintimal angioplasty in the management of crural artery occlusions which is a common presenting feature of patients presenting with critical limb ischaemia. Of the 188 patients, 180 were then prospectively followed up over a period of more than 1 year. Limb salvage rates for patients who had undergone surgery or angioplasty were compared and there was no significant difference in the limb salvage outcome at 1 year.[22]

In a more recent study, 133 severely ischaemic limbs were treated by PTA during 1997 (unpublished results), 78% were successfully treated; 85% of the successfully treated patients had no symptoms of critical ischaemia, and limb salvage rate was 92%, at a median follow up of 16 (12–19) months. The outcome of patients with a failed angioplasty was poor. Of 29 (22%) failed procedures, 14 required bypass surgery, 11 undergoing a major amputation and 32% dying as a result of the procedure.

DISCUSSION

With the continual improvement in the devices and expertise for endovascular interventions, an increasing proportion of patients with critical limb ischaemia can be treated by PTA. In the vascular unit at The Leicester Royal Infirmary, PTA is used as a first-line treatment whenever possible and this has significantly increased the proportion of patients treated by angioplasty. In a previous retrospective study of critical limb ischaemia carried out between 1998 and 1991, only 23% of patients were treated by PTA in comparison with 42% during the year 1994. The difference can be accounted for by the developments of better materials, increasing experience in catheter techniques, and the introduction of subintimal angioplasty for tibial occlusive disease.

Subintimal angioplasty is nowadays a routine procedure in almost all cases of occlusive disease of the femopopliteal, iliac and tibial arteries. There are theoretical reasons why subintimal angioplasty might be advantageous. The subintimal plane is the path of least resistance and the guidewire has therefore a tendency to enter this space, particularly when the occlusion is hard and long. Surgeons who perform endarterectomy are familiar with the ease with which occluding atheroma can be excised in this plane. The occlusion is traversed in an extraluminal plane, and this may explain why the technical success rates are the same for the long and short occlusions. Recanalization in the subintimal plane can be likened to the situation in an acute aortic dissection which either re-enters the true lumen spontaneously or is surgically fenestrated. In this situation, the false lumen is often larger and has a higher blood flow than the true lumen.

Another potential advantage of subintimal angioplasty is that the thrombogenic, crushed atheroma is displaced to one side of the new lumen, whereas with conventional intraluminal angioplasty, the new lumen is entirely surrounded by thrombogenic material. In achieving the new lumen of subintimal angioplasty, there is very little mechanical trauma involved, unlike other modes of recanalization whereby mechanical injury or thermal injury (laser angioplasty) occurs. Such injury is likely to have a tendency to platelet adhesion and a possibility of acute reocclusion or early intimal hyperplasia. The minimal injury that occurs during subintimal angioplasty might be expected to minimize the restenosis rate of angioplasty.

Against these advantages, there is a serious disadvantage of subintimal angioplasty which may make the patient worse rather than better. There is a potential risk of damage to important collaterals distal to the occlusions when these are included in the dissected portion. When important collaterals are compromised without achieving a haemodynamically viable channel in the main artery then the patient's distal circulation will be compromised and urgent bypass surgery will be required to restore circulation to the distal leg. It is therefore crucially important that a dissection is not extended too far distal to the occlusion, particularly early on in one's experience. Also, one should only undertake the procedure of subintimal angioplasty with full knowledge that an experienced vascular surgeon is available, should his or her services be required as a matter of urgency. Primary success rates of over 80% can be expected in any occluded segment with a low complication rate of 1–1.5% of major complications. In the femoropopliteal segment a patency rate of approximately 50% of all successful procedures can be expected at 3 years.

The advantages of PTA are well established for the high risk, elderly patients. There is also the increased advantage of a shorter hospital stay and reduced hospital costs. Whilst the technique of subintimal angioplasty in tibial occlusions is not without complications these tend to be relatively minor in the form of perforations of the artery (usually of no consequence) or distal embolism which can be aspirated percutaneously in the majority of cases.

Subintimal angioplasty of the crural vessels has demonstrated that a large non-elective workload associated with the management of critical limb ischaemia in a vascular unit can be taken care of by minimally invasive means. Non-invasive assessment of these patients with colour Doppler scanning followed by angioplasty allows efficient use of time and resources for the management of critical limb ischaemia. The durability of these revascularization procedures requires further follow-up but initial results appear to indicate a favourable outcome for recannalization of crural vessels in critical limb ischaemia resulting in a haemodynamic and symptomatic patency rates of over 50% at 1 year and limb salvage rates that are comparable with those of distal bypass surgery.

REFERENCES

1. Dotter CT, Judkins MP: Transluminal treatment of arterio-sclerotic obstruction: Description of a new technic and preliminary report of its application. *Circulation* **30:** 654–670, 1964
2. Gruntzig A, Hopff H: Percutane rekanalisation chronischer artererieller verschlusse mit einem neuen dilatationskatheter: modifikation der Dotter Technick. *Deutsch Med Wochenschr* **99:** 2502–2511, 1974
3. Johnston KW, Rae M, Hogg Johnston SA *et al.*: Five year results of a prospective study of percutaneous transluminal angioplasty. *Ann Surg* **206:** 403–413, 1987
4. Johnston KW: Femoral and popliteal artieries: reanalysis of results of balloon angioplasty. *Radiology* **183:** 767–771, 1992
5. Murray RR, Hewes RC, White RI *et al.*: Long segment femoropopliteal stenosis: Successful angioplasty a boon or bust. *Radiology* **162:** 473–476, 1987
6. Krepel VM, Van Andel GJ, Van ERP WF, Breslau PJ: Percutaneous angioplasty of the femoropopliteal artery: initial and long-term results. *Radiology* **156:** 325–328, 1985
7. Capek P, McLean GK, Berkowitz HD: Femoropopliteal angioplasty. Factors influencing long-term success. *Circulation* **83:** 170–180, 1991
8. Pell JP, Whyman MR, Fowkes FGR, Gillespie I, Ruckley CV: Trends in vascular surgery since the introduction of percutaneous transluminal angioplasty. *Br J Surg* **81:** 832–835, 1994
9. Skotnicki SH: The vascular surgeon and transluminal angioplasty. *Eur J Vasc Surg* **2:** 143–144, 1988
10. Motarjeme A: PTA and thrombolysis in leg salvage. *J Endovsac Surg* **1:** 81–87, 1994
11. Bolia A, Miles KA, Brennan J, Bell PRF: Percutaneous transluminal angioplasty of occlusions of the femoral and popliteal arteries by subintimal dissection. *Cardiovasc Intervent Radiol* **13:** 357–363, 1990
12. London NJM, Srinivasan R, Sayers RD *et al.*: Subintimal angioplasty of femoropopliteal artery occlusion: the long-term results. *Eur J Vasc Surg* **8:** 148–155, 1994
13. Reekers JA, Kromhout JG, Jacobs MJHM: Percutaneous intentional extraluminal recanalization of the femopopliteal artery. *Eur J Vasc Surg* **8:** 723–738, 1994
14. Heenan SD, Vinnicombe SJ, Buckenham TM *et al.*: Percutaneous transluminal angioplasty by a retrograde subintimal transpopliteal approach. *Clin Radiol* **49:** 824–828, 1994
15. Nasim A, Sayers RD, Dunlop P *et al.*: Intentional extraluminal recanalization of the femoropopliteal segment following perforation during percutaneous transluminal angioplasty. *Eur J Endovasc* **12:** 246–249, 1996
16. Nasim A, Sayers RD, Bell PRF *et al.*: Recanalization of the native artery following failure of a bypass graft. *Eur J Vasc Surg* **10:** 125–127, 1995
17. Berengoltz Zlochin SN, Mali WP, Borst C *et al.*: Subintimal vesus intraluminal laser assisted recanalization of occluded femoropopliteal arteries: one year clinical and angiographic follow-up. *J Vasc Intervent Radiol* **15:** 689–696, 1994
18. Bolia A, Sayers RD, Thompson MM, Bell PRF: Subintimal and intraluminal recanalization of occluded crural arteries by percutaneous balloon angioplasty. *Eur J Vasc Surg* **8:** 214–219, 1994
19. Nydahl S, London NJM, Bolia A: Technical report: recanalization of all three infrapopliteal arteries by subintimal angioplasty. *Clin Radiol* **51:** 366–367, 1996
20. Nydahl S, Hartshorne T, Bell PRF *et al.*: Subintimal angioplasty of infrapopliteal occlusions in critically ischaemic limbs. *Eur J Vasc Endovasc Surg* **14:** 212–216, 1997
21. Varty K, Nydahl S, Butterworth P *et al.*: Changes in the management of critical limb ischaemia. *Br J Surg* **83:** 953–956, 1996
22. Varty K, Nydahl S, Nasim A *et al.*: Results of surgery and angioplasty for the treatment of chronic severe lower limb ischaemia. *Eur J Vasc Endovasc Surg* **16:** 159–163, 1998
23. Bolia A, Bell PRF: Femoropopliteal and crural artery recanalization using subintimal angioplasty. *Semin Vasc Surg* **8:** 253–264, 1995

24. Reekers JA, Bolia A: Percutaneous intentional extraluminal (subintimal) recanalization: how to do it yourself. *Eur J Radiol* **28:** 192–198, 1998
25. Bolia A: Percutaneous intentional extraluminal (subintimal) recanalization of crural arteries. *Eur J Radiol* **28:** 199–204, 1998
26. The Vascular Surgical Society of Great Britain and Ireland: Critical limb ischaemia: management and outcome. Report of a national survey. *Eur J Vasc Endovasc Surg* **10:** 108–113, 1995

Infrainguinal technical improvements? Luminal endovascular procedures

PA Gaines

INTRODUCTION

My heart sank when I was invited to detail recent advances in the intraluminal recanalization of superficial femoral artery disease. Whilst there are data available to suggest that the increased availability of vascular surgery and balloon angioplasty may reduce major amputation rates,[1] for several reasons the impact of endovascular intervention within the superficial femoral artery has, reasonably, been held open to question. First, with increased experience of angioplasty of the superficial femoral artery, the long-term patency rates of this procedure have been critically appraised. Angioplasty may be suitable for isolated stenoses of the superficial femoral artery, but the patency rates of percutaneous transluminal angioplasty (PTA) of complex or complete occlusions of the superficial femoral artery with poor run-off particularly in the setting of critical limb ischaemia, have been associated with a high reocclusion rate.[2–6] Second, the use and evaluation of exercise therapy in claudication has further limited the practise of infrainguinal endovascular intervention even though it is suitable for only a proportion of patients and the durability following cessation of the programme is limited.

Third there has been a certain lack of energy in the management of claudication within strict the financial constraints of the National Health Service. Overall this has lead to a paucity in clinical research within this area. This situation contrasts sharply with the active research in the priority area of coronary intervention where there is strong financial support and the clinical impact is potentially more important. Such financial prioritization is not only seen within the current health system, but also the within industry where coronary intervention is associated with high profits.

Surely a patent native conduit delivered safely using minimally invasive techniques has much to offer over conventional surgery or exercise therapy and herein lies the rub. The decline in interest and lack of focus upon the infrainguinal vessels makes this a particularly fertile area for opportunities to collaborate between Radiologists, Surgeons, Physicians and Industry. It is not the concept of endovascular infrainguinal intervention that is at fault, rather we have not learnt how to obtain satisfactory results. If endovascular intervention upon the superficial femoral artery could result in both high patency and good long-term health benefit then once again this technique may be acceptable as a useful therapeutic modality.

The superficial femoral artery is an excellent model to use for endovascular research. Not only is there a high event rate following intervention, but the vessel is easy to image and functionally assess by non-invasive techniques. For this reason the superficial femoral artery has been targeted throughout this article. The limitation in patency following PTA of the superficial femoral artery is due to acute closure (up to 10% of cases) and late restenosis. Acute closure may be improved by techniques that are associated with high initial lumen gain and therefore high flow (e.g. stents and stent-grafts) or pharmaceutical manipulation that restricts the acute thrombotic process. Delayed patency within the first year of intervention is associated with restenosis. In the spirit of this text I will describe some of the initiatives being followed to improve intraluminal recanalization, and the areas of opportunity that are available for collaboration between interested parties.

PHARMACEUTICAL MANIPULATION

The platelet plays a pivotal role in atherothrombosis and acute thrombosis following endovascular manipulation. Aspirin has been well demonstrated to reduce death and major vascular events in patients with atherosclerosis through the inhibition of the enzyme cyclo-oxygenase. Whilst there are data to indicate it improves outcome in iliac intervention,[7] the data for infrainguinal intervention are limited. Because aspirin affects only one of the soluble stimulators of platelet activators (thromboxane A_2) it has only a weak effect.

The last few years has seen the introduction of more potent antiplatelet agents including thienopyridine derivatives and IIb/IIIa antagonists. The thienopyridines ticlopidine and clopidogrel irreversibly inhibit the binding of ADP to the platelet receptor and thereby block the activation of the platelet. In the cardiology literature there is evidence that the ticlopidine reduces the risk of coronary stent placement. Unfortunately this drug is complicated by neutropenia in 0.9% of cases. One non-randomized study suggests that clopidogrel and aspirin is as effective as ticlopidine and aspirin after coronary stenting but this remains to be confirmed. Despite this active intervention within the coronary circulation, we have seen virtually nothing to investigate its use in the peripheral circulation following intervention. Clearly any intervention that could improve the initial 10% loss due to thrombosis, particularly in situations of long lesions and limited run-off, would have a marked impact on the value of infrainguinal endovascular intervention.

MODIFIED TECHNIQUE

Subtle changes in technique (e.g. the widespread use of hydrophilic wires and low profile catheters) have increased the primary success rate particularly in crossing occlusions, and have therefore improved the overall success when analysed by intention to treat, but have done nothing to alter the long-term patency.[3]

The most widely recognized angioplasty variation is the use of intentional subintimal angioplasty popularized by the Leicester group (Dr Aman Bolia).[8] As a separate chapter within this text is dedicated to this technique I will not expand further here except to say that, to my knowledge, it has not been shown that subintimal angioplasty has a benefit over intraluminal angioplasty. Whilst we all recognize that a randomized trial would be the ideal way to demonstrate any significant difference, there are major logistical problems to overcome. When intraluminal angioplasty is intended, a large proportion (probably 40–70%) of lesions are crossed in the subintimal plane. It is not surprising then that any trial intended to show a difference between the techniques would probably falter because both limbs of the study would naturally involve a large number of patients who are undergoing subintimal angioplasty. In the long term, neither does it logically appear that subintimal recanalization would have a beneficial effect. The mechanical effects that lead onto restenosis are similar which ever plane the dilatation occurs within.

STENTS

The major advantage of using intravascular stents is to improve the initial lumen gain. Such devices have undergone extensive investigation within the superficial femoral artery (see Table 1). Universally, in well constructed studies, they have been shown to have no advantage over simple angioplasty. Stents are limited by thrombosis and restenosis because because of:

1. the characteristics of the metal and surface properties,
2. the metallic bulk and alinement within the vessel,
3. the associated vessel disruption.

It is shown that attention to detail concerning device placement in the coronary circulation, aided by the use of intravenous ultrasound (IVUS), has improved stent patency and therefore long-term outcome. Such detail may be worth persuing within the peripheries.

In an attempt to reduce thrombosis and restenosis, various coatings and drug attachments have been investigated in animals and to a lesser extent humans. The

Table 1

Author	*No of limbs*	*Technical success %*	*Primary % 1*	*Patency % 3*	*Years % 5*	*Compli-cations %*	*Claud-icants %*
Rousseau 1989[29]	40	100	76	76	—	—	78
Zollikofer 1991[30]	15	93	55	18	—	—	76
Do 1992[31]	26	100	59	—	—	—	85
Sapoval 1992[32]	22	95	49	49	—	5	86
Liermann 1992[33]	48	94	71	—	—	4	65
Henry 1995[34]	126	99	81	72	65	3	93
Martin 1995[35]	96	—	61	—	—	—	77
Strecker 1997[10]	80	100	76	48	—	12	84

BENESTENT II study[9] demonstrated that acute closure of a coronary stent could be significantly reduced by the use of a heparin-coated stent and that anticoagulation was no longer required. No peripheral investigation has yet been undertaken.

Drugs or coatings aimed at reducing thrombosis have not yet been shown to reduce restenosis in the human, probably due to the complex mechanisms involved that do not simply involve platelets and their associated functions.[10] Similarly, no additions have as yet been demonstrated to reduce restenosis, but the future is hopeful. Biodegradable stents have the attraction of not being limited by the adverse characteristics of metal or continued trauma and long-term foreign body reaction. Work has been undertaken in animals particularly with polyphosphate esters and paving but as yet human trial are limited.[11] Removable stents have been investigated for a limited amount away from the femoral artery.[12–15] The attraction lies in maintaining an initial lumen gain without contributing to the mechanical stimulation of restenosis in the long term. The full evaluation of removable stents in the superficial femoral artery has not yet been undertaken.

STENT-GRAFTS

This subject is covered in a separate chapter.

RADIATION THERAPY

The principal limitation of endovascular techniques in the superficial femoral artery is the high restenosis rate. Restenosis is a complex process which involves acute recoil, intimal hyperplasia, and late vascular negative remodelling.[16–19] Ionizing radiation has been successfully used to inhibit cell proliferation both in animal models and is currently used to treat recurrent pterygium, keloid formation and hypertrophic bone formation following hip replacement. The exact mechanism whereby ionizing radiation inhibits restenosis is unknown but several processes have been implicated. Radiation may cause cell death by either a direct effect on nuclear DNA or apoptosis. Downregulation of target cell proliferation and impaired function of cells without cell death have both been demonstrated as has the production of early and late response genes and gene products. In addition, radiation may impair late remodelling by inhibiting the myofibroblasts.

Two techniques have evolved to deliver the radiation to the target area. A delivery system (ribbons, seeds, liquids) may be positioned to deliver treatment over a short defined period immediately after angioplasty or stent placement. Alternatively continuous therapy may be delivered by using a radioactive stent.

The radiation is either gamma or beta. Gamma radiation is difficult to manipulate because it penetrates deep through tissues and is less easy to control for staff. Beta radiation has its effect within a few millimetres of the source and as such may be more appropriate for the therapeutic manipulation of restenosis. Even so, the production of X-rays through bremsstrahlung interaction and scattered radiation from the patients' tissues still makes the use of beta radiation potentially hazardous to staff. It appears that the treatment needs to be delivered shortly after endovascular intervention (day 1) and should deliver between 10 and 15Gy within a few millimetres of the vessel wall. Using such techniques, animal models have been demonstrated to produce a highly significant reduction in intimal proliferation and active research within the coronary circulation has shown a reduction in restenosis in several clinical trials.[20–23]

Within the peripheral circulation, the results are early but encouraging. In Austria, Minar *et al.*[24,25] have conducted a randomized trial of intervention within the superficial femoral artery. Patients were randomized to angioplasty alone or angioplasty plus brachytherapy. At 6 months, the recurrence rate in the angioplasty group is 49% and in the brachytherapy group 24% ($p<0.05$). Liermanns group[26–28] studied 25 patients with in-stent restenosis in the superficial femoral artery. The patients underwent directional atherectomy or balloon dilatation followed by endovascular radiation using an 192-Iridium source to deliver 12 Gy to the vessel wall. At 5 years follow-up the investigators reported a patency rate of 80% without any adverse events. Several trials are ongoing, and if the technique becomes user friendly with demonstrated safety to both the patients and staff, then endovascular radiation may well become a dominant treatment in the future.

REFERENCES

1. Hallet JW, Byrne J, Gayari M M *et al.*: Impact of arterial surgery and balloon angioplasty on amputation: A population-based study of 1155 procedures between 1973 and 1992. *J Vasc Surg* **25:** 29–38, 1997
2. Johnston KW: Factors that influence the outcome of aortoiliac and femoropopliteal percutaneous transluminal angioplasty. *Surg Clin North Am* **72:** 1992
3. Murray JG, Apthorp LA, Wilkins RA *et al.*: Long segment femoropopliteal angioplasty: improved technical success and long-term patency. *Radiology* **195:** 158–162, 1995
4. Pekka JM, Hannu IM, Matti TS *et al.*: Chronic critical lower limb ischaemia: prospective trial of angioplasty with 1–36 months follow-up. *Radiology* **188:** 381–387, 1993
5. Pekka JM, Hannu IM, Ritva LV *et al.*: Femoropopliteal angioplasty in patients with claudication: primary and secondary patency in 140 limbs with 1–3 year follow-up. *Radiology* **91:** 727–733, 1994
6. Pekka JM, IM Hannu, L Markku, J Pekka *et al.*: Impact of risk factors on limb salvage after angioplasty in chronic critical lower limb ischaemia. *Angiology* **45:** 797–804, 1994
7. Nawaz S, Cleveland T, Gaines PA *et al.*: Aortoiliac stenting, determinants of clinical outcome. *Eur J Vasc Endovasc Surg* **17:** 351–359, 1999
8. London NJM, Varty K, Sayers RD *et al.*: Percutaneous transluminal angioplasty for lower limb critical ischaemia. *Br J Surg* **82:** 1232–1235, 1995
9. Serruys PW, van Hout B, Bonnier H *et al.*: Randomised trial of implantation of heparin-coated stents with balloon angioplasty in selected patients with coronary artery disease (Benestent II). *Lancet* **352:** 673–681, 1998
10. Strecker EP, Gabelmann, Boss I *et al.*: Drug releasing stents for the prevention of intimal hyperplasia after stent implantation – an experimental study. *Cardiovasc Intervent Radiol* **20:** (Suppl 1): S88, 1997
11. Skepian MJ, Schindler A: Polymeric endoluminal paving/sealing a biodegradable alternative to intracoronary stenting (Abstract). *Circulation* **78** (S2)**:** II-409, 1988
12. Lierman D, Donnerstag F, Laufer U: Does transient stent implantation improve the results of permanent stents? *Cardiovasc Intervent Radiol* **20** (Suppl 1)**:** S72, 1997
13. Gaspard PE, Didier BP, Delsanti GL: The temporary stent catheter: a non-operative

treatment for acute occlusion during coronary angioplasty (Abstract) *J Am Coll Cardiol* **15:** 118A, 1990
14. Schlansky-Goldberg RD, LeVeen RF, Hillstead MR *et al.*: Temporary vascular stenting (Abstract) *Radiology* **177(P):** 299, 1990
15. Irie T, Furui S, Yamaguchi T, Makita K *et al.*: Relocatable Gianturco expandable metallic stents, *Radiology* **178:** 575–578, 1991
16. Haude M, Erbel R, Issa H *et al.*: Quantitative analysis of elastic recoil after balloon angioplasty and after intracoronary implantation of balloon-expandable Palmaz-Schatz stents. *J Am Coll Cardiol* **21:** 26–34, 1993
17. Consigny PM, Bilder GE: Expression and release of smooth muscle cell mitogens in arterial wall after balloon angioplasty. *J Vasc Med Biol* **4:** 1–8, 1993
18. Mintz GS, Popma JJ, Pichard AD *et al.*: Arterial remodeling after coronary angioplasty. A serial intravascular ultrasound study. *Circulation* **94:** 35–43, 1996
19. Isner JM: Vascular remodeling. Honey, I think I shrunk the artery. *Circulation* **89:** 2937–2941, 1994
20. Condado JA, Waksman R, Orlando G *et al.*: Long-term angiographic and clinical outcome after percutaneous transluminal coronary angioplasty and intracoronary radiation therapy in humans. *Circulation* **96:** 727–732, 1997
21. Serruys PW, Levendag PC: Intracoronary brachytherapy: the death knell of restenosis or just another episode of a never-ending story. *Circulation* **96:** 709–712, 1997
22. Waksman R: Local catheter-based intracoronary radiation therapy for restenosis. *Am J Cardiol* **78** (Suppl 3A): 23–28, 1996
23. Bertrand OF, Mongrain R, Lehnert S *et al.*: Intravascular radiation therapy in atherosclerotic disease, promises and premises. *Eur Heart J* **18:** 1385–1395, 1997
24. Minar E , Pokrajac B, Maca T *et al.*: Brachytherapy for the prophylaxis of restenosis after femoropopliteal PTA of long lesions. *Cardiovasc Intervent Radiol* **20** (Suppl 1): S88, 1997
25. Minar E, Pokrajac B, Maca Th *et al.*: Brachytherapy for prophylaxis of restenosis after femoropopliteal PTA: mid-term results of a prospective randomised study. *Cardiovasc Intervent Radiol* **22** (Suppl 2): S85, 1999
26. Liermann D, Bottcher HD, Kollath J *et al.*: Prophylactic endovascular radiotherapy to prevent intimal hyperplasia after stent implantation in femoropopliteal arteries, *Cardiovasc Intervent Radiol* **17:** 1994
27. Lierman D, Schopohl B, P L Jühling *et al.*: Myointimal hyperplasia and prophylactic endovascular radiotherapy of peripheral vessel, a 6 year follow up. *Cardiovasc Intervent Radiol* **20:** (Suppl 1): S88, 1997
28. Schopohl B, Liermann D, Pohlit L *et al.*: ^{192}Ir endovascular brachytherapy for avoidance of intimal hyperplasia after percutaneous transluminal angioplasty and stent implantation in peripheral vessels: 6 years of experience. *Int J Radiat Oncol Bio Phys* **36:** 835–840, 1996
29. Rousseau HP, Raillat CR, Joffre FG *et al.*: Treatment of femoropopliteal stenoses by means of self-expandable endoprostheses: midterm results. *Radiology* **172**: 961–4, 1989
30. Zollikofer CL, Antonucci F, Pfyffer M *et al.*: Arterial stent placement with use of the Wallstent: midterm results of clinical experience. *Radiology* **179**: 449–66, 1991
31. Do DD, Triller J, Wilpoth BH, Stirnemann P, Mahler F: A comparison study of self-expandable stents vs balloon angioplasty alone in femoropopliteal artery occlusions. *Cardiovasc Intervent Radiol* **15**: 306–12, 1992
32. Sapoval MR, Long AL, Raynaud AC *et al.*: Femoropopliteal stent placement: long-term results. *Radiology* **184**: 844–50, 1992
33. Liermann D, Strecker EP, Peters J: The Strecker stent: indications and results in iliac and femoropopliteal arteries. *Cardiovasc Intervent Radiol* **15**: 298–305, 1992
34. Henry M, Amor M, Ethevenot G *et al.*: Palmaz stent placement in iliac and femoropopliteal arteries: primary and secondary patency in 310 patients with 2–4 year follow-up. *Radiology* **197**: 167–74, 1995
35. Martin EC, Katzen BT, Benanti JF *et al.*: Multicenter trial of the Wallstent in iliac and femoral arteries. *J Vasc Intervent Radiol* **6**: 843–9, 1995

Infrainguinal technical improvements? Remote endarterectomy

Frans L Moll, Gwan H Ho

INTRODUCTION

When the superficial femoral artery is occluded and conservative treatment fails, when, why and where do we look for an alternative for the traditional prosthetic or biological femoropopliteal bypass?

Short occlusions or stenoses of the superficial femoral artery can be treated by percutaneous transluminal angioplasty (PTA), but the long-term patency results of PTA for long (>10 cm) occlusive lesions have been disappointing. The use of stents in combination with angioplasty has not altered the results, despite close surveillance and reintervention; venous bypass has a far better patency rate in fact. It might be the first option for treatment, even when the vein has to be harvested from another extremity than the affected leg as long as it is autogenous vein. The debate begins when new techniques have equal results and the vein can be saved for other procedures. The traditional alternative is the prosthetic or biological bypass in an extra-anatomic route from the common femoral artery to the popliteal artery. The primary patencies of these bypasses at 5 years vary from 60 to 80%. However, over the last 10 years no major improvements have been recorded despite the progress in medical technology. Our aim is to explore and utilize a minimally invasive technique, in an attempt to obtain at least comparable patency results which will shorten the patient's hospital stay and lower the patients morbidity and mortality. One such technique might be a modernized semi-closed endarterectomy. This original technique was described in the late 1950s and early 1960s, but has fallen into disuse. The main reasons are the occurrence of unexpected restenoses and occlusions in the endarterectomized artery, though this is not supported by recent publications that show no significant difference in patency between the endarterectomy and the prosthetic bypass graft. Currently, no data are available from randomized trials. Our reason for a reappraisal of the semi-closed endarterectomy is the availability and application of new intraoperative technology to improve the results from the past, such as intraoperative digital subtraction angiography, angioscopy, and intravascular ultrasonography. With the help of these new modalities the semi-closed endarterectomized artery can be inspected more accurately and endoluminal corrections are possible intraoperatively. Postoperatively, the onset of initial intimal hyperplasia and restenosis can be detected by duplex-scanning. These localized lesions may be treated by angioplasty creating a better primary assisted patency rate.

MODERN TECHNIQUE

With the use of a modified ringstripper which enables the surgeon to cut the endoluminal intima core remotely from the side of entrance, the surgical exposure of the superficial and femoral artery can be limited to a small single arteriotomy at its origin in the groin, and a distal exposure of the popliteal artery at the endpoint of the endarterectomized conduit is unnecessary.

SEMI-CLOSED ENDARTERECTOMY

Semi-closed endarterectomy is currently performed less commonly than it was in the 1960s and 1970s, when it was a popular surgical technique. Reasons for its decline in popularity include the relative difficulty of removing intimal flaps after endarterectomy of the closed compartment as well as the occurrence of early unpredictable restenosis after an apparently perfect technical procedure.

TECHNIQUE

By a vertical groin incision, the common femoral artery, the proximal deep femoral artery or profunda artery, and the proximal part of the superficial femoral artery are exposed. A second medial incision at the distal part of the superficial femoral artery and proximal part of the popliteal artery is made to expose the endpoint of the semiclosed endarterectomy. After a bolus of heparin is administered intravenously, the origin of the superficial femoral artery is clamped in the groin. The blood flow through the usually patent deep femoral artery is uninterrupted. A longitudinal arteriotomy (3cm) of the proximal superficial femoral artery permits dissection of the intimal core inside of the occluded or stenosed superficial femoral artery. This part of the operation is essential and should be performed meticulously. The cleavage plane of the intima core should be between the lamina elastica interna and media (recognizable from the circular fibres of the media) or, preferably, between media and adventitia (which has a featureless smooth appearance [lamina elastica externa]).

After transsection of the intima core in the exposed superficial femoral artery area, most surgeons prefer blunt dissection of the first 2cm or 3cm within the closed artery before using a suitably sized ringstripper. The loop of the ringstripper is advanced distally into the artery with gentle, rotating movements by one hand while grasping the intima core by the other (Fig. 1). In case the ringstripper cannot be passed, fluoroscopy is of great help. Different sizes of ring loops can be tried, or an additional arteriotomy is possible. The intima is dissected to the distal superficial femoral artery or proximal popliteal artery, and an arteriotomy is performed. After transection of the dissected intima core, the ringstripper and the core are removed from the artery. The distal transected intima is then tagged down by U-sutures, and the arteriotomies can either be closed directly or with patches. Care should be taken to remove the entire intima core within the artery, where they might become a source for future

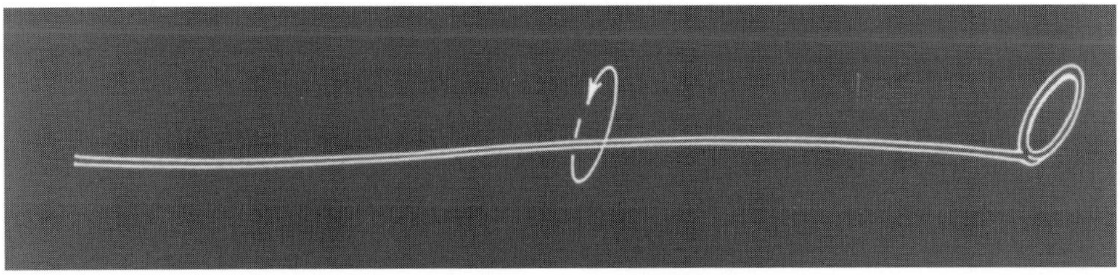

Fig. 1. The loop of the ringstripcutter is advanced distally into the artery with gentle rotating movements.

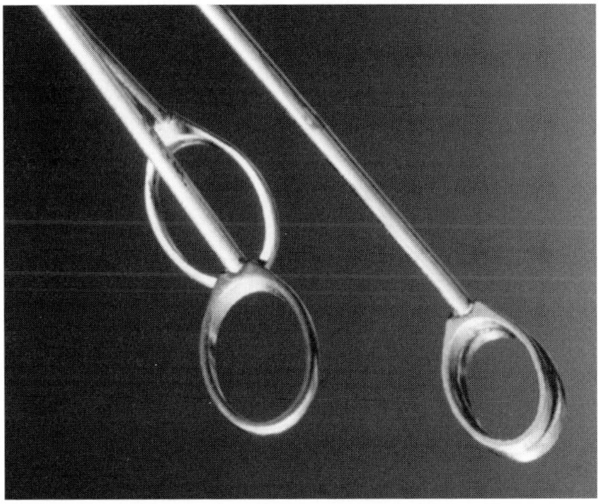

Fig. 2. The ringstripcutter.

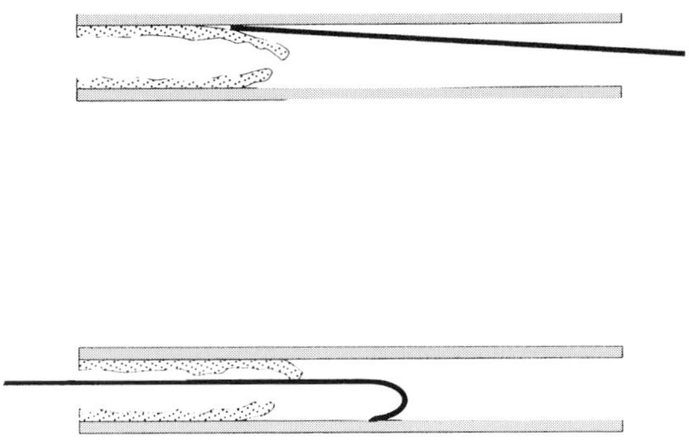

Fig. 3. The guidewire is introduced into the popliteal artery.

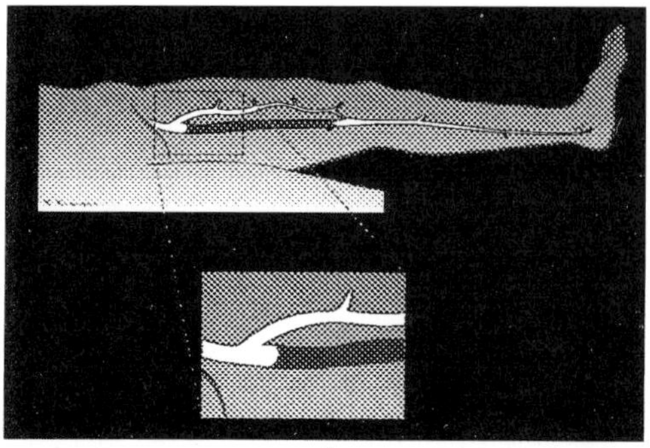

1

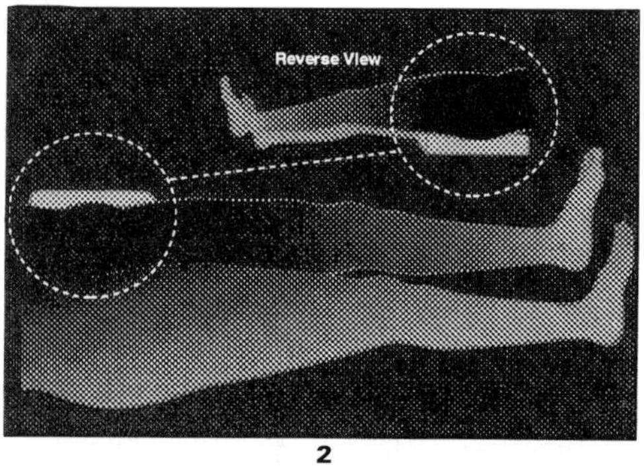

2

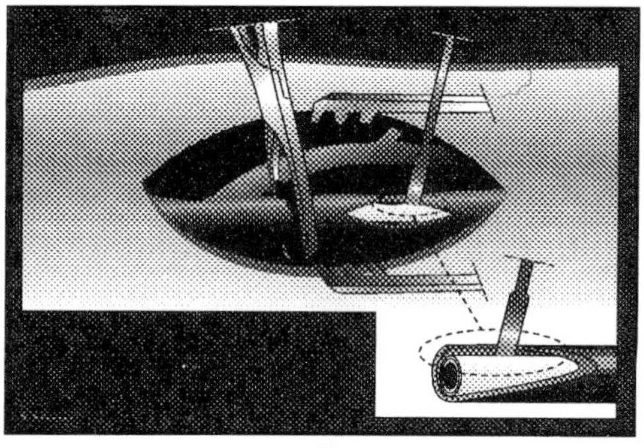

3

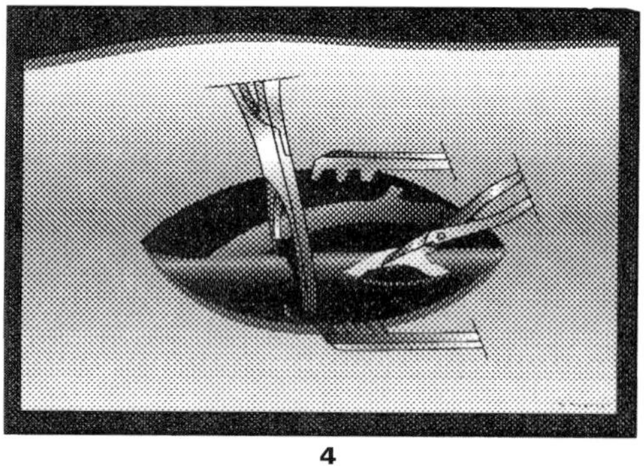

4

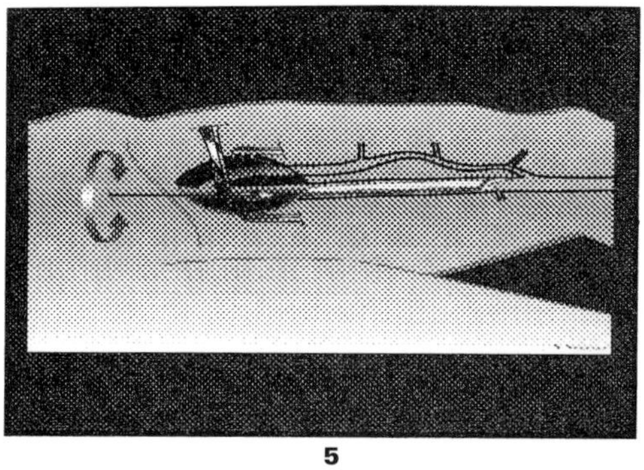

5

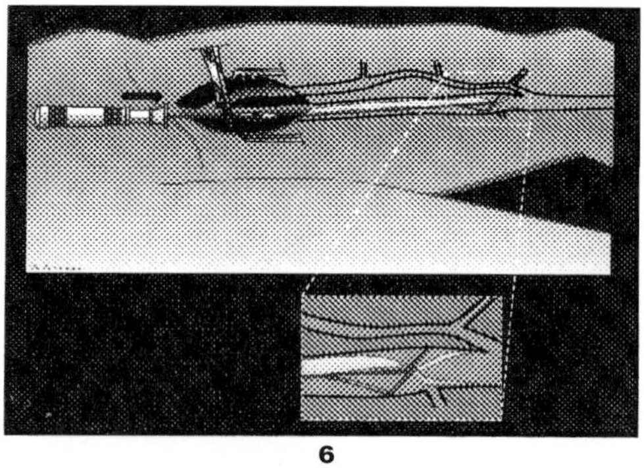

6

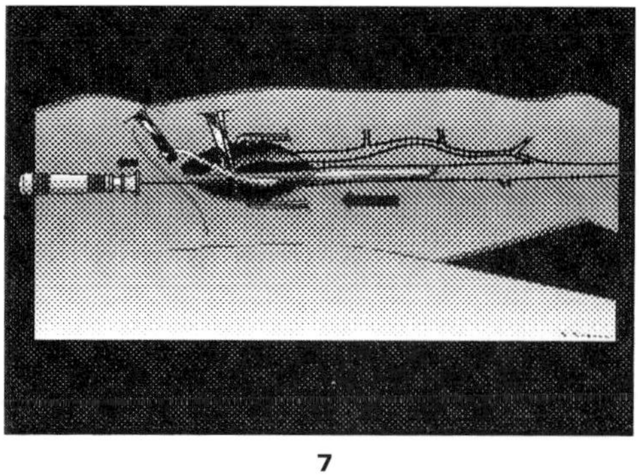

7

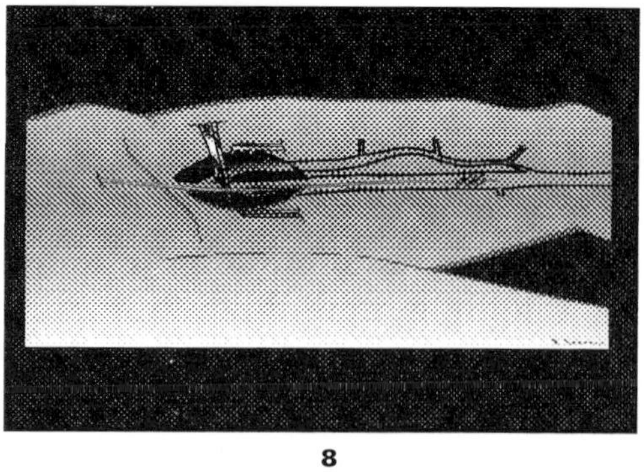

8

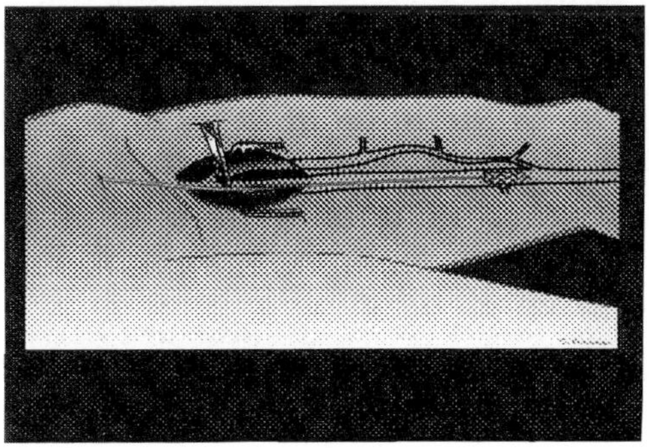

9

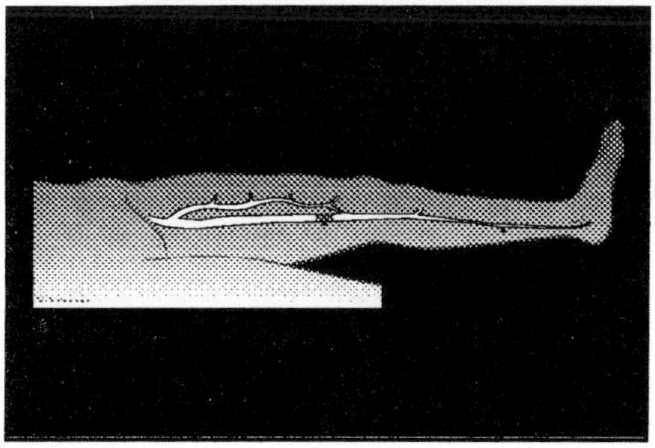

10

Fig. 4. Remote endarterectomy using the ringstripcutter. Technique steps:
1: angiogram of superficial femoral artery occlusion;
2: pillow under the buttock to extend hip – prepare entire extremity circumferentially;
3: expose superficial femoral artery – establish endarterectomy cleavage plain with free elevator;
4: cut atheroma cord;
5: dissection with ringstrippers;
6: cut atheroma cord at distal end-point with ringstripcutter;
7: atheroma cord extraction;
8: remove residual atheroma with graft thrombectomy catheter – visualize entire endarterectomy and distal end-point with angioscope;
9: place stent to secure distal end-point – extend endarterectomy into common femoral artery – close arteriotomy with patch;
10: complete angiogram.

emboli or restenosis. Inspection is possible by angioscopy or intravascular ultrasound. Unfortunately, no studies are available to discriminate clinically irrelevant from relevant incomplete endarterectomies. The decision to accept some technical incompleteness of the procedure remains operator-dependent. In addition to flushing with a heparinized saline solution, a 5 F or 6 F Fogarty graft thrombectomy catheter (Baxter Health Corporation, Irvine, CA) might be of help in removing debris from the closed segment.

RINGSTRIPCUTTER AND REMOTE ENDARTERECTOMY

The ringstripcutter is a modified ringstripper with two shafts instead of one, which telescope into each other and two symmetric single ellipse shaped rings at a 135∞ to the shafts (Vascular Architects, Portola Valley, Ca, USA). It is available in different loop sizes, ranging from 5 to 10 millimeters inner diameter. Both parallel rings have sharpened inner edges and cut like a pair of scissors when both rings shear along each other during telescoping the shafts (Fig. 2). The remote cutting mechanism is activated by a handle at the end of the shafts. The advantage of this endovascular device is a small single groin incision to be sufficient for performing a complete 'remote endarterectomy' of long occlusions of the superficial femoral artery. The operative technique is similar to the semi-closed endarterectomy with the performance of an arteriotomy of the proximal superficial femoral artery. After the initial core is meticulously dissected, a single ringstripper is passed around the intima core and advanced distally to reach the patent popliteal artery under fluoroscopic control. The single ringstripper is then exchanged to the ringstripcutter, which cuts the distal part of the atheroma core endoluminally. The entire intima core and the ringstripcutter are then removed simultaneously. After radiological examination of the reopened artery and the distal renal vessels, an additional part of the intima core can be dissected if necessary, and cut and removed again with the ringstripcutter. Endoluminal stenting of the distal intimal flap with a short endovascular stent prevents any further dissection and provides a smooth transition zone to normal intima. In addition, the minimal loss of compliance and the concentric overpass further resembles normal flow characteristics.[1] A potential risk for further dissection exists if the guidewire will not pass to the open arterial popliteal lumen, but tracks subintimally. As suggested by Whitely *et al.*,[2] the guidewire is introduced into the popliteal artery before the endarterectomy procedure starts (Fig. 3). After removal of the intima core and reaching the open popliteal artery, the guidewire from the distal introduction side may be brought up easily to the groin and facilitates stent placement at the cutting area of the intima, and also allows the procedure to be carried out in the absence of sophisticated angiography with road mapping. See Technique steps 1–10 in Fig. 4.

The minimal invasive approach of remote endarterectomy with the avoidance of a second distal incision and dissection of the popliteal artery, creates less operative trauma and a reduction of postoperative discomfort, leading to earlier recovery and discharge of the patient. The procedure can be performed by the vascular surgeon alone, or in cooperation with the interventional radiologist. Whenever a perforation of the superficial femoral artery or popliteal artery occurs due to technical errors, conversion to regular semi-closed endarterectomy with an additional second incision at the place of perforation always remains possible, as well as recourse to bypass surgery.

In our clinic more than 200 remote endarterectomy procedures have been performed. The indications for surgical intervention were disabling claudication (grade I, category 1–3 Rutherford) in 70% of the patients, and rest pain and/or gangrene (grades II and III, category 4 and 5) in the remaining 30%, sometimes with single vessel run-off. In 95% of all cases the superficial femoral artery was occluded, whereas in 65%, the occlusions extended over more than half of the femoropopliteal segment. The mean length of the endarterectomized segment was 33 centimeters (range 10–45cm). In one patient we did not succeed in passing the ringstripper into the superficial femoral artery. This patient underwent a standard femoropopliteal bypass graft operation. There were complications in 13 cases; perforations occurred in 11 cases, which were restored by inserting a short interposition graft of covered stent without further sequel. In two cases a guidewire could not be inserted into the patent popliteal artery after a successful remote endarterectomy, necessitating a second incision at the distal end-point. One patient died within 30 days of the operation, due to a non-procedure related cardiac arrest. The cumulative 2-year primary, primary-assisted, and secondary patency rates were 73%, 86% and 86%, respectively[3]).

SURVEILLANCE AND MEDICATION

As mentioned previously, routine postoperative surveillance of the endarterectomized superficial femoral artery is mandatory. All patients treated by the remote endarterectomy device in the femoropopliteal artery are entering a duplex scanning surveillance programme, consisting of duplex scanning within 6 weeks postoperatively and after 3, 6, 9 and 12 months. In the authors' series, only 25% of all recurrent stenoses after remote endarterectomy were associated with deterioration of clinical symptoms or a decrease of ankle brachial indices. In 82% of all restenoses, time of onset was within the first year. The locations of these restenoses were equally distributed within the superficial femoral artery and not restricted to the stent or distal superficial femoral artery region. Preliminary studies on the results of revision indicate that early restenoses may be treated successfully with balloon angioplasty.

Recurrent stenoses developing after 1 year seem to have a different natural history and need intervention only for clinical symptoms. Controversy exists with regard to the use of antiplatelet drugs or warfarin. The authors give all patients warfarin postoperatively for at least 6 months. Thereafter, the authors prescribe an antiplatelet drug (aspirin, 100 mg daily).

FUTURE PERSPECTIVES

The ringstripcutter device enables the surgeon to perform a remote endarterectomy of virtually any major occluded artery. The remote endarterectomy procedure can also be performed in iliac and popliteal arteries. Both procedures have already been successfully performed in our institution, using a retrograde approach. The results of this procedure may approach those of grafts for femoral supragenicular popliteal bypasses and can be chosen as a first option for treatment of superficial femoral artery-occlusive disease when minimal invasive procedures are desirable for the individual patient condition. If the occurrence of restenosis in endarterectomies can be reduced, the role of bypass grafting turns into a bail-out procedure for failed minimal invasive techniques.

Currently there are four main areas of research into the prevention of restenosis in endarterectomized superficial femoral arteries: gene and drug therapy, cell seeding of the endarterectomized surface, radiation or brachytherapy, and endoluminal grafting or a combination. Some workers are using balloon expandable polytetrafluoroethylene (e-PTFE). An intravascular ultrasound study showed a better vascular response of the superficial femoral artery with an e-PTFE endolining after endarterectomy than endolining after PTA or partial arterectomy of the superficial femoral artery. In addition, the endoluminal distal transition zone from the endograft to the native artery is haemodynamically more favourable.[4] This finding is also supported by the clinical results of the comparitive study between PTFE femoropopliteal bypasses with distal end-to-side versus end-to-end anastomosis. There was a statistically significant difference in patencies in favour of the end-to-end anastomosis at 1, 5 and 8 years of follow-up (ETE 89/73/68% versus ETS 83/69/55%)[5]).

Recently a European multicentre prospective study has started using the technique of remote endarterectomy of the occluded superficial femoral artery followed by e-PTFE balloon expandable endovascular graft. Undoubtedly more studies will follow hopefully to establish durable alternatives to conventional bypass grafting.

REFERENCES

1. Ho GH, Moll FL, Hedeman Joosten PPhA *et al.*: The Mollring Cutter™ remote endarterectomy: Preliminary experience with a new endovascular technique for treatment of occlusive superficial femoral artery disease. *J Endovasc Surg* **2:** 278–287, 1995
2. Whiteley MS, Magel TR, Torrie EPH *et al.*: Minimally invasive superficial femoral artery endarterectomy: Early experience with a modified technique. *Eur J Vasc Endovasc Surg* **16:** 254–258, 1998
3. Ho GH, Moll FL: Remote endarterectomy in SFA occlusive disease. *Eur J Radiol* **28:** 205–210, 1998
4. Sambeek M van, Gussenhoven E, Hagenaars T: Vascular response in the femoropopliteal artery after implantation of an ePTFE balloon expandable endovascular graft: an intravascular ultrasound study. *Thesis*: Intravascular ultrasound and peripheral endovascular interventions. Ch 5. ISBN 90-9012129-3.
5. Hoedt M, Lugt A van de, Wittens C: Long-term follow-up of femoropopliteal bypasses comparing patencies and complications related to distal end-to-side and end-to-end anastomoses. Presented at the XII Annual Meeting ESVS '98 and accepted for publication *Eur J Vasc Endovasc Surg*.

Infrainguinal technical improvements? Endoluminal grafting

Hero van Urk, Marc RHM van Sambeek

INTRODUCTION

The early surgical solution for the problem of femoropopliteal obstructive disease was discovered by Joao Cid Dos Santos,[1] namely the 'thromboendarterectomy' of the superficial femoral artery. After the introduction of the femoropopliteal venous bypass operation in 1949 by Kunlin,[2] thromboendarterectomy has gradually disappeared, although some institutions continued to perform this operation. The 'semi-closed' technique as devised by Jorg Volmar reduced the impact of the 'open' surgical procedure and therefore could be considered as minimally invasive surgery 'avant la lettre'. The principle of percutaneous treatment by co-axial catheters as developed by Dotter and Judkins[3] in 1964 was the first step to true 'endovascular' treatment, leading to the now commonly used percutaneous balloon angioplasty (PTA) as modified by Grünzig in 1974.[4]

In all of the above-mentioned surgical and interventional procedures the leading parameter for efficacy is: long-term patency. Long-term patency in the femoropopliteal tract is considered to be less than optimal, mainly because of the relatively high incidence of restenosis that occurs in varying degrees but usually leads to re-interventions in up to 40% of the patients.

The introduction of stents raised hopes of better patency through less recoil and less restenosis, based on the theory that stents would better preserve the enlarged vessel lumen. This theory proved right in the iliac area, but proved wrong in the femoropopliteal tract. All in all, the endovascular techniques have not produced a longer patency for femoropopliteal disease, albeit that they are indeed more patient-friendly as a result of their minimally invasive character.

The main cause for restenosis and occlusions in the first 6-12 months is the gradual development of intimal hyperplasia and constrictive fibrosis.[5] Occlusions within the first month are usually considered to be caused by technical failures, either based on the stent-graft material or resulting from deficient surgical or interventional technique. Insufficient inflow or outflow is another reason for early occlusions.

The problem of intimal hyperplasia is multifactorial and universal, and not likely to be solved by correcting one causal factor only. Acceptance of this principle has led to new combinations of different techniques and combinations of different materials.

In the case of femoropopliteal PTA and stenting, it is generally recognized that the process of intimal hyperplasia-formation cannot be stopped by stents. In fact, the stent material itself allegedly triggers intimal hyperplasia-formation. In addition, intimal hyperplasia tends to grow through the interstices of the stent and this process is inadequately compensated for by the wider vessel area (or in-stent area) as measured on cross-sectional images of intravascular ultrasound. Negative remodelling or shrinkage of the vessel wall is another important factor causing restenosis, a fact that was not clinically recognized for a long time but eventually was clearly demonstrated in intravascular ultrasound-studies.[6] Finally, compression of balloon-expandable stents, in particular in the adductor canal area, is probably contributing to the development of restenosis. Similarly, kinking of a graft or stent when the knee joint is flexed is another reason for acute occlusion from external compression forces.

NEWER DEVICES

The recognition of internal hyperplasia growth through the interstices of stents (both balloon-expandable and self-expandable stents) has lead to the concept of 'covered stents'. Covered stents are a combination of a stent and a synthetic vascular graft. The synthetic graft material is used to prevent vascular smooth muscle cells from migrating through the interstices of the stent to the luminal surface of the stent where intimal hyperplasia causes restenosis. Thus, the graft material creates a protective shield against myointimal growth. Stents can be covered on the inside, on the outside or on both sides. The significance of this discrimination lies in the fact that the stent material itself seems to have a triggering effect on intimal hyperplasia-formation. This effect might be abolished if direct contact between stent and arterial wall can be avoided by interposition of an inert material. Polyester and expanded polytetrafluoroethylene (e-PTFE) are known to cause only minimal reaction of the arterial wall, significantly less than stainless steel or metal alloys like nitinol. Covering a stent on the outside thus provides a barrier between stent and arterial wall, while at the same time providing a mechanical barrier against ingrowth of intima hyperplasia.

Stainless steel and 'memory' metals also might cause (acute) thrombosis, as they both are more thrombogenic than either polyester or e-PTFE materials. This is the basis of 'covered stents' with a coating or lining on the inside of the stent. An example of such a covered stent is the Hemobahn™ (WL Gore & Associates, Flagstaff, Arizona, USA) device, consisting of a self-expanding nitinol stent with a thin internal lining of e-PTFE. The combination of the two principles creates – at least theoretically – the best of two worlds namely a stent with internal and external covering. Generally, these covered stents are used in combination with balloon angioplasty. The complete procedure (PTA and stenting) can be performed percutaneously, usually through a 9 Fr introducer sheath.

ENDOLUMINAL GRAFTING

Surgical endarterectomy and PTA have in common that the resulting surface on the inside of the vessel is highly irregular and thrombogenic. Balloon angioplasty has the additional disadvantage of frequently creating plaque rupture and dissection.[7] Calcified plaques are difficult to dilate and frequently lead to restenosis: the original concept of Dotter that plaques could be compressed like 'footsteps in the snow' has long since proven to be not true. The thrombogenic surface may jeopardize early patency of the recanalized artery, especially in low flow situations, for example in patients with occluded crural arteries. At mid-term and long-term follow-up these vessels are at risk for the development of intimal hyperplasia as described above. Several investigators have tried to overcome both problems by inserting – after PTA or endarterectomy – an endoluminal graft in an attempt to cover the raw surface of the vessel with a smoother and biocompatible material, usually e-PTFE; e-PTFE grafts can be balloon-dilated up to about 300% of their original diameter. Goretex® grafts have an outer wrap that provides extra strength to the graft which is meant to prevent aneurysmal dilatation. When this outer wrap is removed, Goretex® grafts can be balloon-dilated like other grafts.* The grafts are usually inserted as a low profile graft (outer diameter 3–4mm) and balloon-dilated to an inner diameter 5–8mm, depending on the size of the balloon used and the size of the reference vessel. The distal end of such an endoluminal graft (or endo-bypass) has to be fixed to the arterial wall, usually by using a short stent. Some authors believe that distal fixation of the graft is not necessary as blood flow and pressure will press the graft against the arterial wall. However, most authors seem to agree that some kind of distal fixation is mandatory to prevent dislodging and migration of the graft.

The proximal end of the graft can also be fixed with a stent (e.g. when inserted percutaneously through an introducer sheath) or anastomosed surgically using a standard surgical suture when introduced through a surgical cut-down in the groin. These endoluminal grafts have been used for short and long stenoses and for superficial femoral artery occlusions. The reported primary and secondary 12-month patencies are quite different and therefore contradictory. Undoubtedly these different patencies are caused by differences in length or severity of stenoses and/or occlusions and also by other factors like clinical indication, inflow- and outflow tracts, and results may be influenced by different peri- and post-procedural antithrombotic regimens. Finally, in most published series a learning curve must be taken into account, as most are performed with new investigational – and frequently 'self-made' – models and techniques. A universal observation is that many additional procedures – both surgical and catheter-based – are necessary to maintain secondary patency.

INDICATIONS FOR AND RESULTS OF ENDOLUMINAL GRAFTING

In the literature ample discussion can be found about indications for above-knee bypass operations, in particular the use of synthetic grafts. The general feeling – not necessarily supported by hard data – is that the result of above-knee synthetic bypasses are inferior to venous bypasses, yet acceptable as these operations are faster, need less extensive incisions, are associated with fewer wound complications and are not prohibitively expensive. The indications for 'endovascular' bypass operations are

* The Gore Company points out that Gore-tex® grafts are not made for this purpose and consequently the company cannot take responsibility for the quality of the graft after removal of the outer wrap.

therefore probably the same as for femoropopliteal synthetic bypasses, provided that the results are comparable. The problem, naturally, is that reported patencies of above-knee synthetic bypasses show considerable variation and are sometimes difficult to interpret. The results of a multicentre randomized prospective trial, as reported by Abott *et al.*[8] can probably be used as an acceptable standard for comparison with endo-bypasses. This study with 244 patients showed a 12-months primary patency rate of 75% and a secondary patency rate of 88%.

On the other hand, results of endoluminal grafting should be compared with results of PTA and stenting, both with bare stents and covered stents. Sapoval *et al.*[9] and Do-dai-do *et al.*[10] reported 1-year secondary patency rates after PTA and Wallstents® of 67% and 89% respectively. Henry *et al.*[11] and Bergeron,[12] using Palmaz® stents, reported a 2-year secondary patency of 95% and 89% respectively. These good results can be achieved with short isolated lesions only; long lesions, multiple lesions and occlusions result in much less favourable patencies, 'long' lesions being longer than 7–10cm.

Spoelstra *et al.*[13] combined recanalization of the occluded superficial femoral artery by PTA or Rotacs catheter (Osypka, Grenzach-Wyhlen, Germany) with a balloon-dilated e-PTFE endoprosthesis and fixed the distal end of the graft with a Palmaz 294 stent (Cordis Endovascular, a Johnson & Johnson Co., Warren, NJ, USA), while using a conventional running end-to-end anastomosis to the common femoral artery at the ostium of the superficial femoral artery. These were long grafts (average length 30cm, range 18–40cm). Primary patency at 1-year follow-up was 73% and secondary patency was 86%.

Rodriguez-Lopez *et al.*[14] reported on 55 endoluminal grafts that were inserted percutaneously for a variety of indications. Recanalization was performed by PTA without the use of atherectomy or endarterectomy. Predilation of the native vessel was performed with a balloon-catheter 1mm larger than the reference diameter to counteract a potential recoil effect. Primary patency after 1 year was 53%, secondary patency was 79%. Causes for failure of these endoluminal grafts were mainly intimal hyperplasia formation (in 20% of occlusions) at the distal and/or proximal end of the graft. Partial retraction of the graft material from the stent, thus exposing the stent to the arterial wall, may have played an important role in this intimal hyperplasia-formation.[15,16] Outflow stenosis in the crural vessels and progression of atherosclerotic disease proximal to the graft was seen in one-third of the failed grafts.

THE ENDURING™ VASCULAR GRAFT

We have experience with a new device for endoluminal grafting of the femoropopliteal artery, the Enduring™ Vascular Graft (Fig. 1). This graft was developed by WL Gore & Associates, Flagstaff, Arizona, USA. The graft consists of e-PTFE material only (contains no metal stent parts) and has integrated rings consisting of denser e-PTFE material (see Fig. 2). The outer diameter of the graft is 3.5mm; it can be balloon dilated to an inner diameter of 5, 6 or 7mm, with a recoil of ±10%. Gold markers are incorporated to allow visualization under fluoroscopy.

The graft is inserted in the superficial femoral artery through a small groin incision

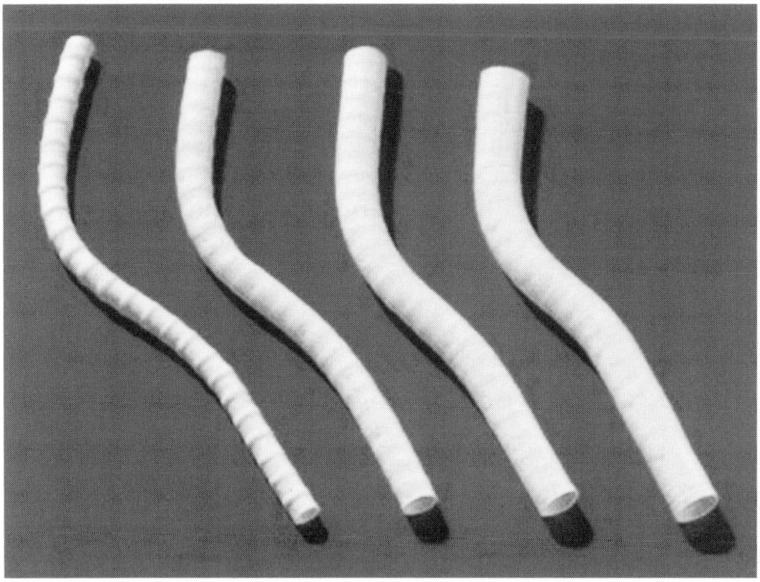

Fig. 1. The different shapes of the enduring graft after balloon dilatation.

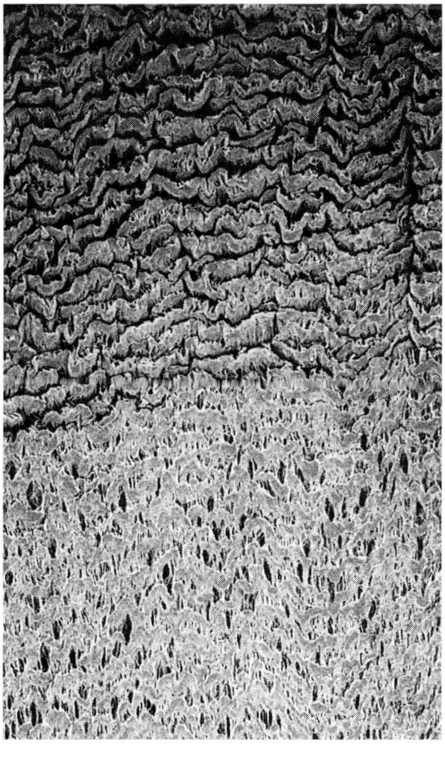

Fig. 2. The microscopic structure of the material. Lower part = denser structure.

and dissection of the femoral artery. Through a longitudinal arteriotomy in the superficial femoral artery a remote endarterectomy is performed, using the Volmar ringstripper and the Moll ringcutter device (Fig. 3) for cutting the atheromatous core at the distal end.

The graft is mounted on a balloon catheter with a pressure of 2 atmosphere and introduced through a long 14 Fr introducer sheath. After withdrawal of the sheath the graft is balloon-dilated with 12 atmospheres of pressure. The denser rings provide kink and compression resistance that is comparable to a Wallstent, while at the same time anchoring the graft against the inner surface of the arterial wall. An overlap of 1½–2cm in the distal 'normal' superficial femoral or popliteal artery is necessary for distal fixation. The graft is available in different lengths of 35, 40 and 45cm. Balloon dilation results in ±10% foreshortening. It is possible the cross the knee joint but until further experience is evaluated we refrain from this. The proximal end of the graft can be cut to the desired length and configuration in order to make a standard end-to-end surgical anastomosis to the origin of the superficial femoral artery using CV-7 e-PTFE sutures.

PRELIMINARY CLINICAL RESULTS

After extensive animal model and human cadaver testing, clinical implantation was started in 1996. After a pilot study using PTA only (without endarterectomy) a prospective multicentre series of 32 patients was performed, always in combination with remote endarterectomy using the Moll ringcutter.

Technical success was achieved in all cases (100%). Procedure-related complications were minimal: two superficial wound infections were seen. Acute thrombotic occlusion was a prominent finding: nine occlusions, of which six occurred

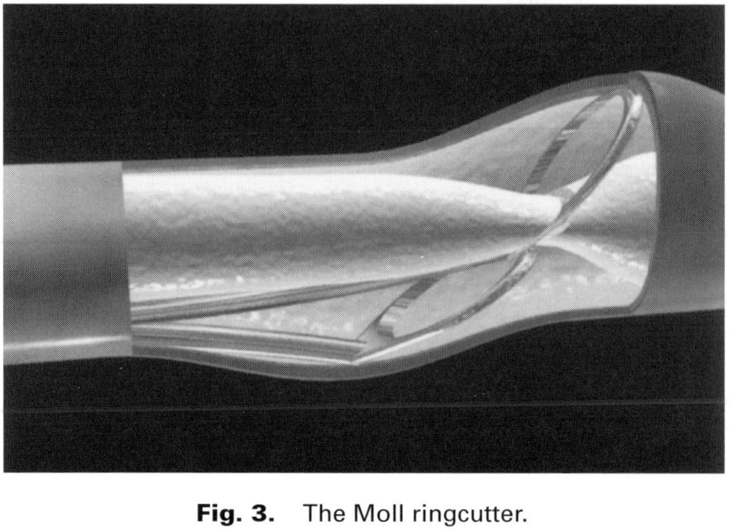

Fig. 3. The Moll ringcutter.

within the first 3 months after implantation. Seven of the nine occlusions were successfully treated with Urokinase, but ten additional procedures were necessary to maintain patency, mainly consisting of PTA (with or without stent) of the distal end of the graft (5 grafts), proximal end (1 graft) or inflow tract (1 graft). After successful fibrinolysis four grafts re-occluded, leading to two open femoropopliteal bypass operations and one amputation.

The primary patency rate at 1 year was 72%, the secondary patency rate 88%. With the restriction that the patient characteristics and indications may be different, these preliminary results seem to be comparable with the results of Spoelstra and Diethrich, while they are not worse than the results of open synthetic above-knee femoropopliteal bypasses.

CONCLUSION

We feel that endovascular devices, specifically designed for endoluminal grafting of the femoral and popliteal arteries, deserve further evaluation and, possibly, refinement. This type of treatment is patient friendly and therefore might be the preferred treatment for femoropopliteal obstructive disease, on condition that their clinical behaviour is at least comparable to 'open' bypass surgery. Further technical improvements in the field of endoluminal grafting are rapidly evolving and may lead to an overall improved performance.

REFERENCES

1. Dos Santos JC: Sur la desobstruction des thromobose arterielles anciennes. *Mem Acad Chir* **73:** 409–411, 1947
2. Kunlin J: Le traitement de l'arterite oblitérante par la greffe veineuse longue. *Arch du mal du coeur* **42:** 371, 1949
3. Dotter CT, Judkins MP: Transluminal treatment of arteriosclerotic obstruction: Description of a new technique and a preliminary report of its application. *Circulation* **30:** 654–670, 1964
4. Grünzig A, Hophoff: Perkuntane Rekanalisation chronischer artieller Verschüsse mit einem neuen Dilatationskatheter. Modification der Dotter-technik. *Dtsch Med Wochenschr* **99:** 2502–2505, 1974
5. Van Lankeren W, Gussenhoven EJ, Kints MJ *et al.*: Stent remodeling contributes to femoropopliteal artery restenosis: An intravascular ultrasound study. *J Vasc Surg* **25:** 753–756, 1997
6. Van Lankeren W, Gussenhoven EJ, Honkoop J *et al.*: Plaque area increase and vascular remodeling contribute to lumen area change after percutaneous transluminal angioplasty of the femoropopliteal artery: an intravascular ultrasound study. *J Vasc Surg* **29:** 430–441, 1999
7. Gerritsen, *et al.*: Intravascular ultrasonography before and after intervention: *in vivo* comparison with angiography. *J Vasc Surg* **18:** 31–40, 1993
8. Abott W, Green RM, Matsumo T *et al.*: Prosthetic above knee femoropopliteal bypass grafting result of a multicenter randomized prospective trial. *J Vasc Surg* **25:** 19-28, 1997
9. Sapoval MR, Long AR, Raynaud AC *et al.*: Femoropopliteal stent placement: Long term results. *Radiology* **184:** 833–839, 1992
10. Do-dai-Do, Triller K, Walpoth BH *et al.*: A comparison study of self-expandable stents vs.

balloon angioplasty alone in femoropopliteal arterial occlusions. *Cardiovasc Intervent Radiol* **15:** 306–312, 1992

11. Henry M, Amor M, Ethevenot G *et al.*: Palmaz stent placement in iliac and femoropopliteal arteries: Primary and secondary patency in 310 patients with 2 to 4-year follow-up. *Radiology* **197:** 167–174, 1995
12. Bergeron P, Pinot JJ, Poyen V, *et al.*: Long-term results with the Palmaz stent in the superficial femoral artery. *J Endovasc Surg* **2:** 161–167, 1995
13. Spoelstra H, Casselman F, Lesceu O: Balloon-expandable endobypass for femoropopliteal atherosclerotic occlusive disease. A preliminary evaluation of fifty-five patients. *J Vasc Surg* **24:** 647–654, 1996
14. Rodrigues-Lopez JA, Soler L, Werner A *et al.*: Long-term follow-up of endoluminal grafting for aneurysmal and occlusive disease in the superficial femoral artery. *J Endovasc Surg* **6:** 270–277, 1999
15. Marin ML, Veith FJ, Cynamon J *et al.*: Effect of polytetrafluoroethylene covering of Palmaz stents on the development of intimal hyperplasia in human iliac arteries. *J Vasc Inerv Radiol* **7:** 651–656, 1996
16. Marin ML, Veith FJ, Cynamon J *et al.*: Human transluminally placed endovascular stented grafts: Preliminary histopathologic analysis of healing grafts in aortoiliac and femorol artery occlusive disease. *J Vasc Surg* **21:** 595–603, 1995

PERIPHERAL ARTERIAL OPPORTUNITIES
Choice of procedure

Angioplasty first for intermittent claudication?

Andries J Kroese, Carl Erik Slagsvold, Tor Flørenes

INTRODUCTION

The natural history of intermittent claudication is relatively benign. In 50–75% of cases symptoms remain stable or improve, with few patients progressing to critical ischaemia, and the risk for amputation is low, approximately 1-2% per year.[1] However, a patient with intermittent claudication usually suffers from a generalized atherosclerotic disease which carries an increased risk of myocardial infarction, stroke and death. Claudicants have an annual mortality of 5–10%, which is two to three times greater than age- and gender-matched asymptomatic groups.[2] Furthermore, the risk of developing intermittent claudication in the contralateral limb is 10–20% per year.[3] Finally, intermittent claudication results in a serious impairment of health-related quality of life.[4]

The increasing demand for treating patients with intermittent claudication is partially due to the ageing of the population and the availability of less invasive techniques, such as percutaneous transluminal angioplasty (PTA). Balloon angioplasty has been popularized in the media as a simple, effective and cheap method which has revolutionized the treatment of peripheral arterial disease. Due to constraints in health care spending, high expectations from patients and a generally greater enthusiasm for treating angiographically suitable lesions with PTA than for supervising a conservative treatment, the use of balloon angioplasty has increased enormously.[4] However, despite the fact that millions of angioplasties have been performed,[5,6] indications to perform PTA are still more based on opinions than scientific data.[7,8]

It is therefore relevant to question on which evidence we select the appropriate treatment for patients with intermittent claudication. Should PTA always be the first choice, because of its low mortality, morbidity and cost, and since it does not preclude subsequent vascular surgery?[9] To answer this question we have to compare aims and results of the three main options to treat patients with intermittent claudication: *conservative treatment*, *angioplasty* and *surgery*.

CONSERVATIVE TREATMENT

Optimal conservative treatment consists of reducing risk factors for atherosclerosis, systematic exercise training and in some cases adjuvant pharmacological treatment. Additionally, co-existing problems such as polycythaemia, anaemia, cardio-pulmonary and other chronic disease have to be managed. Fewer than 10% of claudicants have normal coronary arteries and in 60% significant, correctable coronary obstructions can be found.[10]

Reduction of risk factors

Smoking is the risk factor which is best correlated with both the onset and worsening of intermittent claudication.[11] Smokers have a more than five times greater risk of developing intermittent claudication, whereas the improvement of maximal walking distance is twice as great in patients who stop smoking than in those who continue to do so.[12] Furthermore, the outcome of vascular surgery is significantly better in patients who stop smoking.[13] Last but not least, survival rates even after 1 year are better in non-smokers than smokers.[14] The sole impact of successful smoking cessation on intermittent claudication may be difficult to evaluate since it usually is associated with other lifestyle changes. However, it is the most important prophylactic measure against peripheral atherosclerosis.[15]

Diabetes is associated with a more severe course of atherosclerosis and should therefore be meticulously regulated. The risk of myocardial infarction and stroke are elevated and the amputation rate is increased by as much as seven times.[16]

Hypertension is an independent risk factor for intermittent claudication[11] and requires appropriate treatment, avoiding too great a decrease in blood pressure since this may worsen claudication symptoms.[17]

Lipid risk factors, such as elevated low density lipoprotein cholesterol and triglyceride levels, and low high density lipoprotein cholesterol plasma concentration should be optimized, since this may lead to stabilizing or regression of femoropopliteal atherosclerosis and a reduced mortality.[18] However, the effect of lipid modification by changing diet and/or the use of statins on intermittent claudication has as yet to be proven.

Haematological disorders are more frequently encountered among patients with peripheral arterial disease and have to be diagnosed because hypercoagulability may aggravate the course of the disease.[19]

Increased plasma homocysteine concentration has been shown to be an independent risk factor for peripheral arterial disease.[20] Although the intake of vitamins B12 and B6 may lower the blood levels of homocysteine, the effect on intermittent claudication is not known.

Exercise

Results from treadmill exercise may be difficult to interpret and compare because the reproducibility of results have been unsatisfactory.[21] However, in at least three randomized controlled trials maximum treadmill walking distance was increased in the patients who entered a supervised exercise programme compared with a control group.[22]

A supervised exercise programme may consist of 30-minute sessions, preferably on a treadmill, at least 3 times a week for a period of at least 6 months. Such a programme will most likely imply a better total care of patients with intermittent claudication and is probably more effective than home-based training where compliance may be a problem.[23] However, it still is doubtful whether supervised programmes, being time-consuming and relatively expensive, are sufficiently cost-effective to be generally recommended. Unfortunately, no adequate predictive factors for the outcome of exercise therapy have as yet been identified.[24]

The physiological mechanisms underlying the improvement of intermittent claudication after exercise training are not completely understood. Patients may achieve a significant increase in walking distance without an associated increase in ankle brachial pressure index (ABPI). Possible explanations include improvement of collateral flow, redistribution of blood perfusion, improved oxidative metabolism in ischaemic muscle tissue[25] and a rheological adaptation, e.g. reduced blood viscosity.[26] Raising of pain threshold in the course of a training period may also play a role.[27] Exercise training may encourage patients to reduce weight as part of a change towards a more healthful lifestyle, which in turn may improve intermittent claudication symptoms.[28] Finally, most patients derive a positive psychological benefit from exercise training.

It has recently been suggested that exercise training could be harmful, since an inflammatory response to exercise in ischaemic muscles may have a deleterious effect on atheroslcerotic disease.[29] Until convincing clinical evidence can support this theory, we should, according to the advice from the American Heart Association, 'stop smoking and keep walking'.[30]

Pharmacological treatment

Antiplatelet drugs, such as acetylsalicylic acid[31] and ticlopidine[32] are effective in reducing cardiovascular mortality. Furthermore, daily low-dose aspirin medication has been shown to reduce the need for vascular surgery in apparently healthy men.[33] Although the progression of peripheral atherosclerosis may be slowed down by using a combination of aspirin and dipyridamole,[34] no positive effect of antiplatelet therapy on the symptoms of intermittent claudication has yet been proven. Nonetheless, all patients with peripheral arterial disease should be considered for treatment with an antiplatelet drug to reduce the morbidity and mortality from this disease.[35] The results of trials assessing the effect of aspirin combined with dipyridamole on intermittent claudication are still awaited. However, a randomized, placebo-controlled trial concluded that the use of another platelet inhibitor, ticlopidine, may improve claudication symptoms.[31] Clopidogrel is a promising, effective platelet inhibitor with supposedly fewer side-effects than ticlopidine.

Long-term anticoagulation therapy for intermittent claudication has not been investigated in a prospecitve, randomized fashion.

Pentoxifylline, improving erythrocyte flexibility and several haemorheological factors, and *nafronyl oxalate*, increasing oxygen utilization in ischaemic tissues, are the most commonly used vasoactive drugs in the treatment of intermittent claudication. In randomized studies the efficacy of both drugs was in the order of a 20–60 metre increase in painfree walking distance. Especially because data on quality of life were lacking, these results are hardly clinically relevant. Since the effectiveness of these substances is still a matter of controversy, liberal use is not advocated.[36]

Ketanserin, being a selective serotonin antagonist, causes vasodilation. In addition, it lowers blood viscosity and has antiplatelet properties. However, it is not effective in treating patients with intermittent claudication.[37]

Similarly, the positive effect of prostaglandins and metabolic agents, such as carnitine derivates, on intermittent claudication remains to be convincingly demonstrated. Neither vasodilators such as alpha- and beta- antagonists, calcium channel blockers and angiotensin converting enzyme (ACE-) inhibitors can be recommended for the symptomatic treatment of intermittent claudication. Although antioxidants such as vitamins C, E and beta-carotene may retard the progression of atherosclerosis,[38] their effect on intermittent claudication is still unknown.

PTA

For patients with intermittent claudication the immediate results of PTA have been favourable with an overall technical success rate of 90%, a 1- and 5-year patency rate of 70% and 50%, respectively.[39] Most importantly, the quality of life of patients generally improves following PTA.[40,41] Finally, the periprocedural mortality has been negligible and complications including groin haematoma, false aneurysm and embolism range between 3 and 13%.[42] Due to the better results, it is generally more tempting to perform PTA in iliac arteries than in the femoropopliteal segment.

When indications for PTA are generally restricted to short (<5cm) stenoses or occlusions, only 15–40% of patients with intermittent claudication and clinical indications for invasive treatment are angiographically amenable for PTA.[42] Furthermore, in approximately 5–20% of patients PTA is technically unsuccessful, partly because of the inability to cross the lesion with a guidewire.[43] Although 20–30% of patients treated by PTA need a re-intervention within 3 years, this is not always due to a restenosis or reocclusion. The majority of recurrences are caused by lesions at different locations due to the progression of the underlying disease.[7]

Aortoiliac disease is more common in younger patients who may be impeded in performing their daily work. PTA is angiographically suitable in 75% of cases with aortoiliac atherosclerosis, where stenoses are more than twice as prevalent as occlusions and the majority of stenoses and occlusions are short. The 3-year clinical patency rates for iliac lesions have varied between 60 and 85%.[43] These good results and its low morbidity and mortality make PTA the first choice of treatment in patient with intermittent claudication where conservative treatment has failed.

Femoropopliteal disease is two to five times more prevalant than iliac atherosclerosis. Unfortunately, occlusions occur three times more frequently than stenoses. At centres obtaining 3-year clinical patency rates of 50–60% for femoropopliteal obstructions,[44] it is suggested that PTA is the preferred initial invasive treatment in patients with disabling claudication.[45] In selecting patients for infrainguinal angioplasty one should keep in mind that femoropopliteal patency is adversely affected by diabetes, smoking, long occlusions and low pre- and post-procedural ABPI.[46] Since PTA should preferably be reserved for short (<5cm) lesions, only 30% of patients with femoropopliteal atherosclerosis are candidates for this procedure.

Popliteal and infrapopliteal PTA is rarely performed in patients with intermittent claudication, but may be the first choice of treatment for patients with critical ischaemia.[9] In the hands of a skilled interventionalist primary and secondary patencies at 2-year follow-up may vary between 50 and 80%, comparable with the results achieved with distal bypass surgery.[47] Subintimal angioplasty (S-PTA) as introduced and further developed by Bolia in Leicester, UK, may improve the possibilities of endovascular management of infragenicular atherosclerotic occlusions.[48] We are in the process of publishing the results of treating our first 100 patients with S-PTA, achieving a 75% 24-month primary patency rate.

The exact role of stenting is still unclear. A few trials determining the proper indications for the application of stents are in progress. Due to the greater size of the arteries, stenting may improve patency in the aortoiliac segment. The general use of stents for femoropopliteal lesions provides unacceptably poor results and is therefore not advocated.[49] Presently, stents are used selectively for the management of PTA-induced intimal dissections, eccentric stenoses or restenoses.[50]

SURGICAL TREATMENT

The indications for surgery in patients with intermittent claudication should be strict, due to a greater morbidity and mortality than with alternative treatments. On the other hand, quality of life may be so important for certain patients that they are willing to trade life-expectancy to improve it.[51]

Aortofemoral bypass grafting is rarely indicated to alleviate intermittent claudication, despite the obtainable good long-term results of 80% 10-year patency rates. Similary, extra-anatomic crossover bypass and iliac endarterectomy (ringstripping) are seldomly performed due to the good results after PTA (stent) in this arterial segment.

Femoropopliteal bypass surgery is associated with a 30-day mortality of approximately 1% and increased risk of cardiopulmonary morbidity, and the 1-year amputation rate of 1% is comparable with the natural course of the disease.[52] If it is technically feasible to perform an above-knee bypass, most Scandinavian surgeons would use a prosthetic graft.[53] The resulting 5-year patency rates of 60–80% are similar to those for venous bypass surgery.[54]

The advocates of using an *autologous venous conduit* whenever possible, argue that it offers superior patency rates, whereas the need for a vein for future coronary artery bypass or distal bypass surgery is less than 20% of cases. The saphenous vein is the primary choice for a below-knee femoropopliteal bypass, because prosthetic grafts without the construction of an additional venous patch or cuff at the site of the distal anastomosis, do not perform well at this location. In the absence of an autogenous vein composite bypass grafting is generally reserved for patients with critical limb ischaemia.

Profunda plasty may offer significant relief of symptoms in selected patients with a profunda stenosis, a long occlusion of the superficial femoral artery and good inflow conditions.

COMPARATIVE STUDIES

Treatment strategies should be based on sound research evidence rather than on personal preferences.[55] Results from non-randomized studies are often difficult to compare, since accepted reporting standards are not always being adhered to.[56] They often include patients with intermittent claudication and critical ischaemia and are non-homogenous regarding smoking habits, diabetes and other additional diseases. When choosing between conservative and invasive treatment of patients with intermittent claudication, allocation bias is likely to occur. Patients with more severe symptoms and angiographically more generalized atherosclerosis may more often be treated invasively, thereby contributing to the heterogeneity of patient groups. Finally, the results of treatment have been evaluated by different parameters, including initial technical result, primary and secondary patency of a surgical or endovascular intervention, improvement of ABPI, angiographic or duplex findings, mortality, morbidity, relief of symptoms by increasing pain-free and maximum walking distances. Interestingly, anatomical arterial patency cannot automatically be translated into clinical success, which is also influenced by physiological and psychological factors.[57]

This variety of information may make it difficult to compare the efficacy of different treatment options. Since the aim of all therapy for intermittent claudication is palliation of symptoms, health related quality of life assessment is an indispensible outcome measure.[58] For the estimation of quality of life several well-recognized questionnaires can be used, such as the Nottingham Health Profile and the Short Form Outcomes Questionnaire (SF-36).[59] The advantage of using the EuroQoL (EQ) health questionnaire, is the generation of different profiles of health related quality of life which can be converted into single indices, facilitating comparison between different groups and over time.[60]

Finally, a comparison of different treatment options should include an estimation of cost-effectiveness.

Exercise training alone versus additional PTA

Only two prospective, randomized trials fullfilled the standards set by the Cochrane Review Group,[61] one conducted in Oxford[62] and the other in Edinburgh.[63]

The results from both trials confirmed findings from non-randomized cohort series that there is a short-term benefit from PTA. In the Edinburgh study at 6 months follow-up, walking distances, ABPI, duplex patency rates and quality of life were greater in the PTA group. The Oxford trial found similar early results. However, the clinical benefits of the two treatment modalities, in terms of symptomatology and quality of life, were equalized after 2 years in the Edinburgh trial and at 6 years in the Oxford trial.

In most studies approximately 25% of patients treated by PTA needed some kind of re-intervention, whereas this was necessary in only 10% of the conservatively treated patients.

In conclusion, primary balloon angioplasty and conservative treatment render comparable results in the course of a 2- to 4-year period: between 55 and 80% of patients improve or stabilize their symptoms.[64] Both strategies have advantages and limitations. In contrast to PTA, where a satisfactory result can be obtained during a very short hospital stay, exercise training requires much more time and perseverence. However, a restored arterial patency after PTA does not necessarily imply an improved walking ability. Excercise training may be more effective in increasing quality of life, because in addition to improving local adaptation to muscular ischaemia, it creates better opportunities to modify cardiovascular risk factors such as smoking, diabetes, hypertension, unhealthy dietary habits and overweight.

There is too little scientific evidence to warrant a general conclusion concerning PTA as the primary treatment in patients with intermittent claudication. The treatment of intermittent claudication should be individualized, although it is evident that all patients with intermittent claudication should be treated conservatively for a period of 3-6 months prior to invasive measures are initiated.

Exercise training versus surgery

In a trial of randomizing groups of patients treated to surgery, exercise training or surgery combined with walking training, the results in the surgical group were better than in the group receiving only organized exercise therapy. However, results were best among patients who underwent operation and also participated in physical training, confirming the general notion that exercise training should be an integrated part of treatment for patients with intermittent claudication, regardless of other treatment modalities.[65]

PTA versus surgery

A non-randomized study demonstrated that both PTA and surgical vascular reconstruction can improve quality of life, including pain and physical functioning.[66]

In a Veterans Administration Cooperative Study 263 patients, of whom 73% suffered from intermittent claudication only, were randomly assigned to either surgical treatment or PTA. The initial success rate of angioplasty was lower, but the results of PTA and bypass surgery equalized in the course of 2-3 years.[67] However, 30% of the patients treated by angioplasty needed at least one repeat procedure, increasing costs.[68] This study was criticized for having included patients receiving prosthetic bypass grafts below the inguinal ligament.[69] A smaller randomized trial including only 23 patients with intermittent claudication, did not shed new light on the issue of indications for PTA.[70]

According to a Cochrane review no prospective randomized studies have adequately compared the long-term results of surgery and PTA for patients with intermittent claudication. Recruitment for randomized trials is often difficult, since PTA is mainly used to treat patients with intermittent claudication, whereas bypass surgery is usually indicated for treatment of critical ischaemia.

In conclusion, results for PTA and surgery after 2 years are similar, but the former carries a lower morbidity and does not preclude later bypass surgery. The suggestion of balloon angioplasty being more cost-effective than conventional surgery, may be exagerated, due to the use of expensive catheters and the need for repeat procedures.[71]

Surgery and PTA for intermittent claudication are not mutually exclusive treatments, but rather complimentary with different indications.[52] In patients without major contraindications against surgery and who are angiographically amenable for both PTA and operative treatment, PTA should be tried first. It is less invasive, obtains comparable results with surgery during the first few years and does not exclude a later surgical procedure.

PTA FIRST WHENEVER POSSIBLE?

The main goal of treating patients with intermittent claudication is improving quality of life. To answer the question whether PTA shoul be first choice, the answer is ‘no’ and 'yes'. Since most patients face a reduced life expectancy due to cardiopulmonary disease, diabetes and other chronic ailments, any therapy should carry a minimum of complications. Therefore, optimal conservative treatment for a period of 3–6 months, not PTA, should almost always be initiated. This regimen may slow down the atherosclerotic process and reduce cardiovascular mortality and morbidity. It has been argued that a simple arterial lesion should be treated by PTA as soon as possible, since progression of atherosclerosis may preclude a future attempt with PTA. However, neither this theory nor the role of PTA in enhancing the (local) atherosclerotic process, have ever been scientifically substantiated.

Before proceeding with invasive treatment after conservative measures have failed, a number of factors have to be taken into consideration: the patient´s age, general health, cardiopulmonary status and disability in relation to needs for physical activity in daily life (Fig. 1). In addition to an adequate cardiac examination,

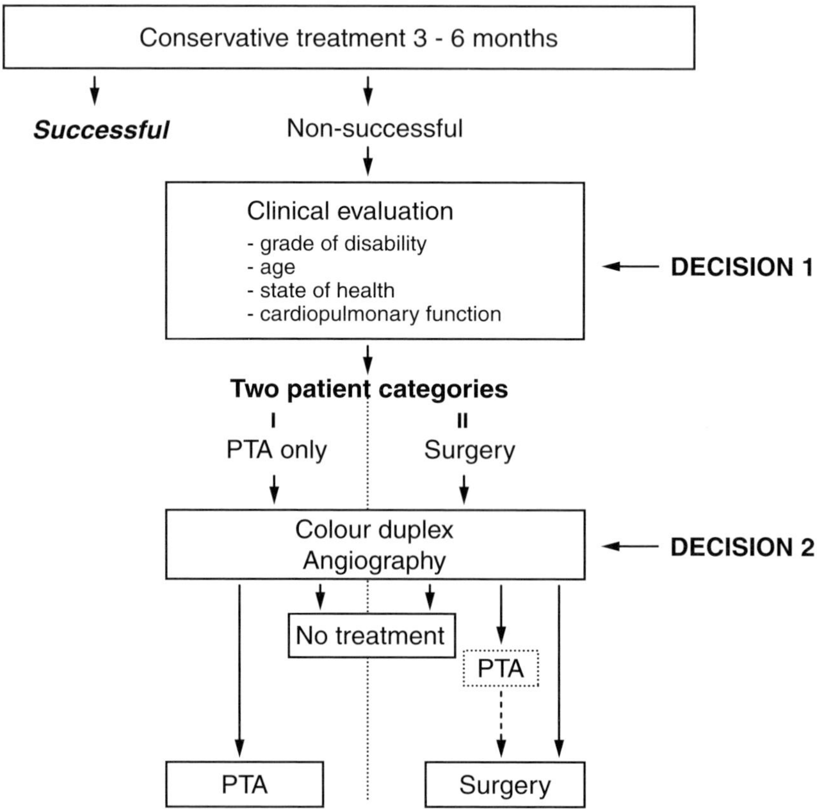

Fig. 1. Therapeutic pathway for patients with intermittent claudication. If 3-6 months of conservative treatment is not successful, the decision to proceed with an invasive intervention, is based on clinical evaluation only. In addition, before the Doppler scan and angiography are performed, it is decided whether the patient belongs to category I: 'PTA only' or category II: 'Surgery if PTA is not feasible'. In all cases which seem angiographically amenable, PTA is the first choice of treatment.

other manifestions of atherosclerosis should be investigated, as 5–10% of patients have a signifcant carotid stenosis and/or an aortic aneurysm.

When a patient is considered eligible for invasive therapy, it should be decided whether this implies 'PTA only' or also surgery if PTA is not feasible (Fig. 1). This decision is also based on a thorough case history and clinical findings and is made before a duplex scan and angiography are performed, to avoid treating attractive angiographic lesions instead of patients. To minimize the use of X-ray contrast medium, a duplex scan may be primarily used to identify whether a patient is suitable for PTA. However, the reliability of this modality is more investigator-dependent.[72]

CONCLUSIONS

At present we still do not know which is the best treatment for individual patients with intermittent claudication. Sufficiently large controlled trials need to be undertaken to find out whether PTA, conservative treatment (including exercise training), or combinations of these will lead to the greatest long-term symptomatic improvement, with the least morbidity and best cost-effectiveness. In the meantime, it is the vascular surgeon´s responsibility to mainly adhere to conservative treatment of patients with intermittent claudication. It may be tempting to use PTA to obtain a quick haemodynamic success. However, there still is little scientific evidence to support its long-term clinical and economic benefits.

In selected patients, after serious attempts of conservative treatment have failed, PTA should be attempted first, whenever feasible, especially in common iliac artery obstructions where results are optimal, provided an experienced interventionalist or a vascular surgeon with endovascular skills is available.

It is important to let our decisions be guided as much as possible by evidence-based information from sources such as the Cochrane Library. Last but not least, sound clinical judgement is a good compass when we are tailoring treatment to suit each patient.

REFERENCES

1. Cronenwett JL, Warner KG, Zelenock GB *et al.*: Intermittent claudication. Current results of nonoperative management. *Arch Surg* **119:** 430–436, 1980
2. Dormandy J, Mahir M, Ascady G *et al.*: Fate of the patient with chronic leg ischaemia: a review article. *J Cardiovasc Surg* **30:** 50–57, 1989
3. Vries SO, Donaldsson MC, Hunink MG: Contralateral symptoms after unilateral intervention for peripheral occlusive disease. *J Vasc Surg* **27:** 414–421, 1998
4. Khaira HS, Hanger R, Shearman CP: Quality of life in patients with intermittent claudication. *Eur J Vasc Endovasc Surg* **11:** 65–69, 1996
5. Coffman JD: Intermittent claudication – be conservative: *New Engl J Med* **325:** 577–578, 1991
6. Whyman MR, Ruckley CVR, Fowkes FGR: Angioplasty for mild intermittent claudication. *Br J Surg* **78:** 643–645, 1991
7. Norgren L: Is balloon angioplasty indicted for intermittent claudication? – Yes. In:

Greenhalgh RM (Ed), *Indications in Vascular and Endovascular Surgery* pp. 285–292. London: W B Saunders, 1999
8. Bradbury AW: Is balloon angioplasty indicated for intermittent claudication? – No. In: Greenhalgh RM (Ed), *Indications in Vascular and Endovascular Surgery* pp. 293–303. London: W B Saunders, 1999
9. Second European Consensus Document on chronic critical leg ischaemia. *Circulation* **84** (Suppl): 1–26, 1991
10. Hertzer NR, Bewen EG, Young JR *et al.*: Coronary artery disease in peripheral vascular patients: a classification of 1000 angiograms and results of surgical management. *Ann Surg* **199:** 223–233, 1984
11. Kannel WB, McGee DL: Update on some epidemiologic features of intermittent claudication. The Framingham study. *J Am Geriat Soc* **33:** 12–28, 1985
12. Quick CRG, Cotton LT: The measured effect of stopping smoking on intermittent claudication. *Br J Surg* **69** (Suppl): 524–526, 1982
13. Smith I, Franks PJ, Greenhalgh RM: The influence of smoking cessation and hypertriglyceridaemia on the progression of peripheral arterial disaese and the onset of critical ischaemia. *Eur J Vasc Endovasc Surg* **11:** 402–408, 1996
14. Jonason T, Bergstrom R: Cessation of smoking in patients with intermittent claudication: effects on the risk of peripheral vascular complications, myocardial infarction and mortality. *Acta Med Scand* **221:** 253–260, 1987
15. McDaniel M, Cronenwett, DeWeese JA: Basic data related to the natural history of intermittent claudication. *Ann Vasc Surg* **3:** 273–277, 1989
16. Dormandy JA, Murray GD: The fate of the claudicant – a prospective study of 1969 claudicants. *Eur J Vasc Surg* **5:** 131–333, 1991
17. Solomon CA, Ramsay LE, Yeo WW *et al.*: Beta-blockade and intermittent claudication: placebo controlled trial of atenolol and nifedipine and their combination. *Br Med J* **303:** 1100–1104, 1991
18. Blankenhorn DH, Azen SP, Crawford DW *et al.*: Effects of colestipolniacin therapy on human femoral atherosclerosis. *Circulation* **83:** 438–447, 1991
19. Ouriel K, Green RM, DeWeese JA: Activated protein C resistence; prevalence and implications i peripheral vascular disease. *J Vasc Surg* **23:** 46–51, 1996
20. Clarke R, Daly L, Robinson K *et al.*: Hyperhomocysteinemia: an independent risk factor for vascular disease. *New Engl J Med* **324:** 1149–1155, 1991
21. Ouriel K, McDonnell AE, Metz CE *et al.*: A critical evaluation of stress testing in the diagnosis of peripheral vascular disease. *Surgery* **91:** 686–693, 1982
22. Hiatt WR, Regensteiner JG, Hargarten ME: Benefit of exercise conditioning for patients with peripheral arterial disease. *Circulation* **81:** 602–609, 1990
23. Regensteiner JG, Meyer TJ, Krupski WC *et al.*: Hospital- vs. home-based exercise rehabilitation to patients with peripheral arterial occlusive disease. *Angiology* **48:** 291–300, 1997
24. Robeer GG, Brandsma JW, Heuvel SP *et al.*: Exercise therapy for intermittent claudication: A review of the quality of randomised clinical trialse and evaluation of predictive factors. *Eur J Vasc Endovasc Surg* **15:** 36–43, 1998
25. Lundgren F, Dahllof A, Schersten T *et al.*: Muscle enzyme adaption in patients with peripheral arterial insufficiency: spontaneous adaption effect of different treatments and consequences on walking performance. *Clin Sci* **77:** 485–493, 1989
26. Ernst EEW, Matrai A: Intermittent claudication, exercise and blood rheology. *Circulation* **76:** 1110–1114, 1987
27. Tsang GMK, Green MA, Crow AJ *et al.*: Chronic muscle stimulaltion improves ischaemic muscle performance in patients with peripheral vascular disease. *Eur J Vasc Surg* **8:** 419–422, 1994
28. Wyatt MG, Scott PM, Scott DJ *et al.*: Effect of weight on claudication distance. *Br J Surg* **78:** 1386–1388, 1991
29. Tisi PV, Shearman CP: The evidence for exercise-induced inflammation in intermittent claudication: should we encourage patients to stop walking? *Eur J Vasc Endovasc Surg* **15:** 7–17, 1988

30. Weitz JI, Byhrne J, Clagett GP *et al.*: Diagnosis and treatment of chronic arterial insufficiency of the lower extremities: A critical review. *Circulation* **94:** 3026–3049, 1996
31. Antiplatelet Trialists´ Collaboration. Secondary prevention of vascular disease by prolonged antiplatelet treatment. *Br Med J* **296:** 320–331, 1988
32. Janzon L, Bergquist D, Boberg J *et al.*: Prevention of myocardial infarction and stroke in patients with intermittent claudication: effects of ticlopidine. Results from STIMS, the Swedish Ticlopidine Multicenter Study. *J Intern Med* **227:** 301–308, 1990
33. Goldhaber S, Manson J, Hennekens C *et al.*: Low-dose aspirin and subsequent peripheral arterial surgery in the Physician´s Health Study. *Lancet* **340:** 143–145, 1992
34. Hess H, Deichsel G, Mietasck A: Drug-induced inhibition of platelet function delays progression of peripheral occlusive arterial disease. A prospective double-blind arteriographically controlled trial. *Lancet* **i:** 415–419, 1985
35. Balsano F, Coccheri S, Libretti A *et al.*: Ticlopidine in the treatment of intermittent claudication: a 21-month double-blind trial. *J Lab Clin Med* **114:** 84–91, 1989
36. Porter JM, Cutler BS, Lee BY *et al.*: Pentoxifylline efficacy in the treatment of intermittent claudication: multicenter controlled double blind trial with objective assessment of chronic arterial occlusive disease patients. *Am Heart J* 104: 66–72, 1982
37. PACK Claudication Substudy Investigators: Randomized placebo-controlled, double-blind trial of ketanserin in claudicants. Changes in claudication distance and ankle systolic pressure. *Circulation* **80:** 1544–1548, 1989
38. Stephens NG, Parsons A, Schofield PM *et al.*: Randomised controlled trial of vitamin E in patients with coronary disease: Cambridge Heart Antioxidant Study (CHAOS). *Lancet* **347:** 781–786, 1996
39. Adar R, Critchfield, GC, Eddy DM A: Confidence profile analysis of the results of femoropopliteal percutaneous transluminal angioplasty in the treatment of lower-extremity ischaemia. *J Vasc Surg* **10:** 57–59, 1989
40. Cooke TA, O´Regan, Galland RB: Quality of life following percutaneous translulminal angioplasty for claudication. *Eur J Vasc Endovasc Surg* **11:** 191–194, 1996
41. Whyman MR, Fowkes FGR, Kerracher EMG *et al.*: Randomized controlled trial of percutaneous transluminal angioplasty for intermittent claudication. *Eur J Vasc Endovasc Surg* **12:** 167–172, 1996
42. Hunick MGM, Donaldson MC, Meyerovitch MF *et al.*: Risks and benefits from femoropopliteal PTA. *Vasc Surg* 17: 183–194, 1999
43. Johnston KW: Iliac arteries: reanalysis of results of balloon angioplasty. *Radiology* **186:** 207–212, 1993
44. Johnston KW: Femoral and popliteal arteries: ranalysis of results of balloon angioplasty. *Radiology* **183:** 167–171, 1992
45. Hunick MGM, Wong JB, Donaldson MC *et al.*: Revascularization for femoropopliteal disease: a decision and cost-effective analysis. *J Am Med Assoc* **274:** 165–171, 1995
46. Capek P, McLean GK, Berkowitz HD: Femoropopliteal angioplasty: factors influencing long-term success. *Circulation* 83 (Suppl 1): 70–80, 1991
47. Varty K, Bolia A, Naylor AR *et al.*: Infrapopliteal percutaneous transluminal angioplasty: a safe and successful procedure. *Eur J Vasc Endovasc Surg* **9:** 341–345, 1995
48. Bolia A, Bell PRF, London N: The durability of subintimal angioplasty. In: RM Greenhalgh (Ed), *The Durability of Vascular and Endovascular Surgery* pp. 3–15, London: W B Saunders, 1999
49. Vroegindewei D, Vos LD, Tielbeek AV *et al.*: Balloon angioplasty combined with primary stenting versus balloon angioplasy alone in femoropopliteal obstructions. *Intervent Radiol* **20:** 420–425, 1997
50. Gray BY, Sullivan TM, Childs MB *et al.*: High incidence of restenosis / reocclusion of stents in the percutaneous treatment of long-segment superficial femoral artery disease after suboptimal angioplasty. *J Vasc Surg* **25:** 74–83, 1997
51. Torrance Q: Measurement of health state utilities for economic appraisal: a review. *J Hlth Econ* **5:** 1–30, 1986
52. Kent KC, Donaldson MC, Attinger CE *et al.*: Femoropopliteal reconstruction for claudication. The risk to life and limb. *Arch Surg* **123**: 1196–1198, 1988

53. Nielsen OM, Jensen LP, Schroeder TV: The Nordic experience of preference for above knee femoropopleteal bypass. In: Greenhalgh RM and Fowkes FGR (Eds), *Trials and Tribulations of Vascular Surgery* pp. 325–331, London: W B Saunders, 1996
54. Veith FJ, Gupta SK, Ascer E *et al.*. Six year prospective multicenter randomized comparison of autologous saphenous vein and expanded polytetrafluoroethylene grafts in infrainguinal arterial reconstructions. *J Vasc Surg* **3:** 104-114, 1987
55. Sheldon TA: Systematic reviews and meta-analyses: the value for surgery. *Br J Surg* **86:** 977–978, 1991
56. Ahn SS, Rutherford RB, Becker GJ *et al.*: The Ad Hoc Subcommittee on Reporting Stnadards of the SVS/North American Chapter of ISCVS. Reporing standards for endovascular procedures. *J Vasc Surg* **17:** 1103–1103, 1993
57. Creasy TS, McMillan PJ, Fletcher EWL: Is percutaneous transluminal angioplasty better than exercise for claudication? – preliminary results from a prospective randomised trial. *Eur J Vasc Surg* **4:** 135–140, 1990
58. Chetter IC, Spark JI, Scott DJ *et al.*: Prospective analysis of quality of life in patient following infrainguinal reconstructions for chronic critical ischaemia. *Br J Surg* 85: 51–551, 998
59. Brazier JE, Harper RM, Baird RN. Validation the SF-36 health survey questionnaire: net outcome measure for primary care. *Br Med J* **305:** 160–164, 1992
60. Chetter IC, Spark JI, Dolan P: Quality of life analysis in patients with lower limb ischaemia; suggestioins for European standardisation. *Eur J Vasc Endovasc Surg* **13:** 597–604, 1997
61. Leng G, Royle E: More reviews and more trials required. *Eur J Vasc Endovasc Surg* **18:** 280–281, 1999
62. Perkins JM, Collin J, Creasy TS: Exercise training versus angioplasty for stable claudication. Long and medium term results of a prospective, randomised trial. *Eur J Vasc Endovasc Surg* **11:** 409–413, 1996
63. Whyman MR, Fowkes FGR, Kerracker EMG *et al.*: Is intermittent claudication improved by PTA? A randomized controlled trial. *J Vasc Surg* **26:** 551–557, 1997
64. Leng GC, Fowkes FGR. The epidemiology of peripheral arterial disease. *Vasc Med Rev* **4:** 5–18: 1993
65. Lundgren F, Dahlløf AG, Lundholm K *et al.*: Intermittent claudication – Surgical reconstruction or physical training? *Ann Sur* **209:** 346–355, 1989
66. Pell JP, Lee AJ: Impact of angioplasty and arterial reconstructive surgery on the quality of life of claudicants. *Scot Med J* **42:** 47–48,1997
67. Wilson SE, Wolf GL, Cross AP: Percutaneous transluminal angioplsty versus operation for peripheral arteriosclerosis. Report of a prospective randomised trial in a selected group of patients. *J Vasc Surg* **9:** 1–9, 1989
68. Wolf GL, Wilson SE, Cross AP for the investigators of Veterans Administration Cooperative Study number 199: Surgery or balloon angioplasty for peripheral vascular disease: a randomized trial. *J Vasc Intervent Radiol* **4:** 639–648, 1993
69. Weitz JI, Byrne J, Clagett *et al.*: Diagnosis and treatment of chronic arterial insufficiency of the lower extremities: a critical review. *Circulation* **94:** 3026–3049, 1996
70. Holm J, Afvidsson B, Jivegård *et al.*: Chronic lower limb ischaemia. A prospective randomised controlled study comparing 1 year results of vascular surgery and PTA. *Eur J Vasc Surg* **5:** 517–522, 1991
71. Gupta SK, Veith FJ, Ascer E *et al.*: Cost factors in limb threatening ischaemia due to infra-inguinal atherosclerosis. *Eur J Vasc Surg* **2:** 151–155, 1988
72. Whyman MR, Gillespie IN, Ruckley CV *et al.*: Screening patients with claudication from femoropopliteal disease before angioplasty using Doppler colour flow imaging. *Br J Surg* **79:** 907–909, 1992

Bypass or angioplasty for severe ischaemia of the leg: the BASIL trial

Jocelyn Bell, Laszlo Papp, Andrew Bradbury

INTRODUCTION

The relative merits of bypass surgery and percutaneous transluminal angioplasty (PTA) in the management of severe limb ischaemia have been the source of debate and controversy for a number of years. Although it has become increasingly commonplace for PTA to be used as first-line treatment for such patients, the practice is not evidence-based. To date, two prospective randomized, controlled trials comparing bypass surgery and PTA in the management of lower limb ischaemia have been reported.[1,2] Although both trials suggested that the two treatments were equivalent in terms of amputation-free survival, they were flawed in a number of important respects; specifically, both studies were small, included claudicants and did not differentiate patients with aortoiliac and infrainguinal disease. It is clear, therefore, that a larger, properly conducted randomized controlled trial is required.[3,4]

BYPASS SURGERY OR PTA FOR SEVERE LIMB ISCHAEMIA?

Many surgeons believe surgical bypass to be the 'gold standard' and advocate it as first-line treatment for severe limb ischaemia wherever technically possible. However, surgery is not without disadvantages; thus:

- impressive long-term anatomic patency rates[5] and functional outcomes[6] typically reported from single, highly resourced and specialized units in North America have not been matched in multicentre UK studies;[7] especially where prosthetic conduits are anastomosed directly to arteries below the knee;
- surgery is associated with an operative mortality as well as an immediate (30-day) technical failure rate of up to 20%;[8] the latter leading to secondary amputation in up to one-third of cases;[9]
- postoperative graft surveillance is considered by many surgeons to be *de rigeur*. However, surveillance is not supported by level I evidence, results in moderate numbers of (possibly unnecessary) secondary interventions,[10,11] and has major resource implications;
- most UK vascular surgeons lack the time and resources to perform sufficient numbers of femorodistal bypasses.

Increasingly, therefore, patients are being treated by PTA on the basis that:

- it may be associated with less immediate mortality and morbidity;

- it may be more easily repeated;
- it may cost less than surgery;
- although surgery may provide a better long-term anatomic patency this may not translate into a superior clinical outcome because:
    - patients may not live long enough to reap the potential long-term patency benefits of surgery;
    - even if a PTA site does re-occlude, the limb may remain viable due to the development of collaterals.[12]

THE BASIL TRIAL

The Bypass versus Angioplasty in Severe Ischaemia of the Leg (BASIL) trial is being funded by the Health Technology Assessment arm of the UK National Health Service (NHS) (Fig. 1). The trial commenced patient recruitment in August 1999 and will run for 5 years. It is intended to recruit 500 patients over 3 years and to follow each patient for median (minimum) of 3 years (18 months). The specific aim of the trial is to determine whether, in patients with severe limb ischaemia amenable to PTA or bypass, adopting a 'PTA first' strategy rather than the traditional 'surgery first' strategy is associated with a better outcome in terms of:

- amputation-free survival (primary endpoint)
- abolition of symptoms, procedure complications, secondary and crossover interventions, minor amputations, quality of life and cost-effective utilization of NHS resources (secondary endpoints)

SUITABILITY FOR SURGERY OR ANGIOPLASTY: THE DELPHI CONSENSUS

It was considered that defining rigid inclusion and exclusion criteria in terms of suitability for surgery or angioplasty would hamper recruitment and prevent the trial from reflecting true variations in clinical practice; as well as the broad range of anatomic patterns of disease observed in patients with severe limb ischaemia. However, it was felt that the views of individual trialists should be reviewed prior to commencement of the study in order to:

- define and quantify the level of agreement/disagreement amongst surgeons and radiologists regarding the preferred surgical and/or endovascular management of severe limb ischaemia;
- examine angiographic and clinical factors that impact upon these treatment preferences;
- establish a 'grey area of clinical equipoise' where patients could be randomized within BASIL.

This was achieved by means of the Delphi Consensus technique[13] whereby a postal questionnaire was sent to 37 surgeons and 31 radiologists who had agreed to participate in the BASIL trial. The questionnaire consisted of 149 diagrams (angiographic representations) (Fig. 2) depicting different combinations of disease patterns in the:

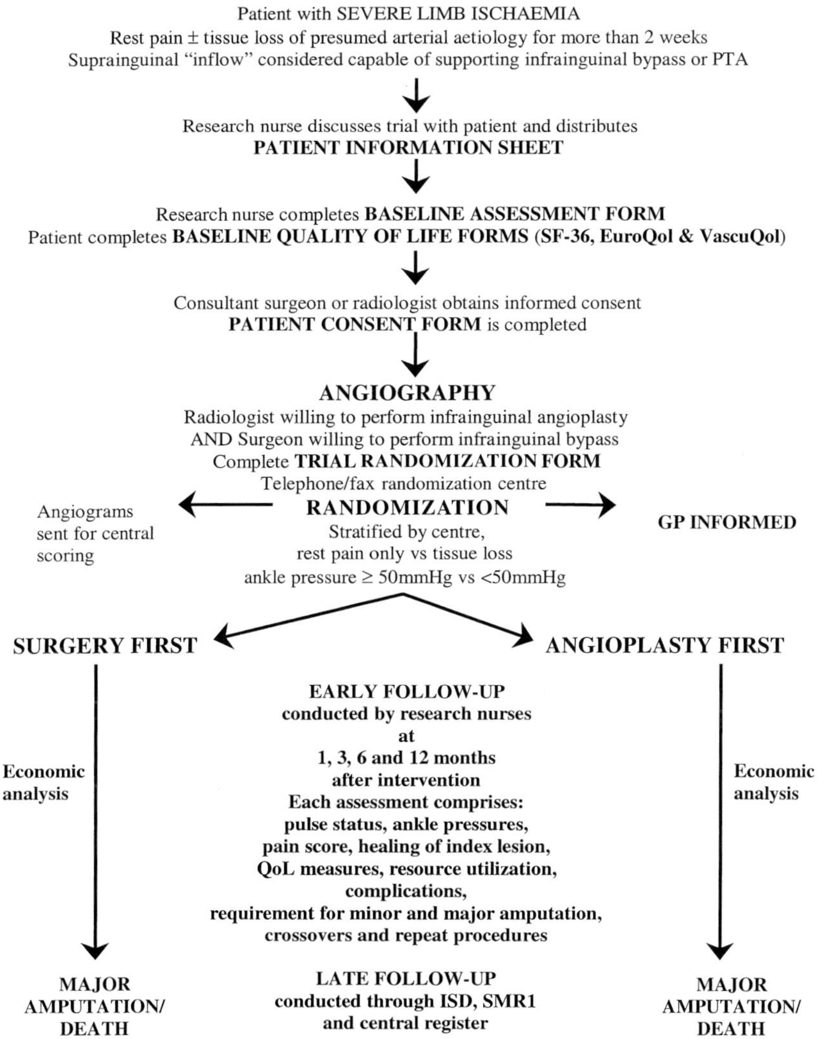

Fig. 1. Outline of bypass versus angioplasty in severe ischaemia of the leg (BASIL) trial.

- superficial femoral artery;
- popliteal artery;
- crural arteries.

Considering the three crural vessels individually would have led to an excessively large number of scenarios. It was therefore decided to ask panellists to consider only that crural vessel which was most amenable to treatment and which would, presumably, be the target outflow vessel for either angioplasty or surgical bypass.

In each segment the severity of disease was presented as either

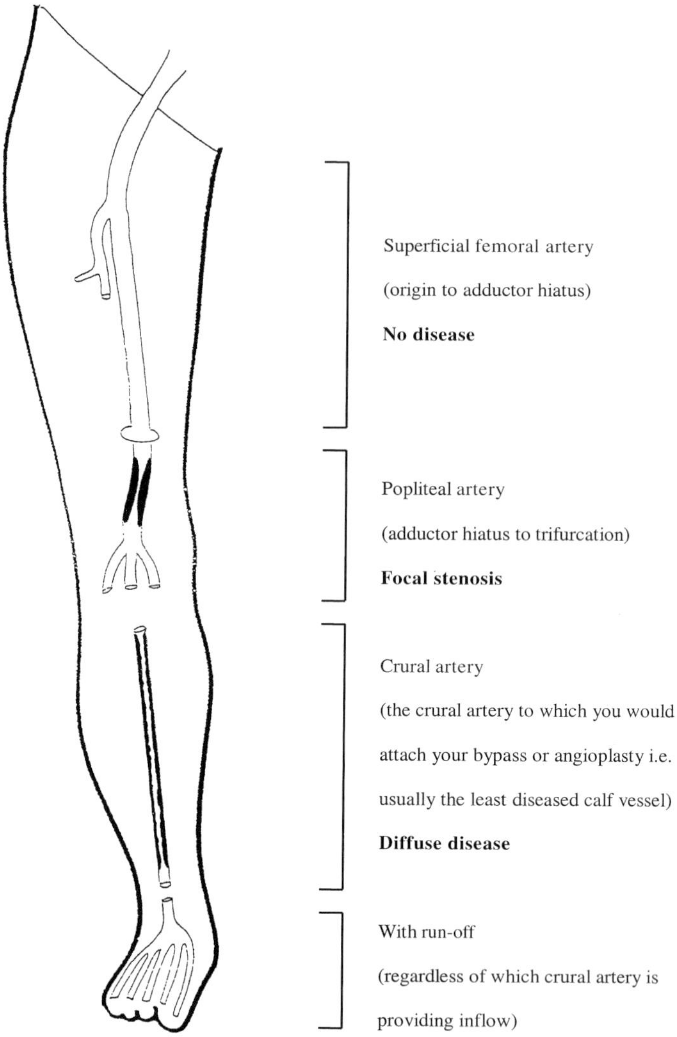

Fig. 2. Delphi consensus. Example of angiographic representation used in questionnaire.

- no haemodynamically significant disease;
- focal (<10cm) non-occlusive haemodynamically significant disease;
- diffuse (>10cm) non-occlusive haemodynamically significant disease;
- short (<10cm) occlusion;
- long (>10cm) occlusion.

No significant disease was present in the pedal vessels apart from scenarios where there was also long occlusion in the crural vessel; these scenarios were presented with and without 'run-off' into the foot.

Panellists were asked to consider each 'angiographic representation' in the presence of either

- rest pain only versus tissue loss (ulcer and/or gangrene);
- suitable vein versus no suitable vein.

This gave a total of 596 disease scenarios. When responding, panellists were asked to assume that:

- patients had received and failed to respond to 'best medical treatment';
- there were no other contraindications to surgery or angioplasty;
- suprainguinal inflow was adequate i.e. there was no significant aortoiliac disease, or it had been successfully treated;
- the patient could not be successfully treated by local treatment to the profunda femoris artery.

For each disease scenario, panellists were asked to decide which of a range of statements (1–8) regarding the appropriateness of surgery, angioplasty or amputation as a first-line strategy most closely agreed with their own personal opinion (Table 1).

DELPHI CONSENSUS – FIRST ROUND RESULTS

Of 68 questionnaires 41 (60%) were returned complete: 21 from surgeons and 20 from radiologists. Both the dispersion and direction of the responses have been considered in the analysis. By convention, the highest 10% and lowest 10% of the responses have been discarded as outliers. The remaining responses were deemed to show agreement if they fell within a 3-point range and disagreement if they did not.

3-point range

1–3	PTA strongly preferred
2–4	PTA preferred
3–5	Appropriate for BASIL
4–6	Surgery preferred
5–7	Surgery strongly preferred
6–8	Surgery/Amputation preferred
Disagreement	Appropriate for BASIL

It was considered that patients could be deemed suitable for BASIL either because there was disagreement about whether PTA or surgery should be used as first-line treatment; or because there was agreement that PTA and surgery were likely to be equally effective. The proportion of scenarios leading to agreement is shown in Fig. 3. Agreement that PTA should be the first-line treatment (scores 123 or 234) was reached in only 44 (7.4%) disease scenarios. These angiographic representations tended to depict minimal disease, which, it could be argued, would be more in keeping with claudication than severe limb ischaemia. Agreement that surgery

Table 1. Dephi consensus study – decision options for each scenario

	1 *Could only be treated by PTA*	2 *Could be treated by PTA or Sx but I strongly prefer PTA*	3 *Could be treated by PTA or Sx but I prefer PTA*	4 *Could be treated by PTA or surgery and I have no preference*	5 *Could be treated by PTA or surgery but I prefer surgery*	6 *Could be treated by PTA or surgery but I strongly prefer surgery*	7 *Could only be treated by Sx*	8 *Not amenable to revascularization – primary amputation*
Rest pain – good vein								
Rest pain – no vein								
Tissue loss – good vein								
Tissue loss – no vein								

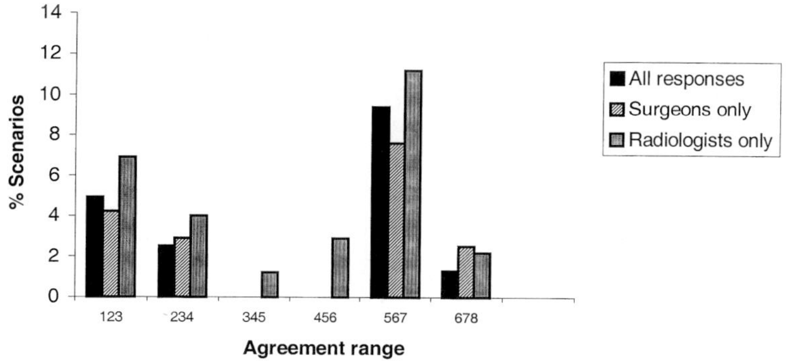

Fig. 3. Proportion of scenarios where agreement was reached.

should be the first-line treatment (scores 456 or 567) was reached in only 56 (9.4%) scenarios. These angiographic representations tended to depict multilevel, occlusive disease; particularly of the superficial femoral artery. Scenarios providing agreement for surgery/amputation (scores 678) were exclusively those where the angiographic representation showed no run-off into the foot. Very few scenarios fell into the middle ground (scores 345). In 488 (81.9%) disease scenarios no agreement was reached. Patients in these latter two categories could be considered to lie in the 'grey area of clinical equipoise' and thus be appropriate for randomization within BASIL. In general, there was a slightly greater level of agreement among radiologists than among surgeons. Perhaps surprisingly, the preferred choice of first-line treatment was unaffected by whether the patient had rest pain only or had tissue loss (with or without rest pain). However, the presence of a suitable vein did influence decision-making by both surgeons and radiologists (Fig. 4).

DELPHI CONSENSUS – SECOND ROUND

First round responses to this Delphi consensus process indicated that there was little agreement between, or among, surgeons and/or radiologists as to the role of bypass and PTA in the management of severe limb ischaemia. Panellist have been provided with feedback on their first-round responses by being shown how their own opinion converges or diverges from that of the group as whole. Each panellist has now been asked to complete the questionnaire again taking into account this information. Responses to the second-round questionnaire will be analysed in the same way and may show that there has been some convergence of views. However, the Delphi study has clearly demonstrated that this is an area where little consensus exists and that the time is right for a randomized controlled trial.

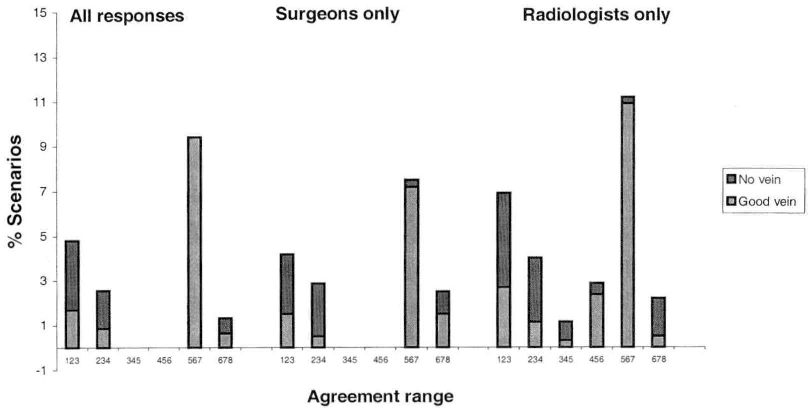

Fig. 4. The effect of availability of vein on preferences for surgery and PTA.

CRITICAL AND SUBCRITICAL ISCHAEMIA

Patients with both critical[14] and subcritical limb ischaemia[15] are eligible for randomization within BASIL provided they have:

- ischaemic rest pain requiring strong (opiate) analgesia for more than 2 weeks, or
- ulceration or gangrene of the foot or toes

At randomization, patients are also being stratified on the basis of their ankle pressure in to groups A, B, C, D:

Clinical presentation	*Ankle pressure ≥50mmHg*	*Ankle pressure <50mmHg*
Rest/night pain only	A	B
Tissue loss ± rest/night pain	C	D

In addition, eligible patients must:

- have no significant suprainguinal disease; although aortoiliac disease can be treated by surgery or PTA (± stent) prior to randomization;
- have given fully informed written consent;
- not have a degree of limb ischaemia, or a co-existing medical or surgical condition, that makes revascularization inappropriate;

- have an angiographic pattern of infrainguinal disease that, in the opinion of the responsible consultant surgeon and radiologist, could be reasonably managed either by surgery or angioplasty in the first instance.

Prior to randomization, relevant baseline information is collected (demographic data, risk factors, relevant past medical history, current medications, clinical status etc) and patients are asked to complete three quality of life questionnaires, the SF-36, EuroQol and a recently developed disease specific instrument for lower limb ischaemia, VascuQol. Patients are randomized to either angioplasty or bypass surgery, according to centre and stratification group, by contacting the co-ordinating centre. Interventions are performed using the normal procedures of the participating centre and relevant details documented.

Patients are followed up at 1, 3, 6 and 12 months after primary intervention either in a hospital-based clinic or by home visit. Should any patient require a secondary or crossover intervention during this follow-up period, details are recorded but the patient continues to be followed-up from the time of primary intervention. At 3, 6 and 12 months patients also complete the three quality of life questionnaires. From 12 months onwards, patients return to normal clinical care but are followed-up through the Information and Statistics Division of the NHS in Scotland or regional Trusts in England.

CONCLUSIONS

Severe limb ischaemia is a major health and socioeconomic problem affecting up to 5000 patients per year in Scotland alone (population about 5 million). It is imperative on both humanitarian and health economic grounds that the treatment of the condition is, as far as possible, evidence-based. The BASIL trial will compare, for the first time, the clinical and cost-effectiveness of PTA and surgery in this condition and, hopefully, allow surgeons and interventional radiologists to make a more informed decisions about the most appropriate treatment for their patients.

REFERENCES

1. Wolf GL, Wilson SE, Cross AP: Percutaneous transluminal angioplasty versus operation for peripheral arteriosclerosis. *J Vasc Surg* **9:** 1–9, 1989
2. Holm J, Arfridsson B: Chronic lower limb ischaemia. A prospective randomised controlled trial comparing the 1-year results of vascular surgery and percutaneous transluminal angioplasty (PTA). *Eur J Vasc Surg* **5:** 517–522, 1991
3. Porter JM: Endovascular arterial intervention: expression of concern. *J Vasc Surg* **21:** 995–997, 1995
4. Bradbury AW, Ruckley CVR: Angioplasty for lower limb ischaemia: time for randomised controlled trials. *Lancet* **347:** 277–278, 1996
5. Pomposelli FB, Marcaccio EJ, Gibbons GW *et al.*: Doralis pedis arterial bypass: Durable limb salvage for foot ischaemia in patients with diabetes mellitus. *J Vasc Surg* **21:** 375–384, 1995
6. Abou-Zamzam AM, Lee RW, Moneta GL *et al.*: Functional outcome after infrainguinal bypass for limb salvage. *J Vasc Surg* **25:** 287–297, 1997

7. Stonebridge PA, Prescott RJ, Ruckley CV for the Joint Vascular Research Group: Randomized trial comparing infrainguinal polytetrafluoroethylene bypass grafting with and without vein interposition cuff at the distal anastomosis *J Vasc Surg* **26:** 543–550, 1997
8. Swedish Vascular Registry: Reoperations, redo surgery and other interventions constitute more than one-third of vascular surgery. *Eur J Vasc Endovasc Surg* **14:** 244–251, 1997
9. Ng RLH, Davies AH, Magee TR *et al.*: Early reoperation rates after arterial surgery. *Eur J Vasc Surg* **8:** 78–82, 1994
10. Cheshire NJW, Noone MA, Wolfe JHN: Re-intervention after vascular surgery for critical leg ischaemia. *Eur J Vasc Surg* **6:** 545–550, 1992
11. Wright MPJ, Davies AH, McGrath C *et al.*: Late reoperation in vascular surgery. *Eur J Vasc Endovasc Surg* **10:** 304–307, 1995
12. Ray SA, Minty I, Buckenham TM *et al.*: Clinical outcome and restenosis following percutaneous transluminal angioplasty for ischaemic rest pain or ulceration. *Br J Surg* **82:** 1217–1221, 1995
13. Fink A, Kosecoff J, Chassin M, Brook RH: Consensus methods: Characteristics and guidelines for use. *Am J Publ Hlth* **74:** 979–983, 1984
14. Second European Consensus Document on Critical Limb Ischaemia: *Eur J Vasc Surg* **6**(Suppl A)**:** 1–32, 1992
15. Wolfe JHN, Wyatt MG: Critical and sub-critical limb ischaemia. *Eur J Vasc Endovasc Surg* **13:** 578–582, 1997

Are infrainguinal angioplasty and surgery comparable?

Jeremy MT Perkins, John HN Wolfe

INTRODUCTION

Vascular surgery has developed since the 1950s. In 1949 Kunlin described the first reversed saphenous vein graft to bridge a superficial femoral artery occlusion,[1] and since then surgical techniques have been refined and the repertoire of infrainguinal bypass grafts expanded to take distal anastomoses ever further down the leg. Artificial materials have been developed as alternative bypass conduits to autologous vein since 1955.[2]

Percutaneous radiological techniques for treating vascular disease arrived in 1964 with Dotter and Judkins description of a rigid coaxial angioplasty catheter system.[3] The great impetus to the widespread introduction of percutaneous angioplasty (PTA) came with the development of the double lumen balloon catheter by Gruentzig in 1974.[4] This ushered in the era of minimally invasive vascular treatment with the perceived benefits of shorter hospital stay, smaller wounds, quicker recovery and return to work, lower mortality and morbidity, and cheaper costs.

With time both surgical and radiological treatment options have increased, as has the ability to treat older and sicker patients. Decision-making is now a complex process and a profusion of data exists to support the appropriateness of each particular treatment. However, much of this information is conflicting, and these data are not robust or free from selection bias. Extrapolation of results from selected series in individual centres to treatment for an individual patient is difficult, and well conducted comparisons of different treatments are few and far between.

This chapter attempts to decide whether, in the 25 years that infrainguinal bypass grafting and percutaneous angioplasty have been available together, we are any closer to deciding which of these treatments is appropriate for specific patients, and whether their results are comparable?

NATURAL HISTORY

Any intervention must be judged against the natural history of the condition being treated. Distinction should be made between intervention for critical ischaemia and for intermittent claudication. The natural history of intermittent claudication is

These authors highlight the absence of quality evidence to indicate whether angioplasty and bypass surgery are comparable techniques. In the future, this evidence will become available, see previous chapter on the BASIL trial. *[Editor: JTP]*

benign, with only approximately 1% of patients progressing to amputation per year.[5,6] Ultimately about 25–30% of patients with claudication will require intervention for worsening symptoms. The minority subgroup of claudicants with critical haemodynamic indices (ankle brachial pressure index (ABPI) <0.35) remain stable in 50% of cases.[7] Progression to limb-threatening ischaemia occurs in the half of the patients, but only 4% require amputation. This benign course of claudication requires that any intervention for this condition must have a low rate of life and limb-threatening complications, and be focussed on a small subgroup that will benefit.

The risk to both life and limb for patients with critical ischaemia is much greater. Procedures which would be inappropriate for the treatment of claudicants, because of associated mortality and morbidity, and risk of limb loss with failure, may be considered suitable for patients with a critically ischaemic limb. Half of these patients (treated or untreated) have died after 3 years, and only 5% of those with tissue loss and and/or an ankle pressure <40mmHg will keep their leg if managed conservatively.[8] Patients with subcritical ischaemia (rest pain and/or an ankle pressure >40mmHg) show a different natural history to the severely critically ischaemic group outlined above, as 27% of patients with subcritical ischaemia will keep their leg within a year if managed conservatively.[8]

Claudicants, and patients with subcritical and critical ischaemia clearly show a different natural history for their disease. Much of the data regarding infrainguinal angioplasty and bypass grafting is confusing and misleading because studies include all three indications together, and often fail to differentiate results according to the indication for intervention.

INTERMITTENT CLAUDICATION

General case series of angioplasty for intermittent claudication have confirmed 3-year clinical patencies of 53–62% for femoropopliteal disease,[9,10] with better results being recorded for shorter lesions,[11,12] and for stenoses rather than occlusions.[11,12] Case series of femoropopliteal bypass grafting solely for claudication are less numerous. The majority of above-knee bypasses recorded use polytetrafluroethylene (PTFE), and report primary patency rates of 48–65% at 5 years.[13,14] Secondary patency rates at 5 years for PTFE are 76–79%.[14,15] The results for autologous vein may be better for above-knee bypass[16] and are definitely better for below-knee bypass. There are a large number of papers reporting the results of below-knee femoropopliteal bypasses, but most of these include claudicants and critically ischaemic patients together and do not discriminate between the two when reporting graft patency. Published primary patency for below-knee femoropopliteal bypasses for claudication vary from 55% at 5 years for PTFE[15] to 77% at 5 years for vein grafts.[13]

Tibial angioplasty or distal surgical bypass for claudication is rarely performed. Only two publications describe femorotibial bypass for claudication[13,17] and one of these includes only three cases in a larger series of aortoiliac procedures and femoropopliteal bypasses.[17] Byrne *et al.* reported on 94 cases of femorotibial bypass performed for disabling claudication in a series of 409 surgical bypasses done for intermittent claudication.[13] The primary patency rate for these tibial bypasses was

79% at 5 years, with a secondary patency rate of 83% at 5 years. Tibial bypasses had better patency rates than the above-knee and below-knee femoropopliteal bypasses. These tibial bypasses performed for claudication represented only 2.1% of all infragenicular bypasses performed at that institution within the same time period. Little detail was given on patient selection, or indeed on outcome other than graft patency.

Tibial angioplasty for claudication is also infrequently performed. Case series highlight the potential success of this technique for severe, lifestyle-limiting claudication, with clinical success achieved in 98% of cases,[18] and primary symptomatic patency at 24 months of 59%.[19] These series report patients with both claudication and critical ischaemia, and offer little rationale for patient selection.

It is tempting to compare these case series and to conclude that the results for surgery and angioplasty are broadly similar. This view would ignore the fact that all these case series are hugely influenced by selection bias according to the interests and policies of the source institutions. There is a tendency for shorter stenoses rather than occlusions to be treated by angioplasty, and less fit patients are also more likely to undergo angioplasty. Patients who are medically unfit in one institution may be standard fare in another. The severity of symptoms also varies from series to series. Methods of assessing patency also show considerable variation from small changes in ABPI (0.1 or 0.15), through change in clinical status, to duplex or angiographic confirmation of vessel stenosis or occlusion.

There are few randomized, trials that compare surgery with angioplasty. One such study compared a mixture of iliac and femoropopliteal disease treated by angioplasty or surgery.[20] An initial screening assessment had shown that 1320 angiograms were performed annually for claudication or critical ischaemia in six Veterans Administration (VA)centres. Over a 4½-year period 263 male patients from nine VA centres were randomized to receive either percutaneous balloon angioplasty (PTA) or surgery for occlusive disease of the iliac, femoral, or popliteal arteries. In all, 255 patients actually received intervention; 126 surgery; 129 PTA. Patients were included who had a stenosis >80% or an occlusion <10cm, with an ABPI of 0.9 or less at rest. Patients with a life expectancy of less than 3 years, or who were unfit for surgery, were excluded. Three-quarters of the patients had claudication, and as a further marker of the moderate nature of the disease treated, over half of the femoropopliteal bypasses performed were above the knee. The results showed that for those patients who had a technically successful PTA, the haemodynamic results, amputations and deaths at a mean follow-up of 2 years, were equal for PTA or surgery.

Despite the admirable intention to randomize similar lesions to each treatment arm, this study has merely confirmed what is intuitively obvious. That is, for lesions that can be treated by either method, the decreased morbidity, mortality and cost of PTA is preferable. The inclusion of both claudicants and critically ischaemic patients weakens the data, as does the small proportion of patients entered into the study from the larger pool of patients investigated in these institutions.

Other non-randomized studies have compared angioplasty with endarterectomy,[21] and with femoropopliteal bypass grafting.[22] A total of 103 limbs with short femoropopliteal occlusions received either endarterectomy (41 patients prior to 1988) or angioplasty (after 1988). The groups were demographically broadly similar, but the surgery group has fewer popliteal occlusions, more run-off vessels, and more severe symptoms. The angioplasty group had more immediate failures (15% versus 2%), and lower 3-year primary patency (46% versus 89%). Taking into account reintervention and bypass grafting, tertiary patency at 3 years was similar in the two groups. Although the cost for each endarterectomy was higher than angioplasty, this higher rate of reintervention in the angioplasty group meant that overall cost-effectiveness was equal.

Femoropopliteal bypass was compared with angioplasty in 179 patients who had already been referred for angiography with a view to surgery.[22] The indication for intervention again included both claudication and critical limb ischaemia . The only reported outcome measure was primary clinical patency, which was similar at 2 years (42% for surgery versus 45% for angioplasty). patency was established using undefined clinical and Doppler pressure measurements. Complication rates in each group were not reported and the results of this study must be viewed with caution. Both of these studies are again subject to selection bias, and applying the results to everyday patients in everyday practice is difficult. They do at least have the merit of comparing patients from the same population treated within the same institution.

For patients with moderate claudication debate centres not so much on whether patients should receive surgery or angioplasty, but on whether conservative treatment is more appropriate than either. Angioplasty has been compared with both conventional medical treatment and supervised exercise training in randomized trials. In Edinburgh patients with discrete iliac or femoropopliteal stenoses, or femoropopliteal occlusions less than 10cm long, were randomized to best medical therapy or PTA.[23] Only 10% of all patients screened were suitable for randomization. At 2 years there was no difference between the groups in walking distance, ABPI, or quality of life.

Supervised exercise training has been compared with PTA for unilateral stable claudicants with a lesion considered suitable for angioplasty.[24,25] Short-term improvement in claudication distance and maximum walking distance was shown only in the exercise training group, despite a significant improvement in the ABPI of the PTA group.[24] In the longer term the improvement in the exercise group was not sustained, but results were similar for both groups at 5 years.[25]

These results support the treatment of mild-to-moderate claudication with non-interventional treatment, rather than by either surgery or angioplasty.

CRITICAL LIMB ISCHAEMIA

The results of both surgery and angioplasty for critical limb ischaemia are worse than for the corresponding intervention for intermittent claudication. Case series of angioplasty for critical limb ischaemia and femoropopliteal disease report 3-year primary patency rates of 35–43%.[9,10] Others report more pessimistic results and patency rates as low as 15% at 1 year for PTA at the femoral popliteal and tibial level for critical limb ischaemia.[26] Reported results for tibial angioplasty vary considerably and the majority of reports include small selected numbers of patients. Clinical success rates vary from 44% at 25 months[27] to a 13% primary patency rate at 1 year.[26]

Distal angioplasty has been shown to be more successful with single stenoses rather than multilevel lesions,[28] and better with short occlusions less than 5cm.[29] Tibial angioplasty may be suitable in only 20–30% of patients presenting with isolated tibial disease.[29] Use of a subintimal technique has been shown in certain centres to provide successful recanalization of occluded tibial vessels with a median length of occlusion of 7cm (range 2–30cm).[30] Technical success was achieved in 82% of limbs and 12-month actuarial haemodynamic and clinical patency was 53%. This technique was used largely in elderly patients unfit for distal surgical bypass.

The results of surgical bypass for limb-threatening ischaemia are similarly diverse. Above-knee femoropopliteal bypass achieves a 4- and 5-year patency of 62–77% for vein grafts[31,32] and 39% at 4 years for PTFE.[33] One wonders also about the criteria in these patients, since above-knee bypass is rarely effective in true critical ischaemia in our experience. Below-knee vein grafts have best 5-year patency rates of 80%,[32] with lower rates for synthetic grafts. Femorodistal bypass patency rates vary from 63 to 82% at 5 years for vein grafts in individual series;[34,35] PTFE grafts onto a vein collar have reported 3-year patency rates of 29–48%.[36,37]

These data from individual centres represent the optimum results that can be obtained, often from centres with a special interest in distal reconstruction. Patency reports are subject to publication bias whereby series reporting good results tend to be published. The above data regarding femorodistal bypass contrast with the results of a multicentre study, which reports a 1-year primary patency of 45% for prosthetic grafts and 52% for vein grafts.[38] These results may be more applicable to vascular surgical practice in general.

No randomized studies comparing angioplasty with surgery have been confined to patients with critical ischaemia. This may suggest that the two techniques are not comparable because either they are treating different lesions and patients, or because experience is too ingrained to allow comparison.

In a retrospective, non-randomized study PTA and surgery for limb-threatening ischaemia were compared.[39] In all, 54 PTAs (superficial femoral and popliteal arteries) were compared with 63 infrainguinal bypasses (29 femoropopliteal, 34 femorodistal). The PTA group showed initial success in 72% of cases, but with a high subsequent failure rate, such that at 2 years patency was 18%. This contrasts with the surgery group, which had 2-year patencies of 68% for femoropopliteal bypass and 47% for femorodistal bypass. Limb salvage was 78% in the PTA group and 90% for femoropopliteal bypass, and 74% for femorodistal bypass. The limb salvage rate in the PTA group was achieved by secondary procedures in 59% of patients, including surgical bypass in 16 patients. Only 35% of limbs were salvaged by a single angioplasty compared with 64% of limbs salvaged by a single bypass graft.

Opportunities exist for collaboration in bypass grafting where proximal angioplasty or stenting are performed to improve inflow prior to or simultaneously with surgical bypass. Multilevel occlusive disease can be treated with a combined endovascular and surgical approach, particularly where iliac arteries show inflow limiting stenoses or occlusions. The use of iliac PTA, with or without stenting, to improve inflow above an infrainguinal reconstruction safely reduces the extent of surgical intervention.[40] Angioplasty of the superficial femoral artery may allow use of autologous vein as a bypass graft where only short segments exist.[41]

CONCLUSION

Are infrainguinal angioplasty and surgery comparable? The short answer is probably no, on a number of counts. When one looks at the available evidence, there simply are not any well conducted, non-biased comparisons of the two techniques. All other series are subject to selection bias in allocation of treatment to one technique or the other, based on a jumbled formula of length of stenosis, site of lesion, severity of symptoms, and an indefinable factor that incorporates institutional prejudice and tradition.

There is a tendency for angioplasty in claudicants to be reserved for those with moderate claudication and short occlusions or discrete stenoses in the femoropopliteal segment. Despite this there is no convincing evidence that femoropopliteal angioplasty in this group is any better than conservative management or non-interventional treatment such as exercise training. Surgery would rarely be considered for these patients.

The more severe the symptoms, and for patients with multilevel or long occlusive segments, there is a preference for surgery to be undertaken, largely based on an unproven assumption that angioplasty is ineffective and potentially dangerous in these patients. Encouraging results for tibial angioplasty and subintimal angioplasty of crural vessel occlusions may translate into more widespread application of these techniques, which currently seem to be frequently reserved only for the elderly and frail patient with critical limb ischaemia.

There is a need for randomized trials of all comers to compare angioplasty and surgery in infrainguinal disease, for both claudication and critical ischaemia. Without adequate data and effective comparisons, we will each continue to answer the question in the title of this chapter in a haphazard and individual manner.

REFERENCES

1. Kunlin J: Le traitment de l'arterite obliterante par la greffe veineuse. *Arch Malad Coeur Vaiss* **42:** 371–372, 1949
2. Edwards WS: Chemically treated nylon tubes as arterial grafts. *Surgery* **28:** 61–70, 1955
3. Dotter CT, Judkins MP: Transluminal treatment of arteriosclerotic obstruction. Description of a new technique and a preliminary report of its application. *Circulation* **30:** 654–670, 1964
4. Gruentzig A, Hopff H: Perkutane rekanalisation chronischer arterieller Verschlusse mit einem neuen Dilatations:katheter. *Deutsche Med Woch* **99:** 2502–2505, 1974
5. Boyd A: The natural course of arteriosclerosis of the lower extremities. *Proc Roy Soc Med* **55:** 591–593, 1968
6. Dormandy JA, Murray GD: The fate of the claudicant – a prospective study of 1969 claudicants. *Eur J Vasc Surg* **5:** 131–133, 1991
7. Fowl RJ, Gewirtz RJ, Love MC, Kempczinski RF: Natural history of claudicants with critical hemodynamic indices. *Ann Vasc Surg* **6:** 31–33, 1992
8. Wolfe JH, Wyatt MG: Critical and subcritical ischaemia. *Eur J Vasc Endovasc Surg* **13:** 578–582, 1997
9. Adar R, Critchfield GC, Eddy DM: A confidence profile analysis of the results of femoropopliteal percutaneous transluminal angioplasty in the treatment of lower extremity ischaemia. *J Vasc Surg* **10:** 57–67, 1989

10. Johnston KW: Femoral and popliteal arteries: reanalysis of results of balloon angioplasty. *Radiology* **183:** 767–771, 1992
11. Krepel VM, van Andel GJ, van Erp WFM, Breslau PJ: Percutaneous transluminal angioplasty of the femoropopliteal artery: initial and long term results. *Radiology* **156:** 325–328, 1985
12. Becquemin JP, Cavillon A, Haiduc F: Surgical transluminal femoropopliteal angioplasty: multivariate analysis outcome. *J Vasc Surg* **19:** 495–502, 1994
13. Byrne J, Darling RC, Chang BB *et al.*: Infrainguinal arterial reconstruction for claudication: is it worth the risk? An anlysis of 409 procedures. *J Vasc Surg* **29:** 259–269, 1999
14. Rosenthal D, Evans RD, McKinsey J *et al.*: Prosthetic above-knee femoro-popliteal bypass for intermittent claudication. *J Cardiovasc Surg* **31:** 462–468, 1990
15. Allen BT, Reilly JM, Rubin BG *et al.*: Femoro-popliteal bypass for claudication: Vein vs. PTFE. *Ann Vasc Surg* **10:** 178–185, 1996
16. Michaels JA: Choice of material for above-knee femoropopliteal bypass. *Br J Surg* **76:** 7–14, 1989
17. Zannetti S, L'Italien GJ, Cambria RP: Functional outcome after surgical treatment for intermittent claudication. *J Vasc Surg* **24:** 65–73, 1996
18. Dorros G, Jaff MR, Murphy KJ, Mathiak L: The acute outcome of tibioperoneal vessel angioplasty in 417 cases with claudication and critical ischaemia. *Cathet Cardiovasc Diagn* **45:** 251–256, 1998
19. Varty K, Bolia A, Naylor AR *et al.*: Infrapopliteal percutaneous transluminal angioplasty: a safe and successful procedure. *Eur J Vasc Endovasc Surg* **9:** 341–345, 1995
20. Wilson SE, Wolf GL, Cross AP: Percutaneous transluminal angioplasty versus operation for peripheral arteriosclerosis. *J Vasc Surg* **9:** 1–9, 1989
21. Vroegindeweij D, Idu M, Buth J *et al.*: The cost effectiveness of treatment of short occlusive lesions in the femoropopliteal artery: balloon angioplasty versus endarterectomy. *Eur J Vasc Endovasc Surg* **10:** 40–50, 1995.
22. Martin EC, Fankuchen EI, Karlson KB: Angioplasty for femoral artery occlusion: comparison with surgery. *Am J Roent* **137:** 915–919, 1981
23. Whyman MR, Fowkes FGR, Kerracher EMG *et al.*: Is intermittent claudication improved by percutaneous transluminal angioplasty? A randomised controlled trial. *J Vasc Surg* **26:** 551–557, 1996
24. Creasy TS, McMillan PJ, Fletcher EWL *et al.*: Is percutaneous transluminal angioplasty better than exercise for claudication? Preliminary results from a prospective randomised trial. *Eur J Vasc Surg* **4:** 135–140, 1990
25. Perkins JMT, Collin J, Creasy TS *et al.*: Exercise versus angioplasty for stable claudication: Long and medium term results of a prospective randomised trial. *Eur J Vasc Endovasc Surg* **11:** 409–413, 1996
26. Parson RE, Suggs WD, Lee JJ *et al.*: Percutaneous transluminal angioplasty for the treatment of limb threatening ischemia: Do the results justify an attempt before bypass grafting? *J Vasc Surg* **28:** 1066–1071, 1998
27. Brown KT, Moore ED, Getrajdman GI, Saddekni S: Infrapopliteal angioplasty: long term follow-up. *J Vasc Intervent Radiol* **4:** 139–144, 1993
28. Bull PG, Mendel H, Hold M *et al.*: Distal popliteal and tibioperoneal transluminal angioplasty: long term follow-up. *J Vasc Intervent Radiol* **3:** 45–53, 1992
29. Schwarten DE: Clinical and anatomical considerations for non-operative therapy in tibial disease and the results of angioplasty. *Circulation* **83** (Suppl 2): 186–90, 1991
30. Nydahl S, Hartshorne T, Bell PRF *et al.*: Subintimal angioplasty of infrapopliteal occlusions in critically ischaemic limbs. *Eur J Vasc Endovasc Surg* **14:** 212–216, 1997
31. John TG, Stonebridge P, Kelman J *et al.*: Above-knee femoropopliteal bypass grafts and the consequences of graft failure. *Ann Roy Coll Surg Engl* **75:** 257–260, 1993
32. Taylor LM, Edwards JM, Porter JM: Present status of reversed vein bypass grafting: five year results of a modern series. *J Vasc Surg* **11:** 193–206, 1990
33. O'Riordain DS, Buckley D, O'Donnell JA: Polytetrafluoroethylene in above knee bypass surgery for critical ischemia. *Am J Surg* **164:** 129–131, 1992
34. Englund R, Harris J, May J: Factors affecting the outcome of 463 femorotibial reconstructions. *Aust NZ J Surg* **58:** 279–283, 1988

35. Hickey NC, Thomson I, Shearman CP, Simms MH: Aggressive arterial reconstruction for critical lower limb ischaemia. *Br J Surg* **78:** 1476–1478, 1991
36. Morris GE, Raptis S, Miller JH *et al.*: Femorocrural grafting and regrafting: does polytetrafluoroethylene have a role? *Eur J Vasc Surg* **7:** 329–334, 1993
37. Cheshire NJ, Wolfe J, Noone MA *et al.*: The economics of femorocrural reconstruction with and without autologous vein. *J Vasc Surg* **15:** 167–175, 1992
38. The Iloprost Bypass International Study Group: Effects of perioperative iloprost on patency of femorodistal bypass grafts. *Eur J Vasc Endovasc Surg* **12:** 363–371, 1996
39. Blair JM, Gewertz BL, Moosa H *et al.*: Percutaneous transluminal angioplasty versus surgery for limb-threatening ischemia. *J Vasc Surg* **9:** 698–703, 1989
40. Brewster DC, Cambria RP, Darling RC *et al.*: Long-term results of combined iliac balloon angioplasty and distal surgical revascularisation. *Ann Surg* **210:** 324–330, 1989
41. Verhelst R, Bruneau M, Nicholas AL *et al.*: Popliteal to distal bypass grafts for limb salvage. *Ann Vasc Surg* **11:** 505–509, 1997

THROMBOLYTIC OPPORTUNITIES

Complications of thrombolytic therapy and their avoidance

Bruce Campbell, Denis Kinsella

INTRODUCTION

The discovery of streptokinase by Tillett and Garner in 1933[1] laid the foundation for thrombolytic therapy, but clinical use of lysis was largely delayed until the 1960s, when reports began to appear of treatment using large doses intravenously.[2] This resulted in modest success rates, quite high incidences of bleeding problems, and occasional deaths. The description by Dotter in 1974[3] of the use of low dose intra-arterial infusion of streptokinase set the scene for safer and more successful thrombolysis, and this has been the basis of lytic treatment for arterial thrombosis and embolism since that time.

The use of any lytic agent poses the risk of haemorrhage, which is the most common and potentially most serious complication of treatment. Bleeding may be minor at the site of catheter insertion, or sufficiently severe to require blood transfusion and to threaten the patient's life: it can cause the catastrophic complication of haemorrhagic stroke (Fig. 1). Other less serious complications

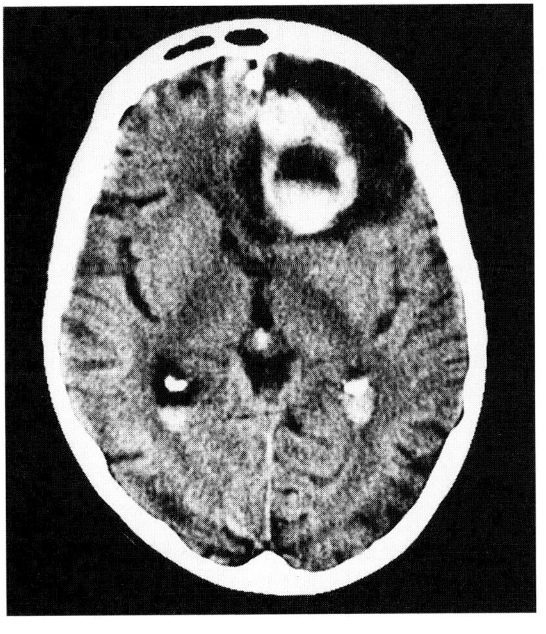

Fig. 1. Intracerebral haemorrhage in the left frontal lobe.

include local problems such as pericatheter thrombosis, distal embolism, arterial perforation and false aneurysm; and general problems such as allergic reactions. Even using low dose intra-arterial infusions there is a small risk of death as a result of thrombolytic therapy. Failure to achieve lysis or to salvage a threatened limb will not be considered a complication for the purposes of this chapter.

Reviewing the literature for complications of thrombolysis is not straightforward. There is great heterogeneity in the techniques used (including the type of thrombolytic agent, the dose, duration of infusion, equipment and techniques employed, and adjuvant treatment), in patient selection, and in the way that results are described. It is important at the outset to describe these variables, not only because they affect the interpretation of published results, but also because they should be considered when trying to minimize complication rates.

Throughout this chapter, the main emphasis will be on thrombolysis for peripheral arterial occlusions (including grafts), with a very brief section on venous thrombolysis: coronary artery thrombolysis will not be dealt with at all.

VARIABLES IN THE PRACTICE OF THROMBOLYSIS

Choice of thrombolytic agent

Streptokinase was the original thrombolytic agent and was in common use until the early 1990s: it is effective and is still used in some hospitals in the UK. Recombitant tissue plasminogen activator (rt-PA) has become increasingly popular since its introduction in the late 1980s: its greater fibrin specificity offered the possibility of a reduced risk of haemorrhage. It was initially very expensive, but is now available in aliquots more appropriate for peripheral thrombolysis at lesser cost. Urokinase is more widely used in the USA.

In a non-randomized comparison of streptokinase and rt-PA, Earnshaw *et al.*[4] found no difference in complication rates. However, a small randomized study comparing streptokinase with rt-PA suggested that the latter was more effective in a dose which was associated with a lesser risk of bleeding complications: this study involved 20 patients in each group, among whom there were three major bleeds with intra-arterial streptokinase and none with rt-PA.[5]

No differences in complication rates have been shown between rt-PA and urokinase, either in the randomized STILE trial (Surgery versus Thrombolysis for Ischaemia of the Lower Extremity)[6] or in a smaller randomized study by Meyerovitz and colleagues.[7] In particular, no differences were observed in bleeding problems.

In summary, there is no good evidence of important differences between the available thrombolytic agents with regard to the risk of bleeding, although there is a suggestion from one small study that the risk with streptokinase may be greater.

Because streptokinase is derived from streptococci, many people have low levels of circulating antibodies to the drug as a result of previous exposure to streptococcal infection. In addition, therapeutic administration of streptokinase causes an antibody response with higher levels of neutralizing antibodies, which remain elevated for some 4 years.[8] The practical significance of these raised antibody levels remains uncertain. There is little evidence that they have an adverse effect on the thrombolytic capacity of streptokinase, and the incidence of serious allergic reactions is low. There is, however, a case for choosing a different agent if a patient requires further thrombolytic treatment within about 4 years of receiving streptokinase.[9] This situation most frequently arises in patients given streptokinase for treatment of myocardial infarction.

There has been a general move away from the use of streptokinase in recent years, based on some evidence of greater effectiveness and more rapid effect of rt-PA, a theoretical yet poorly proven higher risk of bleeding with streptokinase, and the possibility of allergic reactions. We have continued to use streptokinase for most peripheral arterial thrombolysis on our unit, with acceptable complication rates, and early limb salvage rates comparable with published series using other agents.

Route of infusion

Used intravenously, high doses are required for any likely effect on arterial thrombosis[2] and this route has been abandoned almost completely during the last decade, because intra-arterial infusions produce better success rates with a lesser risk of bleeding. Nevertheless, in 1990 Earnshaw *et al.*[10] reported a successful lysis rate of 34% (including about 50% for emboli and graft occlusions but only 6% for arterial thromboses) in 48 patients with acute limb ischaemia. They described just one stroke and one major bleed in this cohort, using 100 000 units/hour of intravenous streptokinase. Berridge *et al.*[5] included intravenous administration of rt-PA as a third arm of their randomized trial comparing intra-arterial rt-PA and streptokinase, and showed a complete or partial lsysis rate of only 45% by the intravenous route (compared with 80–100% intra-arterially) at the expense of three major bleeds (none in the group of 20 patients having intra-arterial rt-PA). It has been suggested that intravenous lysis might be considered when arterial access was impossible, or where radiological expertise and facilities are limited[10] but there seems little doubt that results are poorer and the risk of bleeding is higher.

Dose of thrombolytic agent

In the early years of arterial thrombolysis, a huge range of doses were used – from 1000–100 000 units/hour streptokinase, with total doses of 100 000–1 600 000 units and clinical experience supported the expectation that lower doses caused less haemorrhagic complications.[11]

When rt-PA was introduced a small dose ranging study by Earnshaw *et al.*[12] suggested that an infusion rate of 2.5mg/hour caused more major bleeds than doses of 1mg/hour or less.

Urokinase was studied in Phase I of the TOPAS (Thrombolysis Or Peripheral Arterial Surgery)[13] study, with bleeding complications in 13%, 2%, and 16% respectively of patients receiving 2000 international units (iu)/min, 4000iu/min, and 6000iu/min. These differences were statistically significant, but the authors suggested that the unexpected finding of the lowest rate of bleeding in the intermediate dose group could have occurred by chance.

Dosage schedules have been developed largely on the basis of clinical experience, and still vary to an extent which makes comparison of different series quite difficult.[14]

Radiological and infusion techniques

The methods of adminstering thrombolytic agents have become increasingly diverse.

Type and location of catheter

- Regional intra-arterial infusion. The catheter tip is placed proximal to the occluding thrombus.
- Intra-thrombus infusion. The catheter tip is embedded in the thrombus.
- Intra-thrombus bolusing or lacing. The catheter (often with side holes for delivery of the lytic agent) is passed into the distal part of the thrombus, and withdrawn while infusing a high dose of thrombolytic directly into the thrombus. This may then be followed by a continuous infusion.
- Type of catheter. Depending on the type of infusion planned, catheters may be chosen with a single end hole or side holes of various types. In recent years catheters have mostly been of 5 French size or smaller. Catheters may be used coaxially or with a sheath: although a sheath further enlarges the puncture site, it allows easier access if angioplasty is required following lysis.

Type of infusion

- Continuous infusion. A syringe pump is used to infuse lytic agent at a constant rate.
- Stepwise infusion. Fixed doses of lytic agent are infused, starting in the proximal part of the thrombus, and monitoring the effect radiologically. The catheter is advanced progressively through the thrombus as lysis occurs.
- Graded infusion. Lysis starts with a high dose infusion, then reducing the dose according to a protocol.[15]
- Forced periodic infusion. The lytic agent is injected forcibly into the thrombus using the 'pulse spray' or similar method. Thrombolysis is then continued by continuous infusion.

Pharmacomechanic thrombolysis

Thrombolysis is combined with mechanical disruption of the thrombus using balloons or pulse spray catheters.

Adjunctive procedures

These include catheter suction embolectomy and mechanical thromboembolectomy.

Other variations in radiological technique which might influence the incidence of bleeding are the use of single or double wall arterial puncture, and ipsilateral or contralateral approach for thrombolysis. No good comparisons of these different techniques exist.

Summary

All the alternative types of infusion, and techniques for pharmacomechanic lysis aim to reduce lysis time and/or to improve results compared with the standard continuous infusion, but with an ulterior hope of perhaps reducing the chance of bleeding complications. However, there are no good data to show that the risk of haemorrhage is reduced. A randomized study comparing high dose bolus with low dose infusion of rt-PA showed no significant difference in the rate of major haemorrhage,[16] and analysis of a series of 798 thrombolytic infusions by the Thrombolysis Study Group showed no relationship of any aspect of the radiological technique or infusion method with the incidence of complications.[17]

Adjuvant drugs

The most commonly used are aspirin and heparin, both of which have theoretical potential to increase the incidence and severity of bleeding complications. The Thrombolysis Study Group series of 798 infusions[17] revealed a significantly increased risk of bleeding complications for patients taking aspirin, but no significant association between the use of adjunctive heparin and complication rate. By contrast, heparin was associated with a significantly increased incidence of bleeding in the most recent report of the TOPAS group,[18] and some smaller series have also noted a tendency to increased bleeding complications when heparin was used.[19,20] There are no good experimental data on the risk /benefit aspect of adjuvant heparin.

Patient selection

The Working Group on Thrombolysis in the Management of Limb Ischaemia[14] has published advice on the patients in whom thrombolysis is absolutely or relatively contraindicated, based on the conclusions of the NIH Consensus Development Conference.[21] They have defined three levels of contraindication, with regard to the risk of haemorrhage and its likely consequences:

- Patients with absolute contraindications, including those with recent cerebrovascular events (<2 months), intracranial trauma (<3 months), or neurosurgery (<3 months); those with recent gastrointestinal bleeding (<10 days); and those with bleeding diatheses.
- Patients with relatively major contraindications, including those who have had recent cardiopulmonary resuscitation or major non-vascular surgery or trauma (<10 days), or recent eye surgery (interval unspecified); those with uncontrolled hypertension (systolic >180mmHg or diastolic >110mmHg) or intracranial tumours; and following puncture of an incompressible vessel.
- Patients with minor contraindications, including those with hepatic failure (especially with coagulopathy), bacterial endocarditis, or haemorrhagic diabetic retinopathy; and women who are pregnant.

'Positive' selection criteria (for example shorter duration of ischaemia, a potentially salvageable limb, and the angiographic pattern of occlusion) influence the likely success of thrombolysis. They are unlikely to have an important effect on complication rates, but may well influence risk/benefit considerations.

Age

It is worth adding a comment about age, which may be associated with risk of complications. In the Thrombolysis Study Group series of 798 infusions reported recently,[17] increasing age was significantly associated with higher risk of complications and death, and another recent report by Lambert *et al.*[22] documented an increased complication rate of 40% in patients over 80. On our own unit, deaths associated with thrombolysis have occurred only in patients over 80 years of age.

Other factors

Other factors which might be expected to affect morbidity and mortality rates of thrombolysis include the indication for treatment and the size of the patient.

The indication, for example, may be early acute ischaemia caused by a small embolus, or late acute-on-chronic ischaemia caused by thrombosis. Differences in complication and death rates may therefore be due to the specific conditions and associated comorbidities, rather than the thrombolysis being used to treat them.

The size of the patient might have an influence on bleeding complications because a standard infusion rate of lytic agent will deliver a substantially larger dose relative to body weight to a 45kg patient than a 125kg individual. This suggestion is unproven but worth considering.

Definitions of major and minor complications

Most reports divide bleeding complications into major and minor. These are generally described, but criteria vary, and it seems likely that there are substantial variations between the cases which different authors include – especially among those with minor complications.

INCIDENCE OF COMPLICATIONS OF THROMBOLYSIS

A good indication of the current incidence of complications of peripheral arterial thrombolysis is given by the results of the National Audit of Thrombolysis for Acute Limb Ischaemia (NATALI) database. This is register of cases to dealt with by the Thrombolysis Study Group in the UK, which started in 1990. By early October, 1999 a total of 911 events had been recorded in 794 patients, and the complications are shown in Table 1 (personal communication).

Brief comments about the incidence of various specific complications are as follows:

Major haemorrhage (Fig. 2)

Definitions vary, but the criteria in the recent TOPAS study report[18] are typical and thorough – severe blood loss (>500ml), blood loss requiring transfusion, blood loss causing hypotension, or intracranial haemorrhage. The figure of 8.1% for major haemorrhage from the NATALI database is just a little higher than the 5.1% reported from 19 series reviewed by Berridge *et al.*,[23] and lower than the 12.5 % reported recently the TOPAS study[18] among 255 patients having thrombolysis with urokinase in 113 hospitals in the USA and Europe. Taking account of these and other series, the overall incidence of major haemorrhage is about 10%.

Table 1. Complications associated with 911 thrombolytic infusions reported to the NATALI database of the Thrombolysis Study Group, between 1.1.90 and 11.10.99.

Complication	*Number (%)*
Major bleed	74 (8.1%)
Groin haematoma	58 (6.4%)
Embolization	25 (2.7%)
Stroke	22 (2.4%)
Reperfusion injury	19 (2.1%)
Pericatheter thrombosis	6 (0.7%)
'Other complications'	55 (6.0%)
Death	31 (3.4%)

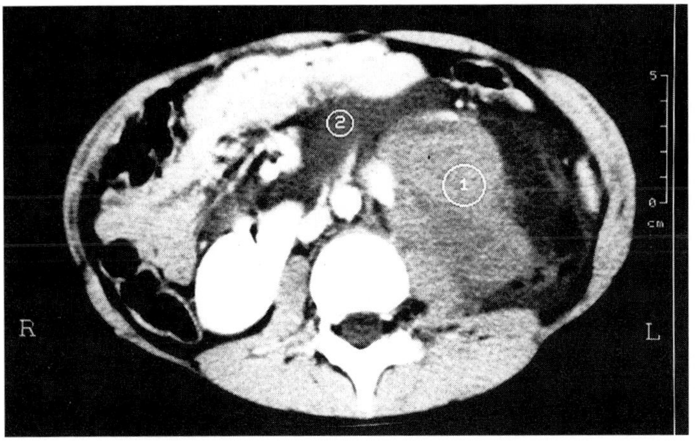

Fig. 2. A left retroperitoneal bleed.

Stroke

This is perhaps the most serious, and certainly the most feared complication of thrombolysis. The three sources cited above (which reflect the experience of a very large number of hospitals over many years) give incidences of 1.0%,[23] 2.4% (NATALI), and 1.6%.[18] It seems reasonable, therefore, to warn patients of a risk of about 2% for stroke.

Although most strokes occurring at the time of thrombolysis are haemorrhagic, not all are caused by intracranial bleeding: for example, the only three strokes (up to 30 days) in a series of 100 patients reported by Armon[24] were due to thrombosis, and one of three in our own series of 81 patients was due to a cerebral embolus.

Minor bleeding

Not surprisingly, reported incidences vary greatly. Whether or not a small groin haematoma is the expected bruising or a minor complication worth recording is highly subjective, and many series do not include a description of minor bleeding complications. Recent studies which have documented the incidences of minor bleeding report rates of 20–25%.[24,25]

Embolization

Distal embolization has been reported in up to 20% patients during lysis:[11] the NATALI figure of 2.7% is rather low compared with reports of 10–15% in other recent series.[18,25] Detection of emboli may well depend on how assiduously they are looked for and recorded, because most cause no serious clinical problem and resolve with continued lysis.[11,18,25]

Reperfusion injury

This was recorded in 2.1% of the NATALI patients, but has not featured at all in other series. It is difficult to know exactly what it means in this context, because reperfusion can be used as an explanation for any clinical deterioration after relief of severe limb ischaemia. The rare occurrence of renal failure after high dose bolus rt-PA[26] may possibly be a manifestation of reperfusion injury.

Allergic reactions

These are uncommon – only one occurred in the NATALI series of 911 treatments. Streptokinase is associated with the greatest risk (discussed earlier) but even series using streptokinase do not document allergic reactions as either frequent or serious:[14] there were none among 136 patients in the series by Hess,[11] just one among 70 patients treated by Walker and Giddings,[27] and one in our own series of 81 patients treated with streptokinase. Low grade febrile reactions were observed with during 5 of 65 streptokinase infusions reported by Katzen.[19] Occasional reactions are seen with urokinase – one among 144 patients (0.7%) in Phase One of the TOPAS Study.[13]

Catheter-related and local complications

These include arterial perforation, intimal damage, pericatheter thrombosis, infection, and false aneurysm formation.[18,25]

Death

Acute limb ischaemia and its associated co-morbidities can be fatal, particularly in the very elderly, so it may be difficult to determine the contribution of thrombolytic therapy to death (except in instances where major or intracranial bleeding is clearly the cause). Related to this is the time interval used for mortality – rates may vary depending upon whether the threshold is for death during the infusion, ensuing 30 days, or the hospital stay. Mortality rates for major series tend to lie in the range 3–5% (TOPAS I,[13] STILE[6] and NATALI) although there are other reports from well recognized experts in thrombolysis with mortalities of 5–10%.[16,25]

Thrombolysis of grafts (including dialysis fistulae) and venous thrombolysis

Bypass grafts and fistulae

Thrombolysis is commonly used as primary treatment of occluded bypass grafts, supported by evidence of reasonable effectiveness and safety.[13,28] Some series have documented a trend towards high complication rates when lysing grafts – especially polytetrafluoroethylene[29] – but there are no really good comparative data. Lysis of haemodialysis shunts appears to be associated with relatively low complication rates.[30]

Thrombolysis for deep vein thrombosis

Based on the recent report of a national multicentre registry in the USA (467 patients), complication rates seem similar to arterial thrombolysis.[31] Major haemorrhage occurred in 11%, and there was minor bleeding in 16%. One fatal intracranial bleed was recorded, and one subdural haematoma – a stroke rate of 0.4%. There was one other death (due to a pulmonary embolus) giving an overall mortality rate of 0.4%. This is rather lower the the mortality rate for arterial thromboslysis, which perhaps emphasizes the high risk to life of acute limb ischaemia, compared with deep vein thrombosis.

AVOIDANCE AND MANAGEMENT OF COMPLICATIONS

In view of the data presented above, it is reasonable to suggest the following.

Patient selection

Careful attention should be paid to the published guidance on contraindications.[14] The balance of risks and benefits must be considered for each patient. If limb loss seems inevitable or the patient is moribund, then lysis is ill advised. If there is no threat to the viability of the limb (for example in acute onset claudication or deep vein thrombosis) then the risks should be considered very carefully. It is essential that the patient is warned of the risk of problems (especially major bleeding and stroke) before embarking on treatment: some patients may decide against thrombolytic therapy when told of these possibilities.

The medical team

The doctors undertaking thrombolysis should be experienced in endovascular work, and skilled in the recognition and management of problems, and in potential adjunctive procedures. The vascular surgical team should be available in case of bleeding or ischaemic problems requiring urgent surgery.

Method of thrombolysis

The precise method of radiological approach, type of catheter, and method of infusion have no proven influence on the incidence of complications, but seems a sensible aim to stop lysis as soon as it becomes clear that no further benefit is likely to be achieved. Many vascular specialists regard rt-PA or urokinase as preferable to streptokinase with regard to the risk of bleeding, but this point is not proven.

Monitoring and care of the patient

Regular monitoring of the patient having thrombolysis is very important, in order to detect complications early and to take appropriate measures. Patients should be nursed in a setting where staff are familiar with thrombolytic infusions. There should be a written protocol for the conduct of the infusion and what to do if problems occur. Patients need regular measurement of pulse and blood pressure, and assessment for level of consciousness and limb movements. The entry site of the catheter should be checked regularly, as should the circulatory state of the ischaemic limb. There is no good evidence that any form of haematological monitoring helps to prevent bleeding complications. Daily monitoring of haemoglobin and renal function seem sensible.[14] Radiological monitoring of progress is essential, but the protocol will depend on local preferences.

Patients should be confined to bed during thrombolysis, because movement increases the risk of catheter displacement and bleeding.

What to do when complications occur

Puncture site bleeding should be treated initially by pressure, and the infusion should be temporarily stopped. Continued bleeding may be dealt with by an increase in catheter size or placement of a sheath. The decision may be made to stop the infusion altogether. Occasionally the affected vessel or graft requires a surgical suture.

If puncture site bleeding is persistent, or if bleeding occurs elsewhere, the first measure should always be discontinuation of the thrombolytic infusion. The coagulation profile and haemoglobin level should be checked, and fresh frozen plasma or cryoprecipitate given if indicated. Blood transfusion may be required. Operation should be reserved for continued bleeding or for evacuation of large haematomata.

Allergic reactions should be managed by discontinuing the infusion, and by administration of an antihistamine and hydrocortisone. It may then be reasonable to recommence thrombolysis using a different agent.

CONCLUSION

All series report an incidence of bleeding and other complications as a result of thrombolysis. The risk of complications is unpredictable for the individual patient, and there are few specific measures which can be taken to reduce their incidence. It therefore seems important to use thrombolysis for those patients with the greatest chance of benefit, so that balance of benefits and risks is maximized. It also seems wise to discontinue treatment as soon as it is clear either that adequate lysis has occurred, or that continuing an infusion is unlikely to achieve further benefit. It is vital that all patients should be properly informed about the risk of complications, and specifically about the small chance of stroke, before starting thrombolysis.

REFERENCES

1. Tillett WS, Garner RL: The fibrinolytic activity of hemolytic streptococci. *J Exp Med* **58:** 485–502, 1933
2. Amery A, Deloof W, Vermylen J, Verstraete M: Outcome of recent thromboembolic occlusions of limb arteries treated with Streptokinase. *Br Med J* **2:** 639–644, 1970
3. Dotter CT, Rosch J, Seaman AJ: Selective clot lysis with low dose streptokinase. *Radiology* **111:** 31–37, 1974
4. Earnshaw JJ, Scott DJA, Horrocks M, Baird RN: Choice of agent for peripheral thrombolysis. *Br J Surg* **80:** 25–27, 1993
5. Berridge DC, Gregson RHS, Hopkinson BR, Makin GS: Randomized trial of intra-arterial recombinant tissue plasminogen activator, intravenous recombinant tissue plasminogen activator and intra-arterial streptokinase in peripherl arterial thrombolysis. *Br J Surg* **78:** 988–995, 1991
6. Weaver FA, Comerota AJ, Youngblood M, Froehlich J *et al.*: and the STILE Investigators. Surgical revascularization versus thrombolysis for nonembolic lower extremity native artery occlusions: Results of a prospective randomized trial. *J Vasc Surg* **24:** 513–523, 1996
7. Meyerovitz MF, Goldhaber SZ, Reagan K *et al.*: Recombinant tissue-type plasminogen activator versus Urokinase in peripheral arterial and graft occlusions: A randomized trial. *Radiology* **175:** 75–78, 1990
8. Lee HS, Cross S, Davidson R *et al.*: Raised levels of antistreptokinase antibody and neutralisation titres from 4 days to 54 months after administration of streptokinase or anistreplase. *Eur Heart J* **14:** 84–89, 1993
9. Jennings K: Antibodies to streptokinase. *Br Med J* **312:** 393–394, 1996
10. Earnshaw JJ, Cosgrove C, Wilkins DC, Bliss BP: Acute limb ischaemia: the place of intravenous streptokinase. *Br J Surg* **77:** 1136–1139, 1990
11. Hess H, Ingrisch H, Mietaschk A, Rath H: Local low-dose thrombolytic therapy of peripheral arterial occlusions. *New Engl J Med* **307:** 1627–1630, 1982
12. Earnshaw JJ, Westby JC, Gregson RHS *et al.*: Local thrombolytic therapy of acute peripheral arterial ischaemia with tissue plasminogen activator: a dose-ranging study. *Br J Surg* **75:** 1196–1200, 1988
13. Ouriel K, Veith FJ, Sasahara AA, for the TOPAS Investigators: Thrombolysis or periheral arterial surgery: Phase I results. *J Vasc Surg* **23:** 64–75, 1996
14. Working Party on Thrombolysis in the Management of Limb Ischemia: Thrombolysis in the management of lower limb peripheral arterial occlusion – A consensus document. *Am J Cardiol* **81:** 207–218, 1998
15. McNamara TO, Fischer JR: Thrombolysis of peripheral arterial and graft occlusions: improved results using high-dose urokinase. *Am J Roent* **144:** 769–775, 1985
16. Braithwaite BD, Buckenham TM, Galland RB *et al.* on behalf of the Thrombolysis Study

Group: Prospective randomized trial of high-dose bolus *versus* low-dose tissue plasminogen activator infusion in the management of acute limb ischaemia. *Br J Surg* **84:** 646–650, 1997
17. Thomas SM, Gaines PA on behalf of the Thrombolysis Study Group: Avoiding the complications of thrombolysis. *Br J Surg* **86:** 710, 1999
18. Ouriel K, Veith FJ, Sasahara AA for the Thrombolysis or Peripheral Arterial Surgery (TOPAS) Investigators: A comparison of recombinant urokinase with vascular surgery as initial treatment for acute arterial occlusion of the legs. *New Engl J Med* **338:** 1105–1111, 1998
19. Katzen BT, Edwards KC, Albert AS, van Breda A: Low-dose direct fibrinolysis in peripheral vascular disease. *J Vasc Surg* **1:** 718–722, 1984
20. Bero CJ, Cardella JF, Reddy *et al.*: Recombinant tissue plasminogen activator for the treatment of lower extremity peripheral vascular occlusive disease *J Vasc Intervent Radiol* **6:** 571–577, 1995
21. NIH Consensus Development Conference: Thrombolytic therapy in thrombosis. *Br Med J* **280:** 1585–1587, 1980
22. Lambert AW, Trkulja D, Fox AD *et al.*: Age-related outcome for peripheral thrombolysis. *Eur J Vasc Endovasc Surg* **17:** 144–148, 1999
23. Berridge DC, Makin GS Hopkinson BR: Local low dose intra-arterial thrombolytic therapy: the risk of stroke or major haemorrhage. *Br J Surg* **76:** 1230–1233, 1989
24. Armon MP, Yusuf SW, Whitaker SC *et al.*: Results of 100 cases of pulse-spray thrombolysis for acute and subacute leg ischaemia. *Br J Surg* **84:** 47–50, 1997
25. Huettl EA, Soulen MC: Thrombolysis of lower extremity embolic occlusions: A study of the results of the STAR registry . *Radiology* **197:** 141–145, 1995
26. Braithwaite BD, Birch PA, Poskitt KR *et al.*: Accelerated thrombolysis with high dose Bolus t-PA extends the role of peripheral thrombolysis but may increase the risks. *Clin Rad* **50:** 747–750, 1995
27. Walker WJ, Giddings AEB: A protocol for the safe treatment of acute lower limb ischaemia with intra-arterial streptokinase and surgery. *Br J Surg* **75:** 1189–1192, 1988
28. Comerota AJ, Weaver FA, Hosking JD *et al.*: Results of prospective, randomized trial of surgery versus thrombolysis for occluded lower extremity bypass grafts. *Am J Surg* **172:** 105–112, 1996
29. Berridge DC, Al-Kutoubi A, Mansfield AO *et al.*: Thrombolysis in arterial graft thrombosis. *Eur J Vasc Endovasc Surg* **9:** 129–132, 1995
30. Beathard GA, Welch BR, Maidment HJ: Mechanical thrombolysis for the treatment of thrombosed hemodialysis access grafts. *Radiology* **200:** 711–716, 1996
31. Mewissen MW, Seabrook GR, Meissner MM *et al.*: Catheter directed thrombolysis for lower extremity deep venous thrombosis: Report of a national multicentre registry. *Radiology* **211:** 39–49, 1999

The role of thrombolysis in acute bypass graft occlusion

TM Buckenham

INTRODUCTION

Until recently there has been considerable confusion over the role of lysis in acute limb ischaemia. The literature abounds with anecdotal series often focussing on technique rather than outcome. The formation of the British Thrombolysis Study Group (TSG) database and its maturation to contain over 1000 events combined with data from prospective randomized trials[1,2] has enabled the risks associated with lytic therapy to be clearly defined. It also has allowed robust criteria for patient selection and outcome determination. Acute limb ischaemia secondary to bypass graft occlusion is an interesting problem and subgroup analysis of the above data enables useful treatment recommendations.

TREATMENT STRATEGIES

Traditionally, open surgical procedures have been used in the management of acute bypass graft occlusion. Surgical management usually involves thrombectomy and local revision or complete graft replacement. Thrombolysis offers the opportunity to revascularize the occluded bypass and associated native vessel occlusion in order to determine the underlying cause of failure. The cause of failure once determined can then be specifically managed with either an endovascular technique at the time of thrombolysis or focal surgical management such as anastamotic revision with a vein patch. Treatment strategies for bypass occlusion must be carefully tailored to the clinical setting. Factors such as the chronicity of occlusion degree of ischaemia and the nature of the occluded conduit allow selection of patients who may benefit from a lysis first-treatment strategy.

PATIENT SELECTION

Careful clinical assessment allows the data accumulated from the Thrombolysis Study Group database to be utilized to select the appropriate patients for treatment with peripheral arterial thrombolysis. The following are significant determinants of outcome and risk.

Severity of ischaemia

It is useful to classify patients according to the modified Rutherford criteria (Table 1). The information given below strongly suggests that groups I and III are unsuitable for initial treatment with lysis.

Acute non-limb-threatening ischaemia

The claudicant

Analysis of the Thrombolysis Study Group database[3] concerning patients presenting with acute onset claudication secondary to bypass graft occlusion is instructive. A total of 52 patients presented with acute onset claudication of less than 2 weeks duration secondary to graft occlusion (Table 2). The majority of the conduits were prosthetic. The immediate outcome of thrombolysis of graft occlusion was thrombus clearance in 48 patients (92%) failed lysis in four patients (8%) and 27 patients (52%) needed a secondary procedure (Table 3). After 30 days four patients (8%) had a major amputation, seven (13%) had died, 32 (62%) were symptom-free and nine (17%) had persistent claudication. Of all patients presenting with intermittent claudication of sudden onset secondary to bypass occlusion and treated with lysis, only 79% were alive with two legs. These outcomes are very similar to those defined for acute limb-threatening ischaemia from native vessel occlusion as reported by the Thrombolysis Study Group and other investigators. These data strongly suggest that acute claudication secondary to bypass occlusion treated with thrombolysis has a poor outcome. The outcomes are considerably worse than those of stable community-based claudicants,[4] although they may not be a comparable group. Patients presenting with acute claudication requiring hospital admission probably represent a different population from those community-based with chronic claudication and the appropriate management of two types of patients may differ. The data were collected prospectively and have been verified to ensure accuracy but lack details of severity of the claudicants, none of the patients had treadmill tests and less than half had ankle brachial pressure indices recorded. Approximately half of the patients had a neurosensory deficit but the outcome of patients with and without neurosensory deficit was similar. The relatively high amputation and mortality rates may be secondary to some of the patients with acute-onset graft-induced claudication actually having poorly defined subcritical ischaemia. The message, however, is clear, patients presenting with sudden onset of bypass graft occlusion resulting in incapacitating claudication who are treated with lysis have the same outcomes as those with established acute limb threatening ischaemia. This is summarized in the International Consensus Document Recommendation 13. Analogous to the indications for operative revascularization, thrombolysis in patients with with bypass graft occlusion should be reserved for those individuals with threatened limb loss and for selected individuals with claudication.[5]

Acute limb-threatening ischaemia

Those in Rutherford category III are inappropriate for lysis and should be considered for primary amputation. Those patients in Group IIB could be considered for lysis

Table 1 Severity of limb ischaemia

						Doppler signals	
	Category	*Description*	*Capillary return*	*Muscle paralysis*	*Sensory loss*	*Arterial*	*Venous*
I	Viable	Not immediately threatened	Intact	None	None	Audible	Audible
IIa	Threatened	Salvageable if treated	Intact/slow	None	Partial	Inaudible	Audible
IIb	Threatened	Salvageable if treated as emergency	Slow/absent	Partial	Partial	Inaudible	Audible
III	Irreversible	Primary amputation frequently required	Absent	Complete	Complete	Inaudible	Inaudible

Table 2. Demographic and clinical details of patients with acute graft occlusions (Thrombolysis Study Group Data)

	Graft (n=52)
Sex ratio (M:F)	33:19
Median (range) age (years)	69 (33–84)
Diabetes mellitus	4
Ischaemic heart disease	20
Previous stroke	1
History of peripheral vascular disease	52
Oral anticoagulation	21
Median (range) duration of symptoms	84 (3h to 2 weeks)
Thrombosis	50
Neurosensory deficit	17
Median ABPI	0.42

ABPI: ankle brachial pressure index

Table 3. Outcome for 52 patients with graft occlusion according to immediate outcome and secondary intervention (Thrombolysis Study Group Data)

	Degree of lysis			
	Complete	*Useful*	*No run-off*	*Failed*
No secondary intervention				
Asymptomatic	12	1		
Claudication	5		2	1
Amputation			1	
Death			2	1
Angioplasty or surgery as secondary procedure				
Asymptomatic	13	6		
Claudication	1			
Amputation			2	1
Death	1	1	1	1

with the proviso that the lytic therapy may fail and an opportunity for revascularization may be lost. Thrombolysis given by a conventional infusion may require procedural times up to 24 hours or longer, this may be unacceptable for those in the IIB Group if a detrimental delay in reperfusion is anticipated. Immediate surgical revascularization may be preferred in this group. Analysis of the Thrombolysis Study Group database for those patients presenting with acute limb threatening ischaemia secondary to bypass graft occlusion is interesting. There are 310 of these patients presenting with a variety of occluded grafts, the majority being polytetrafluoroethylene. Amputation-free survival at 30 days in this group was 75% (amputation=47, death=23). These figures are similar to those achieved in the acute claudicant group.

Information from databases is obviously not perfect; however, the above outcome analysis using the commonly accepted endpoint of amputation and death enable comparison with similar patients managed surgically.

Age

All complications of thrombolytic therapy are age-related, particularly major haemorrhage and cerebrovascular attacks, these increases are particularly apparent in the over-70 age-group.[6]

THROMBOLYSIS VERSUS SURGERY IN THE MANAGEMENT OF ACUTE BYPASS GRAFT FAILURE

The STILE[1] trial published in 1994 gives the best prospective randomized data comparing these two strategies. The STILE investigators randomized 393 patients with limb ischaemia of varying chronicity. In those patients with acute ischaemia 0–14 days who were treated with thrombolysis there was improved amputation-free survival and a shorter hospital stay compared with those treated with surgery. For patients with chronic ischaemia greater than 14 days, surgical revascularization was more effective and safer than thrombolysis. There were no differences in outcomes within treatment groups in patients with native artery or those with occluded bypass grafts.

In surgical patients there was a higher amputation rate in those with occluded bypass grafts and a trend towards high mortality with native arterial occlusion. These outcome differences were not observed in the thrombolysis patients. The results presented in the study support the use of thrombolytic therapy as an initial strategy in the management of acute bypass graft occlusions presenting with acute limb ischaemia. It must be remembered that there was a significant number of technical failures in the thrombolysis group in this study (28%); the specific details as to the number of grafts in this group is not available. It is possible that the superior results of initial management of thrombolysis of occluded bypass grafts is due to the ability of the lytic agent to revascularize the crural vessels and may also be assisted by low pressure reperfusion. If should be noted that the 30-day amputation-free survival rate in the thrombolytic group in the study was around 90%, which is considerably better than has been reported from the Thrombolysis Study Group database.

TECHNIQUES

There has been considerable interest in techniques of administrating lytic agents but few prospective data. A particular problem of technique in dealing with occluded bypass grafts is graft access. Both occluded venous and prosthetic conduits may not be apparent on arteriographic imaging and catheter placement may be blind. This problem is demonstrated in the STILE trial where 28% of the lysis patients were technical failures. Prosthetic conduits may be directly accessed using ultrasound or palpation. However, this technique cannot be applied to venous conduits. Venous conduits tend to collapse on occlusion and if there is no stump visible on angiography, access may prove problematic. Installation of the lytic agent must be intrathrombic and infusion near the suspected origin of the graft is unlikely to be successful. The lytic agent itself may be given in three ways; low dose infusion, high bolusing and pulse spray. There is little evidence that the method of administration makes any difference to the outcome There may be some temporal advantage in using the high dose or pulse spray technique.[7] The Thrombolysis Study Group performed a randomized trial comparing high dose bolusing with recombinant tissue plasminogen activator (rt-PA) with continuous infusion. Outcomes were similar in both groups but the time to reperfusion was considerably shorter in the high dose bolusing group.[8] More important is the successful placement of the perfusion catheter in the occluded segment. The fundamental principle of thrombolysis is that clearance of the occluded conduit and reperfusion of the leg represents only the initial stage of management of the occluded bypass graft. Angiography and more usefully duplex ultrasound must be used in order to determine the likely cause of graft failure. This may allow endovascular repair at the time of thrombolysis or surgical repair shortly thereafter. The failure to address the underlying cause of graft pathology will almost certainly lead to reocclusion.

REFERENCES

1. STILE Investigators: Results of a prospective randomised trial evaluating surgery *versus* thrombolysis for ischaemia of the lower extremity: the 'STILE' trial. *Ann Surg* **220:** 251–268, 1994
2. Braithwaite BD, Richie AWS, Earnshaw JJ: NATALI – a model for National Computer Databases in the investigation of new therapeutic techniques. *J Roy Soc Med* **88:** 511–515, 1995
3. Braithwaite BD, Tomlinson MA, Walker SR *et al.*, on behalf of the Thrombolysis Study Group: Peripheral thrombolysis for acute-onset claudication. *Br J Surg* **86:** 800–804, 1999
4. Dormandy JA, Murray GD: The fate of the claudicants – a prospective study of 1969 claudicants. *Eur J Vasc Surg* **5:** 131–133, 1991
5. Working Party of Thrombolysis in the Management of Limb Ischaemia: Thrombolysis in the management of lower limb arterial occlusion – a consensus document. *Am J Cardiol* **81:** 207–218, 1998
6. Braithwaite BD, Davies B, Birch PA *et al.*: Management of acute leg ischaemia in the elderly. *Br J Surg* **85:** 217, 1998
7. Buckenham TM, George CD, Chester JF *et al.*: Accelerated thrombolysis using pulsed intra-thrombus recombinant human tissue type plasminogen activator (t-PA). *Eur J Vasc Surg* **6:** 237–240, 1992
8. Braithwaite BD, Buckenham TM, Galland RB *et al.*: Prospective randomised trial of high-dose bolus *versus* low-dose tissue plasminogen activator infusion in the management of acute limb ischaemia. Thrombolysis Study Group. *Br J Surg* **84:** 646–650, 1997

Venous thrombolysis lessons

MP Armon, BR Hopkinson

INTRODUCTION

Streptokinase was first used for a venous thrombosis in 1959.[1] More thrombosis occurs on the venous side of the circulation than the arterial side, yet 40 years on, despite this early promise, thrombolysis is used almost exclusively for arterial thrombosis. It is standard first-line treatment for patients with acute myocardial infarction, and enjoys widespread use in the treatment of acute limb ischaemia. But its use for even major deep venous thrombosis (DVT) is negligible. Why is this?

This chapter aims to discuss the reasons commonly given for not using venous thrombolysis and will provide some counter arguments for why it should be given greater consideration as a treatment option.

DEEP VENOUS THROMBOSIS

Deep venous thrombosis is a major health problem with between 2.5 and 5% of the population affected at some time in their lives. Its main complications are pulmonary embolism in the short-term and post-thrombotic syndrome in the long-term. Standard treatment with anticoagulation is aimed purely at the prevention of pulmonary embolism, which it does effectively. However, its extensive use over the last 40 years has made no impact on the long-term complications of post-thrombotic syndrome. Around 50% of patients suffer some degree of pain, swelling, skin pigmentation or venous ulceration after a deep venous thrombosis in the long-term.[2] This is worst in those with proximal thrombosis, with most studies reporting eventual venous ulceration in at least 6% despite treatment with compression bandaging. The prevalence of venous ulcers in the general population is around 2 in 1000 and between 40 and 50% of patients with venous ulcers have evidence of post-thrombotic damage.[3] Because the majority of these patients are managed in the community, and their complications develop many years after their hospital admission, they are conveniently forgotten by the clinicians who dealt apparently successfully with the acute admission.

In this context thrombolysis has theoretical advantages over anticoagulation. By dissolving thrombus in the acute phase, venous valvular function may be preserved, thus preventing post-thrombotic complications in the long-term.

THE EVIDENCE FOR THROMBOLYSIS

Numerous studies of systemic streptokinase versus heparin were carried out in the 1960s and 1970s, and these have largely shaped our thinking today. Goldhaber's pooled analysis of the six randomized trials in this period which used phlebography to confirm the diagnosis and assess therapy is often quoted.[4] This showed that thrombolysis was achieved 3.7 times more often in those treated with streptokinase than those treated with heparin (95% CI 2.5–5.7, p <0.0001). In 1990, Rogers added a further seven studies.[5] All 13 showed much higher rates of lysis in the streptokinase-treated patients (20–70%) compared with those treated with heparin (0–28%). A more recent meta-analysis by Ng and Rivera arrived at similar conclusions showing that streptokinase recipients achieved higher rates of thrombolysis than recipients of heparin alone (Odds Ratio 6.24; 95% CI 3.62–10.78).[6] Thrombolysis works in the short-term.

However, the main reason for using thrombolysis is to prevent post-thrombotic syndrome in the long-term and it is on this that it must be judged. In those studies that had follow-up data, nine showed higher rates of normal venous function with streptokinase (36–92%) compared with heparin (12–50%) at 3–106 months follow-up. Two studies showed no difference. Ng's meta-analysis also showed systemic streptokinase patients were less likely to have post-thrombotic changes at follow-up (OR 0.32; 95% CI 0.12-0.86). The consensus then is that streptokinase is effective both at achieving thrombolysis in the short-term and reducing the incidence of post-thrombotic syndrome in the long-term. This must be balanced against the risk of bleeding.

THE RISK OF BLEEDING

Goldhaber's analysis of the randomized controlled trials available in 1984 found only three studies that provided worthwhile figures for bleeding complications. The combined numbers of patients in these trials were 57 (streptokinase) and 59 (heparin). No trial showed a statistically significant difference on its own, but combined found 2.9 times more bleeding complications in the streptokinase-treated group (95% CI 1.1–8.1, p = 0.04). Rogers, however, put this down to an increased incidence of minor bleeding and concluded that 'major bleeding requiring transfusions occurred equally with streptokinase and heparin.'

The definition of what constitutes a major bleed varies from publication to publication, making comparison between papers difficult. A haemorrhage requiring blood transfusion, or a fall in haemoglobin level of 2g/dl is the definition most frequently, but not invariably used. Fatal haemorrhage and cerebrovascular events are more unequivocal end-points and meaningful comparison of these rates can be made. The Rogers review of 33 studies found that only two of 810 patients treated with streptokinase suffered a fatal haemorrhage (0.2%), and five had an intracranial haemorrhage (0.62%). These figures for fatal haemorrhage and stroke are comparable with those in the major trials of thrombolytic agents in the treatment of acute myocardial infarction. In the ASSET study,[7] a placebo-controlled trial of tissue plasminogen activator (tPA) in over 5000 patients with acute myocardial infarction, the incidence of stroke in tPA-treated patients was 1.1% and fatal haemorrhage 0.4%. There was no difference in the placebo-treated group (1.0% and 0.2% respectively).

Questions have been raised over the exclusion criteria of the early deep venous thrombosis studies. Of the five patients suffering haemorrhagic strokes in the Rogers review, two had thrombophilia and two had a history of previous cerebrovascular events. In Ng's meta-analysis, all but two studies were excluded because of the inclusion of patients who had contraindications to thrombolysis (e.g. major surgery within 7 days), and there was no significant difference in major bleeding between the two (small) groups of streptokinase- and heparin-treated patients that remained.

The concern about the risk of bleeding in thrombolysis is understandable but ultimately based on limited evidence in deep venous thrombosis patients. The established increased risk for patients with acute myocardial infarction and acute limb ischaemia is for a different patient population with an arguably greater risk of stroke due to underlying arterial disease. It could therefore be argued that the bleeding risk in deep venous thrombosis may be lower, and that with careful patient selection, may be safer than previously thought.

PATIENT SELECTION

The main potential benefit of thrombolysis for deep venous thrombosis is the prevention of post-thrombotic syndrome. It follows therefore that those patients most at risk and with a long life-expectancy have most to gain. Young patients with proximal deep venous thrombosis are the ideal candidates. Results of lysis in general seem to be best with fresh thrombus and as valve preservation is the aim, early intervention should be aimed for. There is no good evidence on which to base a time limit for intervention, but lysis should probably be commenced no later than 10 days from the onset of symptoms and ideally within 3-4 days. The earlier the better. Established contraindications include: recent surgery or kidney/liver biopsy (within 2 weeks), cerebrovascular history, active gastrointestinal bleeding, known bleeding diathesis, uncontrolled hypertension and chronic renal, hepatic or metastatic disease.

SUITABILITY FOR THROMBOLYSIS

Markel and colleagues have postulated that only 7% of patients with deep venous thrombosis would be suitable for thrombolysis, based on a retrospective review of 209 case-notes.[8] Our own prospective study of 55 consecutive patients with proximal deep venous thrombosis found that 36% of patients were potential candidates for thrombolysis, the most common contraindications being recent surgery, intracranial pathology and extensive malignancy (Table 1). Much of this difference can be accounted for by our differing criteria for suitability, in particular the safe postoperative time period (Markel deemed patients within 1 month of even minor procedures such as paracentesis to be unsuitable for thrombolysis). We used a cut-off period of 2 weeks post-surgery and successfully lysed two patients within a month of

Table 1. Reasons for unsuitability for thrombolysis

Absolute contraindication	*No.*
Major surgery within 2 weeks	9
Recent cerebrovascular accident/intracranial pathology	5
Extensive malignancy	5
Active gastrointestinal bleeding	1
Thrombocytopenia	1
Phlegmasia cerulea dolens – thrombocytopenia	1
– hepatic failure	2
Relative contraindication	
Previous confirmed ipsilateral deep venous thrombosis	4
History more than 3 weeks	4
Elderly and frail	3
TOTAL	35

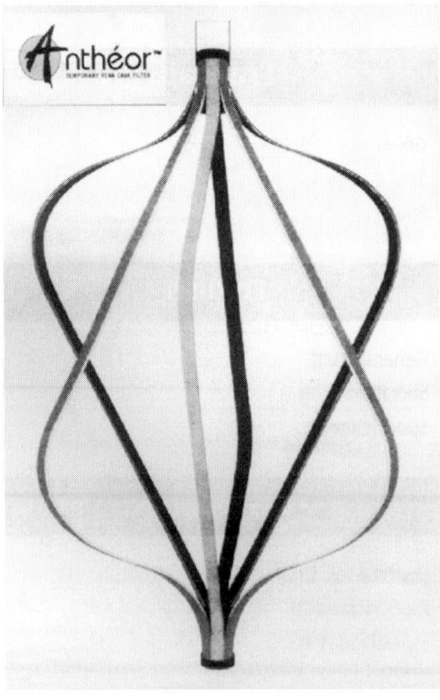

Fig. 1. A temporary vena caval filter (Antheor, Boston Scientific Corporation).

a total hip replacement with no adverse consequences. Conversely, one patient lysed 2 months after a total hip replacement developed a wound haematoma.

CATHETER-DIRECTED THROMBOLYSIS FOR PROXIMAL DEEP VENOUS THROMBOSIS

A regional approach to arterial thrombosis has produced superior results compared with systemic infusion.[9] Such an approach to deep venous thrombosis has yet to be thoroughly evaluated though early reports of catheter-directed thrombolysis have been encouraging.[10,11] We conducted a feasibility study aimed at developing a method of catheter-directed thrombolysis, which if safe and effective could be tested against the current treatment regimen of standard anticoagulation.

Technique

A temporary 'Antheor' vena caval filter (Boston Scientific Corporation) (Fig. 1) was positioned in the inferior vena cava below the renal veins via either the common femoral vein (three cases) or the brachial vein (six cases). A 5 French catheter was inserted into the affected deep veins from either the contralateral femoral vein, the ipsilateral popliteal vein or a posterior tibial vein under ultrasound guidance[12] and an initial venogram taken (Fig. 2). A guidewire was then positioned in the thrombus and

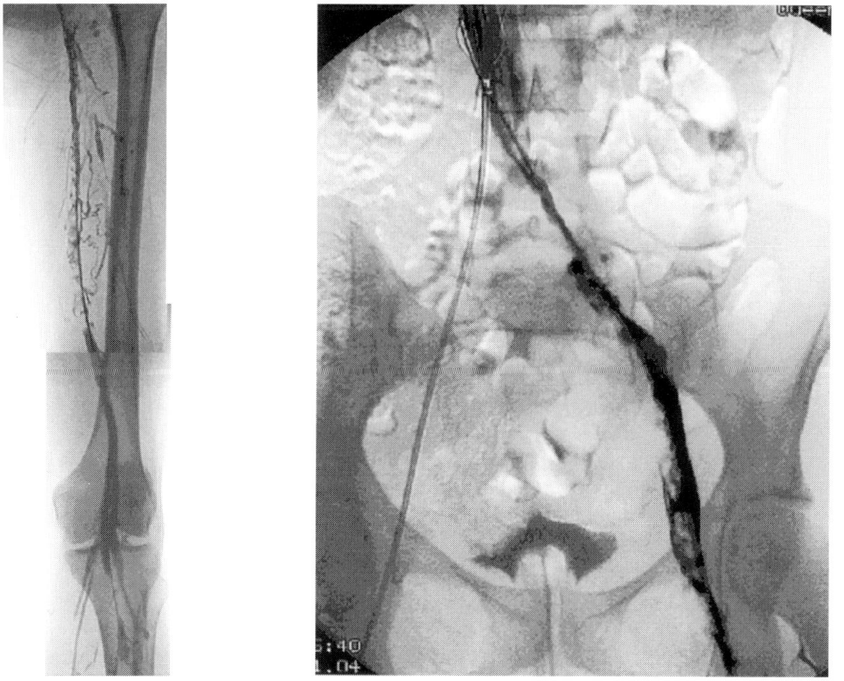

Fig. 2. Venography demonstrating an iliofemoral deep venous thrombosis in a 31-year-old female. A 5F thrombolysis catheter has been inserted via the left posterior tibial vein, and a temporary vena caval filter via the right common femoral vein.

a multi-sidehole pulse-spray catheter advanced over the guidewire and positioned at the proximal end of the thrombus. Pulse spray infusion was commenced with recombinant tissue plasminogen activator (Actilyse, Boehringer Ingleheim, Bracknell Berkshire, UK) (rt-PA) for a maximum of 4 hours. Progress was monitored by regular venography. If lysis was incomplete after 4 hours a low-dose infusion of rt-PA 0.5ml/h was continued for up to 48 hours with venographic review at 24 hour intervals. Angioplasty or stent placement was considered for any underlying stenoses.

Eight patients were treated with catheter-directed thrombolysis. In every case the iliac and common femoral veins were cleared of thrombus. In three patients with thrombus extending below the inguinal ligament in whom a popliteal or femoral vein approach was used, rethrombosis occurred in the superficial femoral and/or popliteal veins despite initial lysis. In the two patients in whom a posterior tibial vein approach was used for infrainguinal thrombosis, complete clearance of the deep venous system was obtained (Fig. 3). The total time taken to achieve lysis was 3.5–50 hours (median 25 hours), and the total dose of rt-PA used was 25–98mg (median 35mg).

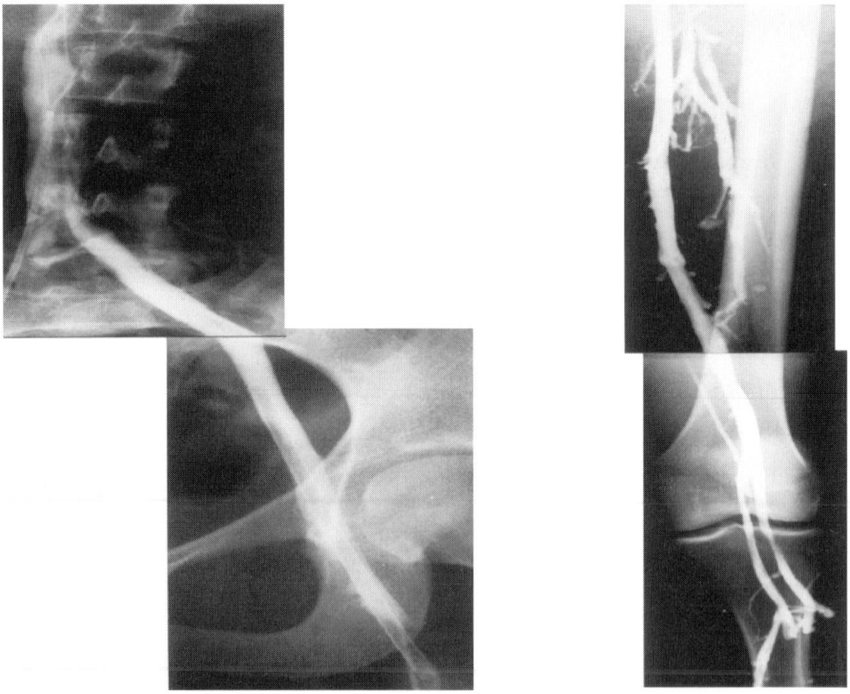

Fig. 3. Venography of the same patient after 24 hours of catheter-directed thrombolysis with 26 mg of rt-PA and insertion of an 8mm Wallstent.

Common iliac vein stenosis

A left common iliac vein stenosis, close to the junction with the inferior vena cava was present in six of nine patients undergoing catheter-directed thrombolysis. Three patients in whom no stenoses were found were all post total hip replacement. One stenosis was iatrogenic in origin, but in five it was an unexpected finding. This led to the abandonment of the procedure in one patient. The remaining five patients were all successfully treated by insertion of a Wallstent with no complications (Fig. 4).

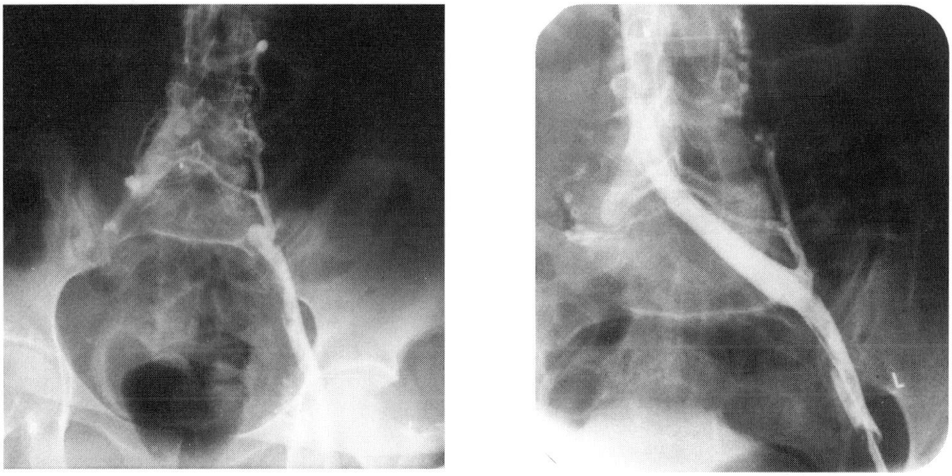

Fig. 4. Venography of a 60-year-old female illustrating a left common iliac vein stenosis discovered during catheter-directed thrombolysis of an iliofemoral deep venous thrombosis, before and after placement of a Wallstent.

Antheor temporary caval filters were left in position for up to 3 days. Thrombus was dislodged into the filter on three occasions following catheter manipulation. On all three occasions the thrombus was successfully treated by a low-dose thrombolytic infusion. One patient developed mild haematuria during thrombolysis and another patient developed a wound haematoma at the site of his 2-month old total hip replacement incision. There were no cases of pulmonary embolus during the course of the procedure either clinically or as assessed by V/Q scans before and after lysis.

Follow-up

In all eight patients treated with catheter-directed thrombolysis the lysed iliofemoral segments remained patent at between 1 and 13 months. Three patients in whom a popliteal or femoral approach to a full-length deep venous thrombosis was used had residual thrombus within the superficial femoral and popliteal veins. One patient had significant reflux, two patients had persistent calf pain and swelling and one had some swelling but no pain. In all three patients the residual symptoms were less severe than before lysis.

CONCLUSIONS

Thrombolysis is an underused treatment modality for venous disease. The sequelae of venous obstruction are considerable and often underestimated. The fear of bleeding complications is based largely on old studies using outdated thrombolytic regimens with poor selection criteria. The risk of fatal haemorrhage and stroke is probably similar to that for anticoagulation, and whilst the overall incidence of bleeding is greater for thrombolysis, this short-term inconvenience needs to be weighed against the long-term consequences of post thrombotic syndrome. With careful patient selection, the additional risks of bleeding may be further reduced. As always, there is a great need for further randomized controlled studies using newer catheter-directed techniques to establish the role of venous thrombolysis in the new millenium.

REFERENCES

1. Johnson AJ, McCarty WR: The lysis of artificially induced intravascular clots in mankind by intravenous infusions of streptokinase. *J Clin Invest* **28:** 173–178, 1959
2. Johnson BF, Manzo RA, Bergelin RO, Strandness DE: Relationship between changes in the deep venous system and the development of the postthrombotic syndrome after an acute episode of lower limb deep vein thrombosis: A one to six year follow-up. *J Vasc Surg* **21:** 307–313, 1995
3. Browse NL, Burnand KG, Irvine AT, Wilson NM (Eds), *Diseases of the Veins.* London: Arnold, 1999
4. Goldhaber SZ, Buring JE, Lipnick RJ, Hennekens CH: Pooled analyses of randomised streptokinase and heparin in phlebographically documented acute deep venous thrombosis. *Am J Med* **76:** 393–397, 1984
5. Rogers LQ, Lutcher CL: Streptokinase therapy for DVT: A comprehensive review of the English literature. *Am J Med* **88:** 389–395, 1990
6. Ng CM, Rivera JO: Meta-analysis of streptokinase and heparin in deep vein thrombosis. *Am J Hlth-Syst Pharm* **55:** 1995–2001, 1998
7. Wilcox RG, van der Lippe G, Orlssonn CG *et al.*: Effects of alteplase in acute myocardial infarction: 6-month results from the ASSET study. Anglo-Scandinavian Study of Early Thrombolysis. *Lancet* **335:** 1175–1178, 1988
8. Markel A, Manzo RA, Strandness E: The potential role of thrombolytic therapy in venous thrombosis. *Arch Int Med* **152:** 1265–1267, 1992
9. Berridge DC, Gregson RHS, Hopkinson BR, Makin GS: Randomized trial of intra-arterial recombinant tissue plasminogen activator, intravenous recombinant tissue plasminogen activator and intra-arterial streptokinase in peripheral arterial thrombolysis. *Br J Surg* **78:** 988–995, 1991
10. Semba CP, Dake MD: Iliofemoral deep venous thrombosis: Aggressive therapy with catheter-directed thrombolysis. *Radiology* **191:** 487–494, 1994
11. Comerota AJ, Aldridge SC *et al.*: A strategy of aggressive regional therapy for acute iliofemoral venous thrombosis with contemporary venous thrombectomy or catheter directed thrombolysis. *J Vasc Surg* **20:** 244–254, 1994
12. Armon MP, Whitaker SC, Tennant WG: Catheter-directed thrombolysis of proximal DVT: A new approach via the posterior tibial vein. *Eur J Vasc Endovasc Surg* **13:** 413–416, 1997

Upper limb venous thrombolysis: The Paget–Schroetter syndrome

Andrew D Platts, Syed A Babar

INTRODUCTION

The Paget–Schroetter syndrome (PSS) of subclavian and axillary vein thrombosis was named after two physicians who independently described the condition, Sir James Paget in 1875 and Von Schroetter in 1884. This condition of primary subclavian thrombosis is also variously described as Primary, Spontaneous, Idiopathic, Effort, Traumatic, Positional and Strain thrombosis. The condition is also occasionally described by the activity that precipitated it e.g. work-out, body-builders', rowers', or pitchers' thrombosis.

There has been a massive increase in the occurrence of upper limb venous thrombosis, the substantial majority of cases are causally related to long-term venous access catheters, or other devices that cause local venous damage including pacemaker leads. Axillosubclavian thrombosis may be secondary to local anatomical venous compression by, for instance, callus from fractured clavicle or rib, local tumour or by non-compressive vein wall damage, for example from radiotherapy. These cases lie outside the scope of this chapter.

Why should the subclavian vein be particularly susceptible to thrombotic occlusion? The factors that lead to thrombosis were described by Virchow and are now called Virchow's triad. These are, changes in the constituents of the blood, changes in the flow of blood and changes in the vessel wall.

Changes in the constituents of the blood include any of the causes of thrombophilia. These conditions are a contributing factor in some patients who develop PSS but do not alter acute management. A thrombophilia screen should be performed in patients who have no identifiable physical cause for the event, have a normal vein after thrombolysis and in those who give a history of previous thrombotic episodes.[1,2]

Changes in the flow of blood are probably the single most important factor in the development of PSS. The subclavian vein passes through a dynamic corridor, the costoclavicular space, where it is liable to extrinsic compression resulting in slowed or obstructed flow. The vein passes between the clavicle and first rib, a space that narrows with arm abduction and external rotation or shoulder depression causing venous compression in a significant proportion of the population. This space is further narrowed by the subclavius muscle that attaches to the undersurface of the clavicle and increases its bulk when contracted in arm abduction and when the muscle hypertrophies with exercise. The vein is restricted posteriorly by the anterior scalene muscle that holds the vein forwards between the bony 'scissors' of the clavicle and first rib. Extrinsic constriction of the subclavian vein becomes worse when the shoulder is depressed and during exercise or activities that involve elevation and abduction of the arm, particularly when load bearing. Many patients present shortly after vigorous sessions in the gym or after the return to some seasonal sport such as tennis or cricket in the summer. Other cases of subclavian vein thrombosis clearly relate to positional occlusion of the vein with patients reporting the onset of symptoms after a period of drink- or drug-induced somnolence, perhaps with the arm draped over a chair.

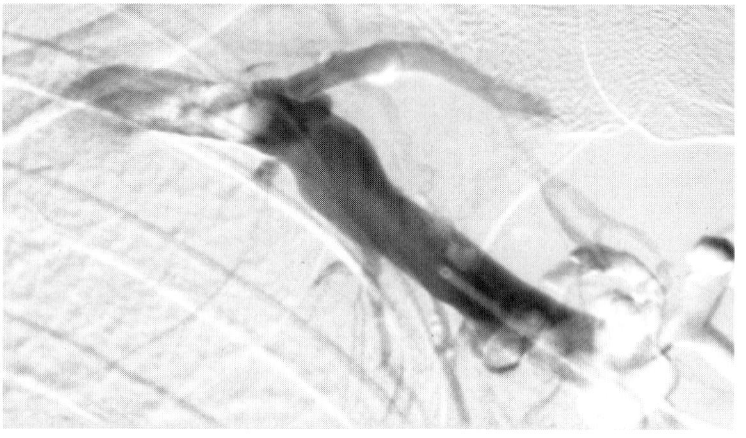

Fig. 1. Catheter venogram demonstrates occlusion of the left subclavian vein, thrombus is outlined within the vessel.

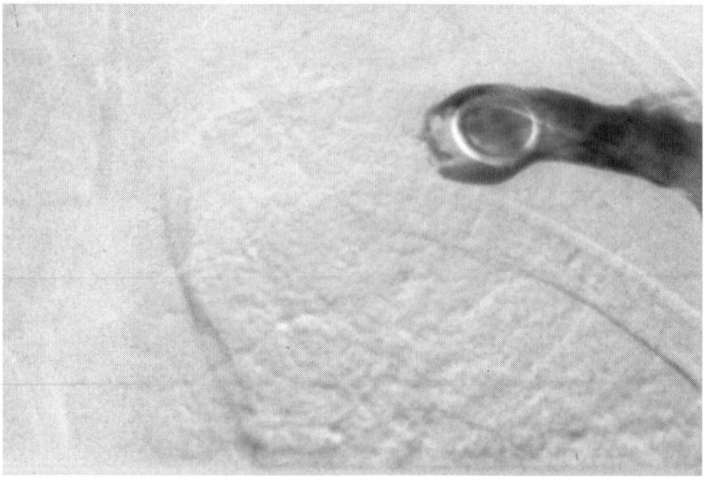

Fig. 2. A guidewire would not easily cross the venous occlusion. A pigtail catheter was advanced into the thrombus and manually rotated to fragment the thrombus. A bolus of 5mg rt-PA was injected.

Case 1 (Figs 1–7): A 28-year-old female presented 18 hours after a vigorous session of swimming with a swollen, painful arm.

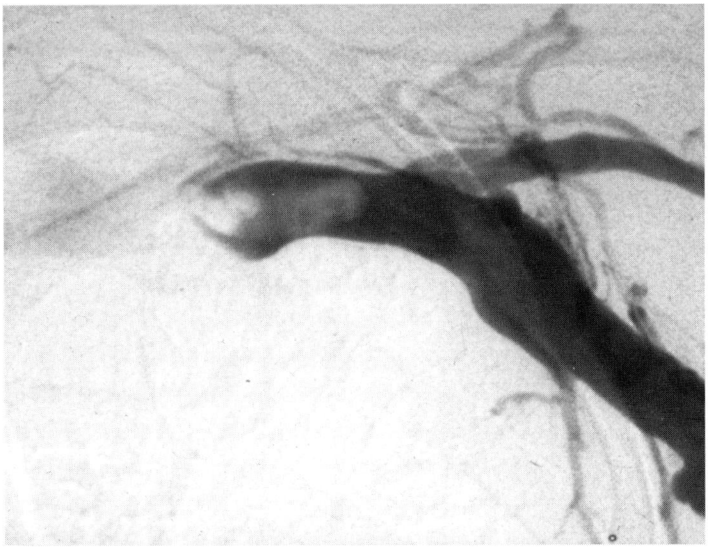

Fig. 3. After 15 minutes the mass of thrombus has reduced in size.

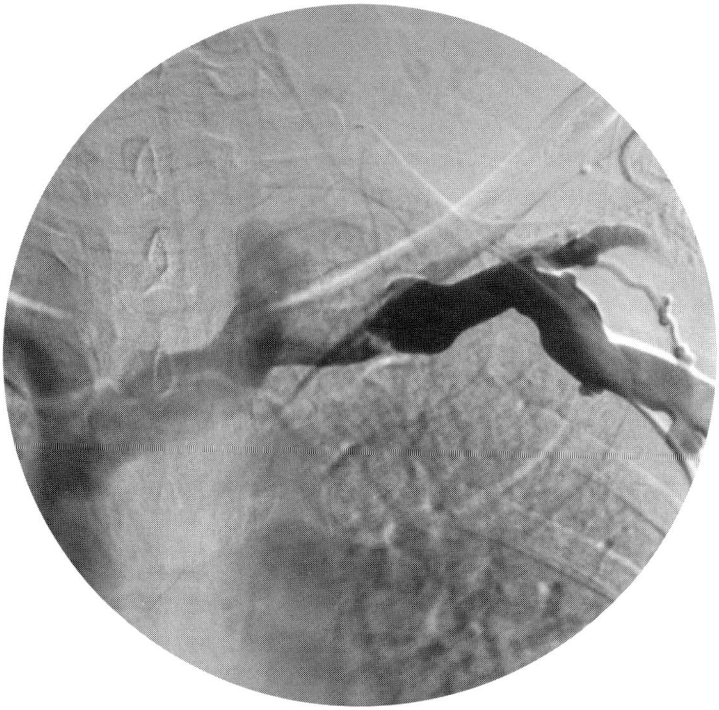

Fig. 4. After a 6-hour infusion of rt-PA at 1mg per hour the thrombus has cleared to reveal the underlying lesion. A markedly thickened and stenosed valve is shown. This lies precisely at the point where the vein is compressed between the clavicle and first rib. This supports the hypothesis that the damage is caused by repeated compression.

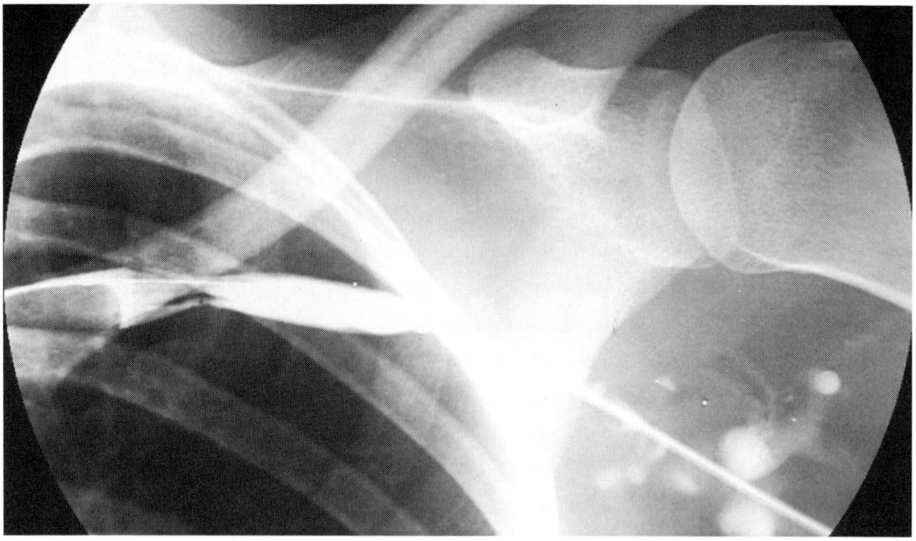

Fig. 5.

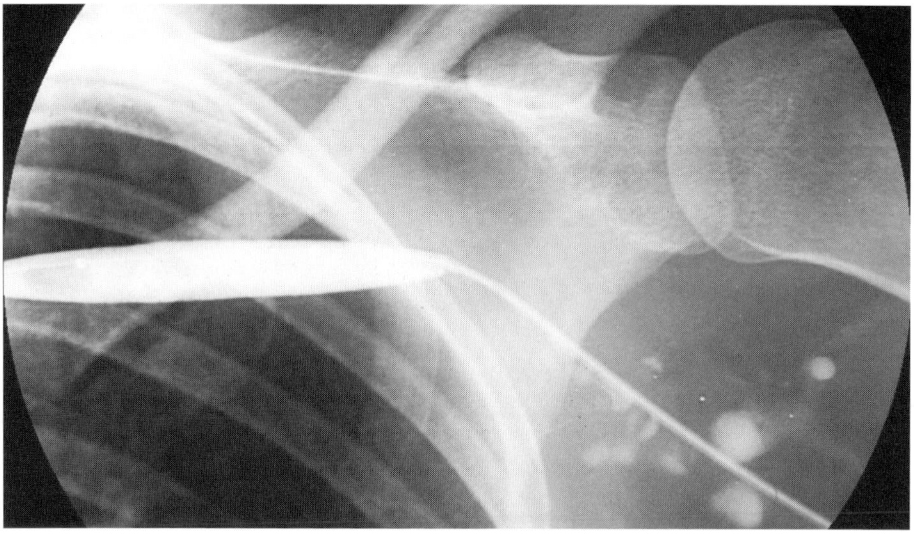

Fig. 6.

Figs 5, 6. Repeated inflation of the angioplasty balloon did not resolve the lesion completely.

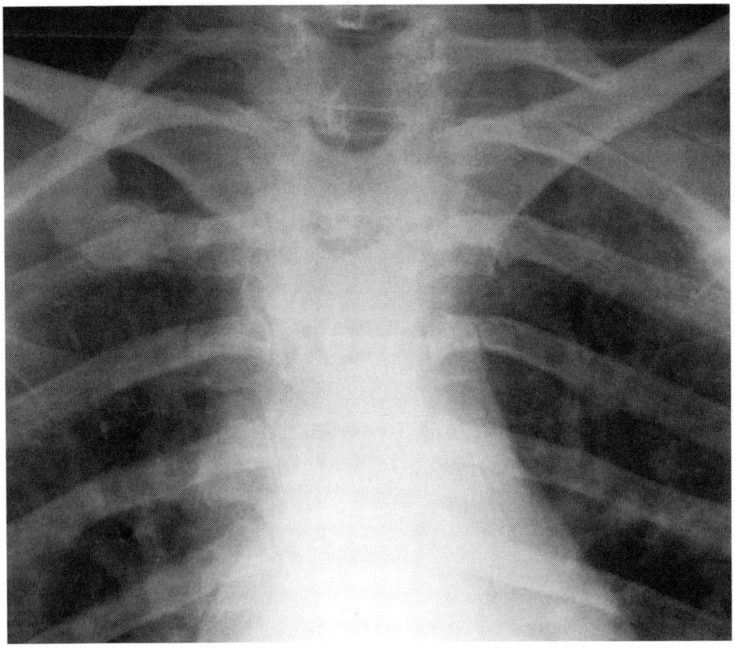

Fig. 7. The first rib was resected, there has been no recurrence of thrombosis. The patient is symptom free at 7 years.

Changes in the vessel wall can be the result of chronic trauma to the vein during repetitive or vigorous arm movement whether occupational or recreational. This leads to thickening and stenosis of the vein wall, the development of intraluminal synechae or damage to a valve. Venous valves occur at variable sites in the subclavian vein but when the valve lies precisely at the position of bony venous compression it may become thickened, dysplastic and stenosed. This is readily demonstrated in some patients who suffer PSS after the thrombus has been cleared (Fig. 4) Repeated acute trauma during vigorous exercise probably causes damage to the vein wall leading to endothelial denudation and vein wall swelling.

Patients typically present in young adulthood to middle age with a short history of arm swelling, arm discomfort, paraesthesia or pruritis. There will be obvious swelling, mild cyanosis of the limb and distended superficial veins. Tender firm veins may be palpable in the axilla. The condition has been most frequently reported in males but females are not spared. The dominant limb is most frequently affected as one would predict with any condition that is related to limb activity.

The diagnosis may be confirmed by any of a wide range of tests that include duplex ultrasound, magnetic resonance venography, computed tomography, and plethysmography. Of course contrast venography offers the advantage of accurate diagnosis combined with the ability to proceed immediately to treatment.

Historical studies have shown that conservative treatment by limb elevation results in considerable long-term morbidity with persisting limb swelling and discomfort.[3] Significant numbers of patients are unable to return to work. Anticoagulation prevents propagation of thrombus into collateral veins and will in itself result in benefit compared with conservative management reducing long-term morbidity.[4,5]

Approximately 10% of patients with upper limb thrombosis develop pulmonary embolism[5] though this may be clinically silent, anticoagulation may improve the prognosis in this group. Anticoagulation will not, by itself, however, result in restoration of normal flow, some veins do recanalize but usually as a late phenomenon. Late recanalization results in a stenosed vessel with abnormal venous flow and a thickened wall caused by the secondary periphlebitis, exactly the conditions likely to lead to recurrent thrombosis.[6–8] The management of patients with PSS must address two issues, namely the acute thrombosis and any underlying local cause. The goal is to restore normal venous flow and prevent recurrent thrombosis. The aim is to prevent the morbidity associated with a chronically swollen, uncomfortable, clumsy or easily fatigued arm that would otherwise be the result. Thrombolysis is consensually proposed to be the preferred treatment,[9] though there are no randomized trials that compare it against treatment by anticoagulation or surgical thrombectomy.

Thrombolysis offers the opportunity for rapid vessel recanalization with restoration of flow. Secondary periphlebitis should thus be limited resulting in less vein wall damage. Underlying venous abnormalities will be revealed when the vein lumen is clear. There is considerable evidence from retrospectively collected data that this is the case.

The technique is straightforward. The site of venous occlusion is confirmed by venography usually as an ascending study via the basilic vein from the affected limb. A guidewire is advanced into the occluded segment. If there is no underlying venous stenosis the wire will pass into the superior vena cava. If the wire does not easily traverse the occluded segment an underlying web is highly likely and this should not be further traumatized by prolonged or vigorous manipulation by guidewire or catheter. A catheter is advanced into the thrombus over the wire and thrombolysis commenced. The thrombus may well be quite bulky and as thrombolysis is a surface effect a simple infusion may take a considerable time, typically 24–36 hours, to clear the clot. It is useful to increase the contact surface between the thrombus and lytic agent either by forced pulsatile injection or by agitation and fragmentation of the thrombus with a shaped catheter. The latter is particularly useful when there is a venous stenosis proximal to the thrombus preventing the thrombus from becoming dislodged. Any effective thrombolytic agents may be used. We have found recombinant tissue plasminogen activator (rt-PA) given by 5mg lacing bolus followed by an infusion at 1mg per hour to be effective usually producing complete lysis within 12–24 hours. Distal injection of the thrombolytic drug without impaction of the delivery catheter into the thrombus is ineffective; the drug simply enters the collateral veins. Urokinase and steptokinase have all been use with good effect. Complications are less frequently reported than when arterial thrombolysis is performed because there is no arterial puncture and the cohort of patients are younger and healthier with fewer comorbidity factors.

When the vein has cleared, venography will show any underlying intrinsic venous pathology. If a venous stenosis, web, or dysplastic valve are shown then clearly the vein has been chronically traumatized by adverse anatomy. This should be corrected by resection of the first rib with release of scalenus anterior. The venous stenosis can be dilated by balloon, some centres have found this to be ineffective alone[8] and it should always be accompanied by sugical decompression. Division of thickened perivenous tissue and surgical venoplasty, with or without a patch, can of course be performed at the time of thoracic outlet decompression.[10]

There are conflicting recommendations regarding the appropriate timing of surgery with advocates both for surgery immediately after thrombolysis and surgery delayed until after 3 months of anticoagulation; both report excellent outcome. Patients treated by immediate surgery need not be anticoagulated but venography should be repeated at 3 months to demonstrate venous stenosis and allow treatment by angioplasty.

Metallic stents can temporarily restore venous patency but should not be deployed between an intact clavicle and first rib,[5] balloon-expanded stents crush irreversibly at this site[11] and self-expanding stents will eventually succumb to fatigue failure. There are numerous anecdotes of stent failure with stent fragmentation, pressure erosion of adjacent bone and local pain all being described to us.

If there is no venous lesion when the thrombus has cleared the situation is perhaps more complex. Where there is an identifiable thrombophilia such as Protein C or S deficiency, or history of oral contraceptive usage then anticoagulation and avoidance of any precipitating activity are effective without surgical decompression. In individuals with an obvious precipitating activity that they are able, and willing to avoid in future such as painting the ceiling, then short-term oral anticoagulation for 3 months without surgery can be advised. When the patient is unable to avoid the provoking activity for occupational reasons, or unwilling to for social reasons, then surgical decompression should be offered in the expectation that recurrent thrombosis is otherwise highly likely to occur.

When this strategy is used, most patients with a duration of symptoms of less than 8 days will achieve a successful result with the substantial majority able to return to normal work and activity.[12] Those with a longer duration of symptoms are less likely to achieve primary success, are more likely to rethrombose and to suffer postphlebitic symptoms that restrict work and recreation.[13]

When postphlebitic symptoms do persist surgical decompression may still be beneficial if it can be shown that there is positional occlusion of collateral veins.

Transaxillary, supraclavicular and infraclavicular approaches to decompression all have advocates and approximately equivalent published outcome. Venous bypass may be accomplished by swinging down the jugular vein with at least temporary benefit in cases that do not respond to, or recur after, thrombolysis.

When acute subclavian thrombosis propagates to the arm it may result in phlegmasia caerulia dolens or progress to venous gangrene. These conditions as almost universally associated with markedly deranged clotting and often with malignancy. The priority is to reverse the coagulopathy by heparinization thereby preventing further propagation of thrombosis into collateral vessels. The condition of the limb can be improved by elevation to reduce swelling. If these measures do not result in rapid improvement then intra-arterial thrombolysis should be considered. Intravenous lysis is unlikely to be effective because in these conditions the thrombosis has propagated retrogradely within the vascular system into the

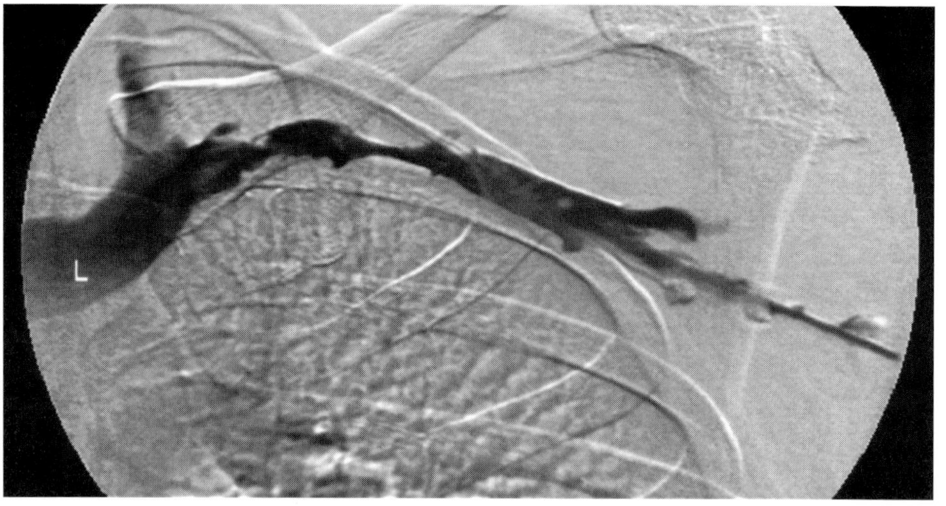

Fig. 8. Venogram after 24 hours of thrombolytic infusion demonstrates a stenosed and irregular vein. This was dilated to 9mm and the patient anticoagulated for 3 months.

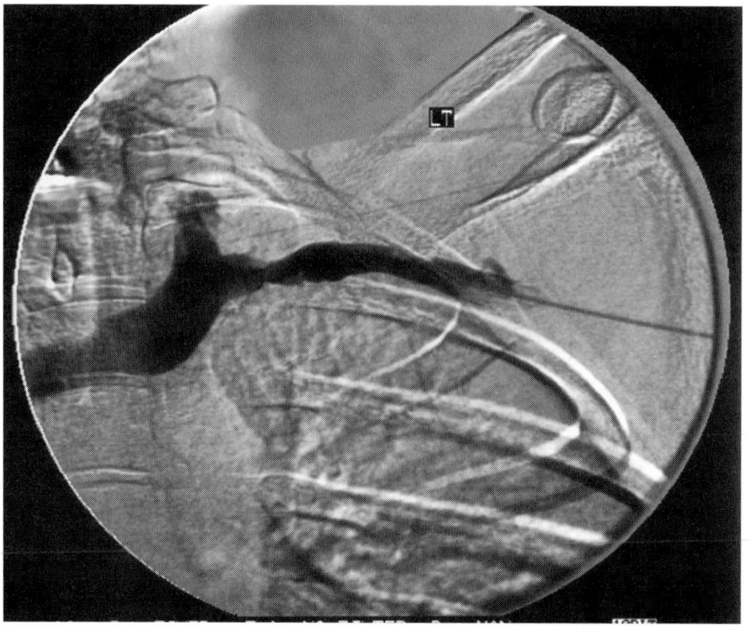

Fig. 9. Venogram at 3 months, prior to planned resection of the first rib shows only minor vein narrowing. The patient refused surgery and stopped anticoagulation because he considered himself cured despite medical advice to the contrary.

Case 2 (Figs 8–10): A 27-year-old male presented 36 hours after the onset of painful arm swelling. He was a work-out enthusiast who self-administered anabolic steroids and attended the gymnasium every day.

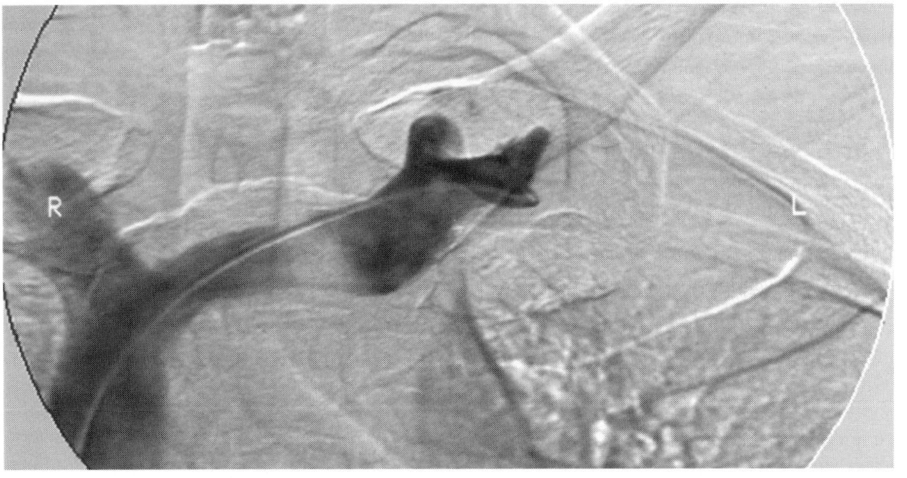

Fig. 10. Repeat venography at 15 months after the initial thrombosis via femoral approach confirms rethrombosis.

postcapilliary venules. Experience in the lower limb has shown that by intra-arterial infusion there will be rapid control of symptoms and improvement in the condition of the limb.[14] It has to be recognized that the long-term prognosis in these patients is poor.

Despite the absence of controlled comparative studies thrombolysis is now extensively used in the treatment of primary subclavian venous thrombosis, PSS. This has been accompanied by general abandonment of primary surgical thrombectomy but with late surgical decompression after thrombus has been cleared and the underlying anatomy demonstrated. If all patients with P-SS were managed by experienced vascular units rather than by general physicians who offer simple anticoagulation there would be reduced morbidity and more patients would resume normal activity and employment. It is incumbent on vascular units to promote improved care by development of local guidelines and to offer an efficient pathway to combined patient management.

REFERENCES

1. Scott DJA, Farmilo W, Horrocks M *et al.*: Venous thrombolysis [letter]. *Eur J Vasc Surg* **2:** 274, 1998
2. Scott DJA, Farmilo W, Taylor P: The place of first rib resection in the management of axillary-subclavian thrombosis [letter] *Eur J Vasc Surg* **1:** 363, 1987
3. Tilney NL, Griffiths HJG, Edwards EA: Natural history of major venous thrombosis of the upper extremity. *Arch Surg* **101:** 792–796, 1970
4. Swinton NW, Edgett JW, Hall RJ: Primary subclavian-axillary vein thrombosis. *Circulation* **38:** 737–745, 1968
5. Adams JT, McEvoy RK, DeWeese JA: Primary deep venous thrombosis of the upper extremity. *Arch Surg* **91:** 29–42, 1965

6. Coon WW, Willis PW: Thrombosis of axillary and subclavian veins. *Arch Surg* **94:** 657–663, 1967
7. Prescott SM, Tikoff G: Deep venous thrombosis of the upper extremity: a reappraisal. *Circulation* **59:** 350–355, 1979
8. Machleder HI: Evaluation of a new treatment strategy for Paget-Schroetter syndrome: spontaneous thrombosis of the axillary-subclavian vein. *J Vasc Surg* **17:** 305–317, 1996
9. Rutherford RB, Hurlbert SN: Primary subclavian-axillary vein thrombosis: consensus and commentary. *Cardiovasc Surg* **4:** 420–423, 1996
10. Thompson RW, Schneider PA, Nelken NA *et al.*: Circumferential venolysis and peraclavicular thoracic outlet decompression for 'effort thrombosis' of the subclavian vein. *J Vasc Surg* **16:** 723–733, 1992
11. Bjarnason H, Hunter DW, Crain MR *et al.*: Collapse of a Palmaz stent in the subclavian vein. *Am J Roent* **160:** 1123–1124, 1993
12. Urschel HC, Razzuk MA: Neurovascular compression in the thoracic outlet. *Ann Surg* **228:** 609–617, 1998
13. Adelman MA, Stone DH, Riles TS *et al.*: A multidiscipline approach to the treatment of Paget-Schroetter syndrome. *Ann Vasc Surg* **11:** 149–154, 1997
14. Wlodarczyk ZK, Gibson M, Dick R *et al.*: Low dose intra-arterial thrombolysis in the treatment of phlegmasia caerulia dolens. *Br J Surg* **81:** 370–372, 1994

First rib resection and the management of Paget–Schroetter syndrome

P Nafteux, DC Kinsella, JF Thompson

INTRODUCTION

Axillosubclavian vein thrombosis is a rare condition with potentially serious sequelae. The acute event is a perfect example of a vascular and endovascular opportunity. If this opportunity is missed the patient may suffer the early complication of pulmonary embolism or the late outcome of disabling venous engorgement in a post-phlebitic upper limb, with subsequent limitations in their everyday life, employment or sporting activities.

Retrospective reviews of the outcome in mixed aetiology groups of patients with axillosubclavian vein thrombosis provide partially reassuring data with which to advise patients with acute thrombosis. We would tell such a patient that they could expect a 50–60% chance that their limb would return to normal after a period of anticoagulation. Prospectively, however, there is no way of predicting those who will have adequate collateral venous channels to achieve this. In a fit, young patient who would like to remain active, in full employment and to continue sport, we believe an aggressive policy of combined endovascular and surgical management yields good results.

Conservative management with anticoagulation should be reserved for older, more sedentary patients and those with clots more than 3–4 weeks old. This is a safe, well established approach with much to commend it.

PATHOPHYSIOLOGY

Acute deep vein thrombosis of the upper limb has many causes, including effort-related (Paget–Schroetter) syndrome, immobilization and thoracic outlet syndrome as primary causes and the following as secondary causes: catheter-related causes, tumour/node compression, radiotherapy, trauma, oral contraceptive, cardiac failure, thrombophilia and paraneoplastic, amyloid, and sarcoid causes. In general it may result from trauma, extrinsic compression or hypercoagulable states such as those associated with malignancy. It is now recognized that central venous catheters frequently cause axillosubclavian vein thrombosis in critically ill or dialysis patients and is a potent source of pulmonary emboli.

Spontaneous or effort-related thrombosis, in a fit young patient is known as Paget–Schroetter syndrome (PSS) – the first two cases being published by these two authors over a century ago. Hughes, who in 1949 collected 320 cases and recognized the distinct entity, coined the eponym.[1] The mechanism of compression leading to PSS is primarily hypertrophy of the subclavius and scalenus anterior muscles with bony exostosis at the scalene tubercle and at the junction of the first costal cartilage and sternum. The first rib is elevated by the hypertrophied scalene muscles, which are of course accessory muscles of respiration, used during exercise. The clavicle borders the compartment superiorly. The clavicle rotates during arm movement so the mechanism of compression is not just a simple scissors type action. There is a constant valve within the subclavian vein, level with the inner border of the first rib, which can be seen quite clearly during transaxillary first rib resection and which has been present in nearly every cadaver we have examined during training courses. Most thromboses start at this point. In addition, repeated trauma to the vein as it

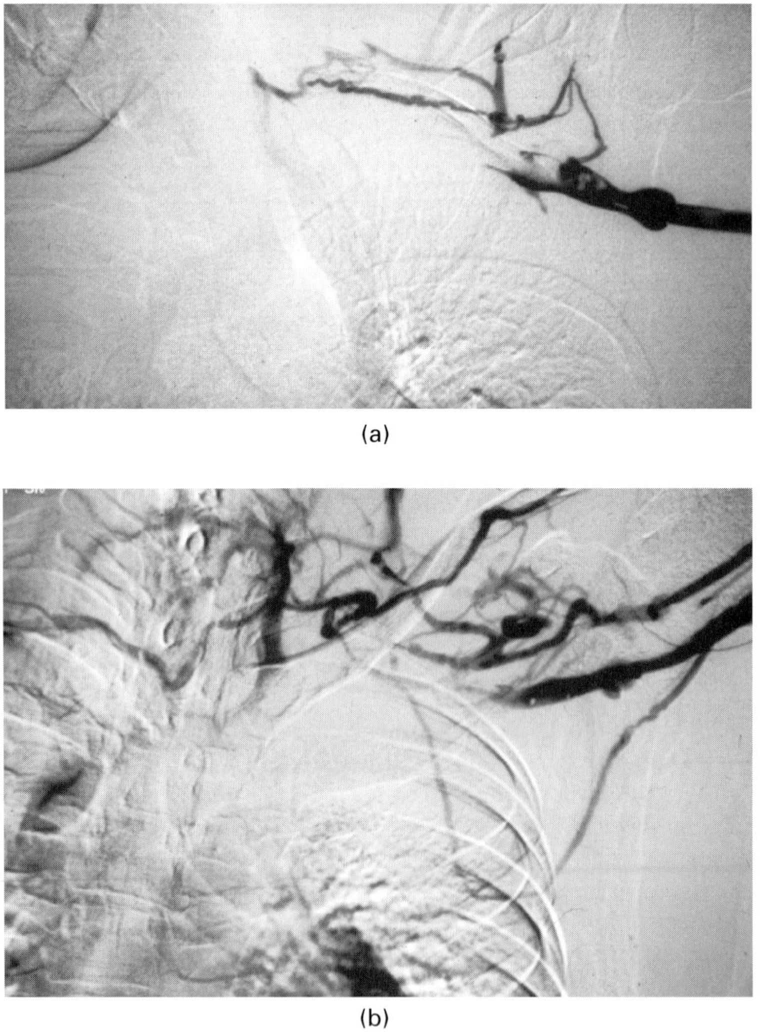

(a)

(b)

Fig. 1. Axillosubclavian vein thrombosis due to Paget–Schroetter syndrome. Loose thrombus is seen within the axillary vein (a). The extensive collateral veins which traverse the thoracic outlet travelling under the clavicle are shown with the arm in abduction in (b).

passes through this narrow tract leads to an hourglass deformity and eventually a rind of fibrous tissue that surrounds the vein like a sleeve.

Eventually a critical event such as vigorous exercise leads to intimal damage and *in situ* thrombosis. The thrombus originates at the site of the valve and propagates centrifugally to the first major collateral tributary, which often accompanies the cephalic vein confluence in the deltopectoral triangle (Fig. 1). In severe cases the brachial and axillary systems may be completely obliterated to the extent that phlegmasia alba dolens can occur. In addition, loose thrombus may lead to pulmonary embolism in approximately 10% of cases.

HISTORY AND EXAMINATION

The typical patient is a young male athlete or tradesman with well-developed upper limb musculature. Acute painless unilateral upper limb swelling occurs, usually without an obvious cause, but a careful history may elicit factors such as a change in exercise regime, a particularly strenuous workout, or carrying a heavy load or backpack. A previous episode may have resolved spontaneously, without medical attention being sought. Patients may report symptoms and signs of pulmonary embolism and on direct questioning there may be evidence of arterial compression, leading to effort-associated brachial ischaemia or irritation of the lower trunk of the brachial plexus with paraesthesia in the ulnar nerve distribution. The key point to the symptoms is their direct relationship to physical effort.

Physical signs include dilatation of the superficial veins over the shoulders (Fig. 2) oedema and swelling, and often a pink congestion of the skin caused by stasis. Arterial and neurological examination is usually normal at rest, but if the arms are elevated to 90 degrees from the trunk and externally rotated (the AER or Roos position), the venous collaterals stand out, the arterial pulse may diminish or disappear and a systolic infraclavicular bruit may be detected. Repeated slow finger clenching in this position may precipitate ulnar paraesthesia.

INVESTIGATIONS

Chest X-ray is usually normal – a cervical rib is rare. This is because the primary mechanism is costoclavicular and involves secondary musculotendinous compression. Blood tests including full blood count, coagulation studies and a thrombophilia screen should be taken before anticoagulation with heparin. Duplex scanning is useful in demonstrating arterial and venous occlusion during provocative manoeuvres (Fig. 3); compression of both the ipsi and contralateral neurovascular bundle points to an anatomical predisposition that led to the thrombosis.

Venography should be carried out via the basilic system as the cephalic vein often feeds supraclavicular veins that bypass the area of interest. Venous access may be difficult in the swollen limb; ultrasound guidance can in our experience be helpful. The extent of the thrombosis can be underestimated by simple venography via the

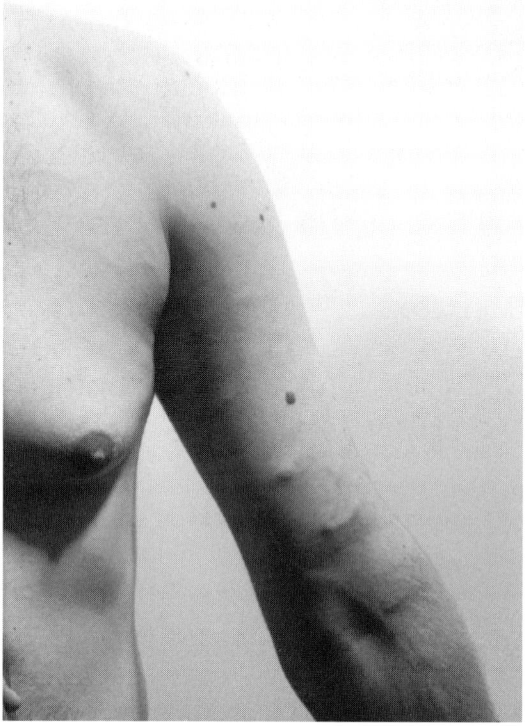

Fig. 2. The same patient as Fig. 1, demonstrating the extensive dilated collateral veins, erythema and swelling associated with Paget–Schroetter syndrome.

forearm veins. More accurate information can be obtained with a catheter placed in the axillary vein. The appearances are pathognomonic as shown in Fig. 3. Once the diagnosis has been established the opportunity should be taken to discuss the case whilst the catheter is in position. Pressure measurements can be made with the arms in the neutral and Roos position, and after repeated finger clenching, using a simple transducer borrowed from the operating theatre. The guidewire test is useful. A guidewire is advanced into the thrombus to determine whether it is soft (and therefore more likely to lyse) and to identify the residual stenosis or valve cusp. We would recommend lysis with tissue plasminogen activator at a dose of 1.0mg/h for fresh clot less than 3 or 4 weeks old.

TREATMENT STRATEGIES

Patients have the options of conservative management, anticoagulation, thrombolysis, angioplasty, stenting or surgical decompression or a combination of

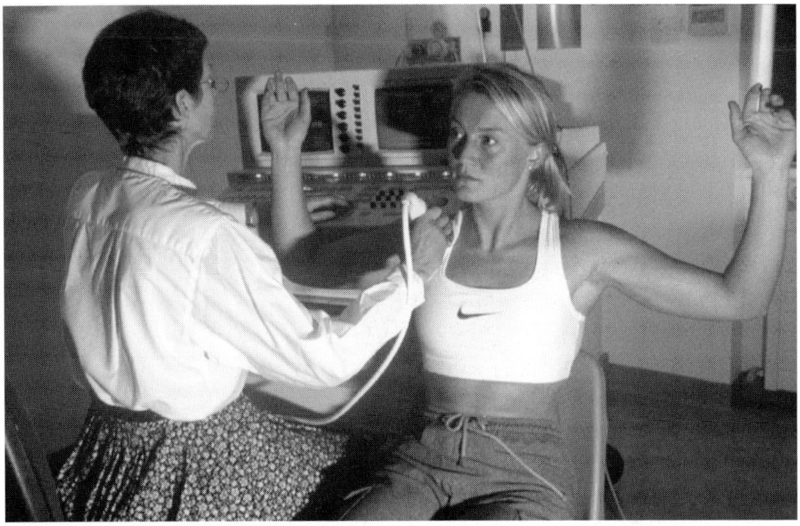

Fig. 3. Duplex scanning is a dynamic investigation and should be performed in various provocative manoeuvres to identify compression of the neurovascular bundle at the thoracic outlet.

modalities. Unfortunately the literature surrounding the subject is confusing and there are no randomized trials. The main problems are:

- trials include patients with different aetiologies such as catheter thromboses as well as PSS;
- few consider the age of the patient or the thrombus;
- none have used duplex scanning to provide evidence of costoclavicular compression to confirm the diagnosis;
- pressure measurements have not been performed to confirm decompression;
- follow-up is subjective, incomplete and usually biased (i.e. performed by the surgeon responsible for the operations).

Conservative management

This has no place in modern practice; conservative management with bed rest and elevation give poor overall results, with approximately 50% of patients developing long-term and disabling symptoms.[2] However, as this condition, has a significant incidence of pulmonary embolism, it should be treated by anticoagulation with heparin and warfarin at the very least, for a minimum period of 6 weeks, in view of the medicolegal implications.

Anticoagulation

Intravenous heparin followed by warfarin is safe, inexpensive and predictable.[3] Several authors have commended this approach but all the reported series are of mixed aetiology, and have included cases with pericatheter thrombosis or malignancy. Lindblad, from Malmo in Sweden reported 120 axillosubclavian thromboses over a 15-year period.[4] Only seven cases of effort thrombosis were found. The specific outcome for this group was not reported. In the primary thrombosis group 25% had mild (occasional pain or restriction of activity) or moderate symptoms (limiting certain activities) which presumably included sport, recreation or more strenuous exercise. In the discussion, the authors commented that they had treated selected patients referred to their department from other areas in southern Sweden. They were not included in the report and were younger patients with a higher frequency of post-thrombotic sequelae and neurovascular complications. This is precisely the group of patients who could benefit from a more aggressive approach, designed to reopen their principal veins and to prevent further episodes. From the University of Toronto, Ameli reported 10 years experience with excellent objective follow-up.[5] Of only seven patients with effort thrombosis six were seen – half had residual symptoms of intermittent oedema and discomfort, albeit mild.

Larger series of patients with pure PSS indicate the incidence of significant and persistent symptoms to be 25–40%.[6–8] The importance of particular symptoms to the individual depends on the questions asked and the length of follow-up, with symptoms generally decreasing slowly over time. Urschel[8], reported 21 of 67 PSS patients to be symptomatic after return to work. Hicken,[5] in a comprehensive review bordering on a meta-analysis, summarized the results of studies involving the treatment of 437 patients with primary thrombosis. Many were of poor quality with small numbers but 38% had persistent symptoms. Taking all of Hicken's patients, with both primary and secondary thromboses, symptoms were present in half of those treated conservatively, 32% of those treated with anticoagulation, 26% who were lysed, 19% who had surgery and lysis and 16% who had surgery alone.

The duration of treatment with warfarin is arbitrarily set at 3 months; unfortunately, radiographically-confirmed rethrombosis may happen in many cases due to the persistence of the underlying lesion.

Thrombolysis

In our experience this treatment is very effective to clear the primary thrombus as long as it is fresh. The history is often an unreliable guide as patients often have a chronically traumatized vein. We have found that the venographic appearance, elevated D-Dimer levels and most importantly the guidewire test to be helpful in identifying fresh clot. We would recommend tissue plasminogen activator (t-PA) as it is more fibrin-specific. Patients are carefully counselled with regard to the risk of this treatment. We quote a stroke risk of less than 1% because these patients are young and fit. In our experience of lysis, complications have only occurred in elderly female patients undergoing treatment for lower limb ischaemia. In this patient group, pericatheter haemorrhage is the only complication that has occurred. Haemorrhage has not been seen at other sites.

Unfortunately, lysis alone has been shown to be followed by unacceptably high rates of rethrombosis. Machleder reported a 34% incidence when lysis was used without surgical decompression and this is supported by several series.[9–10] We cannot see the logic of exposing a patient to the risk of this potentially dangerous treatment without dealing with the underlying lesion, namely the first rib.

Stenting and angioplasty

The failure of percutaneous balloon angioplastry (PTA) and stenting if they are used either before or instead of surgical decompression is easy to understand in relation to the anatomy and pathophysiology of PSS. The underlying lesion is like a retained valve cusp giving rise to a femorodistal vein graft stenosis – it is *not* atheroma, rather an intrinsic venous anomaly with superimposed partly organized thrombus, contained within a vein wall surrounded by fibrosis, repeatedly compressed by a bony nutcracker with a ligamentous fulcrum.

Primary stenting has now been shown to be associated with a high rate of failure due to fracture, distortion and rethrombosis.[11–13] Quite apart from the above-mentioned mechanisms, the distal vein is quite mobile, resulting in relative movement between the stent and subsequent trauma to the vein. In addition these are young patients with many years ahead of them and many doctors would be loathe to introduce an unnecessary prosthesis.

SURGICAL DECOMPRESSION

The literature contains several reliable series documenting the success of surgical decompression in obtaining lasting relief of the symptoms of PSS without the need for long-term anticoagulation.[14–16] Controversy still exists regarding the timing of surgery and the treatment of those with symptomatic chronic occlusion. Azakie *et al.* treated 33 patients with 34 subclavian thromboses, 21 of which were acute and of whom seven had unsuccessful PTA.[17] Eight were chronic occlusions of whom five had undergone nine operative attempts at decompression. Four had high-grade stenoses without thrombosis. Complete venolysis was achieved via 31 first rib resections and 33 scalenectomies. Twenty had complete resolution of their symptoms and full activity was restored. The other was lost to follow-up.

Many other groups have reported similar results and in particular Machleder, who treated 50 patients with an integrated programme of lysis followed by surgery, with an 80% success rate.[18] Four of his patients were symptomatic but still working and six were unable to work.

With regard to patients who present late, with chronic symptoms, is there a role for surgery? This concept has always been promoted by Roos and others and is supported by several small studies in the literature. Darke and Pittam, for example, treated five chronic and one acutely thrombosed patients who remained symptomatic after a period of anticoagulation, using transaxillary first rib resection.[19] Five of seven limbs so treated (one case was bilateral) remained asymptomatic, and crucially, symptoms were not related to the patency of the main subclavian channel. Venous hypertension is more important than the radiographic appearance.

In patients with disabling chronic venous hypertension, jugular vein swingdown operations or various forms of venous bypass graft have been advocated but patency rates are poor and the clinical results disappointing.[20] In addition these are disfiguring operations in a young patient.

Local experience

In the last five years we have performed 150 procedures for thoracic outlet problems and have treated 17 cases of PSS. There were ten males (the male to female ratio for our thoracic outlet series is 1 : 4) and the overall median age was 32 years (range 18–58 years). All were right-handed but ten of the thromboses were on the left. Two patients presented with serious pulmonary emboli, confirmed on ventilation/perfusion scanning. Thrombophilia screens including the factor V Leiden mutation were negative. All the acute episodes were associated with strenuous activity.

Two of the patients had undergone decompression surgery elsewhere. One had her second rib removed erroneously and had also had a surgical sympathectomy. She had neurological, arterial and venous symptoms with high venous pressure measurements. Redo transaxillary first rib resection was performed. Another female had undergone transaxillary first rib and cervical rib resection for PSS elsewhere, complicated by axillary haematoma. She had severe neurological (upper plexus) and venous symptoms. She had a supraclavicular scalenectomy.

Two more patients had long histories, typical duplex and venographic appearances and were prepared to tolerate their symptoms (one was a taxi driver with no sporting aspirations and another a dentist who was prepared to give up squash at the age of 46).

In all, 11 acutely thrombosed limbs were scheduled to receive lysis. Six were successful, three had no access, one was given systemic lysis by the physicians (no effect) and one had lysed spontaneously on heparin overnight.

The rationale behind surgery was explained after primary treatment with lysis and anticoagulation continued with heparin. Three declined (two accepted symptoms, one after failed attempts at venous access). Twelve transaxillary first rib resections were performed. Postoperative venograms showed stenoses treated by PTA in five cases. Two patients had residual occlusions with symptoms after a year. One of these (and the second chronic case) had an 8mm brachial artery/cephalic vein fistula formed. On disconnecting the fistula 6 months later the increased collateral veins rendered the patients asymptomatic and with normal invasive pressures.

Results of treatment protocol for Paget–Schroetter syndrome showed that the overall success rate was 85% for acute cases and 50% for the four chronic cases. Follow-up was at a minimum of 12 months by independent assessor (PN).

Complications

There were no deaths and no transfusions. One patient suffered from persistent intercostobrachial pain finally responding to nerve block. There were two minor haemothoraces that resolved and one that was treated by chest drainage with autotransfusion of the chest drain blood. Following this event, the heparin infusion was discontinued before surgery in the last patient. She rethrombosed the vein postoperatively and it was reopened at 10 days using clot aspiration and t-PA with successful PTA of her residual stenosis.

CONCLUSIONS

An aggressive policy directed towards the treatment of acute PSS by lysis and early decompression provides a safe, durable restoration of full upper limb function in selected patients.[21] PSS should be treated promptly by referral to a centre with combined vascular surgical and interventional radiological expertise so that the opportunity is not lost.

REFERENCES

1. Hughes ESR: Venous obstruction in the upper extremity (Paget-Schroetter's syndrome). *Int Abstr Surg* **88:** 89–127, 1999
2. Swinton NW, Edgett JW, Hall RJ: Primary subclavian-axillary vein thrombosis. *Circulation* **38:** 737–745, 1968
3. Ameli FM, Minas T, Weiis M, Provan JL: Consequences of 'conservative' conventional management of axillary vein thrombosis. *Can J Surg* **3:** 167–169, 1987
4. Lindblad B, Tengeborn L, Bergvqist D: Deep vein thrombosis of the axillary-subclavian veins; epidemiological data, effects of different type of treatment and late sequelae. *Eur J Vas Surg* **2:** 161–165, 1988
5. Hicken GJ, Ameli FM: Management of subclavian-axillary vein thrombosis: a review. *Can J Surg* **41:** 13–25, 1998
6. Adams JT, McEvoy RK, DeWeese JA: Primary deep venous thrombosis of the upper extremity. *Arch Surg* **91:** 29–42, 1965.
7. Lamdercasper J, Gall W, Fischer M *et al.* Thrombolytic therapy of axillary-subclavian venous thrombosis. *Arch Surg* **122:** 1072–1075, 1987
8. Urschel HC, Razzuk MA: Improved management of the Paget-Schroetter syndrome secondary to thoracic outlet syndrome. *Ann Thorac Surg* **52:** 1217–1224, 1991
9. Machleder HI: Evaluation of a new therapeutic stragegy for treatment of Paget–Schroetter syndrome: axillary-subclavian vein thrombosis. *J Vasc Surg* **17:** 305–317, 1993
10. Wilson JJ, Zahn CA, Newman H: Fibrinolytic therapy for idiopathic subclavian axillary vein thrombosis. *Am J Surg* **158:** 208–211, 1990
11. Meier GH, Pollak JS, Rosenblatt M *et al.*: Initial experience with venous stents in exertional axillary-subclavian vein thrombosis. *J Vasc Surg* **24:** 974–981, 1996
12. Rutherford RB: Primary subclavian-axillary vein thrombosis: the relative roles of thrombolysis, percutaneous angioplasty, stents and surgery. *Semin Vasc Surg* **11:** 91–95, 1998
13. Hall LD, Murray JD, Boswell GE: Venous stent placement as an adjunct to the stage, multimodal treatment of Paget–Schroetter syndrome. *J Vasc Intervent Radiol* **6:** 565–569, 1995
14. Adelman MA, Stone DH, Riles TS *et al.* A multidisciplinary approach to the treatment of Paget–Schroetter syndrome. *Ann Vasc Surg* **11:** 149–154, 1997
15. Urschel HS, Razzuk MA. Improved management of the Paget–Schroetter syndrome secondary to thoracic outlet compression. *Ann Thorac Surg* **52:** 1217–1221, 1991
16. Molina JE. Surgery for effort thrombosis of the subclavian vein. *J Thorac Cardiovasc Surg* 1992;**103:** 341–346, 1995
17. Azakie A, McElhinney DB, Thompson RW, *et al.*: Surgical management of subclavian-vein effort thrombosis as a result of thoracic outlet compression. *J Vasc Surg* **28:** 777–786, 1998
18. Machleder HI: Venous compression at the thoracic outlet. In: Machleder HI (Ed), *Vascular Disorders of the Upper Extremity* pp. 227–257. New York: Futura, 1998
19. Pittam, MR, Darke SG: The place of first rib resection in the management of axillary subclavian vein thrombosis. *Eur J Vasc Surg* **1:** 5–10, 1987

20. Sanders RJ, Cooper MA: Surgical management of subclavian vein obstruction including six cases of subclavian vein bypass. *Surgery* **118:** 856–863, 1995
21. Rutherford RB, Hurlbert SM: Primary subclavian-axillary vein thrombosis. Consensus and commentary. *Cardiovasc Surg* **4:** 420–423, 1996

Iliofemoral venous thrombolysis and stenting

MKW Johnston, S Babar, A Watkinson

In this chapter we aim to discuss the current thinking on therapeutic options for the treatment of lower limb venous thrombosis. It is our opinion that lower limb venous thrombosis requires different treatment options, depending on the site of involvement. Iliofemoral thrombosis demands an aggressive interventional approach with catheter-directed thrombolysis with or without stent placement, whilst thrombosis of the superficial femoral vein or popliteal vein can be treated with low molecular weight heparin (Fig. 1). It is important to clearly define the aims of modern therapies in the management of iliofemoral venous thrombosis particularly focusing on symptom control and the prevention of long-term complications.

INTRODUCTION

The conventional treatment for deep vein thrombosis has for many years been initial intravenous anticoagulation with heparin, followed by 3–6 months oral anticoagulation with warfarin. Anticoagulation prevents thrombus propagation but does not significantly contribute to lysis of the clot. The pain and oedema associated with thrombosis are gradually relieved by clot retraction and spontaneous thrombolysis. Advances in techniques in endovascular therapy have seen an increasing role in the management of lower limb thrombotic conditions particularly in the iliofemoral segment.

Predisposing factors to lower limb venous thrombosis include obesity, pregnancy and immobility. There is an increased incidence in patients with thrombophilias including factor V Leiden mutation, Protein-C and Protein-S deficiencies, antithrombin III deficiency, the presence of antiphospholipid antibodies and lupus anticoagulants. There are many anatomical considerations, both congenital and pathological that predispose to venous thrombosis, the most prevalent being May–Thurner syndrome (iliac vein compression syndrome) which may account for up to 25% of patients presenting with iliofemoral thrombosis.[5]

Deep venous thrombosis is amongst the most common postoperative complication. In patients over 40 years, those undergoing pelvic or abdominal surgery for malignant disease and those having lower limb orthopaedic surgery, the incidence of peripheral venous thrombosis is reported as between 40 and 80%, with propagation to involve the proximal veins in 10–30% and embolization to produce a symptomatic pulmonary embolus in 0.3–3%.[13]

The process of thrombus formation commences at the valves where there is increased turbulent flow, often combined with venous endothelial trauma, stasis, and in the postoperative period or thrombophilias, elevated platelet count (Virchow's

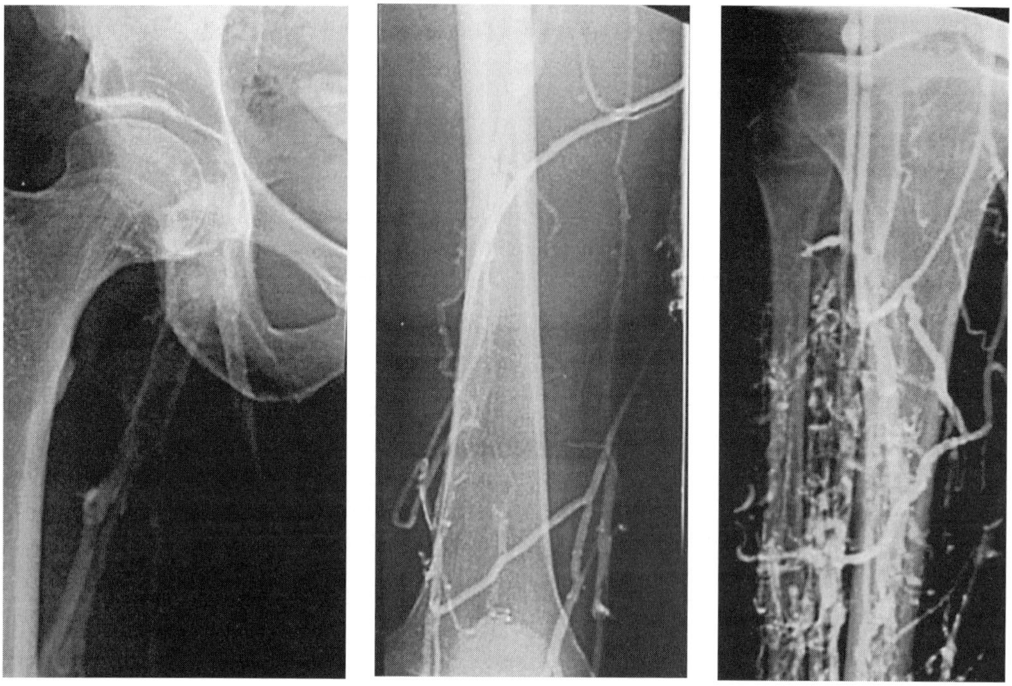

Fig. 1a,b,c. Extensive thrombus involving the right common femoral vein with involvement of the profunda, superficial femoral and popliteal veins. In our institution this would be treated by a conservative approach including intravenous or subcutaneous heparin.

triad). The thrombi grow by successive deposition of alternating bands of platelets and erythrocytes producing the characteristic lines of Zahn. The thrombus is held together with fibrin strands producing the coralline growth pattern. When a primary thrombus has accumulated sufficiently to impede flow, it is augmented by a secondary thrombus consisting of a looser meshwork of erythrocytes and fibrin that propagates rapidly to involve the proximal veins.

The earliest sign of peripheral venous thrombosis is often systemic pyrexia, associated with progressive pain and swelling of the affected limb and a rise in skin temperature. Prolonged thrombosis leads to a combination of obstruction and venous incompetence resulting in leg oedema and, in severe cases, venous eczema and ulceration.[1] In the long-term up to two-thirds of patients with iliofemoral deep venous thrombosis will develop post-phlebitic syndrome and lipodermatosclerosis, with 5% affected by venous ulcers.[2] Damage to venous valves leading to incompetence is the most important cause of post-phlebitic syndrome and when the thrombus fails to recanalize, persistent obstruction leads to venous hypertension.

In approximately 50% of patients in some studies, an anatomical predisposition to iliofemoral thrombolysis is found.[5] In about 25% of patients who undergo thrombolysis, May–Thurner syndrome is seen on the left side on the post-lysis venogram, caused by chronic trauma to the vein wall from pulsation of the overlying artery. A brief review of anatomy explains the higher incidence of iliofemoral deep venous thrombosis on the left. The common iliac vein is formed anterior to the sacroiliac joints by union of the internal and external iliac veins. The left common iliac vein is longer then the right and is crossed by the right common iliac artery, where it is liable to be compressed. A number of patients who develop iliofemoral venous thrombosis are seen to have venous drainage through the lumboazygous collateral system due to absent inferior vena cava (the renal veins drain via the same collateral system). Rarely the inferior vena cava is found to be obstructed, either from previous inferior vena cava thrombosis that has not recanalized, or from inferior vena cava stenosis. Pathological changes in anatomy predisposing to thrombosis can occur following trauma where there is direct damage to the venous endothelium or valves, or following pelvic radiotherapy where vessel fibrosis has been reported.

A rare type of acute iliofemoral thrombosis is phlegmasia caerulea dolens (PCD). This is often seen in association with malignancy (20–40%) or in the presence of a hypercoagulable thrombophilia. It may progress from the classic presentation of blue painful legs to venous gangrene. It is characterized by massive occlusion of the venous drainage of the limb including microvascular collaterals and consequently has a high morbidity, and a mortality reported as high as 20–40%.[6] There is consequent arterial insufficiency associated with PCD, the likely mechanism of which is arteriolar collapse secondary to a decrease in hydrostatic pressure from hypotension (to below 50mmHg), and increased tissue pressure from severe oedema as a result of venous outflow obstruction. PCD has a peak incidence in the fifth and sixth decades, is slightly more common in women and occurs more often on the left. Although amputation is the therapeutic option of choice in about 50% of cases, the role of thrombolysis is evolving and in our hands combined arterial and venous thrombolysis resulted in limb salvage in our first three cases.[10] Subsequent experience has achieved limb salvage with rapid symptomatic improvement in ten further cases.

Phlegmasia alba dolens occurs from relatively slow thrombosis of the iliofemoral veins resulting in painful white legs. It is seen most commonly in medical patients or following pregnancy. The swelling and pain may increase over 2–6 weeks where the pain is initially the result of ischaemia within the vein wall. Venous insufficiency from permanent disruption of the valve system is almost inevitable and thrombolysis has not been shown to have significant results in this subgroup.

In the diagnosis of iliofemoral venous thrombosis, venography is considered the gold standard and is also used in the post-procedure follow-up. Duplex ultrasound, however, is now used more extensively, both as a non-invasive and less time-consuming technique to make the initial diagnosis and as the method of choice for long-term follow-up.[1] Computed tomography (CT) of the pelvis is also performed and is useful in ruling out a pelvic mass as the cause of the thrombosis. The treatment options for iliofemoral thrombosis, therefore include:

1. conventional anticoagulation with heparin and 3–6 months warfarin;
2. systemic infusion of thrombolytic agent;
3. catheter-directed thrombolysis;
4. angioplasty, stent placement or both, with or without catheter-directed thrombolysis;

5. operative techniques: thrombectomy (with or without the formation of an arteriorvenous fistula) and venous bypass procedure.

In order to define the place of thrombolysis in the management of iliofemoral venous thrombosis it is first necessary to assess the aims of treatment, which must be weighed up against the potential risk of complications of the procedure. The benefits of early thrombolysis are in symptom control. The reasoning is that as the vessel is recanalized and venous outflow is restored, the pain is improved and the oedema settles far more rapidly then if lysis is left to the patient's own fibrinolytic system. Long-term, thrombolysis reduces the risk of venous insufficiency from vessel and valve damage and patients are therefore less likely to develop post-phlebitic syndrome and venous ulceration. When administered systemically, thrombolytic agents are superior to standard anticoagulative therapy in achieving early lysis of the thrombus.[8] With conventional anticoagulation, eventual recanalization depends solely on the effectiveness of the patient's own fibrinolytic system. Anticoagulation cannot resolve a massive iliofemoral thrombosis and is slow to relieve pain and lower extremity swelling. Only 6% of patients show complete lysis within 10 days of commencing heparin treatment, and propagation still occurs in 40%.[8] The advantages of thrombolysis, however, must be compared with the risks of haemorrhage (in all its forms) and of embolic disease.

THROMBOLYSIS

Thrombolysis can be achieved either mechanically or by chemical means. Patient selection for thrombolysis is of great importance. In a review of recent studies, 70% of patients selected for thrombolysis had iliofemoral thrombosis,[1] 20–25% had femoropopliteal thrombosis and the remainder had common iliac or inferior vena cava thrombus. Thrombolysis is most effective in the early stages of thrombosis, the best results being achieved with thrombus less than 30 days old, most reviews having a mean of 7–10 days.[3,4] (Iliofemoral thrombosis is classified as 'acute' if it presents less than 10 days after onset of symptoms.)

The thrombolytic agent of choice and perfusion time in the management of iliofemoral thrombosis varies greatly between different centres. There seems to be little difference in thrombolytic efficacy and complication rates between the different agents used, most centres opting for the agent with which they have most experience usually from earlier arterial thrombolytic work. Intravenous heparin is usually continued during the procedure of thrombolysis whichever thrombolytic agent is used. In the largest review from a national multicentre registry in the USA, urokinase was the thrombolytic agent of choice in 287 patients with a dose range of 0.5–44 million international units (iu) (mean of 7.8 million iu) and an infusion time of 2–147 hours (means 53.4 hours).[1] Alteplase (rt-PA) is also commonly used at an infusion rate of 3mg/h with total dose ranges from recent studies of between 45 and 174mg (mean 86mg) and a mean duration of treatment of 29.7 hours.[5] Streptokinase is not used as commonly as the other agents but has shown good thrombolytic efficacy at an infusion rate of 100000 units per hour, the average infusion time being 67.2 hours.[7]

There appears to be a slight preference in the literature for the use of urokinase and this is probably due to the proven efficacy of this agent in arterial thrombolysis and upper limb venous thrombosis. Urokinase has been shown to be marginally more effective at dissolving clots than streptokinase and is also more cost-effective (although more expensive) due to fewer haemorrhagic complications resulting in shorter hospitalization.[8]

Most studies use immediate post-thrombolytic venography to assess the extent of thrombus dissolution and classify it according to percentage lysis (Grade III: 100% lysis, Grade II: 50–99% lysis, Grade I: <50% lysis). A thrombus score can be used to calculate initial and post-treatment thrombus burden in the seven venous segments from popliteal vein to inferior vena cava. Follow-up patency is carried out with duplex ultrasound.

TECHNIQUE

The technique of catheter placement and type of catheter used is also subject to variation. There are several possible routes for local administration of a thrombolytic agent in the treatment of iliofemoral venous thrombosis.[8] Arterial infusion into the affected lower extremity and infusion into a foot vein have both been attempted but with poor results and are no longer favoured techniques of choice except in the management of PCD when a mixed arterial and venous infusion have been used with some success.[6] The transjugular approach has traditionally been the preferred access route.[8] However, increasingly operators are favouring the femoral, ipsilateral popliteal or posterior tibial approach. These approaches have shown an increased efficacy of clot lysis[1] and are more suitable for treating thrombus extending from the inferior vena cava into the superficial femoral vein, for which a transjugular approach is difficult due to the presence of valves or difficulty in passing a guidewire through chronic thrombus.

In the largest American review of thrombolysis techniques, the approach for catheter placement was selected by the physician performing the procedure and reflected personal experience, varying between transjugular, common femoral vein and popliteal vein approaches. As the study progressed, the popliteal venous approach became the access of choice.[1] Popliteal vein puncture is carried out under ultrasound guidance, preferably with an echogenic needle to prevent puncture of the adjacent popliteal artery, which would be a contraindication to administration of thrombolytic agent. The same principle is used in the transjugular approach to avoid carotid puncture. A new approach that is rapidly gaining support is advocated by some authors[4] involving a posterior tibial vein approach (again under ultrasound guidance). This allows the catheter to be pulled back and enables thrombolysis of the more distal tibial veins thus improving venous inflow. It also reduces the risk of damage to the venous valves which is commonly associated with retrograde catheter placement, and there is therefore a theoretical possibility of reducing the incidence of post-phlebitic syndrome.

Most authors recommend the use of a 5 F (or less commonly 4 F) sheath insertion through which subsequent wire and catheter exchanges are performed.

Infusions can be performed using a coaxial catheter and guidwire and/or a double lumen multiple side-hole system. A recent large Belgian study[5] introduced a 5 F straight catheter with ten side-holes using a contralateral femoral or ipsilateral popliteal approach. A common way to position the catheter is by using a 0.035 inch soft-tipped guidewire to cross the thrombosed vein. Once the guidewire has traversed the occlusion a 5 F catheter can be advanced into the thrombus. The use of both the multiside-hole catheter or coaxial system (5 F end-hole catheter with infusion wire) requires the placement of a 5 F side-arm sheath at the venous access site. With the coaxial technique the tip of the infusion wire is placed at the peripheral edge of the thrombus and the end-hole catheter positioned nearer the puncture site. This technique involves the use of two infusion pumps. With the multiside-hole catheter technique, the tip is placed at the distal aspect of the thrombus (Figs 2a, b, c).

The advantage of catheter-directed infusion of thrombolytic agents is the ability to deliver high concentrations directly into the thrombus while possibly minimizing the potential for a systemic fibrinolytic effect, if the agent is assumed to remain in a local distribution. Because thrombolytic agents activate plasminogen in the thrombus, delivery of the drug to that site enhances its efficacy, thus reducing the overall duration of treatment and complication rate. On review of recent studies, catheter-directed thrombolysis for iliofemoral venous thrombosis resulted in Grade III lysis (complete) in 31% of patients, Grade II lysis in 52% (50–99%), and Grade I lysis (<50%) in 17%. Grade III lysis was seen in 34% of acute and 19% of cases of chronic deep venous thrombosis.[8] After lysis, the venographic grade of thrombolysis was a major predictor of long-term patency with significant benefits in completely lysed limbs, irrespective of thrombus location.[3] However, of patients who achieve complete lysis, a significant number will develop abnormal plethysmography and post-phlebitic syndrome in 5 years. During thrombolysis, laboratory parameters are checked regularly. If fibrinogen levels are seen to fall below 150mg/dl the thrombolytic infusion rate is reduced, and if the level falls below 100mg/dl then thrombolysis is stopped and transfusions of FFP given[11] Thrombolysis is routinely stopped when there is no residual thrombus on venography, no further lysis after a predetermined infusion time, or significant complications.

COMPLICATIONS

The major complications of thrombolysis are haemorrhage or the theoretical risk of initiation of pulmonary embolus. Risk factors for haemorrhage are increasing age of

Fig. 2. (a) Inferior vena cava, left common iliac and external venous thrombosis. A temporary filter has been positioned in the lower inferior vena cava from a jugular vein approach. An infusion wire has been advanced into the left common iliac vein. (b) Venogram performed via the infusion catheter in the left common femoral vein. This demonstrates that the thrombus extends into the left common femoral vein but the distal veins are patent. (c) After 48 hours of directed thrombolysis through the infusion wire, there has been recanalization of the left common femoral and left external iliac vein with free flow through a patent inferior vena cava. No underlying abnormality was demonstrated and the temporary inferior vena cava filter was removed.

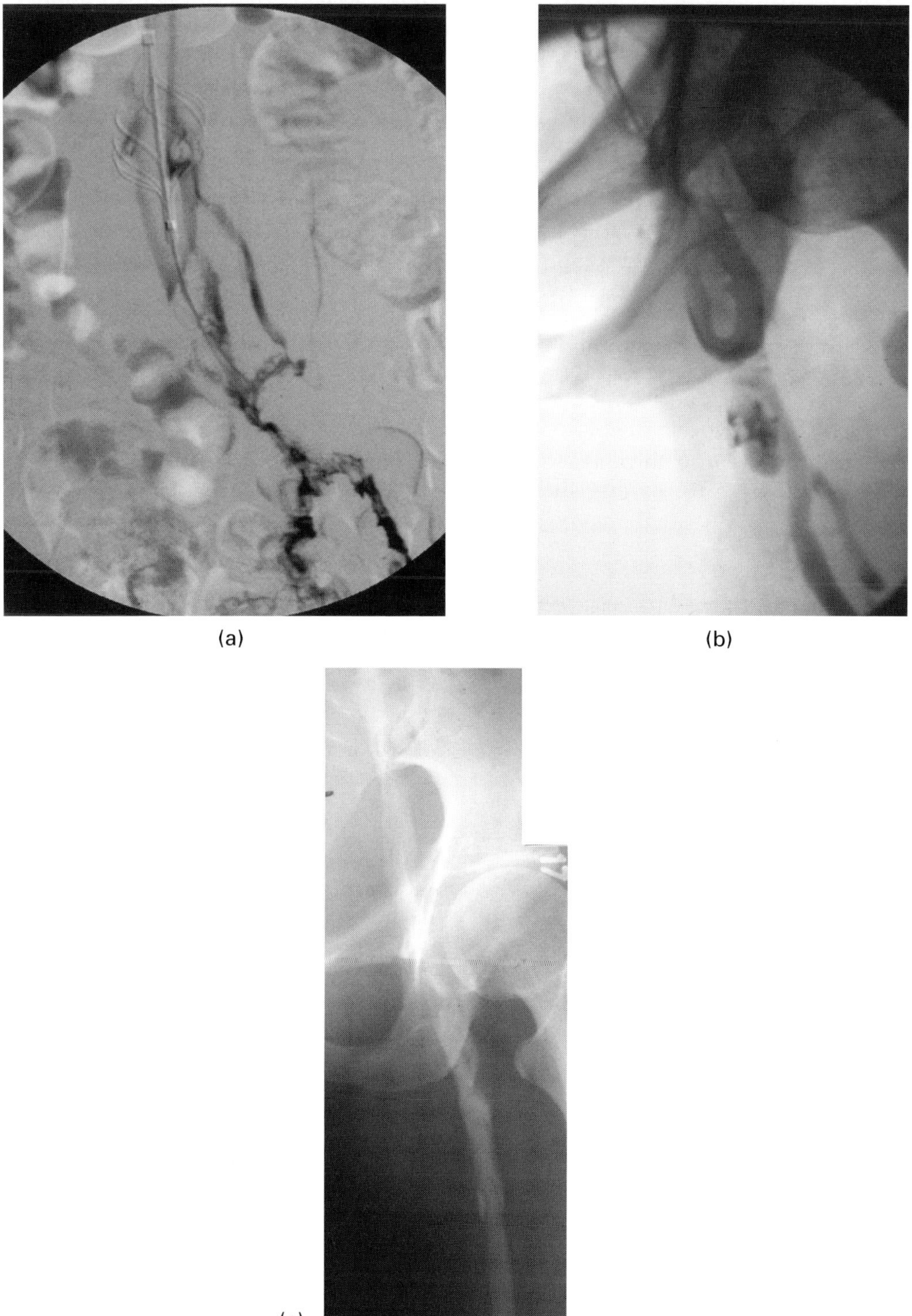

(a) (b)

(c)

Fig. 2.

the patient, increasing dose of thrombolytic infused, and increased duration of infusion. Symptomatic pulmonary embolism is seen in around 1% of patients undergoing thrombolysis.[1] Major haemorrhage occurs in 10%. This includes significant bleeding at the venous puncture site (40%) and retroperitoneal haematomas. Bleeding has been reported from the musculoskeletal, gastrointestinal and urogenital systems or more rarely but often more catastrophic, intracerebral haemorrhage or subdural haematoma. Epistaxis has also been reported during thrombolysis but is usually easily controlled. Puncture site bleeding is considered significant if it leads to a drop in haemoglobin of >2g/dl, or results in the patient requiring blood transfusion. The overall mortality for the largest American review was 0.4%. Interestingly, the incidence of pulmonary embolism during thrombolysis in many trials has been low irrespective of whether or not a temporary inferior vena cava filter was inserted before commencement of infusion.[1] This may indicate that there is a rather overcautious approach to the use of such filters and that with modern techniques the incidence of pulmonary embolism is not as high as previously quoted. Some authors advocate the placement of an inferior vena cava filter only in patients with large, mobile, free floating thrombi within the inferior vena cava, or in patients with compromised cardiac function.[5]

ANGIOPLASTY

Percutaneous transluminal angioplasty can be used as an adjuvant therapy with thrombolysis, and has been advocated as a primary treatment for lower limb venous thrombosis in chronic occlusion. It can be used at follow-up to macerate residual thrombus, and to dilate venous stenosis and occlusions with or without the subsequent insertion of a stent. A stenosis is thought worthy of dilatation if there is a trans-stenotic pressure drop of greater than 3mmHg.[3] Studies have shown that systemic thrombolysis is far from optimal in treating thrombolytic occlusions of the iliac vein in which patency is 20% or less. Up to 80% of totally occluded iliac clots are resistant to systemic thrombolysis and most patients will develop venous sequelae in follow-up.[7] In such situations a guidewire can be passed though the thrombus to the inferior vena cava and multiple balloon inflations carried out. Temporary inferior vena cava filters are commonly placed before angioplasty to reduce the risk of pulmonary embolism, however, research is still inconclusive as to whether this does actually reduce the incidence of symptomatic pulmonary emboli.[3] In recent studies[7] 7F, Prothia or Montrouge inferior vena cava filters have been advocated. However, removable filters are now available (Gunter Tulip filters, Cook UK) that may be used in this role. Once a good channel has been created by percutaneous balloon angioplasty (PTA), systemic thrombolysis is continued to remove residual thrombus; PTA is a valuable adjunct to systemic thrombolysis when it alone fails to completely lyse a thrombus where PTA can produce increased efficacy of the thrombolytic agent in occlusions greater than 80% of vessel diameter. In a study of 18 patients with complete iliac vein occlusion resistant to systemic thrombolysis of between 24 and 48 hours duration, angioplasty enabled complete recanalization in 39% and improved recanalization in 28% after thrombolysis was continued for a further 24–48 hours.[7] In all these studies, angioplasty was used in combination with systemic thrombolysis. The efficacy of angioplasty at improving lysis rates as an adjunct to catheter-directed thrombolysis may be less marked where the thrombolytic agent is infused directly into the thrombus. Angioplasty is also effective in dilating post-thrombotic venous stenoses where improved patency at follow-up is seen. This in turn leads to fewer severe trophic venous sequelae and has obvious health and socioeconomic benefits.[1,7] If angioplasty fails to adequately recanalize the vessel then stent placement is considered. We advocate catheter-directed thrombolysis as the initial treatment of choice for iliofemoral thrombosis. This is followed by PTA for an underlying stenosis. If there is a residual pressure gradient after PTA then we advocate stent placement.

STENTS

It has long been appreciated that the results of thrombolysis can be greatly improved with the use of adjuvant therapies, namely angioplasty and stent insertion for post-thrombolysis venous stenosis. After thrombolysis, underlying venous stenoses may become evident and require further management. Stent placement has been described for post-thrombotic stenoses and May–Thurner syndrome, as well as malignancy, previous surgery or radiotherapy, and trauma. A recent study has demonstrated a venous spur in 54% of patients presenting with left-sided iliofemoral thrombosis.[2] The use of catheter-directed thrombolysis with stent implantation has dramatically reduced the need for surgical thrombectomy and arteriovenous fistula construction.[9] A review of modern techniques shows that traditionally three types of metallic endovascular stent have been used in the management of lower limb venous thrombosis.[9] These include Wallstents, (Boston Scientific) single Palmaz stents (Johnson & Johnson) or Gianturco stents (Cook UK, Bloomington). Wallstents are stainless steel, self expanding, and are flexible. They are deployed with a removable sheath delivery system, with or without subsequent balloon dilatation, and are the commonest stents in the use of venous occlusive disease or stenosis.[9] The Palmaz stent is balloon expandable and ridged and can be preloaded onto a balloon. Gianturco Z stents are self-expanding and placed with a sheath and pusher. Gianturco single stents can be joined (by tying or welding) to produce double or triple stents. Recently, numerous balloon expandable stainless steel and self-expanding nitinol stents have been released onto the market.

Stents can be used as a primary treatment for venous thrombosis but this is usually in the presence of old thrombus not amenable to thrombolysis, or with a contraindication to the infusion of lytic agents. It is common practice to perform initial thrombolysis and assess whether there are any underlying anatomical abnormalities. Angioplasty is routinely attempted to dilate the stenosis and if this is not successful in treating the stenosis then stent placement is considered. All stents should be placed above the inguinal ligament if possible to avoid crushing during hip flexion. Stent placements are considered a success if there is less than 50% residual stenosis following insertion, and less than a 3mmHg pressure gradient across the stent. The formation of an arteriovenous fistula has been advocated,[9] if the peak velocity in the iliac region after thrombolysis and stent placement is less than 25cm/second.

COMPLICATIONS

Major complications following stent placement are seen in 6–8% of patients.[9] Peri- or post-procedural haemorrhage may be serious, particularly in the presence of anticoagulation. Sepsis has been reported in one patient with venous stasis ulcers who was not adequately covered with antibiotics during the procedure. Fractured stents have been noted on follow-up venography, though these small fractures (reported in both Gianturco and Wallstents) are often of no clinical consequence 1 year following stent insertion.[9] They should, of course, be subject to regular review to assess long-term patency. Slippage of stents is seen in about 3.5% of cases at 6-month follow-up[9] and occurs more commonly with the Gianturco single stents. In a review of recent literature, stents were used in approximately 20% of patients undergoing venous thrombolysis; 71% of these iliac stenoses were on the left reflecting the link between May–Thurner syndrome (iliac vein compression syndrome) and the incidence of left iliac vein stenoses. Failure to eliminate the underlying anatomical obstruction to normal flow may lead to recurrence of thrombosis on stopping oral anticoagulation.[5] Questions remain on the rethrombosis risk and potential risk of late arterial erosion. An extensive fibrotic reaction develops at the point of contact between vein and artery in iliac compression syndrome due to the overlying arterial pulsation. The presence of a stent in such an area may lead to late wall erosion and theoretically false aneurysm formation.

Stent placement in the femoropopliteal venous segments has been attempted but has produced very poor patency rates and is therefore not recommended. The primary and secondary 2-year patency rates for implanted left iliac vein stents are 73% and 82% respectively. Overall primary patency for all venous stents is 50% at 1 year , while secondary patency over the same period is 81%

COMPARISON OF RESULTS FOR THROMBOLYSIS AND STENTING

The technique of thrombolysis, combined with the adjuvant therapies of PTA and stent placement, has led to a marked improvement in speed of resolution of symptoms (namely pain and oedema) in the acute stages of iliofemoral venous thrombosis.[1,3] Whether there is a reduction in the incidence of post-phlebitic syndrome is still to be proven. As expected, the best results for thrombolysis with >50% lysis (Grade II and III), occur in patients with acute onset thrombosis and no history of previous deep venous thrombosis. In some of the larger trials there appears to be little difference in outcome for thrombolysis comparing iliofemoral with femoropopliteal thrombosis, although 70% of cases are of the former. Results for systemic thrombolysis are universally poor, conferring only a small increase in clot lysis from patients treated with conventional anticoagulation and with more serious haemorrhagic complications. In the American reviews, primary patency for catheter-directed thrombolysis for all venous segments was 65% at 6 months and 60% at 1 year. Patency at 1 year was more likely to be maintained in patients with iliofemoral deep venous thrombosis. At 1 year, 79% of limbs with initial Grade III thrombolysis (complete) were still patent compared with only 32% of patients with initial Grade I lysis (>50%).[1]

Further improved patency, was seen in patients treated with adjuvant angioplasty and stent placement in the iliac vein (74% patent at 1 year, compared with 53% of patients without stent placement) the exception to this is in patients who received femoropopliteal stents in whom 70–80% had occluded at 1–3 months.

Another advantage of catheter-directed thrombolysis is that it demonstrates anatomical abnormalities that may predispose to thrombosis. In the case of May–Thurner syndrome, this allows stent placement to allow adequate expansion of the common iliac vein. If this anatomical element is taken into account, in addition to the discovery of haematological anomalies, then the incidence of true 'idiopathic' thrombosis is far less than previously thought (possible around 8%).[5]

Phlegmasia caerulea dolens is a rare cause of venous thrombosis and no single technique has produced convincing results. The current management is usually a combination of elevation, rehydration and anticoagulation, thrombolysis (both intravenous and intra-arterial administration have been simultaneously tried with good results in our institution),[10] thrombectomy and amputation. Thrombolysis has produced some promising results but due to the rarity of the condition, further evaluation is required (Fig. 3).

Technical success with stent placement is seen in 90% of patients (resulting in <50% stenosis and <3mmHg pressure gradient). Technical failure is more likely in patients in whom venous occlusions are greater than 5 years old, usually where the occlusion cannot be crossed with a guidewire. There does not appear to be a statistically significant difference in patency rates for stents inserted for stenosis versus thrombotic occlusions, or for left- versus right-sided occlusions.

In conclusion, the benefits of thrombolysis must be carefully weighed up with the risks of potential complications (0.4% mortality in the largest American series of 287 patients). Thrombolysis provides the opportunity for prompt restoration of venous patency thus helping to prevent the long term venous sequelae of deep venous thrombosis. Whether this helps to preserve valve function and thus reduce the incidence of post-thrombotic syndrome is unknown. With catheter-directed thrombolysis, complete lysis is seen in about 70% of patients,[1] with concomitant resolution of symptoms. By focusing the delivery of higher concentrations of the drug with the catheter-directed technique, lysis rates can be improved, the duration of treatment can be reduced and complications associated with the exposure of the patient to systemic thrombolytic therapy may be reduced. The progress of thrombolysis can be monitored with directed imaging techniques and lesions that potentially contribute to the thrombosis can be identified and treated with adjuvant therapies such as endovascular stenting or angioplasty.

Thrombolysis does not seem to promote significant pulmonary embolus and may even have a slight preventative effect. The use of inferior vena cava filters for thrombolysis has not shown any reduction in the prevalence of pulmonary embolisms but they are routinely inserted before stenting or angioplasty where the

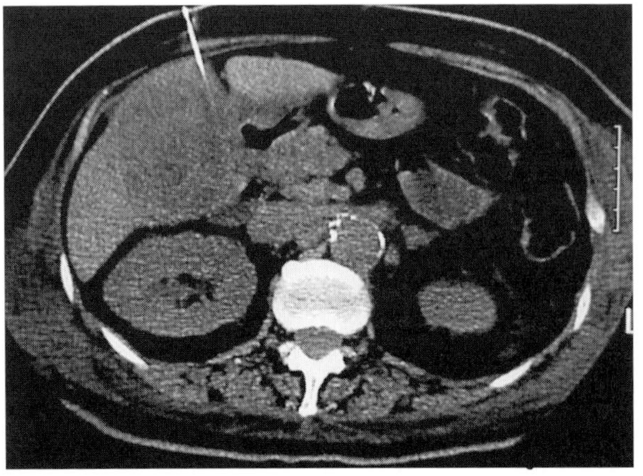

(a)

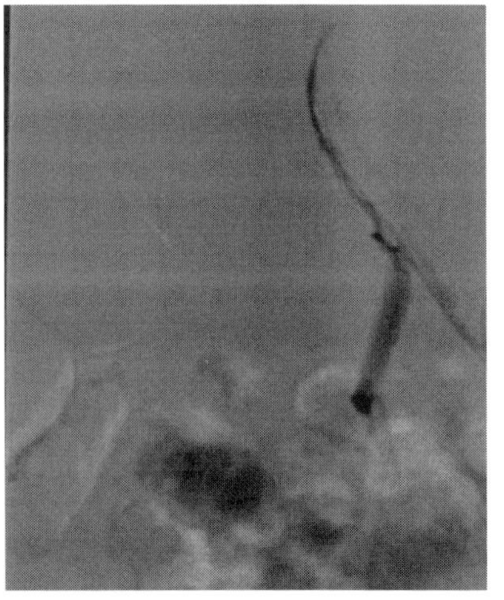

(b)

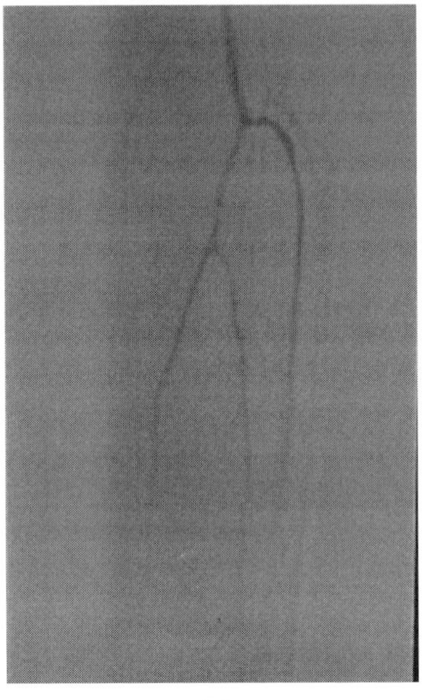

(c)

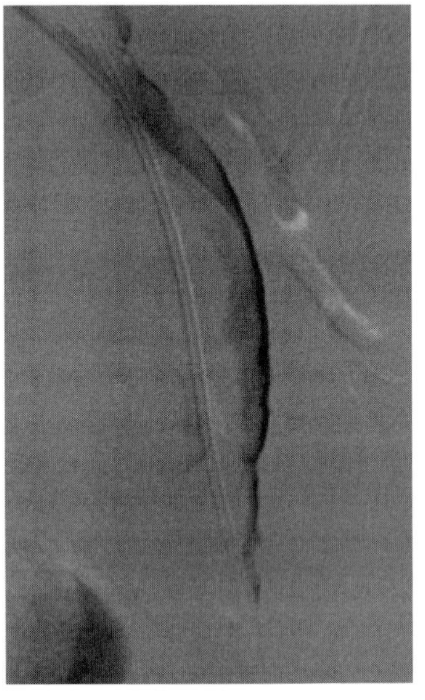

(d)

Fig. 3. (a) 68-year-old female with biopsy proven hepatocellular carcinoma. (b) An infusion wire has been passed via a jugular vein approach, and a temporary filter positioned in the distal inferior vena cava. The tip of the wire is in the left common iliac vein which is filled with thrombus extending into the inferior vena cava proximally, and the left external iliac vein and leg veins distally. (c) Angiogram of the calf vessels. There is markedly delayed passage of contrast; 35 seconds after injection into the left common femoral artery, static flow is noted in the midcalf vessels with no flow distally. This implies thrombosis of the capillary bed. (d) After 24 hours combined arterial and venous thrombolysis via the catheter and infusion wire respectively, there has been little improvement although some flow is seen in the left ascending lumbar vein. The arteriographic catheter has been positioned via a crossover technique with the tip in the region of the left common femoral artery.

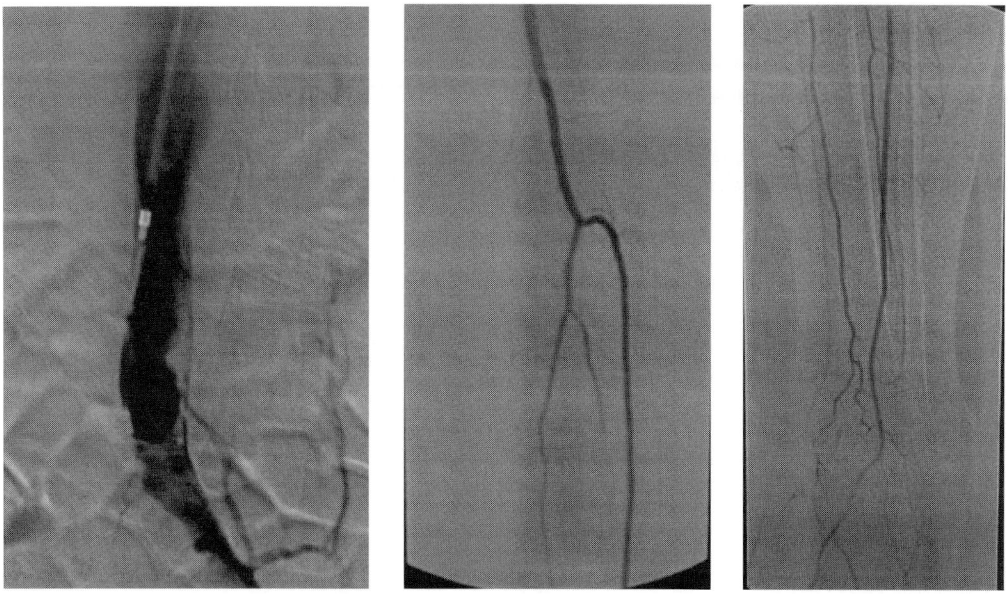

e(i) e(ii) e(iii)

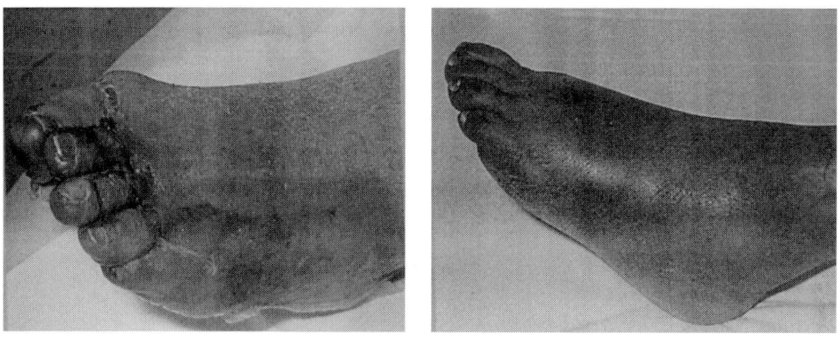

(f) (g)

Fig. 3. (continued) (e) (images i,ii and iii) After 120 hours of combined arterial and venous thrombolysis there has been some clearing of the left common iliac vein and distal inferior vena cava. The arteriographic images now demonstrate rapid flow through the calf vessels into the foot with flow into the anterior plantar arch after 7 seconds. At this point there was marked symptomatic improvement and the procedure was terminated. It should be emphasized that limb salvage was the aim and not radiological resolution of the thrombus. (f) Above patient presenting with phlegmasia caerulea dolens left foot. (g) Post-thrombolysis there is marked improvement in the patient's symptoms and the appearances of the left foot.

risk of embolization is greater. The advent of new temporary filters has led to an increase in usage due to a greater ease of deployment and fewer complications. Catheter-directed thrombolysis has two drawbacks. First, it is a lengthy, labour-intensive procedure, and second it is associated with a not insignificant morbidity or mortality, mostly related to the increased risk of haemorrhage. Puncture site bleeding may start during lysis and its full extent may only be appreciated the day following termination of the procedure.

FURTHER RESEARCH

Further research is needed to determine patency rates of angioplastied and stented venous segments at long-term follow-up, and whether treated limbs have a lower frequency of recurrent deep venous thrombosis. Studies must also look at the incidence of post-phlebitic syndrome in patients undergoing thrombolysis compared with anticoagulation alone, with particular attention paid to post-thrombolysis valve function. Techniques must also be assessed to reduce bleeding complications. Whether a lower infusion rate of thrombolytic would reduce bleeding from the access site requires further comparative trials.

ACKNOWLEDGEMENTS

We would like to thank Mr G Hamilton FRCS and Mr D Baker FRCS, Consultant Vascular Surgeons, Royal Free Hospital, London, for their support and permission to show their illustrated cases.

REFERENCES

1. Mewissen MW, Seabrook GR, Meissner MH *et al.*: Catheter thrombolysis for lower extremity DVT: report of a national multicentre registry. *Radiology* **211:** 39–49, 1999
2. Mickley V, Schwagienek R, Rilinger N *et al.*: Left iliac venous thrombosis caused by venous spur: treatment with thrombectomy and stent implantation. *J Vasc Surg* **28:** 492–497, 1998
3. Bjarnason H, Kruse JR, Asinger DA *et al.*: Iliofemoral DVT: Safety and efficacy outcome during five years of catheter directed thrombolytic therapy. *J Vasc Intervent Radiol* **8:** 405–418, 1997
4. Armon MP, Whitaker SC, Tennant WG: Catheter directed thrombolysis of iliofemoral DVT: A new approach via the posterior tibial vein. *Eur J Vasc Endovasc Surg* **13:** 413–416, 1997
5. Verhaeghe R, Stockx L, Lacroix H *et al.*: Catheter directed lysis of iliofemoral vein thrombosis with use of rt-PA. *Eur Radiol* **7:** 996–1001, 1997
6. Perkins JMT, Magee TR, Gallard RB: Phlegmasia caerulea dolens and venous gangrene. *Br J Surg* **83:** 19–23, 1996
7. Marache P, Asseman P, Jabinet JL, Thery C: Percutaneous transluminal angioplasty in occlusive iliac vein thrombosis resistant to thrombolysis. *Am Heart J* **125:** 362–367, 1993

8. Semba CP, Dake MD: Iliofemoral DVT: Aggressive therapy with catheter-directed thrombolysis. *Radiology* **191:** 487–494, 1994
9. Nazarian GK, Bjarnason H, Dietz C, Hunter D: Iliofemoral venous stenosis : effectiveness of treatment with metallic endovascular stents. *Radiology* **200:** 193–199, 1996
10. Wlodarczyk ZK, Gibson M, Dick R , Hamilton G: Low dose intra-arterial thrombolysis in the treatment of Phlegmasia caerulea dolens. *Br J Surg* **81:** 370–372, 1994
11. Grossman C, McPherson S: Safety and efficacy of catheter directed thrombolysis for iliofemoral venous thrombosis. *Am J Radiol* **172:** 1999

Surgical and radiological correction of arteriovenous fistulae

Matthew Waltham, Allan Irvine, Kevin G Burnand

INTRODUCTION

An arteriovenous fistula is an abnormal communication between an artery and a vein. These can be congenital or are acquired, usually following trauma. The communications are often multiple, and may occur at any site from the large vessels to the capillaries. The length of the abnormal channels may vary from millimetres to centimetres, and there may be abnormal vascular structures interposed. In this chapter the aetiology and pathology of peripheral arteriovenous fistulae are reviewed and the current method of treatment discussed.

HISTORICAL REVIEW

The first recorded clinical case of an arteriovenous fistula was by Guido, personal physician to King Francis I of France in the late sixteenth century.[1] Guido referred the young man with grossly dilated scalp veins to Fallopius in Padua, who declined to operate. In 1676 Sennertus of Wittenburg described an aneurysm that must have been an arteriovenous fistula as it had 'a thrill like boiling water' as well as a bruit.[2] It was not until William Hunter's description of a traumatic arteriovenous fistula in 1757 that the association was made between the physical signs and an abnormal communication between an artery and a vein.[3]

The first good description of a congenital arteriovenous fistula was by John Bell in 1815,[4] with subsequent accounts by Bushe (1827),[5] Adams (1858),[6] Ghérini (1867)[7] and Hewitt (1867).[8] The postmortem anatomy was demonstrated by Warren in 1858[9] and Krause in 1862 who injected the vessels of an amputated arm to show the abnormal connections.[10]

In 1875 Nicoladoni described the slowing of the pulse that followed occlusion of the subclavian artery proximal to a congenital arteriovenous fistula of the arm.[11] He incorrectly believed this to be caused by distension of the subclavian artery compressing the recurrent laryngeal branch of the vagus nerve. Branham, after whom the test is now named, later made a similar observation.[12]

Collected cases of arteriovenous fistulae were described in the early twentieth century. These included works by Halsted and Callender,[13] Osler,[14] Rösler[15] and Lewis.[16] Reid[17] and Stewart[18] described the effect of an arteriovenous fistula on heart size, but most of our understanding of their pathophysiology and natural history is based on the work of Holman.[19]

AETIOLOGY

Arteriovenous fistulae can be classified on the basis of their aetiology into congenital and acquired. Congenital fistulae usually pass undetected in the first year of life with many becoming clinically apparent between the ages of 10 and 40 years.[20–22] They are a consequence of abnormal vasculogenesis but there is little understanding of the underlying mechanism.

The majority of clinically significant acquired arteriovenous fistulas involving the extremities are single and the result of penetrating trauma to blood vessels, for example gunshot wounds or stabbing. Elsewhere in the body other causes have to be considered, for example aortocaval fistula following aortic aneurysm rupture, arteriovenous communication due to erosion secondary to infection, tumour or caval filter placement and iatrogenic fistulae following lumbar disc surgery or femoral artery catheterization.[23] Iatrogenic fistulae from arterial and inadvertent venous cannulation are becoming more common with the increase in interventional endovascular procedures.

Arteriovenous fistulae commonly enlarge over time, which may be the result of dilatation of the communicating channels, or of continuing angiogenesis with the formation of new fistulae.

CLASSIFICATION AND PATHOLOGY

There is a wide variety of combinations of position, size and configuration of arteriovenous fistulae. In acquired fistulae there is usually only one abnormal communication, whereas congenital lesions are usually more complex. Congenital arteriovenous fistulae may be clinically classified into truncal, diffuse or localized.[24]

Truncal

This type of fistula is usually localized and arises from major arterial branches, is haemodynamically active and progressive. The connecting fistulae can be demonstrated on arteriography and are easily defined at operation. They commonly occur on the upper limb and in the head and neck. The interconnections may be very short, with the artery and vein almost adherent. There may sometimes be an interposed bulky malformation (a cirsoid aneurysm) although the main bulk of the malformation usually consists of the dilated inflow and outflow vessels.

Diffuse

These extensive malformations usually arise in the limbs, most commonly the lower limb, and the connections are very small and numerous. Diffuse fistulae tend to be less haemodynamically significant than truncal fistulae, although the limb is usually enlarged and warm to the touch. Machinery murmurs are often heard all over the limb but the connections themselves may not be visible on arteriography or at surgery. When a diffuse malformation is associated with limb hypertrophy and superficial capillary dilation it is known as Parkes–Weber syndrome.

Localized

These mostly consist of a mass of vascular channels without a high flow from the artery. The majority produce few haemodynamic effects because the malformation offers a high resistance to flow. They most commonly occur in the skin but can be found in any organ.

Pathology

An understanding of the haemodynamic effect and natural history of arteriovenous fistulae is necessary to interpret the clinical findings and plan treatment. Blood is shunted from the high pressure arterial circulation into the low pressure venous system. This establishes two circuits: a low resistance circuit through the fistula and a high pressure system through the peripheral capillary bed. As a result of the low resistance through the fistula there is an increase in flow through the feeding artery causing it to become dilated, thickened and tortuous. This often develops a considerable distance upstream of the fistula. Reversed flow in vessels distal to the fistula may produce a parasitic circulation fed by dilated collaterals. This lowers the pressure in the distal vessels and causes ischaemia of the tissues in this territory.

The excess blood flowing into the venous circulation causes the veins to dilate and the flow velocity to increase. The vein wall becomes thickened as a consequence of muscle hypertrophy and increased quantities of connective tissue, known as 'arterialization'. The increase in venous pressure may further compromise blood flow to the distal tissues, and may lead to ulceration and gangrene. Ulcers associated with arteriovenous fistulae may be caused either as a direct result of arterial ischaemia consequent upon a steal from the fistula or from the associated venous hypertension, capillary fibrin cuffing and tissue deprivation of nutrients which causes venous ulceration.[25,26] Turbulence of the arterial blood flowing into the venous side can be palpated as a thrill and heard as a bruit.

CLINICAL PRESENTATION AND INVESTIGATIONS

Acquired arteriovenous fistulae can develop after any major vascular injury. Congenital fistulae are more frequent in the lower limb and in females.[27–30] The clinical manifestations of arteriovenous fistulae depend on their size, length, number and position within the circulation. Large proximal fistulae are more commonly seen in the head, neck, and upper limb and may result in high output cardiac failure, without any ischaemic effect on the distal tissue. Multiple small distal fistulae are more often seen in the lower limb where they can cause gangrene without having a significant effect on cardiac output.

Patients may present with local symptoms and signs from tissue ischaemia or necrosis. They may also display signs of venous hypertension or frank ulceration.

Pain may be the predominant symptom. Carotid-jugular fistulae may cause an annoying bruit heard by the patient. Fistulae can be associated with limb hypertrophy as a consequence of both skeletal and soft tissue overgrowth, and sometimes it may only be the presence of a cutaneous vascular naevus that suggests an underlying malformation.

The reduced peripheral resistance and the associated increase in flow through the fistula must be met by an increase in cardiac output. On examination there may be a tachycardia, cardiac enlargement, and if the fistula is large ultimately it may lead to high output cardiac failure. Signs of venous insufficiency and peripheral ischaemia are common if the fistula is proximal. The temperature of the limb may be raised and varicose veins may be present. Branham's test of slowing of the heart rate when the fistula is occluded may be present. On auscultation a systolic or continuous bruit (machinery murmur) may be heard.

Colour Doppler imaging is a useful preliminary investigation. Accurate measurements of flow, volumes and resistive indices can be helpful in the initial evaluation and for follow-up purposes.[30] Arteriography, however, remains the most important investigation to delineate the vascular anatomy of the malformation and determine whether treatment by embolization or surgery is feasible. Plain radiographs may suggest bone involvement but magnetic resonance (MR) imaging has become the primary imaging tool to evaluate vascular malformations. MR has replaced computed tomography as it can delineate the relationship of the malformation to muscle, nerve, bone and adjacent vessels, and hence show whether complete excision is possible. MR can distinguish between high and low flow malformations, with high flow lesions demonstrating signal void on most sequences. MR can also be used to access the efficacy of treatment.[31,32] Echocardiography may be used to measure cardiac output both to assess the indication for intervention and also to gauge effectiveness of any treatment.

When these investigations have been undertaken, the decision as to whether therapy is warranted can be taken. Any radiological intervention should be carefully planned in conjunction with the surgical specialists with an interest in this field. As it has been estimated that only 20% of patients can be cured by surgery alone, the opportunity for combined surgical and radiological intervention is large.[33]

TREATMENT – PRINCIPLES

Arteriovenous fistulae are often complex and their treatment is difficult and prone to failure. Ligation of the feeding vessels is ineffective, as this does not remove the fistula which will continue to steal blood worsening distal ischaemia. Ligating both proximal and distal vessels ('Hunterian ligation') also commonly fails to help as there are usually alternative feeding vessels which open up and more collaterals form. The fistula must therefore be treated either by excision or occluding all the intercalating vessels by embolization, and a combination of embolization and excision is often the best option. Before this can be performed the anatomy must be clearly defined.

Additional procedures such as equalization of leg length, preferably by epiphysiodesis while the patient is still growing, may also be necessary.

TREATMENT – CONSERVATIVE

When the patient complains of limb heaviness, discomfort after prolonged standing and lipodermatosclerosis, the prescription of graduated compression stockings often brings relief. This may be sufficient to keep the patient symptomless without treating the underlying fistula. Ulceration should be healed by compression bandaging or skin grafting where necessary.

Mild symptoms may need no treatment other than observation. Iatrogenic fistulae following cannulation frequently close spontaneously[34] whereas non-iatrogenic penetrating vascular trauma often has an adverse natural history.[35] Local compression with the probe of a duplex scanner can be shown to occlude flow through many local fistulae and this will often result in thrombotic occlusion providing the patient is not taking anticoagulation medication.

There is no evidence for any benefit of radiotherapy, cryotherapy or sclerotherapy in treating superficial arteriovenous fistulae or associated varices.

TREATMENT – RADIOLOGICAL

Embolization can be undertaken as a single definitive procedure or as a repeated procedure in more complex abnormalities. The majority of vascular malformations are approached by a percutaneous arterial catheter method, but direct injection into the abnormality is sometimes performed.

It is essential that modern digital subtraction angiography, a full range of catheters, microcatheters and guidewires are available. With use of some intravascular occlusive agents, such as Ethanol, pain control will be necessary and in certain circumstances, for example children or large complex lesions, general anaesthesia will be required.

To achieve successful embolization requires a careful choice of embolic material that will result in occlusion of the malformation while preserving the distal vascular bed. This is particularly important if immediate debulking surgery is not contemplated. Ischaemia is more likely if there has been previous surgery, embolization, or radiation therapy or there is coexisting atheromatous disease.

There is a wide range of different embolic agents and devices available, and the radiologist performing the procedure should understand their physical, chemical and biological characteristics. The embolic agent is selected on the basis of whether temporary or permanent occlusion is desirable and whether proximal or peripheral occlusion is the aim. Embolic material can be classified as shown in Table 1.

The agent selected must be appropriate and of a suitable size to occlude vessels without lodging too proximally or passing through the lesion entirely where it may enter another vascular bed, for example the pulmonary circulation. The general principle of embolization, regardless of which material is used, is to occlude the central portion or nidus of the malformation. Once this has been achieved, then feeding vessels can be occluded. In general, proximal occlusion is safer because the collateral circulation is preserved. However, as the nidus of the malformation is not

Table 1. Classification of embolic material

Absorbable materials	
(a)	Autologous blood clot
(b)	Gelfoam
Non-absorbable materials	
(a)	Particulate agents
	Polyvinyl alcohol sponge (PVA)
	Ferromagnetic microspheres
(b)	Fluid, glue and sclerosing agents
	Ethanol
	Hypertonic glucose
	Isobutyl 2 – cyanoacrylate
	Ethibloc
	Boiling contrast media
	Lipiodol
(c)	Non-particulate agents
	Metallic coils
	Detachable balloons

obliterated by this approach persistence of the fistula is inevitable and subsequent embolization becomes much more difficult. Direct injection may be necessary for subsequent treatment if there is no feeding vessel access left.

In part the choice of embolic material will depend on the vulnerability of the target site and the type of malformation. A functional division is as follows:

Type I: Fast flow large vessel arteriovenous malformation
Type II: Fast flow small vessel arteriovenous malformation
Type III: Slow flow venous arteriovenous malformation

In the fast flow large vessel fistulae (Type I) emboli may escape into the lungs. Early large draining veins are visible on angiography. These fistulae are not suitable for particle or liquid embolic agents.

Fast flow small vessel fistulae (Type II) have later filling veins and are ideal for particulate or liquid embolic agents.

In slow flow venous fistulae (Type III) embolization via the arterial route is not possible as the arterial and venous beds are normal. Arteriography is normal in these cases. A retrograde venous approach or direct injection of the arteriovenous malformation may be contemplated.

Poor choice of material or inaccurate assessment of collateral flow can result in ischaemia and infarction. The small particle size Gelfoam powder has resulted in lower limb paralysis in some patients.[36] Poor deployment of coils or overenthusiastic injection of particles and liquid agents with resultant retrograde flow can cause distal embolization. Material can pass up the internal carotid artery following external carotid embolization with disastrous consequences. Other reported areas of inadvertent embolization and subsequent infarction include the bladder, paraspinal muscles and spinal cord.[37–39]

Particulate materials are not suitable for large arteriovenous communications as these will pass through and enter the pulmonary circulation, causing an iatrogenic pulmonary embolism. Particles are therefore suited to fistulae terminating in a small capillary network.

Liquid and sclerosing agents are favoured by some,[40] but these can cause adherence of embolic glue material to the delivery catheter and ischaemic nerve paralysis. Skin necrosis can also develop after Ethanol use. For technical reasons, Ethanol is combined with Lipiodol as an embolic agent. Ethanol toxicity can occur at doses of over 1.0ml/kg body weight, and overdose can result in fatal cardiopulmonary collapse. If liquid agents are employed, external pneumatic blood pressure cuffs and intravascular occlusion balloons may be necessary to provide flow arrest during the embolization.

During the embolization procedure it is not uncommon for the flow dynamics to change as a consequence of arterial occlusion. Occlusion of one feeding vessel may result in reversal of flow in another feeding vessel. If the operator does not appreciate this injected embolic material may then pass away from the fistula and into a vulnerable vascular bed. Repeated angiographic checks during the procedure are necessary to prevent this.

Metallic coils produce permanent occlusion in the deployed vessel. When using coils, it is important not to occlude the vessel too proximally. If this occurs, then collateral feeding vessels will continue to supply the malformation. These vessels may not be accessible percutaneously, resulting in a failure to occlude the central fistula and failure to obliterate the malformation.

An extensive review analysed 137 embolization procedures in patients with systemic arteriovenous malformations. In a number of cases, feeding vessels had been ligated and surgical reconstruction by reanastomosis or venous interposition was necessary before selective catheterization. In twelve of these cases, in whom surgery was considered too dangerous, cardiac output was reduced from a pre-treatment mean of 14 litres/min to 10 litres/min following embolization, but no long-term follow-up was performed.[41,42]

The purpose of embolization prior to surgery is to reduce surgical blood loss, not the extent of surgical resection. In those cases surgical resection should be undertaken within 72 hours of the embolization, prior to the development of an inflammatory post-embolic response. Following the radiological procedure, the patient will require monitoring of vital signs, observation of the puncture site and pain relief if required. The post-embolization syndrome, comprising pain, fever and malaise for 3–5 days following the procedure is self-limiting, but a prolonged fever should raise the possibility of infection.

As might be expected with such a complex procedure, various complications can occur. These are summarized below:

1. General
   - related to general complications of angiography.
2. Specific
   - pain

- embolization and infarction of normal structures
- pulmonary embolus
- infection and abscess formation in an embolized area.

Complication rates range from 10 to 29%.[40] Following therapy, a follow-up with MR and colour Doppler can assess the efficacy of treatment.

It is important to emphasize that a multidisciplinary approach combining both surgical and radiological treatment is necessary in the management of congenital arteriovenous malformations.[43]

Acquired arteriovenous malformations

The major haemodynamic effect of these fistulae is related to size of the communication. With a large communication, there is a low haemodynamic resistance associated with the communication and the volume of the shunt is large. This results in an increased cardiac output and subsequent high output cardiac failure. The peripheral or distal consequences are related to ischaemia from shunting of blood and elevation of venous pressure which can result in ulceration and gangrene. The majority of these communications are treated by surgery, although some authors favour a 'wait and see' policy in the case of post-femoral artery catheterization induced arteriovenous fistula.[44]

Recent advances in endoluminal stenting have led to a new approach to the treatment of arteriovenous communications. A percutaneous intra-arterial covered stent is placed to obliterate an arteriovenous communication. The majority of those reported are in the acquired group of arteriovenous fistula[45-53] with satisfactory treatment of aortocaval, aortoiliac and femorofemoral communications, although the long-term effects are not yet known. The obvious advantages of this form of treatment are the lack of any inadvertent embolic risks as no embolic materials are used and the avoidance of surgery. The development of intimal hyperplasia may however limit the long-term success of such an approach.

TREATMENT – SURGICAL

Surgery can either be used to modify the blood flow through the fistula or radically resect all of the abnormal tissue.[27] Before any surgical procedure is attempted, the detailed anatomy must be defined, using duplex ultrasonography, angiography and MRI.

Resection

Congenital arteriovenous fistulae are almost always more complicated and more difficult to operate on than traumatic fistulae and in practice is it rarely possible to completely excise them. Surgery is difficult for a number of reasons. It can be hard to clearly delineate the extent of the abnormality, as even during contrast angiography there may be undetectable flow in distant vessels. MRI is helpful to predict the involvement of adjacent tissues and hence the feasibility of radical resection, and may also give additional information concerning the nature of the malformation.[31] The anatomy is much harder to see at the time of operation when excessive blood loss can hamper visibility.

Congenital arteriovenous fistulae often transgress tissue planes and the malformation is rarely confined to one muscle compartment when it can be excised en mass. More commonly the fistulae is present in all tissues including muscle, tendon, nerves and bone, all of which may need to be excised to provide a radical cure.[16,54,55]

Surgical treatment may be made easier if embolization is first carried out to reduce the vascularity of the lesion. This is usually performed 24–48 hours beforehand. Proximal and distal control must be achieved prior to excision of the malformation. The use of a tourniquet is not recommended as blood is still able to pass through bone collaterals and the veins can then become progressively distended.

Unfortunately many arteriovenous malformations are either not suitable for surgical treatment or rapidly recur after operation when they have been incompletely excised. In the head, neck or trunk repeated embolization is often the only option, whereas in the limb amputation is sometimes the most appropriate treatment. Intractable pain, ulceration, gangrene or loss of limb function are all relative indications for amputation. In addition cardiac failure or recurrent haemorrhage are more absolute indications for amputation. A more conservative approach can often be taken preserving useful limb function whilst acknowledging that abnormal tissue has to be left in place. For example painful gangrenous distal tissue may be excised to ameliorate symptoms without attempting to excise the full extent of the malformation. Patients may live many more years with symptomless fistulae.[56] Arteriovenous malformations are very variable in the symptoms that they cause and the rate at which they progress, and many patients survive without ever needing amputation.[57]

Haemodynamic procedures

Attempts to impair the blood supply to arteriovenous fistulae by surgery are rarely indicated but are sometimes used when excision is not possible, has failed, or there is significant regrowth after excision. This can be performed by ligating either the main feeding vessels or their tributaries. Sometimes the sheer extent of the abnormality or the size of the fistula makes embolization impossible and surgical skeletonization of the vascular tree can be effective in reducing haemodynamic changes, especially cardiomegaly. Further embolization is then often successful.

Ligating the main feeding vessels to an arteriovenous fistula rarely has a beneficial effect, and can often make ischaemia of the distal tissues worse. This occurs because the lesion is also fed by collateral vessels. When the main supply is lost the flow through these increase further depriving the distal tissues of blood supply. This procedure is also undesirable because it removes access to the fistula for embolization.

Branch artery ligation is sometimes useful to at least slow the enlargement of a fistula. This tends not to have an adverse effect on distal perfusion, but is in effect the surgical equivalent of embolization. It is, however, not as effective as embolization as the interstitial spaces of the fistula cannot be thrombosed at the same time, and thus embolization should be the treatment of choice if the branches are visible on angiography.

Cotton described the process of skeletonization,[58] also known as deafferentiation,[27] whereby all the arterial branches in the region of the malformation are ligated with the exception of the main feeding vessel. This tricky process reduces the blood flow through the fistula without compromising distal blood supply and may help reduce symptoms, especially when it is combined with subsequent embolization.

Amputation

Unfortunately few cases of arteriovenous fistulae are cured and many end up with amputation. This should leave a reasonable stump if a prosthesis is to be effective but the fistulous tissue must by fully excised or the stump itself can cause problems.

CASE EXAMPLES

The following case histories illustrate some of the aforementioned principles.

Case 1: Inappropriate embolization

A 29-year-old female presented with a painful congenital arteriovenous malformation suffered since childhood. Arteriography demonstrated an extensive malformation involving the palm of the hand (Fig. 1a). Percutaneous embolization with Ethanol and Lipiodol was attempted. Digital gangrene ensued resulting in index and middle finger amputation (Fig. 1b). This was the dominant hand and the patient was an artist.

Comment

The arteriogram demonstrates that the digital supply is closely related to the malformation. Liquid embolization was inappropriate because of the likelihood of involvement of adjacent vascular beds.

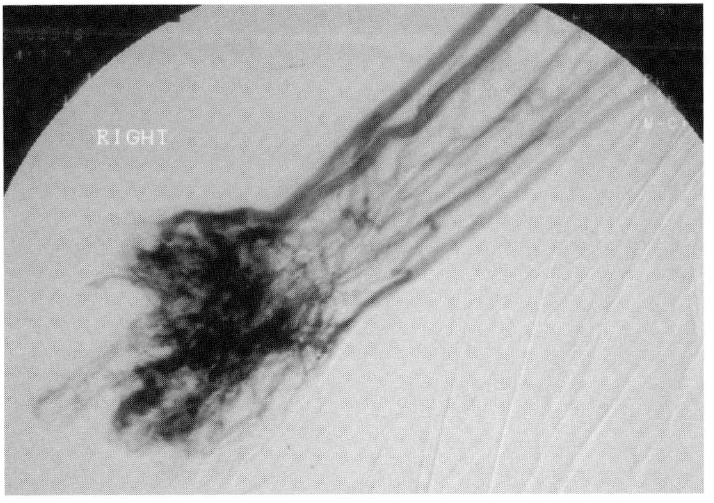

(a)

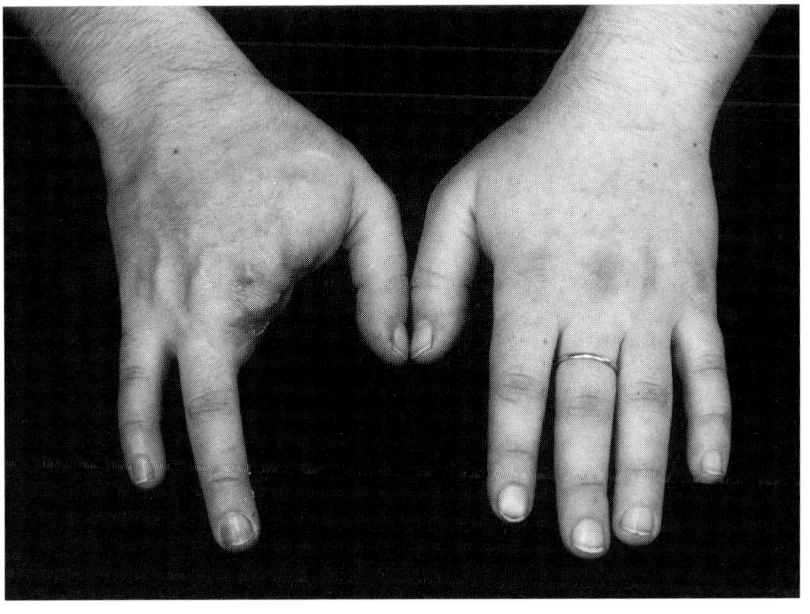

(b)

Fig. 1 (Case 1). (a) Arteriogram demonstrates extensive malformation of the hand. (b) The hand following amputation of two digits.

Case 2: Failure of radiological embolization

An 11-year-old boy presented with a diffuse malformation of the leg due to Parkes–Weber syndrome. A mid-thigh amputation had been performed at the age of 5, but there had been progressive increase in size of the stump since that time rendering the fitting of a leg prosthesis impossible (Fig. 2a). The cardiac output was elevated and the child failed to thrive. Arteriography demonstrated extensive arteriovenous communications from the stump and pelvis (Fig. 2b). Eleven percutaneous embolizations were attempted using a combination of coils and

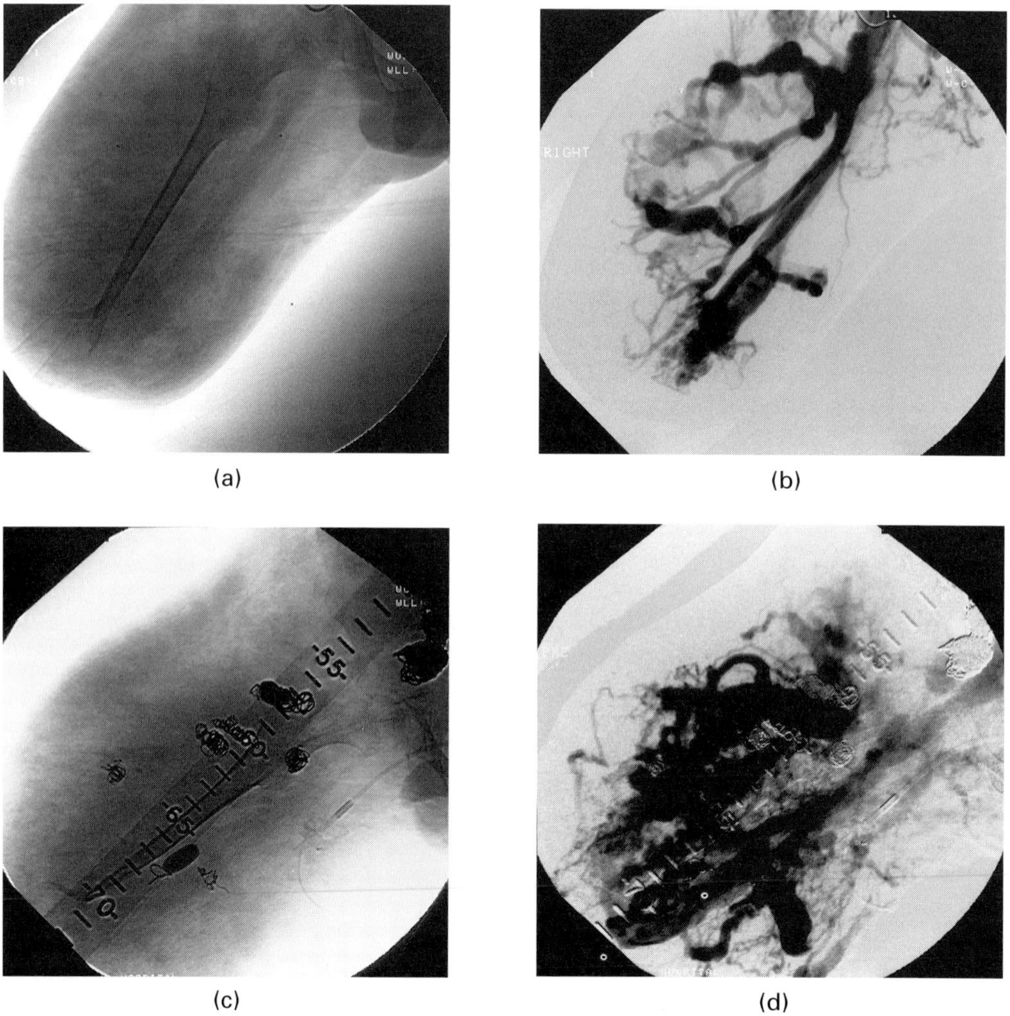

Fig. 2 (Case 2). (a) Pre-embolization shows the amputation stump. (b) An intra-arterial digital subtraction angiogram shows the malformation with large arteriovenous communications. (c) After 2½ years a control film shows multiple coils and a detachable balloon in the amputation stump. (d) A repeat angiogram shows little in the way of change in the malformation despite numerous embolization attempts.

detachable balloons (Fig. 2c). These procedures resulted in some reduction of cardiac output but no reduction of stump size or change in body weight and height (Fig. 2d). Eventually a hindquarter amputation was performed. The child is now gaining weight and height and has a normal cardiac output.

Comment

Percutaneous embolization was never likely to occlude such a diffuse malformation. Mutilating surgery was deferred but became inevitable and proved to be the correct course.

Case 3: Combined treatment

A 22-year-old man presented with a painful congenital arteriovenous malformation on the lateral aspect of his foot. Arteriography demonstrated dominant arterial supply from the posterior tibial artery with some supply from the anterior tibial. The posterior tibial was surgically explored in the lower calf and excised following direct injection of Gelfoam into the artery (Fig. 3a).

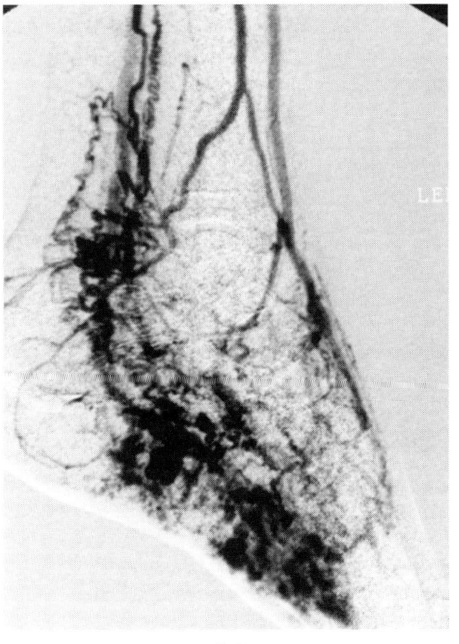

(a)

Fig. 3a (Case 3). (a) A lateral angiogram of the foot demonstrates vascular supply of the malformation predominantly from the anterior tibial and peroneal. The posterior tibial has been ligated just above the ankle with small vessels from this artery supplying the malformation. The proximal surgical ligation has not reduced the malformation.

The malformation transiently became less painful but symptoms soon recurred. Percutaneous embolization with polyvinyl alcohol resulted in symptomatic relief (Figs 3b, 3c).

Comment

Proximal surgical ligation was initially effective but could not occlude the whole abnormality which was supplied by two other vessels. The choice of absorbable Gelfoam was incorrect.

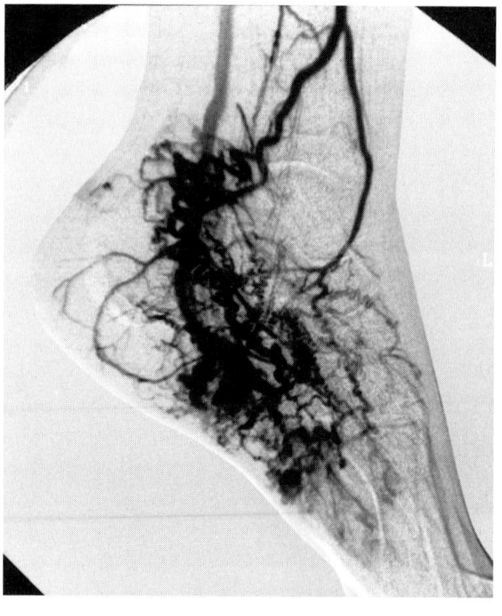

(b)

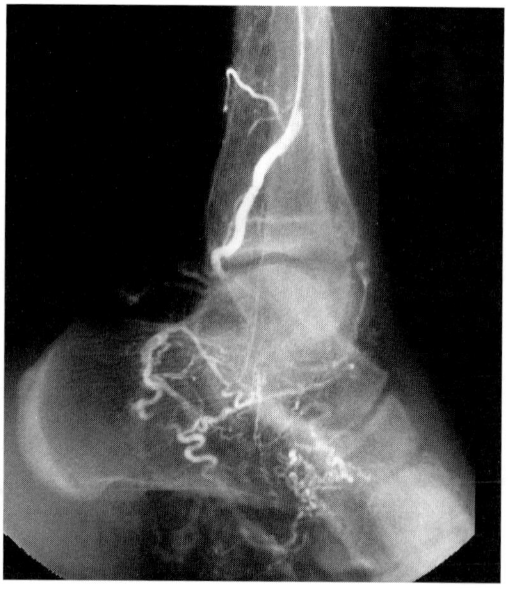

(c)

Fig. 3b,c (Case 3). (b) Preembolization arteriogram with a catheter placed in the posterior division of the peroneal artery. (c) Following polyvinyl alcohol embolization there is a reduction in the size of the malformation.

Case 4: Successful combined surgical and radiological approach

A 66-year-old female presented with a painful congenital arteriovenous malformation of the upper arm (Fig. 4a). Previous surgical intervention had been unsuccessful. Angiography revealed several large arteriovenous communications in the shoulder and upper arm. Percutaneous coil embolization, followed by local excision was undertaken with a good result (Figs 4b, 4c).

Comment

Combined radiological and surgical intervention gave the most effective therapy.

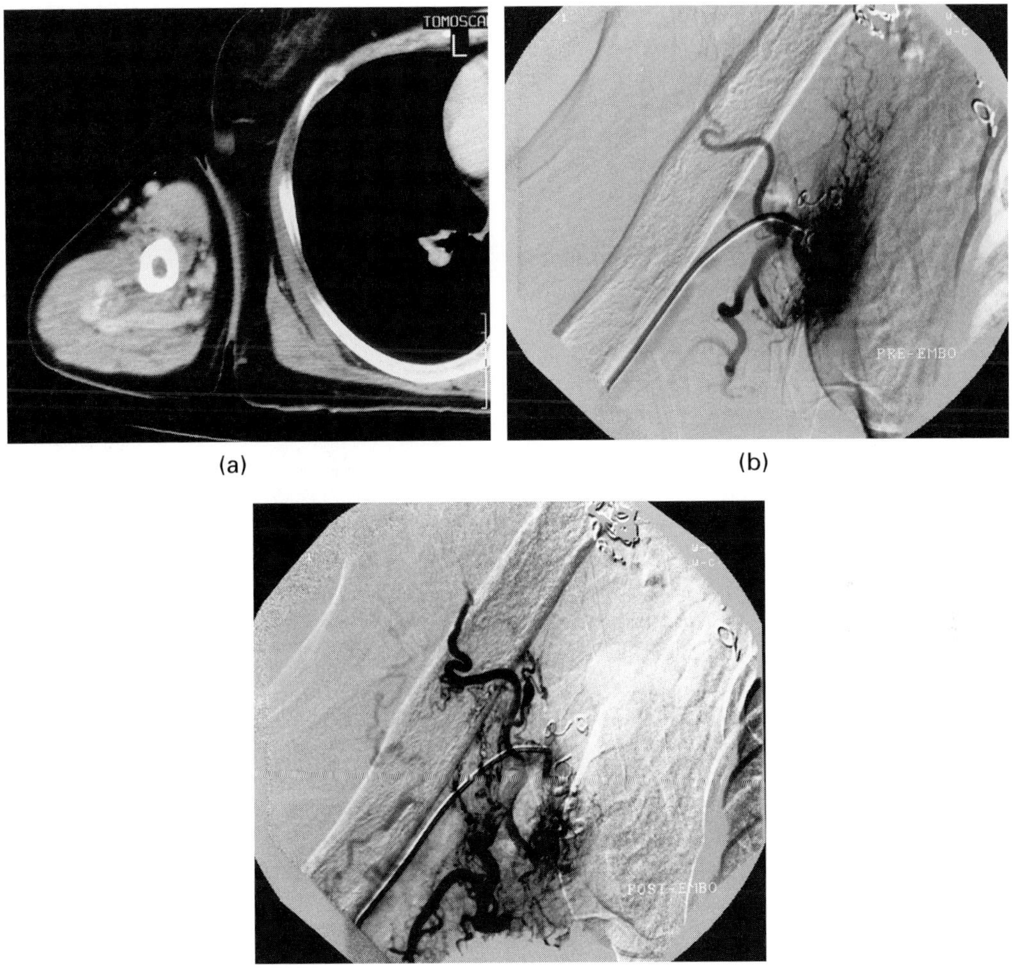

Fig. 4 (Case 4). (a) Axial CT shows the malformation in the upper arm involving the musculature. (b) A retrograde brachial arteriogram demonstrates some of the malformation in the upper arm. Metallic coils are noted from previous embolization attempts. (c) Following embolization with particulate matter, there is reduction in the malformation.The patient subsequently underwent surgical exploration and, with a combined approach, had a satisfactory result.

Case 5: Successful combined surgical and radiological approach

A 41-year-old female presented with a Parkes–Weber malformation involving the whole of the lower limb (Fig. 5a). The affected limb was painful and there was increased cardiac output. Amputation had been offered but refused by the patient. Multiple percutaneous coils had been placed in proximal vessels that had failed to alleviate symptoms or reduce cardiac output. Skeletonization of the superficial femoral artery with repeated particulate embolization of small arteriovenous malformations in the calf was performed with a subsequent reduction in pain and cardiac output (Fig. 5b).

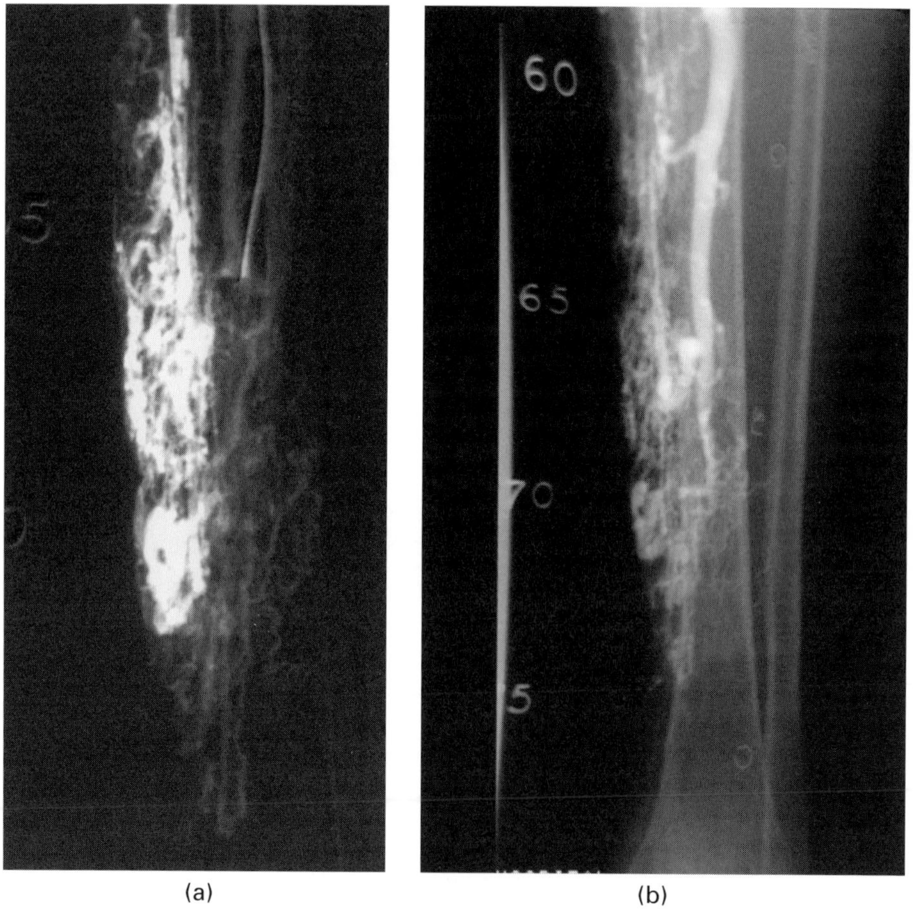

(a) (b)

Fig. 5 (Case 5). (a) Selective study of the posterior tibial artery demonstrates multiple arteriovenous malformations in a patient with Parkes–Weber syndrome. (b) Post-embolization, there is some reduction of the malformation but there is still abnormal flow present. Note metallic coil insertion elsewhere in the leg from previous unsuccessful embolization attempts.

Comment

The combination of skeletonization and particulate embolization was successful in reducing symptoms and cardiac output. Proximal coil placement was time-consuming and failed to produce any useful clinical benefit.

CONCLUSION

The treatment of complicated arteriovenous fistulae can be difficult and they are often best treated by a combined radiological and surgical approach. Unfortunately this is sometimes not successful and then repeated embolization or surgical amputation may be necessary.

REFERENCES

1. Cited in Young AE: Arteriovenous malformations. In: Mulliken JB, Young AE (Eds), *Vascular Birthmarks.* London: WB Saunders, 1998
2. Cited by Osler W: Remarks on arteriovenous aneurysm. *Lancet* **i:** 949, 1915
3. Hunter W: The history of an aneurysm of the aorta with some remarks on aneurysms in general. *Med Obs Soc Phys (Lond)* **1:** 323, 1757
4. Bell J: In: Hurst, Rees *et al. The Principles of Surgery* pp. 456–489. London: Longman, 1815
5. Bushe G: A case, after the excision of an anastomosing aneurysm from the right temple, ligature of the external carotid became necessary to restrain haemorrhage. *Lancet* **ii:** 413, 1827
6. Adams J: Singular case of hypertrophy of the right lower extremity with superficial cutaneous naevus of the same side. *Lancet* **ii:** 140, 1858
7. Ghérini (of Milan): Varice anéurysmatique congénitale. *Gaz ed Hop ed Paris* 27 Juin, 303, 1867
8. Hewitt P: A case of congenital aneurysmal varix. *Lancet* **i:** 146, 1867
9. Warren JM: Extracts from the records of the Boston Society for Medical Improvement – Unusual case of varicose aneurysm. *Boston Med Surg J* **57:** 528, 1858
10. Krause W: Traumatische angiectasie der linken armes. *Arch Klin Surg* **ii:** 142, 1862
11. Nicoladoni C: Phlebarteriectasie der rechten oberen extremität. *Arch Klin Chir* **18:** 252, 1875
12. Branham AA: Aneurysmal varix of the femoral artery and vein following a gunshot wound. *Internat J Surg* **3:** 250, 1890
13. Callender CL: Study of arteriovenous fistula with analysis of 447 cases. *Ann Surg* **71:** 428, 1920
14. Osler W: Remarks on arteriovenous aneurysm. *Lancet* **i:** 949, 1915
15. Rösler H: Über herzvergrösserlung bei angeborener arteriovenöser kommunikation. *Klin Woch* **8:** 1621, 1929
16. Lewis D: Congenital arteriovenous fistulae. *Lancet* **ii:** 621, 680, 1930
17. Reid MR: The effect of arteriovenous fistula upon the heart and blood vessels: an experimental and clinical study. *Bull Johns Hopkins Hosp* **31:** 43, 1920
18. Stewart FT: Arteriovenous aneurism treated by angeiorrhphy. *Ann Surg* **57:** 574, 1913
19. Holman E: *Abnormal Arteriovenous Communications,* 2nd edn. Springfield, IL: Charles C Thomas, 1968
20. Sako Y, Varco R: Arteriovenous fistula: results of management of congenital and acquired forms, blood flow measurements, and observations on proximal arterial degeneration. *Surgery* **67:** 40, 1970

21. Szilagyi DE, Smith RF, Elliott JP, Hageman JH: Congenital arteriovenous malformations of the limbs. *Arch Surg* **111:** 423, 1976
22. Young AE: *Mixed Vascular Malformations*. MChir Thesis, University of Cambridge, 1978
23. Nobbs JU, Carrin AA, Kadwa AM *et al.*: Traumatic arteriovenous fistula: Experience with 202 patients. *Br J Surg* **81:** 1296–1299, 1994
24. Young AE: Arteriovenous malformations. In: Mulliken JB, Young AE (Eds), *Vascular Birthmarks*. London: WB Saunders, 1998
25. Browse NL, Burnand KG: The cause of venous ulceration. *Lancet* **ii:** 243, 1982
26. Burnand KG, Whimster I, Naidod A, Browse NL: Pericapillary fibrin in the ulcer bearing skin of the leg. *Br Med J* **285:** 1071, 1982
27. Malan E, Puglionisi A: Congenital angiodysplasia of the extremities. *J Cardiovasc Surg* **6:** 255, 1965
28. Cotton LT, Sykes BJ: The treatment of diffuse congenital arteriovenous fistulae of the leg. *Proc Roy Soc Med* **62:** 245, 1969
29. Robertson DJ: Congenital arteriovenous fistulae of the extremities. *Ann Roy Coll Surg Engl* **18:** 73, 1956
30. Yakes W F, Stauros AT, Parker SH *et al.*: Color Doppler imaging of peripheral high flow vascular malformations before and after Ethanol embolotherapy. RSNA Presentation. *Radiology* **177:** 156, 1990
31. Rak KM, Yakes WF, Ray RL *et al.*: MR imaging of symptomatic peripheral vascular malformations. *Am J Roent* **159:** 107–112, 1992
32. Saks AM, Paterson FC, Irvine AT *et al.*: Improved MR venography: Use of fast short inversion time inversion recovery technique in evaluation of venous angiomas. *Radiology* **149:** 908–911, 1995
33. Halliday AW, Smith EJ, Jackson J *et al.*: Indications for surgery for arteriovenous malformations., *Br J Surg* **79:** 361–362, 1992
34. Toursarkissian B, Allen BT, Petrinec D *et al.*: Spontaneous closure of selected iatrogenic pseudoaneurysms and arteriovenous fistulae. *J Vasc Surg* **25:** 803–809, 1997
35. Rich NM, Hobson RW, Collins GJ: Traumatic arteriovenous fistula and false aneurysms: a review of 558 lesions. *Surgery* **78:** 817–828, 1975
36. Hare W, Land F, Holland C: Paresis following internal celiac artery embolisation. *Radiology* **146:** 47–51, 1983
37. Hietala S: Urinary bladder necrosis following selective embolisation of the internal celiac artery. *Acta Radiol* **19:** 316–320, 1978
38. Doppman J, Di Chiro G: Paraspinal muscle infarction. A painful complication of lumbar artery embolisation. *Radiology* **119:** 609–613, 1976
39. Gang DE, Dole K, Adelman S: Spinal cord infarction following therapeutic renal artery embolisation. *J Am Med Assoc* **237:** 2641–2642, 1977
40. Yakes, WF, Ross IP, Odink H: Arteriovenous malformation management. Cardiovascular interventional. *Radiology* **19:** 65–71, 1996
41. Allison DJ, Kennedy A: Peripheral arteriovenous malformations. *Br Med J* **303:** 1191–1194, 1991
42. Hemingway AP, Allison DJ: Complications of embolisation. *Radiology* **166:** 669–672, 1988
43. Erdmann MW, Davies DM, Jackson JE: Multidisciplinary approach to the management of head and neck arteriovenous malformations. *Ann Roy Coll Surg* **77:** 53–59, 1995
44. Toursarkissian B, Allen BT, Petrinec D *et al.*: Spontaneous closure of selected iatrogenic pseudoaneurysms and arteriovenous fistulae. *J Vasc Surg* **25:** 803–809, 1997
45. Marian ML, Veith FJ, Panetta TF *et al.*: Percutaneous transfemoral insertion of a stented graft to repair a traumatic femoral arteriovenous fistula. *J Vasc Surg* **18:** 299–302, 1993
46. Parodi JC: Endovascular repair of aortic aneurysms, arteriovenous fistulas and false aneurysms. *World J Surg* **20:** 655–663, 1996
47. Uflacker R, Elliott BM: Percutaneous endoluminal stent-graft repair of an old traumatic femoral arteriovenous fistula. *Cardiovasc Intervent Radiol* **19:** 120–122, 1996
48. Criado E, Marston WA, Ligush J *et al.*: Endovascular repair of peripheral aneurysms, psuedoaneurysms and arterior venous fistulas. *Ann Vasc Surg* **11:** 256–263, 1997
49. Quinn SF, Sheley RC, Semonsen KG *et al.*: Endovascular stents covered with pre-

expanded polytetrafluoroethylene for treatment of iliac artery aneurysms and fistulas. *J Vasc Intervent Radiol* **8:** 1057–1063, 1997

50. Beveridge CJ, Pleass HC, Chamberlain J *et al*.: Aortoiliac aneurysm with arterio caval fistula treated by a bifurcated endovascular stent-graft. *Cardiovasc Intervent Radiol* **21:** 244–246, 1998
51. Ruebben A, Tettoni S, Muratore P *et al*.: Arteriovenous fistulas induced by femoral arterial catheterisation: percutaneous treatment. *Radiology* **209:** 729–734, 1998
52. Parodi JC , Schonholz C, Ferreira LM *et al*.: Endovascular stent-graft treatment of traumatic arterial lesions. *Ann Vasc Surg* **13:** 121–129, 1999
53. Waigland J, Uhlich F, Gross CM *et al*.: Percutaneous treatment of pseudoaneurysms and arteriovenous fistulas after invasive vascular procedures. *Catheter Cardiovasc Intervent* **47:** 157–164, 1999
54. Clay RC, Blalock A: Congenital arteriovenous fistulas in the mandible. *Surg Gyn Obstet* **90:** 543, 1950
55. Nisbet NW: Congenital arteriovenous fistula in the extremities. *Br J Surg* **41:** 658, 1953
56. Flanc C: Congenital arterio-venous fistulas of the extremities. *Austr NZJ Surg* **37:** 222–232, 1968
57. Robertson DJ: Congenital arteriovenous fistulae of the extremities. *Ann Roy Coll Surg Engl* **18:** 73, 1956
58. Cotton LT, Sykes BJ: The treatment of diffuse congenital arteriovenous fistulae of the leg. *Proc Roy Soc Med* **62:** 245, 1969

RENAL ARTERY STENOSIS OPPORTUNITIES

Magnetic resonance angiography of renal artery stenosis

W Gedroyc

IMPORTANCE OF RENAL ARTERY STENOSIS

Renal artery stenosis is an increasingly recognized cause of renal impairment in the elderly and middle aged, often leading to end stage renal failure in the older age group. Few good studies have been performed to assess this, but figures from the only prospective study in this area by Scoble *et al.*[1] suggest that at least 14% of patients over 50 with end stage renal failure have significant renal artery stenosis.

The socioeconomic impact of this condition, which in the elderly is almost invariably due to atheroma, is very large in terms of years on dialysis and transplantation. Two other points, however, are also of great importance in this consideration and they are naturally linked. The first is that reasonably successful minimally invasive and operative treatments for renal artery stenosis do exist. The arguments about which patient should have which form of treatment is outside the scope of this article, but the important fact is that there is treatment available which may, in some patients, improve renal function or in others slow the rate of deterioration[2,3] towards end stage renal failure.

The second important point is that the presence of renal artery stenosis is a marker of severe generalized atheroma (see below) and patients with renal artery stenosis fare particularly poorly on dialysis programmes with overall only a 12% 5-year survival.[4]

EPIDEMIOLOGY

As mentioned above, atheroma is the predominant cause (70%) overall of renal artery stenosis and is often an expression of widespread atheromatous disease. Renal artery stenosis is present in 39% of patients with lower extremity occlusive disease[5] and in 22% of patients with coronary artery disease. In a large postmortem study, renal artery stenosis was identified in 4.3% of all patients and in 8.3% of diabetic patients.[6]

NATURAL HISTORY

Schreiber *et al.*[7] have shown that the severity of renal artery stenosis will deteriorate in 53% of patients leading to renal artery occlusion in at least 16% of patients with atheroma within 2 years. Loss of renal mass is a common accompaniment of this progressive deterioration of arterial flow.

GOALS OF TREATMENT

In view of the common nature of this disease, its known progression to renal arterial occlusion and end stage renal failure, and the existence of reasonably successful treatment if applied early enough, it seems very reasonable to concentrate substantial resources into devising a rapid, non-invasive, successful method of diagnosing this condition. The goal of such an endeavour would be to maintain native renal function for as long as possible, keeping these patients off dialysis and end stage renal failure replacement programmes. Blood pressure maintenance is a relatively minor consideration in comparison with the above in the majority of patients.

WHAT IS REQUIRED

For a test to be of benefit in this difficult area it should ideally fulfil as many as possible of the following criteria:

1. Be as non-invasive as possible.
2. If intravenous contrast is used, the media should be non-nephrotoxic.
3. Aorta and main abdominal vessels should be visualized in relation to renal artery.
4. Be able to produce a clear anatomical depiction of vasculature, plus an assessment of accessory renal arteries.
5. Have potential for producing three-dimensional (3D) reconstruction from these data.
6. Have high sensitivity and specificity.
7. Be cheap.
8. Be operator-independent.

MAGNETIC RESONANCE ANGIOGRAPHY

Magnetic resonance arteriography is starting to meet many of the above criteria and the introduction of ultrafast contrast-enhanced angiography will develop the strength of MR in angiographic imaging, further addressing many of the drawbacks inherent in conventional MRA.

The two basic conventional MRA techniques are time of flight and phase-contrast sequences. Each of these can be acquired in a 2D or 3D format.

Time of flight (TOF) studies image flow secondary to the flow-related enhancement seen when non-saturated spins enter the imaging volume and 3D TOF studies have an intrinsically high spatial resolution and high signal-to-noise which makes them theoretically very attractive for the imaging of renal arteries. The long imaging times required and the substantial in-plane flow saturation limits their application[8] to the imaging of arteries with high velocity within small volumes such as the Circle of

Willis. As a result, 3D TOF images renal arteries poorly and is relatively unsuitable in this application; 2D TOF performs better over a large area, but the tortuosity of the renal arteries placed deep in the abdomen results in significant signal loss due to in-plane saturation effects at vessel bends preventing these sequences from routinely visualizing the whole length of the renal arteries.[9] These problems prevent TOF from assuming a routine place in renal MRA imaging.

Phase-contrast MR sequences work on a different MR principle. In brief, a signal is produced by the phase shift produced by flowing blood in the imaging volume. The greater the velocity, the greater the phase shift and the higher the signal produced. Phase-contrast MRA is much less susceptible to signal fallout at vessel tortuosities, but is severely affected by signal loss in areas of turbulence due to intravoxel dephasing. It has been suggested that turbulence-associated signal loss may be minimized by cardiac gating, but de Haan *et al.*[10] showed that in clinical practice this did not make much difference. The finding of significant signal loss in areas of turbulence has several effects in clinical practice. First, it overestimates vessel stenoses when one interprets the images using criteria learned from conventional angiography. This can be overcome by altering one's reporting pattern and learning a new scale of interpretation for phase-contrast MRA, e.g. mild vessel wall narrowing on phase-contrast MRA = normal; signal loss across full vessel wall diameter on phase-contrast MRA = mild stenosis, etc. Indeed, having mild areas of abnormality overemphasized on MRA does make it less likely that stenoses will be missed, but the problem of false positives is introduced. Sharp vessel junctions and prominent kinks in vessels cause local turbulence which is displayed as loss of signal. Often a clue to the fact that this is purely turbulence is the very good distal signal beyond the area in question. False positives can also be seen when metallic surgical clips[11] are placed close to the renal arteries. The ferromagnetic susceptibility artefact produced by such clips can cause signal loss leading to an erroneous suggestion of a stenosis, again a good distal signal should throw doubt on this diagnosis and a review of the constituent magnitude images may reveal a round area of clip-associated signal loss.

The overall results for phase-contrast MRA in renal artery stenosis have been maintained through multiple papers with sensitivities of 92–94% and specificities of 94%.[12–14] The use of phased array surface coils further improves images with better signal.[15]

The ability to produce multiple views around the renal arteries is a great strength of MRA. Conventional angiography can usually only acquire one angulation per contrast injection and as a result 3D appreciation is limited. This becomes an important limitation when atheromatous renal arteries and abdominal aortas are studied because they are often very tortuous, causing substantial overlap of vessels which is difficult to unwind with only a few planar views. With its greater 3D capabilities, MRA allows a much more complete assessment of the origins and bends of renal arteries making the depiction of complex stenoses and normal but tortuous overlapping vessels much easier and we have described a small group of patients[16] in which the MRA was positive, but in which the initial angiographic study was negative.

Subsequent intra-arterial pressure measurements revealed the stenosed area because the planar nature of the conventional angiography could not depict these complex stenoses.

Conventional MRA studies only image a relatively small area around the main renal arteries and accessory arteries arising from outside this area will not be easily visualized. Similarly, it is not common to visualize renal arteries beyond the renal hilum and abnormalities seen beyond the hilum must be interpreted with much greater caution because of the multiple vessel branches and unsuspected turbulence in smaller vessels.

Vessel occlusions are difficult to differentiate from severe stenoses on conventional MRA. Usually the origin of the vessel is visible, but little signal is seen more distally. This may reflect severe turbulence or no flow beyond an occlusion. This does have therapeutic relevance since a severe stenosis is amenable to intravascular recanalization whereas an occlusion would rarely be treated.

The above description emphasizes how conventional MRA images flow within vessels rather than imaging the anatomic vessel outline which is the situation in intra-arterial angiography. MRA may provide much more haemodynamic information as a result because it images the effects of a stenosis on flow rather than the physical dimensions of the arterial lumen. This does have an important benefit in the following situations. First, if a doubtful area is visualized on a conventional contrast angiogram, normal signal on MRA is a strong indicator that this area is normal. Second, in the follow-up of angioplasty, loss of signal on MRA may be an earlier finding than a change in vessel calibre on contrast arteriography.

Because MRA depicts blood flow in vessels when that flow is low, as seen in patients with poor renal function, the visualized signal from the renal arteries is correspondingly poor, making identification of renal arteries much more difficult. It is of course within this group of patients that it is particularly important to detect any possibility of reversible renal arterial disease ideally without the use of nephrotoxic contrast agents. Definitive examinations are therefore more of a problem in this group and it is in this sort of area that the most recent developments in the use of 3D contrast-enhanced MRA may be particularly helpful, although this new technique will probably have successful applications in a wide variety of areas, both within the abdomen and other body areas.

Little in comparison has been written about the use of MRA in the imaging of renal transplants. Results very comparable[17] with those in native renal arteries can be achieved using 3D phase-contrast. In renal transplants MRA is particularly useful because such transplants often have tortuous blood supplies which are difficult to image conventionally, but which are easily sorted out by the 3D assessment provided by MRA. Otherwise, all of the above discussion applies equally to the renal transplant.

3D MRA CONTRAST-ENHANCED ANGIOGRAPHY

This a relatively recent development in MRA and uses techniques borrowed from computed tomography (CT) angiography which are modified for use in magnetic resonance. These sequences overcome many of the drawbacks of conventional MRA.

The principle of these sequences is to use gadolinium chelates with their T1 shortening effects to provide the predominant signal in the images. Blood flow is not imaged directly as in TOF or phase-contrast sequences but the signal brightening caused by contrast within the vessel in question is used. This has many advantages over conventional MRA. The potential of this technique is great and fulfils many of the requirements initially described at the beginning of this article for successful MRA sequences. A substantial proportion of MRA will be carried out in the future using this method and we believe that this technique and its variations will take over much of the diagnostic work currently performed by conventional angiography (Fig. 1).

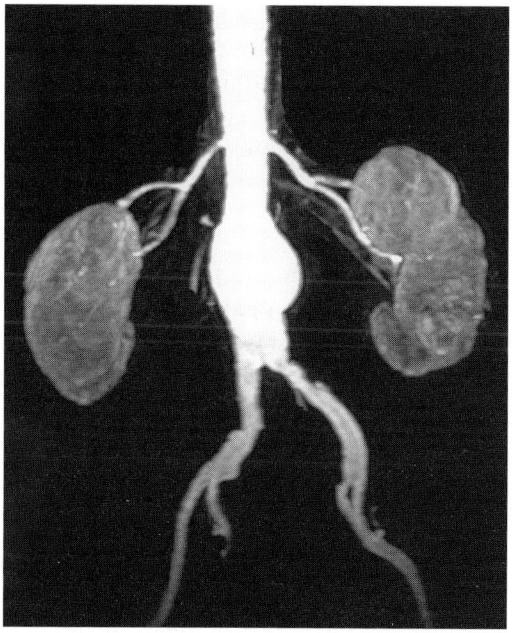

Fig. 1. MRA of the abdominal aorta. Single bilateral renal arteries. No significant stenosis of either renal artery is seen. Note prompt symmetrical nephrograms. Also well visualized is a discrete infrarenal aortic aneurysm and significant but non-stenotic vascular disease of both iliac arteries.

Contrast is infused intravenously so that a high concentration of gadolinium is created in the arterial area being investigated during the scanning time.[18] The images should be acquired as rapidly as possible, ideally in a short breath-hold to minimize respiratory artefacts. A 3D-volume acquisition should be used to allow very thin slices to be acquired within the single breath-hold allowing the highest resolution possible as a result. The 3D sequences also allow a shorter TR to be used allowing large data sets to be gathered. It is immediately obvious that only machines with high performance gradient strength at high field strength are suitable to carry out such sequences.

The most commonly used echo sequences are 3D acquisitions using fast spoiled gradient because they have inherent T1 weighting[19,20] although other T1 sequences, if fast enough, can also be implemented such as MPRAGE (Magnefization Prepared Rapid Gradient echo) or inversion recovery prepared sequences. Ideally, 40–60 slices of 1mm or 1.5mm thickness are acquired within a breath-hold of less than 30 seconds (ideally 20 s). The use of such rapid sequences minimizes the possibility of significant respiratory artefacts degrading the images and allows improved spatial resolution particularly of the smaller more peripheral arteries such as those beyond the renal hilum which in the past were blurred by respiratory motion over the time course of a much longer scan.

The reduction in the overall scan acquisition time means that correct timing of the enhancing contrast bolus is much more critical. The principle is to achieve peak contrast opacification during the time when the central K space lines are being collected. This part of the acquisition defines the low spatial frequencies which are responsible for image contrast as opposed to the peripheral lines of K space with their higher spatial frequencies which play a large role in spatial resolution. Conventional sequences sample this central area in the middle of the acquisition (sequential) and therefore one should aim to produce the peak gadolinium concentration throughout this part of the sequence. Multiple approaches have been developed to achieve this goal[21] but the consensus now is that some form of test bolus is required to measure the injection sites to renal artery time delay.

This period is quite variable between patients depending on a range of factors from state of cardiac output to injection rate. The area of the aorta adjacent to the renal arteries is monitored by repeated sagittal scans and the signal intensity rise of the inflowing test bolus of 4ml is measured. The subsequent imaging scan sequence can then be automatically triggered if appropriate software is used or a calculation is made[22] which will provide the optimal delay between injection and the beginning of the scan. The aim is to minimize venous overlap so that a pure arteriogram is produced. The renal circulation, however, only has a time delay of about 3 seconds between the arterial and the venous stage so correct timing is crucial and one of the above techniques must be implemented. If a best-guess technique is utilized, the success rate of such a procedure is reduced to about 60% as opposed to over 90% using the above.[22] The injection rate most commonly used is between 2 and 3ml per second using a contrast dose of 0.3mmol/kg resulting in volumes between 30 and 50ml approximately.[20]

The echo times used should be as short as possible to minimize T2* decay and signal dephasing, ideally below 3ms; TR should also be kept as short as possible and a typical value used is 4–5ms.

Multiple studies have now been produced examining the renal arteries with this technique (Fig. 2, Fig. 3).[18–23] All these studies have compared the results of 3D MRA with conventional angiography and have produced sensitivity values of 90% and above and specificity values of above 95%. These results are broadly superior to those of conventional MRA in this field. A recent study compared phase-contrast MRA

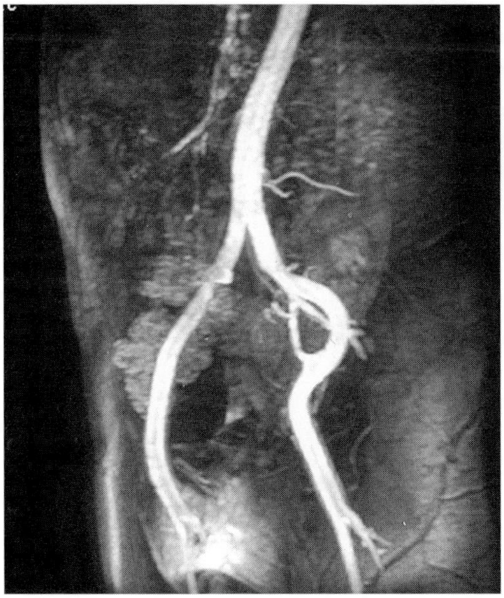

Fig. 2. MRA of abdominal aorta and iliac arteries. This study demonstrates a normal transplant artery arising from the left external iliac artery.

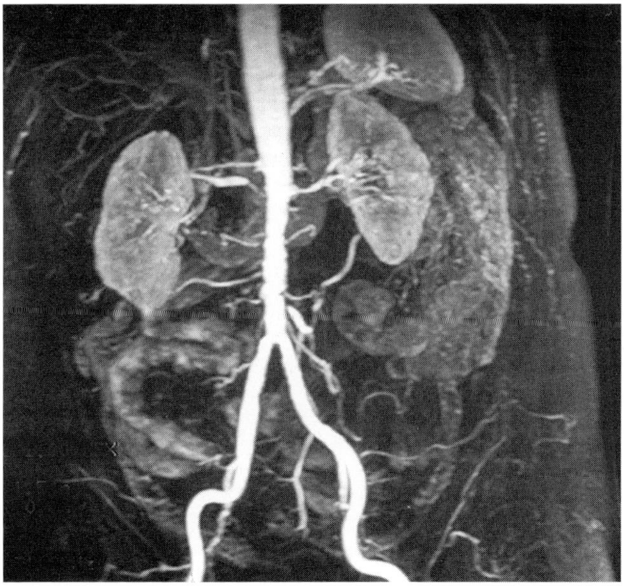

Fig. 3. MRA of abdominal aorta and iliacs; severe stenosis of origin and first part of right renal artery is clearly seen and less severe but also significant stenosis of the first part of the left renal artery also identified. Note severe irregularity of lower abdominal aorta indicating severe atheromatous disease.

directly to 3D contrast MRA and the results are also similar to that described above. In patients with normal renal function, conventional MRA may produce very satisfactory results, but when very tortuous diseased arteries are encountered, particularly in patients with diminished renal function, conventional MRA is much more difficult because of the artefacts and low intrinsic flow of this situation (Figs 4, 5). Such patients commonly have dilated or frankly aneurysmal abdominal aortas which is a further problem for conventional MRA because of the massive turbulence seen in this situation; 3D contrast studies function equally well in this type of patient provided the timing of the sequence is adjusted appropriately. These studies are not affected significantly by turbulence because they purely assess areas of T1 shortening rather like conventional angiography and are therefore much more robust in such problematic areas where excellent imaging is vital to assess the possibility of reversible renal artery stenosis.

At first glance it would appear that this approach is very similar to CT angiography and indeed the first applications of this type of technique were stimulated by the above. However, 3D MRA has many crucial advantages over CT angiography which allow it to become widely accepted as the primary imaging method in a wide variety of body angiography areas. No ionizing radiation is used.

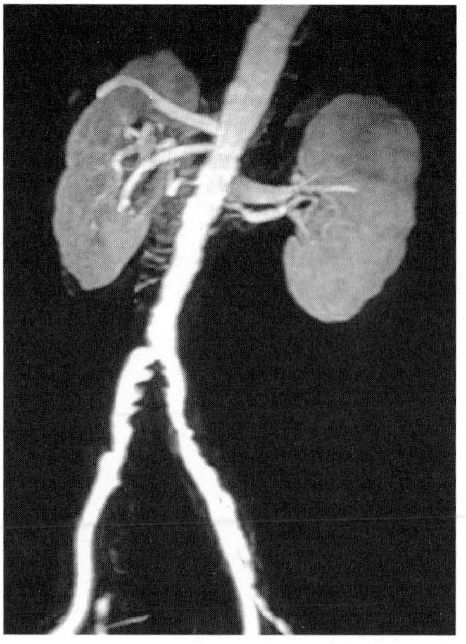

Fig. 4. Abdominal MRA showing severe bilateral renal artery stenosis and extensive atheromatous disease of aorta and iliacs. Note some contrast in an early filling left renal vein but in this obliquity it does not compromise the visualization of the left renal artery.

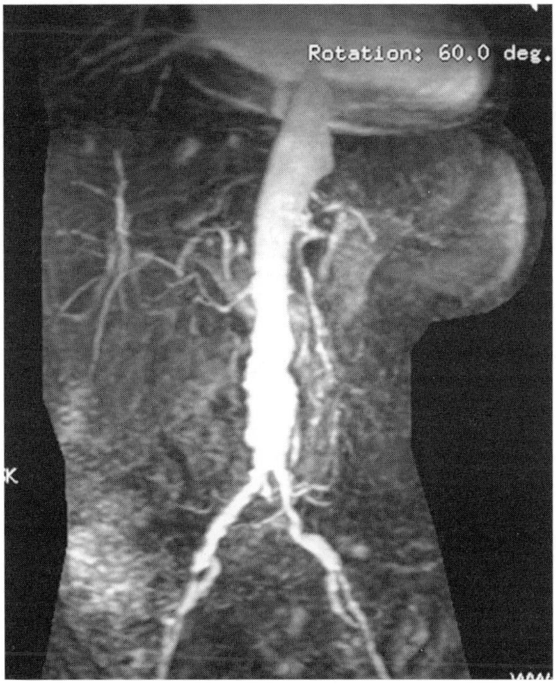

(a)

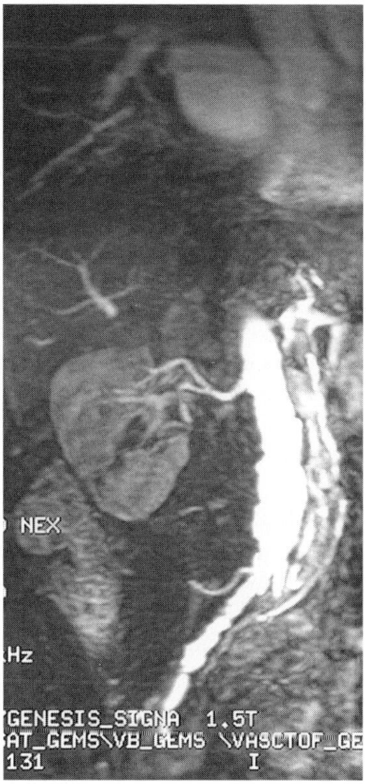

(b)

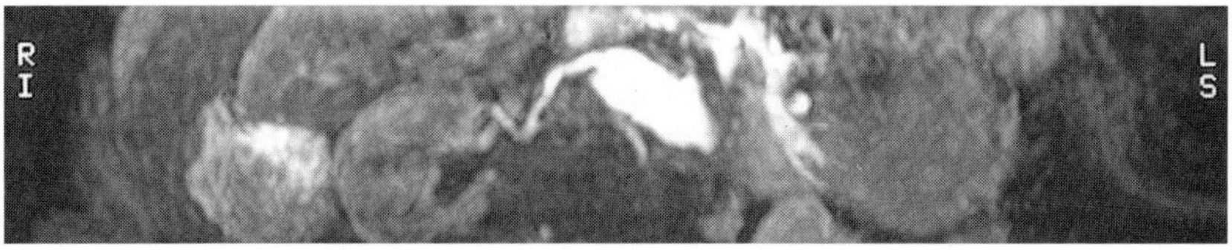

(c)

Fig. 5. MRA of abdominal aorta. (a) Severe disease and low flow in renal arteries with extensive atheromatous disease of aorta and iliacs. This anteroposterior full volume reconstruction suggests the right renal artery is diffusely thinned but with a focal stenosis and the left renal artery is also small. (b) Subvolume oblique reconstructions confirm the lack of stenosis of the right renal artery with an oblique right view. (c) An axial subvolume reconstruction showing the full length of this artery. Such a patient with severe atheromatous disease of the aorta with irregular ectatic vessels is often extremely difficult to examine with conventional angiography but the 3D MRA technique has the ability to examine the vessels from all obliquitys and to carry out subvolume reconstructions to further clarify abnormalities allowing much more reliable visualization of the full length of main arteries in comparison with angiography which is a huge advantage in dealing with high risk patients.

The contrast used in 3D MRA has no nephrotoxic effects and has a lower osmolar load than iodinated media. Large volumes may be acquired at one sitting because coronal plane acquisitions can be used and the reconstruction algorithms are simpler because no high intensity structures such as bone or calcifications have to be removed from the data set.

Further development of this technique is anticipated with more rapid imaging and repeated subtraction of data sets before and after contrast administration allowing improved definition and selection of arterial and venous structures.

SUMMARY

Conventional MRA techniques allow acceptable non-invasive imaging of the renal arteries, particularly using 3D phase-contrast techniques with phased array body coils. The inherent disadvantages, however, of these sequences as regards turbulence and difficulty imaging in low flow situations cause many problems in ciritical cases. Many of these problems are overcome by 3D contrast-enhanced MRA which is particularly useful in the situation where conventional MRA sequences are problematic, as it has the potential to replace conventional MRA in this and many other body areas, allowing vascular visualization comparable with that of intra-arterial angiography with the minimum invasion of an intravenous injection.

REFERENCES

1. Scoble JE, Maher ER, Hamilton G *et al.*: Atherosclerotic renovascular disease causing renal impairment: a case for treatment. *Clin Nephrol* **31:** 119–122, 1989
2. Novick AC, Ziegelbaum M, Vidt DG *et al.*: Trends in surgical revascularisation for renal artery disease: ten years experience. *J Am Med Assoc* 498–501, 1987
3. Novick AC: Atherosclerotic ischaemic nephropathy. *Urol Clin North Am* **21:** 184–186, 1994
4. Mailloux LU, Bellucci AG, Mossey RT *et al.*: Predictors of survival in patients undergoing dialysis. *Am J Med* **84:** 855–862, 1988
5. Olin JW, Melia M, Young JR *et al.*: Prevalence of atherosclerotic renal artery stenosis in patients with atherosclerosis elsewhere. *Am J Med* **188:** 46–51, 1990
6. Sawicki PT, Kaiser S, Heinemann L *et al.*: Prevalence of renal artery stenosis in diabetes mellitus: an autopsy study. *J Int Med* **229:** 489–492, 1991
7. Schreiber MJ, Pohl MA, Novick AC: The natural history of atherosclerotic and fibrous renal artery disease. *Urol Clin North Am* **11:** 383–392, 1984
8. Yamashita Y, Mitsuszaki K, Tang Y *et al.*: Gadolinium-enhanced breath-hold three-dimensional time of flight MR angiography of the abdominal and pelvic vessels: the value of the ultrafast MPRAGE sequence. *J Mag Res Imag* **7:** 623–628, 1997
9. Gedroyc W: Magnetic resonance angiography of renal arteries. *Urol Clin North Am* **21:** 201–214, 1994
10. de Haan MW, Kouwenhoven M, Thelissen GR *et al.*: Renovascular disease in patients with hypertension: detection with systolic and diastolic gating in three-dimensional phase-contrast MR angiography. *Radiology* **198:** 449–456, 1996
11. McCarty M, Gedroyc WM: Surgical clip artifact mimicking arterial stenosis: a problem with magnetic resonance angiography. *Clin Radiol* **48:** 232–235, 1993

12. Gedroyc WM, Neerhut P, Negus R *et al.*: Magnetic resonance angiography of renal artery stenosis. *Clin Radiol* **50:** 436–439, 1995
13. Debatin JF, Spritzer CE *et al.*: Imaging of the renal arteries: value of MR angiography. *Am J Roent* **157:** 981–990, 1991
14. Prince MR, Schoenberg SO, Ward JS *et al.*: Haemodynamically significant atherosclerotic renal artery stenosis: MR angiographic features. *Radiology* **205:** 128–136, 1997
15. De Cobelli F, Mellone R, Salvioni M *et al.*: Renal artery stenosis: value of screening with three-dimensional phase-contrast MR angiography with a phased-array multicoil. *Radiology* **201:** 697–703, 1996
16. Gibson M, Cook G, Gedroyc W: Case report: renal transplant artery stenosis – three cases where magnetic resonance angiography was superior to conventional arteriography. *Br J Radiol* **68:** 89–92, 1995
17. Gedroyc WM, Negus R, Al-Kutoubi A: Magnetic resonance angiography of renal transplants. *Lancet* **339:** 789–791, 1992
18. Holland GA, Dougherty L, Carpenter JP *et al.*: Breath-hold ultrafast three-dimensional gadolinium-enhanced MR angiography of the aorta and the renal and other visceral abdominal arteries. *Am J Roent* **166:** 971–981, 1996
19. Hany TF, McKinnon GC, Leung DA *et al.*: Optimization of contrast timing for breath-hold three-dimensional MR angiography. *J Mag Res Imas* **7:** 551–556, 1997
20. Leung DA, McKinnon GC, Davis CPC *et al.*: Breath-hold contrast-enhanced three-dimensional MR angiography. *Radiology* **201:** 569–571, 1996
21. Wilman AH, Riederer SJ, King BF *et al.*: Fluoroscopically triggered contrast-enhanced three-dimensional MR angiography with elliptical centric view order: application to the renal arteries. *Radiology* **205:** 137–146, 1997
22. Prince MR, Grist TM, Debatin JF: MRA basic concepts. In: *Three-dimensional Contrast MR Angiography*, 2nd edn, pp. 12–18. London: Springer, 1999
23. Snidow JJ, Johnson MS, Harris VJ: Three-dimensional gadolinium-enhanced MR angiography for aortoiliac inflow assessment plus renal artery screening in a single breath-hold. *Radiology* **198:** 725–732, 1996

Endovascular renal interventions in high-risk patients

Tony Nicholson

INTRODUCTION

The majority of renal endovascular interventions in the Western world are the result of atherosclerosis. Arteritis and middle aortic syndrome are seen more commonly in the Indian subcontinent and Asia, occurring in younger patients. In these countries young patients are in a high risk category, but in this chapter I will deal only with those high risk patients in whom the primary indication for revascularization is atherosclerotic renal artery disease causing renal insufficiency.

RATIONALE FOR RENAL REVASCULARIZATION

Renal artery atherosclerosis is very common and affects up to 53% of patients at postmortem.[1] It has also been shown in prospective studies that the cumulative instance of progression from less than 60% stenosis to greater than 60% stenosis of the renal artery is 48% at 3 years, and from greater than 60% stenosis to occlusion, 7% at 3 years (Fig. 1a–c).[2] In the same study, the risk of losing more than 1cm in renal length is 19% at 1 year in kidneys with a greater than 60% stenosis. Atherosclerotic renal artery disease has been recognized as an increasingly important cause of renal insufficiency. The exact incidence of the disease causing renal failure is unknown, but in the elderly age group (50 years +) it may account for 14% of patients on renal replacement programmes.[3] The mortality of patients with atherosclerotic renal artery disease on dialysis is higher than any other group, even diabetics. The 2-year survival of 56% in these patients is mainly due to co-morbid disease and dialysis withdrawal. As dialysis is expensive, costing around £20 000 ($32 000) per year in the UK, the cost benefits of effective renal revascularization to preserve renal function are obvious.[4]

WHAT IS A HIGH RISK PATIENT?

It should be obvious by now that the title of this chapter is something of a misnomer, as all patients undergoing renal revascularization for atherosclerotic disease are at high risk. However, risk is relative. A patient with bilateral renal artery stenosis and normal sized kidneys is at less risk from revascularization than a patient with a single kidney and a 70% stenosis. In turn, that patient is at less risk than a patient with a single kidney and a critical 90%+ stenosis. Patients with acute occlusion of a renal

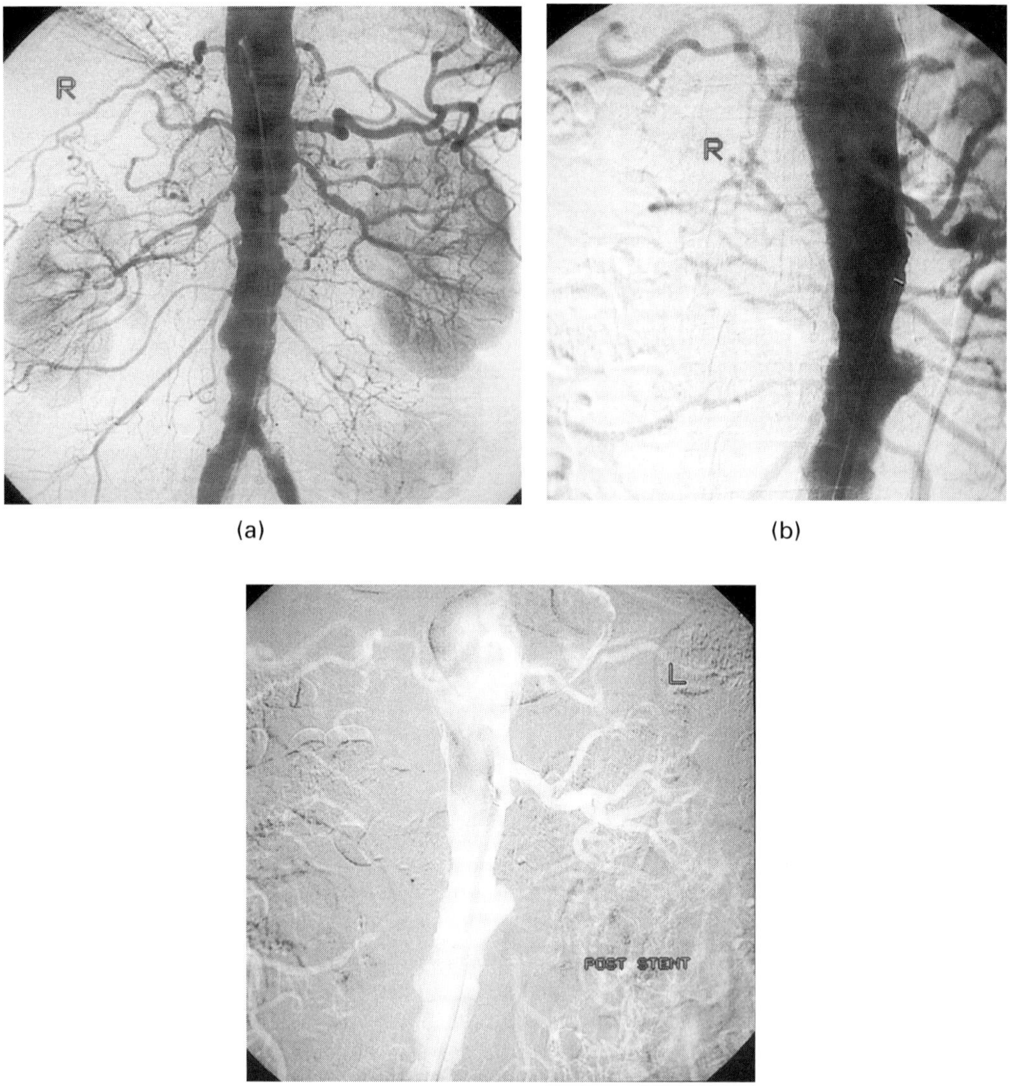

(a) (b)

(c)

Fig. 1. This patient with normal serum creatinine underwent angiography for intermittent claudication. This showed a severe stenosis of the right renal artery and a moderate stenosis of the left renal artery (a). After 3 months he presented with flash pulmonary oedema and poor left ventricular function. Repeat angiography with a view to PTRA demonstrated that the right renal artery had progressed to occlusion (b). Renal size, which had been 8.7cm had decreased to 7.2cm. No attempt was made to cross the lesion. The gradient across the left renal stenosis was 45mmHg and this was stented so that the patient could be prescribed an ACE inhibitor (c).

artery to a single kidney are also at extremely high risk of spending the rest of their lives on dialysis. The patient who has a single kidney with a critically stenosed renal artery and severe atherosclerotic coronary artery and cerebrovascular disease has the highest risk of all. There are some that would argue that these patients should not undergo revascularization, but not to do so is to condemn them to dialysis for the rest of their short lives, with all the economic and quality of life implications that this has.

PRE-PROCEDURAL CONSIDERATIONS

Vascular radiologists are confronted by these high risk patients frequently. In many ways they are the Achilles heel of renal revascularization. They often have longstanding hypertension and renal function that has slowly been deteriorating but which is now accelerating. An accurate test to predict response to revascularization does not exist. The only proof that renal failure and hypertension are renovascular in origin is cure after treatment. This is not a practical screening test. The 'suck it and see' approach is pragmatic but undoubtedly partly explains suboptimal results for endovascular renal revascularization. Although many surgeons would argue that surgery still has a major role, many of the patients who at present undergo endovascular revascularization would not be considered for surgery as this is a rapidly aging atherosclerotic population with a multitude of risk factors (Fig. 2a, b).

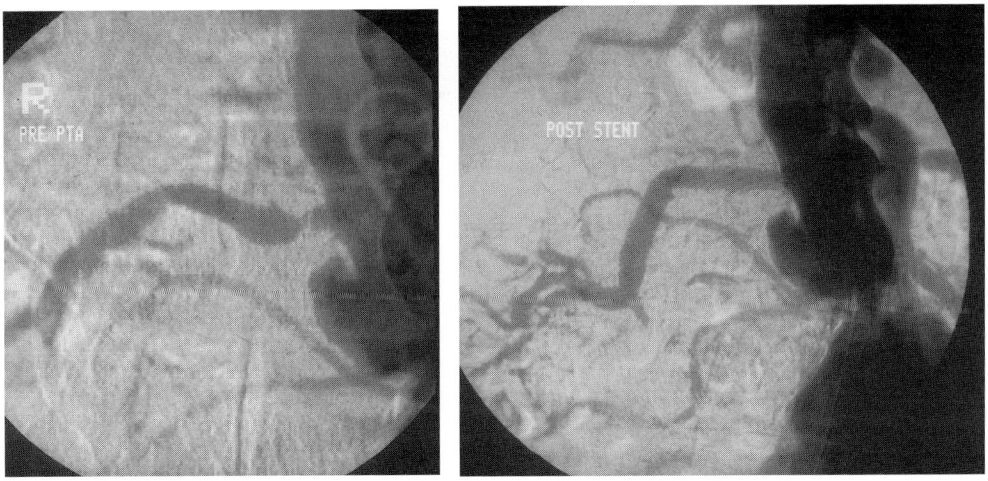

(a) (b)

Fig. 2. This 72-year-old man with severe aortoiliac disease, a chronically occluded left renal artery and a severe stenosis of the right renal artery (a) with small vessel disease causing increasingly deteriorating renal function was considered unfit for surgery because of a myocardial infarction 4 months previously and chronic airways disease. Renal stenting (b) stabilized his renal function and he was never dialysed. He died 4 months later after a further myocardial infarction.

Before considering revascularization other causes of renal insufficiency should be excluded. Significant proteinuria would suggest other non-vascular aetiology. Renal biopsy has been useful in helping to decide whether to revascularize by demonstrating features such as widespread glomerular hyalinization and extensive atheroembolic disease, which indicate irreversible renal damage. However, in my experience renal physicians are wary of biopsy of the single kidney in the type of population described above.

TIMING OF REVASCULARIZATION

Impaired renal function in itself is not an indication for revascularization. It is far more important to monitor a trend and act in the face of deterioration. Timing of renal revascularization is controversial. It may be difficult to justify intervention with only a minor elevation of serum creatinine, yet on the other hand we know that the results are poor once serum creatinine is over 350μmol/litre. It is therefore vital to monitor renal function and renal size. At present most renal physicians monitor at 6- or 12-month intervals. However, this may not be frequent enough in the patient with a single, or dominant kidney and a critical stenosis. In these patients either the disease is static or they will have occluded at acute presentation in crashing renal failure. The monitoring of renal size is mainly done by ultrasound at present but operator error can easily miss a 5 mm change in size and I would suggest that T1 or T2 weighted coronal magnetic resonance imaging (MRI) is the best way of monitoring renal size. Any change in function or size in the wrong direction should precipitate intervention.

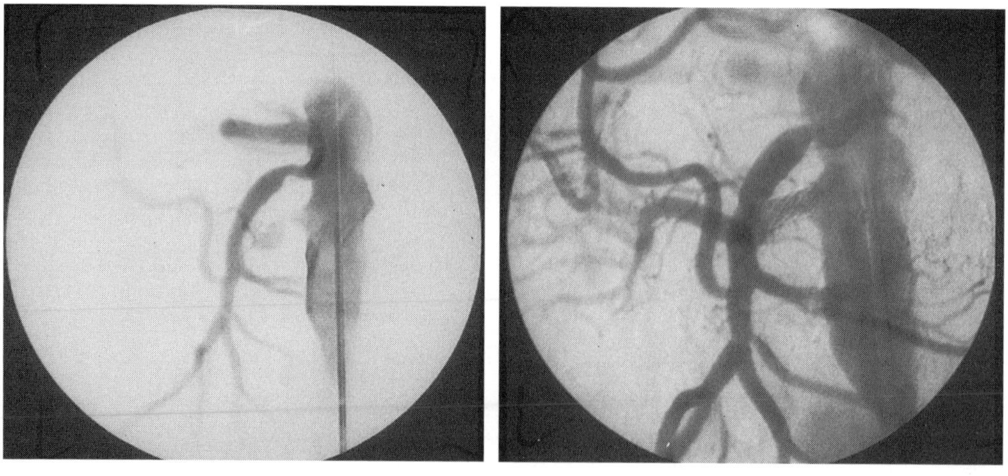

(a) (b)

Fig. 3. This 67-year-old man had only mildly elevated, stable, serum creatinine despite having an occluded left renal artery and a critical stenosis of his left renal artery (a). His left ventricular function was 37%. ACE inhibition was prescribed and renal function deteriorated rapidly. The ostial stenosis was crossed with a coronary balloon and wire and predilated. A 6mm renal stent was then inserted (b) and renal function returned to pre ACE inhibitor levels. The patient is still alive with stable renal function 3 years later.

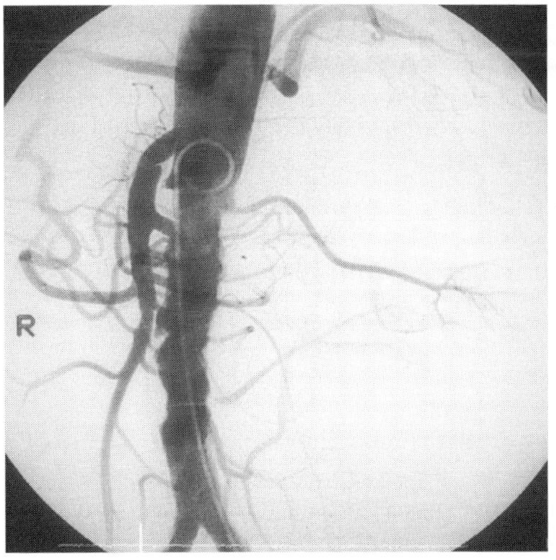

(a)

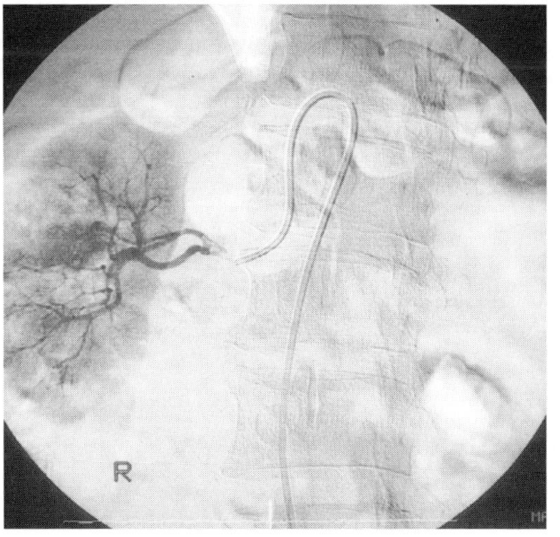

(b)

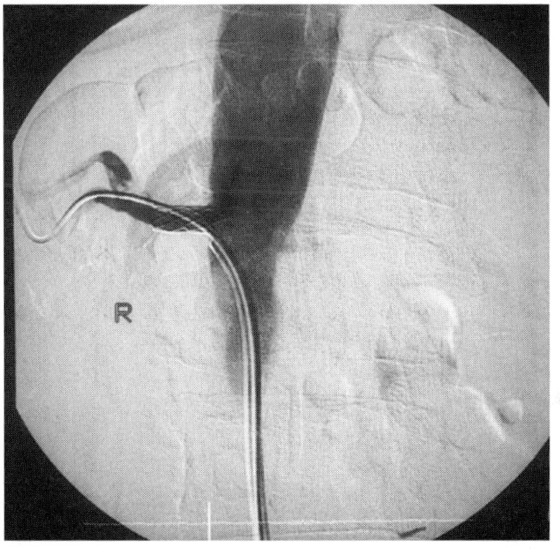

(c)

Fig. 4. A 62-year-old man presented with oliguria due to acute renal failure. Ultrasound revealed a 7.5cm left kidney and a 10.2cm right kidney. Angiography 10 days after admission (a) revealed bilateral renal artery occlusion with just a small polar branch to the left lower pole. The right renal artery ostium was engaged with a Sidewinder 2 catheter (b). Selective angiography revealed an ostial stenosis with thrombus beyond but normal intrarenal arteries. The ostium was stented with a 6mm balloon mounted stent (c) and 2mg of recombinant tissue plasminogen activator injected directly into the artery. Renal function slowly improved and at 1 month he was no longer dialysis-dependant. Renal function remains stable and only slightly elevated at 10 months.

Serum creatinine can be normal even in patients with a single kidney where the artery is stenosed. The decision to intervene under these circumstances is difficult. One good indication is where left ventricular function is poor and angiotensin converting enzyme (ACE) inhibition is required. Percutaneous transluminal renal artery angioplasty (PTRA) and stenting will allow this (Fig. 3a, b).

Where an artery is completely occluded, but there is evidence that the kidney is greater than 8.5cm in length and angiography demonstrates a good collateral supply, it might be possible to revascularize the occluded artery and rescue the patient from renal dialysis (Fig. 4a–c).

ANGIOPLASTY OR STENTING?

The controversy regarding angioplasty and/or stenting revolves around atherosclerotic renal artery disease and particularly ostial disease. The anatomy of atherosclerotic renal artery disease is heterogeneous, with stenoses caused by purely aortic lesions, true renal artery lesions and a mixture of both.[5] Spiral computed tomography (CT) studies have recently shown that lesions within 1cm of the aortic wall on angiography are, in fact, ostial lesions.[6] The implication of this is that a great majority of atherosclerotic renal artery lesions are ostial. Until the development of stents, surgery was the treatment of choice for ostial lesions, as technical success rates

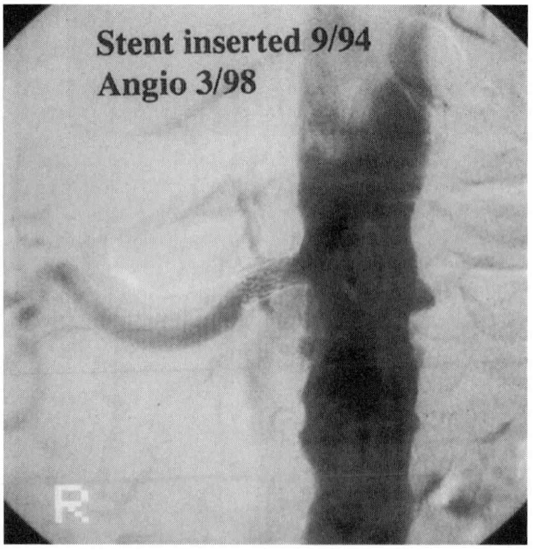

Fig. 5. This balloon mounted stent was inserted into a single stenosed right renal artery for deteriorating renal function. During angiography for claudication 42 months later, the opportunity was taken to image the stent. There is minor, smooth and regular neointimal hyperplasia only. The stent was widely patent and the renal function normal.

for angioplasty with these lesions were as low as 25%. A recent randomized trial comparing stents with angioplasty in ostial renal artery disease has shown a significantly higher procedural success rate and a significant reduction in stenosis rates at 6 months with stents.[7] This randomized study does not give any details about long-term clinical benefits of stenting. Nevertheless, the technical benefits of stenting at the renal ostium and the greater long-term patency (Fig. 5), mean that angioplasty and stenting should be the treatment of choice for the majority of renal arterial disease.

CONTRAST AGENTS AND THE DIAGNOSIS OF RENAL ARTERY STENOSIS IN THE HIGH RISK PATIENT

In this group of patients though ultrasound is useful to measure size, and magnetic resonance angiography (MRA) can diagnose renal artery stenosis with a high sensitivity but moderate specificity, digital subtraction angiography remains the gold standard for diagnosis. However, in high risk patients there is a significant incidence of contrast nephropathy. In a randomized study of patients with abnormal renal function, carbon dioxide angiography and gadolinium angiography were superior to non-ionic contrast media; 5/13 developing deteriorating renal function in the contrast media group and 1/24 in the CO_2/gadolinium group.[8] It is my current preference to use gadolinium but CO_2 angiography is potentially the procedure of choice.

TECHNIQUE IN HIGH RISK PATIENTS

Fully informed consent is vital before any form of renal revascularization is undertaken. Patients should be aware of the high risk nature of their disease. They should be told that although PTRA and stenting are generally safe, the literature evidence at the moment suggests that there is at least a 1% chance of losing a kidney. In the uninephric patient this has obvious implications. Patients with renal insufficiency should be aware of deteriorating renal function following the procedure though an explanation regarding the alternatives of surgery and continuing medical treatment should accompany this.

All patients should be monitored throughout the procedure by electrocardiogram (ECG), blood pressure and pulse oximetry. In addition, it is wise to have an intravenous infusion running slowly, to guard against precipitous falls in blood pressure, especially in patients with concurrent cardiovascular and cerebrovascular disease. It is our practice to catheterize all patients in renal failure in order to have accurate measurements of urine output.

Careful note should be made of the morphology and anatomy of the renal arteries. An extremely ptotic kidney is better approached from the arm than the groin. This can be achieved via 6 or 8F sheaths. At 6F percutaneous puncture is possible but at 8F a cutdown is advised. Our normal technique is to use a curved femorovisceral catheter, such as a Sidewinder, from the groin, or a multipurpose catheter from the arm, together with either a soft tipped Benson 0.035 wire (Mallinkrodt UK), or a curved hydrophilic wire (Fig. 6a–c). However, our technique is modified where there is a critical stenosis (Fig. 7a–c).

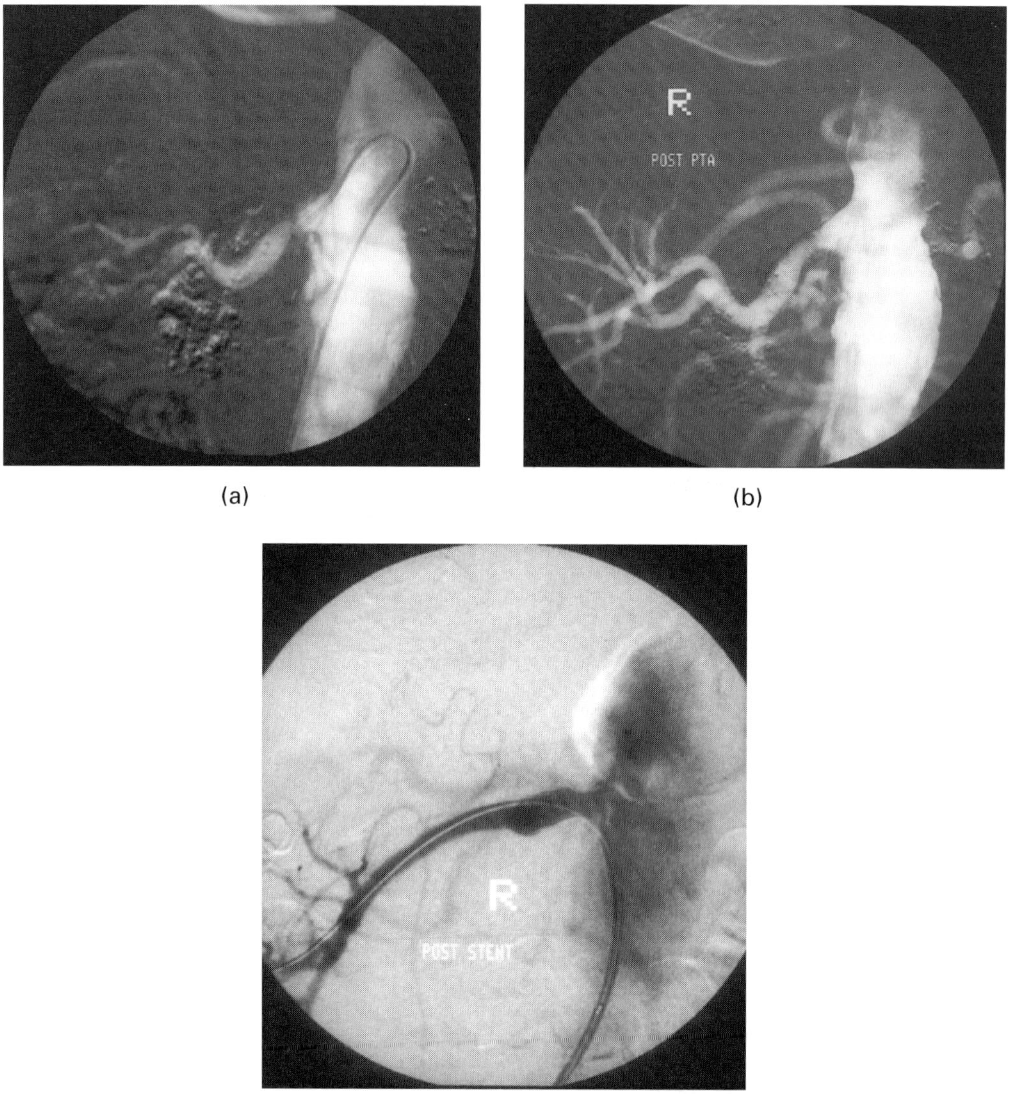

(a) (b) (c)

Fig. 6. A 75-year-old man with a single right kidney presented with deteriorating renal function. Angiography revealed a moderate right renal artery stenosis that could be crossed conventionally with a femorovisceral catheter and wire (a). Balloon angioplasty left a 20–30% residual stenosis (b) and the artery was therefore stented (c) with a good result. Renal function stabilized. Note how the stent has straightened out the right renal artery. The patient died 1 year later after a myocardial infarction.

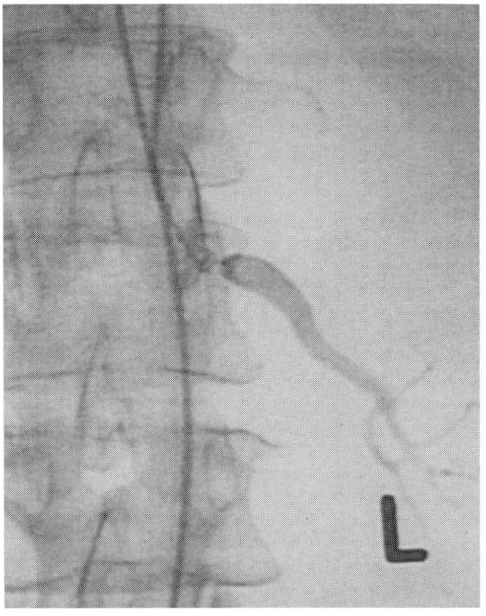

(a)

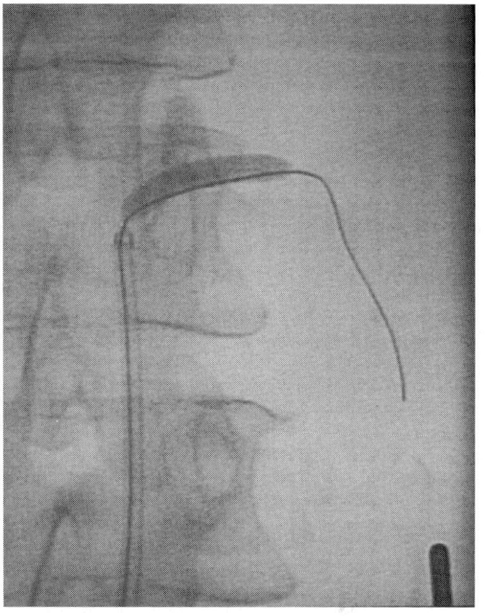

(b)

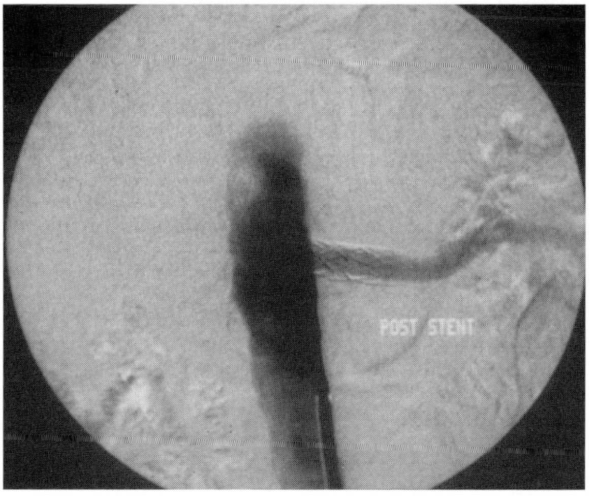

(c)

Fig. 7. A 56-year-old woman presented with acute renal failure and unstable hypertension. Aortography revealed an occluded right renal artery and a faintly visible left renal artery. Selective left renal angiography was performed revealing a critical stenosis. This was crossed with a coronary wire and a 4mm coronary balloon (b). The coronary guide catheter was then passed into the renal artery and a TAD wire inserted. A 7 mm balloon mounted renal stent was then inserted across the lesion straightening out the artery (c). Renal function stabilized and the patient remained dialysis-independent for 3 years. After this time her renal function again deteriorated. Angiography revealed a patent stent but small vessel disease. She died 4 weeks after commencing dialysis following a myocardial infarction.

Ostial plaque can be extremely friable but also occasionally extremely hard. Wires and blunt-ended catheters can dissect the plaque, causing complete occlusion. Occasionally, though a wire crosses the stenosis, the catheter proves too large to go through the opening in the stenosis. It seems logical under these circumstances to use wires and catheters designed to traverse critical stenoses in small tortuous arteries. Such systems have been developed for the coronary arteries. Our preference is the 0.014 extra support wire (ACS Guidant, Indianapolis, USA), whose tip can be shaped to order, over the puncture needle, prior to use. This can be inserted and used to cross the stenosis via a 6F Judkins 4 right coronary guiding catheter (Cordis, UK). Once the wire has been gently manipulated across the stenosis, a low profile monorail 4mm coronary balloon, such as the Worldpass (Cordis, UK) or Rocket (ACS Guidant) can be used to pre-dilate the stenosis. On balloon deflation the patency of the angioplastied site can be checked with 300 strength contrast via the guide catheter and if the stenosis is now widely patent the 6F coronary guide can be passed into the artery over the coronary balloon catheter and guidewire.

Once beyond the stenosis the coronary guidewire and catheter are removed and replaced with a TAD 11 wire (Mallinkrodt, UK). This is a tapered guidewire with a very atraumatic 0.018 platinum tip, which can be placed well out in the kidney without causing spasm. The remainder of the wire rapidly thickens to 0.035 and provides very good support for angioplasty catheters and stent balloon catheters. Once this wire is in position the coronary guide catheter can be removed and a stent deployed. Our preference is for pre-mounted balloon expandable stents of which there are several on the market. Most of these stents are extremely flexible and easy to deploy from a femoral approach, with minimal shortening. They can be deployed with millimeter accuracy. Stent size varies between 6 and 8mm. We usually try to place a stent to the exact size of the renal artery, though this is often difficult to estimate. It is best to be cautious in these patients and by and large 6mm is a good default size. Most patients experience some loin pain during inflation but if this is severe it suggests overdilatation and risks arterial rupture (Fig 8a–c). Once the stent has been deployed, angiography is performed through the long introducer sheath with the wire in place. If all is well, the wire is removed and further check angiography is performed in the anterioposterior and 20° left oblique projection. It is our usual practice to give the patients 5000 units of intra-arterial heparin prior to crossing the stenosis but other than aspirin, no anticoagulants are prescribed following the procedure, providing there are no complications. It is important that the entire lesion is stented. I try to leave approximately 1mm of stent beyond the ostium in the aorta. Clearly it is very difficult to be as accurate as this but it is better to leave a small amount of stent in the aorta than not to cover the whole lesion. It is extremely important before stenting to have the right obliquity on the C-arm so that the renal ostium is seen without any distortion.

WHICH STENT?

There are at least eight different stents on the market that can be used for stenting renal arteries. The ideal stent should be very radioopaque, have no discernible

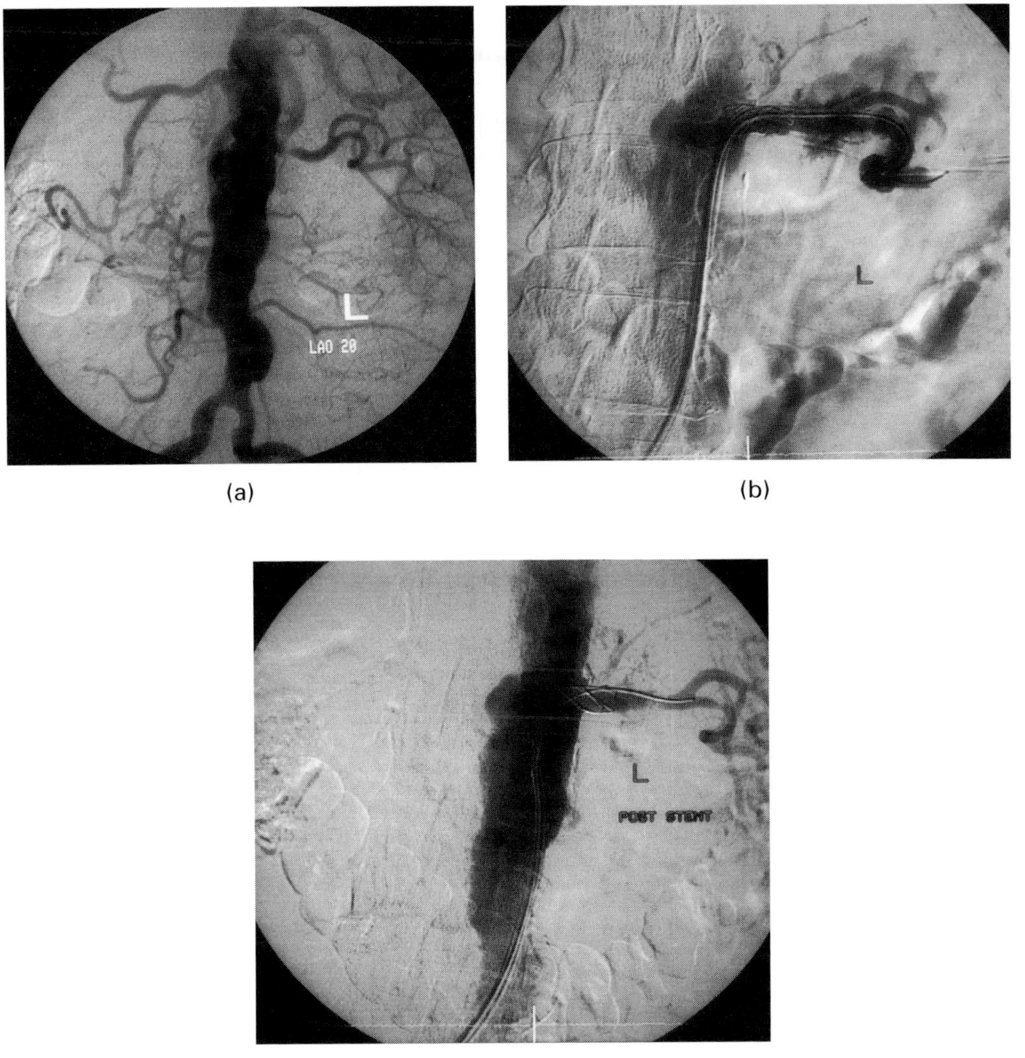

(a) (b)

(c)

Fig. 8. A 68-year-old woman with progressive deterioration in renal function underwent angiography which revealed an occluded right renal artery and a critical stenosis of the left renal artery (a). Predilatation with coronary wire and balloon was uneventful and a 6mm balloon-mounted stent was inserted across the ostial stenosis. The patient experienced great pain as the stent was deployed and as the balloon was deflated, blood pressure dropped precipitously. Check angiography revealed a ruptured renal artery with contrast extravasation (c). After almost 1 hour of balloon tamponade the artery was patent with no further bleeding. Surprisingly, renal function remained stable and there were no immediate sequelae (but see Fig. 10).

shortening, should negotiate tight angles in delivery, have good radial strength, be available in lengths from 12 to 20mm and in diameters from 5 to 8mm. None of the current stents satisfies all of these criteria, though the renal Bridge stent (MedtronicAVE Santa Rosa, USA) and Jostent (Jomed, Malmo, Sweden) come close.

PTRA AND STENTING IN RENAL TRANSPLANTS

Renal artery stenosis in the renal transplant presents several problems. For these patients the loss of a renal artery is a disaster. They have often waited for many years on dialysis for a suitable organ to become available. Increasingly, they have received their transplant from a live donor, most often a relative. The loss of an otherwise healthy transplant kidney due to a renal artery stenosis and revascularization procedure is a disaster of major proportions but patients have to be aware of the possibility. However, in the face of deteriorating renal function, there is very little choice.

Cadaveric transplants are invariably anastomosed end-to-side to the recipient external iliac artery with a Carell patch of donor aorta. True anastomotic stenoses are therefore very rare and the lesion is usually several millimeters into the renal artery beyond the anastomosis (Fig. 9a, b). Live donor transplants are usually anastomosed end-to-end with the recipient internal iliac artery. Prior to any endovascular procedure, comprehensive angiography and multiple projections should be performed to confirm the stenosis and to work out the anatomy fully so that the best approach can be used.

Almost always a live donor transplant is best approached from the contralateral artery across the aortic bifurcation. The more common cadaveric transplant can often be dealt with from an ipsilateral approach (Fig. 9b). Frequently the donor artery is tortuous and much longer than the vein, making the artery very difficult to catheterize. For this reason it has been suggested that flexible stents, such as the Wallstent, are best used in these circumstances. My own preference is to cross the tortuous artery and to try to place a long 8F flexible sheath to the lesion. Again, I prefer deployment of a short balloon mounted stent after pre-dilatation. Most renal transplant stenoses can be crossed with conventional 0.035 wires and catheters. However, where the stenosis is critical and 'pin hole', again I use coronary balloons and wires to pre-dilate the lesion.

ACUTE OCCLUSION OF RENAL ARTERIES

The true incidence of acute renal failure secondary to renal artery occlusion is unknown. Most patients investigated by angiography under these circumstances are usually known to have renal artery stenosis. Ideally, any patient who presents in acute catastrophic renal failure with no obvious cause with a history of arterial disease (claudication/limb ischaemia, angina/previous myocardial infarction or transient ischaemic attacks/stroke) should undergo angiography. Often these patients will have had normal renal function prior to the acute catastrophic event.

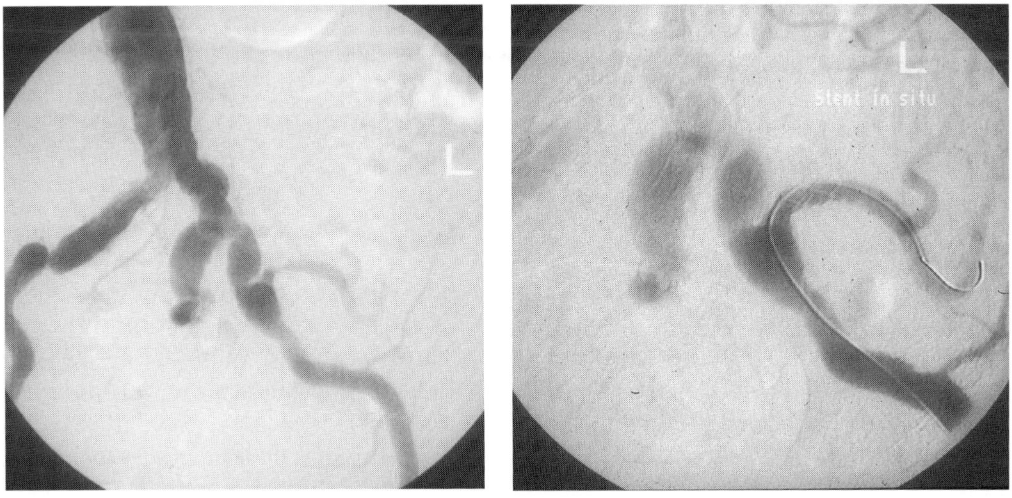

(a) (b)

Fig. 9. Angiography in this 62-year-old man who had undergone cadaveric renal transplantation 4 years previously, but who was now in renal failure and hypertensive, revealed a transplant artery stenosis beyond the anastomosis (a). This was crossed with a hydrophilic wire from the ipsilateral groin and a balloon mounted stent inserted with good and lasting clinical results.

This is due to the development of extensive collaterals over the length of time the stenosis developed. The occlusion usually occurs when blood flow through the collaterals exceeds that through the renal artery. There is usually therefore a plug of thrombus within the stenosis and it is possible to cross the lesion with conventional catheters and guidewires. There is certainly absolutely nothing to lose in attempting such revascularization (Fig. 4 a–c).

Whilst time is an important factor, it should not unduly influence the decision to request angiography and revascularization. Though it is said that the kidney has a 48-hour ischaemia time, this is not based on a large clinical series and successful recanalization of occluded renal arteries with good clinical outcomes have been reported up to 28 days post-occlusion. The collateral supply is all important. We have used a single bolus of thrombolytic into the renal artery to dissolve thrombus after stenting, where there was a considerable thrombus load. There is no good evidence to support this but it seems a reasonable manoeuvre. The result of such intervention in occluded arteries is rarely immediately successful and often it takes a week to a month for renal function to stabilize. However, where the kidney is of good length (greater than 9cm) and where there is no evidence of small vessel disease, a good result with the patient coming off dialysis can be anticipated after revascularization.

RESULTS

In this high risk subset of patients both technical and outcome criteria (restenosis rate and clinical outcome) should be considered when considering the success or otherwise of these procedures.

Technical success

The definition of technical success means that the obstructing lesion is crossed with a balloon and following dilatation the amount of recoil is less than 20%. Recoil is no longer a problem with the introduction of stenting. With balloon angioplasty technical success rates in atherosclerotic renal artery disease have been reported to be as low as 20%[9] but with stents the technical success rate is much higher, all workers reporting a technical success rate of 90%+. Not only is recoil no longer a problem but pressure gradients are also abolished.[10] One randomized study showed a significant difference in procedural success with stents: 88% versus PTRA 57% ($p<0.05$).[7]

Restenosis rate

There are many problems when assessing the data on restenosis with PTRA.

1. Because of ethical problems many studies have no angiographic follow-up.
2. Where angiography is performed it is often only in patients with clinical recurrence.
3. There has been a failure to separate atherosclerotic renal artery disease from fibromuscular hyperplasia and a failure to distinguish the hypertensive patient from the patient in renal failure.
4. The proportion of ostial to non-ostial lesions has not been stated.
5. There is no agreement on what constitutes a restenosis though most use 50% reduction in diameter.

Data for renal stents is much more precise and overall an analysis of the literature suggests an 85% patency rate at 12 months.

Clinical results

Criteria for success are imperfect but it is generally accepted that improvement equals more than 20% reduction in serum creatinine over baseline, stability equals less than 20% increase or decrease and failure equals more than 20% increase in serum creatinine over baseline.

However, in the group of patients described here it should be appreciated that a 20% increase when serum creatinine is slightly elevated represents a greater loss of renal function than when it is 300–400μmol/litre. It is naive to believe that when patients have severe atherosclerosis causing critical stenoses and occlusions, revascularization of the main renal artery prevents the progression of disease at small vessel and glomerular level. It has been shown that the effect of revascularization is to slow down the progression of renal failure and hopefully delay the requirement for dialysis.[11] As stated earlier the cost of dialysis and the life expectancy in this group of patients makes the achievement of this very desirable.

The literature must be interpreted with caution. For instance in many series, patients were taking ACE inhibitors prior to stenting, stopping them afterwards. Improvements in renal function could therefore be due to cessation of ACE inhibition. Nevertheless, the rule of thirds seems to apply equally to successful PTRA and to stenting. That is, approximately 33% improve, 33% are stable and 33% have deteriorating renal function.

Results in our series of PTRA and stenting in 54 patients with single kidneys are consistent with this : 62% improving or remaining stable and 38% deteriorating. At 1-year follow-up 88% were not on dialysis though six had died. The mortality rate in this group of patients from other causes is high.

Overall our experience and that of others is that the initial degree of renal impairment is possibly the most important factor influencing outcome. If the presenting renal function has been allowed to drift to greater than 500μmol/litre, 90% are dialysis-dependent within 3 months. However, this is not an absolute rule and some patients do respond to renal revascularization. In particular patients who acutely occlude their renal arteries and present with serum creatinine between 600 and 1000μmol/litre can be helped.

This is also true of renal transplants. I have personal experience of two patients with long time cadaver transplants, both of whom developed acute renal failure and were dialysis-dependent for 2 and 3 weeks. In both cases function was restored, though in the second case the graft finally failed 12 months post-stent. However, once again in terms of quality of life and simple economics, 12 months dialysis-free life was important to the patient and the health economist.

Transplant renal arterial stenting can be also be performed for renovascular hypertension and deteriorating renal function. In a series of ten patients with transplant renal artery stenoses, stents were inserted in nine, one failing due to difficult anatomy. Blood pressure control was improved significantly in eight (mean systolic blood pressure 186-142mmHg and mean number of antihypertensive drugs from 3.1 to 1.4) and renal function improved in six (mean SeCr 365 to 180μmoles/litre) [personal communication].

Another patient with a live donor transplant underwent stenting of a stenosed transplant artery for deteriorating renal function but this had no effect on serum creatinine. Only when his cytotoxic drugs were stopped did renal function return to normal emphasizing the multifactorial reasons for renal failure.

Complications

Both PTRA and stent series report complications from 0 to 64% in all types of patient and for all clinical indications. In the group discussed in this chapter it is difficult to make meaningful comparisons with the surgical alternative, as many would not be operated upon for anaesthetic reasons.

Procedure-related deaths have been reported and usually result from renal bleeding from ruptured renal arteries (Fig. 8b) or iliac arteries. Perforation of a renal artery is, however, not always catastrophic and can often be managed with balloon tamponade and ice cold saline perfusion (Fig. 8c). Good renal function can be maintained though close follow-up is recommended to detect pseudoaneurysms and further stenoses at the perforation site (Fig. 10a–c).

The literature suggests that renal occlusion, during attempts to cross renal arterial stenoses, occur at a rate of 3%. However, as stated, the literature is not specific for the high risk patient. In the critically stenosed renal artery, occlusion rates may be as high

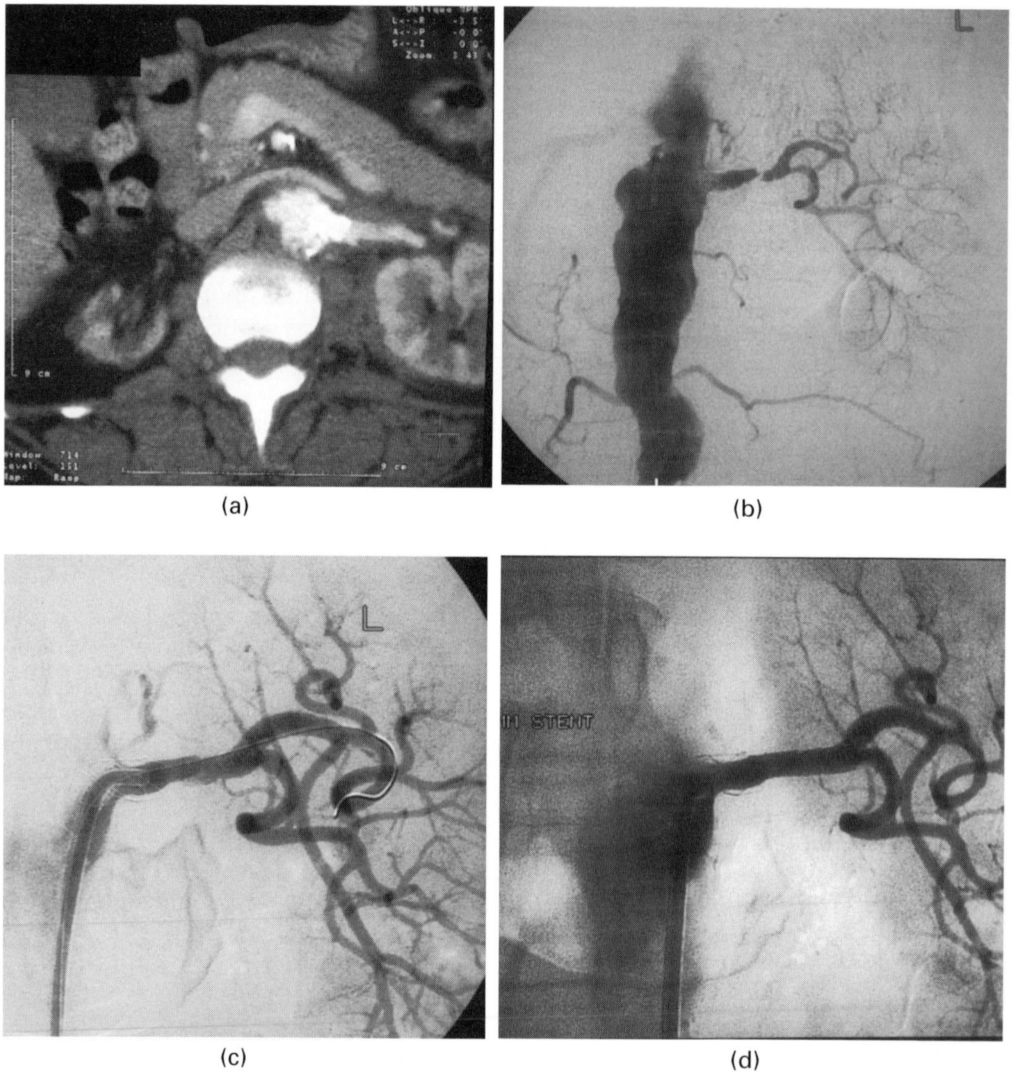

Fig. 10. The patient shown in Fig. 8, underwent a check CT scan 1 week after the PTRA and stent procedure (a). No significant complication was recognized at that time. Though renal function was stable, a check angiogram at 3 months revealed a critical main renal artery stenosis at the site of the iatrogenic perforation (b). After discussion about the surgical possibilities the lesion was crossed using a High Torque Floppy coronary wire (ACSGuidant) and dilated to 4mm. This again produced dissection (c), and therefore a 4mm NIRoyale coronary stent (Boston Scientific, USA) was inserted with a good result (d). Renal function was stable 6 months post-procedure.

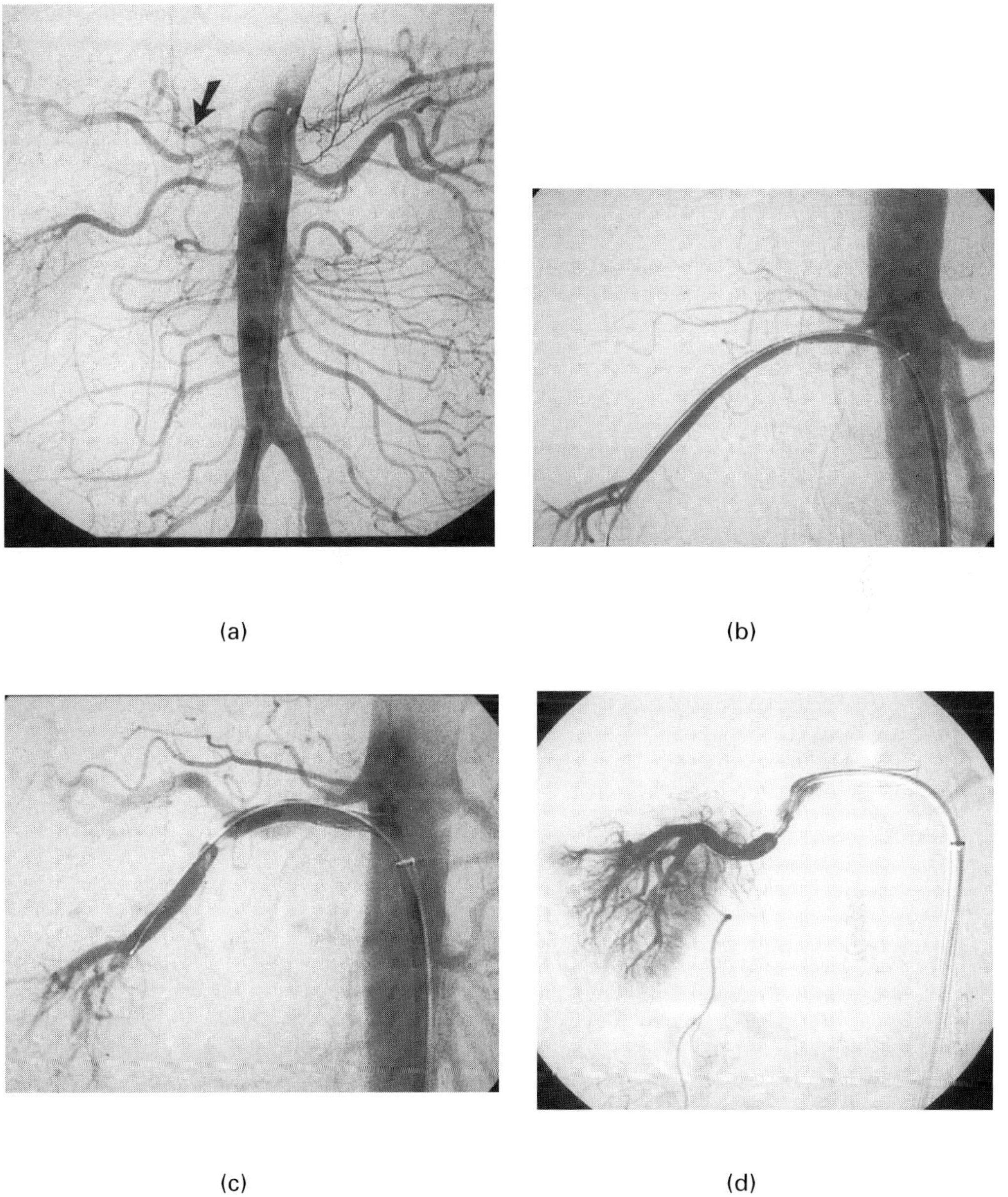

(a) (b)

(c) (d)

Fig. 11. A 38-year-old man with poorly controlled hypertension taking three antihypertensive drugs, underwent angiography (a) which demonstrated an occluded right main renal artery with a well developed collateral circulation (arrow) and a severely stenosed but still patent lower pole branch. The left renal artery was normal. It was not possible to cross the main renal artery occlusion but it was felt that if the stenosis in the lower pole branch was dealt with, ACE inhibition would control his blood pressure. Predilatation caused what was believed to be distal spasm (b). However, after stenting this was clearly an obstructive lesion (c) and attempts to angioplasty the site resulted in further dissection (d). It was not possible to pass a stent across the recently stented ostium. Renal function remained normal and ACE inhibition controlled blood pressure.

as 7–10% (Fig. 11a-d) . In the patient with a single kidney, or the transplant, patient this is catastrophic and often leads to emergency surgery. In our own experience of 54 patients with such lesions we have had no procedure-related occlusions using coronary systems to predilate stenoses and would recommend this technique.

There is a current trend towards primary stenting of renal arterial stenoses. The argument goes that it shortens procedure time, saves the cost of an angioplasty balloon and inserts the stent into a virgin stenosis avoiding dissections and cholesterol emboli. These are all good arguments in favour of this approach. However, a 90%+ stenosis in a 6mm renal artery may have an opening of 0.6mm or less. As the diameter of a 5Fr 6mm balloon catheter with a mounted stent is 2.5mm it is obvious that primary stenting can lead to occlusion, failure to cross (requiring removal of the system) or, if successful, considerable trauma which presumably causes particle embolization. This approach is therefore not to be recommended, in my opinion, in the high risk patient. In the transplant artery where the approach can be tortuous, predilatation is also recommended.

Early thrombosis is reported in 1% of renal arterial stents. This is from early series and is now almost unheard of. Anticoagulation is only recommended where there has been a technical problem and there are doubts about the full expansion of the stent or where there has been dissection distally causing potential run-off problems (Fig. 8c).

In all series permanent and temporary loss of renal function following PTRA and stenting occurs in 4–6%. Early on this may be due to cholesterol embolization or contrast nephropathy. The latter typically occurs within 12–24 hours, deteriorates for 3–5 days and slowly recovers over 7–10 days. The use of CO_2 angiography and/or gadolinium contrast agents is an important new development in this group of patients and can avoid post-procedural deterioration renal function (Fig.12, b). Cholesterol embolization usually reveals itself insidiously over days or weeks. In the future the use of catheters with distal 'trapping umbrellas' to capture emboli during PTRA and stenting will prevent this complication.

SUMMARY

It seems logical to revascularize the kidney where there is a renal artery stenosis in the face of deteriorating renal function. Stenting and PTRA have increased the number and type of patients who can undergo revascularization. Most literature series report a mixed bag of patients with hypertension, varying degrees of renal failure and degrees of stenosis. The patients discussed in this chapter represent the worse end of this spectrum. Technical considerations such as predilatation with small wires and balloons, the use of stents and non-iodinated contrast agents can greatly aid in technical success.

The acutely occluded renal artery should never be written off; PTRA and stenting can be successful after several weeks of apparent ischaemia. All of this applies *par excellence* to the transplant artery the loss of which can be a major catastrophe, leading to dialysis for the patient, bitterness from any live donor and potential successful litigation against the radiologist who has not adopted every precaution to ensure a successful outcome. It goes without saying that these procedures should only be carried out by experienced operators.

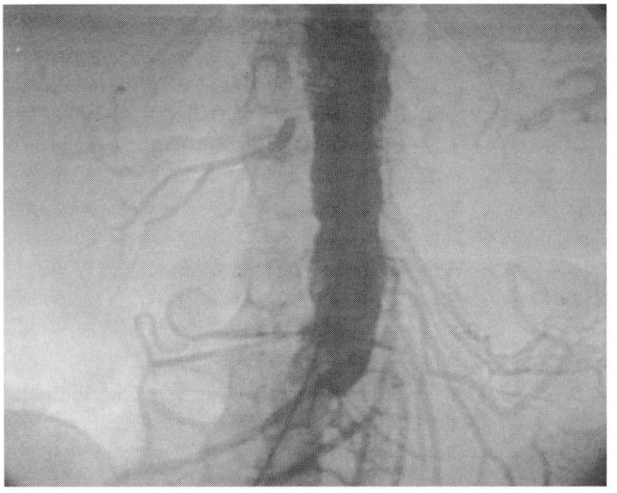

(a)

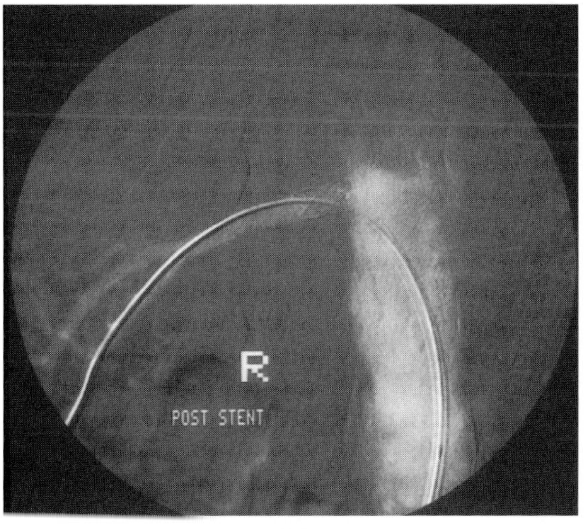

(b)

Fig. 12. A 69-year-old man with deteriorating renal function underwent CO_2 angiography (a) that revealed an occluded left renal artery and a critical stenosis of the right renal artery. This was predilated with a coronary balloon to 4mm and a balloon mounted stent inserted with good technical (b) and clinical results.

REFERENCES

1. Holley KE, Hunt JC, Brown AL *et al.*: Renal artery stenosis: A clinical pathological study in normotensive and hypertensive patients. *Am J Med* **37:** 14–20, 1964
2. Zierler RE, Bergelin RO, Isaacson JA *et al.*: Natural history of atherosclerotic renal artery stenosis: A prospective study with duplex or sonography. *J Vasc Surg* **19:** 250–255, 1994

3. Mailloux LU, Napoliteno B, Belucci A *et al.*: RVD causing end stage renal disease. Incidence, clinical correlates and outcomes: A 20 year experience. *Am J Kidney Dis* **24:** 622–625, 1994
4. Harden PN, Sheppard D, Rodger RSC *et al.*: PTRA in the treatment of chronic renal failure due to renal vascular disease. *J Nephrol* **7:** 186–188, 1994
5. Cicuto KP, McLean GK, Oleaga JA *et al.*: Renal artery stenosis: Anatomical classification for percutaneous transluminal angioplasty. *Am J Roent* **137:** 599–562, 1981
6. Kaate ER, Beek FJA, Verschuyl EJ *et al.*: Atherosclerotic renal artery stenosis, ostial or truncal. *Radiology* **199:** 637–640, 1996
7. Van de Ven PJ, Kaate ER, Beutler JJ *et al.*: Arterial stenting and balloon angioplasty in ostial osteosclerotic renovascular disease: A randomised trial. *Lancet* **353** (9149)**:** 282–286, 1999
8. Spinosa DJ, Angle JF, Hagspiel MD *et al.*: Presented at SCVIR, Orlando March 1999
9. Sos TA, Pickering TG, Sneiderman K *et al.*: PTRA in renovascular hypertension due to atheroma or FMH. *New Engl J Med* **309:** 274, 1983
10. Dorros G, Prince C, Mathiak F: Stenting of renal artery stenosis achieves better relief of obstructive lesions than balloon angioplasty. *Cathet Cardiovasc Diagn* **29:** 191–195, 1993
11. Harden PN, Macload MJ, Rodger RSC *et al.*: Effect of renal artery stenting on progression of renovascular renal failure. *Lancet* **349:** 1133–1137, 1977

The changing face of renovascular disease: a more aggressive attitude and percutaneous intervention

Frank J Criado, Eric P Wilson, Hari Gnanasekeram, Jennifer A Martin, Snehal C Patel

INTRODUCTION

Atherosclerotic renovascular disease has come under close clinical scrutiny over the past 10 years. Current treatment has evolved in parallel with refinements in percutaneous interventional techniques and the availability of endovascular stent devices allowing non-surgical endoluminal revascularization. A better understanding of renovascular disease and its consequences has been another powerful reason explaining the heightened interest in the diagnosis and treatment of this condition;[1] mainly, a clearer appreciation of the natural history of renal artery stenosis, the realization that ischaemic nephropathy is a common and potentially reversible cause of progressive renal failure, and that recurrent 'flash' pulmonary oedema and refractory angina often reflect underlying global renal ischaemia.

Renal artery duplex ultrasonography is currently the most useful non-invasive means of determining the haemodynamic significance of renal artery lesions.[2–4] Despite some limitations (intestinal gas and body habitus), colour-flow duplex ultrasound is now firmly established as the diagnostic modality of choice for screening purposes and natural history studies. Well controlled, large reported series have substantiated its accuracy, with a sensitivity and specificity of more than 95%.[4,5] It is also the ideal method to assess the haemodynamic success (or failure) of renal artery revascularization.[6,7] This is of particular relevance following stent placement as a number of patients are likely to develop restenosis that requires prompt recognition and repeat treatment to avoid possible progression to complete occlusion.

Evidence at hand suggests strongly that untreated renal artery lesions lead to progressive loss of parenchyma and kidney atrophy in a significant proportion of patients.[8] This is particularly true when the degree of renal artery stenosis is severe.[9,10] It is thus pertinent to have a high index of suspicion, and proceed with appropriate screening of patients who are likely to have renovascular lesions (Table 1). Several studies have documented the frequent occurrence of renal artery stenosis in association with coronary artery disease, peripheral arterial disease, and aneurysms.[11,12]

Atherosclerotic renovascular disease typically manifests as ostial lesions that cause stenosis at the origin of the renal artery. These are, essentially, aortic atheromas that 'spill over' into the renal arteries (and other branch vessels). Balloon angioplasty (PTA) alone has a limited role in the treatment of ostial stenoses. The advent of

Table 1. Clinical suspicion of renovascular disease

• Hypertension (medically resistant/uncontrolled)
• Deterioration of renal function precipitated by ACE inhibitors
• 'Unexplained' renal dysfunction – especially when urine shows little or no proteinuria
• Recurrent 'flash' pulmonary oedema
• Generalized, multiorgan atherosclerosis
• Asymmetry of kidneys on ultrasound[a]

ACE: Angiotensin converting enzyme.
[a] Kidney length <8cm predicts (almost universally) non-response to revascularization.

endovascular stent technology has had a major impact with higher technical success rates and, potentially, increased durability after percutaneous revascularization.

INDICATIONS FOR RENOVASCULAR INTERVENTION (TABLE 2)

- *Hypertension*, when medically resistant or poorly controlled, has been the 'classic' indication for revascularization. While renovascular disease is a common cause of secondary hypertension, the mere association of renal artery stenosis with hypertension does not constitute an indication for intervention or predict benefit. Clinical indicators to suggest potentially correctable underlying renovascular disease include onset of diastolic hypertension after age 55, refractory hypertension, development of uncontrolled (with previously well controlled) hypertension, and malignant hypertension.[13] Intervention to treat significant (75%) unilateral or bilateral stenosis is indicated in all such situations.
- *Recurrent flash pulmonary oedema* is often expression of severe bilateral renal artery stenosis or renal artery stenosis to a single-functional kidney. Elevated concentrations of angiotensin II, with direct and indirect effects on the myocardium, are the likely culprit in this setting.[14] Unstable or crescendo angina may also be part of the same syndrome.[15] Diagnosis of renovascular disease should be considered in all such patients, especially when left ventricular function is normal. Revascularization is clearly indicated and often beneficial.
- *Dialysis-dependent end stage renal disease* may be reversible when severe bilateral renal artery stenosis (or severe unilateral stenosis to a single-functional kidney) is present.[16,17] While revascularization can restore renal function and allow discontinuation of dialysis, prognosis is not always favourable. Among others, rapidity of decline of renal function (3 months or less) and kidney size (>8cm) are reasonably good predictors of potential clinical benefit.[18]

Table 2. Indications for renal revascularization

• Hypertension unresponsive to medical treatment
• 'Flash' (episodic) pulmonary oedema
• Progressive renal dysfunction
• 'Prophylactic' critical lesions (>90%)

- *Chronic renal failure* (serum creatinine of >1.8mg/dl) and severe stenosis (>75%) of the arterial supply to the total kidney mass is another situation where renal revascularization can be of benefit. Restoration of renal function is not always predictable, but available information is somewhat encouraging.[19–23] Severe forms of renal insufficiency (creatinine >3.0mg/dl) are less likely to respond.

- *Asymptomatic severe renal artery stenosis* (in the absence of hypertension and renal failure) has implications that are only partially understood at present. While we (and other groups) feel tempted to undertake percutaneous repair of *any* severe renal artery stenosis, such strategy cannot be supported by scientific evidence.[24–25] Very tight, critical lesions (>90%) should probably be considered for intervention to prevent likely progression to occlusion and functional kidney loss. But the practice of 'drive-by' intervention[26] and the policy of 'treating lesions because they exist' must be condemned.

ENDOVASCULAR TECHNIQUES

Endovascular renal artery repair is an advanced-level intervention that should not be attempted without previous significant endovascular experience. The anatomy is quite variable and can be challenging; as emphasized by other authors,[27,28] it is paramount that the correct angle (obliquity) of the fluoroscopic C-arm be determined early on to best visualize the origin and proximal portion of the target renal artery. The femoral approach is preferred in the majority of instances, with a brachial access being anatomically necessary in less than 10% of procedures. The main indications for the brachial approach are steep downward renal artery course, unsuitable iliac artery anatomy, and severe iliac artery disease precluding safe transluminal navigation.

As with other endovascular interventions, different choices and technical approaches exist.

Authors' preferred approach[28]

- *Retrograde femoral puncture*, insertion of 8F introducer sheath.
- *Power-injector contrast aortogram* using a 5F pigtail catheter (Fig. 1). Precise localization and delineation of the renal arteries. If the origin is obscured by the contrast-filled aorta, different angles and repeat injections may become necessary.
- *Selective catheterization of the renal artery* with a 5F diagnostic catheter (Fig. 2). Favorite pre-shaped catheter configurations include: Multipurpose, Cobra, RDC, and Hockey Stick. Additionally, Simmons-type and other catheters should be available for challenging anatomical situations (Fig. 3).
- *Advancement of guidewire and lesion crossing* (if possible) with a Storq (or Wholey) 0.035in guidewire. Complex/tight lesions and very small renal arteries dictate use of a smaller 0.018in guidewire.
- *Selective angiography* is obtained (if necessary) through the 5F diagnostic catheter, before passing the guidewire into the renal artery.

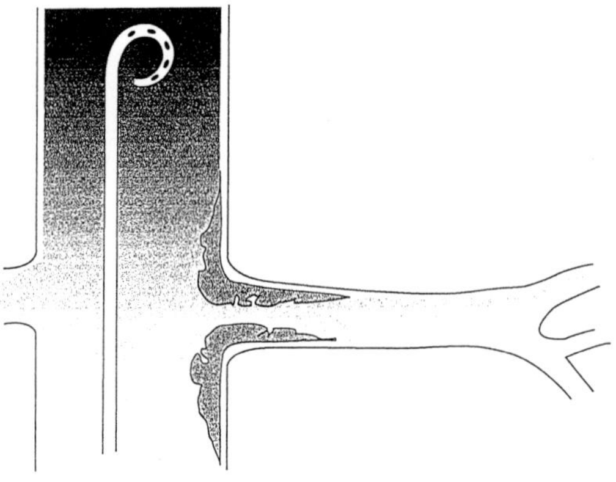

(a)

Fig. 1. (a) The initial step of the intervention consists of diagnostic angiography utilizing a 5F pigtail catheter placed at the T12-L1 level. (b) Alternative technique with a long radiopaque-tip sheath, that can also be used for coaxial-approach renal artery intervention (instead of a guiding catheter).

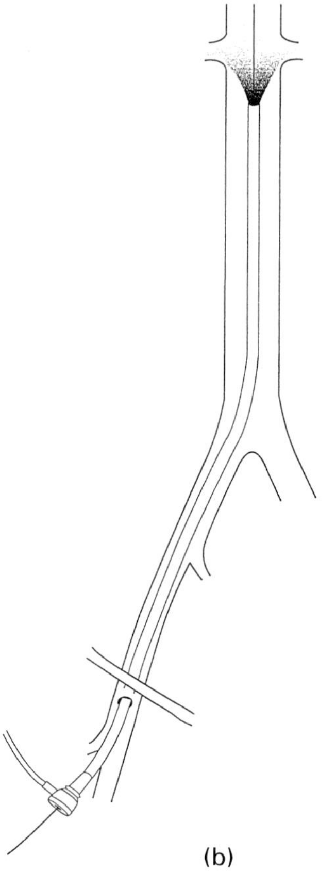

(b)

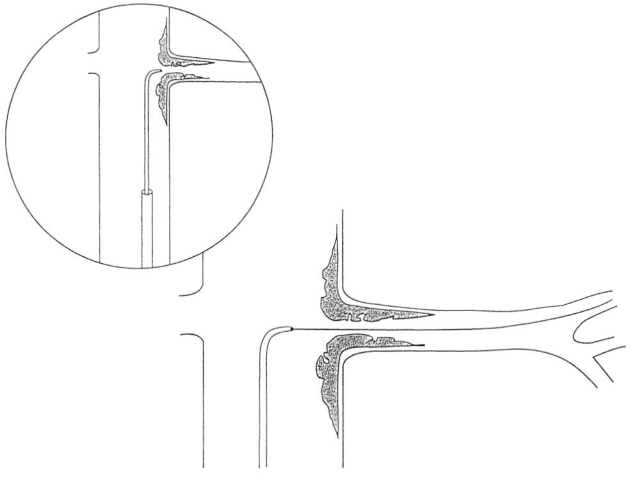

Fig. 2. Selective renal artery catheterization utilizing an appropriately shaped 5F diagnostic catheter. Renal double-curve (RDC) and Cobra (C) configurations are frequently used. The initial guidewire may be a 0.035in Storq or Wholey, or a finer 0.018in wire as advocated by many cardiologists. We only use the latter for extremely tight lesions and small vessels (<5mm). Note position of the 8F guiding catheter in the distal aorta.

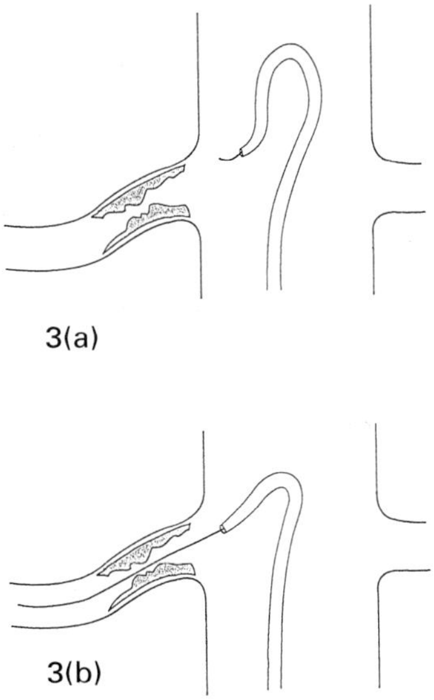

Fig. 3. Use of a Simmons 5F catheter for selective catheterization of a difficult downward-course renal artery. The catheter is allowed to reform its shape in the proximal aorta, and pulled down to a level just above the renal artery. A 0.018in floppy-tip guidewire is 'dangled' into and across the ostium. Next, the catheter is gently manoeuvred (pulled) to engage the artery as it advances over the wire. At times, it is appropriate to select the renal artery directly with the catheter and then pass the guidewire.

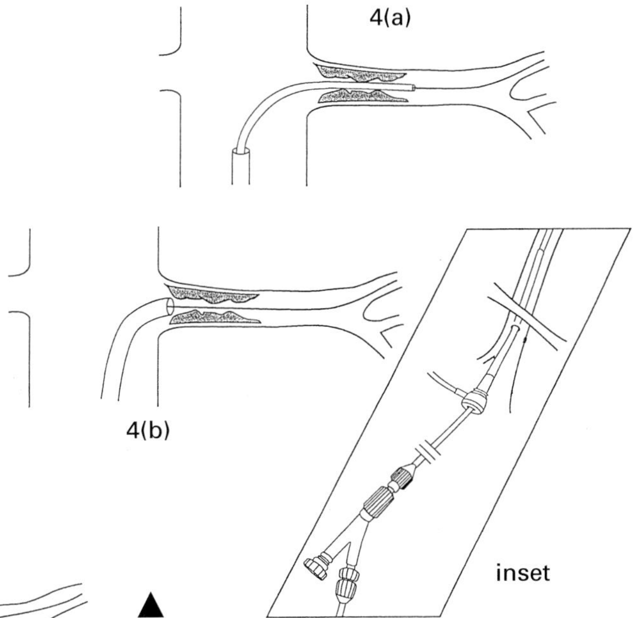

▲

Fig. 4. Guiding catheter is advanced over the wire to the origin of the renal artery (b). The 5F catheter used to select the artery may also be used as the guide over which to advance the larger catheter (a). (Inset): Tuohcy Borst valve/sideport are attached to the guiding catheter before endovascular insertion. It is thus 'converted' into an interventional sheath.

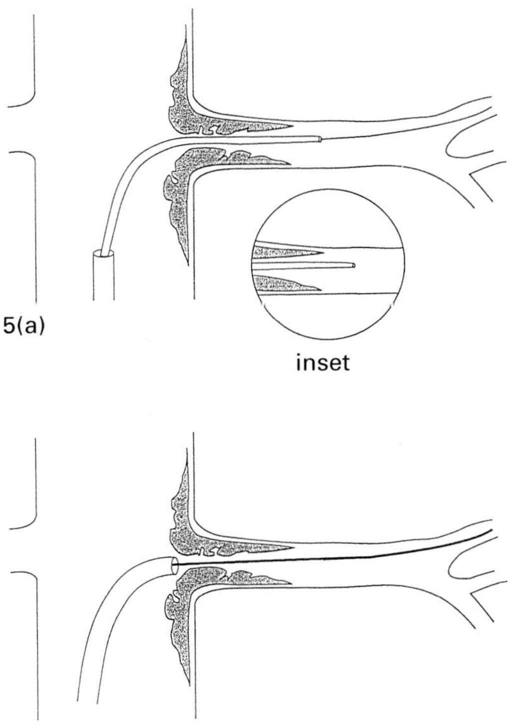

Fig. 5. (a) The 5F catheter has traversed the lesion, over the wire, and it is going to be used for exchange for a larger 0.035 guidewire (inset). (b) Guiding catheter advanced to but not across ostial lesion. Balloon predilatation will be the next step.

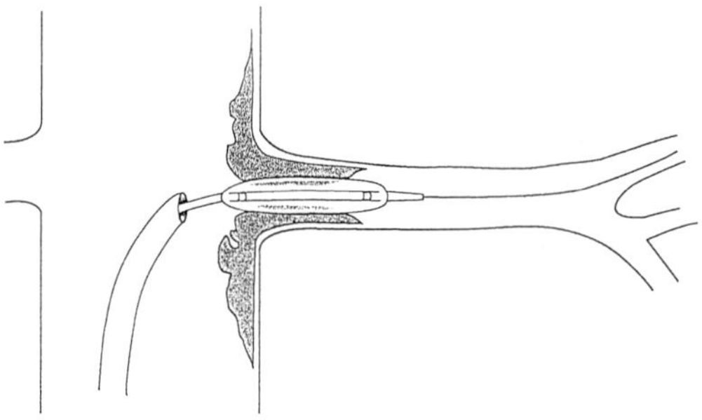

Fig. 6. Predilatation of ostial lesion.

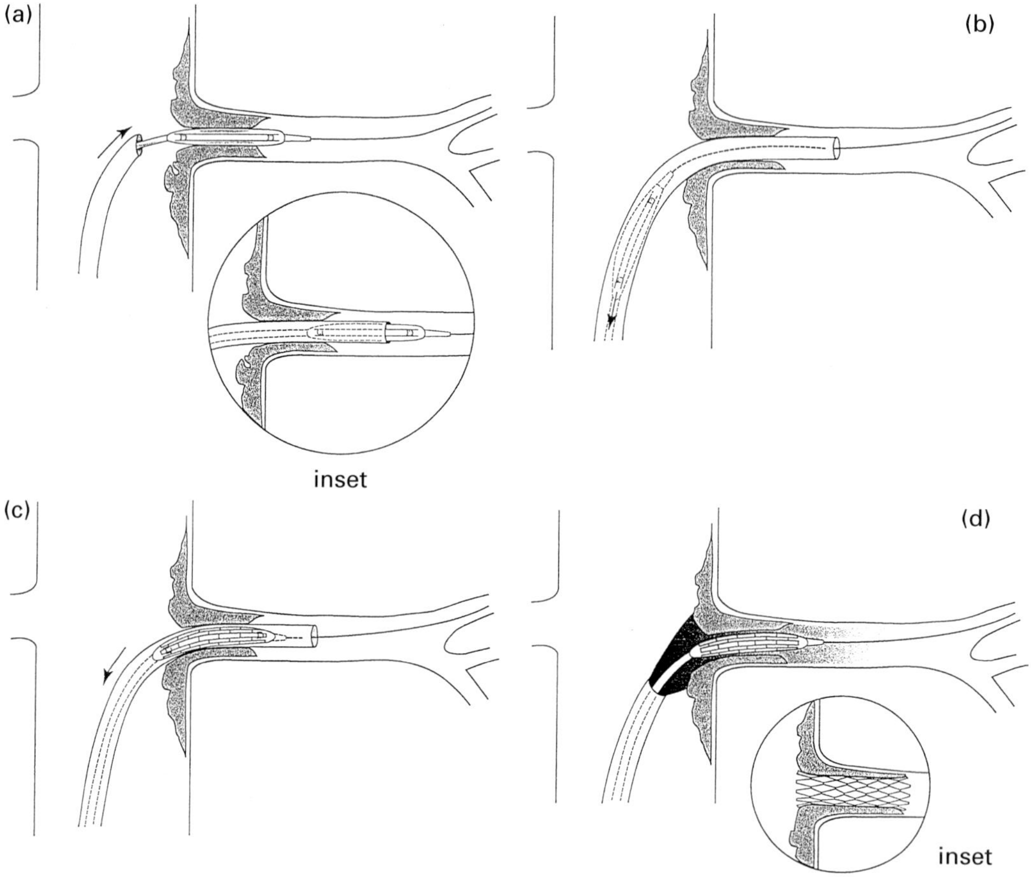

Fig. 7. Guiding catheter is advanced across the lesion over the PTA catheter ((a) and inset). The PTA catheter is removed (b), and the balloon mounted stent advanced through the guider to the desired position (c).The guiding catheter is retracted (d), and a small 'puff' of contrast injected to ascertain anatomical definition of the ostium just prior to balloon-mediated stent expansion. Optimal stent placement involves 1mm protrusion of the device into the aortic lumen (inset).

- *The use of an 8F guiding catheter* (renal double curve or multipurpose (Fig. 4) is recommended to: a) secure an access pathway from puncture site to renal artery; b) provide a protective conduit for stent placement; and c) have access for 'small-puff', repetitive angiographic injections to aid stent deployment and monitor results without need for a full aortogram each time. The guider is tracked over the guidewire to the renal artery origin. When treating a tight ostial lesion, the guider is not passed across the lesion at this time in order to avoid dissection and 'snow-plowing' (Fig. 5).
- *Ostial lesions* 'Pre-dilatation' is useful to test the lesion's response to balloon inflation ('dilatability'), and to open up the way for safer and less traumatic advancement of the guiding catheter (or long sheath) across the lesion. A 2-cm long balloon is used for pre-dilatation (and stent placement) (Fig. 6). We prefer to under-dilate with a 4mm balloon first, and then use a 5–7mm PTA catheter for stent deployment. Other interventionists choose to fully dilate initially, and use the same balloon for expansion of the stent.
- *Non-ostial (mid-renal artery) lesions* Angioplasty with a balloon catheter sized to match the normal artery diameter (5–6mm in most patients) is used as sole therapy (if a good anatomical result is achieved); stent placement always necessary.
- *Stents.* The Palmaz stent (P154 most often) is favoured overwhelmingly for this location. Its high radial force and precise placement characteristics are felt to be important features for renal artery intervention. Other attractive choices include some of the more recently developed devices, i.e. the AVE stent, and the new Corinthian IQ Palmaz device.

Technique of stent placement

First, the guider is advanced across the pre-dilated lesion into the renal artery (Fig. 7). This step can be facilitated by using the PTA catheter (with the balloon deflated) to support and guide the advancing guiding catheter across the lesion (Fig. 7a and inset). The stent is manually crimped onto a nylon balloon (Cordis Opta 5 in our practice), and placed over the wire through the guiding catheter to the desired location. Road-mapping technique is quite useful during this manoeuvre. The guiding catheter is retracted (to uncover the balloon-mounted stent) to a point (in the aortic lumen) near the origin of the renal artery, enabling the administration of a small 'puff' of radiocontrast to outline the ostium and aortic border to enable final adjustments of placement location before stent deployment (Fig. 7d). In the treatment of ostial lesions, 1–2mm of the stent should be left protruding into the aortic lumen. Following balloon-mediated deployment, a repeat angiogram (through the guiding catheter) is obtained for completion assessment. Flaring of the aortic end of the device can be done for 'cosmetic' purposes, but it is of no proven value (Fig. 7d and inset).

Pre-loading is an available technical option that may obviate some of the difficulties encountered with passage of a rigid device (Palmaz stent) across a curved guiding catheter. Technique: an 8F guiding catheter (renal double curve or multipurpose) is preloaded with a 5F shaft balloon (2cm length); a P154 Palmaz stent is mounted onto the balloon, and then backloaded into the guiding catheter and left in its distal-most portion (but totally covered). The preloaded guider, with catheter and balloon-mounted stent within, is introduced over the previously placed 0.035in Storq guidewire through the 8F femoral sheath and into the renal artery. It is noteworthy that the renal artery stenosis must be pre-dilated with balloon over the wire as a preliminary step. The technique of stent deployment proceeds in exactly the same manner as described above.

Brachial artery approach

The transbrachial technique may be used, but it is necessary in less than 10% of patients. It is not employed routinely because the multiply curved, tortuous and very long access pathway to the renal artery combine to create potential technical difficulties. Transfemoral intervention is much simpler and straightforward. The *tools* necessary for transbrachial renal artery intervention must be of *sufficient length*: 90-cm long guide catheter (or sheath), and 120 cm balloon catheter shafts, with 250–300 90cm guidewires. It is our preference to puncture the brachial artery at (or immediately above) the antecubital fossa where the vessel is relatively superficial, and non-mobile; additionally, it can be reliably compressed against the humerus for haemostasis following sheath removal. A 5-F (10–11cm) sheath is placed initially, and guidewire passed retrograde to the abdominal aorta (Fig. 8). A pre-curved (or pigtail) catheter is used to direct the guidewire down the descending thoracic aorta as it emerges retrograde from the subclavian artery (Fig. 9). Fluoroscopic monitoring and guidance are paramount. It cannot be overemphasized that *blind passage* of a guidewire into the arch of the aorta must *never* be practised, as the wire will often go into the ascending aorta and within the heart with potential for causing arrhythmias and other serious complications. Guidewire advancement and manipulations must always be monitored under fluoroscopic visualization.

Initial diagnostic aortogram (Fig. 10), selective catheterization and guidewire crossing of the renal artery lesion proceed much the same way as described for the transfemoral route. Use of an 8F guiding catheter would be optimal for stent placement; however, the brachial artery may not tolerate or allow the use of an 8F sheath. A better alternative may be to use instead a long 90cm 6F or 7F sheath that is flexible enough as to track over the wire into the renal artery.

Newer renal artery interventional systems are now available that allow use of a 6F guider for stent placement. Additionally, coronary systems can be adapted for renal application, but insufficient radial strength of coronary stent devices may constitute a significant disadvantage when treating aortic-ostial lesions.

RESULTS OF RENAL ARTERY INTERVENTION

Surgical revascularization has been documented to be of clinical value in treating renovascular hypertension and improving renal function as well as increasing overall patient survival.[19,29,30] Despite the associated morbidities and mortality with conventional renal bypass or endarterectomy, these methods remain the gold standard with which all subsequent forms of treatment should be compared.[31] Unfortunately, direct comparative studies performed in a prospective manner are not available; therefore, a review of individual techniques and outcomes needs to be performed with a critical eye, lest it is automatically assumed that a percutaneous procedure is a wiser treatment choice.

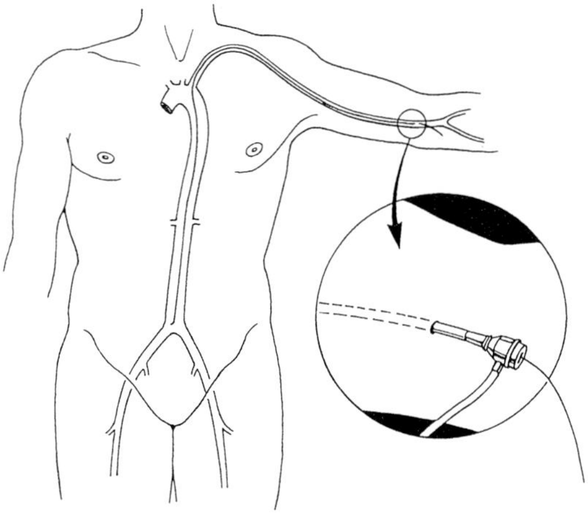

Fig. 8. Percutaneous puncture of left brachial artery at the antecubital fossa with initial insertion of a 5F short introducer sheath. Guidewire is advanced, first retrograde to the aortic arch, and then down to the distal abdominal aorta.

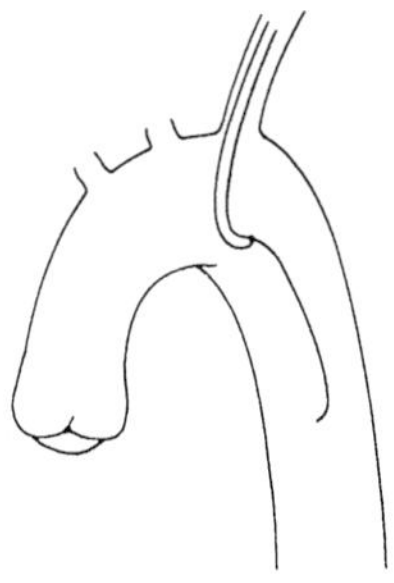

Fig. 9. A curved selective (or the pigtail) catheter is used to direct the guidewire along the correct pathway.

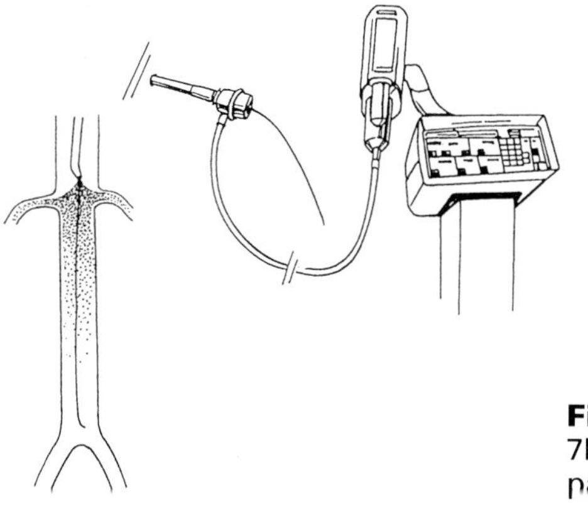

Fig. 10. A 90cm radiopaque-tip interventional 7F sheath is used for initial angiography of the pararenal aorta. Note use of a power injector.

Atherosclerotic renal artery stenosis, which comprises nearly 95% of cases of renovascular hypertension, has been successfully treated by operative means since 1952.[32] In a recent review by Steinbach *et al.*,[31] long-term patency of renal artery bypass was achieved in 90% of patients with an operative mortality of 2.2%. Significant morbidity in the form of bypass graft thrombosis or stenosis occurred in approximately 7% of patients. Long-term cure from hypertension was obtained in 35%, 36% were markedly improved, and only 27% remained unaffected by the treatment. Renal function as measured by postoperative serum creatinine levels revealed improvement in 35%, stabilization in 36%, and deterioration in 28% (with 8% ultimately requiring dialysis). These results, as well as those of Cambria *et al.*[33]

and others, are representative of what is achievable today, and reflect contemporary improvements in surgical techniques, patient election, and perioperative management.

Percutaneous renal artery intervention has evolved dramatically since the introduction of endoluminal stent devices. While PTA alone can produce acceptable results on highly selected patients,[34] ostial lesions are notoriously unresponsive to this modality of treatment. Adjunctive stent placement has clearly revitalized and expanded the role of catheter-based therapy for renovascular disease.[35] Blum *et al.*,in their 1997 study,[36] performed balloon angioplasty in 82 renal arteries. Initial technical success was only possible in 10% of the arteries (by their criteria); the unsuccessfully angioplastied arteries were stented using a Palmaz stent. No major complications were encountered and local haematoma was present in three of 68 patients. Reversal of hypertension was shown in 16% of patients, with an additional 42% obtaining clinical improvement. At 12 and 24-month follow-up, eight of the 74 stented arteries showed evidence of restenosis with a subsequent long-term secondary patency rate of 92% at 5 years. The study clearly demonstrated that ostial atherosclerotic lesions can be successfully treated by stent placement with marked improvement in hypertension. A secondary finding of the study was that although improvement in renal function was not necessarily achieved in the 20 patients with renal dysfunction, there did not appear to be any subsequent worsening in follow-up. The authors also point out that they were able to achieve a lower restenosis rate (10%).

Dorros *et al.* in a 1998 study evaluated the use of balloon angioplasty and stenting for the treatment of atherosclerotic renal artery stenosis.[5] They reported technical success in 99% of patients with procedure-related mortality in under 1%, and contrast-induced renal failure in 13%. They concluded that at 1-year follow-up approximately 1% of patients were 'cured' of their hypertension, with improvement achieved in an additional 42%. Approximately 54% had no improvement. This trend continued for an additional 3 years of evaluation. They were also able to conclude that two-thirds of patients had improved or stabilized renal function, but with one-third continuing to show signs of renal deterioration.

In a recent multiple-study review involving 10 previously published stent trials, the authors conclude that renal artery stenting is 'technically feasible' and can be done without major complications.[37] They also note that ostial stenosis is treatable with stenting. Although a cure for hypertension may be possible in up to 15% of patients, there seems to be a discrepancy in the description of what 'improved' blood pressure control actually means. However, it would seem that the trend towards a drug-sparing effect of renal artery stenting is undeniable. With revascularization, there may also be an increase in the role of ACE inhibitors. Potential for parenchymal and renal function preservation were also noted, and has been further substantiated in other reports.[38] The authors of this review further concluded that surveillance following renal artery stenting is of paramount importance. They base it on the observation of a 10–15% likelihood of restenosis within a year, although secondary patency was achievable in up to 90% during a 5-year follow-up. As in other studies, they remind us that a prospective trial needs to be conducted to compare PTA alone with PTA and stenting. A recently published Dutch study addresses this issue[39] In patients with ostial atherosclerotic lesions, primary patency rates at 6 months were 88% with stenting versus 57% with PTA alone. Restenosis developed over a 6-month period of time in 14% of stented patients and 48% of angioplasty cases. Secondary patency rates were 80% and 51% respectively. Improvement or cure in hypertension occurred in 58% of patients with stenting and 49% of patients with PTA, although this difference was not statistically significant. One additional conclusion by these authors is that primary stenting (during the initial intervention) would seem to be more cost-effective in view of the need for secondary and tertiary interventions otherwise observed in their study.

Renal artery stenting has been shown to be associated with a low procedure-related mortality (<1%) and an overall complication rate of about 10%. Serious morbidity is likely to occur in <5%.

OVERVIEW AND CONCLUSIONS

The prevalence of renal artery stenosis in patients with generalized atherosclerotic disease and hypertension is higher than previously believed. Surgical revascularization remains the best anatomical approach, producing superb long-term results. However, surgery carries significant risks that can be prohibitive for some patients. Percutaneous intervention is very appealing, with results that continue to improve as stent devices become available for repair of aortic-ostial lesions. Renal artery stenting is rapidly becoming the therapeutic approach of choice for most patients with atherosclerotic renovascular disease who present with a clinical indication for intervention. Asymptomatic critical lesions may also be considered for percutaneous repair on carefully selected patients.

It is paramount that vascular surgeons keep pace with rapidly evolving developments in percutaneous revascularization approaches in the renal arteries and other territories. It is undeniable that percutaneous intervention will probably replace conventional surgical reconstruction as the standard of care for treatment of renovascular disease in a significant proportion of patients.

REFERENCES

1. Taylor DC, Kettler MD, Moneta GL *et al.*: Duplex ultrasound scanning in the diagnosis of renal artery stenosis: a prospective evaluation. *J Vasc Surg* **7:** 363–369, 1988
2. Strandness DE: Duplex imaging for the detection of renal artery stenosis. *Am J Kidney Dis* **24:** 674–678, 1994
3. Olin JW, Piedmonte MR, Young JR *et al.*: The utility of duplex ultrasound scanning of the renal arteries for diagnosing significant renal artery stenosis. *Ann Intern Med* **122:** 833–838, 1995
4. Isaacson JA, Zierler RE, Spittell PC *et al.*: Non-invasive screening for renal artery stenosis: comparison of renal artery and renal hilar duplex scanning. *J Vasc Tech* **19:** 105–110, 1995
5. Dorros G, Jaff MR, Jain A *et al.*: Follow-up of primary Palmaz–Schatz stent placement for atherosclerotic renal artery stenosis. *Am J Cardiol* **75:** 1051–1055, 1995
6. Cohn EJ, Benjamim ME, Sandager GP *et al.*: Can intrarenal duplex waveform analysis predict successful renal artery revascularization? *J Vasc Surg* **28:** 471–481, 1998
7. Caps MD, Zierler RE, Polissar NL *et al.*: Risk of atrophy in kidneys with atherosclerotic renal artery stenosis. *Kidney Int.* **53:** 735–742, 1998

8. Dean R, Kieffer RW, Smith BM *et al.*: Renovascular hypertension: anatomic and renal function changes during drug therapy. *Arch Surg* **116:** 1408–1415, 1981
9. Zierler RE, Bergelin RO, Davidson RC *et al.*: A prospective study of disease progression in patients with RAS. *Am J Hypertens* **9:** 1055–1061, 1996
10. Gross CM, Kramer J, Waigand J *et al.*: Relation between arteriosclerosis in the coronary and renal arteries. *Am J Cardiol* **80:** 1478–1481, 1997
11. Olin JR, Melia M, Young JR *et al.*: Prevalence of atherosclerotic RAS in patients with atherosclerosis elsewhere. *Am J Med* **88:** 46N–51N, 1990
12. National High Blood Pressure Education Program Working Group: 1995 update of the working group reports on chronic renal failure and renovascular hypertension. *Arch Intern Med* **156:** 1938–1947, 1996
13. Diamond JR: Flash pulmonary edema and the diagnostic suspicion of occult RAS. *Am J Kidney Dis* **21:** 328–330, 1993
14. Tami LF, McElderry MW, al-Adli NM *et al.*: Renal artery stenosis presenting as crescendo angina pectoris. *Cath Cardiovasc Diagn* **36:** 252–256, 1995
15. Kaylor WM, Novick AC, Ziegelbaum M *et al.*: Reversal of end stage renal failure with surgical revascularization in patients with atherosclerotic renal artery occlusion. *J Urol* **141:** 486–488, 1989
16. Ascer E, Gennaro M, Rogers D: Unilateral renal artery revascularization can salvage renal function and terminate dialysis in selected patients with uremia. *J Vasc Surg* **18:** 1012–1018, 1993
17. Hansen KJ, Thomason RB, Craven TE *et al.*: Surgical management of dialysis-dependent ischemic nephropathy. *J Vasc Surg* **21:** 197–211, 1995
18. Scoble JE, Sweny P, Stansby G *et al.*: Patients with atherosclerotic renovascular disease presenting to a renal unit: an audit of outcome. *Postgrad Med J* **69:** 461–465, 1993
19. Novick AC, Pohl MA, Schreiber M *et al.*: Revascularization for preservation of renal function in patients with atherosclerotic renovascular disease. *J Urol* **129:** 907–912, 1983
20. van Damme H, Jeuserre F, Pans A *et al.*: The impact of renal revascularisation on renal dysfunction. *Eur J Vasc Endovasc Surg* **10:** 330–337, 1995
21. Cambria RP, Brewster DC, L'Italien GJ *et al.*: Renal artery reconstruction for the preservation of renal function. *J Vasc Surg* **24:** 371–382, 1996
22. Losinno F, Zuccala A, Busato F *et al.*: Renal artery angioplasty for renovascular hypertension and preservation of renal function: long-term angiographic and clinical follow-up. *Am J Roent* 162: 853–857, 1994
23. Connolly JO, Higgins RM, Walters HL *et al.*: Presentation, clinical features and outcome in different patterns of atherosclerotic renovascular disease. *Q J Med* **87:** 413–421, 1994
24. Chaikof EL, Smith III RB, Salam AA *et al.*: Empirical reconstruction of the renal artery: long-term outcome. *J Vasc Surg* **24:** 406–414, 1996
25. Tarazi RY, Hertzer NR, Beven EG *et al.*: Simultaneous aortic reconstruction and renal revascularization: risk factors and late results in eighty-nine patients. *J Vasc Surg* **5:** 707–714, 1987
26. White CJ: The renal oculosten(t)otic reflex. *Cathet Cardiovasc Diagn* **37:** 251, 1996
27. Kaatee R, van Leeuwen MS, Mali WPT: Renal artery angle in atherosclerotic abdominal aorta prior to renal stent deployment: assessment with spiral computer tomography angiography. *Cardiol Vasc Intervent Radiol Soc Eur* 1995, Lyon: France (abstract)
28. Criado FJ (Ed): *Endovascular Intervention: Basic Concepts and Techniques* pp. 93–104. Armonk, NY: Futura Publishing Co., 1999
29. Deab RH, Krueger TC, Whitenock JM *et al.*: Operative management of renovascular hypertension: results after a follow-up of 15–23 years. *J Vasc Surg* **1:** 234, 1984
30. Hunt JC, Strong CG: Renovascular hypertension, mechanisms, natural history, and treatment. *Am J Cardiol* **32:** 562, 1973
31. Steinbach F. Novick AC, Campbell S, Dykstra D: Long-term survival after surgical revascularization for atherosclerotic renal artery disease. *J Urol* **158:** 38–41, 1997
32. Freeman NE, Leeds FH, Elliott WG *et al.*: Thromboendarterectomy for hypertension due to renal artery occlusion. *J Am Med Assoc* **156:** 1077, 1954

33. Cambria RP, Brewster DC, L'Italien GJ *et al.*: The durability of different reconstructive techniques for atherosclerotic renal artery disease. *J Vasc Surg* **20:** 76–87, 1999
34. Weibull H. Bergqvist D, Bergentz SE *et al.*: Percutaneous transluminal renal angioplasty versus surgical reconstruction of atherosclerotic renal artery stenosis: a prospective randomized study. *J Vasc Surg* **18:** 841–852, 1993
35. Eldrup-Jorgenson J, Harvey HR, Sampson LN *et al.*: Should percutaneous transluminal renal artery angioplasty be applied to ostial artery atherosclerosis? *J Vasc Surg* **21:** 909–915, 1995
36. Blum U, Krumme B, Flugel P *et al.*: Treatment of ostial renal-artery stenosis with vascular endoprostheses after unsuccessful balloon angioplasty. *New Engl J Med* **336:** 459–465, 1997
37. Isles CG, Robertson S, Hill D: Management of renovascular disease: a review of renal artery stenting in ten studies. *Q J Med* **92:** 159–167, 1999
38. Harden PN, MacLeod MJ, Rodger RSC *et al.*: Effect of renal-artery stenting on progression of renovascular renal failure. *Lancet* **349:** 1133–1136, 1997
39. van de Ven PJG, Kaatee R, Beutler JJ *et al.*: Arterial stenting and balloon angioplasty in ostial atherosclerotic renovascular disease: a randomized trial. *Lancet* **353:** 282–286, 1999

Protected renal artery angioplasty and stenting

Michel Henry, Christos Klonaris, Max Amor, Isabelle Henry, Michèle Hugel

INTRODUCTION

Renal artery stenosis is common in patients with arterial occlusive disease due to the generalized and multifocal nature of atherosclerosis. Its clinical manifestations include secondary hypertension, ischaemic nephropathy and recurrent flash pulmonary oedema. However, it can be an incidental finding during arteriography performed for unrelated indications.[1] When the renal artery stenosis is bilateral or in an anatomic or functional solitary kidney it can reduce the renal function, leading to end stage renal failure.[2] The three major clinical settings in which one must suspect ischaemic renal disease include acute renal failure precipitated by the treatment of hypertension particularly with angiotensin converting enzyme inhibitors; progressive azotemia in a patient with known renovascular hypertension treated medically and unexplained progressive azotemia in elderly patients with refractory hypertension and other evidence of atherosclerotic disease. Also, recurrent unexplained (flash) pulmonary oedema in cases of hypertension and renal failure is indicative of bilateral renal artery stenosis.

A better understanding of the natural history and progressive pattern of renal artery stenosis,[3] and appreciation that it is a potentially correctable cause of secondary hypertension and renal failure suggest that many symptomatic patients (especially with decline in renal function) may benefit from aggressive surgical or interventional treatment with appropriate control of blood pressure and stabilization or improvement of renal function. Medical management of renovascular disease should be reserved for those patients with contraindications or unwillingness to undergo corrective procedures to relieve renal ischemia.[4] Surgical revascularization techniques have documented their efficacy in the management of renovascular hypertension and ischaemic nephropathy with stabilization or reversal of renal function even in patients undergoing dialysis therapy. However, the mortality rate of the surgical approach even in the most recent series remains high, varying between 5% and 10%, due partially to the fact that in many concomitant aortic procedures were performed.[5–8]

Recently, percutaneous transluminal renal angioplasty (PTRA) has become the cornerstone of therapeutic strategy. This technique is currently widely accepted as a treatment of choice in cases of non-ostial atherosclerotic renal artery lesions and in fibromuscular dysplasia. For ostial lesions PTA alone is limited by moderate initial success and high restenosis rates. However, the introduction of stents has dramatically improved its efficacy in ostial stenoses and further reduced the indications for surgical revascularization.[9–13]

In many recent series,[11–17] the positive effects of angioplasty or stenting in patients with renal artery stenosis have been well documented. However, even after successful initial technical results, a decline in renal function has been reported in a considerable number of patients. In a prospective study Dorros *et al.*[13] presented the results of primary stent placement for atherosclerotic renal artery stenosis in 76 patients with 6-month follow-up. Serum creatinine values improved in 30%, remained unchanged in 48% and deteriorated in 22% of the patients. When the baseline creatinine values were less than 1.5mg/dl, deterioration occurred in 5%, but with higher initial values a decline in renal function was seen in 45% of the patients. Recently, Isles *et al.*[14] published a review of 10 studies including 416 stent placement procedures in 379 patients treated for renal artery stenosis. Although technical success was high in all these studies (96–100%), renal function improved in 26%, stabilized in 48% and deteriorated in 26% of the patients.

Many factors may account for this deterioration: contrast media-induced nephrotoxicity, progression of concomitant nephrosclerosis as a part of the natural history of the disease or due to exposure of the diseased glomeruli in higher arterial pressure after successful revascularization, restenosis of the renal artery and atheroembolism during the steps of the procedure.[13] The majority of these factors are iatrogenic in origin[18] and therefore any efforts should be made to eliminate their incidence. Consequently, proper patient selection, application of strict indications for intervention, meticulous techniques and close follow-up are of paramount importance in order to obtain the best outcome. Although many efforts have been made towards more effective and safer endovascular procedures for renal artery stenosis, little attention has been given to the detrimental effects of atheroembolism on renal function for many reasons. This entity is caused by the release of microscopic plaque fragments and cholesterol crystals from the renal artery lesion or the atherosclerotic aorta into the parenchymal renal vasculature during the steps of the procedure.[19–21] Instrumental manipulations on the aortic wall and renal arteries with selective or guiding catheters and guidewires, balloon dilatation of the lesion and stent deployment can result in detachment and embolism of atheromatous debris from ulcerated plaques. The large size of the devices used and the increased length or specific difficulties of the procedure may be promoting factors. There is also evidence that both oral and intravenous anticoagulants and thrombolytic drugs can induce atheroembolism.[22–23] This has particular importance because anticoagulants are commonly used in renal artery interventions to prevent acute thrombosis.

The true incidence of atheroembolism is uncertain. Many patients can have a silent atheroembolism owing to the large functional kidney reserve which allows for normal serum creatinine values despite a significant decline of the total glomerular filtration. Therefore, only the most severe cases, especially in patients with preprocedural renal dysfunction and limited functional reserve are usually detected. Clinical manifestations of the disease are also non-specific. Onset of renal function deterioration after an interventional procedure has been estimated to be between 3 and 8 weeks[24] but earlier intervals have been reported.[25] Eosinophilia is not a common finding.[24] Although proteinuria and nephrotic syndrome represent uncommon manifestations, Haqqie *et al.*[26] reported four patients with documented histopathological atheroembolism who developed nephrotic-range proteinuria and suggested that atheroembolism should be considered in the differential diagnosis of nephrotic syndrome in elderly patients with serious vascular disease. Similar conclusions were made by Greenberg *et al.*,[27] after reviewing the clinical features and histological findings of 24 patients found at renal biopsy to have cholesterol atheroembolism; 19 of them had recently undergone an invasive vascular procedure.

Moreover, even in cases of clinical suspicion, the diagnosis of atheroembolism is difficult to establish using routine laboratory tests. Renal biopsy is the only definite diagnostic tool but its application is difficult to justify for confirmation of a disease amenable to supportive treatment only. For these reasons it is not surprising that atheroembolism after renal artery interventions is often misdiagnosed as contrast-induced nephrotoxicity or is attributed to the progression of nephrosclerosis. There are very few angioplasty studies that address this complication. Boisclair *et al.*[25] reported 4/33 cases of renal artery embolism treated with stent placement for immediate renal angioplasty failure or recurrent stenosis after previous angioplasty, documented by postprocedural renal scintigraphy or arteriography.

Despite difficulties in diagnosis, renal atheroembolism poses a serious risk for renal function deterioration and decreased survival in patients undergoing endovascular procedures for renal artery stenosis. Its importance is clearly demonstrated in a recent work by Krishnamurthi *et al.*[28] who evaluated its impact on morbidity and survival in 44 patients who had surgery for atherosclerotic renal artery stenosis and concomitant intraoperative renal biopsy for detection of atheroemboli and arteriolar nephrosclerosis. Atheroembolic renal disease was identified in the biopsy specimens in 16 patients (36%), and correlated significantly with decreased patient survival. The 5-year survival in this group was 54% versus 85% in patients without atheroembolism ($p=0.011$). In contrast, no association between nephrosclerosis and postoperative survival was found.

ELIMINATING THE RISK OF ATHEROEMBOLISM

Every effort should be made to avoid the occurrence of atheroembolic events during renal interventions. Elderly patients with diffusely diseased aorta, and renal arteries and patients with baseline renal insufficiency represent a high risk category for atheroembolism but their exclusion from treatment protocols may deprive them from possible beneficial effects of the procedure. Although proper indications for renal revascularization are beyond the scope of this chapter we should note here that due to the relative simplicity of endovascular techniques, an enlarging number of patients may undergo interventional therapy based on debatable or inappropriate indications. Such cases could be a unilateral renal artery stenosis in an asymptomatic patient, or a not haemodynamically significant renal artery stenosis in patients with hypertension and normal renal function. In these scenarios, the cost of the procedure outweighs the anticipated benefit and any complication, including atheroembolism, is unacceptable.

From a technical point of view the intervention should be as atraumatic as possible, with utilization of small devices and adaptation of coronary angioplasty techniques.

Recently, Feldman *et al.*[29] reported a 'no-touch' technique consisting of placing a second 0.035 inch J-wire within the guiding catheter during catheterization of the renal artery to prevent the tip of the catheter from rubbing the aortic wall minimizing its contact with atherosclerotic plaques and therefore reducing the potential for embolization. Beyond these technical considerations, in our efforts to eliminate this complication, thus avoiding later deterioration in renal function, we applied the concept of protected renal angioplasty and stenting in the management of patients with severe renal artery stenosis manifested with difficult to control hypertension or renal insufficiency.

PROTECTED ANGIOPLASTY AND STENTING TECHNIQUE

The PurcuSurge™ (PercuSurge Inc. Sunnyvale, CA, USA) protection device consists of the Guardwire temporary occlusion catheter, the Microseal™ Adapter, and the Export aspiration catheter. Initially, an 8 F guiding catheter is placed at the ostium of the renal artery generally via the femoral approach. The Guardwire is then slowly advanced through the guiding catheter. The lesion is crossed and the marker of the protection balloon is placed 2 or 3cm distally. The Microseal™ Adapter is attached and the balloon is slowly inflated to occlude the renal artery flow. On detaching the Microseal™ Adapter the occlusion balloon remains inflated. Angioplasty and stenting are then performed under protection. Any debris generated is removed from the renal artery using the aspiration catheter advanced over the wire at the level of the treated area and close to the protection balloon. The aspirated blood is collected for later analysis. The aspiration catheter is then removed. The Microseal Adapter is reattached to the Guardwire™ and the occlusion balloon is deflated allowing normal vessel flow. If the angiographic result is satisfactory the device is removed. In case of early division of the main renal artery one could use two 0.014 inch Guardwires™ placed in the two arteries to protect the kidney. Peripheral dilatation balloons and stents can be mounted over these two Guardwires and used at the same time.

Since February 1999, 14 patients (males: 10, mean age 71.1 years, range 59–87 years) with ipsilateral or bilateral renal artery stenosis of atherosclerotic origin were treated with the above-described technique. All patients had diagnostic renal duplex scan and intra-arterial digital subtraction angioplasty performed prior to the intervention. Seventeen renal artery angioplasties and stenting procedures were performed under balloon protection (right: 8, left: 9). Four patients underwent bilateral procedures. All had poorly controlled hypertension. Eight patients had normal vessel function (serum creatinine ≤1.4mg/dl), five had moderate renal insuffiency (creatinine between 1.5 and 1.9mg/dl) and one patient severe dysfunction (creatinine 3.7mg/dl). Renal artery stenosis was located at the ostium in 15 cases, mean lesion length was 13.8mm. All stenoses were greater than 70% of the vessel diameter, mean stenosis was 84.4%. Nine patients had diffuse, severe atherosclerosis at the abdominal aorta. Associated coronary artery disease was found in seven, cerebrovascualr disease in four and peripheral arterial disease in seven patients.

All procedures were performed under local anaesthesia and intravenous sedation.

An intravenous bolus of 5000 internation units (IU) of unfractionated heparin was routinely administered at the beginning of the procedure. Postprocedural drug regimen included LMWH (low molecular weight heparin) for 24 hours, and antiplatelet medication.

All stenoses were easily crossed with the Guardwire™. All arteries were treated with stent placement (Figs 1–6). Primary stenting, without previous angioplasty was performed in nine cases. Eighteen stents of different types were implanted, six AVE, five Palmaz P 154, five Herculink and two Corinthian stents. One patient received two stents in the same artery to treat a long lesion. Technical success was obtained for all arteries with good deployment of the stent, no significant residual stenosis and good covering of the lesion. Mean time of renal artery occlusion with the protection balloon was 251 seconds (149–540s).

After angioplasty and stenting aspiration was routinely performed allowing removal of visible particles in all patients. The aspirated blood samples were analysed and studied by optic and electronic microscopic technique. Different particles were isolated and identified. Number of particles varied from 15 to 187 per procedure (mean 68.2) and diameter varied from 45 to 6206µm, (mean 210 5µm) The particles were atheromatous plaques, cholesterol crystals, necrotic cores, fibrin, thrombi, platelets, and macrophage foam cells.

Patients remained in the hospital for 48 hours to monitor serum creatinine levels and adjust blood pressure medications. Renal duplex scan was scheduled at 6 and 12 months and then annually and angiography at 6 months or when restenosis was suspected. Serum creatinine values were measured before and after the procedure at days 1 and 15, at 1 and 2 months, at 6 months and thereafter every 6 months. Mean follow-up period was 19 weeks, range 2–10 months, in all cases was beyond the crucial time required for the development of clinical manifestations of atheroembolism. We observed no deterioration of the renal function in all patients. Three patients with baseline renal insufficiency had improvement after the procedure.

The results of this small study showed that all patients benefited from the procedures with stabilization or improvement of their renal function with no case of deterioration. This may be well attributed to the utilization of the protection system during all steps of intervention. It was very important that visible atherosclerotic debris was extracted in all interventions. In one case we removed a fragment measuring 6mm in its maximum diameter, a size large enough to produce macroembolism or even renal artery occlusion.

The concept of protected renal artery angioplasty and stenting is similar to that of brain protection during angioplasty of the carotid arteries to avoid embolism of atherosclerotic debris into the cerebral circulation during balloon dilatation and stent deployment. Our technique has recently gained popularity worldwide, as a testimony to the suboptimal results of percutaneous procedures in the carotid territory. Our concept was that the same technique could be suitable in the management of renal artery stenosis, eliminating the risk of atheroembolism. Our results are encouraging and larger studies evaluating the future role of protection devices in renal artery interventions are anticipated. Our study raises many questions suitable for future investigations. Is this technique indicated for all patients undergoing endovascular treatment for renal artery stenosis or should it have

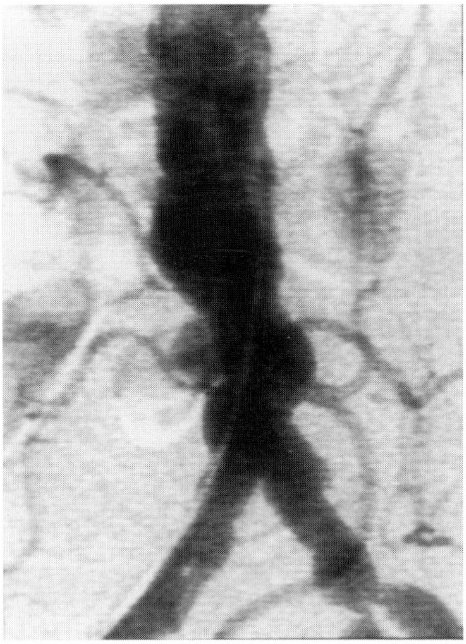

Fig. 1. Diffuse atherosclerotic aorta in a patient with baseline renal insufficiency presenting with blue toe syndrome.

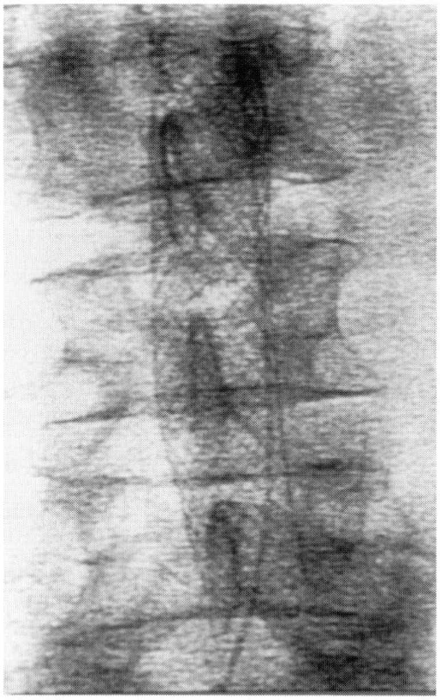

Fig. 2. An Expander self-expandable stent was used to cover a large infrarenal aortic ulcer responsible for the symptoms.

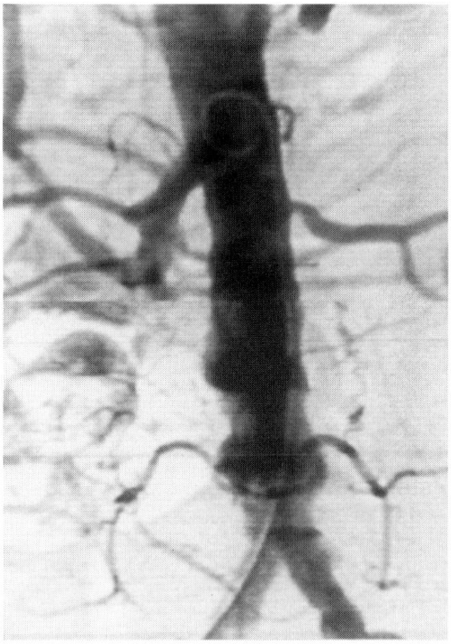

Fig. 3. Result after treatment.

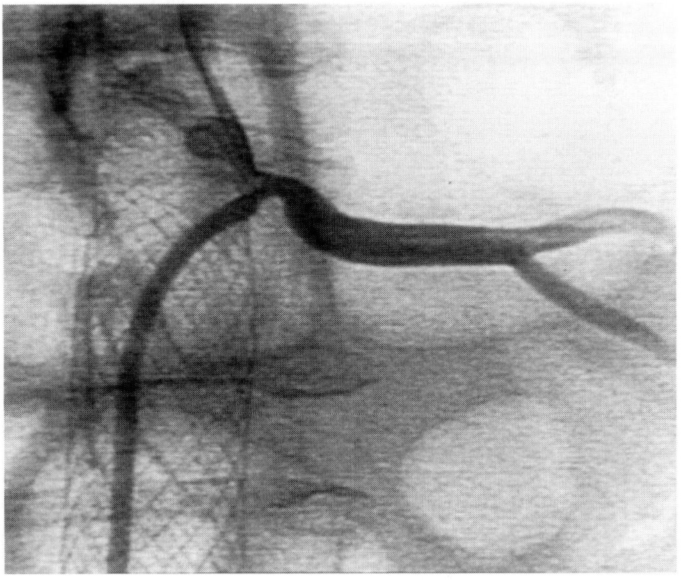

Fig. 4. Selective angiography revealed a severe left renal artery stenosis.

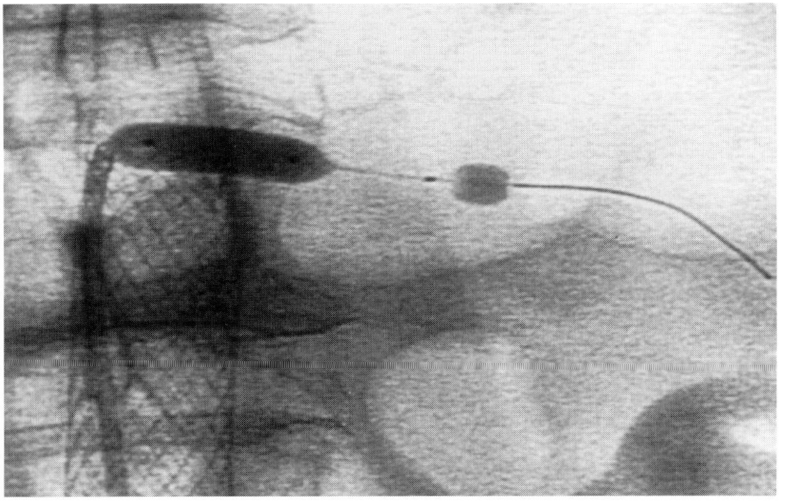

Fig. 5. Angioplasty and stenting of the lesion was performed under protection with the PercuSurge device. The inflated occlusion balloon is shown.

applications in some subgroups like patients with multilevel atherosclerotic disease or with pronounced atherosclerotic aorta or with ostial renal artery lesions? Is there any role for intravascular ultrasound in this area? Should its applicability be restrained in patients with baseline renal insufficiency or extended in those with normal renal function?

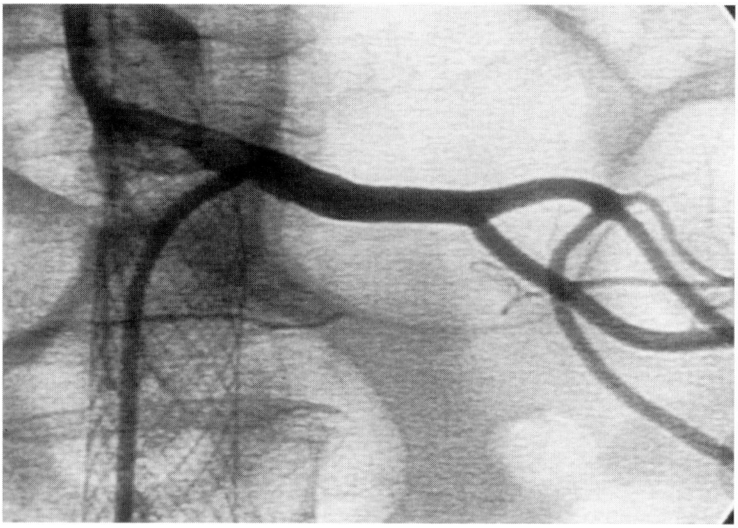

Fig. 6. Final result.

Difficulties in producing the definite diagnosis of atheroembolism by non-invasive means impede the evaluation of its true occurrence and its role in renal function deterioration.

CONCLUSION

Physicians dedicated to the treatment of renovascular disease should be aware of the risk of atheroembolism during interventional procedures for renal artery stenosis. Considering that this entity represents an iatrogenic complication with detrimental effects and no specific treatment, every effort should be made to prevent it. Due to the increasing number of patients with renovascular disease being treated with percutaneous techniques, the cost of possible renal function deterioration might constitute a health problem. Appropriate indications for intervention and meticulous techniques are of paramount importance for the best outcome. Proper utilization of protection devices may offer additional safety and improve the results of renal angioplasty and stenting. Our initial encouraging results provide adequate support to continue further evaluation of this therapeutic strategy.

REFERENCES

1. Canzanello VJ, Textor SC: Noninvasive diagnosis of renovascualr disease. *Mayo Clin Proc* **69:** 1172–1181, 1994
2. Preston RA, Epstein M: Ischemic renal disease: an emerging cause of chronic renal failure and end-stage renal disease [editorial] *J Hypertens* **15:** 1365–1377, 1997

3. Caps MT, Perissinotto C, Zierler RE *et al.*: Prospective study of atherosclerotic disease progression in the renal artery. *Circulation* **98:** 2866–2872, 1998
4. Ram CV, Clagett GP, Radford LR: Renovascualr hypertension. *Semin Nephrol* **15:** 152–174, 1995
5. van Damme H, Rorive G, Limet R: Reversal of acute renal failure by kidney revascularisation. *Eur J Vasc Endovasc Surg* **11:** 134–139, 1996
6. Cambria RP, Brewster DC, L'Italien GJ *et al.*: Renal artery reconstruction for the preservation of renal function *J Vasc Surg* **24:** 371–382, 1996
7. Hallett JW Jr, Fowl R, O'Brien PC *et al.*: Renovascular operations in patients with chronic renal insufficiency: do the benefits justify the risks? *J Vasc Surg* **5:** 622–627, 1987
8. Crinnion JN, Gough MJ: Bilaterial renal artery atherosclerosis: the results of surgical treatment. *Eur J Vasc Endovasc Surg* **11:** 353–358, 1996
9. van de Ven PJ, Kaatee R, Beutler JJ *et al.*: Arterial stenting and balloon angioplasty in ostial atherosclerotic renovascular disease: a randomised trial. *Lancet* **353:** 282–286, 1999
10. Henry M, Amor M, Henry I *et al.*: Stents in the treatment of renal artery stenosis: long-term follow-up *J Endovasc Surg* **6:** 42–51, 1999
11. Henry M, Amor M, Henry I *et al.*: Stent placement in the renal artery: three-year experience with the Palmaz stent. *J Vasc Intervent Radiol* **7:** 343–350, 1996
12. Blum U, Krumme B, Flugel P *et al.*: Treatment of ostial renal-artery stenoses with vascular endoprostheses after unsuccessful balloon angioplasty. *New Engl J Med* **13:** 336, 459–465, 1997
13. Dorros G, Jaff M, Jain A *et al.*: Follow-up of primary Palmaz–Schatz stent placement for atherosclerotic renal artery stenosis. *Am J Cardiol* **75:** 1051–1055, 1995
14. Isles CG, Robertson S, Hill D: Management of renovascular disease: a review of renal artery stenting in ten studies. *Q J Med* **92:** 159–167, 1999
15. Taylor A, Sheppard D, Macleod MJ *et al.*: Renal artery stent placement in renal artery stenosis: technical and early clinical results. *Clin Radiol* **52:** 451–457, 1997
16. Paulsen D, Klow NE, Rogstad B *et al.*: Preservation of renal function by percutaneous transluminal angioplasty in ischaemic renal disease. *Nephrol Dial Transplant* **14:** 1454–1461, 1999
17. Rodriguez-Lopez JA, Werner A, Ray LI *et al.*: Renal artery stenosis treated with stent deployment: indications, technique, and outcome for 108 patients. *J Vasc Surg* **29:** 617–624, 1999
18. Scolari F, Bracchi M, Valzorio B *et al.*: Cholesterol atheromatous embolism: an increasingly recognized cause of acute renal failure. *Nephrol Dial Transplant* **11:** 1607–1612, 1996
19. Meyrier A: Renal vascular lesions in the elderly: nephrosclerosis or atheromatous renal disease? *Nephrol Dial Transplant* **11:** 45–52, 1996
20. Saleem S, Lakkis FG, Martinez-Maldonado M: Atheroembolic renal disease. *Semin Nephrol* **16:** 309–318, 1996
21. Mayo RR, Swartz RD: Redefining the incidence of clinically detectable atheroembolism *Am J Med* **100:** 524–529, 1996
22. Rauh G, Spengel FA: Blue toe syndrome after initiation of low-dose oral anticoagulation. *Eur J Med Res* **17:** 278–280, 1998
23. Belenfant X, d'Auzac C, Bariety J, Jacquot C: Cholesterol crystal embolism during treatment with low-molecular-weight heparin. *Presse Med* **13:** 1236–1237, 1997
24. Thadhani RI, Camargo CA, Xavier RJ *et al.*: Atheroembolic renal failure after invasive procedures. Natural history based on 52 histologically proven cases. *Medicine (Baltimore)* **74:** 350–358, 1995
25. Boisclair C, Therasse E, Oliva VL *et al.*: Treatment of renal angioplasty failure by percutaneous renal artery stenting with Palmaz stents: midterm technical and clinical results. *Am J Roent* **168:** 245–251, 1997
26. Haqqie SS, Urizar RE, Singh J: Nephrotic-range proteinuria in renal atheroembolic disease: report of four cases. *Am J Kidney Dis* **28:** 493–501, 1996
27. Greenberg A, Bastacky SI, Iqbal A *et al.*: Focal segmental glomerulosclerosis associated with nephrotic syndrome in cholesterol atheroembolism: clinicopathological correlations. *Am J Kidney Dis* **29:** 334–344, 1997

28. Krishnamurthi V, Novick AC, Myles JL: Atheroembolic renal disease: effect on morbidity and survival after revascularization for atherosclerotic renal artery stenosis. *J Urol* **161:** 1093–1096, 1999
29. Feldman RL, Wargovich TJ, Bittl JA: No-touch technique for reducing aortic wall trauma during renal artery stenting. *Catheter Cardiovasc Intervent* **46:** 245–248, 1999

Index

ADVANCED ISSUES IN INTERNATIONAL AND EUROPEAN TAX LAW

This book examines recent developments and high-profile debates that have arisen in the field of international tax law and European tax law. Topics such as international tax avoidance, corporate social responsibility, good governance in tax, matters harmful tax competition, state aid, tax treaty abuse and the Financial Transaction Tax are considered. The OECD/G20 project on Base Erosion and Profit Shifting (BEPS) features prominently in the book. The interaction with the European Union's Action Plan to strengthen the fight against tax fraud and tax evasion is also considered. Particular attention is paid to specific BEPS deliverables, exploring them through the prism of European Union law. Can the two approaches be aligned or are there inherent conflicts between them? The book also explores whether, when it comes to aggressive tax planning, there are internal conflicts between the established case law of the Court of Justice and the emerging policy of the European Union institutions. By so doing it offers a review of issues which are of constitutional importance to the European Union. Finally, the book reflects on the future of international and European tax law in the post-BEPS world.

Advanced Issues in International and European Tax Law

Christiana HJI Panayi

·HART·
PUBLISHING
OXFORD AND PORTLAND, OREGON
2018

Hart Publishing
An imprint of Bloomsbury Publishing Plc

Hart Publishing Ltd
Kemp House
Chawley Park
Cumnor Hill
Oxford OX2 9PH
UK

Bloomsbury Publishing Plc
50 Bedford Square
London
WC1B 3DP
UK

www.hartpub.co.uk
www.bloomsbury.com

Published in North America (US and Canada) by
Hart Publishing
c/o International Specialized Book Services
920 NE 58th Avenue, Suite 300
Portland, OR 97213-3786
USA

www.isbs.com

First published in hardback, 2015
Paperback edition, 2018

British Library Cataloguing-in-Publication Data
A catalogue record for this book is available from the British Library.

ISBN: PB: 978-1-50992-109-6
HB: 978-1-84946-695-0

Typeset by Compuscript Ltd, Shannon

To my family,
Zak, Maria & Nicholas Palexas
and my parents
Nikos & Chrystalla HJI Panayi

FOREWORD

International tax law and European tax law have become ever more complex: this book sets out to discuss some of the most complex, recent issues in the fields of international and European tax law. It analyses the background and the development of these issues, and offers the views of the author and of other academics. The focus of the book is largely on corporate taxation, mostly of multinational companies. The dominating theme of the last few years has been the work of the Organisation for Economic Co-operation and Development on base erosion and profit shifting ('the BEPS Project'). Following on from the work of the OECD, there have been various developments within the European Union, some of them targeted at similar issues, such as the state aid investigations. This book explains both the BEPS Project and the recent developments within the European Union.

Some books have only a short-term value: this book is likely to have both a short-term and a long-term value. In the short term, the book is an up-to-date explanation of recent trends and projects. It will be extremely useful for students starting courses on international tax law or European tax law in the next few years. However, this is not simply a student textbook: there are many coming to discussions of international taxation for the first time who would benefit significantly from reading this book. In the longer term, as matters move forward—with the BEPS Project reaching implementation and the EU projects either going somewhere or going nowhere—this book will become useful as an aide memoire as to the position reached by the middle of 2015. At present, nobody could predict with absolute certainty what impact the BEPS Project will have—though I think one can predict confidently that politicians will announce that it has been a success, whether it has actually been a success or not. Similarly, nobody could, with any confidence, anticipate whether some of the European Union's projects, such as the introduction of a Financial Transaction Tax, will ever see the light of day. Books like this provide an important record for the future historian of international taxation to see where we went wrong, or where we might have done better.

Intriguingly, the book starts with a discussion of CSR—Corporate Social Responsibility—which, quite rightly, provides the backdrop for much of the recent discussion of the tax system for multinational companies. This is an intriguing approach; not many tax books would begin with issues of social responsibility, rather than traditional questions of jurisdiction, tax and international tax principles.

The following three chapters explain in summary form the BEPS Project and the outcomes that have been reached by the summer of 2015. Of course, developments in international and European Union tax law are continuous, and there is no perfect point in time where one can stop the camera, freeze the frame, and show the current position. Choosing the middle of 2015 means that the book cannot deal with the outcomes expected in September/October/December 2015. Nor can the book predict what will happen with the discussions about the multilateral instrument. However, one has to write the book as at some point in time, and two-thirds of the way through the BEPS Project is likely to be as good a point as any.

After the outline of the BEPS Project, the book turns from international tax law developments to EU developments. This is where the author's background in EU tax law is evidenced most strongly. Chapter 5 discusses concepts of tax avoidance under EU law. It discusses both developments in direct and indirect taxation through the Court of Justice, as well as work by the European Commission.

Chapter 6, which discusses the compatibility of the BEPS proposals with EU law, contains an especially interesting analysis. Here the author brings together her knowledge, both of European taxation and of international taxation, to raise queries as to the possibility of implementing some of the potential BEPS outcomes in EU Member States. This discussion is particularly significant, though in an ideal world the discussion of EU limits on potential BEPS outcomes would have taken place before the BEPS Project got underway. One of the justified criticisms that many people have voiced over the BEPS Project is that it began with a number of assumptions—the degree of base erosion and profit shifting being one of them—which should have been tested before work was undertaken to try to find solutions to this problem. In a similar way, it would have been helpful if the Member States of the European Union had known what they could or could not do before they participated in the BEPS Project.

Chapter 7 on state aid and tax matters is written at a crucial point in the investigations by the Competition Directorate in the European Commission. At present, there is relatively little in the public domain on this topic other than the opening decisions with which the Commission began its investigations. The outcome of these investigations may have an even greater impact than the work of the OECD on BEPS, and may advance or derail the future course and form of agreement in this area. The chapter is particularly good in analysing from a critical perspective what is currently known about the position of the Competition Directorate on these matters. What comes out from this chapter is the total irrationality of approaching issues relating to international taxation through rules that have not been developed with those principles in mind, and with investigations carried out by people who do not have a strong background in these principles.

The last substantive chapter, chapter 8, may end up being a record of an historical aberration: it discusses efforts of the European Commission supported by some EU Member States only, to introduce a Financial Transaction Tax. Only time will tell whether agreement is ever reached on such a tax, or whether it will eventually be abandoned as a pointless exercise.

The appearance of a book devoted purely to advanced issues of international and EU tax law gives testimony to the complexity of the issues that are now under discussion. A book like this is a well-designed guide for those coming to the area for the first time, as well as a record for the future of the point at which these discussions have reached by the middle of 2015. It is a very welcome addition to the literature in the fields of both international taxation and EU direct taxation.

PHILIP BAKER QC
FIELD COURT TAX CHAMBERS
August 2015

PREFACE

I started writing this book perhaps at the most challenging time in recent tax history—the summer of 2013 when the BEPS project was launched. Most of the chapters of this book had to be completely rewritten with the passing of time and the hurricane of developments that followed. It was not just the quantity of materials that were produced as deliverables of the 15 Actions of the BEPS project. The European Union has also been very active in the area, releasing several important measures and proposals, with the promise of more to come. This book covers all these developments, up to 1 June 2015.

Special thanks are due to a number of people for their help and support. I would like to thank Philip Baker, Joy Svasti-Salee, Margarita Liasi and Luca Cerioni for their invaluable insights and comments on earlier versions of this manuscript. All errors are mine, of course.

This book would not have been written had it not been for my family. I am deeply indebted to my parents for their unconditional love and unwavering support throughout the years. I would like to thank my father for his continuous inspiration and encouragement. I am who I am because of his vision and sacrifices. I would also like to thank my husband and his family for their support. A good amount of baby-sitting and endless hours of watching Peppa Pig had to be endured to enable me to concentrate on my research and write this book in the short timeframe provided. Most of all, I would like to thank my children Maria and Nicholas, for all their sacrifices and the tolerance they have shown, even at this young age, towards the complexities of BEPS and reforming the international and European tax systems.

CONTENTS

TABLE OF CASES

United Kingdom

Court of Justice of the European Union

EFTA Court

TABLE OF LEGISLATION

United Kingdom

European Union

Treaties

TABLE OF INTERNATIONAL INSTRUMENTS

Introduction

The author started writing this book a few months before the launch of the OECD/G20 Base Erosion and Profit Shifting (BEPS) project. Unsurprisingly, both the structure and contents of the book are significantly different from what was originally envisaged. This is understandable given that we are currently in the midst of a large-scale review of the international tax system in an attempt to tackle international tax avoidance, or tax abuse, or aggressive tax planning, or however else it is described. The effort is much more coordinated than ever and the level of political commitment unprecedented. Both of these variables are likely to be short-lived, hence the ambitious agenda of the OECD and the G20 in the BEPS project.

The BEPS project features prominently in this book. It is shown that the project, although ambitious, remains somehow realistic. There is an attempt to capture the parameters of this project and consider its impact not only in the wider international tax community, but also in the European tax community. The interaction with the European Union's Action Plan to strengthen the fight against tax fraud and tax evasion is also considered. Particular attention is paid to specific BEPS deliverables, exploring them through the prism of European Union law.

This book also examines other recent developments and high-profile debates that have arisen in the field of international tax law and European tax law. Topics such as corporate social responsibility, good tax governance, state aid and aggressive tax planning, and the Financial Transaction Tax are also considered.

In Chapter one, there is an overview of the various factors and events that led to the launch of the BEPS project. The rhetoric against harmful tax competition and tax havens is examined. Following that, reported cases of aggressive tax planning by multinationals are considered and the aftermath of these cases in some jurisdictions is reviewed. What seems to be emerging from some of the hearings and investigations that have taken place is the overarching inadequacy of existing principles of international tax law to deal with the internationalisation of business. Standards of morality and fairness are increasingly becoming relevant, sometimes to the detriment of legal certainty. What is also apparent is that notions of corporate social responsibility—as far as companies are concerned—and good governance in tax matters—as far as countries are concerned—are becoming prevalent. Both of these concepts are examined. The link between corporate social responsibility and aggressive tax planning is considered, both internationally and within the European Union. It is questioned whether companies that engage in aggressive tax planning are socially irresponsible. Although there is no conclusive answer to this from the brief overview of some of the important literature on the topic, it is argued that corporate social responsibility implications are likely to become increasingly entrenched in the whole debate.

In Chapters two to four, the BEPS project is considered in greater detail. Actions 1 to 5 are considered in Chapter two, Actions 6 to 10 are considered in Chapter three and Actions 11 to 15 are considered in Chapter four. In these chapters, there is an overview of the various discussion drafts and reports produced in the context of these Action items, their merits and demerits. As will be shown in these chapters, the aim of most of the Action items is to address—or at least to attempt to address, either for the first time or for the umpteenth time—some of the most contentious areas in international tax law. Notwithstanding the expectations that had been raised at the inception of the BEPS project, the OECD does not carry out a holistic review of the international tax regime and does not make drastic recommendations. Most of the deliverables produced are very much imbued with pragmatism.

In Chapter four, there is also a review of the OECD's engagement with developing countries. Developing countries have consistently recognised the importance of addressing BEPS as part of wider measures to increase domestic resource mobilisation and promote stable economic growth. It is questioned whether the BEPS agenda prejudices developing countries and whether their interests are properly reflected in the Action Plan. Steps taken by the OECD to address these concerns are considered.

The next chapters examine the measures taken by the European Union to tackle international tax avoidance, many of which share similarities with the BEPS proposals. In the first part of Chapter five, the judicial response to the concept of tax abuse by the Court of Justice is considered. This is then juxtaposed with the Commission's initiatives and most importantly its Action Plan as a newly-formed policy on international tax avoidance. This chapter sets the background against which, in the next chapter, Chapter six, there is an analysis of the compatibility of the various items of the BEPS Action Plan with European Union law.

In Chapter seven, there is a detailed analysis of the state aid prohibition with an emphasis on fiscal state aids. The role of the Commission and of national tax authorities is considered, as well as the rights of competitors and third parties. There is a review of recent important cases in the area of tax law, as well as the latest legislative and quasi-legislative developments. Finally, the use of the state aid prohibition in tackling some (perceived) examples of aggressive tax planning is examined. The Commission's state aid investigations into Apple, Fiat, Starbucks and Amazon are critically reviewed and thoughts are offered as to the legal credentials of the Commission's 'prudent independent market operator' test.

Chapter eight explores another angle of the debate which preceded the BEPS project—the proposal for a Financial Transaction Tax. There is a consideration of the ongoing efforts by the Commission and Member States to introduce the Financial Transaction Tax. The original Commission proposal and the subsequent proposal to be adopted through enhanced cooperation are analysed. The suitability of the enhanced cooperation procedure as a mechanism of adopting legislative proposals and especially tax proposals is examined and the future of the Financial Transaction Tax considered.

In Chapter nine, the author concludes the book with a general discussion on the themes developed previously and offers some thoughts on the development of international and European Union tax law in a post-BEPS world.

The contents of this book are based on materials available up to 1 June 2015.

1

Aggressive Tax Planning, Good Governance in Tax Matters and Corporate Social Responsibility: The New Themes

Increasingly, the international tax community is dominated by a high-level debate on topics such as tax avoidance, aggressive tax planning, corporate social responsibility, tax governance, transparency and exchange of information. Among others, the European Commission, the OECD and G8/G20 countries have become involved in this debate. The most important recent development has been the launch of the OECD/G20's Action Plan to combat base erosion and profit shifting (BEPS). This chapter examines some of the factors and events that led to the BEPS project.

1.1. Harmful Tax Competition, Tax Havens, Base Erosion and Profit Shifting

Globalisation has increased the possibilities for erosion of the national tax base. The global economic crisis has exacerbated this and placed heavy burdens on government budgets.[1] In recent years, the tax practices of some well-known multinational enterprises (MNEs) have attracted attention for their aggressive tax practices,[2] which although legal, they often lead to very low effective tax rates. The ability to shift profits into low or no tax jurisdictions with little corresponding change in business operations has also been criticised for distorting the allocation of capital and eroding national tax bases, especially of developed countries.

[1] Amir Pichhadze, 'Exposing Unaddressed Issues in the OECD's BEPS Project: What About the Roles and Implications of Contract Interpretation Law and Private International Law in the Transfer Pricing Arm's Length Comparability Analysis?' (2015) 7 *World Tax Journal* 99–167, 103.

[2] The term 'aggressive tax planning' was first described in the OECD's 2008 Intermediaries report, although the definition has now evolved. See *OECD Study into the Role of Tax Intermediaries* (OECD, 2008), available on: www.oecd.org/tax/administration/39882938.pdf. See Glossary to the report, p 87: 'Aggressive tax planning. This refers to two areas of concern for revenue bodies: Planning involving

Aggressive tax practices are also thought to have led to a phenomenon coined as stateless income. Stateless income has been described

> as income derived for tax purposes by a multinational group from business activities in a country other than the domicile of the group's ultimate parent company but which is subject to tax only in a jurisdiction that is neither the source of the factors of production through which the income was derived, nor the domicile of the group's parent company.[3]

In an era when many countries, even those with advanced economies, face a fiscal crisis and budget deficits, stateless income is often criticised for leading to a decline in corporate tax collection.

However, MNE behaviour does not occur in vacuum. Stateless income could be construed as the result of tax competition between nations.[4] Base erosion and profit shifting by MNEs would be largely ineffective 'without countries offering preferential tax rules, including low/no tax regimes for particular taxpayers or income categories and benign provisions on profit measurement'.[5] To an extent, MNE tax avoidance is just the flipside of harmful tax competition.[6]

When one talks about harmful tax competition, traditionally, tax havens and harmful tax practices come into mind. The OECD has already spent a considerable amount of time dealing with the phenomenon of harmful tax competition in the late 90s. The OECD project on harmful tax practices was launched in 1996. The initiative was carried out through the Forum on Harmful Tax Practices. In 1998, the Forum produced its first major report, entitled *Harmful Tax Competition: An Emerging Global Issue*.[7] The report only covered geographically mobile

a tax position that is tenable but has unintended and unexpected tax revenue consequences. Revenue bodies' concerns relate to the risk that tax legislation can be misused to achieve results which were not foreseen by the legislators. This is exacerbated by the often lengthy period between the time schemes are created and sold and the time revenue bodies discover them and remedial legislation is enacted. Taking a tax position that is favourable to the taxpayer without openly disclosing that there is uncertainty whether significant matters in the tax return accord with the law. Revenue bodies' concerns relate to the risk that taxpayers will not disclose their view on the uncertainty or risk taken in relation to grey areas of law (sometimes, revenue bodies would not even agree that the law is in doubt)'.

[3] Edward D Kleinbard, 'Through a Latte Darkly: Starbucks's Stateless Income Planning' (2013) 139 *Tax Notes* 1515, 1517 (24 June 2013). The mechanics of stateless income tax planning include earnings stripping, particularly aided by the US check-the-box rules, transfer pricing with an emphasis on abuses in cost sharing arrangements, aggressive contractual terms in transfer pricing and legal system arbitrage etc. For an analysis of the tax policy issues surrounding stateless income, see Edward Kleinbard, 'Stateless Income' (2011) 11 *Florida Tax Review* 699. Also see article by the same author, 'The Lessons of Stateless Income' (2011) 65 *Tax Law Review* 99.

[4] For a generic analysis, see Mindy Herzfeld, 'The Power of a Name: Stateless Income and Its Failings' (2015) 77 *Tax Notes International* 1019 (23 March 2015). Also see an ACCA report produced by Sinclair Davidson, entitled 'Multinational corporations, stateless income and tax havens', available on: www.accaglobal.com/content/dam/acca/global/PDF-technical/tax-publications/tech-tp-mcsith.pdf.

[5] Hugh J Ault, Wolfgang Schön and Stephen E Shay, 'Base Erosion and Profit Shifting: A Roadmap for Reform' (2014) 68 *Bulletin for International Taxation* 275, 276.

[6] *Ibid.*

[7] OECD, *Harmful Tax Competition: An Emerging Global Issue* (OECD Publications, 1998).

activities such as financial and other service activities, including the provision of intangibles. Special tax incentives directed at manufacturing and foreign direct investment were outside the scope of the report. The concept of harmful tax competition was not defined but its harmful effects were raised.[8]

The report targeted tax havens and preferential tax regimes, though no definitions were given.[9] Criteria were used to identify both tax havens and harmful preferential tax regimes[10] and harmful tax regimes.[11] A number of recommendations were made for domestic legislation, tax treaties and international co-operation. The Forum was responsible for supervising the implementation of the standstill and roll back provisions.

The publication of the report led to intense dialogue aimed at eliminating preferential tax regimes within OECD and non-OECD countries. This report and subsequent reports[12] encouraged—rather forcefully—OECD and non-OECD jurisdictions to strengthen their commitments to the principles of transparency and effective exchange of information. These standards were developed by the Global Forum on Taxation[13] but not all jurisdictions showed the same willingness. Following the 2001 Progress Report, in 2002, the Model Agreement on Exchange of Information on Tax Matters was created and used as the basis for the negotiation

[8] These were: the distortion of investment flows; the threat to the integrity and fairness of the tax systems; the discouragement of taxpayers' compliance; the redesign of the appropriate balance between revenue and public spending; the shift of tax burden to other bases (labour, consumption); and the increase of administrative compliance costs. *Ibid*, pp 22–25.

[9] As far as tax havens were concerned, the report referred to 'countries that are able to finance their public services with no or [only] nominal income taxes and that offer themselves as places to be used by non-residents to escape tax in their country of residence' and those that 'raise significant revenues from their income tax but whose tax system has features constituting harmful tax competition'. The report described harmful preferential tax regimes as countries collecting a significant level of revenue from individual and/or corporate income tax but whose tax systems have preferential features that allow the relevant income to be subject to low or no taxation. It could be both tax havens and high-tax jurisdictions: *ibid*, p 20.

[10] (a) no or only nominal tax (generally or in special circumstances) and self-promotion (or appearance of self-promotion as a place to be used by non-residents to escape their residence country taxes); (b) lack of effective exchange of information; (c) lack of transparency; (d) no substantial activities. *Ibid*, pp 22–34.

[11] (a) no or low effective tax rates; (b) ring-fencing; (c) lack of effective exchange of information; (d) lack of transparency. Also, the artificial definition of the tax base and failure to comply with internationally accepted transfer pricing rules. *Ibid*, pp 22–34.

[12] See, for example, OECD, *Towards Global Co-operation: Report to the 2000 Ministerial Council Meeting* and *Recommendations by the Committee on Fiscal Affairs: Progress in Identifying and Eliminating Harmful Tax Practices*; OECD, *Consolidated Application Note: Guidance in applying the 1998 Report to Preferential tax regimes*; OECD, *The OECD's project on Harmful Tax Practices: The 2001 Progress Report*; OECD, *The OECD's project on Harmful Tax Practices: The 2004 Progress*; OECD, *The OECD's project on Harmful Tax Practices: The 2006 Progress Report*; OECD, *The OECD's project on Harmful Tax Practices: The 2007 Progress Report.*

[13] The Global Forum had established a Sub-Group on Level Playing Field Issues to develop a set of proposals which were endorsed at a Global Forum meeting in Berlin in June 2004. At this meeting the representatives of 42 OECD and non-OECD jurisdictions approved a joint report on how to achieve their common objective of a global level playing field based on high standards of transparency and effective exchange of information. The report contemplated actions of an individual, bilateral and a collective nature.

of many Tax Information Exchange Agreements. Even though the US gradually became less supportive of the OECD's project insisting on certain changes,[14] the project was quite successful and by 2006 all regimes which were identified as generating harmful tax competition were abolished, the last one being the Luxembourg 1929 holding company regime. In the 2006 Progress Report,[15] it was claimed that the project had fully achieved its initial aims and the mandate given by the OECD Council on dealing with harmful preferential tax regimes in member countries was met. It was announced that future work in this area would focus on monitoring any continuing and newly introduced preferential tax regimes identified by member countries.

Much of the discourse on the OECD's harmful tax competition project was eventually linked to the benchmarks of transparency and exchange of information. In the G20 meeting of finance ministers and central bank governors, there was a call 'on financial centres and other jurisdictions within and outside the OECD which have not yet adopted these standards to take the necessary steps, in particular in allowing access to bank and entity ownership information'.[16]

Whilst the general feeling was that the OECD's project on harmful tax competition was being wound up, the global financial crisis which started around 2008 led to a renewed 'attack' on tax havens, and later on to jurisdictions that were perceived as facilitating aggressive tax planning. The G20 Communiqué issued at the London 2009 Summit stated that major failures in the financial sector and in financial regulation and supervision were fundamental causes of the financial crisis. The G20 leaders agreed to take action against non-cooperative jurisdictions, including tax havens, and if necessary to deploy sanctions to protect their public finances and financial systems.[17] The era of banking secrecy was declared to be over and countries were called upon to adopt and implement the international tax standards of transparency and information exchange—standards which had assumed top priority by then. This message was reinforced at the G8 meeting in July 2009 and subsequent G8 and G20 meetings, though no sanctions have yet to be taken.

Since 2009, the OECD has been publishing progress reports on the implementation of the internationally agreed tax standard[18] by jurisdictions surveyed by the

[14] The project was initially supported by the USA. In 2001, the Bush administration acting through its Secretary of the Treasury, Paul O'Neil, raised objections. The OECD project was accused of lacking focus, destroying otherwise beneficial tax competition, interfering with the tax sovereignty of foreign nations etc.

[15] See OECD, *The OECD's project on Harmful Tax Practices: The 2006 Progress Report.*

[16] G20 meeting of Financial Ministers and Bank Governors, Berlin, 20–21 November 2004, para 9. Also see, Jan Wouters and Katrien Meuwissen, *Global Tax Governance: Work in Progress?*, Working Paper No 59—February 2011 (Leuven Centre for Global Governance Studies).

[17] G20 London Summit—*Leaders' Statement*—2 April 2009, para 15.

[18] This is set out in footnote 1 of the *Progress Report on the Jurisdictions Surveyed by the OECD Global Forum in Implementing the Internationally Agreed Tax Standard*, on the progress made as at 2 April 2009. 'The internationally agreed tax standard … requires exchange of information on request in all tax matters for the administration and enforcement of domestic tax law without regard to a domestic tax interest requirement or bank secrecy for tax purposes. It also provides for extensive safeguards to protect the confidentiality of the information exchanged'. www.oecd.org/ctp/42497950.pdf.

Global Forum. In these progress reports, there were three lists of jurisdictions: the white list,[19] the grey list[20] and the black list.[21] In the April 2009 progress report, there were four jurisdictions on the black list[22] and numerous jurisdictions on the grey list. This list has been regularly updated and there are now no countries on the black list. All jurisdictions covered by Global Forum have now committed to the international tax standards and more than half have implemented them. Furthermore, a peer review process has begun to monitor jurisdictions, reviewing the legal and regulatory framework, the actual implementation of standards, their tax treaties and tax information exchange agreements.

Notwithstanding the self-declared successful conclusion of the OECD's harmful tax competition project, tax havens still exist—many mostly reconfigured and with different characteristics. It is a widely made assertion that the existence of tax havens has contributed to the financial crisis and has had a major impact on the fiscal sustainability of countries.[23] Other criticisms focus on the impact of tax havens on developing countries and measure the loss of revenues to such countries only and not on developed countries.[24] These claims are not easily proven though.

One of the endemic problems of the tax havens discourse is that it is still beleaguered by definitional uncertainty. Its scope is also uncertain and ever changing—notwithstanding the work of the OECD, or perhaps *because* of the work of the OECD in this area. In a report commissioned by the Norwegian government in 2008[25] the damaging effect of tax havens was examined. It was argued, inter alia, that tax havens increase the risk premium in international financial markets, that they undermine the tax system and public finances and they increase the inequitable distribution of tax revenues. It was also reported that tax havens reduce the efficiency of resource allocation in developing countries and generally reduce their revenues and damage their growth. They also make economic crime more profitable. Not much empirical evidence was shown to support these conclusions though. Instead, it was conceded that 'economic literature cites a number of positive aspects related to tax havens'.[26]

[19] This list included countries that had substantially implemented the internationally agreed tax standard.

[20] This list included countries committed to the internationally agreed tax standard but that had not yet substantially implemented it.

[21] This list included countries that had not committed to the internationally agreed tax standard.

[22] Costa Rica, Malaysia, Philippines, Uruguay.

[23] See, for example, Sol Picciotto, 'How tax havens helped to create a crisis', *Financial Times*, 5 May 2009 at: www.ft.com/cms/s/0/96ec9414-39a6-11de-b82d-00144feabdc0.html#axzz2uzMLkQmw.

[24] See below.

[25] Commission on capital flight from developing countries: Tax Havens and Development—Status, Analyses and Measures. Report from the Government Commission on Capital Flight from Poor Countries. Appointed by Royal Decree of 27 June 2008. Submitted to Erik Solheim, Minister of the Environment and International Development, on 18 June 2009 (henceforth, the Norwegian study).

[26] See *ibid* p 71 et seq.

In this report, it was emphasised that 'the classic tax havens are not alone in promulgating systems that cause loss and harm to public and private interests in other states'.[27] In other words, tax haven regimes are not the prerogative of small sunny islands with minimal tax rates. High-tax countries could also have regimes which are akin to those of tax havens. In any case, as commented, while offshore financial centres may be relevant to the discredited international financial system, their role tends to be exaggerated or misconstrued.[28]

Advocacy groups, non-governmental organisations (NGOs) and civil society in general have also had an important role in raising public awareness on tax havens as well as on what they perceive to be illegitimate tax planning practices and tax dodgers. For example, the UK Uncut movement, a grass-roots activist group, has conducted demonstrations across the UK targeting alleged tax dodgers. On 25 November 2013, the Tax Solidarity Week of Action took place. This formed part of the Europe-wide 'Stop Tax Dodging' initiative—'an initiative bringing together the voices of civil society in 15 countries across Europe, united in a desire to see an end to tax dodging by multinational companies and more action by European leaders to tackle this problem'.[29] There were actions in Denmark, Finland, Sweden, France, Belgium, Italy, Spain, the UK, Czech Republic, Hungary, Slovenia and Poland, ranging from stunts and petitions to film showings, TV spots and public meetings.

Also, reports and briefing papers were published by several NGOs discussing links between tax evasion and tax havens. In a report published by the Tax Justice Network, it was suggested that US$21 to $32 trillion were hidden in tax havens worldwide.[30] In 2011, ActionAid had published information showing that 98 of the UK's biggest companies, most of which operate in the developing world, were using tax havens. This information was reviewed in May 2013, where it was shown that little had changed.[31] In 2013, Christian Aid published a report on the profit-shifting 'lure' of tax havens for multinationals.[32] The authors of the report concluded that MNEs with connections to tax havens engage in profit shifting

[27] Norwegian study, n 25 above, p 21.

[28] See Geoffrey Loomer and Giorgia Maffini, *Tax Havens and the Financial Crisis* (2009) Project Report. Centre for Business Taxation. Available on: www.sbs.ox.ac.uk/sites/default/files/Business_Taxation/Docs/Publications/Policy_Papers/TaxHavensandtheFinancialCrisis.pdf.

[29] www.christianaid.org.uk/ActNow/blog/november-2013/stop-tax-dodging-campaign-across-europe.aspx.

[30] See James S Henry, 'The Price of Offshore Revisited', *Tax Justice Network*, July 2012. Available on: www.taxjustice.net/cms/upload/pdf/Price_of_Offshore_Revisited_120722.pdf. This was believed to be a conservative estimate. See p 5.

[31] See www.actionaid.org.uk/campaign/ftse-100-tax-haven-tracker. It has been claimed that these figures are misleading as UK companies mostly use Delaware companies, which pay US federal tax at 35%. See Bill Dodwell's testimony at the Public Accounts Committee proceedings, reported in 'This Week', *Tax Journal*, Issue 1156, p 8 (8 February 2013).

[32] See Christian Aid Occasional Paper Number 9: *Multinationals and the Profit-Shifting Lure of Tax Havens* by Petr Janský and Alex Prats, Principal Economic Justice Policy Adviser, Christian Aid (March 2013). Available on: www.christianaid.org.uk/Images/CA-OP-9-multinational-corporations-tax-havens-March-2013.pdf.

more intensively than those MNEs with no tax haven links, due to the greater incentives, mostly low tax rates, and other opportunities on offer such as secrecy provisions.[33]

The rhetoric against tax havens, especially from some NGOs' perspective,[34] is often linked with that of tax dodging and the depletion of resources of developing nations. It is often claimed that tax dodging entrenches poverty,[35] weakens the economies of developing countries and deprives the locals from investment in health, education, infrastructure and good quality basic services.[36] Oxfam[37] and Global Financial Integrity[38] have released reports estimating that developing countries lose an estimated US$100 billion to $160 billion annually to corporate tax dodging. Christian Aid estimates that trade mispricing and false invoicing costs developing countries US$160 billion a year.[39] This is thought to be significantly more than the total aid given to them by the developed countries and much more (thought to be three times more) than the amount required to end hunger on an annual basis.[40]

Whatever the legitimacy of these claims and the definition and scope of a rather elusive underlying problem—either tax havens, or harmful tax competition, or tax avoidance, or tax dodging, or aggressive tax planning—as will be shown in this book, an incredible momentum has built up. This much is undeniable. What the final result will be remains to be seen.

[33] *Ibid*, p 10.

[34] See, for example, information on Christian Aid's website (www.christianaid.org.uk/resources/policy/tax.aspx), on Actionaid's website (www.actionaid.org.uk/campaign/tax-justice-policy), a press release by Eurodad (www.eurodad.org/Entries/view/1546115/2013/12/16/Press-Release-Giving-with-one-hand-and-taking-with-the-other-CSOs-urge-European-leaders-to-take-action-against-tax-dodging) etc.

[35] See, for example, the report entitled *Tax Abuses, Poverty and Human Rights* released on 8 October 2013 by the International Bar Association's Human Rights Institute task force. Available on Tax Analysts Document Service, Doc 2013-23604.

[36] See, eg www.healthpovertyaction.org/policy-and-resources/tax-and-health/tax-dodging-global-health/;www.actionaid.org.uk/campaign/tax-justice-policy#gsFxWtrI3VxFUsoJ.99.

[37] www.oxfam.org/en/pressroom/pressrelease/2013-09-01/tax-evasion-damaging-poor-country-economies.

[38] See 'The Implied Tax Revenue Loss from Trade Mispricing', by Ann Hollingshead, February 2010: www.gfintegrity.org/storage/gfip/documents/reports/implied%20tax%20revenue%20loss%20report_final.pdf.

[39] The accuracy of the 160 billion figure has been questioned. See, for example, written evidence to the House of Commons International Development Committee by the Head of Tax of Rio Tinto, an international mining group. The evidence which was given in February 2012 is available on. www.publications.parliament.uk/pa/cm/201213/cmselect/cmintdev/130/130vw23.htm. Also see statements by Heather Self that '[Christian Aid's] continuing use of unreliable and out of date figures, which exaggerate the extent to which behaviour by multinationals contributes to the problem, harms their case; they require transparency and accuracy from companies and should meet that standard themselves … If reliable estimates are simply not available, they should acknowledge this'. News, *Tax Journal*, Issue 1201, p 2 (24 January 2014).

[40] See Tax Justice Toolkit, *Understanding Tax and Development* (Christian Aid, 2013) p 8, available on: www.christianaid.org.uk/Images/Tax-toolkit-1-understanding-tax-development-September-2013.pdf.

1.2. Aggressive Tax Planning of Multinationals: The Politics of the Debate

As discussed in the previous section, the polemic against tax havens and/or low tax regimes is not something new. It has certainly been ongoing at least since the OECD's 1998 harmful tax competition project. However, it would seem that the focus appears to be shifting away from tax havens—something foreign, afar and difficult to influence. Arguably, even the OECD in the course of its 1998 project began to focus on benchmarks such as transparency and exchange of information, rather than interfering (further) with the sovereignty of alleged tax havens. Lately, some of the world's largest multinationals, such as Vodafone, Amazon, Google, Starbucks and Microsoft have been scrutinised for their (technically) legal but highly aggressive tax planning practices, using transfer pricing, intercompany lending, royalty payments for licencing agreements, cost sharing agreements, group losses etc. Fuelled by media attention,[41] the reporting of these practices has in some countries led to public outcry.

It should be pointed out that the issue is of concern to both residence countries and source countries. To put it simplistically, residence countries are concerned that profits held offshore—which appear to belong to resident companies or controlled foreign entities—remain untaxed. By contrast, source countries are concerned that profits which could be perceived to arise within their jurisdiction go untaxed or are seriously depleted/eroded before being taxed. A combination of inadequate and/or antiquated rules in both the countries of residence and source has led to very low effective tax rates and often stateless income, a concept discussed above. Although this concept has been criticised,[42] it has become a catchy phrase and is often used in describing the desired end-result of some MNE tax practices. In any case, stateless income, however defined and whatever it actually encompasses, faces broader conceptual issues of efficiency, tax-base protection and ultimately, fairness.

Politicians (and governments) in many jurisdictions seemed to have jumped on this bandwagon. In the last few years, senior executives of major multinationals were called upon in the UK to give evidence to Parliament's Public Accounts Committee. This was because despite huge profits generated by these multinationals, very little or nothing was paid as UK corporation tax. This is, arguably, the source country perspective to this problem. A brief analysis of selected hearings will be given in this chapter.

[41] See, for example, a few references: www.theguardian.com/business/taxavoidance, www.mirror.co.uk/news/uk-news/tax-avoidance-soars-35billion-under-2362328, www.independent.co.uk/news/uk/politics/revealed-47bn-corporation-tax-lost-through-evasion-and-avoidance-as-royal-mail-is-sold-for-650m-less-than-it-is-worth-8874873.html.

[42] See analysis in 1.1 above.

Starbucks had paid no income taxes in the UK since 2009. At a Public Accounts Committee hearing in November 2012, Troy Alstead, the Starbucks CFO, had argued, inter alia, that high rental costs and a very competitive market had generated losses for the firm for 14 out of the 15 years it had been operating in the UK. Although investors were told that the UK operations were profitable and business was growing, no income tax had in fact been paid to the UK Exchequer since 2009. It was also reported that Starbucks had paid just £8.6 million in corporation tax in the UK over 14 years.[43] The Committee members challenged these figures, arguing it was highly improbable that anyone running a business would keep it going if it was not making any money.[44] Alstead acknowledged that the UK company had made a number of payments to related companies, reducing the taxable base. The taxable base was further reduced through the use of intercompany loans and the company's transfer pricing practices.[45]

Although there was no illegality involved, nevertheless, fearing a boycott by the public, Starbucks pledged to pay £20 million in UK corporate tax over the next two years (2013 and 2014) regardless of its economic performance.[46] This move has been criticised as reducing corporate tax obligations to voluntary charitable donations.[47] It has also been criticised that the social licence to operate has now expanded beyond labour and environmental issues.[48] In fact, it appears to be above that required by current law and rather governed by vague extra-legal standards. Arguably, '[f]or multinationals, that makes for an uncertain future: one in effect shaped by activist vigilantism'.[49] The Starbucks case illustrates this very well. Following its pledge, UK Uncut staged a number of protests at more than 40 Starbucks shops, 'transforming' Starbucks stores into refuges, crèches and

[43] See special four month investigation reported on Reuters (Special Report: How Starbucks avoids UK taxes, by Tom Bergin, available on: uk.reuters.com/article/2012/10/15/us-britain-starbucks-tax-idUKBRE89E0EX20121015. Also see www.bbc.com/news/business-20288077. For a similar investigation in Greece, see www.forologoumenos.gr/permalink/23636.html.

[44] See Julie Martin, 'UK Puts Executives in Hot Seat Over Transfer Pricing Practices', 2012 *WTD* 221-24 (15 November 2012).

[45] For example, it paid annual royalties for intellectual property up to 6% of sales. Half of that royalty was paid to Starbucks' European headquarters in the Netherlands, which had few employees but which was subject to a private low tax arrangement with the Netherlands government. See Stephanie Soong Johnston, 'UK to Investigate Starbucks's Tax Affairs', 2012 *WTD* 202-2 (18 October 2012); Hans van den Hurk, 'Starbucks versus the People' (2014) 68 *Bulletin for International Taxation* 27–34.

[46] See Randall Jackson, 'Starbucks's U.K. Tax Payment Pledge Reduces Corporate Tax to a Charitable Donation, Critics Say' 2012 *WTD* 237-3 (10 December 2012). Also see www.telegraph.co.uk/finance/newsbysector/banksandfinance/9727048/Starbucks-to-start-paying-more-UK-tax-Kris-Engskov-speech-in-full.html. Technically, Starbucks is thought to have deferred deductions for 2013 and 2014 expenses.

[47] For an overview, see Allison Christians, 'The Big Picture: How Starbucks Lost Its Social License—and Paid £20 Million to Get It Back' (2013) 71 *Tax Notes International* 637 (12 August 2013).

[48] *Ibid*, p 638.

[49] *Ibid*, p 639.

homeless shelters.[50] On 16 April 2014, Starbucks announced that it would move the regional head office representing its European, Middle Eastern and African business from Amsterdam to London at the end of 2014. As a result of the move, Starbucks was expected to pay more tax in the UK. However, it did not specify what kind of additional tax it would pay or how much.[51]

Amazon was faced with similar controversies. In the UK, Amazon's public policy director Andrew Cecil was also asked to appear in the Public Accounts Committee. Amazon was able to minimise its tax liability by transferring ownership of its UK business to Amazon EU SARL, a Luxembourg company, in 2006. This was part of corporate restructuring which took place in 2005–06, to lower the company's effective tax rate over time. Following the reorganisation, Amazon was able to classify its UK business as a sales company. As such, sales made in the UK were billed to Luxembourg and profits made from those sales were taxed in Luxembourg and not in the UK. Nevertheless, there was great disparity in the number of people employed by the Luxembourg office and the UK business, as well as in the turnover of these companies.[52] Also, notwithstanding the claim that the UK business was merely a service facility, books, staff payroll and customers were all based in the UK.

Cecil was accused of being evasive in his responses to the Public Accounts Committee. He claimed no information was available to show the proportion of Amazon's European sales into the UK and in any case such information could not be disclosed publicly. Cecil also claimed he did not know who owned the holding company which owned Amazon EU SARL in Luxembourg. Unsurprisingly, the Public Accounts Committee was not very impressed with his responses.[53] In any case, caving to international pressure, it has been recently reported that Amazon has changed its EU business structure so that from 1 May 2015 it would record retail sales made to customers in the UK and some other EU jurisdictions in those jurisdictions rather than Luxembourg.[54] Incidentally, with this move, Amazon might also avoid the UK's diverted profits tax which is higher than the normal tax due.[55]

[50] See reports on www.telegraph.co.uk/finance/newsbysector/retailandconsumer/9731618/Starbucks-branches-hit-by-tax-protests.html, www.theguardian.com/business/2012/dec/09/starbucks-stores-uk-uncut-protest and many more news outlets.

[51] Stephanie Soong Johnston, 'Starbucks to Pay More UK Tax After Moving Regional Headquarters to London', 2014 *WTD* 74-1 (16 April 2014). Starbucks attributed the reduced sales and the drop in turnover to the closure of several unprofitable stores. See Stephanie Soong Johnston, 'Starbucks Denies U.K. Sales Drop Related to Tax Controversy', 2014 *WTD* 80-4 (25 April 2014).

[52] Kristen A Parillo, 'HMRC Targeting Amazon's U.K. Operations', 2012 *WTD* 67-4 (6 April 2012)

[53] It has been reported that the Public Accounts Committee branded Cecil's responses as 'pathetic', 'insulting to everyone's intelligence' and 'not acceptable'. See report available on: www.thebookseller.com/news/amazon%E2%80%99s-corporation-tax-slammed-hoc-committee.html.

[54] Stephanie Soong Johnston, 'Amazon Changes EU Structure to Book Profits in Local Countries', 2015 *WTD* 101-1 (27 May 2015).

[55] For a discussion on the UK's diverted profits tax, see Ch 9.

Google's encounters with the Public Accounts Committee were encapsulated in a report entitled *Tax Avoidance—Google* (henceforth, the Google Report).[56] The Committee questioned how Google, which generated US$18 billion revenue from the UK between 2006 and 2011, could only pay the equivalent of just US$16 million of UK corporation taxes in the same period.

It was argued that there was an overwhelming disparity between where the profit was generated and where tax was paid. Google used the now defunct 'double Irish' structure. Such a structure was commonly used and allowed companies to shift profits to low or no tax jurisdictions by taking advantage of mismatches in corporate residency rules.[57] Google's subsidiaries in Europe, the Middle East and Africa paid royalties to an Irish limited company which made deductible royalty payments to a Dutch BV. In turn, the Dutch BV made a deductible royalty payment to a dual-resident Irish/Bermuda company. The latter company was only taxable in Bermuda which in fact imposed no corporate income tax. Therefore, effectively, profits earned by Google in royalty-paying jurisdictions remained largely untaxed. Kleinbard described Google's structure as the archetypal example of stateless income.[58]

Google defended its tax position by claiming that its sales of advertising space to UK clients took place in Ireland. The Public Accounts Committee found this argument deeply unconvincing on the basis of evidence that, despite sales being billed from Ireland, most sales revenue was generated by staff in the UK. According to the committee:

> It is quite clear to us that sales to UK clients are the primary purpose, responsibility and result of its UK operation, and that the processing of sales through Google Ireland has no purpose other than to avoid UK corporation tax.[59]

According to the Public Accounts Committee, this elaborate corporate construct had damaged Google's reputation in the UK and undermined confidence in the effectiveness of HMRC. The use of a Bermuda company to ultimately shelter the profits was also criticised.[60]

[56] See Google Report published in 17 June 2013, available on: www.parliament.uk/business/committees/committees-a-z/commons-select/public-accounts-committee/news/tax-avoidance-google/.

[57] On October 2014, the Irish Finance Minister Michael Noonan announced that from 1 January 2015, Ireland would eliminate the ability of new companies to use the double Irish tax arrangement, by changing residency rules to require all companies registered in Ireland to be Irish tax residents as well. It was also announced that a 'knowledge development box' would be introduced in 2016 or when the EU Code of Conduct Group (Business Taxation) completed its review of EU patent box regimes. See Antony Ting, 'Old Wine in a New Bottle: Ireland's Revised Definition of Corporate Residence and the War on BEPS' [2014] *British Tax Review* 237–47; Margaret Burrow, 'Ireland to Stop New "Double Irish" Arrangements in 2015' (2014) 145 *Tax Notes* 279 (20 October 2014); David D Steward, 'Ireland Targets "Stateless" Companies in 2014 Budget', 2013 *WTD* 200-1 (16 October 2013).

[58] Edward Kleinbard, 'Stateless Income', n 3 above, 700.

[59] Google Report, n 56 above, para 1, p 5.

[60] As Bermuda does not impose corporate income taxes, the profits channelled to the Bermuda shell company would not be taxed. See http://www.bloomberg.com/news/articles/2012-12-10/google-revenues-sheltered-in-no-tax-bermuda-soar-to-10-billion.

It was argued that Google's tax structure was highly artificial and primarily served to avoid UK taxes rather than to reflect the substance of the way the business was actually conducted. The Public Accounts Committee found that public confidence in Google would only be restored when it established a corporate structure that ensured Google would pay tax where it generated profit.[61] This had to be addressed as a matter of urgency by Google and other companies with a similar corporate structure. The Public Accounts Committee stated it would continue to pursue this issue over the course of Parliament.

HMRC and HM Treasury were also criticised by the Public Accounts Committee in the Google Report. It was argued that HMRC had not sufficiently challenged the 'manifestly artificial tax arrangements' of multinationals.[62] HMRC was hampered by the complexity of existing laws and international tax treaties that allowed for aggressive exploitation of loopholes. It was acknowledged that international tax rules were complicated and had not kept pace with the way businesses operate globally and through the internet. This was not the first time that HMRC had been scrutinised for its efforts to tackle tax avoidance.[63]

The Public Accounts Committee recommended that

> HMRC and HM Treasury should push for an international commitment to improve tax transparency, including by developing specific proposals to improve the quality and credibility of public information about companies' tax affairs, and use that information to collect a fair share of tax from profits generated in each country.[64]

This data should include full information from companies based in tax havens.

In the Google Report, the Public Accounts Committee also emphasised that the reputation of the big accountancy firms in the UK had suffered from their substantial role in advising their clients on corporate structures and tax planning which served only to help them avoid UK taxes. 'We expect the big accountancy firms to recognise that the public mood on tax avoidance has changed'.[65] It was recommended that these accountancy firms should provide responsible advice to ensure that corporate arrangements reflect the substance of transactions in the UK and to enable their clients to be more transparent about where they make profits and pay taxes.[66] It was also recommended that HM Treasury introduce a

[61] Google Report, n 56 above, para 1, p 5.

[62] *Ibid*, para 2, p 5.

[63] On 5 November 2012, Lin Homer, the HMRC chief executive, appeared before the Public Accounts Committee to defend the tax authority's performance in collecting taxes from multinational corporations. She argued that taxes were collected under laws set by governments, not on the basis of morals. See Julie Martin, 'HMRC Chief Executive Defends U.K. Transfer Pricing Enforcement', 2012 *WTD* 215-3 (6 November 2012). Also see subsequent hearing on 28 October 2013, where HMRC representatives faced fierce questioning on their efforts to curb tax avoidance and the failure to include corporate tax avoidance in their report on the tax gap for 2011-2012. See David D Stewart, 'UK Public Accounts Committee Grills HMRC Over Tax Gap, Avoidance', 2013 *WTD* 209-1 (29 October 2013).

[64] See Google Report, n 56 above, conclusions, para 3. Also see p 11, para 17.

[65] *Ibid*, para 4.

[66] *Ibid*.

code of conduct for tax advisers, setting out what it and HMRC consider acceptable in terms of tax planning.[67]

As regards the role of large accountancy firms in aggressive tax planning, similar concerns had been raised a few months earlier by the Public Accounts Committee. In a report published in April 2013,[68] the Public Accounts Committee argued that HMRC was fighting a battle it could not win, due to lack of resources compared to the large accountancy firms.[69] In fact, firms and tax avoiders appeared to take advantage of HMRC's constraints.[70] What exacerbated the situation was the fact that due to the complexity of the system, there was no clarity over where to draw the line between acceptable tax planning and tax avoidance.[71] Simplicity was the key to fighting tax avoidance. Furthermore, greater transparency over companies' tax affairs would increase the pressure on multinationals to pay a fair share of tax in the countries where they operate.[72] It would also help restore the people's trust in the fairness of the tax system.[73]

In a follow-up report on tax avoidance and the role of large accountancy firms published in February 2015, it was concluded that PwC's activities represented nothing short of the promotion of tax avoidance on an industrial scale.[74] This was relevant to the tax advisory industry and its clients as a whole. It was suggested that the UK Government should introduce a code of conduct for all tax advisers. This follow-up report came out after the Luxembourg leaks.[75] In November 2014, the International Consortium of Investigative Journalists (ICIJ) had published correspondence between PwC and the Luxembourg Inland Revenue, showing

[67] *Ibid*, para 17. Also see: www.kpmg.com/us/en/issuesandinsights/articlespublications/taxnewsflash/pages/beps-taxnewsflash.aspx.

[68] House of Commons Committee of Public Accounts, *Tax Avoidance: The Role of Large Accountancy Firms* (Forty-fourth Report of Session 2012–13), April 2013.

[69] As also mentioned in the main conclusions, the government had to ensure that HMRC was properly resourced to challenge the advice given by the firms to companies and individuals seeking to aggressively avoid tax: *ibid*, p 6. A similar conclusion was drawn in another report. See House of Commons Committee of Public Accounts, *Tax Avoidance: Tackling Marketed Avoidance Schemes* (Twenty-ninth Report of Session 2012–13, HC 788), February 2013.

[70] *Tax Avoidance: The Role of Large Accountancy Firms*, n 68 above, pp 3–4.

[71] *Ibid*, p 3, 5.

[72] *Ibid*, p 5.

[73] *Ibid*, p 13.

[74] See House of Commons Committee of Public Accounts, *Tax Avoidance: The Role of Large Accountancy Firms (Follow-Up)*, (Thirty-eighth Report of Session 2014–15). Available on: www.publications.parliament.uk/pa/cm201415/cmselect/cmpubacc/1057/1057.pdf.

[75] For details of the Luxembourg leaks project, see www.icij.org/project/luxembourg-leaks. It is thought that two people have been charged for the disclosure, one being a former employee of PwC. See William Hoke, 'Second Suspect Charged in 'Lux Leaks' Case', 2015 *WTD* 17-1 (27 January 2015); 'PwC Releases Update on Luxembourg Leaks Case', 2015 *WTD* 8-16 (9 January, 2015). Following the publication of the Luxembourg leaks, the newly appointed European Commission President Jean-Claude Juncker faced demands for an investigation into his role and for his resignation. He had been Luxembourg's Prime Minister at the relevant time. However, on the 27 November 2014 he survived a no-confidence vote in the European Parliament. See Amanda Athanasiou, 'Juncker Facing Calls for Resignation', 2014 *WTD* 224-2 (20 November 2014); Kristen A Parillo, 'Juncker Survives No-Confident Vote in European Parliament', 2014 *WTD* 230-4 (1 December 2015).

that between 2002 and 2010 PwC secured deals with the Luxembourg tax authorities for 343 MNEs. Many of these MNEs were household names: Amazon, IKEA, Vodafone, Pepsi etc. Some of the documents indicated that many companies had effective tax rates of less than one per cent on profits channelled into Luxembourg.

The Public Accounts Committee argued that the Luxembourg leaks contradicted the evidence PwC had given in 2013 that it was not in the business of selling schemes. In fact, the Luxembourg leaks suggested that 'PWC had advised many multinational firms to adopt similar complex financial structures for the purposes of avoiding tax'.[76] The fact that PwC's promotion of these schemes was permitted by its own code of conduct showed a need for the Government to take a more active role in regulating the tax industry, 'as it evidently cannot be trusted to regulate itself'.[77] A new code of conduct for tax advisers was needed. The Public Accounts Committee called on HMRC to challenge the nature of the advice being given by accountancy firms to their clients, so as to ensure that tax liabilities reflect the substance of where companies conduct their business.

In response to the report,[78] PwC stood by the evidence given to the Public Accounts Committee in the past and disagreed with the committee's conclusions. However, it was recognised that 'we need to do more to explain the positive role we play in the tax system and in helping businesses to operate successfully'. The complexity of the tax system was raised, as well as the fact that governments competed for investment and tax revenues. 'We take our responsibility to build trust in the tax system seriously and will continue to support reform'.[79]

The banking giant HSBC has also found itself the subject of investigation by the ICIJ.[80] In February 2015, the ICIJ released information on almost 60,000 files from the bank's Swiss private banking branch, which (allegedly) showed that the bank profited from holding over US$100 billion in accounts on behalf of arms dealers, corporate executives, entertainers, politicians, religious leaders, and royalty worldwide. The files, the contents of which were not fully disclosed or completely accurate, included account information for more than 100,000 individuals and offshore entities from more than 200 countries for the years 1988 to 2007.

As criticised by the ICIJ, HSBC repeatedly reassured clients that it would not disclose details of accounts, even if evidence suggested that the accounts were undeclared to tax authorities in the home country. It was also alleged that bank employees discussed with clients a range of measures that would ultimately allow clients to avoid paying taxes in their home countries.[81]

[76] *Tax Avoidance: The Role of Large Accountancy firms (Follow-Up)* Report, n 74 above, para 3.

[77] *Ibid*, p 3.

[78] See PwC statement on the 38th report of the Public Accounts Committee, available on: pwc.blogs.com/press_room/2015/02/my-entry.html.

[79] *Ibid.*

[80] See ICIJ Swiss leaks project page available on: www.icij.org/project/swiss-leaks.

[81] See Key Findings section in: www.icij.org/project/swiss-leaks/new-countries-seek-hsbc-data-and-undeclared-cash.

In a statement obtained by the ICIJ, HSBC admitted that at the time, the compliance culture and due diligence standards of the bank, as well as the industry in general, were significantly lower than they are today. This was no longer the case because the bank had undergone a radical transformation. HSBC was expected to be called to give evidence at the Public Accounts Committee. Recently, an online group has announced its plans to challenge HMRC for failing to prosecute UK taxpayers whose names were included in a list based on stolen HSBC data and for allowing them to participate in a tax amnesty.[82]

It is not just UK taxpayers (or any source country taxpayers) that are losing out as a result of the depletion of their tax base due to the tax practices of MNEs. Local competitors are also affected. An increasing number of UK businesses have expressed their concerns about the aggressive tax planning of MNEs.[83] The Confederation of British Industry has also issued a set of tax principles for its members, 'to advance the debate on the responsible management of tax by UK business'.[84] These are the Tax Planning principles[85] and the Transparency and Reporting principles.[86] Broadly, pursuant to these principles, UK businesses are

[82] Stephanie Soong Johnston, 'Group Challenges UK Tax Authority on HSBC Tax Scandal', 2015 *WTD* 85-5 (4 May 2015).

[83] For example, the managing director at John Lewis has complained that UK businesses are at a disadvantage compared to those of multinationals. He called on the Treasury to conduct a closer examination on the way foreign multinational corporations pay taxes in the UK. See Stephanie Soong Johnston, 'Government to Tackle "Systematic Abuse" of U.K. Tax System, Business Secretary Says' (2012) 68 *Tax Notes International* 813 (26 November 2012). The CEO of J Sainsbury plc, Justin King, has voiced similar concerns. See interview in *The Daily Telegraph* where he called on the Government to follow the US by introducing a 'marketplace fairness tax' for online retailers. Available at: www.telegraph.co.uk/finance/newsbysector/retailandconsumer/10116437/Sainsburys-boss-Justin-King-calls-for-new-online-sales-tax.html. Furthermore, speaking at the Confederation of British Industry's annual conference in London, Justin King expressed his disagreement with business leaders who suggest that corporations should pay their taxes only based on the letter of the law. He emphasised that his company pays an effective tax rate of 59 per cent, including corporate tax, VAT, and business rates. See Stephanie Soong Johnston, 'UK Business Leader Calls for Transparency, Morality in Corporate Taxation', 2013 *WTD* 215-1 (6 November 2013). In addition, the CEO of Morrisons, Dalton Philips, has argued that the tax imbalance between internet and high street retailers is illogical and is damaging Britain's high streets. He has joined other top retailers in demanding a sales tax on online retailers. See interview in *The Daily Telegraph*, available at: www.telegraph.co.uk/finance/newsbysector/retailandconsumer/10178768/Philips-takes-the-bull-by-the-horns-in-drive-to-modernise-at-Morrisons.html.

[84] See Confederation of British Industry: Statement of principles, available as of 5 November 2013, at: www.cbi.org.uk/media/2051390/statement_of_principles.pdf.

[85] The principles listed are the following: 'UK businesses should only engage in reasonable tax planning that is aligned with commercial and economic activity and does not lead to an abusive result; UK businesses may respond to tax incentives and exemptions; UK businesses should interpret the relevant tax laws in a reasonable way consistent with a relationship of "co-operative compliance" with HMRC. In international matters, UK businesses should follow the terms of the UK's Double Taxation Treaties and relevant OECD guidelines in dealing with such issues as transfer pricing and establishing taxable presence, and should engage constructively in international dialogue on the review of global tax rules and the need for any changes'. *Ibid.*

[86] Inter alia, it is stipulated that: '[UK businesses] should consider how best to explain more fully to the public their economic contribution and taxes paid in the UK. This could include an explanation of their policy for tax management, and the governance process which applies to tax decisions, together with some details of the amount and type of taxes paid'. *Ibid.*

urged to engage only in reasonable tax planning that is aligned with commercial and economic activity and does not lead to an abusive result. They are further encouraged to seek to increase public understanding in the tax system in order to build public trust in that system.

The hearings in the UK Parliament's Public Accounts Committee and other investigations in other jurisdictions[87] so far reflect primarily the source country perspective. The residence country perspective[88] is depicted very accurately in numerous hearings in the US Senate where executives from, inter alia, Microsoft, Hewlett-Packard,[89] Apple[90] and Caterpillar[91] were questioned. An overview of the hearings relating to US technology giant Apple illustrates the problems in this area very well.

Apple was questioned at the US Senate for the company's complex tax practices that reportedly led it to successfully shelter US$44 billion from taxation anywhere in the world.[92] This was the result of a variety of offshore structures, arrangements and transactions to shift billions of dollars in profits away from the United States and into Ireland, where Apple had negotiated a special corporate tax rate of less than two per cent.[93] Their strategy was explained at the US Senate hearings. Overall, the double non-taxation of profits was a result of a combination of factors:[94]

[87] See reports of investigations into Apple's tax planning in both France and Italy. See Teri Sprackland, 'France Joins List of Countries Investigating Apple', 2015 *WTD* 72-2. Also, in October 2014, the Australian Senate Economics References Committee started an inquiry into corporate tax avoidance and is to report back in June 2015. Numerous MNEs, such as Apple, Microsoft and Google, have made representations. See information available on: www.aph.gov.au/Parliamentary_Business/Committees/Senate/Economics/Corporate_Tax_Avoidance Also see several reports of the Australian Senate committee inquiries into corporate tax avoidance, eg by Google Australia (2015 *WTD* 82-15), Apple (2015 *WTD* 82-17) etc. The testimony of the various MNE representatives was recently disputed by the Australian Taxation Office Commissioner. See David D Stewart and Stephanie Soong Johnston, 'Australian Tax Chief Challenges Multinationals' Claims' (2015) 78 *Tax Notes International* 327, 27 April 2015.

[88] See Jane G Gravelle, *Tax Havens: International Tax Avoidance and Evasion* (Congressional Research Service, 7-5700, dated 23 January 2013).

[89] US Senate Permanent Subcommittee on Investigations of the Committee on Homeland Security and Government Affairs, *Hearing on Offshore Profit Shifting and the US Tax Code—Part 1 (Microsoft and Hewlett-Packard)*, 112th Congress Second Session (20 September 2012).

[90] US Senate Permanent Subcommittee on Investigations of the Committee on Homeland Security and Government Affairs, *Hearing on Offshore Profit Shifting and the US Tax Code—Part 2 (Apple Inc)* (21 May 2013) (Apple Hearings).

[91] US Senate Permanent Subcommittee on Investigations of the Committee on Homeland Security and Government Affairs, *Hearing on Caterpillar's Offshore Tax Strategy* (1 April 2014); US Senate Permanent Subcommittee on Investigations of the Committee on Homeland Security and Government Affairs, *Caterpillar's Offshore Tax Strategy*, Majority Staff Report Permanent Subcommittee on Investigations United States Senate—Released in conjunction with the Permanent Subcommittee on Investigations 1 April 2014 Hearing. For commentary, see Jaime Arora, 'Caterpillar and PwC come under Fire at US Senate Hearing' 2014 *WTD* 63-1 (2 April 2014).

[92] For a review of Apple's tax strategy, see Antony Ting, 'iTax: Apple's International Tax Structure and the Double Non-Taxation Issue' [2014] *British Tax Review* 40–71.

[93] Apple Hearings, n 90 above, p 17.

[94] See Apple Hearings, n 90 above, p 5 and Ting, n 92 above, pp 46–55.

namely, the definition of corporate residence in Ireland and the US,[95] transfer pricing rules on intangibles and cost sharing agreements,[96] the US Controlled Foreign Corporations rules[97] and the check-the-box regime,[98] and the low taxes at the source jurisdiction.[99] As Professor Stephen Shay testified: 'Our international tax rules are out of balance. They are too generous to foreign income and not strong enough in protecting against US base erosion by foreign companies investing in the United States. The losers are domestic business'.[100]

[95] This is because a company incorporated in Ireland with central management and control in the US is not tax resident in Ireland, which relies on a central management and control test, nor in the US, which relies on the place of incorporation test. On corporate residency rules, also see Christiana HJI Panayi, 'UK Corporate Residence' in *Residence of Companies under Tax Treaties and EC Law*, EC and International Tax Law Series, vol 5 (IBFD Publications, 2009) pp 817–54. The Apple structure made use of the notorious double Irish tax arrangement which was commonly used to enable companies to shift profits to low or no tax jurisdictions by taking advantage of mismatches in corporate residency rules. It has now been abolished. Also see text in n 57 above.

[96] This is because of the transfer of economic rights of Apple's intellectual property to a low tax jurisdiction under a cost sharing agreement, even though the R&D activities were carried out in the US. See Ting, n 92 above, p 47; Apple Hearings, n 90 above, p 16. Also see Stephen Shay, Hearing before the Permanent Subcommittee on Investigations of the Committee on Homeland Security and Governmental Affairs United States Senate, 112th Congress Session, *Testimony before the US Senate Permanent Subcommittee on Investigations—Hearing on Offshore Profit Shifting and the Internal Revenue Code* (20 September 2012).

[97] This was because of the manufacturing exception of the US CFC regime, whereby CFC income was exempt from immediate taxation if the CFC itself was a manufacturer that added value to the goods. A CFC qualified if it also made a substantial contribution to the goods, without being a manufacturer. Ting, n 92 above, pp 50–51; Apple Hearings, n 90 above, p 16.

[98] The check-the-box rules allowed certain business entities to choose their classification for Federal tax purposes under an elective regime. This allowed Apple to maximise their tax savings. 'By using check-the-box disregarded entities, intercompany transactions within the group of companies that are classified as disregarded entities simply disappear'. Stephen Shay, Hearing before the Permanent Subcommittee on Investigations, n 96 above, p 12. Also see Ting, n 92 above, pp 51–54; Apple Hearings, n 90 above, pp 13–15.

[99] See Apple hearings, n 90 above, p 17. 'One of Apple's more unusual tactics has been to establish and direct substantial funds to offshore entities that are not declared tax residents of any jurisdiction. In 1980, Apple created Apple Operations International, which acts as its primary offshore holding company but has not declared tax residency in any jurisdiction. Despite reporting net income of $30 billion over the four-year period 2009 to 2012, Apple Operations International paid no corporate income taxes to any national government during that period. Similarly, Apple Sales International, a second Irish affiliate, is the repository for Apple's offshore intellectual property rights and the recipient of substantial income related to Apple worldwide sales, yet claims to be a tax resident nowhere and may be causing that income to go untaxed … Apple makes use of multiple U.S. tax loopholes, including the check-the-box rules, to shield offshore income otherwise taxable under Subpart F. Those loopholes have enabled Apple, over a four year period from 2009 to 2012, to defer paying U.S. taxes on $44 billion of offshore income, or more than $10 billion of offshore income per year. As a result, Apple has continued to build up its offshore cash holdings which now exceed $102 billion'.

[100] *Ibid*, p 12. At a later article, Stephen Shay argued that the lockout of unrepatriated offshore earnings of US MNEs does not necessarily lead to such economic harm as to justify shifting to a territorial tax system. See Stephen E Shay, 'The Truthiness of "Lockout": A Review of What We Know' (2015) 146 *Tax Notes* 1393–99 (16 March 2015) and studies cited therein. Under US law, these offshore earnings can be invested in the stock or debt of any unaffiliated US company or in a deposit of any unaffiliated US bank, without triggering a distribution. On the basis of the scant evidence available, he argues

At the US Senate hearings, Apple's CEO Tim Cook emphasised that everything the company did was legal and all taxes owed were paid. As noted in the Subcommittee's report, 'Apple executives told the Subcommittee that the company has no intention of returning those funds to the United States unless and until there is a more favourable environment, emphasizing a lower corporate tax rate and a simplified tax code'.[101]

Senator Carl Levin, the Subcommittee Chairman and the Senator who had proposed the ill-fated Stop Tax Haven Abuse Act in 2007[102] called Apple's quest for lower corporate taxes the Holy Grail of tax avoidance. Arizona Senator and former presidential candidate John McCain, praised Apple for its innovations and for being a major US corporation and taxpayer. However, he argued that Apple had violated at least the spirit if not the letter of the law. McCain stressed Congress was at fault for not simplifying the tax code.[103]

Notwithstanding these statements, it should be stressed that the attitude of the US government over its MNEs is considered rather indulgent, especially after the launch of the BEPS project. The general approach seems to be that if the MNE's double non-taxed income were to be taxed somewhere, then the US, which facilitated its creation, should collect the tax revenue.[104]

Nevertheless, to a large extent, the comments of the Committee members in all these investigations, whether from a source country or a residence country perspective,[105] reflect public opinion. What underpins them is the idea that multinationals should follow the spirit and not just the letter of the law—and pay taxes according to that. This is buttressed by an overriding concept of tax morality or tax justice which trumps black letter law. By contrast, what underpins the

that lockout 'is a problem principally for a small number of the largest multinationals, grouped predominantly in the technology and healthcare sectors, that may be engaging in profit shifting'. Ibid, p 1399. Referring to a 2011 Senate Permanent Subcommittee on Investigations report which conducted a survey of 27 US MNEs, almost half of undistributed earnings were held in US financial institutions (Permanent Subcommittee of Investigations, *Offshore Funds Located Onshore, Majority Staff Addendum* (14 December 2011)). Also see Lee A Sheppard, 'Debunking the Overseas Cash Meme' (2015) 78 *Tax Notes International* 700, 25 May 2015.

[101] Apple Hearings, n 90 above, p 5.

[102] See www.govtrack.us/congress/bills/113/hr1554.

[103] See, press reports in www.theguardian.com/technology/2013/may/20/apple-accused-tax-avoidance-billions-scheme, www.huffingtonpost.com/2013/05/21/apple-senate-hearing-irish-tax-loophole_n_3312575.html, www.usatoday.com/story/money/business/2013/05/21/apple-tax-hearing/2344351/.

[104] See discussion in Ch 9 of this volume. Also see Antony Ting, 'The Politics of BEPS—Apple's International Tax Structure and the US attitude towards BEPS' (2015) 69 *Bulletin for International Taxation* 410–15. Ting argues that this lenient approach is evident in the Caterpillar hearing held on 1 April 2014, n 91 above.

[105] Some jurisdictions could encounter aggressive tax planning on the basis of both perspectives. For example, according to a policy brief by the Progressive Policy Institute, although European politicians have complained that US MNEs are taking advantage of loopholes in foreign countries' tax laws to reduce their liability, foreign companies operating in the US also benefit by paying lower taxes than their American counterparts. Reported in Tax Analysts, 2015 *WTD* 96-22 (18 May 2015).

comments of those chosen or asked to defend the tax planning practices of these multinationals is the idea that legality and illegality is determined according to the letter of the law. Compliance with it should be sufficient. If people disapprove of tax planning practices, whether perceived to be aggressive or not, but still legal, then they (or better, their governments unilaterally or in a coordinated manner) should change the relevant tax laws.

Another issue emerging from these and other hearings is the adequacy and suitability of existing principles of international tax law to deal with the internationalisation of business.[106] Some argue that existing tax rules on jurisdiction to tax, in particular, need to be adapted to new business models such as the digital model. Others argue that the existing principles are sufficient but there is discord as to how tax authorities ought to apply them in some cases. As shown in the following chapter, the OECD, in the development of the BEPS project, has the unenviable task of trying to find solutions to some of these issues.

While the traditional concept of legality as the determining factor of what is acceptable and what is not remains—with the OECD endeavouring to shed light on this through its BEPS project—the reputational question, as vague as it may be, is coming to the fore and in some cases becoming all-pervasive, to the detriment of legal certainty and sometimes efficiency. Arguably, the injection of notions of morality into the debate has added further complexity and uncertainty to an already complicated field. Moreover, whether standards of morality and fairness have a place in corporate taxation is still very much debated.[107] Nevertheless, when advising on or designing the optimum (legal) tax structure, tax advisers are now faced with additional questions. How might this structure be perceived by the public? What will the reputational risk be? Some tax savings may have to be foregone so as not to attract criticism and to 'appease' the public. Overall, tax arrangements are being assessed on an increasingly ill-defined set of criteria.[108]

This has led to the development of notions of corporate tax responsibility—as far as companies are concerned—and good governance in tax matters—as far as countries are concerned. These are examined next.

1.3. Good Governance in Tax Matters

Good governance in tax matters is a concept that is acquiring increasing importance and institutional backing, both internationally and, especially, in the European Union.

[106] Also Ault, Schön and Shay, n 5 above.

[107] See comments of a Canadian tax judge reported by Stephanie Soong Johnston, 'Fiscal Morality a "Nonstarter" for Tax Court Decisions, Canadian Judge Says', 2014 *WTD* 111-3 (10 June 2014).

[108] David D Stewart, 'The Fight Against Tax Avoidance and the Uncertainty of Morality' (2013) 72 *Tax Notes International* 99 (14 October 2013).

The OECD and the UN have called for measures to improve governance through tax reform.[109] In a report published in 2010,[110] the OECD recognised the role of taxation as an important catalyst for state capacity development. The report explored how taxation could improve governance. This was to be done first, by developing a shared interest for economic growth. It was argued that governments which depend on taxes have stronger incentives for promoting economic growth.[111] As a second measure, there should be a development of the state apparatus and tax collection through an improved and functioning administration as well as other agencies. Thirdly, notions of accountability and responsiveness ought to be cultivated further,[112] by improving equity in tax enforcement and administration, as well as improving transparency and strengthening civil society engagement with tax issues.[113] As noted, taxation engages taxpayer-citizens in politics; '[g]overnments which rely on taxes have incentives to improve governance in order to ensure tax compliance'.[114]

The report examined the implications of the latter two processes for tax reform in the developing world. The impact of foreign aid on domestic revenue generation and collection, as well as on the dependence of governments on tax revenue were also considered. It was questioned whether reliance on aid instead of taxation could undermine all three processes listed above. By reducing the dependence of governments on tax revenue, aid could reduce political pressures for greater responsiveness and accountability.[115] Recommendations were made to governments to manage the provision of foreign aid in ways that maximise positive revenue-raising incentives and local accountability.[116]

The overtone of the report was that an effective tax system played a key role in state-building and in developing the economy.[117] For that, broader governance improvements were necessary. In its report, the OECD concluded that measures to improve tax governance and to support more integrated administrative structures were indispensable to any long-term strategy of achieving revenue stability and self-sufficiency.[118]

[109] Alicja Brodzka and Sebastiano Garufi, 'The Era of Exchange of Information and Fiscal Transparency: The Use of Soft Law Instruments and the Enhancement of Good Governance in Tax Matters' (2012) 52 *European Taxation* 394; Gemma Martinez Barbara, 'The Role of Good Governance in the Tax Systems of the European Union' (2011) 65 *Bulletin for International Taxation* 270.

[110] OECD, *Citizen-State Relations: Improving Governance Through Tax Reform* (Paris, 2010).

[111] *Ibid*, p 9.

[112] *Ibid*, pp 9–10.

[113] *Ibid*, pp 10–11.

[114] *Ibid*, p 9.

[115] *Ibid*, p 12.

[116] *Ibid*, ch 4 entitled 'The role of development partners in building tax-governance linkages', pp 51–58.

[117] It was, however, acknowledged in the concluding ch 5 of the report, n 110 above, that further research on the linkage between taxation and state-building was necessary. It was also conceded that in the report there was heavy reliance on case studies from a relatively small number of countries. Furthermore, very few of the suggestions made had been rigorously and specifically tested in practice.

[118] Gemma Martinez Barbara, n 109 above, p 270.

Similarly, in developing fiscal good governance principles, the UN's focus is on supporting tax policies for developing countries, removing obstacles to cross-border operations and fighting tax evasion. Following a UN-led international conference on financing for development in 2008, the Doha conference, the Doha Declaration on Financing for Development was adopted by consensus.[119] The Doha Declaration recognised the importance of strengthening technical assistance and enhancing international cooperation in addressing international tax matters, including in the area of double taxation. Commitments were made to enhance tax revenues through modernised tax systems, and more efficient tax collection. This would help broaden the tax base and effectively combat tax evasion. The Doha Declaration also reaffirmed the Monterrey Consensus[120] and called for a United Nations Conference at the highest level to examine the impact of the world financial and economic crisis on development.

The European Union has also had an active involvement in the development of the concept of good governance. At an ECOFIN meeting in 2008, one of the conclusions of the Council was to promote the principles of good governance in the tax area, described as 'the principles of transparency, exchange of information and fair tax competition, as subscribed to by Member States at Community level'.[121] Good governance in the tax area was seen as an essential means for combating cross-border tax fraud and evasion and for strengthening the fight against money laundering, corruption, and the financing of terrorism.

This task was taken on by the Commission. A series of initiatives had already been undertaken prior to the ECOFIN resolution,[122] which in 2009 culminated in a Communication for the promotion of good governance in tax matters.[123] In this Communication, the Commission suggested measures[124] to strengthen the principle of good governance in the tax area within the European Union and

[119] UN, *Doha Declaration on Financing for Development: Outcome Document of the Follow-up International Conference on Financing for Development to Review the Implementation of the Monterrey Consensus*, 9 December 2008, para 16, pp 8–9.

[120] See *Monterrey Consensus of the International Conference on Financing for Development* (2003). Available on: www.un.org/esa/ffd/monterrey/MonterreyConsensus.pdf.

[121] Press Release, 2866th Council Meeting, Economic and Financial Affairs (8850/08 (Presse 113), Brussels, 14 May 2008) p 22.

[122] See eg Communications on Preventing and Combating Corporate and Financial Malpractice (COM(2006) 611), on Caribbean countries (COM(2006) 86), on Pacific countries (COM(2006) 248), on Hong Kong and Macao (COM(2006) 648), on Governance and Development (COM(2006) 421) and on EU competitiveness (COM(2006) 567).

[123] Communication from the Commission to the Council, the European Parliament and the European Economic and Social Committee, Promoting Good Governance in Tax Matters, 28 April 2009. See Timothy Lyons, 'Promoting Good Governance in Tax Matters' [2009] *British Tax Review* 361; Gemma Martínez Bárbara, n 109 above; Alicja Brodzka and Sebastiano Garufi, n 109 above; Wolfang Schön, 'Tax and Corporate Governance: A legal Approach' in Wolfgang Schön and others (eds), *Tax and Corporate Governance* (Berlin/Heidelberg, Springer-Verlag, 2008).

[124] *Good Governance Communication*, n 123 above, pp 9–10.

internationally. It identified existing internal initiatives, as well as proposals to improve the Mutual Assistance Directive[125] and the Savings Directive.[126]

The Commission urged the Council to give the issue of good governance in the tax area appropriate political priority and to include provisions to that effect in general agreements with third countries.[127] Member States were also encouraged to establish a more unified approach towards third countries, regardless of whether those countries apply the principles of good governance in the tax area.[128] Finally, the Commission reiterated its intention to pursue a constructive dialogue with all stakeholders concerned.[129]

The European Parliament has also adopted a resolution promoting good governance in the area of taxation. In this resolution, the European Parliament condemned the role played by tax havens in encouraging and profiting from tax avoidance, tax evasion and capital flight and urged Member States to make the fight against these phenomena a priority.[130] The resolution also noted the need for an EU policy of good tax governance.[131]

At a subsequent ECOFIN Council meeting, the Commission was given a mandate to initiate dialogue with Switzerland and Liechtenstein, to extend the Code of Conduct on Business Taxation beyond the European Union for the first time.[132] This would facilitate the promotion of the principles of the Code of Conduct in third countries.[133]

In 2012, in furtherance to the Commission's plan to strengthen the fight against tax fraud and evasion, the Commission published two recommendations. One dealt with aggressive tax planning[134] and the other one with measures intended to encourage third countries to apply minimum standards of good governance in tax matters.[135] Arguably, to the Commission these are two sides of the same coin. Member States should tackle aggressive tax planning but at the same time, they should also ensure that they as well as any third countries they interact with,

[125] See proposal COM(2009) 29 of 2 February 2009.

[126] See proposal COM(2008) 727 of 13 November 2008. Also see Christiana HJI Panayi, 'The proposed amendments to the Savings Directive' (2009) 49 *European Taxation* 179.

[127] *Good Governance Communication*, n 123 above, p 10.

[128] *Ibid*, p 13.

[129] *Ibid*, p 14.

[130] See European Parliament resolution of 10 February 2010 on promoting good governance in tax matters (2009/2174(INI)), para 1.

[131] *Ibid*, para 17.

[132] 3020th Council meeting Economic and Financial Affairs, Luxembourg, 8 June 2010, PRESSE 162, 10689/10.

[133] *Ibid*, p 20.

[134] Communication from the Commission to the European Parliament and the Council, *An Action Plan to strengthen the fight against tax fraud and tax evasion*, COM(2012) 722. See extensive analysis in Ch 5 of this volume.

[135] Communication from the Commission to the Council on concrete ways to reinforce the fight against tax fraud and tax evasion including in relation to third countries, COM(2012) 351. See analysis in Ch 5 of this volume.

apply principles of good governance. In the Good Governance Recommendation, Member States were urged to reinvigorate the work of the Code of Conduct on Business Taxation. In fact, in order to encourage third countries to apply minimum standards of good governance in tax matters, Member States were urged to renegotiate, suspend or terminate tax treaties with third countries that do not respect the principles of the Code of Conduct and to place such countries on national blacklists.

As a follow-up, the Commission announced on 23 April 2013 that it would set up a Platform for Tax Good Governance.[136] The Platform was set up to monitor Member States' progress in tackling aggressive tax planning and clamping down on tax havens. Its tasks were, inter alia, to encourage discussion between businesses, civil society and national tax authorities on issues of good governance in tax matters. The term good governance in tax matters was to cover transparency, exchange of information and fair tax competition. The Platform would make suggestions to the Commission on the appropriate means and instruments to achieve progress in these areas. A Call for Application to select the member organisations of the Platform was launched the same day.[137]

The European Union has exerted considerable influence on third countries to support the dialogue on governance. For example, clauses of commitment to good governance in different policy areas have been included in various European Neighbourhood Policy instruments.[138] Also, as far as developing countries are concerned, the Commission provides financial incentives and funding to countries that support and implement governance-related objectives and reforms.[139] In addition, the Enlargement Policy strategy of the European Union is intended to address good governance in tax matters at an early stage of the pre-accession process.

[136] See decision of 23 April 2013, C(2013) 2236 final and European Commission Press Release dated 23 April 2003, reported in Tax Analysts in Doc 2013-9887. Also see Stephanie Soong Johnston, 'Anti-Evasion Initiative Meant to Create "Peer Pressure" Among EU' in 2013 *WTD* 73-2 (24 April 2013).

[137] The first appointment of member organisations was made in June 2013. In line with article 4(2) of the Commission Decision of 23 April 2013, C(2013)2236, Members of the Platform are the tax authorities of all Member States and 15 organisations representing business, civil society and tax practitioners. Some of the selected organisations are Tax Justice Network, Christian Aid, Oxfam International, BusinessEurope, the ACCA, the International Chamber of Commerce and the European Association of Tax Law Professors. The Platform meets approximately three times a year. It is chaired by the Director-General of DG Taxations and Customs Union. The work of the Platform on these issues is still very much in progress. See ec.europa.eu/taxation_customs/taxation/gen_info/good_governance_matters/platform/index_en.htm.

[138] Gemma Martinez Barbara, 'The Role of Good Governance in the Tax Systems of the European Union' (2011) 65 *Bulletin for International Taxation* 270.

[139] See Gemma Martinez Barbara, *ibid*, at p 277, who notes that the European Neighbourhood and Partnership Governance Facility provides funding to partner countries that are assessed as having made the most progress in implementing the governance-related objectives of their agreed reform agenda as set out in their Action Plans. The 10th European Development Fund (EDF, 2008–13) also offers additional funding to support a dialogue on governance and reform, including in respect of taxation.

In February 2013, the Commission issued a consultation paper on the proposal for the development of a European Taxpayer's Code.[140] It was proposed that in order

> to improve tax compliance, the Commission would compile good administrative practices in Member States to develop a taxpayers' code setting out best practices for enhancing cooperation, trust and confidence between tax administrations and taxpayers, for ensuring greater transparency on the rights and obligations of taxpayers and encouraging a service-oriented approach.[141]

By improving relations between taxpayers and tax administrations and by enhancing the transparency of tax rules, tax compliance would be encouraged, leading to more effective tax collection.

Most of the contributions to the consultation paper were in favour of the development of a European Taxpayer's Code, as this would ensure equal treatment of all citizens and a higher level of legal certainty, enhance transparency and harmonise the different legal systems.[142] However, it had also been expressed that a European Taxpayer's Code should in no way be binding, as national tax matters are a highly sensitive issue and there would be a danger of going too far, too fast at European level. Furthermore, any attempt to make a code binding would raise subsidiarity concerns. Other concerns expressed were that such a code would jeopardise legal certainty and merge different principles of different jurisdictions. Finally, such a code would not be an appropriate instrument to tackle tax fraud and tax evasion.[143] A Fiscalis Working Group consisting of national experts was established to discuss and develop a European Taxpayer's Code, in light of these conclusions. Nothing has been reported at the time of writing.

It is obvious that the concept of good governance in taxation is becoming very important not only within the European Union but also internationally. This is also reflected by some of the guidelines and soft law produced lately. Measures promoting good governance in taxation are also seen as part of the polemic against multinationals' aggressive tax planning or tax avoidance—it is the other side of the coin. The international tax community cannot just police 'rogue' taxpayers; it needs to also police and rehabilitate 'rogue' states or states with some questionable regimes or rules. Nevertheless, any concrete developments in this area are likely to require political will. There is certainly scope for more coordinated action by EU Member States, so as to support, streamline and complement international action taken in other fora such as the OECD and the UN. Outside of the European Union, instilling and institutionalising principles of good tax governance may not

140 Consultation Paper, *A European Taxpayer's Code* (Brussels, 25 February 2013, TAXUD.D.2.002 (2013)) 276169. See Ch 5, section 5.3.1 of this volume.

141 *Ibid*, p 2.

142 See *Summary Report on the outcome of the public consultation from DG TAXUD* (Brussels, 12 September 2013 TAXUD.D.2 (Ares 2013) 3252439), p 6.

143 *Ibid*, p 6.

be an easy task, as such principles are likely to be seen as interfering with a state's sovereignty in a much more politically sensitive way than any suggested anti-abuse measures targeted against what appears to be stateless income.

What is also evident from the above is that the idea that taxes are part of state-building is beginning to be engrained. Therefore, taxing powers must be exercised in a certain way by countries. There is also the reverse of that—ie that companies are beginning to be expected to behave in a certain way not only by tax authorities internationally but also by civil society. This is certainly the undertone of the various hearings discussed in section 1.2 above. There seems to be a demand for the political rhetoric to translate to concrete societal benchmarks, which are not necessarily underpinned by existing tax laws. Corporate social responsibility, primarily a management concept whereby companies integrate social and environmental concerns in their business operations and interactions with their stakeholders,[144] is beginning to be used in this field. This is examined below.

1.4. Corporate Social Responsibility and Aggressive Tax Planning

As explained above, initiatives on good governance relate to the tax policies of countries. Corporate social responsibility (CSR) in the tax context relates to the conduct of the tax affairs of companies. It is a relatively new concept, or rather a new application of an old concept. It has been argued that paying taxes is a fundamental and easily measured example of a company's citizenship behaviour. In other words, there is a link between CSR and the payment of taxes, and, as a corollary, CSR and aggressive tax planning or tax avoidance.[145] Although literature

[144] The literature on CSR is vast. See, inter alios, Archie B Carroll, Kenneth J Lipartito, James E Post and Patricia H Werhane, *Corporate Responsibility: The American Experience* (Cambridge University Press, 2012); Michael C Jensen, 'Value Maximization, Stakeholder Theory and the Corporate Objective Function' (2001) *Journal of Applied Corporate Finance* 8–21; Ioannis Ioannou, George Serafeim and Robert G Eccles, 'The Impact of a Corporate Sustainability on Organizational Processes and Performance' (2014) 60 *Management Science* 2835–57 etc.

[145] See, inter alios, Reuven Avi-Yonah, 'Corporations, society, and the state: A defense of the corporate tax' (2004) 90 *Virginia Law Review* 1193; Reuven Avi-Yonah, 'Corporate social responsibility and strategic tax behaviour' and Schön, 'Tax and Corporate Governance: A legal Approach' in Wolfgang Schön (ed), *Tax and corporate governance* (Berlin/Heidelberg, Springer-Verlag, 2008); Reijo Knuutinen, 'Corporate Social Responsibility, Taxation and Aggressive Tax Planning' (2014) 1 *Nordic Tax Journal* 36–75; Mihir Desai and Dhammika Dharmapala, 'CSR and Taxation: The missing Link' (Winter 2006) *Leading Perspectives (Business for Social Responsibility)* 4–5; Grahame R Dowling, 'The Curious Case of Corporate Tax Avoidance: Is it Socially Irresponsible?'(August 2013) *Journal of Business Ethics*; Jasmine M Fisher, 'Fairer Shores: Tax Havens, Tax Avoidance, And Corporate Social Responsibility' (2014) 94 *Boston University Law Review* 337; Moran Harari, Ofer Sitbon and Ronit Donyets-Kedar, 'Aggressive Tax Planning and Corporate Social Responsibility in Israel' (2013) *Accountancy Business and the Public Interest* 1; Grant Richardson, *Corporate Social Responsibility and Tax Aggressiveness*, AAA Conference 6–10 August 2011, Denver, Colorado, USA.

on mainstream CSR is voluminous, there is not much discussion on this specific angle of tax avoidance, which is distinguishable from tax evasion.[146]

First, it is useful to describe what CSR entails or purports to entail from a general perspective. There are many definitions of CSR.[147] For example, CSR has been defined by a UK Government report as 'how business takes account of its economic, social and environmental impacts in the way it operates—maximizing the benefits and minimizing the downsides'.[148] However, the report adds, 'we are not talking about altruism—CSR should be good for long-term business success as well as good for wider society'.[149] In a report produced by SustainAbility in 2006, corporate responsibility was described as an approach to business that embodies 'a commitment to economic, social and environmental accountability, open and transparent business principles and practices, ethical behaviour rooted in clearly defined values and active respect for the full range of stakeholders'.[150]

Earlier definitions also captured the voluntary nature of CSR. For example, Engel argued that CSR refers to the 'obligations and inclinations, if any, of corporations organised for profit, voluntarily to pursue social ends that conflict with the presumptive shareholder desire to maximize profit'.[151] Similarly, in its Green Paper, the European Commission saw CSR as 'a concept whereby companies

[146] Some contributions do not make a distinction between the two concepts in arguing that CSR applies in corporate taxes. The point is also made by Fisher, n 145 above, at p 352 who gives as an example the following articles: John Christensen and Richard Murphy, 'The Social Irresponsibility of Corporate Tax Avoidance: Taking CSR to the Bottom Line' (2004) 47 *Development* 37 and Prem Sikka, 'Smoke and Mirrors: Corporate Social Responsibility and Tax Avoidance' (2010) 34 *Accounting Forum* 153. Also see Christensen and Murphy who state, at p 39, that the 'scale of tax-avoidance activity has become so enormous that it can fairly be described as a shadow economy operating in the majority of globalized sectors…'. For criticism of Sikka's paper see John Hasseldine and Gregory Morris, 'Corporate Social Responsibility and Tax Avoidance: A comment and reflection' (2013) 37 *Accounting Forum* 1–14.

[147] For an interesting historical overview of CSR, see Harwell Wells, 'The Cycles of Corporate Social Responsibility: An Historical Retrospective for the Twenty-first Century' (2002) 51 *Kansas Law Review* 77. Also see Cynthia A Williams, 'Corporate Social Responsibility in an Era of Economic Globalization' (2002) 35 *UC Davis Law Review* 705; Joe W Pitts, 'Corporate Social Responsibility: Current Status and Future Evolution' (2009) 6 *Rutgers Journal of Law & Public Policy* 334; Aviva Geva, 'Three Models of Corporate Social Responsibility: Interrelationships between Theory, Research and Practice' (2008) 113 *Business & Society Review* 1–41 and William Allen, 'Our Schizophrenic Conception of the Business Corporation' (1992) 14 *Cardozo Law Review* 261. For criticism because of the divergent definitions, see Michael Hopkins, 'Criticism of the Corporate Social Responsibility Movement' in R Mullerat (ed), *Corporate Social Responsibility: The Corporate Governance of the 21st Century* 543, 2nd edn (Kluwer Law International, 2011); Michael Hopkins, *Corporate Social Responsibility & International Development* (Earthscan, 2007).

[148] UK Government, *Corporate Social Responsibility: A Government Update*, May 2004, p 3. Available on: www.berr.gov.uk/files/file48771.pdf.

[149] *Ibid.*

[150] SustainAbility report, entitled *Tax Issues—Responsible Business and Tax*, p 10. Available on: www.taxjustice.net/cms/upload/pdf/Sustainability_taxing_issues.pdf.

[151] David L Engel, 'An Approach to Corporate Social Responsibility' (1979) 32 *Stanford Law Review* 1, 5–6.

decide voluntarily to contribute to a better society and a cleaner environment'.[152] In describing the concept, the Commission Green Paper explained that it is a 'concept whereby companies integrate social and environmental concerns in their business operations and in their interaction with their stakeholders on a voluntary basis'.[153] Furthermore, as explained, being socially responsible meant 'not only fulfilling legal expectations, but also going beyond compliance and investing "more" into human capital, the environment and the relations with stakeholders'.[154]

It is noteworthy that in the Green Paper, it was emphasised that CSR should 'not be seen as a substitute to regulation or legislation concerning social rights or environmental standards, including the development of new appropriate legislation'.[155] When such regulations do not exist, 'efforts should focus on putting the proper regulatory or legislative framework in place in order to define a level playing field on the basis of which socially responsible practices can be developed'.[156] In this Green Paper, there was no mention of corporate tax responsibility. Passing reference was once made to 'tax revenues' as one of the contributions that companies make to their communities.[157]

In a later discussion document published in 2011, the Commission renewed its commitment to a CSR policy.[158] It was emphasised that CSR 'concerns actions by companies over and above their legal obligations towards society and the environment'.[159] As the economic crisis and its social consequences 'have to some extent damaged consumer confidence and levels of trust in business',[160] the businesses have focused public attention on the social and ethical performance of enterprises. By renewing efforts to promote CSR now, the Commission aimed to create conditions favourable to sustainable growth, responsible business behaviour and durable employment generation in the medium and long term. The Commission reviewed its pioneering role in the development of CSR and the establishment of the European Multistakeholder Forum on CSR.[161]

[152] Commission, *Green Paper, Promoting a European Framework for Corporate Social Responsibility*, COM(2001) 366 final, para 8, p 4. For commentary, see Kristina K Herrmann, 'Corporate Social Responsibility and Sustainable Development: The European Union Initiative as a Case Study' (2004) 11 *Indiana Journal of Global Legal Studies* 205.

[153] *Ibid*, para 20, p 6. This definition is repeated in Commission, *A renewed EU strategy 2011–14 for Corporate Social Responsibility*, COM(2011) 681 final, Brussels, 25 October 2011, p 3.

[154] *Ibid*, para 21, p 6.

[155] *Ibid*, para 22.

[156] *Ibid*.

[157] See para 43: 'Corporate social responsibility is also about the integration of companies in their local setting, whether this be in Europe or world-wide. Companies contribute to their communities, especially to local communities, by providing jobs, wages and benefits, and tax revenues'.

[158] Communication from the Commission to the European Parliament, the Council, the European Economic and Social Committee and the Committee of the Regions, *A renewed EU strategy 2011–14 for Corporate Social Responsibility*, COM(2011) 681 final, Brussels, 25 October 2011.

[159] *Ibid*, p 3.

[160] *Ibid*, p 4.

[161] *Ibid*, pp 4–6.

The Commission put forward a new definition of CSR as 'the responsibility of enterprises for their impacts on society'.[162] To meet their CSR duties, the Commission urged enterprises to have in place a process 'to integrate social, environmental, ethical, human rights and consumer concerns into their business operations and core strategy in close collaboration with their stakeholders'.[163] The aim was to maximise the creation of shared value for their owners/shareholders and for their other stakeholders and society at large, as well as identify, prevent and mitigate possible adverse impacts.[164]

In this report, the Commission referred to the multidimensional nature of CSR. According to the Commission, the concept at least covers human rights, labour and employment practices, and combating bribery and corruption.[165] For the first time in its CSR discourse, the Commission promoted the three principles of good tax governance in relations between states: transparency, exchange of information and fair tax competition. Enterprises were encouraged, where appropriate, also to work towards the implementation of these principles.[166]

It was highlighted that the development of CSR should be led by enterprises themselves, as appropriate to their circumstances, and that public authorities should play a supporting role.[167] In the remainder of the report, the Commission set out its agenda on how to promote CSR, as well as suggestions for enterprises, Member States, and other stakeholder groups. As far as taxes were concerned, it was merely stated that 'the Commission encourages enterprises to disclose information related to the implementation of good tax governance standards'.[168]

The European Parliament resolution on CSR in 2013 was in the same spirit.[169] It was stressed that businesses could not take over public authorities' responsibility for promoting, implementing and monitoring social and environmental standards.[170] The development of CSR ought to be driven primarily through the multi-stakeholder approach. Businesses had an important role and must be able to develop an approach tailored to their own specific situation.[171]

As for tax planning, the language used in this resolution was much stronger than in the Commission's Communication—'a business's tax policy should be considered part and parcel of CSR and that socially responsible behaviour consequently leaves no room for strategies aimed at evading tax or exploiting tax havens'.[172]

[162] *Ibid*, p 6.
[163] *Ibid*, p.6
[164] *Ibid*, p 6.
[165] *Ibid*, p 7.
[166] *Ibid*.
[167] *Ibid*.
[168] *Ibid*, p 11.
[169] See European Parliament Resolution of 6 February 2013 on corporate social responsibility: accountable, transparent and responsible business behaviour and sustainable growth (2012/2098(INI)).
[170] *Ibid*, para 1.
[171] *Ibid*, para 56.
[172] *Ibid*, para 7.

The importance of transparency was stressed, '[to] combat tax avoidance and illicit money flows'.[173] The European Parliament emphasised the need for any regulatory measures to be drawn up within a robust legal framework and in line with international standards, in order to avoid disparate national interpretations, leading to the emergence of competitive advantages or disadvantages at regional or national level.[174]

This is a very important point. CSR-driven tax standards, as all types of tax standards, will inevitably impact on a company's profitability as certain tax planning strategies will no longer be available. If only some countries adopt these standards and others do not, then this will distort the level playing field. In other words, countries that adopt these standards might lose their competitive edge. A similar problem arises with the proposals made in the BEPS project and is discussed in subsequent chapters. This is an issue that ought to be seriously considered especially in the European Union, which is leading the way with its own Action Plan.[175]

Irrespective of the development of the concept of CSR and the extent to which it actually includes (or should include) tax planning, what is evident from these definitions is the inherent conflict with the idea that a company exists solely to maximise profits for its shareholders, and that corporate social responsibility goes against this primary objective of the company. As Reuven Avi-Yonah claimed, our view of CSR largely depends on our view of the corporation. He explains that historically, three views of the corporation had emerged and rotated in cyclical fashion.[176] The first view is the 'artificial entity' view whereby the corporation is primarily a creature of the state. The second view is the 'real entity' view in that the corporation is an entity separate from both the state and from its shareholders. The third view is the 'aggregate' or 'nexus of contracts' view, whereby the corporation is merely an aggregate of its individual members or shareholders.

As Avi-Yonah explains, each of these three views has different implications for the issue of tax and CSR. Under the first two views—ie the artificial entity view and the real entity view—CSR is encouraged as a means of fulfilling the corporation's obligations to the state. The state is also justified in using the corporate tax as a regulatory device to steer corporate CSR activity. However, under the 'aggregate' or 'nexus of contracts' view, CSR is an illegitimate attempt by managers to tax shareholders without their consent and leads to managers being unaccountable to their shareholders. Pursuant to this view, the management's responsibility is to maximise shareholder profits by minimising corporate taxes as much as possible.

[173] *Ibid*, para 22.

[174] *Ibid*, para 54.

[175] See Ch 5 of this volume. For a discussion on the application of CSR in the EU context, also see Luca Cerioni, 'Corporate Social Responsibility (CSR): Crucial Issues and a Proposed "Assessment" in the European Union Context' (2014) 25 *European Business Law Review* 845–74.

[176] Reuven S Avi-Yonah, 'The Cyclical Transformations of the Corporate Form: A Historical Perspective on Corporate Social Responsibility' (2005) 30 *Delaware Journal of Corporate Law* 767.

The state has no business in encouraging corporations to engage in illegitimate CSR through the tax system. Very representative of this approach, Milton Friedman stated in 1970, that 'there is ... only one social responsibility of business—to use its resources and engage in activities designed to increase its profits'.[177]

Avi-Yonah disagreed with this approach, in that taken to its logical extreme, it is self-defeating. If corporations are not permitted to engage in CSR, then all social responsibility functions devolve to the state. As corporate managers would be required to minimise their tax payments as much as possible, that could mean that the state is left without adequate resources to fulfil its governmental functions, given that, it is argued, the payment of corporate income tax ensures the financing of public goods.[178] Therefore, if CSR is not applicable, neither corporations nor the government can fulfil their responsibilities to society and this would not be an acceptable outcome. Other scholars have also argued that a corporation's tax aggressive policies may have a negative effect on society and may be socially irresponsible.[179] Judith Freedman discussed the concept of enlightened shareholder value which has shifted the emphasis from immediate profit maximisation.[180] 'Longer term and sustainable profit maximisation is not only consistent with paying regard to wider stakeholder interests but is actually dependent upon doing so'.[181]

In an opinion issued on 7 June 2013 by Farrer & Co to Tax Justice Network Ltd,[182] it was stated that it was not possible to construe the directors' statutory duty to promote the success of the company[183] as constituting a positive duty to avoid tax. On the contrary, legislation expressly protected directors from criticism in circumstances where they took decisions based on the kind of factors which would militate against tax avoidance (eg change-of-law risk, reputation, brand impact, relationship with HMRC and community impact). The idea of a strictly fiduciary duty to avoid tax was wholly misconceived, according to the authors of the opinion.

[177] See Milton Friedman, 'A Friedman Doctrine—the Social Responsibility of Business Is to Increase Its Profits', *New York Times Magazine*, 13 September 1970, at p 32 (citing Milton Friedman, *Capitalism and Freedom* (University of Chicago Press, 1962) 133).

[178] Arne Freise, Simon Link, and Stefan Mayer, 'Taxation and corporate governance—the state of the art' in Wolfgang Schön (ed), *Tax and Corporate Governance* (Berlin/Heidelberg, Springer-Verlag, 2008).

[179] See David F Williams, *Developing the Concept of Tax Governance* (KPMG, 2007) and references therein. Also see Urs Landolf, 'Tax and Corporate Responsibility' (2006) 29 *International Tax Review* 6–9; Joel Slemrod, 'The economics of corporate tax selfishness' (2004) 57 *National Tax Journal* 877–99; Bernd Erle, 'Tax risk management and board responsibility' and Wolfgang Schön, 'Tax and Corporate Governance: A legal Approach' in Wolfgang Schön and others (eds), *Tax and Corporate Governance* (Berlin/Heidelberg, Springer-Verlag, 2008).

[180] See Judith Freedman, 'Tax and Corporate Responsibility', *Tax Journal*, Issue 695, 2 June 2003, pp 1–4.

[181] *Ibid*, p 2. Also see John M Conley and Cynthia A Williams, 'Engage, Embed and Embellish: Theory Versus Practice in the Corporate Social Responsibility Movement' (2005) 31 *Journal of Corporation Law* 1.

[182] See 'Fiduciary Duties and Tax Avoidance—Opinion', available on: www.taxjustice.net/cms/upload/pdf/Farrer_and_Co_Opinion_on_Fiduciary_Duties_and_Tax_Avoidance.pdf.

[183] Here, s 172(1) Companies Act 2006.

Arguably, in this opinion, tax avoidance is too widely defined. What is also somehow dubious is the conclusion that the reasoning in the opinion is 'applicable to any specific deliberate course of action that, because of tax, yields a more financially advantageous result than another available course of action which is nonetheless reasonable in the circumstances'.[184] The authors of the opinion state that their conclusions 'are therefore equally applicable across the spectrum from unexceptionable tax planning to criminal tax evasion, although of course it goes without saying that there can be no legal duty to engage in the latter'.[185]

In my view this generalisation is wrong. There should be a better distinction between legitimate tax planning, aggressive tax planning and tax avoidance. Attacking all in the same way, and, even worse, grouping them together with criminal tax evasion cannot help but make readers, especially those with a technical background, sceptical. Moreover, it is one thing to say it is not the directors' statutory duty to avoid tax, and another thing to say that companies (via their directors) that engage in aggressive tax planning are socially irresponsible. This argument is based on too many generalisations and too many assumptions.

Certainly, the intuitive (and political) appeal of the social nature of corporate taxation is undeniable. Nevertheless, there is limited research showing a consistently strong correlation between the CSR activities of a corporation and corporate tax aggressiveness. It is, however, worth considering how the topic has been approached by some economists.

In a seminal paper by Desai and Dharmapala,[186] the authors found that increases in incentive compensation tended to reduce the level of tax sheltering. The report also found the surprising result that firms that were *poorly* governed but where managers had high levels of equity incentives engaged in *less* tax avoidance. Desai and Dharmapala interpreted this result as evidence that tax avoidance and managerial rent extraction were complementary activities. They argued that the level of a firm's tax avoidance increased with the strength of its corporate governance.

Another recent study[187] found that risk-taking equity incentives exhibit a positive relationship with the level of tax avoidance. However, in contrast to Desai and Dharmapala, it was found that corporate governance appears to be related to managers' tax avoidance decisions, but only for high levels of tax avoidance.[188]

184 *Ibid*, para 2.

185 *Ibid*.

186 Mihir A Desai and Dhammika Dharmapala, 'Corporate tax avoidance and high powered incentives' (2006) 79 *Journal of Financial Economics* 145–79.

187 Chris Armstrong et al, *Corporate Governance, Incentives, and Tax Avoidance*, (May 2014) Rock Center for Corporate Governance at Stanford University Working Paper No 136, available on: papers.ssrn.com/sol3/papers.cfm?abstract_id=2252682.

188 For other recent studies, see, inter alios, Fariz Huseynov, Bonnie K Klamm, 'Tax Avoidance, Tax Management and Corporate Social Responsibility' (2012) 18 *Journal of Corporate Finance* 804–27; Roman Lanis and Grant Richardson, 'Corporate Social Responsibility and Tax Aggressiveness: An Empirical Analysis' (2012) 31 *Journal of Accounting and Public Policy* 86–108; Moran Harari et al, n 145 above.

Studies have also found that board composition may influence the level of tax aggressiveness of a corporation. A study by Lanis and Richardson[189] showed that outside directors were more responsive to the needs of society and were thus expected to influence the board of directors away from an aggressive tax policy stance. In a similar vein, Robinson et al[190] also examined the association between incentives and governance for both general and 'risky' tax avoidance—here, in tax havens. They found that the proportion of accounting experts on the board was associated with more general, but less risky tax planning. The level of tax expertise was associated with a lower likelihood of participation in risky tax planning.

The reputational concerns from tax avoidance have also been considered in numerous studies.[191] Interestingly, in a survey by Graham et al,[192] company tax executives were questioned whether the potential for an adverse effect on company reputation significantly constrained incentives to engage in tax planning strategies. In this survey, 69 per cent of the survey respondents, including 72 per cent from publicly traded companies, indicated that reputation concerns were 'important' or 'very important.' Reputation concerns ranked second only to the concern that a tax strategy might not pass the judicial standard of business purpose/economic substance. It was found that publicly traded companies, larger companies, more profitable companies and companies in the retail industry were significantly more concerned about the adverse reputation consequences of tax planning. The data suggested that a company would adopt tax avoidance schemes when the benefits outweighed the risks of harm to the company's reputation.

In another recent study, it was found that tax risk management systems used by large Australian companies did not systematically identify reputational risk as one of the tax risks that needed to be managed, even though tax aggressiveness could have a great impact on a company's reputation. A company that had a comprehensive tax risk management system that identified reputational risk would

[189] Roman Lanis and Grant Richardson, 'The effect of board of director composition on corporate tax aggressiveness' (2011) 30 *Journal of Accounting and Public Policy* 50–70. Also see a later study by these authors which examines the association between CSR and corporate tax aggressiveness. Based on a sample of 408 publicly listed Australian corporations for the 2008/2009 financial year, it is shown that the higher the level of CSR disclosure of a corporation, the lower the level of corporate tax aggressiveness. See Roman Lanis and Grant Richardson (2012), n 188 above.

[190] John R Robinson, Yanfeng Xue and May H Zhang, *Tax planning and financial expertise in the audit committee* (2012), available on: papers.ssrn.com/sol3/papers.cfm?abstract_id=2146003. Also see Sean T McGuire, Thomas C Omer and Dechun Wang, 'Tax Planning: Does Tax-Specific Industry Expertise Make a Difference?' (2012) 85 *The Accounting Review* 975–1003; Burak Guner, Ulrike Malmendier and Geoffrey Tate, 'Financial Expertise of Directors' (2008) 88 *Journal of Financial Economics* 323–54.

[191] Joseph Bankman, 'An academic's view of the tax shelter battle' in Henry J Aaron and Joel Slemrod (eds), *The Crisis in Tax Administration* (Brookings Institution, 2004) pp 9–37; Michelle Hanlon and Joel Slemrod, 'What does tax aggressiveness signal? Evidence from stock price reactions to news about tax shelter involvement' (2009) 93 *Journal of Public Economics* 126–41; Carlo Garbarino, *Aggressive Tax Strategies and Corporate Tax Governance: An Institutional Approach*, SDA Bocconi School of Management (2008).

[192] John R Graham et al, *Incentives for Tax Planning and Avoidance: Evidence from the Field* (MIT Sloan Research Paper No 4990–12, 2013) 26.

make more informed and potentially less aggressive tax decisions than a company that did not have a comprehensive tax risk management system that recognised reputational risk.[193]

Apart from the reputational costs, it has also been noted that complex tax planning produces litigation costs.[194] It may also damage the trust that tax authorities have in a company and have a negative effect on the good relations between the company and the authorities. Furthermore, aggressive tax strategies might generate uncertainty as to the tax liability of the company and, as a corollary, uncertainty for investors regarding the value of the shares of the company. Such tax planning may also lead collectively to the adoption of complex tax legislation to close the loopholes, generating new complexities and new compliance costs for the business.

Other studies have attempted to address the question why some firms engage in tax avoidance enthusiastically while others appear to shun it. This has been described as the under-sheltering puzzle.[195] Rather surprisingly, it could not be proved that the reputational costs of tax avoidance led to under-sheltering.[196]

The above brief review of some of the important literature is certainly not comprehensive. Nevertheless, the variations in the studies seem to suggest that the statement that companies that engage in aggressive tax planning are socially irresponsible is a generalisation. While one may more readily be convinced by arguments that engaging in socially responsible activities produces long-term financial gains in excess of any short-term gains from engaging in socially irresponsible activities,[197] it is submitted that as far as taxes are concerned, the arguments are much more complex and nuanced. For example, a local construction firm in a small town is not in the same position to engage in CSR as far as its tax planning is concerned, as a multinational such as Starbucks, Amazon etc. Arguably, its CSR responsibility would be limited to an obligation not to engage in tax evasion.

Even among larger companies and MNEs, some are more susceptible to reputational harm than others. Companies whose success depends strongly on their

[193] Catriona Lavermicocca and Jenny Buchan, 'Role of Reputational Risk in Tax Decision Making by Large Companies' (2015) 13 *eJournal of Tax Research* 5–50.

[194] Moran Harari et al, n 145 above.

[195] See Mihir Desai and Dhammika Dharmapala, n 186 above; John Gallemore, Edward L Maydew and Jacob R Thornock, 'The reputational costs of tax avoidance and the under-sheltering puzzle' (2013) Contemporary Accounting Research; Carlo Garbarino, n 191 above; Michelle Hanlon and Shane Heitzman, 'A review of tax research' (2010) 50 *Journal of Accounting and Economics* 127–78.

[196] Of course, all the studies were subject to caveats. For example in Gallemore et al, n 195 above, the results were confined to shelters that were implemented by firms and later made public. Another point made was that firms self-selected into tax avoidance, so, arguably, firms that engaged in aggressive tax avoidance already had bad reputations. As such, the reputational effect could not be measured. Also, there could be unidentifiable reputational costs that were not considered.

[197] See, inter alios, Ramon Mullerat (ed), *International Corporate Social Responsibility: The Role of Corporations in the Economic Order of the 21st Century* (Kluwer Law International, 2010) 40; Kash Rangan et al, *Why Every Company Needs a CSR Strategy and How to Build it* (Harvard Business School Working Paper, 2012).

reputation and branding are more likely to eschew a tax avoidance scheme in favour of tax practices that are less likely to attract public scrutiny. However, other companies may not bother. This could be, for example, the case when a company is already unpopular (eg if it belongs in the arms or tobacco industries) or when the product it produces is essential and cannot be substituted (eg some pharmaceuticals). One can easily switch from Starbucks to Costa Coffee or Café Nero, but it may not be so easy to do so with medication for Alzheimer's or cancer. If a company producing the latter views an (arguably) aggressive tax planning technique such as a corporate inversion as not only acceptable but also necessary to fulfil its fiduciary duties to shareholders, there is little that customers/patients or healthcare providers may do about this, short of a government intervention. It is noteworthy that in the European Commission's 2011 discussion document, CSR was seen as a concept to be developed by enterprises primarily, as appropriate to their circumstances.[198] The Commission paper was strongly imbued with the idea of voluntary participation. For taxes, the Commission referred to transparency, exchange of information and fair tax competition as the prerequisites of good tax governance that ought to be followed. Neither tax planning nor aggressive tax planning were mentioned.

Moreover, there could be different levels of CSR and different attitudes towards it. For example, a company (or better, its management) in a high tax jurisdiction may be more justified in 'feeling' that it does not owe anything to society and that it is acceptable to try and minimise its very high taxes and mitigate the impact of worldwide taxation. By contrast, the management of a company in a jurisdiction which does not have such high taxes may not necessarily 'feel' that it owes more to society and that it should refrain from aggressive tax planning. How can CSR proponents dictate the solution? What boundaries can be drawn? Furthermore, what if an MNE has subsidiaries in low and high tax jurisdictions? What should its CSR policy be? Should it be a group CSR policy or more localised?[199]

What compounds the situation is the fact that the distinction between tax avoidance, aggressive tax planning and legitimate tax planning is not clear. Tax avoidance has the connotation of doing something artificial and unlawful. Aggressive tax planning has softer connotations than tax avoidance as it does not entail any illegality. But it may be unclear when tax planning is legitimate and when not—because it is aggressive. Is the dividing line of legitimacy whether tax planning leads to double non-taxation? If there is no double non-taxation, is it because there is a reduction of taxes? But how great a reduction should be considered improper? These are very difficult questions. As a corollary, one should be wary of characterising a company as being socially irresponsible on the basis of its tax planning.

[198] Communication from the Commission to the European Parliament, the Council, the European Economic and Social Committee and the Committee of the Regions, *A renewed EU strategy 2011–14 for Corporate Social Responsibility*, COM(2011) 681 final, Brussels, 25 October 2011.

[199] On this point, also see Luca Cerioni, n 175 above.

In the author's view, it is a slippery slope for a country to expect to raise or increase corporate tax revenues as a result of CSR. What is next? Professional social responsibility of accountants, auditors, lawyers and/or anyone else who advises companies on their tax planning? Incidentally, the Public Accounts Committee in its 2015 follow-up report on the role of large accountancy firms may be going down that route, as it suggested a code of conduct for tax advisers.[200] In any case, notwithstanding the theoretical limitations and legal challenges of linking CSR with aggressive tax planning, this appears to be a popular (perhaps populist) cause for some, which is likely to continue.

Lately, many MNEs voluntarily adopt CSR initiatives and there is a trend towards self-regulation.[201] This also seems to be encouraged by influential NGOs.[202] While these initiatives are laudable, it may not be easy to translate them in the tax context. Here, as shown above, the application of CSR may be more complicated. Obviously, Google and Amazon are not going to set up training centres for tax officials; and Starbucks will not be making charitable donations every year. The difficulty is in how to constrain these MNEs in choosing their tax planning strategies and, most importantly, what tax planning strategies should be constrained. Is it strategies that make use of tax havens? But which country is officially a tax haven—is it only in the eyes of the OECD and its ever-changing tests and benchmarks? Is it strategies that result in very low effective tax rates? But what effective tax rate is adequately high? What if the use of a certain structure leads to higher effective tax rates but low (or no) taxes on profit distributions? Are corporate inversions contrary to the CSR duties of companies? Why are such companies socially irresponsible for wishing to replicate the tax benefits enjoyed by companies in foreign jurisdictions that have a territorial system of taxation?

The international tax system is all about choices. Absent a uniform and harmonised international tax system, why should a company be deemed socially

[200] See section 1.2 above.

[201] See, for example, the CSR report of Walmart which states, inter alia, that it promoted about 190,000 US associates in 2013, '51% of our new hires were women and 49% were people of color'; it delivered on its commitment of US$2 billion in cash and in-kind given to fight hunger in America one year ahead of schedule; it hired more than 32,000 US military veterans; it collaborated with the UN Office for Disaster Risk Reduction, etc. See corporate.walmart.com/global-responsibility/environment-sustainability/global-responsibility-report. Also, following allegations of sweatshops and child labour, Nike, inter alia, helped create the Fair Labor Association, a non-profit group that combined companies, and human rights and labour representatives to establish independent monitoring and a code of conduct, including a minimum age and a 60-hour working week, and encouraged other brands to join. See www.businessinsider.com/how-nike-solved-its-sweatshop-problem-2013-5#ixzz38sUzDj6n. For other company affiliates of the Fair Labor Association, see www.fairlabor.org/affiliates; blog.designedgood.com/unique-examples-of-corporate-social-responsibility/.

[202] See, for example, ActionAid's publication of July 2011, entitled *Tax Responsibility—The Business Case for Making Tax a Corporate Responsibility Issue*, available on www.actionaid.org.uk/sites/default/files/doc_lib/tax_responsibility.pdf. Similarly, see the report by SustainAbility, entitled *Tax Issues—Responsible Business and Tax*, available on: www.taxjustice.net/cms/upload/pdf/Sustainability_taxing_issues.pdf. Also see Business Ethics Briefing, 'Tax Avoidance as an Ethical Issue for Business', Issue 31, April 2013, available on: www.ibe.org.uk/userassets/briefings/ibe_briefing_31_tax_avoidance_as_an_ethical_issue_for_business.pdf.

irresponsible for benefitting from certain choices? If some choices are universally unacceptable, then rules or at least guidance should be put in place by international organisations such as the OECD to abolish them; and countries should duly abolish them. Hopefully, this is what the OECD is or should be doing in the context of its BEPS project; and this is what countries ought to be doing in the post-BEPS world.[203] Selective denounciation of some of these choices does little to deter the 'socially irresponsible' behaviour of multinationals—if at all acknowledged as socially irresponsible.

What makes it even more complicated is the fact that one company may be viewed as a major CSR player but may still be targeted as 'socially irresponsible' in its tax planning.[204] For example, Starbucks has long been considered as a rather ethical company in non-tax circles. The same cannot be said following the recent revelations and denouncement of its tax planning structures. Therefore, there may be different perspectives of CSR depending on the subject-matter (eg taxation, employee rights, environmental protection etc) or even depending on the jurisdiction. For instance, European companies are thought to be more active in the CSR field than US companies.[205] In general, there may be different societal expectations from companies, whether in general, or in specific areas.

Overall, the author believes that how most companies conduct their tax affairs and engage in strategic tax planning should not be (or become) a function of CSR or any other soft law concept transplanted from another context—at least not primarily. Ideally, there should be clear rules and principles. This should be the starting point.[206] In any case, tax avoidance or aggressive tax planning has not up until recently been widely discussed or analysed in the context of mainstream CSR literature. Most notably, in established CSR guidelines issued by international organisations, tax was not mentioned at all,[207] though this is now changing.

203 More on this ch 9.

204 Ironically, Margaret Hodge, an outspoken critic of tax avoidance and aggressive tax planning, who led the Public Accounts Committee hearings discussed in section 1.2 above, has been criticised for taking advantage of a tax amnesty (the Liechtenstein Disclosure Facility) that she had once criticised herself as being too lenient. Technically, she was just a beneficiary to the tax planning and did not drive the tax planning. See Stephanie Soong Johnston, 'UK Politician Under Fire for Tax Affairs' 2015 *WTD* 83-4 (30 April 2015).

205 See, for example, a comparative study of the US and the EU approach in Laura P Hartman, Robert S Rubin and K Kathy Dhanda, 'The Communication of Corporate Social Responsibility: United States and European Union Multinational Corporations' (2007) 74 *Journal of Business Ethics* 373–89. Also see Dirk Matten and Jeremy Moon, '"Implicit" and "Explicit" CSR: A Conceptual Framework for a Comparative Understanding of Corporate Social Responsibility' (2008) 33 *Academy of Management Review* 404–24.

206 Also see the point made in Commission Green Paper, n 152 above para 22, that CSR should not be seen as a substitute to regulation or legislation concerning social rights or environmental standards, including the development of new appropriate legislation.

207 See, for example, the ISO 26000 *Guidance Standard on Social Responsibility*. Section 6.6 on 'Fair Operating Practices' is not specific enough to cover taxes, but covers the ethical behaviour of an organisation in its dealings with other organisations, including relationships between organisations

The OECD Guidelines for Multinational Enterprises, last updated in 2011, now includes a chapter on taxation which sets out several recommendations on tax governance and management.[208] There is a specific chapter on taxation.[209] It is emphasised that corporate citizenship in the area of taxation implies that enterprises should comply with both the letter and the spirit of the tax laws and regulations in all countries in which they operate, co-operate with authorities and make information that was relevant or required by law available to them.[210] Furthermore, as noted in section 1.5 below, the duty of care of the board of directors in the context of aggressive tax planning is also mentioned for the first time in the recent draft update to the OECD Principles of Corporate Governance.[211] Arguably, these changes imply a higher level of socially responsible conduct in relation to tax compliance, compared to previous guidelines. It is only as a result of the recent tax 'scandals' discussed earlier on in this chapter that the topic has become more popular.

In any case, irrespective of the difficulties of proving empirically how less aggressive tax planning—and how much less—will be to the benefit of the company and its shareholders, other than reputation-wise in some cases, CSR implications are likely to become increasingly entrenched in the whole debate.[212] It may, therefore, be useful to attempt to map the contours of a CSR concept more specifically to taxes—arguably, the idea of corporate tax responsibility or how tax should feature in the boardroom agenda. Whilst the author believes CSR is not the solution to the problems faced in the international tax field, it may be used as a (constructive) palliative. Of course, if one were to go down this road, then it would be crucial to align European and global approaches to CSR, to ensure the development of uniform (CSR-derived) standards of transparency in tax matters. Otherwise, some countries would be under greater constraints than others, leading to unintentional tax competition.

and governmental agencies. There is only passing reference to tax in section 6.8 on 'Active Involvement and Community Development', which mentions that governments rely on organisations to comply with their tax obligations to generate the revenue to address critical development issues. See also the ILO Tri-partite Declaration of Principles Concerning Multinational Enterprises and Social Policy, 4th edn (International Labour Office, 2006).This focuses on employment issues. Available on: www.ilo.org/wcmsp5/groups/public/---ed_emp/---emp_ent/---multi/documents/publication/wcms_094386.pdf. Also see the United Nations Guiding Principles on Business and Human Rights (2011) which focus on human rights. on: www.ohchr.org/Documents/Publications/GuidingPrinciplesBusinessHR_EN.pdf

208 OECD Guidelines for Multinational Enterprises (2011). Available on: www.oecd.org/investment/mne/48004323.pdf.

209 *Ibid*, chapter XI.

210 *Ibid*, para 100.

211 OECD Principles of Corporate Governance, Draft for Public Comment—November 2014. See para 104. Available on: www.oecd.org/investment/mne/48004323.pdf.

212 See, for example, Fisher, n 145 above, at p 354, who argues that 'MNCs should treat tax avoidance as they treat environmentally harmful activities or human rights abuses: as a CSR issue that may necessitate the sacrifice of profits to mitigate financial harm to various other stakeholders'.

1.5. Tax in the Boardroom

Until recently, tax was not really an item on the boardroom agenda—at least not such an important one. It is only recently that studies were conducted on the topic of tax in the boardroom. Indicatively, in a study conducted by KPMG in 2004, it was emphasised that tax can no longer remain in the isolation to which its technical nature and its perceived independence from the business have traditionally placed it.[213]

> Tax is embedded in the fabric of the capital markets in which wealth is created and companies compete. A company's policies for tax and its risks need to be as sophisticated, coherent and transparent as its policies in all other areas involving multiple stakeholders, such as suppliers, customers, staff and investors.[214]

The survey noted that initially taxation was not treated as a normal business risk but this attitude has changed, with companies now less inclined to engage in tax planning activities that might be construed as aggressive. While companies examined more closely the potential downside in adopting a certain tax planning strategy, 'it [was] often unclear whether management [were] making a fully informed decision or simply reacting to events'.[215] It was further noted that in some countries such as Australia, the UK and the US, tax authorities were inclined to see a lack of board-level involvement in setting the tax agenda as tantamount to bad management or in some cases negligence.[216]

In explaining the corporate role of tax, it was shown that the company, through its management, must decide how it sees tax; ie its tax philosophy. There were two ends of the spectrum. On the one hand, tax was perceived as a social levy that the company had a duty to pay to the community, so it was payable at whatever level was set. On the other hand, tax was perceived as a normal business cost and the company had a duty to its shareholders to reduce it to the lowest level legally possible. The survey noted that the position taken by most senior managers of companies fell somewhere between the two views,[217] though there was an inclination to adopt a position closer to 'the duty to shareholders' end of the spectrum.[218] It was argued that the reputational risk from aggressive tax planning structures could have material consequences and also increase costs.[219]

[213] KPMG, *Tax in the Boardroom—A Discussion Paper* (2004) p 1. Available on: www.kpmg.com/ca/en/topics/managing-risk-driving-performance/documents/tax%20in%20the%20boardroom.pdf. At the time, it was reported that although there were signs that tax departments were becoming less isolated, there was scant evidence of a formal or comprehensive integration of tax into the mainstream. See p 3. Also see KPMG, *Tax Risk Management in the Financial Sector* (KPMG International, 2004).

[214] KPMG, *Tax in the Boardroom,* n 213 above, p 1.

[215] *Ibid*, p 5.

[216] *Ibid.*

[217] *Ibid*, p 6.

[218] *Ibid*, p 7.

[219] *Ibid*, pp 7–8.

In overseeing the design and monitoring of tax strategies, it was recommended that boards should recognise that the 'contemporary debates about governance, corporate social responsibility and ethics mean that even legal tax-minimisation activity can generate reputational liabilities that can destroy shareholder value'.[220] This might have been exaggerated at the time, but with hindsight it has proved truthful. Overall, it was recognised that company boards were under growing pressure to oversee their tax affairs in ways that reconciled their obligations to shareholders with the expectations of external stakeholders such as governments, pressure groups and very importantly the public.

In 2004, the OECD published a set of corporate governance standards and guidelines, intended

> to assist OECD and non-OECD governments in their efforts to evaluate and improve the legal, institutional and regulatory framework for corporate governance in their countries, and to provide guidance and suggestions for stock exchanges, investors, corporations, and other parties that have a role in the process of developing good corporate governance.[221]

Corporate governance was only part of the larger economic context in which firms operated and depended on the legal, regulatory and institutional environment. Factors such as 'business ethics and corporate awareness of the environmental and societal interests of the communities in which a company operates can also have an impact on its reputation and its long-term success'.[222] These were the OECD's Principles of Corporate Governance.

The 2011 OECD Guidelines for Multinational Enterprises, mentioned in section 1.4 above, included a chapter on taxation which set out several recommendations on tax governance and management.[223] It was noted that an enterprise would comply with the spirit of tax laws if it took reasonable steps to determine the intention of the legislature and interpreted those tax rules consistently with that intention.[224]

> Transactions should not be structured in a way that will have tax results that are inconsistent with the underlying economic consequences of the transaction unless there exists specific legislation designed to give that result. In this case, the enterprise should reasonably believe that the transaction is structured in a way that gives a tax result for the enterprise which is not contrary to the intentions of the legislature.[225]

Another area of corporate citizenship in taxation was co-operation with tax authorities and provision of the information they require to ensure an effective and equitable application of the tax laws.[226] Such co-operation should include

[220] *Ibid*, p 8.
[221] OECD Principles of Corporate Governance (2004), p 11. Available on: www.oecd.org/corporate/ca/corporategovernanceprinciples/31557724.pdf.
[222] *Ibid*, p 12.
[223] OECD Guidelines for Multinational Enterprises (2011), n 208 above.
[224] *Ibid*, para 100.
[225] *Ibid*.
[226] *Ibid*, para 101.

responding in a timely and complete manner to requests for information made by a competent authority. However, it was emphasised that cooperation was not without limitations. There should be a link between the information that should be provided and its relevance to the enforcement of applicable tax laws.[227]

In 2014, the OECD published a revised draft text of these guidelines, reflecting recent developments in the corporate sector and capital markets.[228] What becomes obvious is that tax is increasingly considered an essential part of corporate governance. There was a reference to aggressive tax planning in reviewing the duty of care of board members.[229] In discussing how the board should apply high ethical standards, it was also added that

> jurisdictions are increasingly demanding that boards oversee the tax planning strategies management is allowed to conduct, thus discouraging practices that do not contribute to the long term interests of the company and its shareholders, and can cause legal and reputational risks.[230]

In addition to the forms of internal controls and compliance programmes that companies were advised to establish, it was noted that compliance must also relate to other laws and regulations, as well as relevant international agreements, such as those covering taxation.[231]

The importance of corporate governance tools in deterring non-compliant behaviour has also been emphasised by the OECD in the Final Seoul Declaration,[232] where it was acknowledged that the policy debate 'revealed continued concerns about corporate governance and the role of tax advisors and financial and other institutions in relation to noncompliance and the promotion of unacceptable tax minimization arrangements'. Similar issues were raised in an HMRC-sponsored independent study[233] which canvassed the views of over 500 chairmen of large UK

[227] *Ibid*. As noted, there was a 'need to balance the burden on business in complying with applicable tax laws and the need for tax authorities to have the complete, timely and accurate information to enable them to enforce their tax laws'.

[228] OECD Principles of Corporate Governance (2014), n 211 above. The final version of the revised Principles is scheduled for completion in 2015.

[229] See para 104, addition in italics: 'The duty of care requires board members to act on a fully informed basis, in good faith, with due diligence and care. In some jurisdictions there is a standard of reference which is the behaviour that a reasonably prudent person would exercise in similar circumstances. In nearly all jurisdictions, the duty of care does not extend to errors of business judgement so long as board members are not grossly negligent and a decision is made with due diligence etc., *or to an obligation to pursue aggressive tax avoidance*. The principle calls for board members to act on a fully informed basis'.

[230] *Ibid*, para 106.

[231] *Ibid*, para 117.

[232] OECD, *Final Seoul Declaration* (Third Meeting of the OECD Forum on Tax Administration, 14–15 September 2006) p 3.

[233] HMRC, *Tax on the Boardroom Agenda—The Views of Business* (2006). This was an independent study produced through the HMRC Partnership Enhancement Programme. Also see *2006 Review of Links with Large Business* (Varney Report, 2006) and the papers that followed it in March 2007, *Making a Difference: Delivering the Review of Links with Large Business* (Delivery Plan) and *HMRC Approach to Compliance Risk Management for Large Business* (Risk Management Report). For commentary, see Judith Freedman (ed), *Beyond boundaries: Developing approaches to tax avoidance and tax risk management* (Oxford University Press, 2008).

companies. There, it was concluded, inter alia, that better direct communication channels were needed between businesses and HMRC and a cost effective system of reporting. Lack of trust appeared to be a recurrent theme.[234]

What becomes evident is that even before the whole BEPS project took off, it was becoming increasingly apparent that a purely technical approach to tax planning was 'unlikely to protect companies from charges of irresponsibility and associated reputational damage'.[235] This was irrespective of the theoretical difficulties—legal and economic ones—in linking CSR and tax planning. Nevertheless, with hindsight of the recent developments, it is undeniable that corporate governance and tax are becoming closely interwoven. As accurately depicted in the KPMG study in 2004:

> Tax has changed dramatically in recent years. Its public profile has become much more conspicuous, it has acquired moral, ethical and social dimensions that have never been discussed before and, for these reasons, the business management issues associated with tax have become more complicated, more subtle, more steeped in risk and much more challenging.[236]

Certainly, in evaluating tax planning and risk, the variables have increased. Tax is now not only a corporate governance issue but in some cases, a reputational issue as well. Company managers have recognised that their tax strategy must be appropriate from a commercial and legal perspective but also from a reputational one. Otherwise, tax can present a significant risk to shareholder value. It is now widely accepted that the head of tax in a company must be able to communicate effectively at board level with management, with investors, shareholders and external stakeholders, such as tax authorities, customers, the general business community, employees, NGOs, the media etc.[237] Furthermore, organisations with a global footprint are under increased pressure to adopt a global tax policy and to ensure compliance from a global perspective.

To facilitate compliance especially on a large scale for large corporate taxpayers, in the past decade or so, several countries have established enhanced cooperation regimes subsequently rebranded as cooperative compliance. The importance of enhanced cooperation was highlighted in the OECD's 2008 study into the role of tax intermediaries.[238] In this study, there was an attempt to form the basis for an agreed approach to the management of tax risk by revenue authorities. The OECD report considered the tripartite relationship between revenue bodies, taxpayers and tax advisers (the 'intermediaries' for the purposes of the report) in the context of aggressive tax planning, and the impact of this on tax administration.

[234] HMRC, *Tax on the Boardroom Agenda*, n 233 above, p 18.

[235] SustainAbility report, entitled *'Tax Issues—Responsible Business and Tax'*, p 2. Available on: www.taxjustice.net/cms/upload/pdf/Sustainability_taxing_issues.pdf.

[236] KPMG, *Tax in the Boardroom*, n 213, p 1.

[237] *Tax in the Boardroom—The Implications* (Odgers & Berndtson, 2013) p 5. Available on: www.odgersberndtson.co.uk/fileadmin/uploads/united-kingdom/Documents/tax_in_the_boardroom_board_paper_sept2013.pdf.

[238] OECD, *Study into the Role of Tax Intermediaries* (OECD, 2008).

It was recommended that revenue bodies establish a tax environment in which trust and cooperation could develop leading to enhanced relationships with large corporate taxpayers and tax advisers, with all parties going beyond their statutory obligations. It was noted that risk management was an essential tool for revenue bodies, assisting with the identification and treatment of risks, and facilitating the allocation of resources. Risk management, however, relied on information, very much dependent on disclosure from taxpayers. To encourage disclosure, revenue bodies had to operate using the following five attributes when dealing with all taxpayers: understanding based on commercial awareness; impartiality; proportionality; openness (disclosure and transparency); and responsiveness.[239]

It was emphasised that an enhanced relationship would benefit many taxpayers. Taxpayers who behaved transparently and who presented a lower risk were likely to enjoy a cooperative relationship with revenue bodies and therefore lower compliance costs, and increased certainty. Nevertheless, it was recognised that the availability of an enhanced relationship may not deter all large corporate taxpayers from aggressive tax planning. Several countries have established a form of enhanced relationship or cooperative compliance with taxpayers,[240] some even before the publication of the report.[241]

1.6. Conclusion

What becomes evident is that as far as tax avoidance and aggressive tax planning are concerned, the debate is multifaceted. There is an attack on tax havens and countries that engage in harmful tax competition (however defined), as well as an attack on MNEs that conduct their tax affairs 'immorally' vis-à-vis developed countries and the developing countries. The political rhetoric is buttressed by the development of doctrines of good governance in tax matters and of corporate tax responsibility. Civil society now attaches great weight to the issue of taxation, which could harm the public image of companies that follow aggressive tax

[239] *Ibid*, ch 7. For commentary, see, Judith Freedman, Geoffrey Loomer and John Vella, 'Corporate Tax Risk and Tax Avoidance: New Approaches' [2009] *British Tax Review* 74–116.

[240] Inter alia, Australia, Ireland, Italy, the Netherlands, the UK, New Zealand, Spain and the United States have adopted similar regimes. For commentary, see Eelco van der Enden and Katarzyna Bronzewska, 'International/Australia/Italy/Netherlands/United States—The Concept of Cooperative Compliance' (2014) 68 *Bulletin for International Taxation* 567–72; Asmita Singh, 'Enforcement or Cooperation—An Analysis of the Compliance Psychology of Taxpayers' (2015) 21 *Asia-Pacific Tax Bulletin*. For commentary on the French cooperative compliance regime launched in 2013, see Rudolf Reibel, 'Tax Transparency—How to Make it Work' (2015) 55 *European Taxation* 209, 212.

[241] For example, in the UK, following the Varney Report, n 233 above, a similar approach had been adopted in the context of HMRC's links with large business programme. See Annex 4 of 2008 OECD *Study on Intermediaries*, n 238 above and HMRC reports discussed in n 233 above.

planning practices. This often leads to negative media coverage and consumer backslash. Also, advances in technology have meant that the existing tax rules may no longer be appropriate or may need refinement in order to deal with today's tax strategies.

Finally, transfer pricing is a topic which now features heavily in the international tax community. Over relatively recent years most countries have introduced transfer pricing rules and generally those rules have been based on the OECD's Transfer Pricing Guidelines and on the concept of transactions between connected parties being at an 'arm's length price' within an 'arm's length range'. Transfer pricing rules help to ensure that profits fall in the right country and can themselves be seen as anti-avoidance rules. From the brief review of the tax planning practices of MNEs in section 1.2 above, it is obvious that there is an urgent need for the rules to be refined to cope with the current global trading environment.

The above, not necessarily in chronological order, are some of the factors that have led to BEPS. In any case, the BEPS project is now a reality and at the time of writing close to completion. It is examined in the next three chapters.

2

The OECD/G20 Base Erosion and Profit Shifting Project: Actions 1–5

It seems that tax avoidance, however defined and whatever it encompasses at any moment of time, is always on the agenda one way or another. Certainly in the context of the Base Erosion and Profit Shifting (BEPS) project, there is renewed momentum. The OECD, at the request of the G20 Finance Ministers in 2012, launched an international action plan to combat international tax planning structures used by multinationals to escape taxes. Arguably, the BEPS project is the culmination of a number of other recent initiatives and reports, generally on aggressive tax planning[1] and also on corporate loss utilisation[2] and hybrid mismatch arrangements.[3] However, it has acquired urgency from the political-level visibility of 'the failure of cross-border taxation rules to keep up with the realities of modern commerce and finance'.[4]

[1] OECD, *Tackling Aggressive Tax Planning through Improved Transparency and Disclosure* (2011). Prior to this, there were other reports; eg OECD, *Engaging with High Net Worth Individuals on Tax Compliance* (2009); OECD, *Addressing Tax Risks Involving Bank Losses* (2010) etc.

[2] OECD, *Corporate Loss Utilisation through Aggressive Tax Planning* (2011).

[3] OECD, *Hybrid Mismatch Arrangements: Tax Policy and Compliance Issues* (2012). See Andrei Cracea, 'OECD Actions to Counter Tax Evasion and Tax Avoidance (2013): Base Erosion and Profit Shifting and the Proposed Action Plan, Aggressive Tax Planning Based on After-Tax Hedging and Automatic Exchange of Information as the New Standard' (2013) 53 *European Taxation* 565–74. It should be noted that shortly after the launch of the BEPS Action Plan, the OECD published a report entitled *Aggressive Tax Planning Based on After-Tax Hedging* (OECD, 2013). This report describes features of aggressive tax planning based on after-tax hedging and the strategies used to detect and respond to such planning. The report further highlights a number of challenges from a compliance and policy perspective.

[4] Hugh J Ault, Wolfgang Schön and Stephen E Shay, 'Base Erosion and Profit Shifting: A Roadmap for Reform' (2014) 68 *Bulletin for International Taxation* 275–79.

2.1. Addressing Base Erosion and Profit Shifting

Backed by both G8 and G20 countries,[5] the OECD report *Addressing Base Erosion and Profit Shifting*[6] was released on 12 February 2013. BEPS was described in the FAQs of the OECD website[7] as

> tax planning strategies that exploit gaps and mismatches in tax rules to make profits 'disappear' for tax purposes or to shift profits to locations where there is little or no real activity but the taxes are low resulting in little or no overall corporate tax being paid.

In this report, it was accepted that the practices used by some multinational enterprises to reduce their tax liabilities had become more aggressive over the past decade. The OECD report did not suggest optimal tax rates but was expected to draft an action plan, identifying key pressure areas and providing concrete timelines and methodologies for solutions. The overtone of the report was that international tax standards may not have kept pace with global changes.[8] Measures were needed to address the perceived inequity between multinationals that were able to pay very little taxes and domestic enterprises that could not do the same, as well as the discrepancies between the place where the business was conducted and where taxes were paid.[9]

At a ministerial council meeting in Paris on the 29–30 May 2013, the OECD adopted a declaration on BEPS.[10] It reiterated that BEPS 'constitutes a serious risk to tax revenues, tax sovereignty and the trust in the integrity of tax systems of all countries that may have a negative impact on investment, services and competition, and thus on growth and employment globally'.[11] The declaration emphasised the need for governments to work together to develop methods of addressing asymmetries in domestic and international tax laws that can result in double non-taxation or very low effective taxation. There was a pressing need to address BEPS and to work towards a level playing field in this area.[12]

In July 2013 the OECD launched the BEPS Action Plan, in which it identified specific courses of action to be taken.[13] The OECD recognised that fundamental

[5] See references to statements of heads of States in Martijn Nouwen, 'The Gathering Momentum of International and Supranational Action against Aggressive Tax Planning and Harmful Tax Competition: The State of Play of Recent Work of the OECD and the European Union' (2013) 53 *European Taxation* 491–96.

[6] OECD, *Addressing Base Erosion and Profit Shifting* (OECD Publishing, 2013).

[7] Available on: www.oecd.org/ctp/beps-frequentlyaskedquestions.htm.

[8] Nouwen, n 5 above, p 492.

[9] Shee Boon Law, 'Base Erosion and Profit Shifting—An Action Plan for Developing Countries' (2013) 68 *Bulletin for International Taxation* 41–46, 41.

[10] See OECD, *Declaration on Base Erosion and Profit Shifting Adopted on 29 May 2013*. Available on: www.oecd.org/mcm/C-MIN%282013%2922-FINAL-ENG.pdf.

[11] *Ibid*, p 2.

[12] *Ibid*, p 2.

[13] OECD, *Action Plan on Base Erosion and Profit Shifting* (OECD Publishing, 2013). Available on:www.oecd.org/ctp/BEPSActionPlan.pdf.

changes were needed to effectively prevent double non-taxation, but also cases of no or low taxation 'associated with practices that artificially segregate taxable income from the activities that generate it'.[14] A realignment of taxation and relevant substance was needed, as international tax standards may not have kept pace with changing business models and technological developments.[15] While the Action Plan was not directly aimed at changing the existing international standards on the allocation of taxing rights on cross-border income, it sought to restore both source and residence taxation where cross-border income would otherwise go untaxed or would be taxed at very low rates.[16]

The need for consensus and multilateralism was emphasised. '[I]f the Action Plan fails to develop effective solutions in a timely manner, some countries may be persuaded to take unilateral action for protecting their tax base, resulting in avoidable uncertainty and unrelieved double taxation'.[17]

The BEPS Action Plan, which was fully endorsed by the G20, outlined 15 actions across a range of tax areas, including the digital economy, transfer pricing, coherence of corporate income taxation and transparency. Fundamental changes to the international tax architecture and the current source/residence dichotomy were ruled out. The 15 actions were scheduled to be delivered in three phases: September 2014, September 2015 and December 2015. In general, it seems that the BEPS Action Plan is aimed at integrating or reviving several related on-going OECD projects. The technical work is being undertaken by the Committee on Fiscal Affairs (CFA) through a number of its working parties and other subsidiary bodies.[18]

The BEPS Action Plan was endorsed by the G20 Finance Ministers on 19 July 2013 in Moscow and by the G20 leaders in September 2013, in St Petersburg. To show commitment to this project and to ensure progress would be made, the UK, Germany and France contributed €550,000 to the OECD.[19] Since the endorsement of the Action Plan a number of reports have been published on all

[14] *Ibid*, p 13.

[15] *Ibid*, p 13.

[16] *Ibid*, p 11.

[17] *Ibid*. On this point, see also David D Stewart, 'Unilateral Changes in Anticipation of OECD BEPS Project Risk Fragmenting Tax Rules', 2013 *WTD* 226-2 (22 November 2013).

[18] These are Working Parties 1, 2, 6 and 11, as well as the Forum on Harmful Tax Practices and the Task Force on Digital Economy. Working Party 1 *(Tax Conventions and Related Questions)*, in relation to part of action 2, action 6, action 7 and action 14. Working Party 2 *(Tax Policy Analysis and Tax Statistics)*, in relation to action 11. Working Party 6 in relation to part of action 4, actions 8–10 and 13. Working Party 11 *(Aggressive Tax Planning)*, in relation to part of action 2, action 3, part of action 4 and action 12. The Forum on Harmful Tax Practices, in relation to action 5 and the Task Force on Digital Economy in relation action 1. See www.oecd.org/tax/beps-about.htm.

[19] HM Treasury, HM Revenue & Customs, *Tackling Aggressive Tax Planning in the Global Economy: UK Priorities for the G20-OECD Project for Countering Base Erosion and Profit Shifting* (March 2014). Available on: www.gov.uk/government/publications/tackling-aggressive-tax-planning-in-the-global-economy-uk-priorities-for-the-g20-oecd-project-for-countering-base-erosion-and-profit-shifting.

Action items, as well as comments from interested stakeholders.[20] The reports are examined in this and the following two chapters.

It has been questioned[21] whether the BEPS project will be the starting point for the development of new principles of international tax law or whether it will be the final failure of the OECD to gain consensus on topics, notwithstanding the unprecedented level of political support. It is widely acknowledged that BEPS is a political commitment of the OECD and G20 countries, though as has been argued, it is a commitment to the agenda and 'not a commitment to accept whatever solutions come out of the process'.[22] It may prove impossible to reach consensus on solutions to some problems and/or some solutions adopted by the majority might not be implemented by all countries.[23] The need for coordination is crucial. It is not just the survival of the international tax regime that is at stake here but also 'the relevance of the OECD and its dominant members as the key players in the international tax world'.[24]

2.2. The BEPS Action Plan

The Action Plan appears to be broadly concerned with reform in the following three or four categories.[25]

The first category relates to rules on tax base allocation and, to an extent, the application of the source/residence doctrines to some modern-day transactions. Aligning value creation with taxation appears to be the leitmotif. Topics such as the taxation of the digital economy,[26] the avoidance of the permanent establishment (PE) status,[27] transfer pricing of intangibles and other high risk transactions[28] would appear to fall under this category.

The second category relates to anti-abuse rules tackling base erosion and preventing double non-taxation. These would include rules on hybrids,[29] controlled

[20] A calendar for planned stakeholders' input was revised and released a number of times (27 February 2014, 15 April 2014, etc).

[21] Philip Baker, 'Is there a Cure for BEPS?' [2013] *British Tax Review* 605.

[22] *Ibid.*

[23] *Ibid.*

[24] Yariv Brauner, 'BEPS: An Interim Evaluation' (2014) 6 *World Tax Journal* 10, 13.

[25] The BEPS Action Plan itself groups some of the actions under different headings. For different categorisations, see, for example, Ault, Schön and Shay, n 4 above, who group the action items in the following way: (a) Rules for the digital economy (Action 1); (b) Prevention of double non-taxation (Actions 2, 3, 4, 5, 6); (c) Alignment of economic activity and taxation (Actions 7, 8, 9, 10); (d) Tax Transparency and dispute resolution (Actions 11, 12, 13, 14); (e) Efficient and effective implementation (Action 15).

[26] Action 1.

[27] Action 7.

[28] Actions 8–10.

[29] Action 2.

foreign corporation (CFC) rules,[30] thin capitalisation rules,[31] the countering of harmful tax practices[32] and anti-treaty-shopping rules.[33]

The third category deals with procedural reforms. One set of suggestions is to devise rules on country-by-country reporting for transfer pricing documentation.[34] The Action Plan also suggests rules to collect and analyse data and counteractions.[35] Rules demanding disclosure of aggressive tax planning arrangements[36] are also to be developed.

Suggestions to make dispute resolution more effective[37] and to develop multilateral instruments[38] could be viewed as part of the procedural reforms, or as comprising a fourth category on promoting multilateralism. This category could also encompass some of the proposals under the action item on harmful tax practices.[39]

It would seem that most of the action items, especially those under the first two categories (ie tax base allocation rules and anti-abuse rules), are not really new.[40] In some of the BEPS deliverables the OECD refines its previous work but in a few instances it departs from it. Up to the time of writing, important progress had been made in all areas though nothing was finalised. This chapter examines the outputs on Actions 1–5. The next two chapters examine the outputs on the remaining action items.

2.3. Action 1: Addressing the Tax Challenges of the Digital Economy

Action 1 deals with the challenges that the digital economy poses for the application of existing international tax rules and the possible solutions. The work to be undertaken is described as follows.

> Identify the main difficulties that the digital economy poses for the application of existing international tax rules and develop detailed options to address these difficulties, taking a holistic approach and considering both direct and indirect taxation. Issues to be

30 Action 3.
31 Action 4.
32 Action 5.
33 Action 6.
34 Action 13.
35 Action 11.
36 Action 12.
37 Action 14.
38 Action 15.
39 Action 5.
40 Regarding the overlap with previous initiatives and reports, see, inter alios, Yariv Brauner, 'What the BEPS?' (2014) 16 *Florida Tax Review* 55; Ault, Schön and Shay, n 4 above; Nathan Boidman and Michael N Kandev, 'BEPS: The OECD Discovers America?' (2013) 72 *Tax Notes International* 1017 (16 Dec 2013) etc.

examined include, but are not limited to, the ability of a company to have a significant digital presence in the economy of another country without being liable to taxation due to the lack of nexus under current international rules, the attribution of value created from the generation of marketable location-relevant data through the use of digital products and services, the characterisation of income derived from new business models, the application of related source rules, and how to ensure the effective collection of VAT/GST with respect to the cross-border supply of digital goods and services. Such work will require a thorough analysis of the various business models in this sector.[41]

As has been pointed out, the overall concern in this area is the absence of base creation rather than the existence of base erosion.[42] This is not a new area of concern. In the late 1990s, the digital economy, then in its embryonic form referred to as e-commerce, was considered by the OECD leading up to the adoption of the Ottawa Taxation Framework Conditions which guided governments in their approach to e-commerce.[43] The precursor to this was a joint government and business conference in Finland in November 1997.[44] In this conference, the OECD expressed its support for an environment in which electronic commerce could develop its full potential. At the Ottawa conference[45] held in the following year, a taxation framework was adopted. This was the Ottawa Taxation Framework Conditions, which were also mentioned in the OECD's March 2014 Discussion Draft on Digital Economy.[46]

In the Ottawa Taxation Framework Conditions, it was stated that '[t]he taxation principles which guide governments in relation to conventional commerce should also guide them in relation to electronic commerce'.[47] It was thought that at this stage of development in the technological and commercial environment, existing taxation rules could implement these principles. The broad taxation principles which should apply to electronic commerce were the following: neutrality, efficiency, certainty and simplicity, effectiveness and fairness and lastly, flexibility.[48] The challenges faced by revenue authorities on how to implement these principles

[41] BEPS Action Plan, n 13 above, pp 14–15.

[42] Boidman and Kandev, n 40 above, p 1019.

[43] OECD, *Electronic Commerce: Taxation Framework Conditions—A Report by the Committee on Fiscal Affairs*, as presented to Ministers at the OECD Ministerial Conference, 'A Borderless World: Realising the Potential of Electronic Commerce' on 8 October 1998. Available on: www.oecd.org/tax/consumption/1923256.pdf.

[44] The title of the conference was 'Dismantling the Barriers to Global Electronic Commerce'. See OECD, *Implementation of the Ottawa Taxation Framework Conditions: The 2003 Report*, para 5, p 11.

[45] The title of the Ottawa OECD Ministerial Conference in 1998 was *A Borderless World—Realising the Potential of Electronic Commerce.*

[46] Public Discussion Draft, *BEPS Action 1: Address the Tax Challenges of the Digital Economy*, 24 March–14 April 2014 (henceforth, the Digital Economy Discussion Draft). Available on: www.oecd.org/ctp/tax-challenges-digital-economy-discussion-draft-march-2014.pdf. Also see Tax Analysts, 2014 *WTD* 57-33.

[47] OECD, *Electronic Commerce: Taxation Framework Conditions*, n 43 above, para 4.

[48] *Ibid*, para 9, box 2.

were recognised and rather vague suggestions were made.[49] More work was to be done on a post-Ottawa agenda and process.[50]

In January 1999, the OECD Committee on Fiscal Affairs appointed the Technical Advisory Group (TAG) to examine how the current treaty rules on business profits apply in the context of e-commerce and to consider proposals for alternative rules. Following the publication of a number of discussion drafts,[51] in its final report in 2004, the TAG concluded that existing concepts were sufficient to ensure the tax-neutral treatment of e-commerce and physical transactions. Furthermore, it was thought that there was no 'actual evidence that the communications efficiencies of the Internet have caused any significant decrease to the tax revenues of capital importing countries'.[52] This view is no longer held though.

The rapid evolution of information and communication technologies has led to renewed attempts to address the taxation of the digital economy. As noted in the BEPS Action Plan, the spread of the digital economy poses significant challenges for international taxation.

> The digital economy is characterised by an unparalleled reliance on intangible assets, the massive use of data (notably personal data), the widespread adoption of multi-sided business models capturing value from externalities generated by free products, and the difficulty of determining the jurisdiction in which value creation occurs. This raises fundamental questions as to how enterprises in the digital economy add value and make their profits, and how the digital economy relates to the concepts of source and residence or the characterisation of income for tax purposes. At the same time, the fact that new ways of doing business may result in a relocation of core business functions and, consequently, a different distribution of taxing rights which may lead to low taxation is not per se an indicator of defects in the existing system. It is important to examine closely how enterprises of the digital economy add value and make their profits in order to determine whether and to what extent it may be necessary to adapt the current rules in order to take into account the specific features of that industry and to prevent BEPS.[53]

[49] See para 11, box 3, for a number of recommendations. Inter alia: (i) Revenue authorities should make use of the available technology and harness commercial developments in administering their tax system to continuously improve taxpayer service. (ii) Revenue authorities should maintain their ability to secure access to reliable and verifiable information in order to identify taxpayers and obtain the information necessary to administer their tax system. (iii) Countries should ensure that appropriate systems are in place to control and collect taxes. (iv) International mechanisms for assistance in the collection of tax should be developed, including proposals to insert language in the OECD Model Tax Convention, etc.

[50] For an excellent summary of the post-Ottawa developments in this field, see Digital Economy Discussion Draft, n 46 above.

[51] The TAG produced discussion drafts on 'Attribution of Profit to a Permanent Establishment Involved in Electronic Commerce Transactions', which was released in February 2001, and 'Place of Effective Management Concept: Suggestions for Changes to the OECD Model Tax Convention', released in May 2003.

[52] OECD, *Are the Current Treaty Rules for Taxing Business Profits Appropriate for E-Commerce? Final Report* (2004), para 350, p 72.

[53] BEPS Action Plan, n 13 above, p 10.

On 24 March 2014 the OECD released its first discussion draft on Action 1, the Digital Economy Discussion Draft.[54] The Digital Economy Discussion Draft was developed by the Task Force on Digital Economy.[55] The Digital Economy Discussion Draft was largely descriptive of the current situation and did not make any specific recommendations.

The first half of the Digital Economy Discussion Draft contained a comprehensive examination of the evolution of the digital economy and the creation of new business models,[56] without really defining the concept of digital economy. Thereafter, there was a general discussion of the common features of tax planning structures that create opportunities for BEPS with respect to both direct and indirect taxes. Part VI of the report was entitled 'Tackling BEPS in the Digital Economy'. However, it was very difficult to deduce from the analysis any specific recommendations. Here, overlap with other Action items was identified. Confusingly, in discussing most[57] of the overlaps, the Digital Economy Discussion Draft used the terms 'market jurisdiction' and 'market country' as if they were synonymous with source-based taxation[58] and source country[59] respectively. This has been criticised for creating a tension between possible new rules of tax nexus for each of the concepts but mainly for market jurisdiction.[60]

The broader tax challenges were grouped into four categories. The first category looked at the appropriateness of the rules on nexus, due to the limited need for extensive physical presence in order to carry on business.[61] The second category considered how to attribute value created from the generation of data through digital products and services, and how to characterise for tax purposes a person or entity's supply of data in a transaction.[62] The third category examined the characterisation of payments made in the context of new business models for the provision of products or the delivery of services, such as 'cloud' computing.[63] In the fourth category, there was an examination of how to modify the VAT rules to improve the administration of the system.[64]

[54] Digital Economy Discussion Draft, n 46 above.

[55] On the various working groups looking into BEPS issues, see n 18 above.

[56] Digital Economy Discussion Draft, n 46 above, parts I–III.

[57] In discussing the overlap with the action item on CFCs, the discussion paper uses the term 'source country' and not 'market jurisdiction'. *Ibid*, paras 167–69.

[58] See, for example, *ibid*, p 48, heading in 2.1 ('*Measures that will restore taxation in the market jurisdiction*') which is immediately followed by the text of paragraph 147: 'A number of measures of the BEPS Action Plan will in effect restore source taxation, in particular…'.

[59] See, for example, p 49, para 150: 'The treaty definition of permanent establishment may limit the application of domestic law rules applicable to the taxation of the business profits of non-resident companies derived from sources in the market country. The work done with respect to Action 7 aims at preventing the artificial avoidance of the treaty threshold below which the market country may not tax'.

[60] Mindy Herzfeld, 'The BEPS Digital Economy Draft—Struggling for Consensus', 2014 *WTD* 96–2 (19 May 2014). Also see *Business Europe* comments, 19 April 2014.

[61] Digital Economy Discussion Draft, n 46 above, pp 56–57.

[62] *Ibid*, pp 57–58.

[63] *Ibid*, pp 58–59.

[64] *Ibid*, pp 59–62.

As mentioned, the Digital Economy Discussion Draft did not make any concrete recommendations—rather it made several suggestions in the last part of the report, Part VII. Even here, there was merely a broad overview of these suggestions, with the promise of a more thorough analysis in the final report.[65]

The first suggestion was to modify the exemptions in paragraph 4 of Article 5 of the OECD Model—ie the preparatory or auxiliary exemptions from the PE status—when such activities of a business constituted core functions.[66] The second suggestion was to establish a new nexus based on significant digital presence. When an enterprise engaged in certain 'fully dematerialised digital activities' it would have a permanent establishment if it maintained a 'significant digital presence' in the economy of another country.[67] The third suggestion was to establish a virtual PE.[68]

The last two suggestions were more general in nature and did not interfere with the current structure and scope of Article 5 of the OECD Model. The creation of a withholding tax on digital transactions was considered: imposing a final withholding tax on certain payments made by residents of a country for digital goods or services provided by a foreign e-commerce provider.[69] Lastly, consumption tax options were reviewed, such as an exemption for imports of low-valued goods.[70]

As expected, the Digital Economy Discussion Draft attracted great interest—and criticism. Many business groups and NGOs made representations.[71] NGOs tended to favour radical changes to the current rules, whereas the business sector adopted a more conservative approach, lobbying for limited changes to the existing rules and urging the OECD to hold back in making recommendations until the rest of the BEPS project was completed.[72] At the core of the matter lies the disagreement whether the business models arising from the digital economy

[65] *Ibid*, p 63.

[66] *Ibid*, pp 64–65. This could be done by eliminating paragraph 4 entirely, or eliminating subparagraphs (a) through (d), or making them subject to the overall condition that the character of the activity conducted be preparatory or auxiliary in nature, rather than one of the core activities of the enterprise in question. *Ibid*, p 65. Also see analysis of Action 7 in Ch 3, section 3.2 of this volume.

[67] For suggested guidelines on the interpretation of these terms, see Digital Economy Discussion Draft, n 46 above, pp 64–65.

[68] *Ibid*, para 267, p 66.

[69] *Ibid*, pp 66–67.

[70] *Ibid*, pp 67–68.

[71] See comments received on the Digital Economy Discussion Draft, published on the OECD website, available on: www.oecd.org/tax/comments-action-1-tax-challenges-digital-economy.htm.

[72] Herzfeld, 'The BEPS Digital Economy Draft—Struggling for Consensus', n 60 above. Also see KPMG, Comments on the OECD Discussion Draft on the Tax Challenges of the Digital Economy (14 April 2014) at p 4: 'We strongly endorse the Task Force's conclusion stated above and encourage the OECD to develop solutions through other aspects of the BEPS Action Plan to address the tax challenges of the digital economy—challenges manifest more clearly through innovative and modern business models adopted across all sectors'. Reported in Tax Analysts, 2014 *WTD* 75-15 (14 April 2014). Similarly, see Opinion Statement FC 7/2014 of the CFE on the OECD Discussion Draft: Addressing the tax challenges of the digital economy (BEPS Action 1). The Opinion was prepared by the CFE Fiscal Committee and submitted to the OECD in April 2014. Reported in Tax Analysts, 2014 *WTD* 76-30 (18 April 2014).

are so unique as to require new 'tailor-made' international tax rules, or not.[73] The OECD, through its discussion draft, does not seem to take a position on this issue. The fact that there was nothing in the report supporting the conclusion that the digital economy should be treated differently from other businesses suggests that there was no preference for the development of a special set of rules. Moreover, it was argued that many of the tax challenges mentioned in the Digital Economy Discussion Draft were the result of advances in technology and were either outside the framework of BEPS altogether or fell under other Action items.[74]

The same lack of consensus on how to tackle the digital economy was also reflected at governmental level. This became evident at the OECD public consultation meeting held on 23 April 2014. Some countries, such as France, favoured the taxation of digital commerce in the country of residence of the customer because the product was transformed when the customer used it. India and China also favoured the modification of the taxable nexus rules in light of the evolution of the digital economy.[75] Other countries, most notably the US, argued that digitisation was ubiquitous and that there should be no special rules for particular industries.[76]

A second version of the report was issued on 16 September 2014, along with the reports on six other deliverables. The Digital Economy Revised Discussion Draft[77] largely followed the initial discussion draft and confirmed its conclusions. It revisited the key features of the 'new' business models in the digital economy, how these features may exacerbate BEPS risks and how these issues should be addressed.

[73] See, for example, the comments submitted by the BEPS Monitoring Group in favour of revisiting the PE definition to address the shift to a digitalised economy. Available on: bepsmonitoringgroup.files.wordpress.com/2014/04/bmg-digital-economy-submission-2014.pdf.

Also reported in Tax Analysts, 2014 *WTD* 75-16 (17 April 2014). For the contrary view, see, for example, a comprehensive letter from the United States Council for International Business to the OECD, dated 11 April 2014, which endorses 'wholeheartedly the conclusion that there should not be a separate taxation regime for the "digital economy", however defined'. Reported in Tax Analysts, 2014 *WTD* 76-29 (11 April 2014). See, furthermore, David D Steward, 'Silicon Valley Concerned About OECD Digital Economy Draft, Practitioner Says', 2014 *WTD* 75-1 (18 April 2014) and 'OECD Members Divided Over Need for Unique Tax Treatment of Digital Economy', 2014 *WTD* 81-2 (28 April 2014). Also see a PwC Tax Policy Bulletin which also raises the point that the different treatment of digital economy transactions might give rise to state aid problems. Reported in Tax Analysts on 16 May 2014, 2014 *WTD* 96-23.

[74] See comments of the Business and Industry Advisory Committee to the OECD and comments of the Chartered Institute of Taxation submitted on 14 April 2014, and reported in Tax Analysts on 18 April 2014, at 2014 *WTD* 76-28 and 2014 *WTD* 76-31 respectively. In its comments to the OECD, Deloitte suggested the setting up of a Working Group to continue investigating the broader taxation issues specifically attributable to the digital market, outside the scope of the BEPS project. Reported in Tax Analysts, 2014 *WTD* 76-27 (18 April 2014). Also see comments of the Digital Economy Group, discussed in Herzfeld, 'The BEPS Digital Economy Draft—Struggling for Consensus', n 60 above.

[75] *Ibid.*

[76] See Kristen A Parillo, 'OECD Digital Economy Draft Lays Out Reform Options', Tax Analysts, 2014 *WTD* 57-2 (25 March 2014).

[77] OECD, *Addressing the Tax Challenges of the Digital Economy, OECD Publishing* (henceforth, Digital Economy Revised Discussion Draft). Available on: www.keepeek.com/Digital-Asset-Management/oecd/taxation/addressing-the-tax-challenges-of-the-digital-economy_9789264218789-en#page3.

The OECD continued to acknowledge that it would be impossible to ring-fence the digital economy for the purposes of creating separate tax rules '[b]ecause the digital economy is increasingly becoming the economy itself'.[78] Attempting to isolate the digital economy 'would inevitably require arbitrary lines to be drawn between what is digital and what is not'.[79] Furthermore, as the digital economy is in a continuous state of evolution, 'possible future developments need to be monitored to evaluate their impact on tax systems'.[80] On the basis of the fundamental principles of taxation discussed in a new chapter,[81] the options for reform to address the broader tax challenges raised by the digital economy were reviewed in the final chapter. It was obvious that developments on other BEPS items would be intertwined.

Similar to the Digital Economy Discussion Draft, the revised discussion draft suggested that the PE exceptions need to be refined to ensure that core activities would not inappropriately benefit. As such, work on Action 7 ought to be expanded to consider whether certain activities that were previously considered preparatory or auxiliary might be significant components of business in the digital economy.[82] Several suggestions were made most of which were repeated in the discussion draft on Action 7.[83]

The Digital Economy Revised Discussion Draft also considered the importance of intangibles, the use of data and the impact on transfer pricing practices. There was a strong suggestion that transfer pricing allocation methodologies for global value chains in this context should be reviewed. In the taxation of these business models, heavy reliance on collection, analysis and monetisation of data should be factored in.[84] Similarly to the Digital Economy Discussion Draft it was also suggested that CFC rules should be adapted to the digital economy. Income from digital products and services provided remotely was often not caught by CFC rules. Such income may be particularly mobile due to the importance of intangibles in this context and the relatively few people needed to carry out online sales activities.

The Digital Economy Revised Discussion Draft furthermore examined how to deal with tax planning by businesses engaged in VAT-exempt activities.[85] The suggestion was to focus on administrative procedures to collect business to consumer VAT type taxes rather than make changes to VAT regimes.[86] As regards

[78] *Ibid*, p 12.
[79] *Ibid.*
[80] *Ibid.*
[81] See ch 2, entitled 'Fundamental Principles of Taxation'. Also see review of prior work on this topic and especially the Ottawa Taxation Framework Conditions, set out in Annex A.
[82] See ch 8 and pp 153–54.
[83] See section 3.2 in Ch 3 of this volume.
[84] Digital Economy Revised Discussion Draft, n 77 above, pp 129–32. Also see pp 116–19.
[85] *Ibid*, pp 133–34.
[86] *Ibid*, pp 135–38.

cross-border compliance matters, non-OECD countries participating in the BEPS project should be included on equal footing with OECD countries.[87] Working Party 9 had already been working on the issue for its international VAT/GST Guidelines. It was also recommended that the OECD work with all BEPS participants to clarify the characterisation under current treaty rules of payments for cloud computing services, including infrastructure-as-a-service, software-as-a-service and platform-as-a-service transactions.[88]

It was stated that as the recommendations on the other Actions items were to be finalised, the OECD would evaluate how the outcomes affected the broader tax challenges mentioned in the Digital Economy Revised Discussion Draft and would complete an evaluation of the options for addressing them. Overall, a wait-and-see approach was recommended for many issues that may be addressed elsewhere in the BEPS project.[89]

Apart from the OECD's work on the digital economy, the topic has also been considered within the European Union. This is examined in Chapter five, where the work of the Group on Digital Economy is reviewed.[90] Also, as a response to one of the conclusions of the Digital Economy Revised Discussion Draft, further progress on the drafting of the OECD International VAT/GST Guidelines was achieved.[91] On 18 December, the OECD published a joint discussion draft dealing with two new elements to be included in these Guidelines, relating to the place of taxation of business-to-consumer supplies of services and intangibles, and provisions to support the application of the Guidelines in practice.[92]

[87] *Ibid*, p 152.

[88] *Ibid*, p 159.

[89] Kristen A Parillo, Amanda Athanasiou, Margaret Burow, Ajay Gupta and David D Steward, 'OECD Releases BEPS Reports Ahead of G-20 Meeting', 2014 *WTD* 180-1 (17 September 2014).

[90] See section 5.5 of this volume.

[91] The CFA had already been working on the International VAT/GST Guidelines to address issues of double taxation and unintended non-taxation resulting from inconsistencies in the application of VAT in international trade. The first three chapters of these Guidelines were approved in January 2014 and were endorsed as a global standard at the second meeting of the OECD Global Forum on VAT on 17–18 April 2014 in Tokyo.

[92] Discussion Drafts for Public Consultation, *International VAT/GST—Guidelines on Place of Taxation for Business-to-Consumer Supplies of Services and Intangibles Provisions—Provisions on Supporting the Guidelines in Practice* (18 December 2014–20 February 2015). Available on: www.oecd.org/ctp/consumption/discussion-draft-oecd-international-vat-gst-guidelines.pdf.

The discussion draft of the B2C Guidelines presents a set of common principles for determining the place of taxation for B2C supplies of services and intangibles, in accordance with the destination principle. It also presents the recommended approach for collecting the VAT/GST on these supplies, focusing in particular on supplies by non-resident suppliers. It is recommended that non-resident suppliers should be required to register and remit the VAT/GST in the jurisdiction of taxation and that countries should implement a simplified registration and compliance regime to facilitate compliance for non-resident suppliers. There is an analysis of the possible key features of such a simplified regime. The draft supporting provisions present approaches for facilitating the proper and consistent

2.4. Action 2: Neutralise the Effects of Hybrid Mismatch Arrangements

Action 2 under the OECD has called for the development of instruments to neutralise the effects of hybrid mismatch arrangements.

> Develop model treaty provisions and recommendations regarding the design of domestic rules to neutralise the effect (e.g. double non-taxation, double deduction, long-term deferral) of hybrid instruments and entities. This may include: (i) changes to the OECD Model Tax Convention to ensure that hybrid instruments and entities (as well as dual resident entities) are not used to obtain the benefits of treaties unduly; (ii) domestic law provisions that prevent exemption or non-recognition for payments that are deductible by the payor; (iii) domestic law provisions that deny a deduction for a payment that is not includible in income by the recipient (and is not subject to taxation under controlled foreign company (CFC) or similar rules); (iv) domestic law provisions that deny a deduction for a payment that is also deductible in another jurisdiction; and (v) where necessary, guidance on co-ordination or tie breaker rules if more than one country seeks to apply such rules to a transaction or structure. Special attention should be given to the interaction between possible changes to domestic law and the provisions of the OECD Model Tax Convention. This work will be co-ordinated with the work on interest expense deduction limitations, the work on CFC rules, and the work on treaty shopping.

On 19 March 2014, the OECD released two discussion drafts in connection with Action 2. The first discussion draft (the Domestic Law Discussion Draft) made recommendations on domestic law.[93] The second discussion draft (the Treaty Discussion Draft) examined treaty issues and made recommendations to the OECD Model.[94]

In the Domestic Law Discussion Draft, it was recognised that the problematic nature of hybrid mismatch arrangements had been discussed in a number of previous OECD reports.[95] A hybrid mismatch arrangement was described as a profit shifting arrangement that utilised a hybrid element in the tax treatment of an entity or instrument to produce a mismatch in tax outcomes in respect of a payment that was made under that arrangement.[96]

implementation of the principles of the Guidelines in national legislation, as well as their consistent interpretation by tax administrations. See OECD website: www.oecd.org/tax/consumption/release-of-discussion-drafts-of-two-new-elements-of-the-oecd-international-vat-gst-guidelines.htm.

[93] OECD, *BEPS Action 2: Neutralise the Effects of Hybrid Mismatch Arrangements (Recommendations for Domestic Laws) 19 March 2014–2 May 2014* (henceforth, the Domestic Law Discussion Draft).

[94] OECD, *BEPS Action 2: Neutralise the Effects of Hybrid Mismatch Arrangements (Treaty Issues) 19 March 2014–2 May 2014* (henceforth, the Treaty Discussion Draft).

[95] Domestic Law Draft, paras 1–15, referring to OECD, *Addressing Tax Risks Involving Bank Losses* (OECD, 2010); OECD, *Corporate Loss Utilisation through Aggressive Tax Planning* (OECD, 2011); OECD, *Hybrid Mismatch Arrangements: Tax Policy and Compliance Issues* (OECD, 2012).

[96] Domestic Law Discussion Draft, n 93 above, para 17.

The two principal mismatches identified were payments that are deductible under the rules of the payer and not included in the income of the recipient (deduction/no inclusion outcomes—D/NI) and payments that give rise to duplicate deductions from the same expenditure (double deduction—DD outcome).[97] Arrangements were defined to involve payments. Therefore unilateral deductions granted by domestic law which did not involve a payment, such as notional interest deductions for equity capital, were not covered[98]—something which has attracted criticism.[99]

The Domestic Law Discussion Draft set out design principles for the proposed domestic rules that should be developed to neutralise the effect of hybrid mismatch arrangements. In particular, it was suggested that the rules should operate to eliminate the mismatch without requiring the jurisdiction applying the rule to establish that it has 'lost' tax revenue under the arrangement; they should be comprehensive; they should apply automatically; they should avoid double taxation through rule co-ordination, they should minimise the disruption to existing domestic law; they should be clear and transparent in their operation; they should facilitate coordination with the counterparty jurisdiction while providing the flexibility necessary for the rule to be incorporated into the laws of each jurisdiction; they should be workable for taxpayers and keep compliance costs to a minimum; and they should be easy for tax authorities to administer.[100]

It seems that according to the design principles, the domestic rules would eliminate the mismatch without a distinction between intended and unintended mismatches and without targeting the tax benefit in the particular jurisdiction where it arises. Therefore, there would be no need for any 'purpose or intention test', but merely an analysis of tax outcome. This aspect of the proposals has also been criticised because inadvertent results may arise from applying purely mechanical rules.[101]

The overall approach adopted in the Domestic Law Discussion Draft was to identify and categorise hybrid mismatch arrangements based on the particular hybrid technique that produced the profit shifting. Recommendations were set out for domestic rules that would neutralise the effect of these arrangements. The specific categories of hybrid mismatch arrangements considered were the

[97] *Ibid*, para 20.

[98] *Ibid*, paras 21–22.

[99] See PwC Tax Policy Bulletin, *OECD releases two discussion drafts on hybrid mismatch arrangements* (21 March, 2014). Available on: www.pwc.com/en_GX/gx/tax/newsletters/tax-policy-bulletin/assets/pwc-oecd-releases-two-discussion-drafts-hybrid-mismatch-arrangemen.pdf.

[100] Domestic Law Discussion Draft, n 93 above, para 27.

[101] See, for example, the PwC Tax Policy Bulletin, dated 21 March 2014.

following: hybrid financial instruments and transfers,[102] hybrid entity payments,[103] reverse hybrid and imported mismatches.[104]

The Domestic Law Discussion Draft recommended changes to domestic laws designed to reduce the incidence of hybrid mismatches, and linking rules that specifically target the mismatch in tax outcomes under hybrid mismatch arrangements.[105] In order to minimise the risk of double taxation, two linking rules were recommended: a primary rule and a secondary or defensive rule. The primary rule would apply whenever a hybrid mismatch arose, and the secondary or defensive rule would only apply in circumstances where the primary rule did not apply in the jurisdiction of the counterparty. 'The choice of primary and defensive rules is based on ensuring that the hybrid mismatch rules are effective and relatively easy to apply, rather than looking to compensate the jurisdiction that has lost tax revenue under the arrangement'.[106]

For each category of hybrid arrangements identified above, the Domestic Law Discussion Draft provided detailed descriptions of arrangements and examples, domestic law recommendations to be adopted, technical tax discussions, and the application and scope of the rules.[107]

The second discussion draft, the Treaty Discussion Draft, specified that it complemented the first discussion draft but also considered the interaction between the recommendations of the two. The Treaty Draft also made recommendations for amendments to the OECD Model, in order to address the following two problems: the use of dual resident entities to obtain the benefits of treaties unduly; and the use of transparent entities to obtain the benefits of treaties unduly.

[102] This is where a deductible payment made under a financial instrument is not treated as taxable income under the laws of the payee's jurisdiction. See Domestic Law Discussion Draft, n 93 above, para 49. Also see fuller description in para 60, where this is described as any financing arrangement that is subject to a different tax characterisation under the laws of two or more jurisdictions such that a payment under that instrument gives rise to a mismatch in tax outcomes. Domestic Law Discussion Draft, para 60.

[103] This is where differences in the characterisation of the hybrid payer result in a deductible payment being disregarded or triggering a second deduction in the other jurisdiction: *ibid*, paras 49 and 163.

[104] The Domestic Law Discussion Draft, n 93 above, states, in para 49 that these cover payments made to an intermediary payee that are not taxable on receipt. There are two kinds of arrangements targeted by these rules: (i) arrangements where differences in the characterisation of the intermediary result in the payment being disregarded in both the intermediary jurisdiction and the investor's jurisdiction (reverse hybrids); (ii) arrangements where the intermediary is party to a separate hybrid mismatch arrangement and the payment is set-off against a deduction arising under that arrangement (imported mismatches). As discussed in paras 50 and 206–7, reverse hybrids are treated as a subset of the broader category of imported mismatch arrangements. Imported mismatch arrangements are hybrid structures created under the laws of two jurisdictions where the effects of the hybrid mismatch are imported into a third jurisdiction. Imported mismatches rely on the absence of effective hybrid mismatch rules in the investor and intermediary jurisdictions in order to generate the mismatch in tax outcomes which can then be 'imported' into the payer jurisdiction.

[105] Domestic Law Discussion Draft, n 93 above, para 52.

[106] *Ibid.*

[107] There is a summary of the recommendations in para 58, *ibid.*

As regards the recommendations on dual resident entities, it was suggested that these should be included in the discussion draft on Action 6. They were in fact partially addressed by a proposed change to Article 4(3) of the OECD Model, which would allow the competent authorities of the Contracting States to determine the residence of dual resident taxpayers on a case-by-case basis. However, this proposal would not address all BEPS-related concerns (such as deductible hybrid payments made by dual resident companies)[108] and other issues that could arise from dual residence where no bilateral tax treaty was involved.[109] Comments were invited on these points.

As far as transparent entities were concerned, the Treaty Discussion Draft proposed a change to Article 1(2) of the OECD Model and corresponding additional commentary to provide a rule for fiscally transparent entities.[110] Under this rule, income derived by or through an entity or arrangement that was treated as wholly or partly fiscally transparent under the tax laws of either Contracting State should be considered to be income of a resident of a Contracting State, but only to the extent that the income was treated, for purposes of taxation by that State, as the income of a resident of that State. The suggested new Commentary would focus on applying the rule to partnerships and was consistent with the principles of the 1999 OECD report on the Application of the OECD Model Tax Convention to Partnerships.

In the third part of the Treaty Discussion Draft, the interaction with the Domestic Law Discussion Draft and its recommendations was considered. Most specifically the recommendations to deny deductions or force income inclusions in the context of hybrid financial instruments and hybrid entity payments were examined.[111] It was recognised that the deductibility of payments was mainly an issue to be dealt with under domestic law and the only tax treaty provisions that might be relevant were Articles 7 and 24 of the OECD Model.[112] In the Treaty Discussion Draft, it was questioned whether the anti-hybrid provisions would be incompatible with Article 7 of the OECD Model where they lead to the imposition of tax on a non-resident without a permanent establishment in the taxing state.[113] It was also questioned whether they would be incompatible with Article 24 of the OECD Model. Apart from these issues, it was noted in the Treaty Discussion Draft that there does not seem to be a potential conflict with the OECD Model.

These discussion drafts and especially the Domestic Law Discussion Draft, have attracted a lot of criticism. It is obvious that the Domestic Law Discussion Draft attempts to neutralise hybrid mismatch arrangements on a unilateral basis. Nevertheless, the ultimate test of success would be the extent to which these domestic law proposals are broadly and uniformly adopted. Coordination of the

[108] Treaty Discussion Draft, n 94 above, para 8.
[109] *Ibid*, para 9.
[110] *Ibid*, paras 10–11.
[111] *Ibid*, para 12.
[112] *Ibid*, paras 14–15.
[113] *Ibid*, para 15, citing para 9 of the Domestic Law Discussion Draft, n 93 above.

treatment of a hybrid arrangement in two or more countries is key to the OECD's proposals. It has been recommended that domestic General Anti-Abuse Rules (GAARs) should be made inapplicable to hybrid arrangements that are covered by the proposals[114] but at the same time, the recommended rules should not interfere with other regulatory regimes at a domestic or multilateral level. In addition, there should also be internal consistency, as far as the BEPS project is concerned. It was emphasised in some of the comments by stakeholders that the OECD should not finalise its work on hybrids in advance of its work on CFCs, interest deductions and harmful tax practices.[115]

Another issue already mentioned is the absence of any subjective purpose or intention or motive test. It was argued that this might lead to double taxation. As noted by some of the stakeholders,

> [o]bjective mechanical tests such as those recommended in the proposals may offer certainty, but such tests do not take into account situations that are not abusive but happen to fall within the defined parameters. If the OECD seeks to ensure that global commerce operates without distortion resulting from income tax considerations, then such unintended applications of mechanical tests would be counter-productive.[116]

It has also been suggested that the OECD should take into account the broader economic impact of the proposals[117] and that it may be useful to perform an impact assessment.[118] It is likely that there will be an increased incentive for multinationals to document the tax treatment of each cross-border intercompany transaction in two or more jurisdictions, generating compliance costs.[119]

Much more critically, the BEPS Monitoring Group argued that the OECD should 'end this pointless and wasteful game'[120] and deal with the root of the problem and

[114] 'EY Urges OECD to "Act Cautiously" on Hybrid Mismatch Arrangements', reported in Tax Analysts, 2014 *WTD* 91-26 (9 May 2014) pp 4–5.

[115] See, inter alios, comments of the European Business Initiative on Taxation in 'International Cooperation Paramount in Hybrid Mismatch Issues, Corporate Tax Group Tells OECD', 2014 *WTD* 96-25 (15 May 2014); 'EY Urges OECD to "Act Cautiously" on Hybrid Mismatch Arrangements', n 114, 'Japanese Business Federation Wants OECD to Ensure "Normal Business Activities" in Hybrid Mismatch Draft', reported in Tax Analysts 2014 WTD 96-28 (15 May 2014) etc.

[116] 'PwC Fears "Disproportionate Consequences" of Hybrid Mismatch Recommendations', reported in Tax Analysts, 2014 WTD 92-24 (12 May 2014). For an overview of some of the comments, see Amanda Athanasiou, 'OECD's Hybrid Mismatch Proposals Too Drastic, Commentators Say', 2014 *WTD* 94-1 (15 May 2014); Amanda Athanasiou, 'Pessimism Marks Hybrid Mismatch Consultation', 2014 WTD 97-4 (20 May 2014).

[117] 'Deloitte Tells OECD to Take "Broader Economic Impact" of Hybrid Mismatch Draft Into Account', reported in Tax Analysts, 2014 *WTD* 92-25 (12 May 2014).

[118] 'U.S. Business Council Suggests OECD Perform Impact Assessment in Hybrid Mismatch Response', reported in Tax Analysts, 2014 *WTD* 92-26 (12 May 2014).

[119] See Ernst & Young, *Global Tax Alert*, 7 April 2014.

[120] See comments in the submission of the BEPS Monitoring Group on Hybrid Mismatch Arrangements, p 3, available on: bepsmonitoringgroup.files.wordpress.com/2014/05/bmg-hybrid-mismatches-submission.pdf.

the strong motivation for BEPS which is created by the separate entity principle. Many of the proposals considered in the BEPS project, including these relating to hybrids, attempt to counteract some base erosion techniques by overriding the separate entity principle, but only in specifically defined circumstances. As such, 'they can at best hope to provide only temporary palliatives to a system which desperately needs a more fundamental cure'.[121]

In September 2014, the OECD released its revised discussion draft on this deliverable.[122] The Hybrids Revised Discussion Draft broadly followed the March discussion document. As such, the principle of automatic application with no motive or purpose test, as well as the hierarchical linking rules were preserved.[123]

Hybrid payments were broadly defined and could include royalties or even payments for goods but still did not include deemed payments, eg interest deductions. There was clarification of the reverse hybrid and imported mismatch rules, making them consistent with other recommendations. The Hybrids Revised Discussion Draft treated payments deferred for an 'unreasonable' amount of time as giving rise to a hybrid mismatch, though there was no guidance as to what was a reasonable or an unreasonable amount of time. The Hybrids Revised Discussion Draft provided that reasonable differences in the timing of the recognition of payments did not constitute a mismatch in tax outcomes.[124] However, there was no guidance as to what was a reasonable or an unreasonable difference in the timing of recognition. It was stated in the Hybrids Revised Discussion Draft that further details would be agreed in the Commentary on the circumstances and requirements for 'establishing permissible differences in the timing of recognition of payments under the hybrid financing instrument rule'.[125] Further on it was established that in some circumstances, 'a timing mismatch will be considered permanent if the taxpayer cannot establish to the satisfaction of a tax authority that a payment will be brought into account within a defined period'.[126]

A bottom-up approach was favoured for the purposes of scoping the application of the hybrid financial instrument rules.[127] The rules were restricted to related parties, structured arrangements or controlled groups. Rules against deductible dividends and double deduction situations were proposed to have unrestricted scope.

[121] *Ibid*, p 1.

[122] OECD/G20 Base Erosion and Profit Shifting Project, *Neutralising the Effects of Hybrid Mismatch Arrangements*—Action 2: 2014 Deliverable (henceforth, Hybrids Revised Discussion Draft). Available on: www.oecd-ilibrary.org/docserver/download/2314261e.pdf?expires=1422995216&id=id&accname=guest&checksum=26AD343B4D9DE9B0FFCC3564C452ABA3.

[123] See commentary in Kristen A Parillo, Amanda Athanasiou, Margaret Burow, Ajay Gupta and David D Steward, 'OECD Releases BEPS Reports Ahead of G-20 Meeting', 2014 *WTD* 180-1, (17 September 2014); Reinout de Boer and Otto Marres, 'BEPS Action 2: Neutralising the Effects of Hybrid Mismatch Arrangements' (2015) 43 *Intertax* 14–41.

[124] Hybrids Revised Discussion Draft, n 122 above, para 61, p 36 and p 72.

[125] *Ibid*, para 61.

[126] *Ibid*, ch 7, Key Terms, p 72.

[127] *Ibid*, para 119, p 67.

In the Domestic Law Discussion Draft, the OECD had proposed a 10 per cent ownership threshold for relatedness,[128] but in the September 2014 Hybrids Revised Discussion Draft, the threshold was raised to 25 per cent. Two persons were related if one person held, directly or indirectly, 25 per cent or more of the voting rights or the value of any equity interests in another. In addition, two persons in the same control group were related if they fulfilled certain conditions. Also, instruments or arrangements between two persons may fall within the scope of the hybrid instrument rules if the persons were acting together, under certain conditions.[129]

There were no substantive changes to the treaty recommendations of the Treaty Discussion Draft. As far as the OECD Model was concerned, the Hybrids Revised Discussion Draft repeated recommendations regarding dual resident entities[130] and transparent entities.[131] There was a suggestion to include in the OECD Model a new provision in Article 1 and changes to the Commentary to ensure that income of fiscally transparent entities was treated in accordance with the principles of the OECD's Partnership Report 1999.[132] The last part of the Hybrids Revised Discussion Draft examined potential treaty issues that could arise from the recommended domestic law changes and made various proposals.

Some issues are still unresolved. The Hybrids Revised Discussion Draft does not address whether or under what circumstances income included under CFC regimes is to be treated as included in ordinary income for the purposes of these proposals. Moreover, the Hybrids Revised Discussion Draft notes that there are some specific areas where further refinements in the recommended domestic law rules may be needed; for example in the treatment of hybrid regulatory capital that is issued intra-group, for certain capital market transactions (such as on-market stock lending and repos), in the treatment of imported hybrid mismatches and the application of the imported hybrid mismatch rule.[133] It is anticipated that the output on Action 2 will be finalised in September 2015. The report is likely to be in the form of commentary and transitional rules.

The proposals of the revised discussion draft were again criticised by the BEPS Monitoring Group for being still rather limited and not dealing with the underlying problem of the separate entity approach and interest deductibility.[134] For example, they did not deal with Belgium's notional interest deduction regime

[128] Domestic Law Discussion Draft, n 93 above, para 128.

[129] See definitions for 'structured arrangements', 'related persons', 'control group' and 'acting together' in ch 6. The Hybrids Revised Discussion Draft, n 122 above, at p 70 provides a potential exception for collective investment vehicles under common management, to ensure that such vehicles managed by the same manager would not be treated as acting together for the purposes of the legislation.

[130] Hybrids Revised Discussion Draft, n 122 above, ch 8.

[131] *Ibid*, ch 9.

[132] OECD, *The Application of the OECD Model Tax Convention to Partnerships,* Issues in International Taxation, No 6 (OECD Publishing, 1999).

[133] Hybrids Revised Discussion Draft, n 122 above, para 7.

[134] BEPS Monitoring Group, OECD BEPS Scorecard, pp 5–6. Available on: bepsmonitoringgroup.files.wordpress.com/2014/10/oecd-beps-scorecard.pdf.

which provided an allowance for corporate equity—this was to be dealt with (if at all) as a 'harmful tax practice'. What was needed, according to the Group, was a more comprehensive and coherent approach which would enable each country to limit deductions by treating a multinational's debt on a consolidated basis, and to apportion it to entities in each country by an appropriate criterion such as EBITDA. This proposal, while notable, is unlikely to be adopted, since it requires a level of consensus that clearly does not exist for the time being.

The OECD's deliberate attempts to address the problem of hybrids through a series of unilateral domestic rules rather than a supra-national instrument have also been criticised.[135] As a result of the proposals, domestic tax laws are likely to become much more contingent and structurally dependent on the policies and practices of other governments, thus, to an extent, surrendering some of their tax sovereignty. It has been claimed that so far, the deliverables in Action 2 and the design principles therein are 'agnostic as to who should be collecting tax from situations involving inconsistent government choices'.[136] Overall, there could be a significant departure from the BEPS mantra of taxing income where it is earned.

2.5. Action 3: Strengthen CFC Rules

Under Action 3 of the BEPS Action Plan, the OECD is to:

> Develop recommendations regarding the design of controlled foreign company rules. This work will be co-ordinated with other work as necessary.

On 3 April 2015, the OECD published the discussion draft on strengthening CFC rules.[137] It was emphasised that this was not a consensus document. The CFC Discussion Draft considered all the constituent elements of CFC rules and put them into categories of 'building blocks' that were necessary for effective CFC rules.[138] These building blocks would allow countries without CFC rules to implement recommended rules directly and countries with existing CFC rules to modify their rules to align them more with the recommendations. The majority of these building blocks included recommendations. One building block—that on the definition of a CFC—did not yet include any recommendations but there was a discussion of the possible options. Specific questions were identified for which input was required in order to advance the work on CFC rules.

[135] See analysis by Graeme S Cooper, 'Some Thoughts on the OECD's Recommendations on Hybrid Mismatches' (2015) 69 *Bulletin for International Taxation* 334–49.

[136] *Ibid.*

[137] OECD, *Public Discussion Draft, BEPS Action 3: Strengthening CFC Rules* (henceforth, the CFC Discussion Draft). Available on: www.oecd.org/ctp/aggressive/discussion-draft-beps-action-3-strengthening-CFC-rules.pdf.

[138] The building blocks considered were the following: (1) definition of a CFC; (2) threshold requirements; (3) definition of control; (4) definition of CFC income; (5) rules for computing income; (6) rules for attributing income; and (7) rules to prevent or eliminate double taxation.

The recommendations discussed were designed to combat BEPS. However, it was recognised that some countries design their CFC rules to achieve wider policy objectives. Jurisdictions could choose to adopt CFC rules that applied more broadly than the recommendations as long as these were consistent with other international legal obligations. Such wider aims were not within the scope of Action 3.[139] The work was to be completed by September 2015, and interested parties were invited to send comments by 1 May 2015.

The first chapter of the CFC Discussion Draft briefly addressed the policy considerations. There were fundamental policy considerations that needed to be considered when designing CFC rules such as how to strike a balance between the need to tax foreign income and the need to maintain competitiveness,[140] how to limit administrative and compliance burdens while ensuring that CFC rules were effective, and the avoidance of double taxation. The CFC Discussion Draft also considered the role of CFC rules, the scope of base stripping prevented by CFC rules, and the interaction between transfer pricing rules and CFC rules.

The obligations for Member States of the European Union were also considered. It was acknowledged that whilst recommendations developed under Action 3 needed to be broad enough to be effective in combatting BEPS, they also had to be adaptable where necessary, to enable Member States to comply with EU law.[141] The CFC Discussion Draft referred to the *Cadbury Schweppes* case[142] and the wholly artificial arrangements test, as the litmus test.[143] It was also argued that on the basis of the *Thin Cap GLO* case,[144] a CFC rule in a Member State that targeted income earned by a CFC that was not itself wholly artificial may nevertheless be justified so long as the transaction giving rise to the income was at least partly artificial. Reference was also made to the *SGI*[145] and *Oy AA*[146] cases as supporting the argument that a CFC regime may not be limited to wholly artificial arrangements, if the regime explicitly ensured a balanced allocation of taxing power. This position is considered in greater detail and criticised in Chapter six of this volume.

It was also noted that under EU law, a CFC rule would only be found inconsistent with the freedom of establishment if the rule itself discriminated against non-residents. Therefore, if a CFC rule treated domestic subsidiaries the same as cross-border subsidiaries, there would be no discrimination. Of course, CFC regimes tend to apply to non-resident subsidiaries. The CFC Discussion Draft acknowledged the concern that non-EU-based multinational groups could be put at a competitive disadvantage compared to groups within the EU if the latter were subject to less vigorous CFC rules under EU law.

139 *Ibid*, para 4.

140 *Ibid*, para 10.

141 *Ibid*, para 11.

142 Case C-196/04 *Cadbury Schweppes plc and Cadbury Schweppes Overseas Ltd v Commissioners of Inland Revenue* [2006] ECR I-7995.

143 CFC Discussion Draft, n 137 above, para 14.

144 Case C-524/04 *Test Claimants in Thin Cap Group Litigation Order* [2007] ECR I-2107.

145 Case C-311/08 *Société de Gestion Industrielle (SGI) v Belgian State* [2010] ECR I-0487.

146 Case C-231/05 *Oy AA* [2007] ECR I-6373.

The following chapters of the CFC Discussion Draft set out the building blocks. Chapter 2 looked at how to define a CFC but no specific suggestion was made. Rather, it was recommended to broadly define a CFC so that in addition to including corporate entities, CFC rules would also apply to partnerships, trusts, and PEs when those entities were either owned by CFCs or treated in the parent jurisdiction as taxable entities separate from their owners.[147] It was further recommended to include a modified hybrid mismatch rule that would prevent entities from circumventing CFC rules by being treated differently in different jurisdictions.[148]

Threshold requirements were considered in chapter 3. It was recommended to include a low-tax threshold where the tax rate calculation was based on the effective tax rate. The low-tax threshold should also use a tax rate that was meaningfully lower than the tax rate in the country applying the CFC rules.[149]

The definition of control was examined in chapter 4. Two different determinations were recommended: (i) of the type of control that was required; and (ii) of the level of that control. The recommendation for control was that CFC rules should at least apply both a legal and an economic control test so that satisfaction of either test resulted in control. Countries might also include de facto tests where they achieved the same effect. Secondly, a CFC should be treated as controlled where residents held, at a minimum, more than 50 per cent control, although countries that wanted to achieve broader policy goals or prevent circumvention of CFC rules might set their control threshold at a lower level. This level of control could be established through the aggregated interest of related parties or unrelated resident parties, or the aggregated interest of any taxpayers that were found to be acting in concert. Additionally, CFC rules should apply where there was either direct or indirect control.[150]

The building block of defining CFC income was considered in chapter 5 of the CFC Discussion Draft but there were no recommendations. The chapter discussed several possible options that jurisdictions could implement in order to accurately attribute income that raised BEPS concerns. First, general features that would likely be included in effective CFC rules were outlined, including a form-based analysis and several different versions of a substance analysis. Then there was a discussion of how CFC rules should attribute the categories of income that raise the most challenges for existing rules. These categories of income included dividends, interest and other financing income, insurance income, sales and services income, royalties and other IP income. Two possible approaches were considered that could accurately attribute these categories of income, whether implemented separately or in combination with each other. There was also a discussion of whether CFC rules should take a transactional or entity approach to attributing income.

[147] CFC Discussion Draft, n 137 above, para 30.
[148] *Ibid*, para 31.
[149] *Ibid*, para 43.
[150] *Ibid*, para 65.

Comments were invited about the form of recommendations for the building block on the definition of CFC income.

Chapter 6 of the CFC Discussion Draft examined rules for computing income. It was recommended that computing the income of a CFC required two different determinations: first, which jurisdiction's rules should apply; and secondly, whether any specific rules for computing CFC income were necessary. Regarding the first determination, the recommendation was to use the rules of the parent jurisdiction to calculate a CFC's income. Regarding the second determination, the recommendation was for jurisdictions to have a specific rule limiting the offset of CFC losses so that they can only be used against the profits of the same CFC or against the profits of other CFCs in the same jurisdiction.[151]

The rules for attributing income were reviewed in chapter 7. The following issues were addressed.[152] First, how to determine which taxpayers should have income attributed to them. Here, it was recommended that the attribution threshold should be tied to the minimum control threshold when possible, although countries could choose to use different attribution and control thresholds depending on the policy considerations underlying CFC rules. Secondly, how to determine how much income should be attributed. Here, it was recommended that the amount of income to be attributed to each shareholder or controlling person should be calculated by reference to both their proportion of ownership and their actual period of ownership or influence.

Other issues considered were how to determine when the income should be included in the returns of the taxpayers and how the income should be treated. Here, it was recommended that jurisdictions could determine these issues so that CFC rules operated in a way that was coherent with existing domestic law. As for the tax rate that should apply to the income, it was recommended to apply the tax rate of the parent jurisdiction.

Finally, chapter 8 considered rules to prevent or eliminate double taxation. It was noted that jurisdictions were primarily[153] concerned with at least three situations where double taxation might arise: first, situations where the attributed CFC income was also subject to foreign corporate taxes; secondly, situations where CFC rules in more than one jurisdiction applied to the same CFC income; and thirdly, situations where a CFC actually distributed dividends out of income that had already been attributed to its resident shareholders under the CFC rules, or a resident shareholder disposed of the shares in the CFC.[154] In addressing the first two situations, it was recommended to allow a credit for foreign taxes actually paid, including CFC taxes assessed on intermediate companies. As for the third

[151] *Ibid*, para 131.

[152] *Ibid*, paras 142–43.

[153] It was stated that double taxation concerns could arise in other situations, for instance where there had been a transfer pricing adjustment between two jurisdictions and a CFC charge arose in a third jurisdiction.

[154] *Ibid*, para 154.

situation, it was recommended to exempt dividends and gains on disposition of CFC shares from taxation if the income of the CFC had previously been subject to CFC taxation, but the precise treatment of such dividends and gains could be left to individual jurisdictions so that provisions were coherent with domestic law.[155]

In the end, there were three annexes with tables outlining how existing CFC rules currently address several of the issues dealt with in the CFC Discussion Draft, including how countries' de minimis and low-tax thresholds work, and how they define attributable income from insurance.

It has been argued that the principal motivator of the CFC Discussion Draft, but also to some extent the entire BEPS project, is the US check-the-box regime.[156] The acknowledgement of the limitations under which EU Member States operate also suggests that the CFC Discussion Draft is really addressed to the US. As noted by Mitchell Kane,

> [h]ybridity regarding payments, residence and entity characterization has taken a prominent place in the analysis of CFC rules, due, in no small part, to the effects of US law on hybridity, especially an elective rule on entity characterization, a highly formalistic rule on corporate residence, a highly non-formalistic rule on the debt-equity distinction and the impressive creativity of the US tax bar.[157]

Certainly, the lack of consensus suggests fundamental disagreements and a deep political split among OECD countries as to how strict the CFC rules should be. The lack of consensus on the CFC rules can also be attributed in part to countries' self-interest and a misconception that transfer pricing rules can do the job.[158] Furthermore, countries may choose not to have CFC rules so as to attract companies and capital. The most likely outcome of Action 3 of the BEPS project will be a menu of approaches, or suggestions of best practice, or both. This could give a competitive advantage to companies in countries with more relaxed regimes and as a corollary could generate more tax competition which could exacerbate rather than mitigate base erosion and profit shifting.

There have also been criticisms in that, notwithstanding the substantial overlap with the other BEPS actions, the lack of consensus among countries in the CFC Discussion Draft raises the question of what role CFC rules should play in the BEPS project altogether and whether CFC rules might in fact be unnecessary in addressing base erosion and profit shifting.[159] The BEPS Monitoring Group argued that post-BEPS CFC rules must be set at a high standard and be coordinated because

[155] *Ibid*, para 155.

[156] See comments, in Amanda Athanasiou, 'OECD's CFC Rule Draft Likely to Spur Controversy', 2015 *WTD* 65-5 (6 April 2015). See also, Amanda Athanasiou, 'Lack of Consensus on CFC Rules Likely Here to Stay' (2015) 78 *Tax Notes International* 207, 20 April 2015.

[157] Mitchell Kane, 'The Role of Controlled Foreign Company Legislation in the OECD Base Erosion and Profit Shifting Project' (2014) 68 *Bulletin for International Taxation* 321–26, 326.

[158] Amanda Athanasiou, 'Competitive Interests Preventing Consensus on CFCs, Stack Says' 2015 *WTD* 96-3 (19 May 2015).

[159] See comments of the Tax Executive Institute on the CFC Discussion Draft, in 'TEI Criticizes OECD's Strengthening CFC Rules Discussion Draft', 2015 *WTD* 85-19 (30 April 2015).

'a weak standard which is left to states to implement would be counter-productive, as it would encourage source states to reduce their tax rates, and hence worsen the race to the bottom in corporate tax'.[160] Strong CFC rules could give the BEPS project a better chance of success and a better chance of ensuring that MNEs are taxed where economic activities take place and value is created. Weak rules would mean failure.

The adoption of a full inclusion approach was recommended by the BEPS Monitoring Group, under which the home country would tax all CFC income, with a credit for foreign taxes paid.[161] An alternative approach was a substance test based on the proportion of profit to employees, determined by payroll costs. It would apply if the effective tax rate in the CFC's country of residence was below 95 per cent of that of the home country. The preferred response was to adopt a more explicitly unitary approach to MNEs, 'for example by systematizing and regularizing the profit split method with defined concrete allocation factors and weightings for all commonly used business models'.[162] By apportioning profits according to appropriate measures of real economic activity, this would leave countries free to set their corporate tax rates, balancing encouragement of investment in real activities with optimising tax revenues.[163]

Whilst the expectation for an international unitary approach to be applied to MNEs is currently unrealistic, in the European Union, the Common Consolidated Corporate Tax Base (CCCTB)[164] proposal *does* contain CFC rules in a unitary context. However, these CFC rules would only apply to subsidiaries resident in third countries. To the Commission, there could only be CFCs established in third countries—there could never be non-CCCTB CFCs within the European Union. In any case, in a CCCTB discussion draft on the proposed anti-abuse rules for the purposes of the CCCTB,[165] the Commission, referring to its earlier Communication on anti-abuse measures,[166] commented that 'if CFC rules were to be introduced in the CCCTB they should be in line with the recent ECJ rulings'.[167] This meant that

> [t]o comply with the ECJ law either CFC rules are only to be applied in relation with third countries or CFC rules are also to be applied within the EU but, in this case, the rules should be targeted at wholly artificial arrangements only.[168]

160 BEPS Monitoring Group, 'Comments on BEPS Action 3: Strengthening the Rules on Controlled Foreign Corporations (CFCs)', available on: bepsmonitoringgroup.files.wordpress.com/2015/05/ap3-controlled-foreign-corporations.pdf.

161 *Ibid*, page 4, para 6.

162 *Ibid*, page 4, para 3.

163 *Ibid.*

164 Brussels, COM(2011) 121/4, 2011/0058 (CNS); SEC(2011) 316 final. See discussion also in sections 5.2.2 and 8.1 of Chs 5 and 8 of this volume respectively.

165 CCCTB/WP065\doc\en: '*CCCTB: Anti-Abuse rules*' (14–15 April 2008). See discussion in part 6, Christiana HJI Panayi, *The Common Consolidated Corporate Tax Base and the UK* (Institute for Fiscal Studies, 2011).

166 Commission Communication on Anti-Abuse Measures, COM(2007) 785. See discussion in section 5.2.1 of this volume.

167 CCCTB/WP065\doc\en, n 165 above, para 29.

168 *Ibid.*

Perhaps a post-BEPS proposal on the CCCTB, which seems to be likely following recent Commission announcements in the context of the Tax Transparency Package,[169] would now not set the threshold for CFC rules so high.

2.6. Action 4: Limit Base Erosion via Interest Payments and Other Financial Payments

Action 4 mandates the OECD to:

> Develop recommendations regarding best practices in the design of rules to prevent base erosion through the use of interest expense, for example through the use of related-party and third-party debt to achieve excessive interest deductions or to finance the production of exempt or deferred income, and other financial payments that are economically equivalent to interest payments. The work will evaluate the effectiveness of different types of limitations. In connection with and in support of the foregoing work, transfer pricing guidance will also be developed regarding the pricing of related party financial transactions, including financial and performance guarantees, derivatives (including internal derivatives used in intra-bank dealings), and captive and other insurance arrangements. The work will be co-ordinated with the work on hybrids and CFC rules.

On 18 December 2014 the OECD released its discussion draft on interest deductions and other financial payments.[170] The primary concern appeared to be that multinational groups may be able to claim total interest deductions that significantly exceed their actual third-party interest expense. As explained in the Interest Expense Discussion Draft, such deductible payments can give rise to double non-taxation in both inbound and outbound investment scenarios.

> From an inbound perspective, concerns focus on excess interest deductions reducing taxable profits in operating companies even in cases where the group as a whole has little or no external debt. From an outbound perspective a company may use debt finance to produce tax exempt or deferred income, thereby claiming a deduction for interest expense while the related income is brought into tax later or not at all. Similar concerns are raised by payments under financial instruments such as guarantees and derivatives.[171]

The Interest Expense Discussion Draft reiterated the OECD's intention to develop recommendations for a best practice approach or approaches to address concerns

[169] See analysis in Ch 5, section 5.4 of this volume.

[170] OECD, *BEPS Action 4: Interest Deductions and Other Financial* Payments (henceforth, the Interest Expense Discussion Draft). Available on: www.oecd.org/ctp/aggressive/discussion-draft-action-4-interest-deductions.pdf. For commentary, see Amanda Athanasiou and Lee A Sheppard, 'BEPS Action 4 Draft Outlines Options for Interest Expense Deductions', 2014 *WTD* 244-1 (19 December 2014); Emilio Cencerrado Millan and Maria Teresa Soler Roch, 'Limit Base Erosion via Interest Deduction and Others' (2015) 43 *Intertax* 58–71; Jan Vleggeert, 'Public Discussion Draft on Interest Deductions Proposes Worldwide Interest Allocation Rules' (2015) 69 *Bulletin for International Taxation* 297–305.

[171] Interest Expense Discussion Draft, n 170, p 2.

about BEPS through interest expense. There was a review of existing approaches used by countries to address this problem and a discussion of a series of issues that were relevant to any approach chosen.

It was noted that a rule must apply not only to interest but also to payments that were economically equivalent to interest, as well as other expenses incurred in connection with the raising of finance.[172] There was a non-exhaustive list of examples of types of payment that should be covered by such a rule,[173] but it was left to each country to determine how this should be reflected within its domestic law.[174] In deciding whether a payment is economically equivalent to interest, the focus should be on its economic substance rather than its legal form.

It was suggested that an interest deductibility rule should apply to companies and other entities in three different scenarios: first, when they formed part of a corporate group; secondly, when they were under common control, but were not part of a corporate group (eg when a fund, individual or trust exercised the common control); and thirdly, when the parties were (otherwise) related, using a 25 per cent common ownership test, or in the case of a structured arrangement.[175]

It was questioned whether a rule should operate by reference to the level of interest expense in an entity or the level of debt. It was also questioned whether a rule should focus on an entity's gross position (ie only its interest expense or debt liabilities) or its net position (ie also taking into account interest income or debt assets).[176] Factors in favour of each method were considered.

There was also a discussion on whether there should be a de minimis threshold, in order to reduce the level of compliance burden on entities and the administrative burden on tax authorities. Certain entities may pose a sufficiently low risk that excluding them from a rule would be appropriate. The Interest Expense Discussion Draft considered two ways to set a threshold below which entities would not be expected to apply the rule: based on an entity's size (a size threshold) or its level of net interest expense (a monetary threshold). It was not proposed that a threshold would be required as part of a best practice recommendation—it was up to countries to decide so.[177] Where a threshold was introduced, it should be set at an appropriate level, taking into account the economic and interest rate environment in the country. In addition, it was preferable that the threshold should apply to the total level of net interest expense in the local group, to avoid groups fragmenting into multiple entities each applying a separate threshold.[178]

[172] *Ibid*, Part IV.

[173] For example, profit participating loans, imputed interest on convertible or zero-coupon bonds, foreign exchange gains and losses connected with the raising of finance, guarantee fees with respect to financing arrangements and loan arrangement or similar fees. *Ibid*, para 35.

[174] *Ibid*.

[175] *Ibid*, Part V. This scoping rule is similar to that used in the Hybrids Revised Discussion Draft, n 122 above, released by the OECD in September 2014.

[176] *Ibid*, Part VI.

[177] *Ibid*, para 57.

[178] *Ibid*.

The Interest Expense Discussion Draft examined various methods of limiting taxpayers' excessive interest expense deductions. The methods included general interest limitation rules which set an overall limit on the amount of interest expense in an entity, by linking interest deductibility to the position of a group or to fixed ratios, as well as targeted interest limitation rules which address specific base erosion and profit shifting risks. The Interest Expense Discussion Draft focused primarily on two approaches: first, a group-wide rule, which would limit a company's net interest deductions to a proportion of the group's actual net third-party interest expense; and secondly, a fixed-ratio rule, which would apply irrespective of the level of debt of a group and which would limit a company's interest deductions to an amount determined by applying a fixed benchmark ratio to an entity's earnings, assets or equity. Certain combinations of these two approaches and the use of more targeted approaches were also discussed.

Other approaches were rejected, although it was acknowledged that some rules, such as targeted anti-abuse rules, might be helpful in defined circumstances. For example, a fixed debt-to-equity ratio test was not to be included because of the perceived manipulability and efficacy concerns. Also, the arm's length test was not recommended as the sole general rule, as it would be ineffective and/or burdensome to apply and enforce. The imposition of withholding taxes on interest payments was also rejected as a solution in part because the EU's Interest and Royalty Directive would make it very difficult for Member States to impose withholding taxes on interest payments made within the European Union. It was noted that each of these provisions could play a useful role within an overall approach.

Under the group-wide approach, the aim was to align individual entities' interest expenses with the overall group's interest expenses.[179] This would prevent the group from claiming relief for interest expense in excess of its actual interest costs, and could reduce the risk of profit shifting when taxable income was separated from economic activity, according to the draft. There would be allocation of a group's net third-party interest expense between group entities in accordance with their economic activity, measured by earnings or asset values. This could operate by either allocating to each entity a portion of the group's net third-party interest expense or limiting each entity's interest expense to a portion of the group's net third-party interest expense. There was also a group ratio rule, which would compare the relevant financial ratio of an entity—its net interest to earnings or net interest to asset values—with the equivalent ratio of the entity's worldwide group to establish a limit on the net interest expense the entity would be allowed to deduct.

Under the fixed-ratio approach, an entity would be entitled to deduct net interest expenses up to a specified proportion of its earnings, assets or equity. The Interest Expense Discussion Draft noted a perception that even the lower 25 per cent and 30 per cent ratios currently used by other countries might be too high to address BEPS concerns. This approach was more rigid and did not account for the

[179] *Ibid*, Part VIII.

fact that different sectors require different amounts of leverage. However, it was thought to be administratively less cumbersome.

The Interest Expense Discussion Draft described another two approaches that combined elements of the above approaches,[180] so as to reduce administrative and compliance costs and offer certainty to companies. Each of these combined approaches included a general rule and then a carve-out from the general rule. 'Approach 1' was a general group-wide interest allocation rule with a carve-out for entities meeting a low fixed-ratio test, to help alleviate the compliance costs in lower-risk situations. 'Approach 2' was a fixed-ratio rule with a carve-out for entities that might permit them to deduct additional interest expense when the group's overall ratio exceeded the standard fixed ratio.

Targeted rules may be needed to address specific situations, such as for interest paid to connected or related parties, stapled stock, interest accrued on excessive debt push-downs and interest used to fund or acquire tax-exempt or tax-deferred income-yielding assets.[181] The Interest Expense Discussion Draft did not recommend any specific targeted rules but opened up the topic for further discussion. The special issues presented by banking and insurance companies, as well as groups in other sectors were recognised—it was recommended that there should be separate rules for these.[182]

The Interest Expense Discussion Draft acknowledged the interaction with the other BEPS action items, especially Actions 2, 3 and 4, but focused on the need for coordination rather than ranking.[183] In general, although the Interest Expense Discussion Draft did not adopt a specific approach, if seen in the context of other Action items, especially Actions 8–10, there is, arguably, a subtle shift away from separate entity accounting and a move towards a more unitary approach, with less respect for contracts. It has been criticised that BEPS represents a slippery slope towards formulary apportionment.[184]

Written comments by industry and business representatives had denounced the OECD's groupwide approach and its rejection of the arm's length test. Also, at the public consultation on 17 February 2015, it was argued that the proposed group-wide allocation would engender complexity and difficulties for both taxpayers and tax administrators. The proposal was also problematic, due to the temporal volatility in earnings, the unique circumstances of individual constituent entities, and the proposal's perverse incentive for increasing group indebtedness.[185]

[180] *Ibid*, Part X.

[181] *Ibid*, Part XI.

[182] *Ibid*, Part XIII.

[183] *Ibid*, Part XIV.

[184] David D Steward, 'BEPS Presents Slippery Slope Toward Formulary Apportionment', 2015 *WTD* 29-1 (12 February 2015). For an endorsement of the OECD's suggestions, see Chloe Burnett, 'Interest Deductions and Multinational Enterprises: Goldilocks and the Brave New World' (2015) 69 *Bulletin for International Taxation* 326.

[185] Ajay Gupta, 'BEPS Action 4: Keeping Formulary Apportionment at Bay', 2015 *WTD* 45-3 (9 March 2015). Also see review of comments by Amanda Athanasiou and David D Stewart in 'OECD Action 4 Draft Consultation Focuses on Fixed Ratios', 2015 *WTD* 32-1 (18 February 2015).

The leverage and interest ratios between entities may vary depending on the nature of their business, their stage in the business cycle, their size, the market in which they operate etc.[186] Furthermore, due to the differences in tax and accounting in different countries, applying the test might be a complex and cumbersome exercise.

Moreover, given that the discussion draft provides a series of options of best practices rather than definite proposals, the inconsistent implementation of a group-wide rule could lead to double taxation. As countries will have some discretion, they may implement different versions of the rule. 'All this would elevate the compliance burden and related costs to an unprecedented level'.[187] A group-wide approach would also likely incentivise groups to increase third-party funding, which could create further economic distortions. There was overwhelming preference for a fixed-ratio test, though it has also been argued that a combined approach with a fixed-ratio rule as the general rule and group-wide approach as the exception might be more sensible than all.

It has been reported that the OECD may be retracting its tentative steps towards adopting an apportionment regime for interest expense, going back to approaches based on separate entity accounting.[188] The renunciation of the arm's length standard as a solution and the proposals based on group-wide tests were bound to raise problems.

> That an MNE should be treated as an integrated firm for deductibility of interest purposes would surely have been perceived by business interests as going beyond just disavowing arm's length tests to opening the door to some sort of formulary apportionment.[189]

Endorsing the group-wide tests in an unequivocal way would have represented 'an unabashed embrace of unitary taxation'.[190]

2.7. Action 5: Counter Harmful Tax Practices More Effectively, Taking into Account Transparency and Substance

Action 5 of the BEPS Action Plan commits the Forum on Harmful Tax Practices (FHTP) to:

> Revamp the work on harmful tax practices with a priority on improving transparency, including compulsory spontaneous exchange on rulings related to preferential regimes,

[186] Oliver R Hoor and Keith O'Donnell, 'BEPS Action 4: When Theory Meets Practice' (2015) 78 *Tax Notes International* 643 (18 May 2015).

[187] *Ibid.*

[188] Gupta, 'BEPS Action 4: Keeping Formulary Apportionment at Bay', n 185 above.

[189] *Ibid.*

[190] *Ibid.*

> and on requiring substantial activity for any preferential regime. It will take a holistic approach to evaluate preferential tax regimes in the BEPS context. It will engage with non-OECD members on the basis of the existing framework and consider revisions or additions to the existing framework.

Whilst the bulk of the work under the BEPS Action Plan is directed at the position and actions of taxpayers, this Action item—and arguably also Actions 14 and 15—focus on the actions of countries. Under Action 5, the FHTP was to deliver on three outputs: first, the finalisation of the review of member country preferential regimes; secondly, a strategy to expand participation to non-OECD member countries; and thirdly, consideration of revisions or additions to the existing framework. The OECD deliverable on Action 5 was released for the first time in September 2014.[191] The Harmful Tax Practices Discussion Draft outlined the progress made on the delivery of these outputs and discussed progress on the first output at length. Almost half of the discussion draft was devoted to the OECD's previous work on harmful tax practices—the 1998 Harmful Tax Competition Report[192] and its aftermath. The work under Action 5 was seen as an extension of this. The FHTP was now asked to 'revamp' its work on harmful tax practices, with a priority and renewed focus on requiring substantial activity for any preferential regime and on improving transparency through compulsory spontaneous exchange of rulings related to preferential regimes.

Emphasis was placed on elaborating a methodology to define a substantial activity requirement in the context of intangible property.[193] This is understandable given that the taxation of intangible property is at the heart of the BEPS project.[194] The OECD recognised that there has been a shift by countries from creating ring-fenced tax regimes towards introducing more broadly-based corporate tax reductions for particular types of income, such as financial activities or intangibles.[195]

In defining substantial activity, the Harmful Tax Practices Discussion Draft focused primarily on the nexus approach.[196] This looked at whether an

[191] OECD, *Countering Harmful Tax Practices More Effectively, Taking into Account Transparency and Substance, OECD/G20 Base Erosion and Profit Shifting Project* (OECD Publishing, 2014) (henceforth, Harmful Tax Practices Discussion Draft). Available on: www.oecd-ilibrary.org/docserver/download/2314271e.pdf?expires=1422733878&id=id&accname=guest&checksum=DFD58772A6E26FAA92CFD6974A8A8B51.

[192] OECD, *Harmful Tax Competition: An Emerging Global Issue* (OECD Publishing, 1998). See Ch 1 of this volume.

[193] Harmful Tax Practices Discussion Draft, n 191 above, p 28.

[194] *Ibid*, p 28.

[195] *Ibid*.

[196] Other approaches considered were the value creation approach and the transfer pricing approach. The value creation approach required taxpayers to undertake a set number of significant development activities. The transfer pricing approach would allow a regime to provide benefits to all the income generated by the IP if the taxpayer had located a set level of important functions in the jurisdiction providing the regime, if the taxpayer was the legal owner of the assets giving rise to the tax benefits and used the assets giving rise to the tax benefits, and if the taxpayer bore the economic risks of the assets giving rise to the tax benefits: *ibid*, pp 28–29. The third approach, the nexus approach, was preferred.

intellectual property (IP) regime made its benefits conditional on the extent of research and development (R&D) activities of taxpayers receiving benefits. Under this approach, expenditures act as a proxy for substantial activities.[197] The nexus approach sought to build on the basic principle underlying R&D credits and similar 'front-end' tax regimes that apply to expenditures incurred in the creation of IP. It extended this basic principle to 'back-end' tax regimes that apply to the income earned after the creation and exploitation of the IP. Therefore, the initially proposed nexus approach would allow countries to extend their jurisdiction beyond IP regimes that only provide benefits directly to the expenditures incurred to *create* the IP, permitting jurisdictions to provide benefits to the income arising out of that IP—so long as there is a direct nexus between the income receiving benefits and the expenditures contributing to that income.

The nexus approach applied a proportionate analysis to income, under which the proportion of income that may benefit from an IP regime was the same proportion as that between qualifying R&D expenditures and overall R&D expenditures.[198]

Calculations under the formula would be treated as a rebuttable presumption.[199] The purpose of this approach was to grant benefits only to income that arises from IP where the actual R&D activity was undertaken by the taxpayer itself. This goal was achieved by defining 'qualifying expenditures' in a way that prevented mere capital contribution or expenditures for substantial R&D activity by parties other than the taxpayer from qualifying the subsequent income for benefits under an IP regime. The various concepts were analysed extensively in the discussion draft.

Taxpayers wanting to benefit from an IP regime must track expenditures, IP assets, and income to ensure that the income receiving benefits did in fact arise from the expenditures that qualified for those benefits. Each jurisdiction had to establish procedures for tracking and tracing based on consistent criteria capable of objective measurement.[200]

There was some criticism of the approach used by the OECD in delineating substantial activity, in that it had 'a tenuous link to a complex reality'.[201] Expenses that may in some cases produce a significant return may sometimes result in no meaningful assets. Having one standard for all intangible-based businesses was

[197] *Ibid*, p 29.

[198] *Ibid*. For complex business models with multiple strands of income and expenditure, a more complicated formula was recommended:

$$\frac{\text{Qualifying expenditures incurred to develop IP asset}}{\text{Overall expenditures incurred to develop IP asset}} \times \text{Overall income from IP asset} = \text{Income receiving tax benefits}$$

[199] Harmful Tax Practices Discussion Draft, n 191 above, p 30.

[200] *Ibid*, p 34.

[201] Mindy Herzfeld, 'Defining Harmful Patent Boxes', 2014 *WTD* 202-2 (20 October 2014).

unlikely to be effective. Also, the test may be difficult to apply. While it may be easier to link a tax credit to an expense, it may be more difficult to link an income item to an asset generated by a previously incurred expense.[202] The framework arguably offered a formulaic view that was unlikely to recognise the complexities of tracing expenses to income-generating assets.

There was also criticism that through this formula, 'the OECD gives its blessing to a global tax system that allows countries with large pools of skilled labour to provide tax incentives'.[203] This was likely to favour OECD member countries but not developing countries that tend to lack the labour pools to generate research expenses. It was also lamented that this approach would leave little room for IP management entities set up in small open economies to coordinate R&D activities of MNEs conducted in other jurisdictions.[204]

The BEPS Monitoring Group was very much against the basic premise of the substantial nexus approach—the linkage with expenses.[205] The Group argued that tax allowances were an adequate reward for R&D. 'The argument that companies deserve even greater contributions from the taxpayer if an investment in R&D generates exceptional income seems hard to justify'.[206] Innovating companies already make exceptional profits, especially as a result of patent protection which is a state grant of monopoly.

> To grant on top of this a low tax rate, especially on income which could reduce the tax base resulting from economic activities (including marketing and sales) taking place in other countries, is a direct encouragement for firms to devise BEPS strategies.[207]

The Harmful Tax Practices Discussion Draft also set out a framework for compulsory spontaneous exchange of taxpayer-specific rulings related to preferential regimes.[208] The framework did not extend to general rulings, ie rulings that apply to types of taxpayers or that may be given in relation to a defined set of circumstances or activities. A ruling must be specific to an individual taxpayer and that taxpayer must be entitled to rely on it. The suggested framework was to apply

202 *Ibid.* By way of example, Herzfeld referred to the complexities of the much simpler US research credit. She argued that the proposed substantial nexus regime multiplied the problems. Also see Gary Guenther, *Research Tax Credit: Current Law and Policy Issues for the 113th Congress* (Congressional Research Service, 3 October 2014). Available on: nationalaglawcenter.org/wp-content/uploads/assets/crs/RL31181.pdf.

203 *Ibid.*

204 Ajay Gupta, 'Modifying the Modified Nexus Approach—Behind Closed Doors', 2015 *WTD* 60-1 (30 March 2015).

205 See BEPS Monitoring Group, OECD BEPS Scorecard, n 134 above.

206 *Ibid*, p 8.

207 *Ibid.*

208 Harmful Tax Practices Discussion Draft, n 191 above, ch 4. The term 'compulsory' was understood to introduce an obligation to spontaneously exchange information whenever the relevant conditions were met. The term 'spontaneous exchange of information' referred to a situation in which one country was aware of information that could be of relevance to another country, but the information had not been requested by the second country. *Ibid*, p 36.

to member country preferential regimes and at a later stage associate countries' preferential regimes. There were four key design questions:[209]

(1) When does the obligation to spontaneously exchange information on rulings arise?
(2) Who must information be exchanged with?
(3) What information must be exchanged?
(4) What is the legal basis for the spontaneous information exchange?

Some of the other issues which were also considered in this framework were, inter alia, the time limits for compulsory spontaneous information exchange, the relevance of reciprocity, protection of confidentiality of the information exchanged and the implementation of the framework.[210]

In assessing whether the obligation to spontaneously exchange information on rulings arises, a number of filters were recommended. These would ensure that the framework was targeted and that tax authorities' discretion was reduced. The first three filters limited the obligation to rulings related to (i) preferential regimes that (ii) are within the scope of work of the FHTP and that (iii) meet the no or low effective tax rate factor. If a ruling passed all of these three filters, there were additional filters.[211]

Under the filter approach, only a ruling that passed through all of the filters would be subject to compulsory spontaneous information exchange.[212] The obligation to spontaneously exchange would arise for rulings related to *any* preferential regime. There was no prerequisite for the ruling to have been reviewed or to have been found to be potentially or actually harmful within the meaning of the 1998 OECD Harmful Tax Competition Report.[213]

It was stated in the Harmful Tax Practices Discussion Draft that countries with preferential regimes that had not yet been reviewed by the FHTP would need to self-assess whether the first three filters (and the other filters provided in the discussion draft) were satisfied. Regimes that had been reviewed by the FHTP and that were found to meet the first three filters would be added to a compilation to be occasionally updated by the FHTP.

The Harmful Tax Practices Discussion Draft also presented the status of the review of member country regimes and the progress made on the review of preferential regimes of associate countries. In a table showing the status of the review for 30 preferential regimes, 15 of these were IP regimes. Nine of the regimes were found to be 'not harmful', but the remaining regimes, all being IP regimes, were still

[209] *Ibid*, pp 38–39.
[210] *Ibid*, p 39.
[211] For a comprehensive analysis of the filters, see pp 40–44 of the Harmful Tax Practices Discussion Draft, n 191 above. Also see the flowchart in Annex A which explained how these filters were intended to work.
[212] *Ibid*, p 39.
[213] See n 192 above.

under review.[214] Henceforth, all preferential regimes would need to be considered in light of the elaborated transparency factor.

Going forward, it was stated that the FHTP would complete the work under the first output of Action 5 and commence work on the second output by engaging with other non-OECD member countries. The deadline for the delivery of the second output was September 2015. The review of preferential regimes of associate countries would also continue. It was noted at an earlier juncture that any member and associate country can request at any time a review of any existing preferential tax regime.[215] It was emphasised that the goal was to achieve a level playing field and to avoid the risk of the work on harmful tax practices displacing regimes from OECD member and associate countries to other countries, giving them an unwarranted competitive advantage and limiting the effectiveness of the whole exercise.[216]

The revamping of the OECD's work on harmful tax practices was never going to be a straight-forward task—like most of the deliverables under the BEPS Action Plan. While the overarching focus of the Action Plan is on aligning taxation with value creation and the substance of transactions, determining the location of substantial activity in the context of Action 5 was inevitably going to be a subjective exercise—and one to generate a lot of disagreement. However, the proposals on the remaining aspects of Action 5 are more likely to go forward and be considered a success. Especially as regards the proposal for compulsory spontaneous exchange of rulings, there is already a legal basis for this in tax treaties which can be used.[217] It also fits in with the latest global trends for greater automatic exchange of information. The European Commission has made similar but more wide-ranging proposals to allow for automatic exchange of all tax rulings, not just those relating to preferential regimes. The Commission proposals in the context of its Tax Transparency Package are considered in Chapter five of this volume.[218]

On 11 November 2014, Germany and the UK announced a proposal to modify the OECD's nexus approach,[219] which would also curb the UK patent box regime.[220] This was subsequently endorsed by all OECD and G20 countries.

214 Harmful Tax Practices Discussion Draft, n 191 above, pp 58–59.

215 *Ibid*, p 56.

216 *Ibid*, pp 63–64.

217 Art 26 of the OECD Model.

218 See section 5.4.

219 See Germany–UK Joint Statement, available on: www.gov.uk/government/uploads/system/uploads/attachment_data/file/373135/GERMANY_UK_STATEMENT.pdf.

220 Under the UK regime, companies could apply a lower rate of corporation tax (10%) to profits earned after 1 April 2013 from their patented inventions. A company could benefit from the patent box if it owned or exclusively licensed-in patents granted by the UK Intellectual Property Office, the European Patent Office and several EEA countries (namely, Austria, Bulgaria, Czech Republic, Denmark, Estonia, Finland, Germany, Hungary, Poland, Portugal, Romania, Slovakia and Sweden). See HMRC guidance available on: www.gov.uk/corporation-tax-the-patent-box. Therefore, benefits were given even if the qualifying IP was developed outside of the UK. This was very much resented by Germany, as a number of patents obtained in the UK by German-based companies had significantly increased since

The agreed modified nexus approach[221] maintains the underlying principle of the nexus approach proposed in the September 2014 Harmful Tax Practices Discussion Draft but makes some important amendments, following the UK-Germany proposal.

Pursuant to the modified nexus approach, a 30 per cent uplift would be allowed to increase the value of the eligible R&D expenditure proxy for outsourcing or acquisition costs. The 30 per cent uplift to the qualifying expenditures would reflect expenditures for R&D activities outsourced to related parties and IP acquisition costs.[222] Broadly, the revised formula would allow the IP box company, when calculating benefits due under the preferential regime, to take into account related party outsource expenditure (and any IP acquisition costs), subject to a cap on actual expenditure. This provision was introduced to reduce the negative impact of an IP box company choosing to outsource R&D activities to group companies.[223]

Existing regimes would be closed to new entrants (for both products and patents) by June 2016. Countries with IP regimes that are inconsistent with the modified nexus approach would be expected to take steps to amend those regimes and the process to do this should commence in 2015. In addition, there would be no new entrants to such IP regimes after 30 June 2016. There would be a long grandfathering period, under which benefits could continue to be claimed until June 2021. The FHTP would work to reach agreement by June 2015 on a practical and proportionate tracking and tracing approach that can be implemented by companies and tax authorities. It would also work on developing practical methodologies that companies and tax authorities could adopt.

The OECD stated that it would develop more detailed guidance on how businesses can track expenditure and income to ensure that the nexus approach was being correctly applied. It would also consider safeguards to prevent taxpayers from inappropriately using the transitional period to get tax benefits under existing IP regimes. More guidance would also be developed on what would be regarded as a qualifying IP asset. In an accompanying explanatory paper,[224] the OECD committed to completing the work on this guidance by 30 June 2015.

the UK patent box was introduced in 2011. See Mindy Herzfeld, 'Political Developments in BEPS and the EU' (2014) 76 *Tax Notes International* 653, 24 November 2014. For an overview, see Fabian Mang, 'The (In)Compatibility of IP Box Regimes with EU Law, the Code of Conduct and the BEPS Initiatives' (2015) 55 *European Taxation* 78–87.

[221] See *Explanatory Paper—Agreement on Modified Nexus Approach for IP Regimes*, available on: www1.oecd.org/ctp/explanatory-paper-beps-action-5-agreement-on-modified-nexus-approach-for-ip-regimes.pdf. For the full report, see *Action 5: Agreement on Modified Nexus Approach for IP Regimes* (OECD 2015), available on: www.oecd.org/ctp/beps-action-5-agreement-on-modified-nexus-approach-for-ip-regimes.pdf.

[222] Gupta, 'Modifying the Modified Nexus Approach—Behind Closed Doors', n 204 above.

[223] See Jonathan Bridges, 'The Q&A: The UK/German proposal for preferential IP regimes', *Tax Journal*, Issue 1240, p 8 (21 November 2014).

[224] See *Explanatory Paper—Agreement on Modified Nexus Approach for IP Regimes*, n 221 above.

A final formulation for implementing the agreed modified nexus approach would be included in the 2015 deliverable on Action 5.

In a joint statement released on 10 March 2015 by the Federation of German Industries and the Confederation of Dutch Industry and Employers, the modified nexus approach was criticised for being too restrictive.[225] Limiting the tax benefits for outsourced R&D may be problematic, as due to the 'increasingly work-sharing environment it is nearly impossible to provide only local R&D'.[226] The modified nexus approach was also criticised for limiting the benefits of IP regimes to patents and other functionally equivalent IP assets that are legally protected and subject to approval and registration processes. As trademarks and other marketing-related IP assets could not qualify for benefits, this approach would lead to a discrimination of industry sectors, where certain inventions might not be patentable, or are not patented due to commercial considerations (eg trade secrets). It might also discriminate against small and medium-sized enterprises, for which registering a patent often entails a high administrative and/or financial burden.[227] It was recommended that 'where a taxpayer can demonstrate that [it] has borne the expenses of developing the IP, the fruits of such IP should be allowed to benefit from the IP box regime'.[228] Also, there should be some flexibility in the documentation requirements to accommodate IP which was developed out of experience or by chance, where it was difficult to trace the costs retrospectively. It was argued that the final recommendations ought to be effective in stimulating R&D and minimising the administrative burdens but at the same time they should provide a level playing field for all taxpayers, regardless of size or sector.

Other stakeholders made similar comments vis-à-vis the revised draft guidance. It was argued that the nexus approach should be flexible on the definition of qualifying IP assets to include unpatented IP. Limiting benefits to one type of IP asset would create distortions in the type of IP developed and fail to account for the value and expense associated with unpatented IP. It was noted that a significant amount of R&D expenses were devoted to developing unpatented IP assets such as know-how.

Stakeholders also recommended that the OECD should broaden the scope of qualifying R&D expenditures, and procedures for tracking and tracing of expenditures.[229] Regarding qualifying R&D expenditure, as described above, there was a rebuttable presumption in the September 2014 discussion draft that the amount of IP income that qualifies for IP regime benefits should be proportionate to the ratio of qualifying IP expenditures to overall IP expenditures. This should remain a rebuttable presumption, to ensure there were no unfair and inconsistent results

[225] The joint statement is available in Tax Analysts, 2015 *WTD* 48-16 (10 March 2015).
[226] *Ibid*, p 1.
[227] *Ibid*, p 2.
[228] *Ibid*.
[229] See Margaret Burow, 'Stakeholders Seek Flexibility in OECD IP Nexus Approach', 2015 *WTD* 48-2 (12 March 2015).

'particularly when the element of IP essential to bring the product to the market constitutes only a small portion of overall IP expenditures in a multinational group'.[230]

Regarding the obligation to track and trace IP income and expenditures asset by asset to receive IP benefits, this was criticised as it did not reflect the way businesses develop their IP. Stakeholders noted that IP innovations tended to be interconnected and so were the processes to develop them. Pooling of expenditures was essential.

Whilst most of the industry representatives were in favour of expanding the scope of the modified nexus approach, by contrast, in its comments, the BEPS Monitoring Group was very critical. Repeating some of its earlier criticisms, the Group argued that the patent box was unnecessary and undesirable, as encouragement for R&D could already be easily provided through investment allowances.[231] It was thought that the OECD approach would simply legitimise 'innovation box' regimes and supply a legal mechanism for profit shifting. It would be particularly damaging to developing countries, which may be used as manufacturing platforms, but their tax base would be drained by this mechanism.

The BEPS Monitoring Group argued that a better approach would be an extension of the profit split method. The use of such a method, applied with concrete and easily determinable objective allocation keys, would be much easier to administer and less intrusive both for countries and enterprises. It would also leave countries free to decide their own tax rates, as well as investment allowances.

The BEPS Monitoring Group also criticised the secrecy around the work that had already been undertaken by the FHTP in reviewing member country regimes. Although this was in an attempt to insulate the FHPT's work from business pressures, it also hindered the public debate. It was essential to have a widespread public debate about the legitimacy and validity of tax regimes which could be regarded as harmful. The Group recommended that these reviews should be conducted as openly and transparently as other aspects of the BEPS project.[232]

To an extent, any nexus approach which focuses on economic presence to justify income in a country poses the risk of worsening any adverse economic effects of tax competition, as it creates an incentive for taxpayers to move people and activities from high-tax to low-tax jurisdictions. This could be harmful as well. Although the issue was raised even before the revision of the nexus approach,[233] unfortunately, it has not been addressed in the discussion documents. Whether or not the modified nexus approach will reconfigure the parameters of the tax competition debate in such a way as to be deemed to create more rather than less tax-induced relocations and economic distortions remains to be seen.

The remaining BEPS deliverables are examined in the next two chapters.

230 *Ibid.*

231 BEPS Monitoring Group, *Response to Action 5: Harmful Tax Practices: Agreement on the Modified Nexus Approach*. Available on: bepsmonitoringgroup.files.wordpress.com/2015/02/ap5-htps-modified-substance.pdf.

232 *Ibid*, p 3.

233 Amanda Athanasiou, 'The Cost of BEPS', 2015 *WTD* 9-1 (14 January 2015).

3

Tax Treaty Abuse, Permanent Establishments and Transfer Pricing Rules: Actions 6–10

In the previous chapter, the launch of the BEPS Action Plan was considered. Then Action items 1 to 5 were reviewed in greater detail. The focus of this chapter is on Action items 6 to 10. The deliverables on these Action items have produced some of the most contentious proposals of the BEPS project as a whole.

3.1. Action 6: Prevent Treaty Abuse

Action 6 of the Action Plan mandates as follows:

> Develop model treaty provisions and recommendations regarding the design of domestic rules to prevent the granting of treaty benefits in inappropriate circumstances. Work will also be done to clarify that tax treaties are not intended to be used to generate double non-taxation and to identify the tax policy considerations that, in general, countries should consider before deciding to enter into a tax treaty with another country. The work will be co-ordinated with the work on hybrids.

The first discussion draft, which set out the main parameters of the proposals, was published in March 2014 (henceforth, the Treaty Abuse Discussion Draft).[1] There was a second discussion draft in September 2014 (henceforth, the Treaty Abuse Revised Discussion Draft)[2] and a follow-up report in November 2014 (henceforth, the Treaty Abuse Follow-Up Report).[3] A second revised discussion draft was issued in May 2015.

The Treaty Abuse Discussion Draft was composed of three sections. The first section examined the development of model treaty provisions and recommendations

[1] OECD, *BEPS Action 6: Preventing the Granting of Treaty Benefits in Inappropriate Circumstances*—14 March–9 April 2014. Available on: www.oecd.org/ctp/treaties/treaty-abuse-discussion-draft-march-2014.pdf.

[2] OECD/G20 Base Erosion and Profit Shifting Project, *Preventing the Granting of Treaty Benefits in Inappropriate Circumstances—Action 6: 2014 Deliverable* (OECD, 2014). Available on: www.oecd-ilibrary.org/docserver/download/2314281e.pdf?expires=1433339357&id=id&accname=guest&checksum=B5EBBB1C513F73A6C49C3D79ECAC8E12.

[3] OECD, *Follow Up Work on BEPS Action 6: Preventing Treaty Abuse*. Available on: www.oecd.org/ctp/treaties/discussion-draft-action-6-follow-up-prevent-treaty-abuse.pdf.

regarding the design of domestic rules to prevent the granting of treaty benefits in inappropriate circumstances. In the second section, the need to clarify that tax treaties were not intended to be used to generate double non-taxation was assessed. The third section sought to identify the tax policy considerations that, in general, countries should consider before deciding to enter into a tax treaty with another country.

The overall recommendations were summed up in paragraph 9 of the Treaty Abuse Discussion Draft. Very importantly, it was recommended 'to include in the title and preamble of tax treaties a clear statement that the Contracting States, when entering into a treaty, wish to prevent tax avoidance and, in particular, intend to avoid creating opportunities for treaty shopping'.[4] Also, the Treaty Abuse Discussion Draft proposed the inclusion of an anti-abuse rule based on the Limitation-on-Benefits (LOB) provision found in most US tax treaties, as well as the inclusion of a more general anti-abuse rule designed to address other forms of treaty abuse, not covered by the LOB. This 'would provide a more general way to address treaty avoidance cases, including treaty shopping situations that would not be covered by [the suggested LOB]'.[5] Other recommendations would also assist in preventing treaty shopping.[6]

The first section contained some of the most important recommendations. As far as the LOB provision was concerned, the Treaty Abuse Discussion Draft set out the suggested wording, much of which resembled versions of the LOB article used in US treaties.[7] The title of this anti-abuse proposal was *Entitlement to benefits—Article X*. Where it diverged from the US LOB provisions was in the final paragraph, paragraph 6, which introduced a general anti-abuse rule (GAAR), based on a main purpose test, discussed below. A detailed Commentary was to explain the main features of the LOB.[8] The possibility of inclusion of a 'derivative benefits' clause was indicated, with its merits and demerits.[9] Comments were invited.[10]

From paragraphs 18 onwards, the Treaty Abuse Discussion Draft analysed the suggested main purpose test. This test read as follows:[11]

> Notwithstanding the other provisions of this Convention, a benefit under this Convention shall not be granted in respect of an item of income if it is reasonable to conclude, having regard to all relevant facts and circumstances, that obtaining that benefit was one of the main purposes of any arrangement or transaction that resulted directly or indirectly in that benefit, unless it is established that granting that benefit in these circumstances would be in accordance with the object and purpose of the relevant provisions of this Convention.

[4] Treaty Abuse Discussion Draft, n 1 above, para 9, p 4.
[5] *Ibid*, para 10.
[6] *Ibid*, para 10.
[7] *Ibid*, para 11.
[8] *Ibid*, para 12.
[9] *Ibid*, paras 13–16.
[10] *Ibid*, para 17.
[11] *Ibid*, para 18, on p 10.

Again, the new main purpose test would be supplemented by a detailed Commentary which would include examples. Comments were invited on what should be covered by the Commentary[12] but a few explanatory points were included. The main purpose test was meant to supplement the LOB. As such, when a benefit was denied under the LOB it would not be subject to analysis there. Conversely, a benefit allowed under the LOB could be denied under the main purpose test.[13]

In determining whether the main purpose test applied, 'it is important to undertake an objective analysis of the aims and objects of all persons involved in putting that arrangement or transaction in place or being a party to it'.[14] This would be a question of fact.[15] All the evidence would be weighted to determine whether it was reasonable to conclude that an arrangement or transaction was undertaken or arranged for such purpose.[16] Obtaining the benefit under the tax treaty need not be the sole or dominant purpose of a particular arrangement or transaction.[17] 'It is sufficient that at least one of the main purposes was to obtain the benefit'.[18]

The Treaty Abuse Discussion Draft also reviewed specific situations when a person seeks to circumvent treaty limitations.[19] While a general anti-abuse rule may be helpful in addressing such situations, it was suggested that 'targeted specific anti-abuse rules would provide greater certainty for both taxpayers and tax administrators'.[20] Some of these specific situations were discussed.

For example, it was proposed that the reduced rates of withholding tax under Article 10 of the OECD Model applicable to non-portfolio dividends be restricted to shareholdings that are owned throughout a period of months. Comments were sought on what the number of months should be.[21] Furthermore, the Treaty Abuse Discussion Draft proposed the abolition of the 'place of effective management' tie-breaker clause for determining the treaty residence of persons other than individuals. This would be replaced by a requirement that the competent authorities of the two countries endeavour to determine residence, by reference to a number of factors such as the place of effective management, the place of incorporation/constitution etc.[22] There were also suggestions to counter triangular situations involving a third country permanent establishment (PE).[23]

[12] *Ibid*, para 19.
[13] *Ibid*, paras 22–23.
[14] *Ibid*, para 29.
[15] *Ibid*.
[16] *Ibid*, para 30.
[17] *Ibid*, para 31.
[18] *Ibid*.
[19] *Ibid*, para 34.
[20] *Ibid*.
[21] *Ibid*, paras 41–43.
[22] *Ibid*, paras 50–53.
[23] *Ibid*, paras 54–56. A new treaty clause was proposed to restrict relief from withholding taxes on payments attributable to a third country PE of a treaty resident. This would apply if the profits of the PE were subject to a combined aggregate effective tax rate in the PE and residence countries which was less than 60% of the general rate of company tax applicable in the residence country: *ibid*, para 56.

Furthermore, the Treaty Abuse Discussion Draft addressed cases where a person tried to abuse the provisions of domestic tax law using treaty benefits. Here, it was argued, the threat to the national tax base was not caused by the tax treaties but it may have been facilitated by them.[24] There was a list of avoidance strategies that were thought to fall into this category (eg thin capitalisation, transfer pricing, arbitrage etc). Many of these strategies were to be addressed through other items of the BEPS Action Plan.[25] It was also reiterated that tax treaties did not prevent the application of specific domestic law provisions that would hinder such transactions.[26] In order to prevent interpretations intended to circumvent the application of a country's domestic anti-abuse rules, a 'savings clause', often used by the USA should be adopted.[27] This clause would confirm the country's right to tax its residents without regard to the provisions of any tax treaty, other than those provisions that were clearly intended to apply to residents.[28]

In the second section, which sought to clarify that tax treaties are not intended to be used to generate double non-taxation, the Treaty Abuse Discussion Draft made several recommendations. It was suggested that the 'title' of the OECD Model should be amended to state clearly that the prevention of tax evasion and avoidance is a purpose of tax treaties.[29] This should also be reflected in a preamble which 'provides expressly that States that enter into a tax treaty intend to eliminate double taxation without creating opportunities for tax evasion and avoidance', including a specific reference that treaty shopping arrangements are an example of tax avoidance that should not result from tax treaties.[30] The OECD believed that a clear statement of the intention of the signatories that appeared in the preamble would be relevant to the interpretation and application of the treaty.[31]

The last section addressed the third part of the mandate—ie to identify the tax policy considerations that, in general, countries should consider before deciding to enter into a tax treaty with another country. Here, the Treaty Abuse Discussion Draft proposed additional paragraphs to the introduction of the OECD Model. The policy considerations set out in these new paragraphs would help countries explain their decisions not to enter into tax treaties with low-tax or no-tax jurisdictions but they would also be relevant in deciding whether a country should modify, replace or terminate an existing treaty. It was recognised that there were many other non-tax factors that may also be relevant and states had a sovereign right to decide whether to do so.[32]

[24] *Ibid*, para 57 et seq.
[25] *Ibid*, para 58.
[26] *Ibid*, para 59.
[27] *Ibid*, para 69.
[28] *Ibid*.
[29] *Ibid*, para 75.
[30] *Ibid*, para 75.
[31] *Ibid*, para 76.
[32] See paras 79–81. The suggested wording is set out in para 81.

In the proposed addition to the Commentary, a number of considerations were raised. The primary tax policy concern would be 'the existence of risks of double taxation resulting from the interaction of the tax systems of the two States involved'.[33] Where a state levied no or low taxes, other states should consider whether there were risks of double taxation justifying a tax treaty. States should also consider whether there were elements of another state's tax system (eg ring-fenced tax advantages) that could increase the risk of non-taxation.[34] Another tax policy consideration set out was the risk of excessive taxation that may result from high withholding taxes in the source state.[35] In considering whether to enter into a tax treaty, various features of tax treaties that encourage and foster economic ties between countries (eg non-discrimination, greater taxpayer certainty, mutual agreement procedures, arbitration etc)[36] as well as the effective implementation of administrative assistance provisions should be considered.[37]

In general, this discussion draft called for a significant rewrite of both the OECD Model Tax Convention and its Commentary. One of the main recommendations, the main purpose test, proved to be very controversial.[38] The main purpose test was criticised for not striking the right balance in providing legitimate businesses with treaty protection while preventing treaty shopping.[39] It undermined the clarity and predictability principles that were intended by the inclusion of the LOB.[40] The US also voiced its disagreement with the new test, due to its subjective connotations.[41]

It was not just the main purpose test that had attracted criticism. Many stakeholders identified the need for more guidance in various places—for instance, in obtaining discretionary benefits under the suggested LOB.[42] Pursuant to this provision, the competent authorities of a Contracting State could allow a resident of another Contracting State not otherwise entitled to benefits to obtain them if the competent authority found no principal purpose of tax avoidance. The OECD

33 See suggested para 15.2 of the Introduction to the OECD Model, set out in para 81 of the Treaty Abuse Discussion Draft.

34 *Ibid*.

35 *Ibid*, suggested para 15.4.

36 *Ibid*, suggested para 15.5.

37 *Ibid*, suggested para 15.6. It was conceded that administrative assistance could be achieved through more targeted agreements such as the conclusion of a Tax Information Exchange Agreement or participation in the Multilateral Convention on Mutual Administrative Assistance in Tax Matters. Therefore, absent of any actual risk of double taxation, these administrative provisions would not be a sufficient basis for entering into a tax treaty.

38 For a review of the comments submitted to the OECD, see Amanda Athanasiou, 'Stakeholders Weigh In on OECD's Treaty Abuse Discussion Draft', Tax Analysts, 2014 *WTD* 73-1 (16 April 2014).

39 See comments made by Deloitte Tax LLP, reported in Tax Analysts, 2014 *WTD*, 71-22 (9 April 2014). Also see comments made by the National Foreign Trade Council, reported in Tax Analysts, 2014 *WTD* 71-25 (9 April 2014).

40 See comments from the Organisation for International Investment (OFII) reported in Tax Analysts, 2014 *WTD* 71-26 (9 April 2014).

41 See Amanda Athanasiou, 'Doubling Down on Treaty Shopping', 2014 *WTD* 72–3 (15 April 2014).

42 See suggested para 4 of Article X.

was urged to develop guidance on this point.[43] Furthermore, in order to address possible abuse and undue pressure on tax authorities, the BEPS Monitoring Group recommended that 'tax authorities publish a yearly overview of all persons/entities involved in transactions qualifying under this article (not necessarily the items of income or amounts).[44] Most of these concerns were met in the Treaty Abuse Follow-Up Report in November 2014.

Some criticised the proposal to broaden the purpose of treaties by the inclusion of various references to the prevention of tax avoidance and evasion in the title of treaties, as well as the addition of references to the tax policy considerations of Contracting States. Some States might be encouraged to the view that 'even after the application of the various anti-avoidance tests there remains a further residual anti-abuse principle based on this new wording'.[45] At a more general level, it was thought that the Treaty Abuse Discussion Draft went too far and had the potential of eroding international trade and investment, and interfering with the proper functioning of tax treaties.[46] It was suggested that the uncertainty of some of the proposed rules could be mitigated by provisions allowing proper administrative processes and procedures—not just administrative clarity.[47] Albeit more radically, the BEPS Monitoring Group criticised the Treaty Abuse Discussion Draft for the absence of a domestic anti-avoidance rule that would allow source-country tax authorities to disallow treaty benefits unilaterally, quickly and at low cost.[48]

Others have not been so critical of the OECD's proposals. For example, Michael Lang has argued that these proposals reflect current trends, especially within

[43] Amanda Athanasiou, 'Stakeholders Weigh In on OECD's Treaty Abuse Discussion Draft', n 38 above. Also see comments made by David Rosenbloom, reported by David D Stewart and Kristen A Parillo, 'OECD's LOB Approach Needs Refinement, Practitioners Say' (2014) 74 *Tax Notes International* 111 (14 April 2014). Also see Kristen A Parillo and Lee A Sheppard, 'OECD Panel Explores BEPS Treaty Abuse', 2014 *WTD* 106-3 (3 June 2014). The US dislike of a 'main purpose' test was also evident from the US Senate's refusal to approve the ratification of negotiated treaties that contained such a test, making the ratification conditional on the deletion of the main purpose test. See Michael Lang, 'BEPS Action 6: Introducing an Antiabuse Rule in Tax Treaties' (2014) 74 *Tax Notes International* 655, 664, 19 May 2014. Citing Kristen A Parillo, 'Italy-US Tax Treaty Enters Into Force', 2009 *WTD*, 241-2 (18 December 2009).

[44] See BEPS Monitoring Group, *Preventing the Granting of Treaty Benefits in Inappropriate Circumstances*. Available on: bepsmonitoringgroup.files.wordpress.com/2014/04/bmg-treaty-abuse-submission.pdf, pp 3–4. The BEPS Monitoring Group also commented that because the wording of the whole LOB provision is complex and difficult to understand, it should be simplified as much as is possible, 'and in any case properly explained in the Commentary; for example, explanations should be given, with examples, of what constitutes "active conduct of trade or business" and "income derived from … that trade or business", particularly to clarify that it does not cover income from unrelated business': *ibid*, p 3.

[45] See PwC, 'OECD releases discussion draft on the use of treaty benefits in inappropriate circumstances', p 4 (17 March 2014). Available on: www.pwc.com/en_US/us/tax-services/publications/insights/assets/pwc-oecd-releases-discussion-draft-use-treaty-benefits.pdf.

[46] See PwC's comments on Action 6, reported in Tax Analysts, 2014 *WTD* 7-23 (11 April 2014) and Ernst & Young's comments, reported in Tax Analysts 2014 *WTD* 71-24 (11 April 2014).

[47] Amanda Athanasiou, 'Stakeholders Weigh In on OECD's Treaty Abuse Discussion Draft', n 38 above. Also see comments of BEPS Monitoring Group, n 44 above, p 6.

[48] BEPS Monitoring Group, n 44 above, p 6.

the European Union, where many countries have recently introduced general anti-avoidance rules.[49] In fact, as explained in Chapter five, in its Action Plan to Strengthen the Fight against Tax Fraud and Tax Evasion, the European Commission has explicitly recommended the adoption of GAARs by Member States. Such clauses also feature in draft directives which have been recently proposed, such as the Common Consolidated Corporate Tax Base proposal[50] and the Financial Transaction Tax proposal[51] as well as in amendments of existing directives such as that of the Parent-Subsidiary Directive.[52] As Lang notes, not only do these proposals vary in detail but in fact little international consensus exists on how these rules must be designed and whether they are useful at all.[53] He argues that the criticism contained in the statements submitted to the OECD is directed against the design of the rule, unilaterally geared towards the interests of tax administrations, but not against such a rule altogether.[54]

The Treaty Abuse Revised Discussion Draft,[55] published in September 2014, offered a more nuanced approach to treaty abuse. It was recognised that countries have developed different tax treaty policies to reflect their constitutional or other legal capabilities and administrative capacities.[56] Because of this, a number of alternatives were set out aimed at reaching a common goal that was 'to ensure that States incorporate in their treaties sufficient safeguards to prevent treaty abuse, in particular as regards treaty shopping'.[57] For that reason, the Treaty Abuse Revised Discussion Draft recommended a minimum level of protection that should be implemented. The need for further refinements in the objective tests was recognised, particularly in view of constitutional or EU law restrictions that prevent some states from adopting the exact wording of the model provisions recommended in the discussion draft.[58] Overall, the model provisions and related Commentary suggested were to be considered as drafts subject to improvement before their final versions were released in September 2015.

A distinction was made between two types of cases: where a person tries to circumvent limitations provided by the treaty itself; and where a person tries to circumvent the provisions of domestic tax law using treaty benefits.

[49] Michael Lang, 'BEPS Action 6: Introducing an Antiabuse Rule in Tax Treaties', n 43 above, p 655.

[50] Proposal for a Council Directive on a Common Consolidated Corporate Tax Base (CCCTB) COM(2011) 121/4, at 48. For further analysis, see Christiana HJI Panayi, *European Union Corporate Tax Law* (Cambridge University Press, 2013), ch 3.

[51] Proposal for a Council Directive implementing enhanced cooperation in the area of financial transaction tax COM(2013) 71, at 30. See Ch 8 of this volume.

[52] See section 5.3.2 in Ch 5 of this volume.

[53] Michael Lang, 'BEPS Action 6: Introducing an Antiabuse Rule in Tax Treaties', n 43 above, p 656.

[54] *Ibid*, p 663.

[55] OECD/G20 Base Erosion and Profit Shifting Project, *Preventing the Granting of Treaty Benefits in Inappropriate Circumstances—Action 6: 2014 Deliverable* (OECD). For commentary, see Kristen A Parillo, 'BEPS Action 6 (Treaty Abuse): US Gets Its Way', 2014 *WTD* 180-3 (17 September 2014).

[56] Treaty Abuse Revised Discussion Draft, n 55 above, para 6.

[57] *Ibid.*

[58] See Executive Summary, p 11 and para 13, *ibid*. For an analysis of the compatibility of the proposals, see Ch 6, section 6.6 of this volume.

The Treaty Abuse Revised Discussion Draft recommended a three-step approach to be used to address treaty shopping arrangements, as a minimum standard of protection through a flexible approach. First, similarly to the Discussion Draft it was recommended that treaties include in their title and preamble a clear statement of a common intention that the Contracting States, when entering into a treaty, intend to avoid creating opportunities for non-taxation or reduced taxation through tax evasion or avoidance, including through treaty shopping arrangements. Secondly, again similarly to the Discussion Draft, it was recommended to include in tax treaties a specific anti-abuse rule based on the US LOB provisions. Thirdly, to address other forms of treaty abuse not covered by the LOB, it was recommended to add to tax treaties a more general anti-abuse rule based on the principal purposes of transactions or arrangements (principal purposes test or PPT rule).[59] Effectively, the following variations were suggested; first, LOB plus PPT; or, secondly, PPT alone; or, thirdly, LOB plus a restricted PPT rule applicable to conduit financing arrangements, or domestic anti-abuse rules or judicial doctrines that would achieve a similar result.

The 'new' PPT is in fact identical to the previous main purpose test of the Treaty Abuse Discussion Draft, other than the obvious substitution of 'main purposes' with 'principal purposes'.[60] It was argued that the PPT rule incorporated principles already recognised in the Commentary on Article 1 of the OECD Model.[61] The PPT rule was accompanied by Commentary and examples that illustrated the application of the rule.[62]

It was recognised that the combination of the proposed LOB and PPT rules had strengths and weaknesses and might not be appropriate for all countries.[63] For instance, the LOB tests were based on objective criteria that provided more certainty than the PPT, which required a case-by-case analysis based on what could reasonably be considered to be one of the principal purposes of transactions or arrangements. It was also stipulated that these rules may require adaptations, for example, to take account of constitutional or EU law restrictions.[64]

In addition, the revised LOB included a 'derivative benefits' provision that allowed certain entities owned by residents of other Contracting States to obtain

[59] See paras 11–16 of Treaty Abuse Revised Discussion Draft, n 55 above. For commentary, see Luc De Broe and Joris Luts, 'BEPS Action 6: Tax Treaty Abuse' (2015) 43 *Intertax* 122–46; Jack Bernstein, 'BEPS Action 6—Trying to Curtail Treaty Shopping' (2014) 76 *Tax Notes International* 1035 (15 Dec 2014).

[60] The PPT reads as follows: 'Notwithstanding the other provisions of this Convention, a benefit under this Convention shall not be granted in respect of an item of income or capital if it is reasonable to conclude, having regard to all relevant facts and circumstances, that obtaining that benefit was one of the principal purposes of any arrangement or transaction that resulted directly or indirectly in that benefit, unless it is established that granting that benefit in these circumstances would be in accordance with the object and purpose of the relevant provisions of this Convention'. See Executive Summary, p 12. Also see Luc de Broe and Joris Luts, n 59 above, pp 131–34.

[61] Treaty Abuse Revised Discussion Draft, n 55 above, p 12. Also see para 17.

[62] *Ibid*, pp 66–74.

[63] See para 12.

[64] *Ibid*, para 13.

treaty benefits that these residents would have obtained if they had invested directly.[65] Furthermore, following stakeholder comments, a one-year minimum shareholding period for reduced withholding taxes was adopted.

Overall, the Treaty Abuse Revised Discussion Draft watered down the anti-treaty shopping proposals of the initial discussion draft, making them more flexible. It gave countries a choice between the PPT and the LOB rule, supplemented by a domestic anti-abuse rule. The Treaty Abuse Revised Discussion Draft recommended the inclusion of both the LOB rule and the general anti-abuse rule. Neither the US Treasury nor businesses wanted the open-ended treaty abuse clauses suggested in the previous Treaty Abuse Discussion Draft,[66] so this was considered a significant improvement.

The Treaty Abuse Revised Discussion Draft also included recommendations to deal with a number of other situations such as the splitting up of contracts,[67] the hiring out of labour cases,[68] transactions intended to avoid dividend characterisation,[69] certain dividend transfer situations (usufruct and similar transactions),[70] transactions designed to circumvent the application of Article 13(4) of the OECD Model,[71] the tie-breaker rule for determining the treaty residence of dual-resident persons other than individuals;[72] and anti-abuse rules for PEs situated in third states.[73] Further work was needed with respect to the precise contents of the provisions and the implementation of the minimum standard, as well as with respect to the policy considerations relevant to treaty entitlement of collective investment vehicles (CIVs) and non-CIV funds.[74]

The Treaty Abuse Revised Discussion Draft also addressed cases where persons try to abuse domestic tax law using treaty benefits, such as through thin capitalisation, dual residence strategies, transfer pricing, arbitrage transactions and transactions that abuse double tax relief mechanisms. It was recognised that tax treaty anti-abuse rules were not sufficient to address these strategies. These must be addressed through domestic rules, also in light of the other Action items. 'The main objective … is to ensure that treaties do not prevent the application of specific domestic law provisions that would prevent these transactions'.[75] Additional guidance to the OECD Commentary was suggested to clarify that the incorporation of

[65] See para 4 of the LOB clause, set out in para 16 of the Treaty Abuse Revised Discussion Draft.

[66] Kristen A Parillo, 'BEPS Action 6 (Treaty Abuse): US Gets Its Way', Tax Analysts, 2014 *WTD* 180-3 (17 September 2014).

[67] Treaty Abuse Revised Discussion Draft, n 55 above, paras 20–21.

[68] *Ibid*, para 22.

[69] *Ibid*, paras 23–24.

[70] *Ibid*, paras 25–31.

[71] *Ibid*, paras 32–35.

[72] *Ibid*, paras 36–39.

[73] *Ibid*, paras 40–43.

[74] The proposed LOB rule includes a place-holder allowing for the Contracting States to negotiate a provision specific to resident CIVs and non-CIV funds.

[75] See para 45 and the examples given of when this might occur.

the PPT principle would not affect domestic anti-abuse rules and the interaction between treaties and domestic anti-abuse rules.[76] Similarly to the initial discussion draft, the Treaty Abuse Revised Discussion Draft recommended adding a US-style 'savings clause' to the OECD Model.[77]

There was also reference to departure or exit taxes. The Treaty Abuse Revised Discussion Draft clarified that tax treaties do not prevent such taxes, '[t]o the extent that the liability to such a tax arises when a person is still a resident of the State that applies the tax and does not extend to income accruing after the cessation of residence'.[78] However, the application of these taxes could lead to double taxation. A possible approach to resolving this would be for the competent authorities of the two states involved to agree, through the mutual agreement procedure, that each state should provide relief as regards the residence-based tax that was levied by the other state on the part of the income that accrued while the person was a resident of that other state, except to the extent that the new state of residence would have had source taxation rights at the time that income was taxed.[79]

In addressing the second part of this Action item's mandate—ie that it must be clarified that tax treaties are not intended to be used to generate double non-taxation—the Treaty Abuse Revised Discussion Draft sets out the same recommendations as in the Treaty Abuse Discussion Draft. In addressing the third part of the mandate—ie to identify the tax policy considerations that, in general, countries should consider before deciding to enter into a tax treaty with another country—again, the same recommendations were made as in the previous discussion draft.

On 21 November 2014, the OECD released its follow-up report on Action 6.[80] Issues to be addressed included the LOB and the PPT test, treaty entitlement of collective investment vehicles and non-CIVs and other technical issues. Inter alia, suggestions were sought on the guidance that could be included in the Commentary on the discretionary relief provision of the LOB, on the derivative benefits clause, as well as alternative LOB provisions that might be needed to accommodate EU Member States.

As criticised, in the Treaty Abuse Follow-Up Discussion Draft, there was essentially no new guidance on the important issues that remain to be resolved. Rather the discussion draft was simply a solicitation of comments on the various open issues.[81] As far as the discretionary relief provision of the LOB or the PPT tests was concerned, it was recommended that it be restricted and/or applied with

[76] *Ibid*, para 49, with the suggested commentary.

[77] *Ibid*, paras 51–53.

[78] *Ibid*, para 55.

[79] *Ibid*, para 57.

[80] OECD, *Follow Up Work on BEPS Action 6: Preventing Treaty Abuse*. For commentary, see Luc De Broe and Joris Luts, 'BEPS Action 6: Tax Treaty Abuse' (2015) 43 *Intertax* 122–46.

[81] See ICC comments, available on: www.iccwbo.org/Advocacy-Codes-and-Rules/Document-centre/2015/ICC-comments-on-the-OECD-Discussion-Draft-Follow-up-Work-on-BEPS-Action-6-Preventing-Treaty-Abuse-%282015%29-21474824286/.

maximum transparency.[82] The exercise of discretionary relief could also have state aid repercussions.[83]

The BEPS Monitoring Group has criticised the Treaty Abuse Revised Discussion Draft,[84] as well as the follow-up report.[85] Although there were advantages and disadvantages to both proposed measures (LOB and PPT), the Group argued that the failure to agree on a single effective measure was problematic. The targeted LOB provision was detailed and complex but offered possibilities for circumvention, while the PPT was more flexible but also more discretionary and as such likely to be arbitrary and potentially more prone to abuse. The BEPS Monitoring Group argued that a 'belt and braces' approach seems the only solution, combined with a minimum standard as proposed. OECD and G20 countries were urged to comply with their commitment to adopt suitable provisions promptly, and complement these with spontaneous exchange of information by the state of residence. Closer coordination with developing countries was essential.[86]

The BEPS Monitoring Group also claimed that the suggested statement in the preamble was too weak, as such statements were rarely used to counter what may seem to be a rational literal interpretation of a substantive treaty provision. Tax treaties should begin with an article which clearly states that their purpose is to ensure that persons and companies are taxed where their economic activities take place and value is created. One or more suitable anti-abuse clauses can be helpful, but, as argued, it was unrealistic to expect them to carry too much weight, especially if the substantive provisions were ineffective.

In its submission on the Treaty Abuse Follow-Up Report, the BEPS Monitoring Group emphasised, inter alia, that effective implementation was crucial to put pressure on key states with extensive treaty networks to accept inclusion of anti-abuse provisions in their treaties. Some countries were used as global treaty-shopping platforms. If these countries did not cooperate to implement Action 6, it would be severely undermined. Treaty abuse could only be effectively addressed if all relevant countries cooperated. A political commitment through the G20 was necessary.

A report by KPMG Ireland raised another important general concern from the perspective of small countries. The proposals under Action 6 appear to be heavily biased against small countries and will potentially damage legitimate economic

[82] See BEPS Monitoring Group, *Follow-Up Work On BEPS Action 6: Preventing Treaty Abuse*, available on: bepsmonitoringgroup.files.wordpress.com/2015/01/bmg-ap-6-submission-treaty-abuse-2015.pdf.

[83] See analysis in Chs 6 and 7 of this volume.

[84] BEPS Monitoring Group, *OECD BEPS Scorecard*, pp 9–10. Available on: bepsmonitoringgroup.files.wordpress.com/2014/10/oecd-beps-scorecard.pdf.

[85] BEPS Monitoring Group, *Follow-Up Work On BEPS Action 6: Preventing Treaty Abuse*, n 82 above.

[86] It was suggested that if a non-G20 developing country had a strong preference for a specific provision, this choice should be decisive in determining the type of provision in its treaties with OECD and G20 partners. Expecting developing countries to have to apply a range of different anti-abuse measures would unnecessarily strain their administrative capacity.

activity in those countries.[87] To an extent, the Action 6 proposals are partly aimed at denying treaty benefits where one of the main purposes of being located in a particular country is access to tax treaties. 'Clearly, there will always be stronger non tax commercial reasons for locating in a large economy with a large domestic market'.[88] It could lead to circumstances where treaty access may be denied to businesses operating in small countries without causing any similar difficulties for businesses operating in large countries.[89]

At the public consultation in Paris on 22 January 2015, several representatives of US MNEs had argued that the working group should refrain from resolving the complex issues that drafting the text of a model LOB would require and simply provide a general statement of principles on how an LOB could satisfy the OECD's minimum standard.[90] This suggestion was followed-up in the latest OECD revised discussion draft (the Treaty Abuse Second Revised Discussion Draft)[91] published on 22 May 2015.

In the Treaty Abuse Second Revised Discussion Draft, there was a new proposal for an alternative simplified LOB rule that would be supplemented by guidance in the model Commentary, instead of a fully drafted provision. Several other proposals were made, including new proposals for treaty rules intended to address concerns related to special tax regimes and to changes to domestic law made after the conclusion of a treaty.

It was agreed that this approach was consistent with the minimum standard described in the Treaty Abuse Revised Discussion Draft, which may be satisfied by the inclusion of any form of LOB combined with the PPT. The original LOB was considered more appropriate for countries that would prefer to meet the minimum standard through the combination of an LOB rule and a mechanism dealing with conduit arrangements. It was important to ensure that the non-application of the simplified LOB in a given case should not be interpreted in any way as suggesting that the PPT would not be applicable to that case either. In incorporating the simplified LOB into the OECD Model, this could be done by describing the main features of the LOB in the Model and presenting the alternative formulations

[87] See KPMG Ireland report, December 2014, *Action 6: Preventing the Granting of Treaty Benefits in Inappropriate Circumstances, Fairness for Small Countries.* Reported in Tax Analysts, 2014 *WTD* 238-20 (10 December 2014).

[88] *Ibid*, p 2.

[89] *Ibid.* A suggestion made in this report is that for the purposes of the LOB active business test, business support activities should suffice even where those activities are provided for the benefit of related group parties and where there are no or limited sales of the relevant group products/services in the small country concerned. It was also suggested that if there is a dispute on the interpretation or application of a tax treaty, there should be a right of appeal to an independent international tribunal staffed by respected, qualified and independent jurists. See pp 7–8. Also see analysis in Ch 6, section 6.6 of this volume.

[90] Kristen A Parillo, 'OECD Proposes "Skeletal" LOB Article in Treaty Abuse Draft', 2015 *WTD* 100-4 (26 May 2015).

[91] OECD, *Revised Discussion Draft—BEPS Action 6: Prevent Treaty Abuse* (henceforth, Treaty Abuse Second Revised Discussion Draft) available on: www.oecd.org/tax/treaties/revised-discussion-draft-beps-action-6-prevent-treaty-abuse.pdf.

of each paragraph in the Commentary.[92] As stated in a footnote to the proposed LOB,[93] the drafting of such an article in bilateral treaties would depend on countries' preferences for implementing the minimum standard.[94]

The rest of the discussion draft outlined proposals to address the particular LOB and PPT issues identified in the follow-up report, such as the application of the LOB and treaty entitlement to collective investment vehicles or other funds.[95]

Further commentary on the discretionary relief provision of the LOB rule was also provided. More guidance was given regarding the factors that should be taken into account by a competent authority considering a request for discretionary relief.[96] In the amended Commentary,[97] there is, inter alia, a stipulation that the availability of clear non-tax business reasons should also be taken into account by the competent authority of the state from which benefits are sought. Also treaty benefits may be extended where the allowance of benefits would not otherwise be contrary to the purposes of the Convention. It was also added that in the case of a resident subsidiary company with a parent in a third state,

> whilst the fact that the relevant withholding rate provided in the Convention is not lower than the corresponding withholding rate in the tax treaty between the State of source and the third State would be a relevant factor, that fact would not, in itself, be sufficient to establish that the conditions for granting the discretionary relief are met.[98]

There is emphasis on substantial relationship with the state. The competent authority that receives a request for relief should process that request expeditiously.

As far as the LOB rule was concerned, it was noted that it may need to be adapted to reflect certain EU law requirements. The author has argued[99] that in the current state of the case law, a derivative benefits test is not required for EU law purposes. The comment was (anonymously) acknowledged in the Treaty Abuse Second Revised Discussion Draft but in any case, proposals were made to amend the Commentary to address specific EU issues related to the publicly-listed entity and pension fund exceptions of the LOB rule.[100]

[92] The Annex in p 42 et seq included an example illustrating how that approach would work in the case of the publicly-listed entity provision.

[93] See Annex, p 42.

[94] As noted, countries would have three options. 'This could be done either through the adoption of paragraph 7 only, through the adoption of the detailed version of paragraphs 1 to 6 that is described in the Commentary on Article [X] together with the implementation of an anti-conduit mechanism as described in paragraph [x] of that Commentary, or through the adoption of paragraph 7 together with any variation of paragraphs 1 to 6 described in the Commentary on Article [X]'. Treaty Abuse Second Revised Discussion Draft, n 91 above.

[95] *Ibid*, pp 7–10.

[96] *Ibid*, para 31.

[97] *Ibid*, para 32 on proposed changes to para 63.

[98] *Ibid*.

[99] See Ch 6, section 6.6 of this volume. Also see ch 5 in Christiana HJI Panayi, *Double Taxation, Tax Treaties, Treaty Shopping and the European Community* (Kluwer, 2007).

[100] Treaty Abuse Second Revised Discussion Draft, n 91 above, paras 36–40.

Following the previous discussion drafts, the OECD had been asked to ensure that the inclusion of a derivative benefits provision would not raise BEPS concerns and that it would contribute to the work on other parts of the Action Plan. During the discussion of issues, the US delegate made two proposals that would deal with special tax regimes and would make a tax treaty responsive to certain future changes in a country's domestic tax laws. It was argued that these proposals could address some of the objections to the addition of a derivative benefits provision in the LOB rule. These proposals have been incorporated in the Treaty Abuse Second Revised Discussion Draft for the first time.[101] Recommendations were also made regarding 'dual-listed company arrangements', timing issues related to the various provisions of the LOB rule and the 'active business' provision, the latter again influenced by a previous proposal of the US delegate.[102]

The second part to this discussion draft dealt with issues related to the PPT rule. It dealt with issues such as how the PPT rule applies where benefits are obtained under different treaties;[103] the suggestion in the Commentary that countries should consider establishing some form of administrative process ensuring that the PPT is only applied after approval at a senior level;[104] the possibility of discretionary relief provisions;[105] the drafting of the alternative 'conduit-PPT rule'[106] etc. Four more examples were added in the Commentary on the PPT rule.[107]

The remainder of this discussion draft focused on miscellaneous issues. For example, it was suggested that in the Commentary on the new tie-breaker provision, it should be clarified that the fact that a dual-resident entity would not be entitled to treaty reliefs under the new provision will not prevent the person from being considered a resident of each Contracting State for the purposes of the provisions of the Convention that do not provide reliefs to that entity. It was also agreed that the competent authorities should be encouraged to address as quickly as possible requests made under the new provision.[108]

There were also proposals relating to the design and drafting of the rule applicable to PEs located in third states.[109] As regards the previously proposed Commentary on the interaction between tax treaties and domestic anti-abuse rules, this was to be further discussed due to the potential for domestic law anti-abuse provisions to override tax treaties.

[101] *Ibid*, para 53 containing proposal 1 regarding new treaty provisions on 'special tax regimes' and proposal 2 regarding a new general treaty rule intended to make a tax treaty responsive to certain future changes in a country's domestic tax laws.

[102] The proposal was to change paragraph 3 of the LOB rule in order to prevent a resident from aggregating activities of a connected person enjoying a special tax regime and in order to provide that the resident and any connected persons must be in the same or a similar line of business before their activities may be aggregated: *ibid*, para 72.

[103] *Ibid*, paras 73–75.

[104] *Ibid*, paras 76–79.

[105] *Ibid*, paras 87–90.

[106] *Ibid*, paras 91–95.

[107] *Ibid*, paras 96–98.

[108] *Ibid*, paras 99–102.

[109] *Ibid*, paras 103–107.

The final report on Action 6 is likely to be produced after a June 2015 meeting with the working group.

3.2. Action 7: Prevent the Artificial Avoidance of PE Status

As regards the action on preventing the artificial avoidance of PE status, the Action Plan set out the following:

> Develop changes to the definition of PE to prevent the artificial avoidance of PE status in relation to BEPS, including through the use of commissionaire arrangements and the specific activity exemptions. Work on these issues will also address related profit attribution issues.[110]

On 31 October 2014, the OECD released its first discussion draft on the topic (the PE Discussion Draft)[111] with the preliminary results of the work carried on by the Focus Group on the Artificial Avoidance of PE Status. There were no major surprises in this discussion draft and some of the proposals/discussions were foreshadowed in the discussions over Action 1.[112] Proposals for changes to the PE definition in the OECD Model were suggested in order to prevent abuse of the PE threshold through commissionaire arrangements and the specific activity exemptions.[113] Some of the suggestions have the potential to significantly widen the definition of PE, as well as leave room for uncertainty and potentially conflicting tax claims.

As far as commissionaire arrangements were concerned, changes to paragraphs 5 and/or 6 of Article 5 were suggested to address the problem. A commissionaire arrangement was loosely defined as an arrangement though which a person sells products in a given state in its own name but on behalf of a foreign enterprise that is the owner of these products.[114]

> As a matter of policy, where the activities that an intermediary exercises in a country are intended to result in the regular conclusion of contracts to be performed by a foreign enterprise, that enterprise should be considered to have a sufficient taxable nexus in that country unless the intermediary is performing these activities in the course of an independent business.[115]

[110] Action Plan, pp 19–20.

[111] Public Discussion Draft, *BEPS Action 7: Preventing Artificial Avoidance of PE Status* (OECD, 2014). Available on: www.oecd.org/tax/treaties/action-7-pe-status-public-discussion-draft.pdf.

[112] See analysis in Ch 2, section 2.3 of this volume.

[113] For an excellent review, see Arthur Pleijsier, 'The Agency Permanent Establishment in BEPS Action 7: Treaty Abuse or Business Abuse?' (2015) 43 *Intertax* 147–54.

[114] PE Discussion Draft, n 111 above, para 6, p 10.

[115] *Ibid*, para 10, p 11.

Otherwise, there would be a shift of profits out of the country where the sales take place without a substantive change in the functions performed in that country.

Four alternative options were set out in the PE Discussion Draft.[116] Although the alternative options had some variations in the wording of suggested paragraphs 5 and 6, they also had some common elements. For example, all alternatives would have the effect of finding a PE when the commissionaire or other agent had substantial input in contract negotiation so that ratification by the principal would be a certainty. Furthermore, all options would clarify that a person cannot be an independent agent when it acts exclusively or almost exclusively on behalf of one enterprise or associated enterprises.[117]

As regards amending the specific activity exemption of the PE provision, this was anticipated following the OECD's earlier reports in addressing the tax challenges of the digital economy. There were concerns because under Article 5(4) of the OECD Model, a PE was deemed not to exist where a place of business was used solely for activities listed in that paragraph. It was proposed to modify this provision to make it clear that all the activities listed therein are subject to the condition that the activity be preparatory or auxiliary.[118] Alternatively, more targeted changes were suggested, such as deleting the word 'delivery' in subparagraphs (a) and (b) of paragraph 4 so that the use of facilities for delivery and the maintenance of merchandise for delivery would not fall under the exceptions.[119] Another proposal made was as regards the exception for purchasing goods or merchandise or collecting information, in paragraph 4 of Article 5. Here, it was suggested either to delete the exception for purchasing or to delete paragraph 4 altogether.[120]

[116] The options which are set out in pages 11–14 are the following:

'Option A: Add a reference to contracts for the provision of property or services by the enterprise; replace "conclude contracts" by "engages with specific persons in a way that results in the conclusion of contracts"; strengthen the requirement of "independence".

Option B: Add a reference to contracts for the provision of property or services by the enterprise; replace "conclude contracts" by "concludes contracts, or negotiates the material elements of contracts"; strengthen the requirement of "independence".

Option C: Replace "contracts in the name of the enterprise" by "contracts which, by virtue of the legal relationship between that person and the enterprise, are on the account and risk of the enterprise"; replace "conclude contracts" by "engages with specific persons in a way that results in the conclusion of contracts"; strengthen the requirement of "independence".

Option D: Replace the phrase "contracts in the name of the enterprise" by "contracts which, by virtue of the legal relationship between that person and the enterprise, are on the account and risk of the enterprise"; replace "conclude contracts" by "concludes contracts, or negotiates the material elements of contracts"; strengthen the requirement of "independence"'.

[117] See Kristen A Parillo and Lee A Sheppard, 'OECD lays out option on preventing artificial avoidance of PE status', 2014 *WTD* 212-1 (3 November 2014).

[118] Option E was to amend Article 5(4) so that all its subparagraphs were subject to a 'preparatory or auxiliary' condition. See suggested wording in pp 15–16, para 15.

[119] See Option F and paras 16–20. It is notable that the word 'delivery' is absent from the corresponding provisions of the United Nations Model Double Taxation Convention between Developed and Developing Countries. Although this suggestion was originally focused on electronic trading, it could have much wider application.

[120] PE Discussion Draft, n 111 above, paras 21–28 and Options G and H.

The PE Discussion Draft also attempted to address concerns on the application of paragraph 4 where activities were fragmented between related parties.[121] It was noted that the OECD Model Commentary already addressed this point by clarifying that a (single) enterprise 'cannot fragment a cohesive operating business into several small operations in order to argue that each is merely engaged in preparatory or auxiliary activity'.[122] The PE Discussion Draft sought to go beyond this, given the ease with which subsidiaries may be established.[123] A rule was suggested to take account not only of the activities carried on by the same enterprise at different places but also of activities carried on by associated enterprises at different places or at the same place. Two alternative versions of this rule were suggested.[124]

In order to address the splitting up of contracts to circumvent the restrictions imposed by paragraph 3, it was suggested that there should be an automatic rule to take account of any activities performed by associated enterprises or that this could be caught under the general anti-abuse rule (the principal purpose test) proposed as a result of the work undertaken on Action 6.[125]

Overall, BEPS concerns around the PE rules could not be addressed successfully without coordination between the work on PE status and the work on other aspects of the Action Plan, especially Actions 4, 8 and 9.[126] The question of attribution of profits was a key consideration in determining which changes should be made to the definition of PE. Certainly a potential expansion of the definition of PE would have an impact on the application of the authorised OECD approach. This may prove to be challenging, especially when there is fragmentation of activities and/or splitting up of contracts.[127]

The PE Discussion Draft did not propose changes to the OECD Model Commentary. It is uncertain whether the Commentary would be refined in a future model update or whether the changes are to be introduced through the multilateral instrument proposed under Action 15.

[121] *Ibid*, p 19 and paras 29–31.

[122] See para 27.1 OECD Model Commentary.

[123] PE Discussion Draft, n 111 above, para 31, p 19.

[124] Under Option I, the anti-fragmentation rule would be extended to cases where complementary business activities were carried on by associated enterprises, at the same location, or by the same enterprise or by associated enterprises at different locations. For the rule to apply, a group of associated enterprises must have at least one fixed place of business that satisfied the PE threshold and the activities concerned must be complementary functions that were part of a cohesive business operation. Option J was similar except that it would apply where none of the places to which it referred constituted a PE but the combination of the activities at the same place or at different places went beyond what was preparatory or auxiliary. PE Discussion Draft, n 111 above, pp 20–21.

[125] *Ibid*, Options K and L in paras 32–34.

[126] *Ibid*, paras 43–45. The same point was made in the example of insurance activities used to artificially avoid the PE status. The PE Discussion Draft proposed two alternative approaches to deal with BEPS concerns. However, it was emphasised that insurance and re-insurance raised difficult issues as regards the question of where profits that represent the remuneration of risk should be taxed. The work had to be coordinated with the work in Actions 4 and 9 of the Action Plan: *ibid*, paras 35–42.

[127] Parillo and Sheppard (2014), n 117 above.

The PE Discussion Draft and its options have been widely criticised for their subjectivity and for creating additional sources of controversy.[128] For example, it would be difficult to reconcile the continued exemption for storage with the removal of the exemption for delivery. If the option to remove the exemption for the delivery of goods is adopted, the OECD Model Commentary will need to make clear when storage/display ends and when delivery (which would create a PE) starts, in order to bring certainty.[129] It was also argued that it was unreasonable to conclude that delivery in a jurisdiction connotes a substantial economic activity, such as manufacturing.[130] Similar arguments were made as regards the suggested changes to Article 5(6) of the OECD Model. In fact, it has been reported that the United States might take the unprecedented step of entering a reservation on the change to Article 5(6), something it has never done in the past.[131]

As regards the anti-fragmentation options, it is thought that these may lead to a material increase in uncertainty and subjectivity. How would a 'cohesive operating business' be interpreted and would these options enable source countries to pierce or ignore the separate legal personality of substantive legal entities? It has also been argued that the splitting rules need to be qualified, to prevent the situation whereby a range of different activities within a single multinational group might be aggregated, in the absence of any abuse.[132] An overall criticism of business groups was that MNE transactions were being implicated as abusive simply because they took place among related members.[133] It appeared that the OECD had 'failed to understand and properly take into account the commercial drivers for many common cross-border structures'.[134]

The PE Discussion Draft has also been criticised for going beyond the scope of the BEPS project. It has been argued that the proposals do not seem primarily focused on addressing questions of artificial avoidance of PEs but rather just attempt to lower the PE threshold. This is an arbitrary (and inefficient) way of addressing the identified problems. Some of the changes suggested affect routine

[128] See Pleijsier (2015), n 113 above; Mindy Herzfeld, 'The Upcoming Clash over PE Rules', 2015 *WTD* 12-1 (20 January 2015). Also see proceedings at the public consultation meeting held on 22 January 2015, reported in Ajay Gupta, 'Business Groups Resist Lower PE Thresholds During OECD Consultation', 2015 *WTD* 15-2 (23 January 2015).

[129] See PwC, 'Release of BEPS Discussion Draft: Preventing the Artificial Avoidance of PE Status', dated 3 November 2014. Available on: www.oecd.org/ctp/treaties/action-7-pe-status-public-discussion-draft.pdf. Also published in Tax Analysts on 8 January 2015 (2015 *WTD* 6-17).

[130] Gupta, 'Business Groups Resist Lower PE Thresholds During OECD Consultation', n 128 above. Also see comments made by Paul Morton of the Reed Elsevier Group to the effect that, the ability to transact business across several jurisdictions via the internet, with relatively little or no local activity, could result in options E through H posing severe practical difficulties in non-abusive cases: *ibid.*

[131] See Lee Sheppard, 'Stack's BEPS update', 2015 *WTD* 75-1 (20 April 2015).

[132] See the example given in p 4 of the PwC commentary to Action 7, n 129 above, of specialist technicians visiting a site to conduct feasibility studies in advance of a local subsidiary acting as contractor. It was noted that this (referring to Option K) could be a particular challenge for an MNE group that was diversified and decentralised, as they may be unaware of all the activities of the MNE group. There was similar criticism of Option L.

[133] Herzfeld, 'The Upcoming Clash over PE Rules', n 128 above.

[134] *Ibid.*

business structures for which BEPS has not been and should not be a concern.[135] The vague changes suggested in the PE Discussion Draft are likely to lead to a substantial increase in disputes and a significant reduction in cross-border investment and economic growth.[136] As commented, 'it looks like the mission of the Focus Group [on the Artificial Avoidance of PE Status] is to prevent normal business instead of fighting treaty abuse'.[137] It was suggested that there should be a transitional period or grandfathering provision for the implementation of a new PE definition in Article 5. The transitional period should be a minimum of three years, preferably longer.[138]

Another omission is that in the PE Discussion Draft there was no significant discussion on the related PE profit attribution issues. Failure on the part of the OECD to analyse the specific profit attribution implications of each of the various options for amending the PE definition would inevitably lead to unrealistic expectations by governments as to the revenue potentially to be derived from those changes.[139] 'That will in turn lead to ill-considered decisions about whether to make those changes and ultimately to a long period of costly disputes'.[140]

It has been rightly noted that the question of attribution of profits to a PE can be just as contentious and uncertain as the preliminary question of whether a PE exists. There could be many practical difficulties. For example, many countries would readily accept an attribution of profits to a PE within their jurisdiction as a result of such an analysis, but would be reluctant to accept a share of attributed losses to the same PE under the same analysis.[141] This issue was not addressed and it was uncertain whether there would be an official update of the Authorised OECD Approach. Follow-up work on this point was promised in the Revised PE Discussion Draft, analysed below.

The BEPS Monitoring Group, although supporting the shift to source country rights, criticised the proposals for being minimalist and only dealing with a few specific types of abuse.[142] Contrary to what most commentators thought, the Group argued that the proposed rules did not go far enough in addressing fundamental problems in this area.[143] The Group advocated for a more ambitious approach to

[135] See comments from the Business and Industry Advisory Committee to the OECD, reported by Herzfeld, 'The Upcoming Clash over PE Rules', n 128 above.

[136] See TEI Comments—BEPS Action 7, dated 23 December 2014, p 18.

[137] Pleijsier (2015), n 113 above, p 149.

[138] See TEI Comments—BEPS Action 7, n 136 above, p 17.

[139] See comments of the International Alliance for Principled Taxation reported by Herzfeld, 'The Upcoming Clash over PE Rules', n 128 above.

[140] *Ibid.*

[141] See TEI Comments—BEPS Action 7, n 136 above, p 17.

[142] See BEPS Monitoring Group, *Comments on BEPS Action 7: Preventing Artificial Avoidance of PE Status*, para 2. Available on: bepsmonitoringgroup.files.wordpress.com/2015/01/bmg-ap-7-submission-pe.pdf.

[143] The Trade Union Advisory Committee to the OECD (TUAC) held similar views. See Herzfeld, 'The Upcoming Clash over PE Rules', n 128 above.

be adopted, which would entail a reconsideration of not only paragraphs 4 to 6 of Article 5 but also paragraph 7.[144] The Group suggested a revision of Article 5(7) of the OECD Model, so that a controlled entity of an integrated MNE would constitute a PE of the controlling MNE. The Group suggested the reversal of the presumption that the fact that two companies are under common control should not of itself create a taxable presence for the multinational as a whole. It also suggested that to align income from sales with expenses, greater use should be made of the profit split method in transfer pricing, or the apportionment approach which is still allowed for a PE in most treaties, especially with developing countries. Another criticism levelled against the proposals was that the current OECD Model provisions made no distinction between small businesses working through unaffiliated entities in foreign jurisdictions and a globally integrated MNE. As such, the existing rules allowed MNEs to hide behind small businesses.[145]

It has been argued that the PE Discussion Draft seems to 'reflect a reaction to the unwillingness or inability of residence countries to actually impose their tax on multinationals'.[146] While it is unlikely that it will lead to a shift to the UN Model approach as hoped by some interest groups, the proposals are certainly going to be controversial for those refusing to move away from the traditional standards and uncertain for those who wish to see true reform of the international tax system.

On 15 May 2015 the OECD published a revised discussion draft on Action 7 (henceforth, the PE Revised Discussion Draft).[147] This new discussion draft reflected the proposals that resulted from the previous discussion draft. As regards the proposed changes to the wording of paragraphs 5 and 6 of Article 5 of the OECD Model to address commissionnaire structures and similar arrangements, it was concluded that Option B was preferable.[148] There was general support for the changes proposed to the independent agent exception of Article 5(6). It was agreed, however, that the concept of 'associated enterprises' used in Article 5(6) should be replaced by a narrower concept and that Article 5(6) should not automatically exclude an unrelated agent acting exclusively for one enterprise. Additional Commentary guidance on these changes would be provided.[149] Regarding the transfer

[144] See BEPS Monitoring Group, *Comments on BEPS Action 7: Preventing Artificial Avoidance of PE Status*, n 142 above, para 5 et seq.

[145] See comments made in the public consultation by Sol Picciotto on behalf of the BEPS Monitoring Group, reported by Gupta, 'Business Groups Resist Lower PE Thresholds During OECD Consultation', n 128 above. He called for Article 5(7) of the OECD Model to be reconsidered, as per the Group's submissions. The expansion of Article 5(5) and 5(6) envisaged by all four options could then be seen as reinforcing that presumption.

[146] Parillo and Sheppard (2014), n 117 above.

[147] OECD, '*Revised Discussion Draft, BEPS Action 7: Preventing the Artificial Avoidance of PE Status, 15 May 2015—12 June 2015*'. Available on: www.oecd.org/tax/treaties/revised-discussion-draft-beps-action-7-pe-status.pdf.

[148] See options set out in n 116 above.

[149] PE Revised Discussion Draft, n 147 above, paras 9–23 and the suggested changes to paras 5–6 of Article 5 as well as the corresponding changes to the OECD Model Commentary.

of risks between related parties through low-risk distributor arrangements, Article 5(5) of the OECD Model was not to address these. Rather, these concerns would be best addressed through the work on Action 9 (Risks and Capital).

As regards changes to the specific activity exemptions in Article 5(4) of the OECD Model, it was concluded that Option E was preferable and that Article 5(4) should be modified so that each of the exceptions included in that paragraph would be restricted to activities that are otherwise of a 'preparatory or auxiliary' character. Additional Commentary guidance would be given regarding the meaning of the phrase 'preparatory or auxiliary'.[150]

As regards the anti-fragmentation rule, Option J was preferred, which would apply whenever the relevant business activities exceeded the threshold of preparatory or auxiliary, regardless of whether any of the enterprises had a PE.[151] As regards the splitting-up of contracts, it was useful to add an example in the OECD Model Commentary on the PPT rule (as proposed under Option L) which would deal appropriately with the splitting-up of contracts issue. It was also agreed that a more automatic rule based on Option K but with some changes should be included in the OECD Model Commentary as a provision to be used where countries, unable to address that issue through domestic anti-abuse rules, would not include the PPT in a treaty or would want expressly to address concerns related to the splitting-up of contracts.[152]

The PE Discussion Draft included two options (Options M and N) aimed at situations where foreign insurance companies do large-scale business in a state without having a PE in that state. In the PE Revised Discussion Draft it was noted that no specific rule was necessary and the general rules under paragraphs 5 and 6 of Article 5 should apply.[153]

As mentioned, it had been acknowledged in the initial discussion draft that, although the existing rules on Article 7 of the OECD Model would be appropriate for determining the profits of any additional PE arising under the suggested options, more guidance was needed on how these rules would apply, taking also into account the results of work in other Action items. In the PE Revised Discussion Draft, it was decided that follow-up work on the attribution of profits would be carried on after September 2015 with a view to providing the necessary guidance before the end of 2016, which is the deadline for the negotiation of the multilateral instrument that would implement the results of the work on Action 7.[154]

The remainder of this chapter reviews the deliverables on Actions 8 to 10 which deal with transfer pricing rules—a very important part of the BEPS Action Plan. Broadly, the aim of these deliverables is to develop rules to assure that transfer pricing outcomes are in line with value creation. Through Actions 8 to 10, the OECD

[150] *Ibid*, paras 24–32, with the suggested changes to the OECD Model and Commentary.
[151] *Ibid*, paras 33–41 with the suggested changes to the OECD Model and Commentary.
[152] *Ibid*, paras 42–47, with the suggested changes to the Commentary.
[153] *Ibid*, paras 48–52.
[154] *Ibid*, paras 53–37.

attempts to tackle 'high-risk' transactions. It is mainly in these areas that MNEs have been able to use contractual arrangements which facilitated base erosion and profit shifting, often leading to what has been described as 'stateless income'.[155]

3.3. Action 8: Intangibles

Action 8 reads as follows:

> Develop rules to prevent BEPS by moving intangibles among group members. This will involve: (i) adopting a broad and clearly delineated definition of intangibles; (ii) ensuring that profits associated with the transfer and use of intangibles are appropriately allocated in accordance with (rather than divorced from) value creation; (iii) developing transfer pricing rules or special measures for transfers of hard-to-value intangibles; and (iv) updating the guidance on cost contribution arrangements.

Intangibles are at the heart of the BEPS project. The topic has long been considered as one of the most challenging subjects of transfer pricing. The OECD wants to define the concept of intangibles broadly, with the aim of discouraging transfers to tax havens, while continuing to recognise self-serving contracts between multinational affiliates. The overall aim is to allocate returns to where value is created.[156] The mantra used in the BEPS project is that taxable profits (and in this specific item, taxable intangible returns) should correspond to value creation. But how is this to be done given the perceived difficulties of evaluating intangibles?[157] As noted, '[t]he identification of a correct transfer price for intangibles depends on the assumption that there is an intrinsic market value of a given intercompany transaction and this highlights one of the logical weaknesses of the transfer pricing approach'.[158]

Given the difficulties in evaluating intangibles, one can appreciate how hard it is to design rules that correctly allocate intangible related returns. One suggestion is to use proxies to risk-taking, but this would require 'rethinking current methods and perhaps accepting innovations'.[159] There have been suggestions for

[155] Edward D Kleinbard, 'Stateless Income' (2011) 11 *Florida Tax Review* 699. See discussion in Ch 1 of this volume. Also see Georg Kofler, 'The BEPS Action Plan and Transfer Pricing: The Arm's Length Standard Under Pressure?' [2013] *British Tax Review* 646.

[156] Lee A Sheppard, 'Twilight of the International Consensus: How Multinationals squandered their tax Privileges' (2014) 44 *Washington University Journal of Law & Policy* 61, 77.

[157] See Yariv Brauner, 'Value in the Eye of the Beholder: The Valuation of Intangibles for Transfer Pricing Purposes' (2008) 28 *Virginia Tax Review* 79, 161–62. In this excellent article, Brauner explains how the transfer pricing rules produce a range of acceptable prices and how such range is available only to MNEs and more so to intangible-extensive MNEs to minimise their effective taxation unrelated to other tax planning.

[158] Carlo Garbarino and Mario D'Avossa, 'The OECD Intangibles Project and the Concept of "Intangible Related Return"' (2015) 55 *European Taxation* 12–15, 12.

[159] Yariv Brauner, 'What the BEPS?' (2014) 16 *Florida Tax Review* 55, 101.

partial reform so that the arm's length principle is replaced by formulary methods in areas such as intangibles, but this has remained an academic exercise.[160] Agreement would still be needed on when the arm's length principle applies and when it does not apply—this is likely to prove difficult.

Have the BEPS deliverables in this area advanced the discussion? While BEPS negotiators are in agreement that MNEs should not be able to shift valuable intangibles to tax havens, there is still no agreement on the tools to prevent this practice, nor on the locus of value creation and which affected country could tax it.[161]

3.3.1. Transfer Pricing Aspects of Intangibles

An initial discussion draft on intangibles was produced in 2012,[162] which was considered to be too vague.[163] A revised discussion draft (henceforth, the Intangibles Revised Discussion Draft) was released on 30 July 2013,[164] shortly after the announcement of the BEPS Action Plan. Some important points arose from this draft. The Intangibles Revised Discussion Draft advocated for rules aligning taxable intangible returns with value creation, inter alia, based on the concept of important functions. Contractual relationships between related parties would continue to serve as a starting point but the location of material functions related to intangible assets was considered crucial.

The focus was on value-creating functions, rather than the bearing of risk through contractual arrangements, or the implications of legal rights on remuneration. It was stated that funding and risk-taking were integrally related—a funding party often bears the risk of loss of funds.[165] 'Nonetheless, they can and should be analysed separately because there is no standard set of risks assumed in the

[160] Partial reform is not impossible. See arguments by Reuven S Avi-Yonah and Ilan Benshalom, 'Formulary Apportionment—Myths and Prospects: Promoting Better International Tax Policies by Utilizing the Misunderstood and Under-Theorized Formulary Alternative' (2011) 3 *World Tax Journal* 371–98; Reuven S Avi-Yonah, 'Between Formulary Apportionment and the OECD Guidelines: A Proposal for Reconciliation' (2010) 2 *World Tax Journal* 4–18; Reuven S Avi-Yonah and Kimberley A Clausing, 'Reforming Corporate Taxation in a Global Economy: A Proposal to Adopt Formulary Apportionment' in *Path to Prosperity: Hamilton Project Ideas on Income Security, Education and Taxes* (Brookings Institution Press, 2008) p 319; Susan C Morse, 'Revisiting Global Formulary Apportionment' (2010) 29 *Virginia Tax Review* 593; Julie Roin, 'Can the Income Tax Be Saved? The Promises and Pitfalls of Adopting Worldwide Formulary Apportionment' (2008) 61 *Tax Law Review* 169. Also see more recent contribution by Mitchell A Kane, 'Transfer Pricing, Integration and Synergy Intangibles: A Consensus Approach to the Arm's Length Standard' (2014) 6 *World Tax Journal* 282–314.

[161] See Amanda Athanasiou and Lee Sheppard, 'OECD's Discussion Draft on Transfer Pricing Goes Beyond Arm's Length' (2015) 77 *Tax Notes International* 44 (5 January 2015).

[162] OECD, *Revision of the Special Considerations for Intangibles in Chapter VI of the OECD Transfer Pricing Guidelines and Related Provisions* (2012). Available on: www.oecd.org/tax/transfer-pricing/50526258.pdf.

[163] Martin Zetter, 'The OECD's Action Plan on Base Erosion and Profit Shifting', *Tax Journal*, Issue 1181, p 20 (9 August 2013).

[164] OECD, *Revised Discussion Draft on the Transfer Pricing Aspects of Intangibles* (30 July 2013). Available on: www.oecd.org/ctp/transfer-pricing/revised-discussion-draft-intangibles.pdf.

[165] *Ibid*, para 83.

funding of intangible development, enhancement, maintenance, or protection'.[166] Rather, the risks assumed would vary, based, for example, on contractual terms and the conduct and solvency of group members. The risks must be determined considering all the facts and circumstances of the relationship among such group members.

Rules would be developed for risk and capital allocation to match returns with activities rather than contractual arrangements. It was stated that bearing a funding risk without the assumption of any further risk and without any control over the use of the contributed funds or the conduct of the funded activity, generally would entitle the funder to a risk-adjusted rate of anticipated return on its capital invested, but not more.[167] According to the discussion draft, the key questions in each case would be the following: (i) what is the financial risk assumed by the funding entity? (ii) does it have the financial capacity to bear the risk? (iii) how and by whom is that financial risk controlled? (iv) what are the financing options realistically available to the parties? and (v) what is the anticipated arm's length compensation for assuming the financial risk in question?

As summed up later on in the Intangibles Revised Discussion Draft, the legal owner of an intangible would be entitled to all returns attributable to the intangible only if: in substance, it performed and controlled all of the important functions related to the development, enhancement, maintenance and protection of the intangibles; it controlled other functions outsourced to independent enterprises or associated enterprises and compensated those functions on an arm's length basis; it provided all assets necessary to the development, enhancement, maintenance, and protection of the intangibles; and bore and controlled all of the risks and costs related to the development, enhancement, maintenance and protection of the intangible.[168]

To the extent that one or more members of the MNE group other than the legal owner performed functions, used or contributed assets, or assumed risks or costs related to the development, enhancement, maintenance, and protection of the intangible, returns attributable to the intangible must accrue to such other members through arm's length compensation reflecting their anticipated contribution to the intangible value. This may, depending on the facts and circumstances, constitute all or a substantial part of the return attributable to the intangible.[169] The implications of this were that an intangible could generate a return much higher than a normal return on the capital invested in creating the intangible. As such, a group company other than the legal owner of the intangible, which had performed the value-creating functions, could be rewarded by a share of the return from the intangible asset, rather than a cost-plus fee.

As criticised, there may be difficulties in the application of this test. For example, when an intangible is completely designed and perfected in one country but is

166 *Ibid.*
167 *Ibid*, para 84.
168 *Ibid*, para 89.
169 *Ibid*, para 90.

solely exploited in a second country, then it may be difficult to ascertain where value is created and how the two jurisdictions should split the value creation. It may also be difficult to ascertain where value is created, when the value exists for the MNE group but is not controlled by a single member of the group.[170] The implementation of the rules has no chance of success without enhanced collaboration in assessment and enforcement.[171] Another criticism is that the OECD lumps together all intangibles despite some very significant differences between them.[172] Some of these differences may lead to different patterns of value creation. It is noteworthy that in some circumstances where it was not possible to identify reliable comparable uncontrolled transactions, it was suggested in the Intangibles Revised Discussion Draft that a transactional profit split method could be utilised to determine the arm's length conditions for a transfer of intangibles or rights to intangibles.[173] Some examples of situations were given.[174]

Very importantly, the Intangibles Revised Discussion Draft opens the door to treating transactions structured in a given way as if they were different transactions for transfer pricing purposes. It has been criticised that the Intangibles Revised Discussion Draft creates confusion and will generate uncertainty for both taxpayers and tax authorities. Apart from the widespread re-characterisation of transactions involving intangibles, it may also lead to re-characterisation for withholding tax purposes, notwithstanding the fact that the Intangibles Revised Discussion Draft is not intended to have relevance for other tax purposes.

Following the Intangibles Revised Discussion Draft, guidelines were published on this topic in a report published in September 2014 (henceforth, the Intangibles Second Revised Discussion Draft).[175] The Intangibles Second Revised Discussion Draft proposed the deletion and reinstatement of the whole of Chapter VI of the OECD Transfer Pricing Guidelines to be entitled 'Special Considerations for Intangible Property'. Parts of the new text were not finalised on the basis that they were interlinked with other material to be released in 2015. These were the guidelines on ownership of intangibles, on intangibles whose valuation was uncertain at the time of the transaction, the use of unspecified methods and the use of profit split methods.

170 KPMG, *OECD Invitation to Comment on the 'Revised Discussion Draft on Transfer Pricing Aspects of Intangibles'*.

171 Brauner (2014), n 159 above.

172 Intangibles Revised Discussion Draft, n 164 above, paras 100–101.

173 *Ibid*, para 166.

174 For example, with the sale of full rights in intangibles (para 167) or with transfers of partially developed intangibles (para 168) or where limited rights in fully developed intangibles are transferred in a licence or similar transaction, and reliable comparable uncontrolled transactions cannot be identified, a transactional profit split method could often be utilised to evaluate the respective contributions of the parties to earning combined income (para 170).

175 OECD, *Guidance on Transfer Pricing Aspects of Intangibles* (2014). Available on: www.oecd-ilibrary.org/docserver/download/2314291e.pdf?expires=1422449883&id=id&accname=guest&checksum=8E117AD9FC4D4A195249EE598C02B286. For commentary, see Jens Wittendorff, 'More Black Smoke From the OECD's Chimney—Third Draft on Intangibles' (2015) 77 *Tax Notes International* 167, 12 January 2015.

Overall, the new guidelines broadly followed the suggestions in the Intangibles Revised Discussion Draft. There was similar discussion on location savings, assembled workforce, and group synergies. There were additional examples in the annex, taking the total number of examples to 33. The guidance on intangibles included the definition of intangibles from the Intangibles Revised Discussion Draft and similar discussions on ownership of intangibles, use or transfer of intangibles and valuation issues.

Some of the stakeholders' concerns were addressed. For example, the definition of marketing intangibles was further refined,[176] as it was thought to be confusing in the previous version. Also, in a section on the ownership of intangibles and transactions involving the development, enhancement, maintenance, protection and exploitation of intangibles, a paragraph was added which explained the challenges of exploiting intangibles according to the principles of the OECD Transfer Pricing Guidelines.[177] Some of the identified challenges related to collaborative value creation; ie how a valuable intangible may be developed in an iterative process. The Intangibles Second Revised Discussion Draft failed to develop any robust theory on how to deal with these.[178]

Another issue where there was a lot of disagreement but which was eventually left unaddressed was that of location savings and location rents.[179] In the Intangibles Second Revised Discussion Draft, location savings were excluded from the definition of intangibles. It was indicated that where reliable local market

[176] *Ibid*, para 6.16, p 32. It is '[a]n intangible (within the meaning of paragraph 6.6) that relates to marketing activities, aids in the commercial exploitation of a product or service, and/or has an important promotional value for the product concerned. Depending on the context, marketing intangibles may include, for example, trademarks, trade names, customer lists, customer relationships, and proprietary market and customer data that is used or aids in marketing and selling goods or services to customers'. Cf definition in para 50 of the Intangibles Revised Discussion Draft, n 164 above.

[177] Intangibles Second Revised Discussion Draft, n 175 above, para 6.32. There may be lack of comparability of the intangible related transactions between related and independent enterprises; lack of comparability between the intangibles in question; the ownership and/or use of different intangibles by different associated enterprises within the MNE group; the difficulty of isolating the impact of any particular intangible on the MNE group's income; the fact that various members of an MNE group may perform activities relating to the development, enhancement, maintenance, protection and exploitation of an intangible; the fact that contributions of various members of the MNE group to intangible value may take place in years different than the years in which any associated returns are realised; and the fact that taxpayer structures may be based on contractual terms between associated enterprises that separate ownership, the assumption of risk, and/or funding of investments in intangibles from performance of important functions, control over risk, and decisions related to investment in ways that are not observed in transactions between independent enterprises and that may contribute to base erosion and profit shifting.

[178] See Ajay Gupta, 'BEPS Action 8 (Intangibles): Arm's Length is Still the Mantra', 2014 *WTD* 180-4 (17 September 2014).

[179] Ajay Gupta, 'Rough Road Ahead for OECD Intangibles Project', 2014 *WTD* 200-4 (16 October 2014). Also see Leonard Wagenaar, 'The Effect of the OECD Base Erosion and Profit Shifting Action Plan on Developing Countries' (2015) 69 *Bulletin for International Taxation* 84–92. For a discussion on location savings, see Pankaj Jain and Vikram Chand, 'Location Savings: International and Indian Perspective' (2015) 43 *Intertax* 192–98.

comparables were available and could be used to determine arm's length prices, specific comparability adjustments for location savings should not be required.[180] There was disagreement on this point with developing countries and especially India and China. Their argument was as follows: there were economic gains from moving existing operations to a low tax jurisdiction. The MNE's ability to capture those savings constituted an intangible asset, the gains from which should accrue at least in part to the new host country. However, OECD countries and the business community were not very keen on this concept as it would be tantamount to an entry tax and might open the gateway for other ancillary advantages to be construed as intangible assets.[181] Location savings remains a key issue for MNEs operating in low-cost jurisdictions, so the exclusion of this concept from the definition of intangibles was expected. Interestingly, an Indian tribunal has recently followed the OECD approach on location savings.[182]

There was a discussion on ex ante and ex post remuneration. The former referred to 'the future income expected to be derived by a member of the MNE group at the time of a transaction'.[183] The latter referred to 'the income actually earned by a member of the group through the exploitation of the intangible'.[184] As explained, the compensation that must be paid to members of the MNE group that contributed to the development, enhancement, maintenance, protection and exploitation of intangibles was generally determined on an ex ante basis. Such compensation may be fixed or contingent.[185] Guidance was given on how to determine the appropriate arm's length remuneration to members of a group. In applying the arm's length analysis, difficult cases were identified.[186]

It was concluded[187] that if the legal owner of an intangible in substance performed and controlled all of the functions related to the development, enhancement, maintenance, protection and exploitation of the intangible and if the legal owner provided all assets, including funding, necessary to these functions and bore

[180] See suggested para 1.83, p 14 of the Intangibles Second Revised Discussion Draft, n 175 above.

[181] See, for example, the discussion at IFA seminar entitled '*Tax Issues Relating to Intangibles*' held at the 68th annual Congress of IFA in Mumbai, where it was sarcastically suggested that good weather should also be seen as an intangible. Gupta, 'Rough Road Ahead for OECD Intangibles Project', n 179 above.

[182] See appeal before the Income-tax Appellate Tribunal in India, *Watson Pharma Pvt Ltd* (ITA No 1423/Mum/2014 and 1565/Mum/2014)). Here, the Tribunal ruled in favour of the taxpayer, rejecting the Indian tax administration's views on location savings and adopting the OECD's approach under Action 8. No adjustment was necessary on account of location savings when the arm's length price was determined on the basis of appropriate comparables.

[183] Intangibles Second Revised Discussion Draft, n 175 above, para 6.44.

[184] *Ibid.*

[185] *Ibid*, para 6.54.

[186] *Ibid*, paras 6.47–6.48. Eg where intangibles were self-developed by an MNE group, where acquired or self developed intangibles served as a platform for further development or where there were other aspects, such as marketing or manufacturing that were particularly important to value creation.

[187] *Ibid*, para 6.68.

and controlled all of the risks, then it would be entitled to all of the anticipated, ex ante, returns derived from the MNE group's exploitation of the intangible. To the extent that one or more members of the MNE group other than the legal owner performed functions, used assets, or assumed risks related to the development, enhancement, maintenance, protection, and exploitation of the intangible, such member(s) would be entitled to a share in the anticipated returns derived from the exploitation of the intangible by receiving arm's length compensation.

The entitlement of any member of the MNE group to ex post profits or losses as a result of unanticipated events[188] would depend on the terms and conditions of the relevant contracts and on the functions performed, assets used and risks assumed in connection with these events. The Intangibles Second Revised Discussion Draft introduced an analysis of unexpected ex post returns,[189] though it did not answer the question of what to do with these returns.[190] Arguably, this decision was deferred to countries.[191]

The Intangibles Second Revised Discussion Draft reiterated the section on the application of profit split methods on intangibles, when comparables could not easily be found.[192] This was among the parts of the discussion draft yet to be finalised. It has been criticised that using the terms 'transactional profit split method' is oxymoron.[193] Characterising this method as yet another transactional approach under the benign shade of the arm's length standard, 'only ends up shrouding the method in a dense mist'.[194] This was likely to generate confusion to tax administrators and taxpayers on how to apply the method in real-life cases. The fact that the OECD provided little guidance on how the method was to be applied exacerbated the problem.

It has been argued that the OECD's partial endorsement of the profit split method as an acceptable method when comparables are not sufficient suggests that the profit split method could in the future become the rule rather than the exception for transactions involving intangibles.[195] This endorsement was anticipated for a long time 'and is somewhat widely accepted as the best way for the OECD to abandon arm's length in the transfer pricing for intangibles without losing too much face'.[196] Both the Intangibles Revised Discussion Draft and the subsequent discussion draft have been criticised for the vague language used

[188] See examples given in para 6.66 in Intangibles Second Revised Discussion Draft, n 175 above.

[189] *Ibid*, paras 6.66–6.67.

[190] See also criticism of US Treasury official on this point, report by Margaret Burrow, 'Distinguishing Ex Ante–From Ex-Post Returns', 2014 *WTD* 190-5 (1 October 2014).

[191] It has been argued that this proposal contradicts the US cost-sharing regulations in which contractual terms play a key role. In any case, such important changes to the transfer pricing rules would be subject to the consent of national parliaments. See Jens Wittendorff, 'More Black Smoke From the OECD's Chimney—Third Draft on Intangibles', n 175 above.

[192] Intangibles Second Revised Discussion Draft, n 175 above, paras 6.145–1.149.

[193] See Gupta, 'Rough Road Ahead for OECD Intangibles Project', n 179 above.

[194] *Ibid.*

[195] Yariv Brauner, 'Transfer Pricing in BEPS: First Round—Business Interests Win (But, Not in Knock-Out' (2015) 43 *Intertax* 72–84.

[196] *Ibid*, p 78.

as regards the implementation of the rules. There was no guidance as to when comparables were inadequate so that one can eschew the arm's length principle and resort to profit split methods. Yariv Brauner has argued that this was the result of the pressure that the OECD faces but 'it leaves a magnitude of discretion that can annihilate the reform'.[197] Arguably, the commentary in the Profit Split Discussion Draft could be used for guidance in this area too.[198]

As the BEPS Monitoring Group also noted, much work needs to be done to develop recommendations for common tax accounting standards, and define suitable allocation keys for the application of the profit split method.[199] The OECD was criticised in that it still religiously proclaimed its adherence to the arm's length principle, even though it allows methods of application which differ widely.[200] This incoherence of transfer pricing rules 'remains the most blatant indicator of the crisis of the current system'.[201] The Group warned that unless a better approach could be developed, the BEPS project would have to be judged a failure.

Arguably, this is a risk that the OECD is willing or forced to take. It certainly seems politically easier than admitting to the fact that perhaps it is time for formulary methods to be explored. Addressing intangibles, or appearing to do so, is crucial to the BEPS project.[202] As stated in the executive summary to the Intangibles Second Revised Discussion Draft,[203] the OECD planned to finalise the intangibles guidance in 2015 in conjunction with the BEPS work on risk, re-characterisation and hard-to-value intangibles. Some of the suggestions in these deliverables have also proved quite controversial.

3.3.2. Cost Contribution Arrangements

On 29 April 2015, the OECD published a discussion draft under Action 8 as part of the requirement to update the guidance on cost contribution arrangements in Chapter VIII of the OECD Transfer Pricing Guidelines.[204] The guidance suggested in the CCA Discussion Draft also took into account the draft guidance suggested in the Risk and Re-characterisation Discussion Draft.[205]

The CCA Discussion Draft acknowledged the need to simplify the measurement of contributions and to ensure that contributions are commensurate with the benefits received under a CCA. Broadly, the revisions to the OECD Transfer Pricing Guidelines on CCAs supported the use of value contributed over the costs

[197] *Ibid*, p 79.

[198] See section 3.4.2 below.

[199] BEPS Monitoring Group, OECD BEPS Scorecard, n 84 above, p 11.

[200] *Ibid.*

[201] *Ibid.*

[202] J Scott Wilkie, '*Intangibles and Location Benefits (Customer Base)*' (2014) 68 *Bulletin for International Taxation* 352–60, at 360.

[203] See page 11 of Intangibles Second Revised Discussion Draft, n 175 above.

[204] OECD, *BEPS Action 8: Revisions to Chapter VIII of the Transfer Pricing Guidelines on Cost Contribution Arrangements (CCAs)* (henceforth, the CCA Discussion Draft).

[205] See analysis in section 3.4.4 below.

incurred. The CCA Discussion Draft reinforced the notion that the contribution of each participant to a CCA should be reflective of value contribution.

A CCA was defined as 'a contractual arrangement among business enterprises to share the contributions and risks involved in the joint development, production or the obtaining of intangibles, tangible assets or services with the understanding that such intangibles, tangible assets or services are expected to create direct benefits for the businesses of each of the participants'.[206] The definition reveals, once again, the central character of intangibles as part of the BEPS project.[207]

The CCA Discussion Draft emphasised that a CCA was a contractual arrangement rather than necessarily a distinct juridical entity or fixed place of business of all the participants.[208] While the CCA could streamline the flows of intercompany transactions, it did not affect the appropriate valuation of the separate contributions of the participants. The outcomes for transfer pricing purposes for CCA participants 'should be consistent with those which would have arisen had the parties made similar contributions on similar terms outside of a CCA mechanism'.[209]

The CCA Discussion Draft described two common types of CCAs: those established for the joint development, enhancement, maintenance, protection or exploitation of intangibles or tangible assets (development CCAs) and those for obtaining services (services CCAs). The former were expected to create ongoing, future benefits for participants, while the latter would often create current benefits only. In some cases, a CCA for obtaining current services may also create or enhance an intangible which provided ongoing benefits.[210]

The expectation of mutual and proportionate benefit was fundamental to the acceptance by independent enterprises of an arrangement for pooling resources and skills. For a CCA to satisfy the arm's length principle, each participant's proportionate share of the overall contributions to the CCA should be consistent with the participant's proportionate share of the overall expected benefits.[211]

The first step was to determine the participants of the CCA. Since a CCA was premised on all participants sharing not only contributions but also the risks of the CCA activities, to qualify as a participant in a CCA an entity must have the capability and authority to control the risks associated with the risk-bearing opportunity under the CCA in accordance with the definition of control of risks set out in Chapter I of the OECD Transfer Pricing Guidelines. In particular,

> this means that a CCA participant should have the capability to make decisions to take on the risk-bearing opportunity, to make decisions on how to respond to the risks, and

[206] CCA Discussion Draft, n 204 above, para 3.

[207] See PwC comments on the CCA Discussion Draft, available on Tax Analysts, 2015 *WTD* 86-21 (1 May 2015). It was noted that, contrary to the 2010 OECD Transfer Pricing Guidelines, only direct benefits were encompassed under the definition in the CCA Discussion Draft.

[208] CCA Discussion Draft, n 204 above, para 3.

[209] *Ibid*, para 6.

[210] *Ibid*, para 8.

[211] *Ibid*, para 11.

to assess, monitor, and direct any outsourced measures affecting risk outcomes under the CCA.[212]

It was emphasised that there was no rule that could be universally applied to determine whether each participant's proportionate share of the overall contributions to a CCA activity was consistent with the participant's proportionate share of the overall benefits expected to be received under the arrangement. The goal was to estimate the share of benefits expected to be obtained by each participant and to ensure that their contributions were in the same proportions. This may require that participants' contributions be adjusted using balancing payments.[213]

For each participant it was necessary to estimate the expected benefits from the CCA. The shares of expected benefits might be estimated based on the anticipated additional income generated or costs saved or other benefits received by each participant. In practice, a relevant allocation key such as sales; units used, produced, or sold; or number of employees might be appropriate to reflect the participants' proportionate shares of expected benefits.[214] Whatever the method used to evaluate participants' relative shares of expected benefits, adjustments to the measure used may be necessary to account for differences between the expected and actual benefits received by the participants.

For the purpose of determining whether a CCA satisfied the arm's length principle, it was necessary to measure the value of each participant's contributions to the arrangement.[215] Under the arm's length principle, the value of each participant's contribution should have been consistent with the value that independent enterprises would have assigned to that contribution. The CCA Discussion Draft makes it clear that contributions to CCAs are to be based on their arm's length value rather than on their cost.[216] It was, however, acknowledged that sometimes the value of services contributed to a CCA corresponds to the costs associated with providing those services—eg for low value-added services. In that case, it was recommended for practical reasons to value contributions at cost.[217]

Where the value of a participant's contributions was not consistent with its share of expected benefits, balancing payments might be required.[218] As CCAs can often be long-term projects, making minor or marginal adjustments or generally adjustments based on evidence from a single year may be inappropriate.[219] Furthermore, while costs are to be allocated based on expected benefits, it was emphasised that all participants to the CCA must have substance and the ability to exercise some form of control over their investments. Absent such substance, the

212 *Ibid*, para 13.
213 *Ibid*, para 15.
214 *Ibid*, para 16.
215 *Ibid*, para 20.
216 *Ibid*, para 23.
217 *Ibid*.
218 *Ibid*, paras 27–30.
219 *Ibid*, para 30.

CCA can be disregarded.[220] There was no concrete guidance as to the implications of this position. It was generically noted that guidance in Chapter VI on Hard to Value Intangibles might equally apply in situations involving CCAs and that in relevant circumstances 'it may be appropriate for a tax administration to disregard the CCA in its entirety in accordance with the principles for non-recognition of the delineated transaction set out in Chapter I'.[221]

Contributions, including any balancing payments and any buy-in or buy-out payments, by or for a participant of the CCA would continue to be treated for tax purposes in the same manner as would apply under the rules of the tax system applicable to each participant if the contributions were made outside a CCA. The character of the contribution would depend on the nature of the activity being undertaken by the CCA, and would determine how it was treated for tax purposes.[222] The discussion draft goes on to provide examples of scenarios in which balancing payments could be required.

Changes in the membership of a CCA may trigger a reassessment of the proportionate shares of participants' contributions and expected benefits.[223] In the case of new entrants contributing to a CCA, arm's length compensation would be required for such contribution in the form of a buy-in payment.[224] Furthermore, an entrant withdrawing from a CCA may be entitled to a buy-out payment to reflect a disposal of its interest. Again, these payments would be based on value rather than cost.

The guidance remained broadly unchanged in terms of its recommendations for structuring and documenting CCAs. These included conditions for participants eligible to join a CCA, terms to be included and information that should be documented at the beginning and throughout the duration of the CCA.[225]

In general, whilst the requirement for participants in a CCA to have the capability and authority to control the risks associated with the risk-bearing under the CCA was consistent with the overall BEPS theme of aligning taxation with value creation and substance, this is a fundamental change for CCAs. Cost contribution arrangements might become a misnomer, as contributions to CCAs would be based on their arm's length value rather than on their cost.[226] For a CCA participant to be entitled to the returns from a CCA linked with an intangible, controlling risks and developing, exploiting and maintaining the intangible will become essential. Participants only providing funding to the CCA would receive only limited returns. Furthermore, tax authorities are expressly authorised to check the commercial reality of the arrangement and re-characterise part or all of the terms of a CCA.

220 *Ibid*, paras 31–32.
221 *Ibid*, para 32.
222 *Ibid*, para 33.
223 *Ibid*, para 36.
224 *Ibid*, paras 37–41.
225 *Ibid*, paras 42–45.
226 See also PwC comments, n 207 above.

It has been argued that the approach taken by the OECD will potentially increase compliance burdens and controversy. It will also often lead to double taxation due to disagreements in terms of value measurement.[227] The compliance burden of designing and administering a CCA would also be increased. No guidance was given as to how control functions could be valued on an arm's length basis. Furthermore, the fact that it was acknowledged that each participant's contributions may vary with time could make it very difficult to accurately monitor and value the relative contributions of each participant on a continuous basis. Coupled with the right to re-characterise the terms of a CCA on the basis of the vague notion of commercial reality, the powers of tax authorities seem to have incrementally expanded.

3.4. Actions 9 and 10: Risks and Capital and Other High Transactions

Actions 9 and 10 read as follows:

> Develop rules to prevent BEPS by transferring risks among, or allocating excessive capital to, group members. This will involve adopting transfer pricing rules or special measures to ensure that inappropriate returns will not accrue to an entity solely because it has contractually assumed risks or has provided capital. The rules to be developed will also require alignment of returns with value creation. This work will be co-ordinated with the work on interest expense deductions and other financial payments.
>
> Develop rules to prevent BEPS by engaging in transactions which would not, or would only very rarely, occur between third parties. This will involve adopting transfer pricing rules or special measures to: (i) clarify the circumstances in which transactions can be recharacterised; (ii) clarify the application of transfer pricing methods, in particular profit splits, in the context of global value chains; and (iii) provide protection against common types of base eroding payments, such as management fees and head office expenses.

On 3 November 2014, the OECD released a discussion draft in the context of Action 10 relating to low value-adding intra-group services. Modifications to Chapter VII of the OECD Transfer Pricing Guidelines were proposed. The aim was to reduce the scope for base erosion through excessive management fees and head office expenses.

On 16 December, 2014 the OECD issued two further discussion drafts under Action item 10, the first addressing the use of the transactional profit-split method, and the second dealing with transfer pricing for commodity transactions.

[227] David D Stewart, 'OECD Cost Contribution Arrangements Draft Emphasises Value', 2015 *WTD* 83-1.

On 19 December, 2014 a more general discussion draft was issued under Action items 8, 9, and 10, with guidelines on how to ensure that transfer pricing outcomes are in line with value creation. These discussion drafts will be considered in sections 3.4.1–3.4.4 chronologically—according to their dates of release.

3.4.1. Low Value-Adding Intra-Group Services

The Discussion Draft on low value-adding intra-group services[228] (henceforth, the Intra-Group Services Discussion Draft) fully rewrote Chapter VII of the OECD's Transfer Pricing Guidelines on intercompany services. Very importantly, it included a definition of 'low value-adding intra-group services' and provided a 'simplified method' for such services.[229] The simplified approach was elective. Under this approach, the arm's length price for such services would be closely related to costs. Taxpayers that did not elect to apply it would continue using the existing guidance of Chapter VII. The US and the European Union had adopted similar simplified rules on group services to deal with base erosion.[230]

The Intra-Group Services Discussion Draft defined low value-adding intra-group services as those that were of a supportive nature and were not part of the core business of an MNE group.[231] This was an important element of the definition.[232] Furthermore, such services did not require the use of unique and valuable intangibles and did not lead to the creation of such intangibles. They also did not involve the assumption of control of substantial or significant risk and did not give rise to the creation of significant risk.[233] The guidance was not applicable to services that would ordinarily qualify as low value-adding intra-group services where such services were rendered to unrelated customers of MNE members. 'In such cases it can be expected that reliable internal comparables exist and can be used for determining the arm's length price for the intra-group services'.[234]

There was a list of services that would not qualify as low value-adding services eligible for the simplified approach. These included services constituting the core business of the MNE group, research and development (R&D) services, manufacturing, sales, marketing, distribution and corporate senior

[228] *Public Discussion Draft—BEPS Action 10: Proposed Modifications to Chapter VII of the Transfer Pricing Guidelines relating to Low Value-Adding Intra-Group Services*, 3 November 2014—14 January 2015 (OECD). Available on: www.oecd.org/ctp/transfer-pricing/discussion-draft-action-10-low-value-adding-intra-group-services.pdf.

[229] Some other important contributions of the Intra-Group Services Discussion Draft concern the expansion of the list of examples of shareholder services and what to do in the situation of a duplication of services between a service provider and a recipient. These would not be considered further: *ibid*, paras 7.11–7.12.

[230] Jens Wittendorff, 'The OECD's Simplified Approach to Pricing Low-Value-Adding Services' (2015) 77 *Tax Notes International* 793 (2 March 2015).

[231] See suggested para 7.46 in Intra-Group Services Discussion Draft, n 228 above.

[232] Also see, *ibid*, para 7.49 where a number of helpful examples were given.

[233] See suggested para 7.46.

[234] *Ibid*.

A 'global value chain' was described as the full range of firms' activities, from the conception of a product to its end use and beyond. It included activities such as design, production, marketing, distribution and support to the final consumer.[249] It was noted that one-sided methods may not be able to reliably account for the interdependence of key functions and risks in global value chains, and transactional profit split methods may be more appropriate. There was a discussion of the circumstances in which profit split methods might be the most appropriate for determining arm's length pricing. For example, this might be the case when both parties to a transaction made unique and valuable contributions, or when there was fragmentation of functions within a value chain, making it difficult to find reliable comparables. Profit split methods might also be used when an MNE's business operations were highly integrated such that strategic risks were jointly managed and controlled by more than one party. Generally, profit split methods might be used when there was a potential lack of reliable comparables for a one-sided method.

It was conceded in the Profit Split Discussion Draft that transactional profit split methods may be viewed as a means of achieving closer alignment between profits and value creation. In practice, these methods were typically applied using one or more allocation keys or factors to split the profits, based on the outcome of a functional analysis that determines how value is created in the MNE group.[250] The OECD Transfer Pricing Guidelines urged for the factors to be used in an economically valid way that approximated the division of profits that would have been agreed at arm's length.[251] However, it was recognised that transactional profit split methods suffer from subjectivity—'allocation keys can be difficult to verify from objective evidence'.[252]

Through several scenarios, the Profit Split Discussion Draft examined how to develop objectivity in profit split factors so that transfer pricing outcomes were firmly aligned with value creation.[253] It also examined how transactional profit split methods may provide a way to address significant differences between ex ante and ex post results, as an appropriate way to deal with unanticipated events where strategic risks were effectively shared between associated enterprises.[254] The Profit Split Discussion Draft also considered whether profit split methods may be applied in a different way when there were losses to split instead of profits.[255]

Overall, the Profit Split Discussion Draft did not provide recommendations or suggest policy changes, but rather directed the discussion to important issues. In fact, it has been characterised as almost exploratory in nature.[256] Numerous

[249] Profit Split Discussion Draft, n 246 above, para 5, referring to OECD report *Interconnected Economies: Benefitting from Global Value Chains*.

[250] Profit Split Discussion Draft, n 246 above, para 34.

[251] See para 2.108 of OECD Transfer Pricing Guidelines.

[252] Profit Split Discussion Draft, n 246 above, para 35.

[253] *Ibid*, paras 33–43.

[254] *Ibid*, paras 45–49.

[255] *Ibid*, paras 50–53.

[256] Amanda Athanasiou, 'Observers Question BEPS Transfer Pricing Drafts', 2015 *WTD* 61-4 (31 March 2015).

questions were posed on how to apply the transactional profit split method in the context of global value chains, when this method would be the appropriate method to apply and the treatment of losses. A general criticism was that wider adoption of the transactional profit split method would lead to a further shift away from the arm's length standard, and closer to an apportionment system.

Indeed, the BEPS Monitoring Groups in its comments on the use of profit splits[257] suggested that the fiction of separate legal personality should be replaced in situations where it does not reflect economic substance 'with a holistic approach which treats corporate groups in accordance with the business reality that they are run as integrated enterprises'.[258] The Group argued that the continuous evocation of the mantra of the arm's length principle was aimed at reassuring traditionalists that no significant changes were intended, but in reality the proposals suggested a shift from the traditional approach.[259] It was argued that the term 'transactional profit split' was contradictory and confusing, and should not be used. 'It should be made explicit that profit split is a method of apportioning profits to ensure outcomes that are in line with the location of economic activities and value creation'.[260]

3.4.3. The Commodities Discussion Draft

The Commodities Discussion Draft[261] acknowledged that intercompany commodity transactions may be particularly relevant for commodity-dependent developing countries where a major source of economic activity, employment, revenues, and income growth was related to the commodity sector. One of the main issues addressed was transfer pricing oriented tax base erosion resulting from cross-border controlled transactions the object of which was the sale or purchase of commodities. This was a problem acutely felt by tax administrations of commodity-dependent developing countries.[262]

More specifically, countries have reported the following issues. First, the use of pricing date conventions which appeared to enable the adoption by the taxpayer of the most advantageous quoted price. Secondly, significant adjustments

[257] See BEPS Monitoring Group, *Comments on BEPS Action 10: The Use of Profit Splits in the Context of Global Value Chains*. Available on: bepsmonitoringgroup.files.wordpress.com/2015/02/ap10-profit-split.pdf.

[258] *Ibid*, p 2, para 2.

[259] *Ibid*, para 3.

[260] *Ibid*, p 3, para 5.

[261] OECD, *BEPS Action 10: Discussion Draft on the Transfer Pricing Aspects of Cross-Border Commodity Transactions*. Available on: www.oecd.org/ctp/transfer-pricing/discussion-draft-action-10-commodity-transactions.pdf. For commentary, see David D Stewart and Margaret Burow, 'OECD Issues Drafts on Profit-Split Method and Commodity Transactions', 2014 *WTD* 242-1 (17 December 2014).

[262] Commodities Discussion Draft, n 261 above, paras 1–2. The term 'commodities' was defined as physical products for which a quoted price was used by independent parties to set prices. See para 12.

to the quoted price or charging of significant fees to the taxpayer in the commodity-producing country by other group companies in the supply chain (eg processing, transportation, distribution, marketing); and, the involvement in the supply chain of entities with apparently limited functionality, which may be located in tax opaque jurisdictions with nil or low taxation.[263]

It was explained that some countries had acted unilaterally to develop approaches for pricing commodity transactions in response to these concerns. The emergence of such approaches had highlighted the need for clearer guidance on the application of transfer pricing rules to commodity transactions. The Commodities Discussion Draft made a number of alternative proposals.[264]

First, the guidance in Chapter II of the OECD Transfer Pricing Guidelines should be clarified so that the Comparable Uncontrolled Price (CUP) method should be an appropriate transfer pricing method for commodity transactions between associated enterprises.[265] It was also proposed that quoted or publicly available prices could be used under the CUP method as a reference to determine the arm's length price for a controlled commodity transaction.[266] It was acknowledged that the price-setting policy for controlled commodity transactions should be included in the transfer pricing documentation of an MNE.[267]

Secondly, there was a proposal to include additional guidance regarding the adoption of a deemed pricing date for commodity transactions between associated enterprises in the absence of evidence of the actual pricing date agreed upon by the parties to the transactions.[268] It was recommended that, absent reliable evidence of the actual pricing date agreed by the associated enterprises, tax administrations may deem the pricing date for the commodity transaction to be the date of shipment as evidenced by the bill of lading or equivalent documents, depending on the means of transport.[269]

Thirdly, it was recommended that there should potentially be additional guidance on comparability adjustments to the quoted price.[270] The Commodities Discussion Draft did not provide guidance regarding what adjustments would be performed if differences arose, or how to perform them. Certain adjustments may be based on information and costings which were transparent or industry standard.[271] The OECD requested stakeholders to provide information regarding common adjustments or differentials applied to quoted prices and the sources of information used to determine such adjustments or differentials.[272]

263 *Ibid*, para 2.
264 *Ibid*, para 3.
265 *Ibid*, paras 4 and 8–12.
266 *Ibid*.
267 See para 12 and suggested new para 4.
268 *Ibid*, paras 13–15.
269 *Ibid*, para 15 and suggested new para 5.
270 *Ibid*, paras 16–17.
271 *Ibid*, para 16.
272 *Ibid*, para 17.

In general, the proposed guidance seeks to ensure that pricing reflects value creation, thereby protecting the tax base of commodity-dependent countries. It tries to ensure that parties performing value-adding functions in relation to the commodity being transferred are remunerated with arm's length compensation. Although the Commodities Discussion Draft primarily focuses on the base erosion concerns of developing countries—and as such gives credence to the OECD's pronouncements that developing countries ought to have a larger role in the BEPS project[273]—it also highlights the issues faced by taxpayers from the lack of resources in many developing country tax administrations.

At a public consultation meeting held at the OECD on 20 March 2015, participants warned against the urge to oversimplify the transfer pricing of commodities. It was argued that the CUP method may not always be the best method and that the discussion draft did not take into account commodities traded in illiquid markets. Furthermore, the deemed pricing date was criticised for not reflecting the realities and practices in the commodities industries. A preferable method was a system of contract registration that would record the relevant terms of commodity transactions. Such contract registration would also provide both tax authorities and taxpayers with certainty about the contract's terms.[274]

3.4.4. Risk and Re-Characterisation Discussion Draft on Actions 8, 9 and 10

On 19 December 2014 the OECD issued a more general discussion draft under Action items 8, 9, and 10—the Risk and Re-characterisation Discussion Draft.[275] This discussion draft dealt with the recognition to be given to the related parties' allocation of risk and the re-characterisation of transactions. It also considered the appropriateness of the adoption of special measures outside normal transfer pricing rules. The Risk and Re-characterisation Discussion Draft was divided into two parts.

Part I contained a proposed revision to Section D of Chapter I of the OECD Transfer Pricing Guidelines. The proposals focused on the importance of accurately delineating the actual transactions, and included guidance on the relevance and allocation of risk. There was also guidance on determining the economically relevant characteristics of controlled transactions and on re-characterisation

[273] See analysis in Ch 4, section 4.6 of this volume.

[274] David D Stewart, 'Simplicity Versus Flexibility Argued in OECD Transfer Pricing Consultations', n 245 above.

[275] OECD, *Public Discussion Draft—BEPS Actions 8, 9 and 10: Discussion Draft on Revisions to Chapter I of the Transfer Pricing Guidelines (Including Risk, Recharacterisation, and Special Measures)*. Available on: www.oecd.org/ctp/transfer-pricing/discussion-draft-actions-8-9-10-chapter-1-TP-Guidelines-risk-recharacterisation-special-measures.pdf.

or non-recognition of transactions. This formed the basis for comparison with uncontrolled transactions under the existing guidance found in Chapters II and III of the OECD Transfer Pricing Guidelines.

Part II provided options for some special measures, with regard to intangible assets, risk and over-capitalisation. A series of questions relating to all options was set out and responses to these questions were to be taken into account when considering the appropriateness and design of each option.

In order to delineate a controlled transaction, the Risk and Re-characterisation Discussion Draft focused on identifying the actual conduct of the parties. The process of identifying the actual conduct—ie, the actual commercial and financial relations between the parties—in order to accurately delineate the transaction involved identifying the economically relevant characteristics of the transaction. These included the contractual terms of the transaction, the functions performed, the characteristics of the property transferred, the economic circumstances of the parties and their business strategies. There was detailed discussion of these characteristics.

The Risk and Re-characterisation Discussion Draft added a substantially new section on identifying risks in commercial or financial relations between controlled parties to a transaction. There was a discussion on the nature and sources of risk, the allocation of risks in contracts, how risks were assumed, the potential impact of risk, risk management, and identifying the actual conduct of the parties related to risk.[276]

Several issues core to identifying risk in commercial and financial relations between parties were discussed. These issues involved the extent to which associated enterprises could be assumed to have different risk preferences while they were also in fact acting collaboratively in a common undertaking under common control.[277] The issues were broadly grouped into two categories to be considered in the context of the established framework of the arm's length principle.

The first category contained issues around the term 'moral hazard'. This referred to the lack of incentive to guard against risk when one was protected from its consequences. The term was used 'to introduce the concept that unrelated parties would seek to avoid moral hazard that may arise in situations where one party assumes a risk without the ability to manage the behaviour of the party creating its risk exposure'.[278] The concept was thought to extend to the safeguards or incentives that unrelated parties may incorporate into contracts between them.[279] Comments were invited on the implications of moral hazard for the arm's length principle.

[276] The discussion on risk seemed to borrow concepts from Chapter IX of the OECD Transfer Pricing Guidelines on business restructurings, in particular, the concepts of control over risk and allocation of risk.

[277] Risk and Re-characterisation Discussion Draft, n 275 above, para 40, Additional Points.

[278] *Ibid*, p 14.

[279] *Ibid.*

The second category contained issues grouped around the term 'risk–return trade-off'. This concept implied the equivalence on a present value basis between a higher but less certain stream of income and a lower but more certain stream of income. According to the Risk and Re-characterisation Discussion Draft, the principle supported the associated notion that it was economically rational to take on (or lay off) risk in return for higher (or lower) anticipated nominal income. There were several questions on the implications of risk–return trade-off under the arm's length principle.[280] Comments were again requested on distinctions to be made in the guidance on risk transfers applicable to the financial services sector.[281]

Furthermore, the Risk and Re-characterisation Discussion Draft added a substantially new section on non-recognition.[282] It was noted that in exceptional circumstances the transaction may be disregarded for transfer pricing purposes.[283] The concept of fundamental economic attributes of arrangements between unrelated parties was introduced.[284] There could be non-recognition when the transaction did not have the fundamental economic attributes of arrangements between unrelated parties. The term non-recognition was intended to convey the same meaning as that understood to be conveyed by the term re-characterisation.[285] The Risk and Re-characterisation Discussion Draft attempted to delineate the criteria for non-recognition,[286] emphasising that every effort should first be made to determine the actual nature of the transaction and apply arm's length pricing to the accurately delineated transaction. Non-recognition should not be used simply because determining an arm's length price was difficult.[287]

There was a section on specific considerations which included losses, the effect of government policies and the use of customs valuations. Further, the Risk and Re-characterisation Discussion Draft added, with no changes, the section on location savings and local market features, previously released under the Intangibles Second Revised Discussion Draft.[288]

[280] *Ibid.*

[281] *Ibid.*

[282] *Ibid*, paras 83–93.

[283] *Ibid*, para 83.

[284] See more fully para 83: 'In order for the transaction as accurately delineated to be recognised for transfer pricing purposes, the transaction should exhibit the fundamental economic attributes of arrangements between unrelated parties. An arrangement exhibiting the fundamental economic attributes of arrangements between unrelated parties would offer each of the parties a reasonable expectation to enhance or protect their commercial or financial positions on a risk-adjusted (the return adjusted for the level of risk associated with it) basis, compared to other opportunities realistically available to them at the time the arrangement was entered into. If the actual arrangement, viewed in its entirety, would not afford such an opportunity to each of the parties, or would afford it to only one of them, then the transaction would not be recognised for transfer pricing purposes. In applying the criterion, it is relevant to consider whether there exists an alternative for one or more of the parties, including the alternative of not entering into the transaction, which does provide the opportunity to enhance or protect their commercial or financial positions. It is also a relevant pointer to consider whether the MNE group as a whole is left worse off on a pre-tax basis'. Risk and Re-characterisation Discussion Draft, n 275 above.

[285] *Ibid.*

[286] *Ibid.*

[287] *Ibid*, para 84.

[288] Intangibles Second Revised Discussion Draft, n 175 above.

In the second part of the Risk and Re-characterisation Discussion Draft,[289] options for potential special measures to address residual BEPS risks[290] were considered. One of the largest sources of disagreements in the BEPS project had been whether special measures should be proposed to address abuses outside the arm's length standard.[291] The Risk and Re-characterisation Discussion Draft proposed five alternative special measures[292] and invited comments.

In general, the Risk and Re-characterisation Discussion Draft unequivocally suggests a reconsideration of the role of risk allocation among related group members.

> It shines a spotlight on the tensions inherent in the arm's length principle—namely, the challenges in comparing a transaction between related parties that share a common economic goal with one between independent parties that often pursue competing economic goals.[293]

The Risk and Re-characterisation Discussion Draft reduces the importance of contractual allocations of risk while raising the importance of functions such as managing and controlling risks.[294] It is evident from the proposals that lesser weight would be given to written contractual agreements and greater weight to the parties' commercial or financial relations. Written contracts between related parties would no longer be the starting point for the analysis. Prioritising the conduct of risk management functions over legal arrangements seems to go beyond the current understanding of the arm's length principle and is likely to lead to more disputes.[295] Henceforth, businesses are likely to put significant emphasis on aligning substance with contracts.[296]

The Risk and Re-characterisation Discussion Draft certainly seeks to widen the re-characterisation doctrine and expand the test of commercial rationality which underpins the existing test. This is likely to lead to more subjectivity, increase

[289] Risk and Re-characterisation Discussion Draft, n 275 above, pp 38–45.

[290] These residual risks mainly related to information asymmetries between taxpayers and tax administrations and the relative ease with which taxpayers could allocate capital to low-tax entities with minimal functions. This capital could be invested in assets used within the MNE group, creating base eroding payments to the low-tax entities: *ibid*, p 38, para 3.

[291] See Amanda Athanasiou, 'Experts Disagree on Transfer Pricing Special Measures', 2014 *WTD* 242-3 (17 December 2014).

[292] The following special measures were set out: (1) special measures for hard-to-value intangibles; (2) dealing with a capital-rich, asset-owning company that depends on another group company to generate a return from the asset; (3) 'thick capitalisation rule' based on a pre-determined capital ratio; (4) special measures focusing on a level of functionality that, where lacking, would cause the profits of that entity to be reallocated; (5) ensuring appropriate taxation of excess returns. See Risk and Re-characterisation Discussion Draft, n 275 above, pp 41–45.

[293] Mindy Herzfeld, 'BEPS—Phase II' (2015) 77 *Tax Notes International* 14(5 January 2015).

[294] See David D Stewart, 'OECD Risk and Recharacterization Draft Could Boost Controversy', 2015 *WTD* 19-4 (29 January 2015), who notes that the Risk and Re-characterisation Discussion Draft diminishes the importance of capital as a driver of returns.

[295] Richard Collier, 'BEPS: New Thinking on Risk, Excess Capital and Recharacterisation', *Tax Journal*, Issue 1246, p 20 (16 January 2015) pp 20–21.

[296] See comments made by US expert in that companies are enquiring whether they need to move executives to the country of residence of the residual risk-taking entity. David D Stewart, 'US Treasury Official Suggests Refined Message for OECD Risk Draft', 2015 *WTD* 3104 (17 February, 2015).

uncertainty and controversy, and potentially lead to more double taxation. It is feared that the breadth of the definition of fundamental economic attributes will give a lot of discretion to tax authorities to reclassify a transaction on grounds that another transaction would have resulted in more taxable income arising in the jurisdiction.[297] The special measures introduced in the second part of the discussion draft may also cause uncertainty and make the system worse.[298] There is very little guidance, with many open-ended questions for stakeholders to provide an input. The United States has indicated that it is not prepared to support the current version of the Risk and Re-characterisation Draft but it is 'working hard to find consensus that could also resolve conflicts on related drafts'.[299]

It has been argued that the Risk and Re-characterisation Discussion Draft effectively proposes a new enhanced functional analysis to determine how value is generated by a multinational group as a whole, and each entity's capabilities and contribution to value creation.[300] The new analysis reflects the nature of the interdependencies of the functions performed by entities in a multinational group, how commercial activities are coordinated, and group synergies. It requires multinational groups to calculate which entity actually performs management activities. However, the fact that the Risk and Re-characterisation Discussion Draft fails to define value makes it difficult to determine its creation, especially in the context of a multinational group.[301]

Nevertheless, despite the OECD's continued loyalty to the arm's length standard for pricing transactions between related enterprises, the arm's length standard that will emerge in the post-BEPS world is likely to be modified. Part of the challenge is that there is no well-established definition of what value creation means. Value creation is a vague term—what this entails, where it occurs and its valuation are difficult issues to be addressed. Without agreement on these, it is very difficult to find solutions. What broadly seem to emerge from the transfer pricing BEPS deliverables so far, are undeveloped suggestions and a series of vague concepts that add undue complexity to administration and compliance.[302]

In an interview with Tax Analysts on 22 January 2015, OECD representatives admitted that additional work was necessary in order for the proposals to

[297] Amanda Athanasiou, 'Definition of BEPS Fundamental Economic Attributes Too Broad, Practitioners Say', 2015 *WTD* 34-3 (20 February 2015).

[298] Amanda Athanasiou, 'Experts Disagree on Transfer Pricing Special Measures', n 291 above.

[299] David D Stewart, 'Breakthrough on BEPS Risk Draft Could Lead to Larger Consensus', 2015 *WTD* 46-1 (10 March 2015).

[300] See Margaret Burow, 'OECD Draft Challenges Intragroup Risk Allocations', 2015 *WTD* 21-9 (2 February 2015). She discussed comments made by Alan Shapiro of Deloitte Tohmatsu Tax Co during a Deloitte webcast on 30 January 2015.

[301] *Ibid.* It was questioned whether sales revenue, income profits, competitive advantage, synergies, economic power, asset ownership, or other measures should be considered value.

[302] Amanda Athanasiou and Lee Sheppard, 'OECD's Discussion Draft on Transfer Pricing Goes Beyond Arm's Length', 2014 *WTD* 245-7 (22 December 2014). For criticism, also see David Stewart, 'ABA Meeting: U.S. Troubled by Aspects of OECD Risk Draft', 2015 *WTD* 21-4 (2 February 2015); Margaret Burow, 'OECD Draft Challenges Intragroup Risk Allocations', n 300 above.

produce coherent and workable changes to the existing rules.[303] It was important to coordinate the implications of the transfer pricing analysis with a more general legal analysis, such as the interpretation of contracts. It was argued that the discussion draft simply clarified transfer pricing best practices and made no radical changes to existing rules, nor was there a departure from the arm's length standard.

Although the importance of legal contracts in a transfer pricing analysis was arguably diminished by giving tax authorities more discretion to disregard them, the scope of this was played down in the interview. It was argued that the language of the Risk and Re-characterisation Discussion Draft simply emphasised that the legal contracts must be in line with the parties' behaviour under those contracts to be an accurate reflection of how the parties actually operated. 'The contracts definitely play a role … But paper reality is not what we are pricing. We are pricing the business reality of the transaction'.[304] Contracts and conduct were both very important elements of looking at the actual transaction, and had to be seen together in the context of the commercial and financial relationships between the group members.

A tenuous distinction between delineating a transaction and re-characterising it was made. Re-characterisation differed from accurately delineating the transaction and applied when the transaction had been accurately delineated and the analysis was factually correct, but the transaction did not seem to make economic sense. This has been criticised for ignoring the fact that a transfer pricing analysis allows for some variability in determining pricing. It also appears to provide tax authorities with extensive latitude to substitute their own interpretation of the facts for the taxpayer's.

There was limited approval of the Risk and Re-characterisation Discussion Draft from the BEPS Monitoring Group.[305] This was because, although the discussion draft identified many of the difficulties caused by the separate entity principle which the Group had in the past heavily criticised, the discussion draft did not clearly articulate an alternative. The Group again expressed its support for the profit split method, regularised and systematised 'by clarifying the methodology for defining the aggregate tax base to be split and specifying definite, concrete and easily determinable objective allocation keys for all commonly used business models'.[306]

The remaining items of the Action Plan are examined in the next chapter. There is also an overview of how the BEPS project affects developing countries, as well as their involvement in the consultation process.

[303] Mindy Herzfeld, 'Input Needed on Transfer Pricing Drafts', 2015 *WTD* 21-2 (2 February 2015). The interview was with Marlies de Ruiter and Andrew Hickman of the OECD's Centre for Tax Policy and Administration. See, also, Andrew Velarde, 'BEPS Transfer Pricing Draft Struck Nerve, Official Says', 2015 *WTD* 34-1 (20 February 2015).

[304] *Ibid.*

[305] See BEPS Monitoring Group, *Comments on BEPS Actions 8, 9, and 10: Revisions to Chapter I of Transfer Pricing Guidelines (including Risk, Recharacterisation, and Special Measures)*. Available on: bepsmonitoringgroup.files.wordpress.com/2015/02/ap8-9-10-risk-special-measures.pdf.

[306] *Ibid*, p 2.

4

Procedural Rules, Country-by-Country Reporting, Dispute Resolution, Multilateralism and Developing Countries: Actions 10–15

The previous chapters examined Action items 1 to 10 of the BEPS Action Plan. Most of the remaining items of the Action Plan considered in this chapter deal with procedural reforms, the most prominent one being Action 13, on country-by-country reporting and transfer pricing documentation. In Action 11, there is an attempt to establish methodologies to collect and analyse data and counteractions. Rules on disclosure of aggressive tax planning arrangements are reviewed in Action 12. Suggestions to make dispute resolution more effective and to develop multilateral instruments are the final Action items, Actions 14 and 15, considered in this chapter. The chapter concludes with a brief review of the role of developing countries in the consultation and decision-making processes of the BEPS project and the overall impact that the project may have had on them.

4.1. Action 11: Establish Methodologies to Collect and Analyse Data on BEPS and the Actions to Address it

Action 11 mandates as follows:

> Develop recommendations regarding indicators of the scale and economic impact of BEPS and ensure that tools are available to monitor and evaluate the effectiveness and economic impact of the actions taken to address BEPS on an ongoing basis. This will involve developing an economic analysis of the scale and impact of BEPS (including spillover effects across countries) and actions to address it. The work will also involve assessing a range of existing data sources, identifying new types of data that should be collected, and developing methodologies based on both aggregate (e.g. FDI and balance

of payments data) and micro-level data (e.g. from financial statements and tax returns), taking into consideration the need to respect taxpayer confidentiality and the administrative costs for tax administrations and businesses.

In the summer of 2014, a short briefing paper was published by the OECD on Action 11, which summarised the issues on which it requested input from stakeholders.[1] There were four categories. First, recommendations were sought on indicators of the scale and economic impact of BEPS, including identifying and assessing a range of existing data sources. Secondly, recommendations were also sought on the development of an economic analysis of the scale and impact of BEPS (including spillover effects across countries) including developing methodologies based on both aggregate and micro-level data. Furthermore, the OECD asked for recommendations on how to develop an economic analysis of the effectiveness and impact of actions to address BEPS. Lastly, there was an enquiry as to the necessary tools to monitor and evaluate the effectiveness and economic impact of the actions taken to address BEPS on an ongoing basis, including identifying and assessing new types of data needed for the tools.[2]

On 7 October 2014, the OECD published the comments received on Action 11. Compared to other Action items, few inputs were provided, including responses from two governments such as China and Costa Rica and the BEPS Monitoring Group. The topic was considered rather academic. It was suggested that there should be another opportunity to comment when the OECD set forth proposed BEPS metrics in a future consultation document.[3] The BEPS Monitoring Group argued that the main problem was the lack of suitable data and problems of access to such data when they do exist.[4] Efforts to quantify the scale and impact of BEPS, and hence the effects of anti-BEPS measures, could only be properly explored if researchers all over the world and the public at large had access to suitable data. Furthermore, it was argued that all existing data sources had critical shortcomings, mainly because of the limited number of countries they covered or the limited amount of detail they provided. The BEPS Monitoring Group emphasised that the data generated by the country-by-country reporting of multinational enterprises should become publicly available to enable research on BEPS.

[1] OECD, *Request for input—BEPS Action 11: Establish methodologies to collect and analyse data on BEPS and the actions to address it*. Available on: www.oecd.org/ctp/public-request-for-input-beps-action-11.pdf.

[2] *Ibid*, para 5.

[3] See PwC commentary, available on: www.pwc.com/gx/en/tax/tax-policy-administration/beps/data-and-methodologies.jhtml.

[4] BEPS Monitoring Group, *Action 11: Establishing Methodologies to Collect and Analyse Data on BEPS and the Actions to Address It*. Available on: bepsmonitoringgroup.wordpress.com/the-oecd-beps-action-plan/.

On 16 April 2015, the OECD released its discussion draft on improving the analysis of BEPS.[5] This set out the context and background to the work on Action 11, and included three chapters that focused on key areas.

In chapter 1, there was an assessment of existing data sources relevant for BEPS analysis, describing the available data and their limitations for measuring the scale and impact of BEPS and BEPS countermeasures. The data included macroeconomic sources (eg national accounts, balance of payments and foreign direct investment) as well as microeconomic sources (eg corporate income tax return information, customs data and company financial information). This chapter concluded that the significant limitations of existing data sources meant that, at present, attempts to construct indicators or undertake an economic analysis were severely constrained and, as such, should be heavily qualified.

Chapter 2 considered potential indicators of the scale and economic impact of BEPS and their various strengths and limitations. While there was a large and growing body of evidence of the existence of BEPS, through empirical analysis and specific information that had emerged from numerous legislative and parliamentary enquiries, the scale of BEPS and changes over time were difficult to measure. It was suggested to have a dashboard of indicators because no single indicator could present a snapshot of the existence and scale of BEPS.[6] This chapter outlined a number of potential indicators that might assist in tracking the scale and economic impact of BEPS over time. These could only provide 'general indications' and the interpretation of any such indicators had to be heavily qualified by numerous caveats.

In chapter 3, there was a consideration of existing empirical analyses of BEPS. Two complementary approaches to estimating the scale of BEPS were proposed as alternatives. One approach was to estimate an overall revenue effect of BEPS by extrapolating from studies of profit shifting using the estimated tax responsiveness of shifted financial profit to tax rate differentials (the aggregate tax rate differential approach). Another approach was to estimate the revenue effects by reference to the individual BEPS channels focusing on Actions 2 to 10 (the specific BEPS channels approach). Both approaches had advantages and disadvantages, and could be drawn upon as part of the economic analysis to be undertaken under Action 11.

Overall, the options included in this discussion draft did not represent conclusions on the assessments or proposed measures, but were intended to provide

[5] See OECD, 'BEPS Action 11, Improving the Analysis of BEPS', available on: www.oecd.org/ctp/tax-policy/discussion-draft-action-11-data-analysis.pdf. For commentary, see PwC analysis of the discussion draft, reported by Tax Analysts, 2015 *WTD* 77-25 (21 April 2015).

[6] The seven potential indicators were the following: concentration of high levels of net foreign direct investment (FDI) relative to GDP; differential profit rates compared to effective tax rates; differential profit rates between low-tax locations and worldwide MNE operations; domestic vs foreign profit rate differentials; differential profit rates between MNE group domestic and foreign operations; differential effective tax rates between MNE affiliates and comparable domestic firms; concentration of high levels of royalty payments received relative to R&D spending; interest expense to income ratios of MNE affiliates in high-tax locations: see para 78 et seq of Action 11 discussion draft, n 4 above.

stakeholders with substantive options for analysis and comment. The discussion draft identified specific questions where input was required in order to advance the work on Action 11.

This discussion draft was met with mixed reactions. Some praised the OECD for tackling a difficult topic and others criticised it for not addressing the topic more thoroughly before launching the BEPS project in 2013.[7] It was generally recognised that the OECD's task in this Action item was incredibly challenging. It was readily conceded that economists do not 'always agree on fundamental questions such as what activities generate profits and how to distinguish between the artificial and natural separation of profits from activities'.[8] How legal rules could be fairly devised to address these issues when there is a wider underlying disagreement by economists is highly questionable. Arguably, there should have been an attempt to quantify the size and scale of BEPS first before devoting so many resources into solving it.[9]

Another criticism was that the discussion draft focused mainly on measuring BEPS for MNEs. The same approach may not work on small and medium-sized enterprises. Furthermore, the inherently difficult task of obtaining data for purely tax-driven structures was mentioned. It was recommended that there should be a broader review of the effects of BEPS on economic growth to determine the actual impact of BEPS actions—ie whether they are improving or worsening economic welfare.

> A broader assessment should also take into account compliance and administrative costs as well as possible unintended consequences of the BEPS project, such as the increased risk of double taxation and of companies moving people and assets into tax havens in response to BEPS rules that align profits with tangible activities.[10]

4.2. Action 12: Require Taxpayers to Disclose their Aggressive Tax Planning Arrangements

Action 12 reads as follows:

> Develop recommendations regarding the design of mandatory disclosure rules for aggressive or abusive transactions, arrangements, or structures, taking into consideration the administrative costs for tax administrations and businesses and drawing on experiences of the increasing number of countries that have such rules. The work will use a modular design allowing for maximum consistency but allowing for country specific needs and

[7] See Stephanie Soong Johnston, 'OECD Draft on Measuring BEPS Receives Mixed Reactions', 2015 *WTD* 78-2 (23 April 2015).

[8] Ibid.

[9] Ibid, see comments by Heather Self.

[10] Ibid, see comments by Peter Merill.

risks. One focus will be international tax schemes, where the work will explore using a wide definition of 'tax benefit' in order to capture such transactions. The work will be co-ordinated with the work on co-operative compliance. It will also involve designing and putting in place enhanced models of information sharing for international tax schemes between tax administrations.

In this Action item, the OECD attempts to examine the usefulness of disclosure initiatives in addressing the lack of comprehensive and relevant information on tax planning strategies available to tax authorities. The Mandatory Disclosure Discussion Document[11] was published by the OECD on 30 March 2015. It provided an overview of mandatory disclosure regimes, based on the experiences of countries that had such regimes, and set out recommendations for a modular design of a mandatory disclosure regime, including recommendations on rules designed to capture international tax schemes. The design recommendations would take into account the role played by other compliance and disclosure initiatives such as the initiative on co-operative compliance.[12]

Both initiatives were intended to improve transparency, risk assessment and ultimately taxpayer compliance, although co-operative compliance programmes often focused on the largest corporate taxpayers. It was argued that mandatory disclosure could reinforce the effectiveness of a co-operative compliance regime by ensuring that there was a level playing field in terms of the disclosure and tax transparency required from all taxpayers.[13]

The Mandatory Disclosure Discussion Draft sought to set out a standard framework for a mandatory disclosure regime that would ensure consistency while providing sufficient flexibility to deal with country-specific risks, allowing tax administrations to control the quantity and type of disclosure.

Following the introduction, there was an overview of the key features of a mandatory disclosure regime and a consideration of its interaction with other disclosure initiatives and compliance tools. In the next chapter, the framework and features for the modular design of a mandatory disclosure regime were set out. It was noted that there were other disclosure and information exchange initiatives being considered in the Action Plan, such as country-by-country reporting under Action 13 and the work on spontaneous exchange of rulings as part of the work on Action 5. Also, the Forum on Tax Administration was developing a framework for cooperation between tax administrations. Recommendations for the design of enhanced models of information sharing would need to take into account the outcome of these initiatives and developments.

[11] OECD, *BEPS Action 12: Mandatory Disclosure Rules*. Available on: www.oecd.org/ctp/aggressive/discussion-draft-action-12-mandatory-disclosure-rules.pdf.

[12] See, for example, reports listed in paras 8–9: *Study into the role of Tax Intermediaries* (OECD, 2008); *Tackling Aggressive Tax Planning through Improved Transparency and Disclosure* (OECD, 2011); *Co-operative Compliance: A Framework—From Enhanced Relationship to Co-Operative Compliance* (OECD, 2013).

[13] Mandatory Disclosure Discussion Draft, n 11 above, para 10.

The objectives of existing different mandatory disclosure rules were summarised as follows: to obtain early information about tax avoidance schemes in order to inform risk assessment; to identify schemes, and the users and promoters of schemes in a timely manner; and to act as a deterrent, to reduce the promotion and use of avoidance schemes.[14]

There were a number of key design principles. First, mandatory disclosure rules should be clear and easy to understand. Secondly, mandatory disclosure rules should balance additional compliance costs to taxpayers with the benefits obtained by the tax administration. Thirdly, mandatory disclosure rules should be effective in achieving the intended policy objectives and accurately identify relevant schemes. Fourthly, information collected under mandatory disclosure should be used effectively.[15]

It was emphasised that the design of a mandatory disclosure regime had to be flexible to the needs and risks of countries—that is why a modular approach was preferred. It was noted that existing mandatory disclosure regimes could be described as falling into two basic categories: a transaction-based approach and a promoter-based approach. The transaction-based approach, adopted by the US, first identified transactions that the tax administration considered as giving rise to tax revenue or policy risks (a reportable scheme) and then required disclosure from taxpayers who derived a tax benefit from it, and any person who provided material assistance in relation to that reportable scheme. The promoter-based approach had a greater focus on the role played by promoters of tax planning schemes but it also considered what types of reportable scheme promoters and taxpayers were required to disclose.[16]

In reality, the distinction between transaction and promoter-based approaches may not be that significant, because none of the existing mandatory disclosure regimes followed a purely transaction or promoter-based approach.[17] While acknowledging the differences between regimes, the design recommendations in the Mandatory Disclosure Discussion Draft were based on the core features common to all these regimes.[18]

Certain important design features had to be considered for either approach, such as who reports, what information they report and when.

The question of 'who has to report' was reviewed first.[19] Two options were considered: either both the promoter and the taxpayer have the obligation to disclose separately or, either the promoter or the taxpayer has the obligation to disclose.[20] Countries had to decide whether or not they would introduce a dual reporting requirement that applied to the promoter and taxpayer, or whether they would

[14] Ibid, para 16.
[15] Ibid, paras 19–24.
[16] *Ibid*, para 57.
[17] *Ibid*, para 59.
[18] *Ibid*, para 60.
[19] *Ibid*, para 61–75.
[20] *Ibid*, para 76.

introduce a reporting obligation that falls primarily on the promoter.[21] Where the primary reporting obligation fell on the promoter, it was recommended that the reporting obligation would switch to the taxpayer where the promoter was offshore, or where there was no promoter or the promoter asserted legal professional privilege. Countries were free to introduce their own definition of promoter or advisor but some guidelines were given.[22]

As for the question of 'what has to be reported', countries could adopt a single-step approach or a multi-step or threshold approach in defining the scope of a disclosure regime.[23] A de minimis filter was also considered as an alternative to, or in addition to, a broader threshold test and could operate to remove smaller transactions, below a certain amount. This would narrow the ambit of the mandatory disclosure regime and reduce the risk of over-disclosure.[24]

The Mandatory Discussion Draft analysed the concept of the hallmark as a tool to identify the features of schemes that tax administrations were interested in. There could be both generic and specific hallmarks. Generic hallmarks would target features that were common to promoted schemes, such as the requirement for confidentiality or the payment of a premium fee. Generic hallmarks would be used to capture new and innovative tax planning arrangements that might be easily replicated and sold to a variety of taxpayers. Specific hallmarks would be used to target known vulnerabilities in the tax system and techniques that were commonly used in tax avoidance arrangements such as the use of losses.[25] Generic hallmarks might increase the amount of reportable transactions and as a corollary taxpayer costs. By contrast, specific hallmarks or listed transactions would allow tax administrations to target known or common areas of risk and provide flexibility in terms of enabling a tax administration to strike a balance between costs and capacity issues.[26]

In introducing mandatory disclosure regimes, countries had the option to use either a single-step approach or a multi-step/threshold approach. It was, however, recommended that mandatory disclosure regimes should include a mixture of generic and specific hallmarks.[27] Countries could choose whether or not to adopt a hypothetical approach or adopt purely factual objectives tests.[28] When a scheme or transaction triggered one hallmark, that should be sufficient to require disclosure.[29]

[21] *Ibid.*
[22] *Ibid*, para 77 referring to principles set out in para 71.
[23] *Ibid*, paras 78–86.
[24] *Ibid*, paras 87–90.
[25] See paras 91–92 et seq.
[26] *Ibid*, para 132–33.
[27] *Ibid*, para 135. It was noted that generic hallmarks should include a confidentiality and premium/contingent fee hallmark. A country may also want to adopt additional generic hallmarks such as the one applying to standardised tax products.
[28] *Ibid*, para 136.
[29] *Ibid*, para 137.

As for the question of 'when information should be reported', there were two suggested options. There could be a timeframe linked to the availability of a scheme or a timeframe linked to its implementation.[30] It was recommended that where the promoter had the obligation to disclose, then the timeframe for disclosure should be linked to the availability of the scheme. A short timescale for reporting a scheme was recommended.[31] Where a taxpayer had the obligation to disclose it was recommended that the disclosure should be triggered by the implementation rather than the availability of a scheme.[32]

As far as the consequences of compliance and non-compliance with the reporting requirements, it was recommended that countries should be explicit in their domestic law about the consequences of reporting a scheme or transaction under a disclosure regime ie that this does not imply acceptance of the scheme or its purported benefits. Furthermore, in order to enforce compliance with mandatory disclosure rules, countries should introduce financial penalties that would apply if there was failure to comply with any of the obligations introduced. Countries were free to introduce penalty provisions (including non-monetary penalties) aligned with their general domestic law provisions.[33]

Thereafter, there was a comprehensive analysis of procedural and tax administration matters. Recommendations were made as to what information tax administrations should require a promoter or taxpayer to disclose.[34]

As for international tax schemes, changes to the design of a disclosure regime were recommended in order to better target cross-border tax planning. Inter alia, hallmarks should be developed which focus on the specific risks posed by cross-border tax planning but which are wide enough to capture different and innovative tax planning techniques (cross-border outcomes). There should be a broad definition of arrangement that would treat any arrangement involving a domestic taxpayer as a reportable scheme where that arrangement included a cross-border outcome (regardless of the jurisdiction where that outcome arose). Threshold conditions may need to be removed. There was a comprehensive review of the suggestions in chapter IV of the Mandatory Disclosure Discussion Draft.[35]

The final work on Action 12 was to be completed by September 2015. Interested parties were invited to send comments on this discussion draft.

[30] *Ibid*, para 140.

[31] *Ibid*, para 156.

[32] *Ibid*, para 157. If only the taxpayer disclosed (ie because there was no promoter or the promoter was offshore) the timescale for reporting was recommended to be short to maximise the tax administration's ability to act against a scheme quickly.

[33] *Ibid*, paras 174–200.

[34] *Ibid*, paras 220–222. It was recommended that the information should include: the identification of promoters and scheme users; the details of the provisions that make the scheme reportable; a description of the arrangements and the name by which they are known (if any); details of the statutory provisions on which the tax advantage was based; a description of the tax benefit or advantage; a list of clients (promoter only) where domestic law allows it, and the amount of expected tax benefit. In addition, any mandatory disclosure provisions would need to be supported by information powers necessary to enable a tax administration to enquire into the reasons for a failure to disclose, or enquire into the identity of promoters and intermediaries or request follow-up information etc.

[35] *Ibid*, paras 223–74.

It has been argued that an effort should be made so that mandatory disclosure rules do not just focus on small and medium-sized enterprises and wealthy individuals, but also cover MNEs. Existing domestic rules tend to target standard schemes which are widely marketed by promoters, whereas MNEs generally use arrangements tailored to their specific needs, even if based on standard techniques. The BEPS Monitoring Group gave as an example the tax clearances arranged by PwC in Luxembourg over a period of eight years for 343 MNEs that were not notified under the UK's disclosure regime.[36] The Group has urged for any disclosure rules to be adapted to international corporate tax avoidance and to include hallmarks to that effect. 'Like all methods of improving compliance, mandatory disclosure must balance deterrence with cooperation. However, there should be safeguards against the pitfalls experienced by some forms of "cooperative compliance", which have led to public concerns about "sweetheart deals"'.[37] Provisions for access to information derived from notification by a wide range of other tax authorities, and standards for reporting to the public of information and data from disclosure arrangements would help.[38] Such measures would not only improve transparency but also facilitate the independent evaluation of the effects of mandatory disclosure schemes.

4.3. Action 13: Re-Examine Transfer Pricing Documentation

Under Action 13 of the Action Plan, the OECD is to:

> Develop rules regarding transfer pricing documentation to enhance transparency for tax administration, taking into account the compliance costs for business. The rules to be developed [would] include a requirement that MNEs provide all relevant governments with needed information on their global allocation of the income, economic activity and taxes paid among countries according to a common template.

In January 2014, the OECD released a discussion draft on a proposed template for country-by-country reporting to tax authorities—the CbC Discussion Draft.[39] This elaborated on the OECD's White Paper on Transfer Pricing Documentation[40] which had been released on 30 July 2013. The CbC Discussion Draft contained an initial draft of the revised guidance on transfer pricing documentation and

[36] BEPS Monitoring Group, *Comments on BEPS Action 12: Mandatory Disclosure Rules*, available on: bepsmonitoringgroup.files.wordpress.com/2015/05/ap12-mandatory-disclosure-rules.pdf.

[37] *Ibid*, p 1.

[38] *Ibid*.

[39] OECD, *Discussion Draft on Transfer Pricing Documentation and CbC Reporting* (30 January 2014). Available on: www.oecd.org/ctp/transfer-pricing/discussion-draft-transfer-pricing-documentation.pdf.

[40] OECD, *White Paper on Transfer Pricing Documentation*. Available on: www.oecd.org/ctp/transfer-pricing/white-paper-transfer-pricing-documentation.pdf.

country-by-country reporting, and was intended to replace Chapter V of the existing OECD Transfer Pricing Guidelines. As reflected in earlier proposals, the OECD followed a two-tier approach that would involve a global master file, together with local country files.

In the CbC Discussion Draft, it was proposed that the master file should include comprehensive information about the global operations of an MNE and should contain standardised information relevant to all MNE group members.[41] Although the country-by-country data required in the master file may be helpful for risk assessment processes, nevertheless, such information should not be used as a substitute for a detailed transfer pricing analysis of individual transactions and prices.[42]

The local country files would include transactional information relevant to each country. As a result, MNEs would be required to provide extensive information for each entity in the group. The information required in the local file would supplement the master file and would be relevant to the transfer pricing analysis. Such information would include relevant financial information, a comparability analysis and the selection and application of the most appropriate transfer pricing method.[43] Although the CbC Discussion Draft provided for the country-by-country template to be included in the master file, it sought stakeholders' comments on whether the template should instead be provided to tax authorities as a separate document.[44]

In the CbC Discussion Draft it was recommended that transfer pricing documentation requirements should include specific materiality thresholds.[45] Also, the documentation ought to be periodically reviewed, probably annually, in order to determine whether functional and economic analyses are still accurate and relevant and to confirm the validity of the applied transfer pricing methodology.[46]

As a general matter, the CbC Discussion Draft recommended that the master file should be prepared and submitted to all tax administrations in English. However, it was noted that transfer pricing documentation must be useful to local country tax administrations seeking to undertake a risk assessment, so at least the

[41] As stated in paragraph 19 of the CbC Discussion Draft, n 39 above, the information required in the master file would provide a 'blueprint' of the MNE group and contain relevant information that can be grouped in five categories: (a) the MNE group's organisational structure; (b) a description of the MNE's business or businesses; (c) the MNE's intangibles; (d) the MNE's intercompany financial activities; and (e) the MNE's financial and tax positions. See, also, suggested template in Annex I.

[42] CbC Discussion Draft, n 39 above, para 21.

[43] See para 23 and the suggested template in Annex II of the CbC Discussion Draft, n 39 above.

[44] *Ibid*, para 20.

[45] *Ibid*, para 29. These materiality requirements should take into account the size and nature of the local economy, the importance of the MNE group in that economy, and the size and nature of local operating entities, in addition to the overall size and nature of the MNE group.

[46] *Ibid*, para 33. In order to simplify the compliance burden, it was suggested that when operating conditions remain unchanged, the searches in databases for comparables supporting part of the local file should be updated every three years rather than annually. However, financial data for the comparables should nonetheless be updated every year. See para 34 in CbC Discussion Draft, n 39 above.

local file should be prepared in the relevant local language.[47] The use of penalties for non-compliance was also recommended,[48] as well as compliance incentives such as penalty protection or a shift in the burden of proof.[49]

As far as confidentiality was concerned, tax administrations were encouraged to ensure that there was no public disclosure of trade secrets, scientific secrets, or other confidential information. Tax administrations were also encouraged to use discretion in requesting this type of information and to assure taxpayers that the information presented in the documentation would remain confidential.[50] Transfer pricing documentation requirements were features of local law and should continue to be so. Therefore, in order to implement the recommended two-tiered approach, countries would have to modify their domestic laws in line with these recommendations[51] to adopt consistent and uniform formats.[52]

Comments were requested regarding the most appropriate mechanism for making the master file and country-by-country reporting template available to relevant tax administrations.[53] Possibilities included the direct local filing of information by MNE group members subject to tax in the jurisdiction, or the filing of information in the parent company's jurisdiction and the sharing of it under treaty information exchange provisions or some combination of the above.

During the consultation period,[54] the CbC Discussion Draft was criticised in that it would generate compliance costs and that the reporting standards went beyond what governments needed for transfer pricing risk assessment. The business community complained about the enormous quantity of data requested. It was argued that much of the data requested was not relevant to a transfer pricing analysis based on the arm's length standard. Moreover, it was feared that by providing local tax administrations with all this data, it would 'lead to individual tax authorities applying a formulary apportionment standard, rather than the arm's-length standard'.[55] It was recommended that the country report be limited to high-level data only, which was required to establish the footprint of an MNE.[56]

[47] *Ibid*, para 35.

[48] *Ibid*, paras 36–40.

[49] *Ibid*, para 40. Also see para 38, where countries were discouraged from imposing sizeable documentation-related penalties on taxpayers that made a reasonable effort, in good faith, to demonstrate through reliable documentation that their controlled transactions satisfy the arm's length principle.

[50] *Ibid*, para 41.

[51] *Ibid*, para 44.

[52] *Ibid*, para 45.

[53] *Ibid*.

[54] See, generally, comments received on the CbC Discussion Draft, published by the OECD. Available on: www.oecd.org/ctp/transfer-pricing/comments-discussion-draft-transfer-pricing-documentation.htm.

[55] Lee A Sheppard, 'OECD BEPS Country-by-Country Reporting Is Too Burdensome, HMRC Official Says', 2014 *WTD* 28-1 (11 February 2014). Also see Mindy Herzfeld, 'Country-by-Country Reporting—Drawing the Battle Lines', 2014 *WTD* 46-2 (10 March 2014); Mindy Herzfeld, 'Country-by-Country Reporting—The Debate Rages on', 2014 *WTD* 101-2 (27 May 2014).

[56] Margaret Burow, 'Stakeholders Find Common Ground on OECD Country-By-Country Reporting Draft', Tax Analysts, 2014 *WTD* 51-3 (17 March 2014).

In addition, most of the business community were in favour of a materiality threshold but stressed the importance of a clear definition of materiality. It was also suggested that for some EU headquartered MNEs, the compliance burden was exacerbated by the differences between the EU transfer pricing standards and the OECD standards.[57]

Confidentiality was also a concern, if the master file and the country-by-country reporting template were to be shared with a local tax authority. This was because some tax authorities have no confidentiality provisions under their local laws, or under tax treaties, if there are any. Some of the data in the country-by-country template might be sensitive and as such its disclosure ought to be limited, protected and monitored. The preference by multinationals was for this type of information to be shared under the exchange of information provisions of treaty networks. It was argued by many that the best place to file the master file and country-by-country template was with the home taxing authority and should only be shared through the exchange of information provisions.[58] Businesses also showed concerns as to how the contents of the country-by-country report would be used and how disputes would be resolved to avoid multiple layers of taxation.[59]

By contrast, several advocacy groups and NGOs argued that the OECD did not go far enough in mandating disclosure of information that would reduce cross-border tax evasion.[60] There was preference for a general disclosure standard for all large transnational corporations.[61] Confidentiality ought to be restricted only to information crucial for business operations and success. It was even argued that it should be made as easy as possible for local tax authorities to obtain access to information and for the information provided to be allowed to be used for purposes other than income tax reporting.[62] China also advocated direct filing to countries as the preferred alternative.[63]

In March 2014, it was revealed that to ease the compliance burden, the OECD would change the proposed country-by-country reporting template to require aggregate country-wide reporting instead of entity-by-entity reporting.[64]

[57] Herzfeld, 'Country-by-Country Reporting—Drawing the Battle Lines', n 55 above. On the EU standards, see section 6.7 in Ch 6 of this volume.

[58] *Ibid.* Also see Dana Glenn, 'Costs and Confidentiality Are Biggest Concerns With OECD Discussion Draft, Practitioners Say', 2014 *WTD* 32-2 (18 February 2014).

[59] Margaret Burow, 'Dispute Resolution Tops Business Community's Concerns with Country-By-Country Reporting', Tax Analysts, 2014 *WTD* 108-7 (5 June 2014).

[60] Herzfeld, 'Country-by-Country Reporting—Drawing the Battle Lines', n 55 above.

[61] See, for example, comments of the BEPS Monitoring Group, *Response to OECD Discussion Draft on Transfer Pricing and Documentation and Country-by-Country Reporting*, pp 1–2. Available on: bepsmonitoringgroup.files.wordpress.com/2014/03/bmg-cbc-response1.pdf.

[62] Also see comments from Christian Aid and Oxfam, reported in Tax Analysts, respectively, by Herzfeld, 'Country-by-Country Reporting—Drawing the Battle Lines', n 55 above and Stephanie Soong Johnston, 'Stakeholders Lock Horns Over Execution of OECD's CbC Reporting Proposal', 2014 *WTD* 97-3 (20 May 2014).

[63] Herzfeld, 'Country-by-Country Reporting—The Debate Rages on', n 55 above.

[64] William R Davis, 'Changes Coming to OECD Country-by-Country Reporting Template', 2014 *WTD* 62-1 (1 April 2014).

Furthermore, in May 2014, the OECD held a public consultation which helped address some of the concerns of various stakeholders. It was reported[65] that taxpayers would be given flexibility in the sources of data they can use in preparing the recommended transfer pricing documentation. The amount of information requested by the templates would be reduced, and small and medium-sized enterprises would be excluded from the more burdensome filing requirements. Information would be requested only on a consolidated basis by country[66] and the master file and country-by-country report would be kept separately. All other issues remained unresolved.[67]

What was certain was that the evolution of the process of developing reporting requirements and mechanisms was perceived to be critical to advancing the BEPS project.[68] While it might also benefit transfer pricing practitioners and tax administrators,[69] there were doubts as to whether in fact country-by-country reporting would discourage MNEs from profit shifting.[70] There were also concerns that the costs of country-by-country reporting would exceed the benefits. In fact, country-by-country reporting could become particularly expensive if it was based on a new set of reporting rules very different from existing financial and tax accounting rules and if companies considered it necessary to justify and explain extensively their reports to the public.[71]

With hindsight of the comments received, in its subsequent report released on 16 September 2014 (the CbC Revised Discussion Draft),[72] the OECD moved from a two-tier to a three-tier approach. The three-tier approach comprised a master file, a local file, and a separate country-by-country template that had been proposed

[65] It was reported that the OECD released confidential copies of a revised draft on Action 13 in advance of the 19 May 2014 public consultation. See Margaret Burow, 'Tax Analysts Exclusive: Revised Transfer Pricing Discussion Draft Kept under Wraps', 2014 *WTD* 103-1 (29 May 2014).

[66] As noted by Burow, there was a new paragraph in the revised draft stating that taxpayers would have the option to prepare the master file either for the MNE group as a whole or by line of business or product group, depending on which presentation would provide the most relevant transfer pricing information to tax administrators. Burow, 'Tax Analysts Exclusive: Revised Transfer Pricing Discussion Draft Kept under Wraps', n 65 above.

[67] Regarding the issue of the language for the local file, see Amanda Athanasiou, 'Language for Local File Lost in Translation at Consultation on Transfer Pricing Discussion Draft', 2014 *WTD* 101-1 (27 May 2014).

[68] Marie Sapirie, 'A Preview of Country-by-Country Reporting', 2013 *WTD* 203-2 (21 October 2013).

[69] Mindy Herzfeld, 'An Alternative View of Country-by-Country Reporting', 2014 *WTD* 76-3 (21 April 2014).

[70] Maria Theresia Evers, Ina Meier and Christoph Spengel, 'Transparency in Financial Reporting: Is Country-by-Country Reporting Suitable To Combat International Profit Shifting?' (2014) 68 *Bulletin for International Taxation* 296.

[71] *Ibid*, citing Michael Devereux, *Transparency in Reporting Financial Data by Multinational Corporations*, Project Report, Oxford University Centre for Business Taxation, p 24 et seq (2011).

[72] See OECD, *Guidance on Transfer Pricing Documentation and Country-by-Country Reporting* (2014). Available on: www.oecd.org/tax/guidance-on-transfer-pricing-documentation-and-country-by-country-reporting-9789264219236-en.htm. For commentary, see inter alia, Andrew Casley, Kevin Norton and Michael Krhoda, 'The OECD's New Transfer Pricing Documentation Standard: An Overview and Possible UK Implementation' (2015) 22 *International Transfer Pricing Journal* 3–10.

in the OECD's earlier work on this topic. The country-by-country information was to be reported to tax authorities at a very high level and for risk assessment only. The amount of information being requested for risk assessment purposes was significantly curtailed and the standards for transfer pricing documentation were revised under the CbC Revised Discussion Draft.

MNEs would be required to file a master file containing a high-level overview of their global operations and transfer pricing policies. This would be available to all relevant country tax administrations.[73] It is obvious that the OECD steered the master file towards being a high-level general document.

There would also be a local file which provides detailed information concerning specific intercompany transactions. The requirements of the local file have also been refined. The local file would focus 'on information relevant to the transfer pricing analysis related to transactions taking place between a local country affiliate and associated enterprises in different countries and which are material in the context of the local country's tax system'.[74] In determining what transactions would need to be part of the local file, tax jurisdictions had to draft materiality standards that were objective, commonly understood and accepted in commercial practice.

The description of the local file requirements was refined. The detailed data requirements for each 'material category of controlled transactions' of the local entity now required, inter alia, copies of material intercompany agreements, copies of advance pricing agreements and other tax rulings to which the local tax authority was not a party, an indication of the most appropriate transfer pricing method with regard to the category of transaction, a summary of the important assumptions made in applying the transfer pricing methodology, etc.[75]

The country-by-country report would be based on a common template and would give all countries a broad picture of how a company operated. It required aggregate tax jurisdiction-wide information on the global allocation of the MNE's income, taxes paid, and certain indicators of the location of economic activity within the MNE group. It also required MNEs to report their total employment capital, retained earnings and tangible assets in each tax jurisdiction. Furthermore, MNEs had to identify each entity within the group doing business in a tax jurisdiction and to provide an indication of the business activities each entity was engaged in.[76]

It was expressly stated that the country-by-country report would be used as a high-level risk assessment tool and not as the basis to propose transfer

[73] See paras 18–21 of new Chapter V of OECD Transfer Pricing Guidelines, set out in the CbC Revised Discussion Draft, n 72 above.

[74] *Ibid*, para 22 of new Chapter V of OECD Transfer Pricing Guidelines.

[75] See Annex II to Chapter V Transfer pricing documentation—Local file, set out in p 31 et seq in the CbC Revised Discussion Draft, n 72 above.

[76] *Ibid*, paras 24–26 of new Chapter V of OECD Transfer Pricing Guidelines.

pricing adjustments using a global formulary apportionment of income.[77] Tax administrations should also take reasonable steps to ensure that the information was not released to the public.[78]

Arguably, the final version of the template was designed to highlight those low-tax jurisdictions where a significant amount of income was allocated, without some 'proportionate' presence of employees.[79] There was likely to be increased pressure to ensure that profit allocations to a particular jurisdiction were supported by the location in that state of sufficient and appropriately qualified employees, making a substantial contribution to the creation and development of intangibles.[80]

Also, transfer pricing documentation was to be submitted to tax administrations in the language established under local laws, but tax jurisdictions were encouraged to permit filing in commonly used languages if this did not compromise the usefulness of the documents.[81] Where tax administrations believed that translation of documents was necessary, they should make specific requests for translation and provide sufficient time to make such translation as comfortable a burden as possible.[82]

It was uncertain and open for discussion how the master file and country-by-country report, once prepared, would be shared among participating country tax authorities. Concerns had already been noted about the confidentiality of the data. The CbC Revised Discussion Draft stipulated that tax administrations should take all reasonable steps to ensure that there was no public disclosure of confidential information and other commercially sensitive information contained in the documentation package. Tax administrations should also assure taxpayers that the information presented in transfer pricing documentation would remain confidential.[83] This stipulation was in rather vague terms and did not meet the concerns of stakeholders for more certainty. The CbC Revised Discussion Draft referred to the OECD Guide 'Keeping It Safe' on the protection of confidentiality.[84] This contained useful guidelines which were more suitable to bilateral scenarios and not necessarily tailored to the multi-jurisdictional reporting context envisaged in the CbC Revised Discussion Draft. There were indications that information would

[77] *Ibid*, para 25 of new Chapter V of OECD Transfer Pricing Guidelines. For a discussion of the concerns that the information provided under country-by-country reporting might lead to formulary apportionment see Maria Amparo Grau Ruiz, 'Country-by-Country Reporting: The Primary Concerns Raised by a Dynamic Approach' (2014) 68 *Bulletin for International Taxation* 557–66.

[78] See paras 18–21 of new Chapter V of OECD Transfer Pricing Guidelines, set out in the CbC Revised Discussion Draft, n 72 above.

[79] Richard Collier and Philip Greenfield, 'Thoughtful commentary—by tax experts, for tax experts', *Tax Journal*, Issue 1232, p 8 (26 September 2014) pp 10–11.

[80] *Ibid*.

[81] See CbC Revised Discussion Draft, n 72 above, para 29.

[82] *Ibid*, para 39.

[83] *Ibid*, para 44. Where disclosure was required in public judicial decisions, every effort should be made to ensure that confidentiality would be maintained and that information would be disclosed only to the extent needed.

[84] *Ibid*, para 45. The OECD Guide 'Keeping It Safe' is available on: www.oecd.org/ctp/exchange-of-tax-information/keeping-it-safe-report.pdf.

only be exchanged pursuant to treaty or tax information exchange agreement provisions.[85]

The above new guidelines were to be reviewed before the end of 2020 to determine their effectiveness and whether to add transactional reporting of payments of interest, royalties and service fees between associated enterprises. This was something requested by Argentina, Brazil, China, India, South Africa, Turkey and other emerging economies.

On 6 February 2015, the OECD released a follow-up report on Action 13 (the CBC Follow-Up Discussion Draft), which provided some much-anticipated guidance on the implementation of country-by-country reporting.[86] It dealt with the following four issues: (i) the timing of preparation and filing of the country-by-country report; (ii) which MNE groups should be required to file the country-by-country report; (iii) the necessary conditions underpinning the obtaining and the use of the country-by-country report by jurisdictions; and (iv) the framework for government-to-government mechanisms to exchange country-by-country reports, together with the work plan for developing an implementation package.[87]

As regards filing, periods within the scope of country-by-country reporting would be those beginning on or after 1 January 2016. As companies would have 12 months to file the report, the first filings would be due by 31 December 2017.[88] There was an exemption for groups with an annual consolidated group revenue of less than €750 million. There were no other exemptions. The threshold would be reviewed in the overall 2020 review.[89]

Three conditions were outlined for countries obtaining and using the country-by-country report: confidentiality, consistency and appropriate use.[90] Countries should have in place and enforce legal protections for the confidentiality of the reported information.[91] They should use the template provided in the CbC Revised Discussion Draft—they should not require more or less information than in the template. Countries were reminded of the appropriate use of the

[85] See PwC Tax Policy Bulletin, 'OECD finalises guidance on transfer pricing documentation and country-by-country reporting', p 5, available on: download.pwc.com/ie/pubs/2014 pwc ireland oecd guidance-tp-and-cbc-reporting-25-09-2014.pdf.

[86] *Action 13: Guidance on the Implementation of Transfer Pricing Documentation and Country-by-Country Reporting.* Available on: www.oecd.org/ctp/beps-action-13-guidance-implementation-tp-documentation-cbc-reporting.pdf. For commentary, see Amanda Athanasiou, 'OECD Releases Implementation Guidance for CbC Reporting', 2015 *WTD* 26-3 (9 February 2015).

[87] CbC Follow-Up Discussion Draft, n 86 above, para 4.

[88] *Ibid*, para 7.

[89] *Ibid*, paras 8–12.

[90] *Ibid*, para 13.

[91] As noted in para 13, '[s]uch protections would preserve the confidentiality of the CbC Report to an extent at least equivalent to the protections that would apply if such information were delivered to the country under the provisions of the Multilateral Convention on Mutual Administrative Assistance in Tax Matters, a TIEA or a tax treaty that meets the internationally agreed standard of information upon request as reviewed by the Global Forum on Transparency and Exchange of Information for Tax Purposes. Such protections include limitation of the use of information, rules on the persons to whom the information may be disclosed, ordre public, etc'.

country-by-country report: it should only be used to assess high-level transfer pricing risk.

The guidance indicated that the ultimate parent of the group that meets the revenue threshold would be required to file the report in its home state. This home state would exchange the information on an automatic basis with other countries in which the MNE operates and that meet the above conditions. If a country failed to provide information to another jurisdiction that meets the conditions, a secondary mechanism would be accepted as appropriate, through local filing or by moving the obligation of requiring the filing of the country-by-country reports and automatically exchanging these reports with the next tier parent country.[92]

As part of an implementation package, the OECD has agreed to develop further guidance on the key elements of statutory legislation that countries would be able to adopt for use in their own legal systems. It would also develop implementing arrangements for the automatic exchange of the country-by-country reports under international agreements, bilateral and multilateral.[93]

While these clarifications were welcomed, country-by-country reporting was still criticised for the complexity it would bring to corporate tax departments. Notwithstanding some of the refinements made, the proposed measures continue to be heavily skewed towards tax authorities. There is a concern that country-by-country reporting will be further expanded, particularly in developing countries. Furthermore, sensitive information may still be leaked to the public and some jurisdictions may not have the capability to use and understand the information. In fact, confidentiality risks are higher when large volumes of information are exchanged.[94] There are concerns that the US might stop sending information if EU law were changed to make tax information not confidential.[95] It has also been noted that new reporting requirements are likely to change taxpayer behaviour. For example, as advance pricing agreements must be reported in the master file, they may not remain an attractive option for taxpayers.[96] Moreover, it has been argued that data gathered through country-by-country reporting would not suffice to give a full picture of the size and scope of BEPS. Action 11 is likely to be crucial to the success of the overall BEPS project.[97]

Another issue that still remains to be clarified is how an MNE group would be defined. Again, there does not seem to be a clear consensus on the meaning of an

[92] *Ibid*, para 14.

[93] *Ibid*, para 15. For a discussion on the challenges that the OECD will face in getting the USA and other jurisdictions to implement country-by-country reporting, see Mindy Herzfeld, 'Implementing CbC Reporting (or Not) in the United States', 2015 *WTD* 35-2 (23 February 2015).

[94] Marie Sapirie, 'US Expresses Concerns About Country-By-Country Reporting', 2015 *WTD* 37-3 (25 February 2015). Also see Mindy Herzfeld, 'Implementing CbC Reporting (or Not) in the United States', n 93 above.

[95] Lee A Sheppard, 'BEPS Overwhelming Tax Administration', 2015 *WTD* 74-1 (17 April 2015).

[96] See Margaret Burow, 'BEPS could be a "nightmare" for corporate tax departments', 2015 *WTD* 31-5 (17 February 2015).

[97] Stephanie Soong Johnston and David D Stewart, 'CbC Reporting a Good Start but Not Enough to Analyse BEPS', 2015 *WTD* 96-1 (19 May 2015).

MNE, not just in the context of Action 13 but also in the context of the whole of the BEPS project.[98] If the new transfer pricing documentation requirements are to apply to MNEs solely on the basis of national laws and, to an extent, national definitions of control, then any benefits that might accrue to tax authorities and businesses from country-by-country reporting would be greatly diminished. Different definitions of control might lead to divergent reporting needs in different jurisdictions—double reporting or double non-reporting. That would render the deliverables under Action 13 a Pyrrhic victory.

4.4. Action 14: Make Dispute Resolution Mechanisms More Effective

Action 14 considers how to improve dispute resolution mechanisms. It reads as follows:

> Develop solutions to address obstacles that prevent countries from solving treaty-related disputes under MAP [Mutual Agreement Procedure], including the absence of arbitration provisions in most treaties and the fact that access to MAP and arbitration may be denied in certain cases.

Unlike the other Action items, Action 14 does not deal with problems of base erosion and profit shifting, but instead with taxpayer problems which in the post-BEPS world are likely to increase and require improved dispute resolution mechanisms. The Action Plan recognises that the actions to counter BEPS must be complemented with actions to ensure certainty and predictability for businesses. The OECD had looked at this issue previously, resulting for example in its Manual on Effective Mutual Agreement Procedures (MEMAP).

On 18 December 2014, the OECD released a discussion draft examining how to make dispute resolution mechanisms more effective.[99] The Dispute Resolution Discussion Draft recognised that the BEPS project presented a unique opportunity to make a difference in this area and to overcome traditional obstacles. Although there was no consensus on moving towards universal mandatory binding arbitration, it was recommended that complementary solutions should be provided which would have a practical, measurable impact.[100]

This Dispute Resolution Discussion Draft was the preliminary result of the work done to identify comprehensively the obstacles that prevented countries from resolving disputes through the mutual agreement procedure (MAP) and

[98] Mindy Herzfeld, 'What is an MNE Group? The Scope of CbC Reporting' (2015) 78 *Tax Notes International* 204 (20 April 2015).

[99] OECD, *BEPS Action 14: Make Dispute Resolution Mechanisms more Effective.* Available on: www.oecd.org/ctp/dispute/discussion-draft-action-14-make-dispute-resolution-mechanisms-more-effective.pdf.

[100] *Ibid*, para 3.

to develop possible measures to address these obstacles. It must be read in the broader context of the intention to introduce a three-pronged approach designed to represent a step change in the resolution of treaty-related disputes through the MAP. This three-pronged approach would consist first, in political commitments to effectively eliminate taxation not in accordance with the Convention; secondly, provide new measures to improve access to the MAP and improved procedures; and thirdly, establish a monitoring mechanism to check the proper implementation of the political commitment.[101]

It was expected that the work on Action 14 would result in a political commitment to substantially improve the MAP process. The political commitment and the measures through which it would be implemented would be guided by the following four principles:

1. Ensuring that treaty obligations related to the mutual agreement procedure are fully implemented in good faith.
2. Ensuring that administrative processes promote the prevention and resolution of treaty-related disputes.
3. Ensuring that taxpayers can access the mutual agreement procedure when eligible.
4. Ensuring that cases are resolved once they are in the mutual agreement procedure.

For each of the above four principles, the Dispute Resolution Discussion Draft listed obstacles that might prevent the principle from being fully implemented and put forward options as to how these obstacles could be addressed.

It was stated that specific measures would constitute a minimum standard to which participating countries would commit.[102] Also, the final results of the work on Action 14 would include additional measures that some countries may commit to adopt in order to address obstacles to an effective MAP in a more comprehensive way. There would be monitoring of the overall functioning of the MAP process, including assessment of the measures to which countries had committed.[103]

One obstacle to ensuring that treaty obligations related to MAP were fully implemented in good faith was the absence of an obligation to resolve MAP cases under Article 25. The importance of resolving cases under MAP could be clarified in the treaty commentary.[104] Another potential obstacle was the absence of paragraph 2 of Article 9 of the OECD Model in some treaties, which caused some countries to take the position that they were not obliged to make corresponding adjustments following a primary transfer pricing adjustment by a treaty partner. Thus, treaties could be amended to specifically include Article 9(2).[105]

[101] *Ibid.*
[102] *Ibid*, para 7.
[103] *Ibid*, para 8.
[104] *Ibid*, para 10.
[105] *Ibid*, para 11.

Moreover, the effectiveness of MAP may be undermined by a variety of factors, such as the lack of independence of the competent authority and inappropriate influence of considerations related to the negotiation of possible treaty changes,[106] lack of resources,[107] or inappropriate performance indicators for the competent authority function and staff.[108] In addition, competent authorities may not actively use their authority under Article 25(3) of the OECD Model to try reaching a mutual agreement on matters of a general nature involving treaty interpretation or application.[109] Finally, field auditors in some countries may seek to enter into audit settlements requiring a taxpayer to forego access to MAP, and some countries may not have implemented bilateral advance pricing arrangement programs.[110] Addressing each of these shortcomings could help ensure an environment in which competent authorities are able to fully and effectively carry out their mandate.

It was important to ensure that taxpayers could access MAP when eligible. Obstacles to MAP access included, inter alia, the complexity and lack of transparency of the procedures to access and use MAP,[111] excessive or unduly onerous documentation requirements,[112] time limits to access MAP[113] and the requirement that the disputed tax be paid in order to access MAP.[114] Also, the right to access MAP might be unclear when domestic or treaty-based anti-abuse rules or remedies have been applied. MAP access might also be denied by the unilateral decision of one competent authority that a taxpayer's objection was not justified.

Certain of the main obstacles to the resolution of treaty-related disputes through MAP were issues related to MAP processes—'i.e. procedural and other blockages that impede the timely and effective resolution of MAP cases that have been accepted for bilateral competent authority consideration'.[115] These included the lack of a principled approach to the resolution of MAP cases,[116] lack of co-operation, transparency or good competent authority working relationships,[117] and the absence of a mechanism, such as MAP arbitration, to ensure the resolution of all MAP cases.[118] In addition, it was questioned how to address issues related to multilateral MAPs and APAs which deviated from the traditionally bilateral MAP.[119] Issues related to the consideration of interest and penalties in MAP were also of significant importance.[120]

[106] *Ibid*, paras 14–15.
[107] *Ibid*, para 16.
[108] *Ibid*, para 17.
[109] *Ibid*, para 18.
[110] *Ibid*, paras 19–23.
[111] *Ibid*, para 25.
[112] *Ibid*, paras 26–27.
[113] *Ibid*, para 34.
[114] *Ibid*, para 33.
[115] *Ibid*, para 36.
[116] *Ibid*, paras 37–38.
[117] *Ibid*, para 39.
[118] *Ibid*, paras 41–45.
[119] *Ibid*, paras 58–59.
[120] *Ibid*, para 60.

The Dispute Resolution Discussion Draft explored various options for improving these issues within the MAP process, though it refrained from making any strong recommendations. The solutions proposed were primarily in the form of suggestions for amending the treaty commentary or statements regarding what different tax administrations could commit to, in order to advance dispute resolution procedures.[121] Furthermore, the monitoring process would include assessment of the measures to which countries had committed. It was envisaged that an appropriate forum of competent authorities could be responsible for such monitoring. Such a forum would also facilitate experience sharing and capacity building and, more generally, work to foster co-operative and collaborative competent authority relationships.[122]

The various options suggested were criticised as being under-developed.[123] Perhaps the disappointing aspect of the Dispute Resolution Discussion Draft was that there was no consensus on moving towards mandatory arbitration.[124] Enhanced dispute resolution options such as administrative appeals, mediation and arbitration, as well as alternative means of preventing and resolving disputes and audits should also have been developed. Without such changes, there is a real prospect of a dramatic increase of disputes leading to double taxation.

The BEPS Monitoring Group[125] welcomed the statement that disputes should be resolved in a 'principled, fair and objective manner', but urged for these criteria to be explained in more detail in the Commentary.[126] Transparency, including publication of decisions, was very important. Also, the rules themselves should be capable of being applied consistently and objectively, rather than leave wide scope for interpretation. 'Rules which give decision makers wide scope for interpretation, or which permit a variety of acceptable alternatives, do not lend themselves to

[121] It was also noted that administrative processes that promoted the prevention and resolution of treaty-related disputes were being comprehensively examined in the parallel work being undertaken by the Forum on Tax Administration's MAP forum.

[122] See para 8 of the Dispute Resolution Discussion Draft, n 99 above.

[123] For a comprehensive analysis, see the KPMG submission, available on: www.kpmg.com/Global/en/IssuesAndInsights/ArticlesPublications/taxnewsflash/Documents/kpmgcomments-beps14-jan19-2015.pdf.

For all the comments received on this action, see OECD website: www.oecd.org/tax/dispute/public-comments-action-14-make-dispute-resolution-mechanisms-more-effective.pdf.

[124] Kristen A Parillo, 'OECD Proposes Improvements to Treaty Dispute Resolution Process', 2014 *WTD* 244-2 (22 December 2014).

[125] See BEPS Monitoring Group, *Comments on BEPS Action 14: Make Dispute Resolution Mechanisms More Effective*. Available on: bepsmonitoringgroup.files.wordpress.com/2015/01/ap-14-dispute-resolution.pdf.

[126] The suggested explanation to accompany these criteria was the following: '*principled*: this requires that outcomes should take the form of reasoned decisions, based on analysis of the facts of the case, the applicable rules and how they have been interpreted and applied to the specific case; *fair*: like cases should be treated alike, and decisions should be published, to ensure consistency; *objective*: decision-makers should be independent of the disputing parties and have no vested interests or conflicts of interest; and rules to be applied should be formulated so as to be easily applicable to specific cases based as far as possible on their facts rather than requiring value-judgments': *ibid*, p 1.

objective decision-making'.[127] According to the Group, highest priority should be given to ensuring that international tax rules were agreed which were simple, concrete, and clear to apply. This was more important than strengthening the existing dispute resolution mechanism. As an immediate response, the G20 should consider 'a transition mechanism, to supervise the process of implementation of the BEPS reforms, monitor the way the rules are introduced by states, and provide advice and perhaps even interpretations'.[128] The fact that the BEPS project also included developing countries with very limited competent authority resources makes this an imperative.

What is undeniable is that BEPS will increase the issues under dispute, many of which are of high value. Also, the disputes are likely to be multinational and involve economic double taxation more than legal double taxation. For Action 14 to be successful, dispute resolution has to be swift and effective. Also, the right of taxpayers to intervene in the dispute resolution process needs to be ensured. So far, this right has been neglected.[129]

During the public consultation meeting on 23 January 2015, the fact that the Dispute Resolution Discussion Draft did not recommend specific dispute resolution measures but merely outlined possibilities was found to be disappointing.[130] Stakeholders criticised the failure to endorse mandatory binding arbitration for mutual agreement procedure cases. Arbitration could be designed in different ways to suit countries' preferences. The US baseball-style arbitration approach may not be the right choice for all countries. It was argued that taking a quasi-judicial approach, offering expedited access to arbitration, or giving arbitration decisions precedential value could make arbitration more appealing to countries that did not like the baseball-style approach. A US Treasury representative suggested that there should be an in-depth study of the various types of arbitration to examine the pros and cons of each approach and determine whether any of the approaches would exacerbate the concerns some countries have.

It was noted that MAP case requests had almost doubled and many businesses saw this Action item 'as the linchpin that [would] make everything else in the BEPS project work'.[131] It was recognised that there was an alarmingly large and growing number of outstanding MAP cases. The key to preventing treaty-related disputes would be a comprehensive review of all phases of the dispute resolution process, starting with the tax examinations that gave rise to disputes.[132]

[127] *Ibid*, p 2.

[128] *Ibid*, p 6.

[129] Jacques Malherbe, 'The Issues of Dispute Resolution and Introduction of a Multilateral Treaty' (2015) 43 *Intertax* 91, 93.

[130] Kristen A Parillo and Ajay Gupta, 'Business Sector Decries OECD's Lack of Support for Arbitration', 2015 *WTD* 16-2 (26 January 2015).

[131] *Ibid*. As also noted by one of the industry representatives, businesses and their advisers were already drowning in MAP cases, and BEPS was a river about to be diverted in their direction.

[132] *Ibid*.

There was talk of 'bad' institutional behaviour giving rise to double taxation, such as tax authorities making transfer pricing adjustments too readily. Other 'bad' institutional behaviour included the lack of empowerment among some competent authorities to actually relieve double taxation, undue influences that may be exercised on competent authorities and the limited resources available. It was also noted that the Dispute Resolution Discussion Draft's proposals seem to put unrealistic expectations on the ability of some countries, particularly smaller or developing countries to deal with tax disputes. The MAP Forum, established in 2013 by the competent authorities in the OECD Forum on Tax Administration member states, was recommended as the most effective place for addressing these problems and evaluating fundamental tax administration policies and practices.

In February 2015, the OECD announced that it would issue a 'strengthened' follow-up draft with more specific proposals to address the impediments to resolving mutual agreement procedure cases.[133] The follow-up draft would include a range of options that recognise the different views among various countries on how to improve MAP—particularly on the question of moving towards universal mandatory binding arbitration provisions. At the same time, the follow-up draft would reflect the common goal of finding ways to improve the effectiveness and efficiency of dispute resolution mechanisms. Although the next draft may contain stronger language recommending mandatory arbitration, the proposal still faces considerable opposition from many countries.

It has since been reported that about 25 countries have expressed an interest in implementing mandatory arbitration provisions through a multilateral instrument as part of BEPS. The US is in favour of mandatory arbitration but is reluctant to include GAAR disputes as being eligible for arbitration.[134] Developing countries also seem to be reluctant to endorse arbitration, mainly due to the high costs of arbitral proceedings in comparison to MAP.[135] At an interview with Pascal Saint-Amans, the head of the Centre for Tax Policy and Administration at the OECD, the continuing difficulty of convincing other countries to accept arbitration was reiterated. It was hinted that monitoring and peer reviewing were likely to

[133] Kristen A Parillo, 'OECD Will Add "Muscle" to Next BEPS Dispute Resolution Draft', 2015 *WTD* 30-1 (13 February 2015).

[134] Kristen A Parillo, 'About 25 Countries Interested in Treaty Arbitration, Rolfes Says', 2015 *WTD* 52-2 (18 March 2015) and David D Stewart, 'Post-BEPS Priority is Improving Tax Administration, Stack Says', 2015 *WTD* 57-1 (25 March 2015). It has been reported that the US is trying to educate other countries about what mandatory arbitration means, in the hope that education can ultimately lead to acceptance. See Mindy Herzfeld, 'Status Check on BEPS' (2015) 77 *Tax Notes International* 1125 (30 March 2015).

[135] See Jasmin Kollmann, Petra Koch, Alicja Majdanska and Laura Turcan, 'Arbitration in International Tax Matters' (2015) 77 *Tax Notes International* 1189 (30 March 2015). It has been reported that the UN is planning to release a paper on arbitration for developing countries. See David D Stewart, 'UN Work Needed to Add Credibility to Transfer Pricing Rules', 2015 *WTD* 61-5.

be the only available options.[136] These options are, however, also challenging due to the subjective nature of the task.[137]

4.5. Action 15: Develop a Multilateral Instrument

Action 15 of the BEPS Action Plan explores the feasibility of developing a multilateral instrument to address treaty-related BEPS issues. The Action item reads as follows:

> Analyse the tax and public international law issues related to the development of a multilateral instrument to enable jurisdictions that wish to do so to implement measures developed in the course of the work on BEPS and amend bilateral tax treaties. On the basis of this analysis, interested Parties will develop a multilateral instrument designed to provide an innovative approach to international tax matters, reflecting the rapidly evolving nature of the global economy and the need to adapt quickly to this evolution.

The first discussion draft on this Action item was released in September 2014.[138] The Multilateral Instrument Discussion Draft analysed the tax and public international law issues related to the development of a multilateral instrument without infringing sovereign autonomy in tax matters. Such an instrument would enable countries to implement treaty-based BEPS issues in a quicker and more efficient way. In the absence of any special measures, BEPS-related changes through bilateral tax treaties would take many years to introduce across the network of double tax treaties, as individual treaties would need to be renegotiated. As noted, 'globalisation makes the bilateral approach obsolete: the mobility of factors and the existence of global value chains are likely to generate multi-country disputes and require multilateral MAP, which could better be addressed in a multilateral treaty'.[139]

As far as next steps were concerned, the OECD recommended convening an international conference in early 2015 to develop the multilateral instrument. An international conference would negotiate the content and actual text of the multilateral instrument and would be open to all interested countries, under the aegis of the OECD and the G20. The mandate of the conference would be limited in scope

[136] 'Conversations: Jeffrey Owens and Pascal Saint-Amans' (2015) 77 *Tax Notes International* 797 (2 March 2015).

[137] It has been reported that the Action 14 working group had been considering how to implement the discussion draft's proposed peer review process for monitoring countries' adherence to their political commitment to improve MAP and the minimum standard for operating their treaty dispute resolution program. See Parillo, 'About 25 Countries Interested in Treaty Arbitration, Rolfes Says', n 134 above.

[138] OECD/G20 Base Erosion and Profit Shifting Project, *Action 15: A Mandate for the Development of a Multilateral Instrument on Tax Treaty Measures to Tackle BEPS*. Available on: www.oecd.org/ctp/beps-action-15-mandate-for-development-of-multilateral-instrument.pdf.

[139] Jacques Malherbe, 'BEPS: The Issues of Dispute Resolution and Introduction of a Multilateral Treaty' (2015) 43 *Intertax* 91–95, 94.

(implementing the BEPS Action Plan) and in time (no more than two years).[140] As an example of a successful multilateral instrument, the Convention on Mutual Administrative Assistance in Tax Matters was mentioned.[141]

Some issues relating to the development of a multilateral instrument were identified. It was suggested that the development of such an instrument was desirable as it would overcome the hurdle of cumbersome bilateral negotiations and produce important efficiency gains. This would especially enable developing countries to reap the benefits from the BEPS project more fully, without having to exhaust themselves with tax treaty negotiations or re-negotiations.[142]

Furthermore, a multilateral instrument would increase consistency and help ensure the continued reliability of the international tax treaty network, providing additional certainty for businesses. It was argued that such an instrument would focus the attention of a large number of highly-qualified treaty negotiators on a single document that could incorporate the language deemed most appropriate by all countries. At the same time, it was noted that flexibility, respect for bilateral relations and a targeted scope were crucial; otherwise the process would stagnate or would involve too few countries. Broad participation was also essential to success—in order to ensure a level playing field.[143]

It was acknowledged that developing a multilateral instrument posed several challenges, although the OECD was positive in that legal mechanisms existed to address these challenges. The most promising approach was to have a multilateral instrument that would co-exist with bilateral tax treaties. 'Like existing tax treaties, this instrument would be governed by international law and would be legally binding on the parties'.[144] It was later on clarified that the instrument would follow established negotiating processes and ratification would require conventional domestic procedures. However, rather contradictorily to the previous statement as to the binding effect of the instrument, it was stated that the relationship between parties to a multilateral instrument that were not parties to a bilateral tax treaty between themselves would not be affected—'a multilateral instrument will only govern the relationship between parties that have concluded bilateral tax treaties amongst themselves'.[145] In other words, a multilateral treaty was not envisaged as a stand-alone instrument.[146] The only possible exception would be a multilateral dispute resolution mechanism.

This rather pragmatic stance, arguably reflective of the difficulties of achieving full consensus in this area, raises many issues. To an extent, this position nullifies the possible (intended) impact of the multilateral instrument, if it only has an

140 Multilateral Instrument Discussion Draft, n 138 above, p 14.
141 *Ibid.*
142 *Ibid*, pp 15–16.
143 *Ibid*, p 17.
144 *Ibid*, p 17.
145 *Ibid*, p 18.
146 Malherbe (2015), n 139 above, p 94.

impact on countries that are already covered by a tax treaty. Even when bilateral tax treaties do exist, there would also be a number of technical challenges. For example, there could be variations in scope between similar provisions of existing bilateral treaties, or linguistic discrepancies. For these, there should be compatibility clauses or primacy clauses in the multilateral instrument,[147] or superseding language,[148] defining its relationship with prior, or even future, bilateral treaties. Mechanisms to resolve the technical challenges that might arise and relevant precedents in other areas of international law were described in more detail in the Annex to the Multilateral Instrument Discussion Draft, which included a 'toolbox' for a multilateral instrument for the swift implementation of BEPS measures.[149]

It was emphasised that the multilateral instrument should be highly targeted and efficient,[150] yet it was later on conceded that 'a flexible approach will be paramount'.[151] In fact, it was suggested that the multilateral instrument 'should allow for the tailoring of the level of certain commitments towards all the other parties and/or depending on the partner country'.[152]

In chapter 2 of the Discussion Draft there was an analysis of possible BEPS-related themes that could lend themselves to multilateral application: multilateral MAP, dual-residence structures, hybrid mismatch arrangements, triangular cases involving PEs in third states and treaty abuse.[153] It was stated that such treaty-related BEPS measures could be drafted and implemented as stand-alone measures but could also be included in a multilateral instrument that complemented and co-existed with bilateral tax treaties. It was conceded, however, that some treaty-related BEPS measures may implicate concerns that were bilateral in nature which would require additional flexibility.[154] Later on in the discussion draft it was stated that '[f]or the moment, it is important to keep the multilateral instrument narrowly targeted, and at the same time start a reflection on what further incremental opportunities may be available'.[155] Again, this seems like a pragmatic conclusion suggesting multilateralism à la carte.

Interestingly, the Multilateral Instrument Discussion Draft also recommended close examination of the relationship of a multilateral instrument with EU law and other multilateral agreements such as the Nordic tax treaty.[156] The possible implications of this, vis-à-vis EU law, are considered in Chapter six of this volume.[157]

What seems to emerge from the Multilateral Instrument Discussion Draft is that strict uniformity is likely to give way to optionality and flexibility. This is a

[147] Multilateral Instrument Discussion Draft, n 138, p 19.
[148] *Ibid*, p 20.
[149] *Ibid*, p 29 et seq.
[150] See, for example, p 18.
[151] *Ibid*, p 21.
[152] *Ibid*.
[153] *Ibid*, pp 23–26.
[154] *Ibid*, p 25.
[155] *Ibid*, p 26.
[156] *Ibid*, p 21.
[157] See analysis in section 6.7 of this volume.

pragmatic outcome. There is likely to be a variable amount of clarity and certainty to which businesses could adjust to. There would—presumably—be some core provisions universally applicable and other provisions which would be optional (opt-outs and opt-ins). However, there are no indications as to what is likely to be optional and what is likely to be compulsory. While it is understandable that the OECD wishes to streamline the implementation of BEPS-induced changes in the international tax treaty landscape, multilateralism—certainly a dynamic and innovative solution—may not be as easy to achieve, at least not immediately.

It has been argued that too much optionality would weaken the multilateral instrument and make it as complex as a series of protocols amending bilateral treaties.[158] Furthermore, reservations to a multilateral treaty raise practical difficulties as the instrument loses its uniformity between Contracting States. If a Contracting State's reservations are too great, other Contracting States may refuse to allow the multilateral treaty to enter into force vis-à-vis the Contracting State making those reservations. In other words, the multilateral treaty would risk becoming 'fractioned' or 'divisible'. Therefore, rather than allowing reservations, it is arguably preferable, especially when divergences are too strong, to have two or more multilateral agreements and/or for these instruments to be limited to a given sector.

The above analysis suggests that multilateralism, at least in its pure sense, is unlikely to be applicable in the international context, even post-BEPS. What we might see develop is a watered down version of multilateralism. Apart from established areas dealing with exchange of information and administrative assistance, bilateral tax treaties would still rule the day, with all their limitations. Let us not forget that in the European Union, the bilateralism of tax treaties has survived the Court of Justice following the *D* case.[159]

While there have been a few examples of multilateral instruments addressing procedural rules (eg exchange of information or administrative assistance), with the exception of the Nordic treaty, this would be the first time that a multilateral instrument of such a scale addresses substantive rules. The goal is certainly laudable but rather disappointingly, the Multilateral Instrument Discussion Draft does not give any specific guidance as to how such multilateral instrument is to be developed, drafted, implemented and, in the future, revised or amended.[160] Perhaps input should be sought not just from tax lawyers but also from experts in public international law and treaty law.

[158] Malherbe (2015), n 139 above, pp 94–95.

[159] See Case C-376/03 *D v Rijksbelastingdienst* (*D* case) [2005] ECR I-5821. Also see analysis in Ch 6, section 6.7 of this volume.

[160] Malherbe (2015), n 139 above, at pp 93–94, makes a number of suggestions as to how a multinational instrument could be implemented. One solution would be a mere adjustment of the OECD Model Commentary. Arguably, this would not be binding and if binding, there would be issues with tax treaties already signed. Another more unrealistic solution would be to sign a general multilateral treaty replacing the network of bilateral treaties. Alternatively, there could be a framework multilateral treaty to which various countries could adhere by declaration without modifying its terms. There could

On 6 February 2015, the OECD and the G20 agreed to a mandate to begin negotiations on a multilateral instrument to streamline implementation of treaty-related BEPS measures. The formation of a negotiating ad hoc group hosted by the OECD was authorised. The group would be open to participation from all states and would hold its first meeting by July 2015. The goal was to finalise the drafting of the instrument by the end of 2016.[161] On 28 May 2015, it was announced that an ad hoc group of over 80 countries had begun work on developing a multilateral instrument. Substantive work was scheduled to begin at an inaugural meeting in November 2015.[162]

4.6. BEPS and Developing Countries

It is undeniable that BEPS affects developing countries. According to the OECD, engagement with developing countries has been extensive since the beginning of the project.[163] Over 80 developing countries and other non-OECD/non-G20 economies have been consulted through at least four in-depth regional consultations and five thematic global fora, attended by more than 110 jurisdictions as well as representatives from civil society and the business community. The input received from developing countries has been fed into the development of the BEPS Action Plan by the technical groups carrying out the work on BEPS. Developing countries have contributed to the discussion on most of the deliverables and have provided influential input especially as regards the template for country-by-country reporting for the purposes of Action 13 and the work on treaty abuse under Action 6. The OECD's engagement with development countries is also buttressed by the signing of several memoranda of understanding (MOUs) with international and regional organisations.[164]

In addition to including developing countries in the consultation and decision-making process, the OECD has also published a number of papers on topics directly affecting developing countries.

also be a binding multilateral treaty amending bilateral treaties but on which countries could formulate reservations. Malherbe, at p 95, also discusses some of the issues that could arise with the drafting of the treaty and its future amendments. He questions whether the revision of the treaty would require unanimity or consent by majority. If the latter, then minority states may want to withdraw: *ibid.*

[161] See first steps towards implementation of OECD/G20 efforts against tax avoidance by multinationals, and *OECD Secretary-General Report to G20 Finance Ministers* (Istanbul, Turkey, February 2015). Available on: www.oecd.org/tax/oecd-secretary-general-tax-report-g20-finance-ministers-february-2015.pdf.

[162] See announcement published in Tax Analysts, 2015 *WTD* 103-18 (28 May 2015).

[163] See www.oecd.org/tax/beps-about.htm.

[164] An MOU was signed between the Centre de rencontres et d'études des dirigeants des administrations fiscales (CREDAF) and the OECD on 16 March 2015. CREDAF joined the African Tax Administration Forum (ATAF) and the Center for Inter-American Tax Administrators (CIAT) which already have MOUs with the OECD aimed at strengthening the partnership to improve tax policy, and helping build greater capacity within the respective regions. See report in Tax Analysts, 'OECD Global Forum Welcomes Participation by Developing Countries', 2015 *WTD* 57-14 (24 March 2015).

In March 2014, the OECD published a consultation document in response to a call from the G8 to find ways to address the concerns expressed by developing countries on the quality and availability of information on comparable transactions that was needed to administer transfer pricing effectively. The paper considered transfer pricing comparability data and developing countries.[165] It provided some useful ideas for dealing with practical difficulties in benchmarking returns for parties in developing countries.[166]

Furthermore, in the summer of 2014, the OECD published a two-part report that sought to map out the impact of BEPS on low income countries.[167] The report highlighted the numerous challenges faced by developing countries in tackling BEPS. It was noted that some developing countries lack the necessary legislative measures needed to address BEPS and any measures they have are often hindered by lack of information. Furthermore, developing countries faced difficulties in building the capacity needed to implement highly complex rules and to challenge well-advised and experienced MNEs. This was likely to lead to simpler, but potentially more aggressive tax avoidance than is typically encountered in developed economies.

As part of its interim conclusions, in the first part of this report it was recognised that BEPS had the potential to have a considerable impact on domestic resource mobilisation in developing countries. The second part to this report was meant to provide guidance to developing countries to meet the challenges of the most relevant BEPS issues they face. Some generic guidance was indeed given, though most issues were referred for further consideration. Inter alia, it was noted that political-level engagement on BEPS issues in many developing countries was at an early stage. It was important for this engagement to be improved. Furthermore, it was recommended that G20 countries should analyse the spillover effects of changes to the design of their own tax systems on those of developing countries, also considering tax incentives.

Concerns were reiterated as to the importance of capacity building on BEPS issues. It was recommended that guidance should be drawn from the extensive experience not only of the OECD's Task Force on Tax and Development but also of other organisations such as the IMF and the World Bank Group, as well as the experience of other developing countries. It was also suggested that the

[165] See OECD Public Consultation, *Transfer Pricing Comparability Data and Developing Countries* (2014). Available on: www.oecd.org/ctp/transfer-pricing/transfer-pricing-comparability-data-developing-countries.pdf.

[166] Four possible approaches were set out to address these concerns: expanding access to data sources for comparables, more effective use of data sources for comparables, approaches to identifying arm's length prices without reliance on direct comparables and advance pricing agreements and mutual agreement proceedings.

[167] See Parts 1 and 2 of *A Report to G20 Development Working Group on the Impact of BEPS in Low Income Countries*, published in July 2014 and August 2014 respectively. Available on: www.oecd.org/ctp/tax-global/part-1-of-report-to-g20-dwg-on-the-impact-of-beps-in-low-income-countries.pdf and www.oecd.org/g20/topics/taxation/part-2-of-report-to-g20-dwg-on-the-impact-of-beps-in-low-income-countries.pdf.

OECD, IMF, UN, World Bank Group and regional organisations should consider developing practical toolkits to help developing countries implement key BEPS actions, without creating separate or alternative norms or standards.

For the project to succeed, it was necessary to ensure that BEPS solutions were relevant to, and effective for, developing countries. At the same time, developing countries had to be fully engaged to ensure that the suggested solutions take into account the information and capacity gaps they frequently face. The OECD promised to strengthen its involvement with developing countries. Moreover, it was noted that a multilateral instrument, as envisaged by Action 15 of the BEPS Action Plan, might prove to be an important tool for developing countries that have a tax treaty network. G20 countries were urged to engage in dialogue with developing countries on the design and potential benefits of a multilateral instrument.

Following this report, the OECD continued to seek ways to ensure developing countries were better integrated into the BEPS project. On 12 November 2014, the OECD published its strategy for deepening the engagement of developing countries.[168] Guidance was given on how to strengthen their involvement in the decision-making process and bring them to the heart of the technical work. It was reiterated that capacity building to address BEPS issues was imperative.

In the summary of proceedings of an Eurasian BEPS meeting held on 4–5 March 2015, participants welcomed the new OECD/G20 strategy to strengthen the involvement of developing countries into the BEPS project. This made the entire process more inclusive and provided a unique opportunity to enhance the dialogue.[169] The BEPS project was welcomed as a means of updating the international standards to the economic realities of globalisation. However, concerns were expressed mostly about implementation and the transitional costs of BEPS measures, as well as the need for a coordinated approach to prevent double taxation.

Notwithstanding the OECD's attempts to be more inclusive in the BEPS project, there is still a general concern that the BEPS agenda prejudices developing countries and that their interests are not properly reflected in the Action Plan.[170] One could argue that efforts to align the arm's length principle to reflect value creation are there only to temporarily appease developing countries. These countries face substantial challenges especially as regards the implementation of transfer pricing regimes in their economies: the cost of commercial databases, the difficulties of hiring and retaining specialised auditors, as well as the lack of comparable data and other transitional costs.[171] Some of the proposals in the discussion drafts, for example the proposals under the Risk and Re-characterisation Discussion Draft,

[168] Available on: www.oecd.org/tax/strategy-deepening-developing-country-engagement.pdf.

[169] See 'OECD Releases Eurasian BEPS Meeting Summary', 2015 *WTD* 47-15 (5 March 2015). Also see comments made by Pascal Saint-Amans at the Global Forum on Transfer Pricing meeting on 16-17 March 2015, where developing countries were welcomed as vital participants in the BEPS project. See report in Tax Analysts 2015, n 164 above.

[170] Shee Boon Law, 'Base Erosion and Profit Shifting—An Action Plan for Developing Countries' (2013) 68 *Bulletin for International Taxation* 41–46.

[171] See OECD Releases Eurasian BEPS Meeting Summary, n 169 above.

depend on the availability of experts with specialised knowledge of many industry sectors and business models, which is an unrealistic expectation for many developing countries. As noted by the BEPS Monitoring Group, '[e]ven the most developed OECD members struggle to match the resources of the private sector, as seen by the recent decision of the US IRS to pay $2m to consultants to help with its audit of Microsoft'.[172]

Furthermore, while procedurally the OECD appears to have integrated developing countries much more than in any previous initiative, the extent to which these countries have actually influenced the final product remains to be seen. The discussion drafts of the deliverables produced so far, as analysed in this and in previous chapters, suggest limited influence.[173] Perhaps this can be attributed to the fact that the scope of the BEPS project itself is rather limited—it is (or supposed to be) about reform of existing rules. By contrast, as suggested by NGO representatives, for developing countries, more radical proposals might be appropriate such as taxation on a unitary basis or general application of the profit split method.[174] Of course, adoption of such proposals by the OECD and universal implementation by countries is a near impossibility—hence why the gap between the demands of developing and developed countries is unlikely to be ever fully bridged.

In any case, it has been argued that cooperation is not necessarily good and its consequences are not always desirable. International taxation has thus far been based on cooperation that serves OECD countries rather than all countries. Tsilly Dagan has referred to this as cartelistic cooperation.[175] Her arguments seem to counter the conclusions of the BEPS initiative that a shift to cooperation is a prerequisite for the survival of the international tax regime. Whilst this may be to the benefit of OECD countries, it might not necessarily serve other countries such as the BRICS (ie Brazil, Russia, India, China and South Africa). Although these countries have a unique position of power in today's global economy and this position grants them increasing influence and great potential, nevertheless, for the time being, BRICS countries face many limitations in transforming the international tax landscape. It might be best if these and other developing countries embrace

[172] BEPS Monitoring Group, *Summary of Evaluations of BEPS Action Plan Proposals*. Available on: bepsmonitoringgroup.files.wordpress.com/2015/03/summary-march-2015.pdf.

[173] As Sol Picciotto argued, while the OECD has had some engagement with developing countries on BEPS issues, it has not adopted their views, such as the inclusion of location-specific advantages as intangibles. See analysis in section 3.3 of Ch 3 of this volume. Although the OECD has tried to consult developing countries, the most it has been able to do is alert them to the issues. See David D Stewart, 'Sol Picciotto—BEPS and the Developing World' (2014) 76 *Tax Notes International* 1060 (22 December 2014).

[174] See Tax Justice Network, *Briefing on Base Erosion and Profit Shifting (BEPS) Implications for Developing Countries (February 2014)*. Available on: www.taxjustice.net/wp-content/uploads/2013/04/TJN-Briefing-BEPS-for-Developing-Countries-Feb-2014-v2.pdf.

[175] See Tsilly Dagan, 'BRICS: Theoretical Framework and the Potential of Cooperation' in Yariv Brauner and Pasquale Piston (eds), *BRICS and the Emergence of International Tax Coordination* (IBFD, 2015). The concept was developed in her previous work. See, eg Tsilly Dagan, *The Costs of International Tax Cooperation*, University of Michigan Law, Public Law Research Paper 13 (2002); Tsilly Dagan, 'Just Harmonisation' (2010) 42 *University of British Columbia Law Review* 331.

the BEPS project and participate in the consultations, to try and ensure as far as possible that their concerns are taken into account.

In general, in the current state of the international tax system, it is only through proper engagement in the BEPS discourse that some tangible benefits could accrue to developing countries and their interests and agenda promoted. Therefore, however cynical one is of the BEPS project, for developing countries there is something to be gained. If efforts to streamline the arm's length principle with value creation do reach fruition, even partially, then this could have important implications for the tax base of developing countries.

At the time of writing this book, the final versions of some of the BEPS proposals were not yet released. As already explained in the introduction to this book, this and the previous chapters on BEPS analyse material available up to 1 June 2015. There is an overview and a general critique of the proposals in the final chapter to this book. The next chapters examine the measures taken by the European Union to tackle international tax avoidance. It is noted that some of the EU measures share similarities with the BEPS proposals. The compatibility of some of the BEPS proposals with the general principles of EU law are also considered later on in this book.

5

International Tax Avoidance and European Union Law

In order to understand the European Union's response to aggressive tax planning and MNEs engaged in such tax planning, it is important to consider the background against which some of the relevant initiatives unfolded. Up until very recently, there was not much of an official policy on tax avoidance, let alone aggressive tax planning. In fact, most of the case law of the Court of Justice seemed to be devoted to the unravelling of domestic anti-abuse rules on the basis of incompatibility with the various fundamental freedoms under EU law.

The first part of this chapter considers the judicial response to the concept of tax abuse, mainly by the Court of Justice. This is then juxtaposed with the European Commission's initiatives and its Action Plan to Strengthen the Fight against Tax Fraud and Tax Evasion as a newly-formed policy on international tax avoidance. This chapter sets the background against which, in the next chapter, there is an analysis of the compatibility of the various items of the BEPS Action Plan with EU law.

5.1. The Judicial Development of A Principle of Abuse of Tax Law

For some time, it has been debated whether there is one coherent principle of abuse of EU law and, as a corollary, whether Member States are entitled or under an obligation to combat abusive *tax* practices. As discussed elsewhere, in the current state of the Court's jurisprudence, it is difficult to conclude that the concept of tax abuse has been de-nationalised and that there is now an EU principle of tax abuse.[1] Not only is the terminology inconsistent, with the Court using the

[1] See ch 8 in Christiana HJI Panayi, *European Union Corporate Tax Law* (Cambridge University Press, 2013). Contrast with the position of Paolo Piantavigna, 'Tax Abuse in European Union Law: A Theory' (2011) 20 *EC Tax Review* 134 and Adolfo Martin Jimenez, 'Towards a Homogeneous Theory of Abuse in EU (Direct) Tax Law' (2012) 66 *Bulletin for International Taxation* 270.

terms 'abuse', 'evasion', 'avoidance' and 'fraud' interchangeably in the tax case law but there are also linguistic discrepancies in the translations of the judgments.[2] Furthermore, the various terms may have different meanings in different jurisdictions and/or their boundaries may be unclear.[3]

Overall, recent case law suggests that EU law does not provide a general principle of abuse of rights in the field of direct taxation. Whilst a principle of abuse of rights may be deduced from some cases in the area of VAT, it does not apply in a non-harmonised area.

In *Halifax*,[4] the Court of Justice first showed signs of accepting a free-standing principle of abuse of law in the VAT context.[5] This case dealt with an aggressive and complex VAT planning scheme intended to locate the place of supply of services outside the EU. The UK tax authorities challenged this scheme. Eventually, a reference was made to the Court of Justice to interpret the rules of the Sixth VAT Directive on the place of supply of services. More importantly, the Court of Justice was also asked to determine whether there was a principle of abuse of rights disallowing such schemes.

The Court of Justice decided that the transactions encompassed supplies of services for the purposes of the VAT legislation and therefore were subject to it. In any case, the application of Community legislation could 'not be extended to cover abusive practices by economic operators, that is to say transactions carried out not in the context of normal commercial operations, but solely for the purpose of wrongfully obtaining advantages provided for by Community law'.[6] In this context, an abusive practice occurs where first, the transaction results in a tax advantage which would be contrary to the purpose of the provisions formally applied, and secondly, the essential aim of the transaction was to obtain a tax advantage.[7] To the Court of Justice, objective criteria and respect of legal certainty were essential.[8] For the purposes of the second part of the test, the Court of Justice stated that, in determining the real substance and significance of the transactions, national courts could consider factors such as the purely artificial nature of those transactions and the legal, economic and/or personal links among

[2] Opinion Statement of the CFE ECJ Task Force on the Concept of Abuse in European Law, based on the Judgments of the European Court of Justice Delivered in the Field of Tax Law (November 2007).

[3] What is mainly disputed in different jurisdictions is whether or not a certain transaction constitutes legitimate tax planning or (illegitimate) tax avoidance.

[4] Case C-255/02 *Halifax plc, Leeds Permanent Development Services Ltd and County Wide Property Investments Ltd v Commissioners of Customs & Excise* [2006] ECR I-1609.

[5] In the non-tax context, the origins of such a principle are traced back to earlier cases and mainly Case C-110/99 *Emsland-Stärke GmbH v Hauptzollamt Hamburg-Jonas* [2000] ECR I-1569. See Rita de la Feria, 'Prohibition of Abuse of (Community) Law: The Creation of a New General Principle of EC Law through Tax' (2008) 45 *Common Market Law Review* 395, 408.

[6] *Halifax*, n 4 above, para 69.

[7] *Ibid*, paras 74–75.

[8] *Ibid*, para 72.

operators involved in the tax avoidance scheme.[9] If an abusive practice was found to exist, then the transactions involved had to be redefined so as to re-establish the situation that 'would have prevailed in the absence of transactions constituting that abusive practice'.[10]

Although the *Halifax* case was hailed as a ground-breaking decision for the purposes of VAT legislation, it was not entirely clear whether guidance could be derived from it for other areas such as direct tax law. Later cases seem to confirm the idea that the principle would only be relevant to VAT cases.

In *Part Service*, another VAT case,[11] the *Halifax* two-pronged test was applied and refined. The Court of Justice clarified that to find an abusive practice for the purposes of the Sixth VAT Directive it was enough when the accrual of a tax advantage was the *principal* aim of the transaction or the transactions in question, and not the *sole* aim pursued, to the exclusion of other economic objectives.[12] This was for the national court to assess.[13]

Similarly, in *Weald Leasing*,[14] the Court of Justice dealt with an asset-leasing transaction, the purpose of which was the deferment of the VAT liability through its spreading on rental payments. Here, the existence of the tax advantage was not enough. It had to be shown that this advantage was contrary to the purposes of the VAT legislation.[15] The Court of Justice emphasised that a taxable person could not be criticised for choosing a leasing transaction which procured him the advantage of spreading the payment of his tax liability.[16] A finding that there was an abusive practice was inferred from the object and effects of the impugned transactions, as well as their purpose.[17] The fact that the undertaking did not usually engage in such transactions was irrelevant.[18] If the transaction was abusive, then it had to be redefined so as to re-establish the situation that would have prevailed in the absence of the elements of those contractual terms which were abusive.[19] *Weald Leasing* is important as the Court of Justice openly embraced the arm's length principle as a means of delineating elements that could go towards establishing the abusive nature of a transaction.[20] It also clarified that a finding of abuse does not nullify the transaction but paves the way for its re-characterisation.

[9] *Ibid*, para 81.
[10] *Ibid*, para 94.
[11] Case C-425/06 *Ministero dell'Economia e delle Finanze, formerly Ministero delle Finanze v Part Service Srl, company in liquidation, formerly Italservice Srl* [2008] ECR I-897.
[12] *Ibid*, para 45.
[13] *Ibid*, para 62.
[14] Case C-103/09 *The Commissioners for Her Majesty's Revenue and Customs v Weald Leasing Ltd* [2010] ECR I-13589.
[15] *Ibid*, para 33.
[16] *Ibid*, para 34.
[17] *Ibid*, para 44.
[18] *Ibid*, para 45.
[19] *Ibid*, para 53.
[20] Also see para 50 in Case C-277/09 *The Commissioners for Her Majesty's Revenue & Customs v RBS Deutschland Holdings GmbH* [2010] ECR I-13805, where the fact that the various transactions concerned took place between two parties which were legally unconnected was decisive.

More recently, in the *Ocean Finance* case[21] the Court of Justice seems to have shifted away from the more objective element of the *Halifax* test.[22] By focusing on the artificiality of the transaction, it gave emphasis to the more subjective second test. In *Ocean Finance*, it was stated that the consideration of economic and commercial realities was a fundamental criterion for the application of the common system of VAT. These may be more decisive than the contractual terms for identifying the recipient of a supply of services. This language is very reminiscent of the language used by the OECD in its Risk and Re-characterisation Discussion Draft, reviewed in Chapter three of this volume.[23]

In this case, Paul Newey, a UK loan broker supplied VAT-exempt broking services. At the same time, he received advertising services for the promotion of his business, which were subject to VAT in the UK. In consequence, the VAT paid for the advertising services was not recoverable. Mr Newey entered into complex arrangements[24] with an offshore subsidiary to mitigate a substantial amount of irrecoverable input VAT. The UK tax authorities challenged this structure, arguing that the aim of going offshore was to avoid paying VAT on taxable advertising services. The essence of the questions referred was whether the contractual terms were to be considered as decisive in determining the supplier and recipient in a supply of services for VAT purposes.

The Court of Justice found that contractual terms, although an important factor to be taken into consideration, were not decisive. Sometimes, contractual terms did not wholly reflect the economic and commercial reality of the transactions.[25] 'That is the case in particular if it becomes apparent that those contractual terms constitute a purely artificial arrangement which does not correspond with the economic and commercial reality of the transactions'.[26] Referring to previous case law and to the objective of the Sixth VAT Direct, the Court of Justice recalled that 'the effect of the principle that the abuse of rights is prohibited is to bar wholly artificial arrangements which do not reflect economic reality and are set up with the sole aim of obtaining a tax advantage'.[27]

Contractual terms could be disregarded if it became apparent that they did not reflect economic and commercial reality. This was for the referring court to ascertain.[28] If indeed this was the case, then 'those contractual terms would have to be redefined so as to re-establish the situation that would have prevailed in

[21] Case C-653/11 *HM Revenue & Customs v Paul Newey, trading under the business name Ocean Finance* [2013] ECR I-409.

[22] Ie whether the transaction resulted in a tax advantage which would be contrary to the purpose of the provisions formally applied.

[23] See section 3.4.4 of this volume.

[24] *Paul Newey*, n 21 above, paras 17–28.

[25] *Ibid*, paras 43–44.

[26] *Ibid*, para 45.

[27] *Ibid*, para 46.

[28] *Ibid*, para 49.

the absence of the transactions constituting that abusive practice'.[29] In this case, the Commissioners could legitimately regard Mr Newey as actually being the supplier of the loan broking services and the recipient of the supplies of advertising services at issue.[30]

This case seems to strengthen the position of the tax authorities in their fight against tax fraud and abusive practices. For businesses, it makes it imperative to have comprehensive and well-structured documentation reflecting the economic reality. Substance over form has become crucial. To an extent, the Court's judgment seems to be aligned with recent trends whereby artificiality and other objective factors are the main ingredients of proposed anti-abuse rules, thus also catching unintentional mismatches and double non-taxation. However, it is not certain whether the Court is reverting to the *Halifax* sole purpose test, in which case, the onus of proof for the tax authorities would seem to be higher than the 'one of the principal purposes' test of later case law. If that is the case, then arguably, the amendment to the Parent-Subsidiary Directive discussed below, which relies on 'one of the principal purposes' test is more empowering for tax authorities—as an abuse of tax law test—than what seems to be provided for in the area of VAT.[31]

Apart from VAT cases, the idea of a general principle of abuse of tax law was explored in some cases under the Merger Directive.[32] Although the Court's statements in these cases suggested a free-standing principle of abuse of rights, in *3M Italia*[33] the Court of Justice rejected this view, concluding that a general principle of abuse of rights did not apply to unharmonised taxes. To the Court, it was clear that no general principle existed in EU law which might entail an obligation on the Member States to combat abusive practices in the field of direct taxation.[34] To an extent, the Court's judgment put to rest arguments that there is a general anti-avoidance rule—ie a GAAR—for the purposes of EU tax law;[35] which renders the insertion of a GAAR in the Parent-Subsidiary Directive even more perplexing.

Nevertheless, a finding of abuse of tax laws or tax avoidance is not completely irrelevant as far as the compatibility of national tax legislation in non-harmonised areas is concerned. Depending on the term used by Member States or the Court, the prevention of tax abuse or tax avoidance or tax evasion is often advanced as a justification for national measures restricting fundamental freedoms.

[29] *Ibid*, para 50.

[30] *Ibid*, para 51.

[31] See also analysis in section 5.3.2 below.

[32] See Case C-321/05 *Hans Markus Kofoed v Skatteministeriet* [2007] ECR I-5795, para 38 and Case C-126/10 *Foggia—Sociedade Gestora de Participações Sociais SA v Secretário de Estado dos Assuntos Fiscais* [2011] ECR I-10923. Cf the Court's decision in Case C-352/08 *Modehuis A Zwijnenburg BV v Staatssecretaris van Financiën* [2010] ECR I-4303. See ch 7 in HJI Panayi (2013), n 1 above.

[33] Case C-417/10 *Ministero dell'Economia e delle Finanze, Agenzia delle Entrate v 3M Italia SpA* [2012] ECR I-184.

[34] *Ibid*, para 32.

[35] See analysis in ch 8, HJI Panayi (2013), n 1 above.

Sometimes it is enough to justify the restriction but sometimes it is not. This is an essential point to grasp in assessing the compatibility of some of the BEPS deliverables, especially the pure anti-abuse measures, with EU law. The compatibility assessment should arguably be done in conjunction with the European Union's official policy on aggressive tax planning, to avoid contradictory results. At the time of writing, this policy is still largely a work in progress. The various stages of development of this policy are described next.

5.2. The EU Policy on Tax Abuse and Aggressive Tax Planning

It is difficult to delineate the European Union's policy in this area. As already mentioned, initially the emphasis was not so much on the prevention of international tax avoidance but rather on the prevention of overtly restrictive domestic anti-abuse rules which hindered the single market. There was no discussion on double non-taxation[36] or aggressive tax planning.

5.2.1. Commission Communication on Anti-Abuse Measures

The 2007 Commission Anti-Abuse Communication[37] on the application of anti-abuse measures placed emphasis on intentional tax abuse, though there was mention of adopting coordinating solutions in close cooperation with Member States so as to reduce potential mismatches resulting in inadvertent non-taxation. In this Communication, it was stated that the notion of 'anti-abuse regulations' covered numerous laws, measures and practices in Member States. This Communication called for a more targeted and better coordinated application of these rules. There had to be a just balance between the public interest in tackling abuse and the need to avoid restrictions on cross-border activities within the European Union.

The Commission went on to reiterate the principles under the case law which had arisen at the time. The need to prevent tax avoidance or abuse[38] could

[36] See for example the IFA 2004 conference topic on double non-taxation for which there was no EU report. Similarly, there were very few references to EU law in the General Report. Double non-taxation was not an issue for the European Community at the time; rather measures to curb it were. See IFA Cahiers 2004—Vol 89a, 'Double non-taxation', General Report by Michael Lang.

[37] Commission Communication of 10 December 2007 to the Council, the European Parliament and the European Economic and Social Committee entitled 'The application of anti-abuse measures in the area of direct taxation—within the EU and in relation to third countries' (COM(2007) 785 final) (henceforth, Commission Anti-Abuse Communication).

[38] Rather confusingly, in many places, the Commission used the terms tax avoidance and abuse as if they were synonymous, as far the analysis was concerned.

constitute an overriding reason in the public interest capable of justifying a restriction on fundamental freedoms. The Commission added that the notion of tax avoidance is limited to 'wholly artificial arrangements aimed at circumventing the application of the legislation of the [Member States] concerned'.[39] In order to be lawful, national tax rules must be proportionate and serve the specific purpose of preventing wholly artificial arrangements.

As in the case law, the Commission emphasised that the mere fact that a subsidiary was established in another Member State could not, of itself, be treated as giving rise to tax avoidance.[40] Similarly, the fact that the activities carried out by a secondary establishment in another Member State could just as well be pursued by the taxpayer from within the territory of its home Member State did not warrant the conclusion that there was a wholly artificial arrangement.[41] The objective of minimising one's tax burden was in itself a valid commercial consideration as long as the arrangements entered into with a view to achieving it did not amount to artificial transfers of profits. In so far as taxpayers had not entered into abusive practices, Member States could not hinder the exercise of their freedoms simply because of lower levels of taxation in other Member States.[42] The detection of a wholly artificial arrangement amounted in effect to a substance-over-form analysis.[43]

As far as proportionality was concerned, again, the Commission, echoing case law, noted that in order to ensure that genuine establishments and transactions were not unduly sanctioned it was imperative that where the existence of a purely artificial arrangement was alleged, the taxpayer was given the opportunity, without being subject to undue administrative constraints, to produce evidence of any commercial justification that there may have been for that arrangement. This would be determined on a case-by-case basis[44] and would be subject to an independent judicial review. The Commission Anti-Abuse Communication also offered some guidance regarding adjustments; these should be limited to the extent that was attributable to the purely artificial arrangement. 'With regard to intra-group transactions that means adherence to the arm's length principle, i.e. the commercial terms as would have been agreed upon between unrelated

[39] Commission Anti-Abuse Communication, n 37 above, p 3.

[40] *Ibid*, p 3.

[41] *Ibid*.

[42] *Ibid*. Citing Case C-294/97 *Eurowings Luftverkehrs AG v Finanzamt Dortmund-Unna* [1999] ECR I-7447, para 44. Interestingly, at pp 3–4, the Commission stated that distortions to the location of business activities due to state aid that was incompatible with the EC Treaty and to harmful tax competition did not entitle Member States to take unilateral measures intended to counter their effects by limiting freedom of movement. Rather they need to be resolved at source through the appropriate judicial or political procedures. Citing Advocate General Léger in Case C-196/04 *Cadbury Schweppes plc and Cadbury Schweppes Overseas Ltd v Commissioners of Inland Revenue* [2006] ECR I-7995, paras 55–60.

[43] Commission Anti-Abuse Communication, n 37 above, p 4.

[44] *Ibid*, p 5. In addition, the Commission considered that the burden of proof should not lie solely on the side of the taxpayer and that account should be taken of the general compliance capacity of the taxpayer and of the type of arrangement in question.

parties'.[45] Member States were not prevented from imposing penalties on taxpayers who had made use of abusive schemes to avoid tax. Later on in the Communication, the Commission applied these conclusions in the context of CFC and thin capitalisation rules.[46]

The same conclusions applied as regards EEA States, except in situations where there was no adequate information exchange relationship with the relevant EEA State.[47] As far as third countries were concerned, in the context of CFC and thin capitalisation rules, the Commission stated that the gravity of these rules 'lies clearly within freedom of establishment'[48] to the extent that they involve definite influence and control. Member States should therefore not be precluded from applying CFC and thin cap rules in relation to third countries. 'Community law does not impose any particular requirements on the legitimacy of the application of such legislation to transactions outside the EU'.[49] However, should the application of those rules not be confined to situations and transactions between companies in a corporate group (or otherwise related parties where one has definite influence over the other), they would need to comply with the free movement of capital.

Although the emphasis of this Communication was on tax abuse and the compatibility of anti-abuse measures with EU law, there was recognition of the importance of such measures for Member States, in protecting their tax bases. The Commission identified the need for a general review of Member State anti-avoidance rules.[50] It was important for Member States to improve the coordination of anti-abuse measures within Member States and in relation to third countries. Inter alia, Member States were encouraged to establish common definitions of the notions of abuse and purely artificial arrangements, to improve administrative cooperation to detect and neutralise fraudulent fiscal practices, to exchange best practices compatible with Community law and to reduce overlaps, which can result in unintended non-taxation.

Unintentional non-taxation was also mentioned earlier on in the Commission Anti-Abuse Communication, where it was noted that Member States need 'to be able to operate effective tax systems and prevent their tax bases from being unduly eroded because of inadvertent non-taxation'.[51] As further on elaborated, lack of concerted interaction between Member State tax systems could result in unintended non-taxation and provide scope for abuse, thus undermining the

[45] *Ibid.*
[46] *Ibid*, pp 6–7.
[47] *Ibid*, pp 5–6.
[48] *Ibid*, p 8.
[49] *Ibid.*
[50] *Ibid*, pp 8–9.
[51] *Ibid*, p 5.

fairness and balance of these systems.[52] To an extent, this could be perceived as the precursor of some of the actions subsequently taken at EU level not only to deal with tax abuse but also double non-taxation and later on aggressive tax planning. The shift in the Commission's priorities, while barely noticeable at the time of the 2007 Commission Anti-Abuse Communication, was clearly evident in subsequent years.

5.2.2. From Double Taxation to Double Non-Taxation

A Communication on double taxation was published on 11 November 2011.[53] In this Communication, the Commission expressed its determination to address double taxation problems. It was acknowledged that in the current state of the law, in the absence of an EU initiative, Member States were not obliged to prevent juridical double taxation, since this phenomenon fell outside the scope of fundamental freedoms.[54] Citing also Commission consultations produced the previous year,[55] it was reiterated that EU taxpayers remained significantly concerned by double taxation issues and the double taxation problem was significant: on average more than 20 per cent of the reported cases were above €1 million for corporate taxpayers and more than 35 per cent were above €100,000 for individuals.[56]

[52] *Ibid*, p 6. Specific examples of mismatches giving rise to non-taxation were discussed in p 6. 'Mismatches may arise, for example, in relation to the qualification of debt and equity. One [Member State] may consider a transaction to be an equity injection and thereby exempt the income derived from it (as profit distribution), whereas another [Member State] may consider the same transaction to be a loan and allow tax deductibility for the consequent payments (as interest). This may result in a deduction in one [Member State] without corresponding taxation in another [Member State]. The same is true of hybrid entities, i.e. entities which are regarded as corporate bodies by one [Member State] and as transparent entities by another. This difference in qualification may lead to double exemptions or double deductions. Such problems are best tackled at source, by reducing the occurrence of mismatches. Failing that, it is desirable to improve administrative co-operation to detect situations in which such mismatches are exploited abusively. The Commission proposes to discuss these issues with [Member States] in more detail to examine what scope there is for possible coordinated solutions in this area'.

[53] See Communication from the Commission to the European Parliament, the Council and the European Economic and Social Committee, *Double Taxation in the Single Market*, COM(2011) 712 final—henceforth, the Commission Double Taxation Communication.

[54] *Ibid*, p 5. See also ch 5 in HJI Panayi (2013), n 1 above.

[55] See Public Consultation Paper, *Double Tax Conventions and the Internal Market: factual examples of double taxation cases with a follow-up questionnaires for experts, corporate and individuals*. Also see the summary of the responses received available on: ec.europa.eu/taxation_customs/resources/documents/common/consultations/tax/summary_report_consultation_double_tax_conventions_en.pdf. Also see Public Consultation Paper, *Consultation on possible approaches to tackling cross-border inheritance tax obstacles within the EU* (2010) and Public Consultation Paper, *Consultation on Taxation of cross border interest and royalty payments between associated companies* (2010). Available on: ec.europa.eu/taxation_customs/common/consultations/tax/2010_04_doubletax_en.htm; ec.europa.eu/taxation_customs/common/consultations/tax/2010_06_inheritance_en.htm; ec.europa.eu/taxation_customs/common/consultations/tax/2010_08_royalty_en.htm.

[56] See Commission Double Taxation Communication, n 53 above, p 6.

Existing instruments were insufficient to address many of the remaining double taxation situations.[57] The Interest and Royalties Directive was limited in scope. Also, tax treaties did not cover all taxes relevant from an internal market perspective; nor did they provide for the removal of double taxation, especially in triangular or multilateral cases. Moreover, tax treaty provisions were not interpreted and implemented consistently by all Member States. The time needed to conclude mutual agreement procedures under either the Arbitration Convention or tax treaties was too long and these procedures often did not succeed in solving the problems submitted.

As an immediate step, the Commission referred to its proposal for a Common Consolidated Corporate Tax Base (CCCTB)[58] and the proposal for a recast of the Interest and Royalties Directive.[59] In addition, the Commission expressed its willingness to adopt further measures, such as possible solutions to tackle cross-border inheritance tax obstacles as well as the double taxation of dividends paid to portfolio investors.[60] Other suggestions were the creation of a forum on double taxation for purely EU tax matters, a proposal for a code of conduct on double taxation and the feasibility of an efficient dispute resolution mechanism. The Commission also expressed its concerns about double non-taxation and said that it was reviewing the situation with a view to proposing appropriate action.[61]

Indeed, shortly thereafter, the Commission issued a public consultation document on double non-taxation.[62] The scope of the double non-taxation consultation only included cases of cross-border double non-taxation, ie cases where the tax rules of two countries combined led to non-taxation. It was limited to direct taxes, such as corporate income taxes, non-resident income taxes, capital gains taxes, withholding taxes, inheritance taxes and gift taxes. It was stated that double non-taxation had potentially harmful effects in terms of fairness of the tax systems and distortion of the internal market.[63] The Commission noted that avoidance of double non-taxation had 'an enhanced importance in the present Economic Crisis context'.[64]

[57] *Ibid.*

[58] Brussels, COM(2011) 121/4, 2011/0058 (CNS); SEC(2011) 316 final. This was accompanied by a detailed impact assessment. See Commission Staff Working Document Impact Assessment Accompanying document to the Proposal for a Council Directive on a Common Consolidated Corporate Tax Base (CCCTB), Brussels, 16 March 2011, SEC(2011) 315 final. Also see Commission Staff Working Paper, *Summary of the impact assessment—Accompanying document to the proposal for a Council Directive on a Common Consolidated Corporate Tax Base (CCCTB)*, SEC(2011) 316 final.

[59] Proposal for a Council Directive on a common system of taxation applicable to interest and royalty payments made between associated companies of different Member States, COM(2011) 714 final.

[60] Commission Double Taxation Communication, n 53 above, p 11.

[61] *Ibid*, p 8.

[62] Staff working paper, *The internal market: factual examples of double non-taxation cases: Consultation document* (Brussels, TAXUD D1 D(2012)).

[63] *Ibid*, p 4.

[64] *Ibid.*

The Commission sought consultation on a number of situations leading to double non-taxation, pointing out that the list was not exhaustive.[65] Interested parties were invited to submit their contributions by 30 May 2012. The Commission then published a summary of the responses received.[66] Overall, it was noted that there were fewer contributions compared to previous consultations. While having full regard to the principle of subsidiarity, the Commission reiterated the need to establish more coherence between Member States' individual positions in the international tax arena. 'This requires a greater degree of coordination at EU level so as to ensure that the momentum towards a more open and constructive tax co-operation continues at a global level'.[67]

It was noted that the business community expressed concerns on the scope of the consultation. In fact, many of the contributors did not provide answers to the specific questions of the consultation document, instead they provided broader and more general comments on the issues raised. One general criticism was that the consultation was vague. There was no clear distinction between actual double non-taxation (eg due to mismatches of hybrid entities and hybrid instruments) and tax competition (low taxation). A definition of 'double non-taxation' was needed.[68]

It was stressed that direct taxation falls within the competence of the Member States' sovereignty. Several contributors found that any measures against double non-taxation should be handled at Member State level, while others found some coordination appropriate (eg to avoid mismatches). Others argued that the issue of double non-taxation should not be addressed separately from that of double taxation, as the two were considered as two sides of the same coin.[69] There was support for the CCCTB as a measure to deal with some of these issues.

The double non-taxation issue which most contributors found least acceptable was double non-taxation due to mismatches of countries' qualifications of hybrid entities and hybrid financial instruments. Several contributors also argued that application of tax treaties sometimes led to double non-taxation. This was an issue also to be considered in the future. It was overwhelmingly stressed that double taxation and double non-taxation were two sides of the same coin and should

[65] The following 10 situations were considered: mismatches of entities, mismatches of financial instruments, application of double tax treaties leading to double non-taxation, transfer pricing and unilateral Advance Pricing Arrangements, transactions with associated enterprises in countries with no or extremely low taxation, debt financing of tax exempt income, different treatment of passive and active income, double tax treaties with third countries, availability of relevant information for detection of double non-taxation.

[66] Commission, *Summary report of the responses received on the public consultation on factual examples and possible ways to tackle double non-taxation cases* (Brussels, 5 July 2012, TAXUD D1 D(2012)). Available on: ec.europa.eu/taxation_customs/resources/documents/common/consultations/tax/double_non_tax/summary_report.pdf.

[67] *Ibid*, p 2.

[68] *Ibid*, p 3.

[69] *Ibid*, p 3.

both be addressed by the Commission. Furthermore, it was noted that measures against double non-taxation had an adverse impact on European economic competitiveness. Therefore, it was preferable to coordinate the EU's initiatives with other initiatives at EU and international level that addressed similar aspects of double (non-) taxation.[70]

Furthermore, building on the positive experiences of the Joint Transfer Pricing Forum (JTPF), it was suggested to set up a Forum on double taxation for purely EU tax matters and perhaps to cover double non-taxation. The Commission revealed its intention to publish a Communication on good governance in the tax area in relation to tax havens and aggressive tax planning before the end of 2012. These were indeed published, under slightly different titles, in the context of a wider Action Plan to reinforce the fight against tax fraud and tax evasion.

5.2.3. The EU Pre-Action Plan Communication

Since 2012, the EU institutions are taking a much more active role in the fight against tax fraud and tax evasion. On 2 March 2012, the European Council called on the Council and the Commission to rapidly develop concrete ways to tackle this issue, including in relation to third countries and to report by June 2012. On 19 April of that same year, the European Parliament adopted a resolution echoing the urgent need for action in this area.[71]

Following this, on 27 June 2012, the Commission adopted a Communication on concrete ways to reinforce the fight against tax fraud and tax evasion including in relation to third countries.[72] In this Communication, it was suggested that the problems posed by tax fraud and evasion must be tackled at three levels. First, tax collection within each Member State had to be improved. Secondly, there was a need to enhance cross-border cooperation between Member States' tax administrations. Thirdly, it was important for the European Union to have a clear and coherent policy vis-à-vis third countries in order to promote its standards at international level and ensure a level playing field.

The Communication outlined how tax compliance could be improved and fraud and evasion reduced, through a better use of existing instruments and the adoption of pending Commission proposals. It also identified areas where further legislative action or coordination would benefit the European Union and

[70] At the time, it was the EU Code of Conduct Group's reports and the (pre-BEPS) OECD report on Hybrid Mismatches. See OECD, *Hybrid Mismatch Arrangements: Tax Policy and Compliance Issues* (OECD, 2012).

[71] European Parliament resolution of 19 April 2012 on the call for concrete ways to combat tax fraud and tax evasion (2012/2599(RSP)).

[72] Communication from the Commission to the European Parliament and the Council on concrete ways to reinforce the fight against tax fraud and tax evasion including in relation to third countries, COM(2012) 351 final of 27 June 2012.

Member States. It was suggested that such action should not only target fraudulent activity and tax evasion but also aggressive tax planning.[73] As such, the term aggressive tax planning was formally introduced and described as follows: 'Aggressive tax planning includes the use of artificial operations or structures and the exploitation of mismatches between tax systems with the effect of undermining Member States' tax rules and exacerbating the loss of tax revenues'.[74]

The importance of tax policy for fiscal consolidation and growth was noted,[75] as well as the fact that fair and ambitious fiscal consolidation was impaired by inefficient and ineffective tax collection mechanisms. For many Member States there were substantial problems of tax evasion often linked to poor administrative capacity.[76]

The Commission suggested amending and strengthening existing instruments.[77] At the same time, it had to be ensured that established good governance principles in the tax area, such as transparency, exchange of information and fair tax competition, were promoted in a more consistent manner, not just within the European Union but with third countries as well.[78] Coherence between EU policies was essential. Good governance principles in the tax area should continue to be included in all relevant EU-level agreements with third countries[79] as well as promoted through development cooperation incentives as outlined in previous Communications.[80] Furthermore, it was suggested that cooperation with other international organisations should be improved and synergies should be explored.[81]

[73] *Ibid*, p 3.

[74] *Ibid.*

[75] This was recognised in the process of the European Semester (Commission Communication on the Annual Growth Survey 2012—COM(2011) 815 final of 25 November 2011—17229/11; Council conclusions of 16 February 2012 (6353/1/12 Rev.1)) and the Euro Plus Pact (Council conclusions of 16 February 2012 (6404/1/12 Rev.1)). See p 4 of the Commission Communication on concrete ways to reinforce the fight against tax fraud and tax evasion, n 72 above.

[76] *Ibid*, p 4.

[77] Eg the Savings Directive, the Mutual Assistance Directive on exchange of information. There was also discussion of the possible use of the Tax Identification Number, the Quick Reaction Mechanism on VAT fraud etc: *ibid*, pp 6–9.

[78] *Ibid*, p 9.

[79] *Ibid*, p 11.

[80] Communication from the Commission to the European Parliament and the Council, *Promoting Good Governance in Tax Matters*, COM(2009) 201 final of 28.4.2009 and Communication from the Commission to the European Parliament and the Council, *Tax and Development—Cooperating with Developing Countries on Promoting Good Governance in Tax Matters*, COM(2010) 163 final of 21 April 2010.

[81] Commission Communication on concrete ways to reinforce the fight against tax fraud and tax evasion, n 72 above, p 11. It was noted that the European Union participates actively in other international forums such as the OECD, the International Organisation for Tax Administration (IOTA), the Inter American Center of Tax Administrations (CIAT), the International Tax Dialogue (ITD), the International Tax Compact (ITC), and the African Tax Administration Forum (ATAF).

As far as tax havens were concerned, the Commission briefly reviewed the ongoing work of the OECD.[82] It was recognised that important progress was made through the almost universal adoption of strong rules on information exchange and transparency following the successful re-launching of the OECD's Global Forum on Transparency and Exchange of Information for Tax Purposes. One criticism raised was that the Forum did not consider the question of 'fair tax competition', a principle which the European Union upheld internally via the Code of Conduct for business taxation.[83] 'Promoting such a concept to third countries is relevant both for the OECD and the EU'.[84] The Commission added that the burden of additional compliance costs due to uncoordinated actions by Member States to protect their tax bases against tax havens fell on all taxpayers. Such compliance costs would be reduced if there was a coordinated action.

The Commission discussed possible policy responses. This was a precursor to the Commission's detailed Action Plan to strengthen the fight against tax fraud and tax evasion. This Action Plan would seek to set out concrete steps to enhance administrative cooperation and to support the development of the existing good governance policy, the wider issues of interaction with tax havens and of tackling aggressive tax planning. The Action Plan, accompanied by two recommendations, was released in December 2012. By that time, the concept of aggressive tax planning was beginning to be firmly established and concerns about it widely shared in the international tax community.

5.2.4. Action Plan to Strengthen the Fight Against Tax Fraud and Tax Evasion

The Commission Communication on an Action Plan to strengthen the fight against tax fraud and tax evasion[85] set out the parameters of the scope of action to be taken. In this Communication, the Commission presented the initiatives it had already taken or had already discussed in its previous Communication[86] and new initiatives. The Action Plan contained practical actions which could deliver concrete results to all Member States.[87] In a remarkably different tone than in

[82] *Ibid*, pp 11–12.

[83] Conclusions of the ECOFIN Council meeting on 1 December 1997 concerning taxation policy ([1997] OJ C2/1 of 6 January 1998).

[84] Commission Communication on concrete ways to reinforce the fight against tax fraud and tax evasion, n 72 above, p 12.

[85] Communication from the Commission to the European Parliament and the Council, *An Action Plan to strengthen the fight against tax fraud and tax evasion*, COM(2012) 722 final of 6 December 2012.

[86] Commission Communication on concrete ways to reinforce the fight against tax fraud and tax evasion, n 72 above.

[87] Action Plan, n 85 above, p 3.

earlier communications it was noted that, taking into account the freedoms awarded to Member States when operating in the internal market, businesses may structure arrangements with such jurisdictions via the Member State with the weakest response to these issues. 'This does not only erode Member States' tax bases but also endangers fair competitive conditions for business and, ultimately, distorts the operation of the internal market'.[88]

Two recommendations were mentioned in the Communication. These were the Recommendation on measures intended to encourage third countries to apply minimum standards of good governance in tax matters (henceforth, the Recommendation on Good Governance)[89] and the Recommendation on Aggressive Tax Planning.[90] The Recommendations were published separately at the same time as the Communication but their essence was summarised in the Communication.

The Recommendation on Good Governance sought to provide Member States with a set of criteria to identify third countries that did not meet minimum standards of good governance in tax matters and a 'toolbox' of measures in regard to third countries according to whether they comply with those standards, or are committed to complying with them. As far as the Recommendation on Aggressive Tax Planning was concerned, the Commission referred to complex and artificial tax planning leading to the relocation of the tax base to other jurisdictions within or outside the European Union, as well as mismatches in national laws leading to double non-taxation and the exploitation of tax rates. The Commission also noted that aggressive tax planning could be considered contrary to the principles of Corporate Social Responsibility.[91] Therefore, concrete steps were needed to address the problem.[92] This was an interesting link to draw—one that is increasingly discussed, as shown in Chapter one of this volume.

The Commission expressed its willingness to contribute to the work of international tax fora such as the OECD. Initiatives mentioned were, inter alia: the development of international standards to address the complexities of taxing electronic commerce; the creation of a Platform for Tax Good Governance; improvements in the area of harmful business taxation; promoting the Code of Conduct for business taxation in selected third countries; ensuring the Directives do not lead to double non-taxation; and continuing to develop standard forms for exchange of information in the field of taxation etc.[93]

[88] *Ibid*, p 5.

[89] Commission Recommendation of 6 December 2012 regarding measures intended to encourage third countries to apply minimum standards of good governance in tax matters (C (2012) 8805 final).

[90] Commission Recommendation of 6 December 2012 on Aggressive Tax Planning (C (2012) 8806 final).

[91] Communication on a renewed EU strategy 2011–14 for Corporate Social Responsibility—COM(2011) 681 final of 25 October 2011.

[92] Action Plan, n 85 above, p 6.

[93] *Ibid*, pp 7–8.

The remainder of the Communication set out specific measures to be taken in the short term,[94] medium term[95] and long term[96] to tackle the problems mentioned. This was the Commission's self-proclaimed 'general contribution to the wider international debate on taxation and [which was] aimed at assisting the G20 and the G8 in its on-going work in this field'.[97]

In the Recommendation on Good Governance, the Commission reiterated the importance of setting out minimum standards of good governance in tax matters. This was a practical but essential first step in aligning the attitudes taken by Member States vis-a-vis jurisdictions not applying minimum standards.

It was stipulated that a third country would only be complying with minimum standards of good governance in tax matters where it had adopted legal, regulatory and administrative measures intended to comply with the standards of transparency and exchange of information,[98] where it effectively applied those measures and did not operate harmful tax measures in the area of business taxation.[99] Tax measures which provided for a significantly lower effective level of taxation, including zero taxation, were to be regarded as potentially harmful.[100] Such a level of taxation could operate by virtue of the nominal tax rate, the tax base or any other relevant factor.

[94] This would include, inter alia, the revision of the Parent-Subsidiary Directive and the anti-abuse provisions of the other Directives, promoting the standard of automatic exchange of information in international fora and the EU IT tools, a European Taxpayer's Code, reinforcing cooperation with other law enforcement bodies, promoting the use of simultaneous controls and the presence of foreign officials for audits, obtaining an authorisation from Council to start negotiations with third countries for bilateral agreements on administrative cooperation in the field of VAT etc: *ibid*, pp 9–11.

[95] This would include the development of a computerised format for automatic exchange of information on income from employment, directors' fees, life insurance products, pensions and on ownership of and income from immovable property, pursuant to Art 8(1) of the Mutual Assistance Directive 2011/16/EU, the use of an EU Tax Identification Number (TIN), the development of guidelines for tracing money flows, extending EUROFISC (a system of rapid exchange of information on cases of fraud in the VAT area) to direct taxation, creating a one-stop-shop approach in all Member States, developing motivational incentives including voluntary disclosure programmes, a tax web portal, an EU Standard Audit File for Tax etc: *ibid*, pp 11–14.

[96] This would include a methodology for joint audits by dedicated teams of trained auditors, the development of mutual direct access to national databases, a single legal instrument for administrative cooperation for all taxes: *ibid*, pp 14–15.

[97] *Ibid*, p 15.

[98] These were set out in the Annex of the Recommendation on Good Governance, n 89 above, p 8.

[99] *Ibid*, pp 4–5.

[100] When assessing whether such measures are harmful, account should be taken of inter alia: (a) whether advantages are accorded only to non-residents or in respect of transactions carried out with non-residents, or (b) whether advantages are ring-fenced from the domestic market, so they do not affect the national tax base, or (c) whether advantages are granted even without any real economic activity and substantial economic presence within the third country offering such tax advantages, or (d) whether the rules for profit determination in respect of activities within a multinational group of companies departs from internationally accepted principles, notably the rules agreed upon within the Organisation for Economic Co-operation and Development, or (e) whether the tax measures lack transparency, including where legal provisions are relaxed at administrative level in a non-transparent way. In applying these criteria, the Recommendation urged Member States to take account of the conclusions reached by the Code of Conduct Group on Business Taxation on this issue: *ibid*, p 5.

A number of measures would be taken vis-à-vis third countries, with a view to encouraging those countries to comply with those standards. It was recommended that Member States should publish blacklists of third countries not complying with the minimum standards set out above.[101] Furthermore, Member States that had already adopted national blacklists should include in such lists third countries not complying with these minimum standards. Member States were encouraged to renegotiate, suspend or terminate tax treaties with non-compliant third countries, as well as initiate bilateral negotiations for tax treaties with compliant third countries. Member States should consider offering closer cooperation and assistance to third countries, especially developing ones, which were committed to complying with the minimum standards. Such closer cooperation would assist those third countries in their fight against tax evasion and aggressive tax planning.[102]

In the Recommendation on Aggressive Tax Planning,[103] aggressive tax planning was described as consisting in the taking advantage of the technicalities of a tax system or of mismatches between two or more tax systems for the purpose of reducing tax liability. It could take a multitude of forms. Its consequences included double deductions and double non-taxation.[104] It was emphasised that, with a view to moving to a better functioning of the internal market, it was necessary to encourage all Member States to take the same general approach towards aggressive tax planning.[105] Situations leading to double non-taxation could 'lead to artificial capital flows and movements of taxpayers within the internal market and thus harm its proper functioning as well as erode Member States' tax bases'.[106]

Member States were, inter alia, urged to introduce a subject-to-tax requirement both in their unilateral double tax relief rules and in their bilateral tax treaties with other EU Member States and with third countries Also, Member States were encouraged to incorporate GAARs in their national legislation.[107] The following wording was suggested:

> An artificial arrangement or an artificial series of arrangements which has been put into place for the essential purpose of avoiding taxation and leads to a tax benefit shall be ignored. National authorities shall treat these arrangements for tax purposes by reference to their economic substance.

[101] *Ibid.*

[102] *Ibid*, p 6. 'To this end, they could second tax experts to such countries for a limited period of time. When judging third countries' commitment to complying with those minimum standards, Member States should take into account all concrete indications to this effect, in particular steps towards compliance already taken by the third country concerned'. See para 6.1.

[103] Recommendation on Aggressive Tax Planning, n 90 above. See also definition of term in Commission Communication on concrete ways to reinforce the fight against tax fraud and tax evasion, n 72 above, discussed in section 5.2.3.

[104] Recommendation on Aggressive Tax Planning, n 90 above, p 2.

[105] *Ibid.*

[106] *Ibid.*

[107] *Ibid*, p 4.

It was explained in the Recommendation that an 'arrangement' meant any transaction, scheme, action, operation, agreement, grant, understanding, promise, undertaking or event. An arrangement could comprise more than one step or part. An arrangement was considered artificial where it lacked commercial substance.[108]

The Commission emphasised the risk for countries seeking to tackle the problem alone—the companies would simply relocate. An EU-wide response was needed to close loopholes and ensure that no country lost out financially for addressing the problem. The Commission was committed to monitoring the implementation of these recommendations and putting pressure on countries whose progress was slow.

It is undeniable that the concept of aggressive tax planning, as developed through these Commission initiatives goes beyond the EU concept of abuse discussed in section 5.1 above. In fact, some of the Commission's recommendations such as the GAAR run contrary to the Court of Justice's refusal to acknowledge, in *3M Italia*,[109] the existence of a general principle of abuse of rights which would impose an obligation on the Member States to combat abusive practices in the field of direct taxation. Not only is such a measure now recommended—albeit in a technically non-binding manner—but the scope of abusive practices is expanded to cover legal gaps or mismatches leading to double non-taxation[110] and harmful tax regimes.

Notwithstanding the questionable legality of some of these recommendations, as time goes by, they are increasingly seen as irreversible, especially due to the similarities they share with the BEPS project which, in principle and as an idea, enjoys almost universal support. The question of compatibility of some of the Commission's Action Plan proposals with EU law will further be addressed when considering the compatibility of the BEPS deliverables in Chapter six.

[108] *Ibid*, pp 4–5. In determining whether the arrangement or series of arrangements was artificial, national authorities were invited to consider whether they involved one or more of the following situations: (a) the legal characterisation of the individual steps which an arrangement consisted of was inconsistent with the legal substance of the arrangement as a whole; (b) the arrangement or series of arrangements was carried out in a manner which would not ordinarily be employed in what was expected to be a reasonable business conduct; (c) the arrangement or series of arrangements included elements which had the effect of offsetting or cancelling each other; (d) transactions were circular in nature; (e) the arrangement or series of arrangements resulted in a significant tax benefit but this was not reflected in the business risks undertaken by the taxpayer or its cash flows; (f) the expected pre-tax profit was insignificant in comparison to the amount of the expected tax benefit. The purpose of an arrangement or series of arrangements consisted in avoiding taxation where, regardless of any subjective intentions of the taxpayer, it defeated the object, spirit and purpose of the tax provisions that would otherwise apply. It was useful to consider whether one or more of the following situations occurred: an amount was not included in the tax base; the taxpayer benefitted from a deduction; a loss for tax purposes was incurred; no withholding tax was due; foreign tax was offset.

[109] Case C-417/10 *3M Italia*, n 33 above.

[110] See Ana Paula Dourado, 'Aggressive Tax Planning in EU Law and in the Light of BEPS: The EC Recommendation on Aggressive Tax Planning and BEPS Actions 2 and 6' (2015) 43 *Intertax* 42–57.

5.3. The Aftermath of the Action Plan

5.3.1. Improving Standards and Soft Law

Following the publication of the Action Plan, the Commission has moved forward with several of the recommendations outlined.

On 25 February 2013, the Commission launched two consultations: one on the European Taxpayer's Code[111] and one on the European Taxpayer Identification Number (the EU TIN).[112]

In the first consultation, the Commission proposed to develop a European Taxpayer's Code which would embed a core but comprehensive set of common tax principles and taxpayers' rights and obligations. Member States would then be in a position to establish or adapt their own codes by reference to these common and generally agreed standards. As far as cross-border operations were concerned, a European Taxpayer's Code might not only lead to improved access to the internal market but could also help raise the overall standards of tax administration.[113] Through its questionnaire, the Commission assessed the situation in Member States and examined existing experience with national taxpayer's codes or similar instruments.[114]

In the second consultation on the EU TIN, it was noted that the absence of a common approach to the identification of taxpayers impaired the efficiency of administrative cooperation and (automatic) exchange of information in particular. Although almost all Member States used some form of national TIN, these were built according to national rules which differed considerably among countries. These differences made it difficult to correctly identify, register and report foreign TINs. The introduction of an EU TIN could resolve these difficulties and facilitate the proper identification of taxpayers engaged in cross-border operations. A unique EU TIN would maintain rather than replace the existing national TINs. As far as the design of an EU TIN, the Commission put forward a number of questions for consultation.[115]

On 23 April 2013, the Commission launched the Platform for Tax Good Governance, to discuss best practices in the fight against tax evasion, tax avoidance and

[111] Consultation Paper—A European Taxpayer's Code—Brussels, 25 February 2013 (TAXUD.D. 2.002 (2013) 276169). See Luca Cerioni, 'The Possible Introduction of a European Taxpayer Code: Objective and Potential Alternatives' (2014) 54 *European Taxation* 392-403.

[112] Consultation Paper—Use of An EU Tax Identification Number—Brussels, 25 February 2013 (TAXUD.D.2.002 (2013) 276134).

[113] Consultation Paper—A European Taxpayer's Code, n 111 above, p 3.

[114] For the questions and the summary report of the contributions, see Summary Report on the outcome of the public consultation from DG TAXUD—A European Taxpayer's Code, Brussels, 12 September 2013, (TAXUD.D.2 (Ares 2013) 3252439).

[115] See ec.europa.eu/taxation_customs/common/consultations/tax/2013_eutin_en.htm.

tax havens.[116] This platform would monitor Member States' progress in tackling aggressive tax planning and clamping down on tax havens, in line with the aforementioned Recommendations. The Commission's work on good governance was discussed in Chapter one in reviewing international initiatives on the topic.[117]

In its plenary session in May, 2013, the European Parliament approved its 'Report on Fight against Tax Fraud, Tax Evasion and Tax Havens'.[118] Many issues were raised in this Report. The European Parliament emphasised that the European Union should take the leading role in discussions on the fight against tax fraud, tax avoidance and tax havens in the OECD, the Global Forum on Transparency and Exchange of Information for Tax Purposes, the G20, the G8 and other relevant multinational fora. The importance of international cooperation in this fight was raised, as well as the need to

> persuade non-EU countries to build up and improve the efficacy of their respective tax collection systems by subscribing to the principles of transparency, automatic exchange of information and abolition of harmful tax measures, and to assist them in doing so.[119]

The European Parliament also welcomed the Foreign Account Tax Compliance Act (FATCA) as a first step towards an automatic exchange of information between the European Union and the US to fight cross-border tax fraud and tax evasion, criticising the fact that a bilateral/intergovernmental approach had been taken in the negotiations with the US rather than a common EU negotiating position.[120] It also criticised the lack of full reciprocity in the exchange of information.[121]

The European Parliament called on Member States, as a matter of priority, to close the loopholes of the Savings Directive and welcomed the international discussions on the updating of the OECD guidelines on transfer pricing[122] and the measures suggested in the Action Plan.[123] The European Parliament called for a common EU approach towards tax havens but also asked the Commission to adopt a clear definition and a common set of criteria to identify tax havens.[124] A public European blacklist of tax havens was necessary.[125]

There is certainly a lot of focus on transparency now. On 9 April 2013, five EU Member States (Germany, France, Spain, Italy and the UK) announced their

[116] Commission Decision of 23 April 2013 on setting up a Commission Expert Group to be known as the Platform for Tax Good Governance, Aggressive Tax Planning and Double Taxation, Brussels, 23 April 2013 (C(2013) 2236 final).

[117] See Ch 1, section 1.3 of this volume.

[118] Report on Fight against Tax Fraud, Tax Evasion and Tax Havens (2013/2060(INI)), Committee on Economic and Monetary Affairs, 2.5.2013. Available on: www.europarl.europa.eu/sides/getDoc.do?pubRef=-//EP//TEXT+REPORT+A7-2013-0162+0+DOC+XML+V0//EN.

[119] *Ibid*, para 8.

[120] *Ibid*, para 15.

[121] *Ibid*.

[122] *Ibid*, paras 46–47.

[123] *Ibid*, paras 48–63, 67–75.

[124] *Ibid*, paras 64–65.

[125] *Ibid*, para 66.

intention to co-operate on a pilot multilateral exchange facility. This would be based on the Model inter-governmental agreement for the implementation of FATCA. Through this, they would exchange the same type of information among themselves as they would exchange with the US under FATCA. Arguably, with the advent of the OECD's Common Reporting Standard and with the amendments to the Mutual Assistance Directive 2011/16/EU discussed in 5.3.2, this arrangement is likely to be obsolete.[126]

In June 2013, the new Accounting Directive[127] was enacted which introduced an obligation for large extractive and logging companies to report country-by-country the payments made to governments, and also on a project-basis. The obligation to publish the accounts is for tax years beginning on or after 1 January, 2016. There are several exemptions for small and medium-sized enterprises.[128] Increased transparency is also manifest in the Extractive Industries Transparency Initiative.[129] Furthermore, the Revised Capital Requirements Directive[130] aims to improve transparency in the activities of banks and investment funds in different countries, particularly regarding profits, taxes and subsidies in different jurisdictions.[131]

More recently, there is a move towards cracking down on anonymous shell companies. On 12 January 2015, the Council issued a proposal designed to combat money laundering and terrorist financing.[132] This proposal revised the fourth anti-money laundering directive to include a specific reference to tax crimes, as well as require Member States to store beneficial ownership information in central registers which would be accessible to the public. Legal professional privilege would be preserved.[133] To access a register, a person would in any event have to demonstrate a 'legitimate interest' in suspected money laundering, terrorist

[126] See OECD report on Standard for Automatic Exchange of Financial Account Information in Tax Matters and model agreement. Available on: www.oecd.org/ctp/exchange-of-tax-information/automatic-exchange-financial-account-information-common-reporting-standard.pdf.

[127] Directive 2013/34/EU of the European Parliament and of the Council of 26 June 2013 on the annual financial statements, consolidated financial statements and related reports of certain types of undertakings, amending Directive 2006/43/EC of the European Parliament and of the Council and repealing Council Directives 78/660/EEC and 83/349/EEC.

[128] See Arts 30–32 of Directive 2013/34/EU.

[129] For more information, see: eiti.org/.

[130] Directive 2013/36/EU of the European Parliament and of the Council of 26 June 2013 on access to the activity of credit institutions and the prudential supervision of credit institutions and investment firms, amending Directive 2002/87/EC and repealing Directives 2006/48/EC and 2006/49/EC.

[131] For commentary, see Rudolf Reibel, 'Tax Transparency—How to Make it Work' (2015) 55 *European Taxation* 209–12.

[132] See Proposal for a Directive of the European Parliament and of the Council on the prevention of the use of the financial system for the purpose of money laundering and terrorist financing. See release on 12 January 2015, available on: data.consilium.europa.eu/doc/document/ST-5116-2015-ADD-2/en/pdf.

[133] See *ibid*, para 7 of preamble: 'There should, however, be exemptions from any obligation to report information obtained either before, during or after judicial proceedings, or in the course of ascertaining the legal position of a client. Thus, legal advice should remain subject to the obligation of professional secrecy unless the legal counsellor is taking part in money laundering or terrorist financing, the legal advice is provided for money laundering or terrorist financing purposes or the lawyer knows that the client is seeking legal advice for money laundering or terrorist financing purposes'.

financing and in 'predicate' offences that might help to finance them, such as corruption, tax crimes and fraud. The persons who are able to demonstrate a legitimate interest should have access to information on the nature and extent of the beneficial interest held.[134] The European Parliament and Council agreed on this proposal on 27 January 2015.[135]

On 20 April 2015 the Council approved the revision to the fourth anti-money-laundering directive, including a requirement for all Member States to create central registers of beneficial ownership information for companies, other legal entities, and trusts incorporated in their respective territories.[136] Member States must ensure that the registers are available to competent authorities, financial intelligence units, and 'obliged entities', such as banks conducting due diligence tasks. A person must show a legitimate interest in alleged money laundering, terrorist financing, and predicate offences such as tax crimes to be able to access the beneficial ownership details.[137] For trusts, central beneficial ownership information registers will be used when the trust generates tax consequences. It is up to the discretion of Member States to decide whether to make their beneficial ownership registers public.[138]

More instruments are likely to follow. On 7 May 2015, the European Parliament Legal Affairs committee approved the Shareholders' Rights Directive,[139] a draft law that would require, inter alia, large undertakings and public-interest entities to publish country-by-country information on profits or losses before tax, taxes on profits or losses and public subsidies received. The draft law aims to improve transparency and foster shareholders' commitment to companies which should in turn improve their competitiveness and sustainability.[140]

5.3.2. Amendments to Direct Tax Directives

Following the momentum created by the OECD/G20 BEPS Action Plan and the EU Action Plan, the Commission seized on the opportunity to amend several

[134] See *ibid*, para 11 of preamble.

[135] See 2015 *WTD* 18-14 (27 January 2015).

[136] See Position of the Council at first reading with a view to the adoption of a Directive of the European Parliament and of the Council on the prevention of the use of the financial system for the purposes of money laundering or terrorist financing, amending Regulation (EU) No 648/2012 of the European Parliament and of the Council, and repealing Directive 2005/60/EC of the European Parliament and of the Council and Commission Directive 2006/70/EC, Brussels, 8 April 2015 (OR. en). Also see regulation, available on: 2015 *WTD* 76-20. For commentary, see Stephanie Soong Johnston, 'EU Council Approves Beneficial Ownership Register Rules' 2015 *WTD* 76-1 (21 April 2015).

[137] The details to be accessed are name, month and year of birth, nationality, country of residence, and nature and approximate extent of held beneficial interest.

[138] See Draft Statement of the Council's Reasons, Brussels, 27 March 2015, available on: 2015 *WTD* 76-22.

[139] For a background to the Commission's initiatives to amend the Shareholders' Rights Directive 2007/36/EC, see: ec.europa.eu/internal_market/company/shareholders/indexa_en.htm.

[140] See Stephanie Soong Johnston, 'EU Parliamentary Committee Backs CbC Reporting Measure', 2015 *WTD* 89-1 (8 May 2015).

direct tax directives.[141] Some of the proposed amendments, such as those to the Savings Directive,[142] were long overdue.

On 25 November 2013, the Commission made a proposal to amend the Parent-Subsidiary Directive to tackle hybrid loans and mismatches.[143] The proposal also required Member States to adopt a common general anti-abuse clause to prevent them from extending the benefits of the directive to arrangements that did not reflect economic reality. This would replace the existing anti-abuse provision found in Article 1(2) of the Directive.

At the ECOFIN meeting on 6 May 2014 there was no agreement by Member States. Regarding the hybrid loans aspect of the proposal, there was broad agreement but Sweden requested further assurance on certain technical aspects. The Member States also did not agree with the proposed general anti-abuse clause. There were concerns that the formulation was too broad and could lead to different interpretations in different Member States, creating uncertainty for businesses. Discussions on the proposed amendments continued.

At the ECOFIN meeting on 20 June 2014,[144] Member States finally reached an agreement but only on the hybrid element of the proposal. Article 4(1)(a) of the Directive would be amended to provide that where a parent company, by virtue of its association with its subsidiary, receives distributed profits, the Member State of the parent company shall refrain from taxing such profits to the extent that such profits are not deductible by the subsidiary of the parent company. It was confirmed that this provision would be applicable in situations of double non-taxation resulting from mismatches in the tax treatment of profit distributions between Member States which generate unintended tax benefits. Member States would have until 31 December 2015 to transpose the amendment into national law. There was no agreement on the common anti-abuse provision—the Council agreed to split it from the broader proposal in order to allow early adoption of the new rule on hybrid loans.

On 9 December 2014, it was announced that the Council finally approved the general anti-abuse provision which would replace the existing anti-abuse provision. Broadly, this provision would allow Member States not to grant the benefits of the Directive to

> an arrangement or a series of arrangements that, having been put into place for the main purpose or one of the main purposes of obtaining a tax advantage which defeats the

[141] Measures have also been taken in the VAT field, where new instruments were introduced to better fight VAT fraud, eg the Quick Reaction Mechanism and the Reverse Charge Mechanism. Also see Commission Proposal for a Council Directive amending Directive 2006/112/EC on the common system of value added tax as regards a standard VAT return, COM(2013) 721 of 23.10.13. See also the Implementation Plan (SWD/2013/ 428), the Impact Assessment (SWD/2013/427) and its summary (SWD/2013/426). These measures and proposals are not considered further in this book.

[142] See ch 2 in HJI Panayi (2013), n 1 above.

[143] See IP/13/1149.

[144] See announcement available on: www.consilium.europa.eu/uedocs/cms_data/docs/pressdata/en/ecofin/143274.pdf.

object or purpose of this Directive, are not genuine having regard to all relevant facts and circumstances.

An arrangement could comprise more than one step or part—ie it can be a series of arrangements. Also an arrangement or a series of arrangements would be regarded as not genuine to the extent that it was not put into place for valid commercial reasons which reflect economic reality. Member States were entitled to continue applying their domestic or agreement-based provisions required for the prevention of tax evasion, tax fraud or abuse.[145]

The Commission welcomed this breakthrough agreement. As Commissioner Moscovici said, '[t]he agreement on the anti-abuse provisions of the Parent-Subsidiary Directive ensures a level-playing field for honest businesses in the EU's Single Market and it closes down loopholes that could be exploited for aggressive tax planning'.[146]

Arguably, there are a few issues with these amendments. First, the hybrid loan aspect of the proposal raises similar concerns to the linking rules of Action 2 of the Action Plan, because of the mechanical nature of the rule and its expansive scope beyond wholly artificial arrangements. The compatibility of the BEPS linking rules is discussed in greater detail in the next chapter. There are, however, differences between the two anti-hybrid rules which ought to be pointed out. It would seem that the Parent-Subsidiary Directive amendment *allows* the Member State of residence of the recipient not to exempt the profits received—it does not impose an obligation to do so.[147] Furthermore, there is no obligation on the Member State of source (ie the state of residence of the payor of profit distributions) to act in a certain way. Of course that Member State can use the common anti-abuse provision to take further punitive action. But the fact remains that it is within the discretion of either Member State to take any action at all. If some Member States exercise this discretion and others not, then it can lead to jurisdiction shopping. The same result would ensue if Member States in principle set out to enforce this provision but in practice interpret it very laxly.

[145] Art 1(2) would be replaced by the following: '2. Member States shall not grant the benefits of this Directive to an arrangement or a series of arrangements that, having been put into place for the main purpose or one of the main purposes of obtaining a tax advantage which defeats the object or purpose of this Directive, are not genuine having regard to all relevant facts and circumstances. An arrangement may comprise more than one step or part. 3. For the purposes of paragraph 2, an arrangement or a series of arrangements shall be regarded as not genuine to the extent that they are not put into place for valid commercial reasons which reflect economic reality. 4. This Directive shall not preclude the application of domestic or agreement-based provisions required for the prevention of tax evasion, tax fraud or abuse'. See No doc: 16435/14 FISC 221 ECOFIN 1157. For commentary, see Luc De Broe, 'At Last, Some Output on the Fight against Double Non-Taxation' (2014) 23 *EC Tax Review* 310–12.

[146] See STATEMENT/14/2501, available on the Commission's website: europa.eu/rapid/press-release_STATEMENT-14-2501_en.htm.

[147] For a contrary view, see Evgenia Kokolia and Evgenia Chatziioakeimidou, 'BEPS Impact on EU Law: Hybrid Payments and Abusive Tax Behaviour' (2015) 55 *European Taxation* 149–56; Filip Debelva and Joris Luts, 'The General Anti-Abuse Rule of the Parent-Subsidiary Directive' (2015) 55 *European Taxation* 223.

By contrast, the rules devised under Action 2 of the BEPS Action Plan rely on action which is *required* to be taken by either jurisdiction in which the mismatch arises. The aim is for the mismatch to be neutralised by either jurisdiction. As a result of the primary and defensive rules which apply automatically and in a hierarchical manner, there is an obligation on *either* jurisdiction to take action. The amendment in the Parent-subsidiary Directive relies on unilateral discretionary action, whereas the linking rules under Action 2 rely (or will aim to rely) on bilateral obligatory action. Notwithstanding these differences, it would seem that the same analysis as to compatibility with EU law applies. The fact that a measure is at the discretion of a Member State does not cure any potential incompatibility with EU law.

There is a further issue with the new anti-abuse rule of the Parent-Subsidiary Directive. The new rule incorporates a main purpose test, akin to that of Action 6 of the BEPS Action Plan. The compatibility of such tests with EU law is considered in the following chapter. However, as has already been pointed out,[148] even if this clause is compatible with the principles set out by the Court of Justice in the *Halifax* line of cases,[149] unlike VAT, this is an area of law remaining largely unharmonised. Therefore, where the main rules are not themselves harmonised, it is rather odd to have harmonisation of anti-abuse rules—ie the exception to the rules.[150]

As a result of the impetus, the Savings Directive was also finally adopted. Although a proposal to amend the Savings Directive had been pending since 2008,[151] up until recently there was no consensus to adopt it.[152] On 24 March 2014, the EU Council of Ministers finally adopted the revised version of the Savings Directive.[153] Changes were made to close existing loopholes and better prevent tax evasion. Inter alia, a look-through approach based on 'customer due diligence' was implemented which would have prevented individuals from circumventing the Directive by using an interposed legal person (eg foundation) or arrangements (eg trust) situated in a non-EU country which did not ensure effective taxation.

[148] See discussion in section 5.2.4 above.

[149] See analysis in section 5.1 above.

[150] As Hans van den Hurk noted, '[a]s the Member States are unwilling to agree on harmonization of the rules, harmonisation of the exception to such rules is unlikely to be accepted'. See Hans van den Hurk, 'Proposed Amended Parent-Subsidiary Directive Reveals the European Commission's Lack of Vision' (2014) 9 *Bulletin for International Taxation* 488, 493.

[151] Proposal for Council Directive amending Directive 2003/48/EC on taxation of savings income in the form of interest payments: COM(2008) 727 final. This proposal was again discussed in the ECOFIN Council on 14–15 February 2011. See also Council of the European Union, 6514/11, Provisional Version, PR CO 6, 3067th Council meeting, ECOFIN, Brussels, 15 February 2011. Reported at 2011 *WTD* 33-16.

[152] Notwithstanding Member States' reluctance to amend the Savings Directive, the Commission continued with its mandate to re-negotiate stronger savings tax agreements with Switzerland, Andorra, Monaco, San Marino and Liechtenstein. The main purpose of re-negotiating these agreements was to ensure the continued equivalence of the measures applied by these countries with those applied internally within the European Union. See MEMO/12/353.

[153] [2014] OJ L155/50 of 15 April 2014.

The provisions of the Savings Directive were also refined to ensure that individuals would not circumvent the Directive by using an interposed legal person situated in an EU Member State. National rules transposing the revised Savings Directive should be adopted by Member States by January 2016.[154]

Ironically, just when the amendments to the Savings Directive have finally been approved, the whole Directive is likely to be repealed in the near future. This is because of the all-encompassing changes to the Mutual Assistance Directive 2011/16/EU which Member States agreed to at the ECOFIN meeting in October 2014. In this important meeting, Member States agreed on a Commission proposal to apply the widest possible scope of automatic exchange of information within the European Union, to mirror the global standard of automatic information exchange agreed by the G20.[155] It was agreed that from 2017, Member State tax authorities would automatically exchange information with each other on most categories of income and capital held by private individuals and certain entities. Austria was to be given an additional year to apply the new rules, so as to have sufficient time to make the necessary technical adaptations. The revised Mutual Assistance Directive would cover a wide scope of income and capital—including most of what was already covered by the revised Savings Directive. In order to have just one standard of automatic information exchange and to avoid legislative overlaps, the Commission recommended the repeal of the Savings Directive to ensure that no loopholes are created or left for tax evaders.

In December 2014, the newly-appointed EU Tax Commissioner Pierre Moscovici announced that the Commission would unveil a directive on the automatic exchange of information on tax rulings in the first quarter of 2015 and would examine additional anti-avoidance proposals.[156] Automatic exchange of tax rulings was, inter alia, one of the proposals that the OECD made in the context of Action 5 of the BEPS project,[157] as discussed in Chapter two of this volume.[158]

In February 2015 the Commission announced that it would soon present a Tax Transparency Package, including a legislative proposal for the automatic exchange of information on tax rulings[159] and a proposal for a Common Consolidated Corporate Tax Base (CCCTB).[160] This would set a foundation for a fairer and more transparent approach to taxation in the European Union. The Tax Transparency Package was to be based on the Commission's commitment in its Work

[154] See ec.europa.eu/taxation_customs/taxation/personal_tax/savings_tax/revised_directive/index_en.htm.

[155] See n 126 above.

[156] Stephanie Soong Johnston, 'EU to Unveil Directive for Tax Rulings Info Exchange in Early 2015', 2014 *WTD* 232-1 (3 December 2014).

[157] See OECD, *Countering Harmful Tax Practices More Effectively, Taking into Account Transparency and Substance—Action 5: 2014 Deliverable.*

[158] See analysis of Action 5, in Ch 2, section 2.7.

[159] See Press Release on 18 February 2015, IP/15/4436 available on: europa.eu/rapid/press-release_IP-15-4436_en.htm.

[160] Teri Sprackland, 'Now Is the Time for Action on Transparency, EU Tax Commissioner Says', 2015 *WTD* 37-4 (25 February 2015).

Programme in December 2014 to clamp down on tax evasion and tax avoidance and to ensure that taxes are paid in the country where profits were generated.[161] Indeed, not long after that announcement, the Commission released its tax transparency package, which is discussed in greater detail below.

5.4. The Tax Transparency Package

On 18 March 2015, the Commission presented its Tax Transparency Package—the latest initiative of its ambitious agenda to tackle corporate tax avoidance and harmful tax competition in the European Union. A key element was the proposal to introduce the automatic exchange of information between Member States on their tax rulings. The problem with tax rulings was that Member States shared very little information with one another about their tax rulings and it was at their discretion to decide whether a tax ruling might be relevant to another EU Member State. As a result, Member States were often unaware of cross-border tax rulings issued elsewhere in the European Union which might impact their own tax bases. This lack of transparency was exploited by certain companies in order to artificially reduce their tax contribution.

As noted in the Commission Communication on tax transparency,[162] tax rulings which result in a low level of taxation in one Member State may entice companies to artificially shift profits to that jurisdiction. 'Not only can this lead to serious tax base erosion for other Member States, but it can further incentivise aggressive tax planning and corporate tax avoidance'.[163]

Under the existing Mutual Assistance Directive 2011/16/EU, information on tax rulings can be exchanged on a spontaneous basis under certain circumstances.[164] The Member State granting the tax ruling is, however, the only one to decide whether, and for whom, this information may be relevant. Moreover,

[161] See Press Release on 16 December 2014, IP/14/2703 available on: europa.eu/rapid/press-release_IP-14-2703_en.htm. Among the 23 initiatives see the initiative entitled 'A Fairer Approach to Taxation' which sets out the following: *An Action Plan on efforts to combat tax evasion and tax fraud, including measures at EU level in order to move to a system on the basis of which the country where profits are generated is also the country of taxation; including automatic exchange of information on tax rulings and stabilising corporate tax bases.*

[162] Communication from the Commission to the European Parliament and the Council on tax transparency to fight tax evasion and avoidance, COM(2015) 136 final (Brussels, 18 March 2015), p 4.

[163] *Ibid.*

[164] For example, if the country has grounds for assuming that there may be loss of taxation in another Member State and this information would be foreseeably relevant for the enforcement of the income tax law of that other Member State, or if a person liable to tax obtains a reduction in, or an exemption from, tax in one Member State which would give rise to an increase in tax or to liability to tax in the other Member State, or if the competent authority of a Member State has grounds for supposing that a saving of tax may result from artificial transfers of profits within groups of enterprises etc. See Art 9(1) of existing Mutual Assistance Directive 2011/16/EU, which sets out the scope and conditions of spontaneous exchange of information.

it can refuse to spontaneously exchange information on the basis of its commercial secrecy laws or public policy. To address this situation, the Commission proposed new provisions on exchange of tax rulings to be built into the existing legislative framework for information exchange, through amendments to the Mutual Assistance Directive.[165] This would enable the rapid implementation of automatic exchange of information on tax rulings, as the procedures and processes to do so were already in place.

This is not the first time that automatic exchange of tax rulings was considered within the European Union. During 2012, the Code of Conduct Group for Business Taxation had reviewed developments in Member States' procedures regarding tax rulings. The Group had identified the types of cross-border rulings on which information should be exchanged spontaneously, and recommended the development of a Model Instruction that could be used by Member States for internal application.[166]

Obviously, the scope of the Commission's proposal under the Tax Transparency Package is much more empowering than this. When the Commission's proposal is adopted, Member States would be required to *automatically* exchange information on their tax rulings. Every three months, national tax authorities would have to send a short report to all other Member States on all cross-border tax rulings and advance pricing agreements[167] that they have issued after the date of entry into force of the suggested Directive, including those which were issued during the last 10 years but remain valid on 1 January 2016. Member States would then be able to ask for more detailed information on a particular ruling.

The exchange of information is expected to be carried out using a standard form that will be produced by the Commission. The Commission will develop a database where information may be recorded and centralised for other Member States to detect certain abusive tax practices by companies and take the necessary

[165] See Proposal for a Council Directive amending Directive 2011/16/EU as regards mandatory automatic exchange of information in the field of taxation, SWD(2015) 60 final, COM(2015) 135 final, 2015/0068 (CNS) Brussels, 18 March 2015. The proposed Directive would also update the rules in the existing Directive concerning the provision of feedback, the practical arrangements for information exchange and the evaluation of administrative cooperation so as to extend them to the automatic information exchange on advance cross-border rulings and advance pricing arrangements.

[166] See Document 10903/12 FISC 77, mentioned in the proposal, p 3.

[167] Under para 5 of the proposed Art 8a of the Directive (Scope and conditions of mandatory automatic exchange of information on advance cross-border rulings and advance pricing arrangements) the information to be communicated shall, as a minimum, include the following: (a) the identification of the taxpayer and where appropriate the group of companies to which it belongs; (b) the content of the advance cross-border ruling or advance pricing arrangement, including a description of the relevant business activities or transactions or series of transactions; (c) the description of the set of criteria used for the determination of the transfer pricing or transfer price itself in the case of an advance pricing arrangement; (d) the identification of the other Member States likely to be directly or indirectly concerned by the advance cross-border ruling or advance pricing arrangement; (e) the identification of any person, other than a natural person, in the other Member States likely to be directly or indirectly affected by the advance cross-border ruling or advance pricing arrangement.

action in response.[168] After the initial exchange, a Member State may request more details or the full text of the document if it can demonstrate that the information is foreseeably relevant.

The concepts of advance tax ruling and advance pricing agreement are broadly defined to ensure there are no divergent interpretations which could enable Member States to circumvent their obligations.[169] Tax rulings and advance pricing agreements that cover purely domestic transactions or cross-border rulings that exclusively concern the tax affairs of natural persons are outside the scope of the proposal. It should be noted that the cross-border element does not seem to be restricted to EU Member States. To an extent, whether or not a transaction is a cross-border one does not appear to be well-defined.[170]

The Mutual Assistance Directive provides for a general limitation, according to which the provision of information may be refused by Member States where it would lead to the disclosure of a commercial, industrial or professional secret, or of a commercial process, or of information the disclosure of which would be contrary to public policy.[171] Under the proposal, this limitation would not apply with respect to the exchange of information on advance tax rulings and advance pricing agreements.[172] The Commission considers that such interests would be adequately protected under EU law and that the limited nature of the information that is required to be shared with all Member States should ensure sufficient protection of those commercial interests.

In its Communication accompanying the proposals of the Tax Transparency Package, the Commission argued that this initiative would encourage healthier tax competition, as tax authorities would be less likely to offer selective tax treatment to companies if this was open to scrutiny by their peers.[173] Moreover, the automatic exchange of information on tax rulings would enable Member States to detect certain abusive tax practices by companies and take the necessary action in response.

In the Communication, the Commission also repeated its proposal to repeal the Savings Directive, as this text had since been overtaken by more ambitious EU legislation, which required the widest scope of automatic information exchange on financial accounts, including savings-related income. Repealing the Savings Directive would also create a streamlined framework in this context and prevent any legal uncertainty or extra administration for tax authorities and businesses.

[168] See para 6 of proposed Art 8a which enables the possible creation by the Commission of a secure central directory concerning information communicated in the framework of this proposal.

[169] See proposed paras 14–15 of Art 3.

[170] See amendment to Art 3 of the existing Directive—insertions of paras 14–15. Cross-border transaction is defined as follows: '[t]he cross-border transaction may involve, but is not restricted to, the making of investments, the provision of goods, services, finance or the use of tangible or intangible assets and does not have to directly involve the person receiving the advance cross-border ruling'.

[171] See Art 17(4) of the existing Directive.

[172] See proposed Art 8a(9). Also see preamble, para 5.

[173] Communication from the Commission to the European Parliament and the Council on tax transparency to fight tax evasion and avoidance, COM(2015) 136 final (Brussels, 18 March 2015), p 4.

The Commission outlined a number of other initiatives to advance the tax transparency agenda in the European Union. New transparency requirements for multinationals would be assessed, such as the public disclosure of certain tax information by multinationals. The Commission would consider the benefits, costs and necessary safeguards in terms of data protection, protection of business secrets, etc. It would also examine how it would affect international competitiveness. Impact assessment work would be launched to analyse the various possible options. The OECD's BEPS work on transparency requirements would also need to be considered, as well as the costs and benefits of transposing such rules into European Union law.[174]

Also, the Code of Conduct on Business Taxation was to be reviewed. It was noted that over the past years, the Code had become less effective in addressing harmful tax regimes as its criteria did not take into account more sophisticated corporate tax avoidance schemes. The Commission would therefore work with Member States to review the Code of Conduct as well as the mandate of the Code of Conduct Group in order to make it more effective in ensuring fair and transparent tax competition within the European Union.[175]

Further work would also be undertaken towards the better quantification of the tax gap.[176] The Commission, along with Eurostat, would work with Member States to see how a reliable estimate of the level of tax evasion and avoidance can be reached. The Commission would also continue to promote greater transparency internationally, furthering the OECD's efforts through its BEPS project.

As a follow-up, two legislative proposals would be submitted to the European Parliament for consultation and to the Council for adoption. It was hoped that Member States would agree on the proposal for automatic exchange of tax rulings by the end of 2015, so that it can enter into force on 1 January 2016. It was also announced that before the summer, there would also be an Action Plan on Corporate Taxation. This second Action Plan would focus on measures to make corporate taxation fairer and more efficient within the single market. The re-launch of the CCCTB would also be considered as well as ideas for integrating some of the BEPS proposals at EU level.

The EU's Tax Transparency package has been hailed as revolutionary by Commissioner for Taxation Pierre Moscovici, but also by the OECD Secretary-General Angel Gurria, who urged Member States to resist aggressive lobbying to weaken the legislation.[177] At a joint hearing by members of the Special Tax Rulings Committee and the Economic and Monetary Affairs committees of the European

[174] *Ibid*, p 5.

[175] *Ibid*, p 6.

[176] *Ibid*, p 6. It was explained that the tax gap is the difference between tax that is due and the amount actually collected by national authorities. Tax evasion and avoidance were not the only contributors to the tax gap—administrative errors and bankruptcies also played a role.

[177] Stephanie Soong Johnston, 'OECD Chief Hails EU Tax Transparency Package as "Revolutionary"', 2015 *WTD* 62-1 (1 April 2015).

Parliament, Moscovici repeated calls for measures ensuring tax fairness in the European Union.[178] He called for a single market for taxation.

The European Union has certainly been living up to its pledge of tackling tax evasion and aggressive tax planning. Whether the measures on enhanced transparency will improve Member States' capacity to address harmful tax practices and profit shifting beyond EU borders, without having a detrimental impact on the international competitiveness of EU companies, remains to be seen.

There is obviously an appetite within the European Union to tighten corporate tax rules against aggressive tax planning. Various groups and working parties have been examining specific topics which are also on the BEPS agenda. They are examined next.

5.5. The Group on Digital Economy

In October 2013, a High-Level Expert Group on Taxation of the Digital Economy (henceforth, the Group on Digital Economy) was appointed to examine taxation issues linked to the digital economy, looking at both indirect taxes such as VAT and direct corporate taxation.[179] The Group was asked to identify key problems and solutions, as well as improvements in the current way of taxing the digital economy in the European Union, in order to enable the Commission to develop an appropriate tax framework.

In a report published on 28 May 2014, the EU Digital Economy Report,[180] the Group on Digital Economy reached a number of important conclusions. First, it noted that special rules for the digital economy were not needed. Rather, the general rules should be applied or adapted so that digital companies were treated in the same way as others. The role of digitisation in lowering the costs for small and medium-sized enterprises to access the internal market was considered. The importance of having simple and predictable rules to promote increased growth was emphasised.

> [A] well-coordinated tax system, simple to comply with and to administer and inspired by best practices becomes a necessary condition for digital technology to realise its Single Market potential. Tax barriers for small and medium sized enterprises (SME) operating in the Single Market should be removed.[181]

[178] See comments made at Special Tax Rulings Committee and the Economic and Monetary Affairs Committees. Available on: www.europarl.europa.eu/news/en/news-room/content/20150330IPR39428/html/Moscovici-Corporate-profits-should-be-taxed-where-value-is-created.

[179] The Group included seven representatives from business and academia. The first meeting of the group took place on 12 December 2013 and it was mandated to report back to the Commission in the first half of 2014.

[180] *Report of the Commission Expert Group on Taxation of the Digital Economy*, 28 May 2014, p 5. Available on: ec.europa.eu/taxation_customs/resources/documents/taxation/gen_info/good_governance_matters/digital/report_digital_economy.pdf.

[181] *Ibid*, p 5.

The Group on Digital Economy expressed a firm belief 'that the digital economy offers great opportunities for Europe including solutions and opportunities to radically simplify tax administration and collection'.[182] However, it also posed new challenges to which the tax systems needed to adapt.[183] The Group on Digital Economy recognised that the increased mobility associated with digital technologies exacerbated challenges faced by the existing tax systems. In the substantive part of the report, it was reiterated that the high-profile cases that led to the BEPS agenda concerned digital companies. 'There is a perception, supported by some of the publically available data, that BEPS is especially prevalent in the digital economy'.[184]

The Group on Digital Economy endorsed the work of the OECD/G20 on BEPS and emphasised that it was in the best interests of the European Union for Member States to speak with one voice in the project and to have common positions.[185] At the same time, there was a tacit recognition of the limitations of the BEPS project: how it was bound by its mandate and timeline; and how it took the existing international rules as a given.

By contrast to the OECD's deliverables on Action 1 which made no recommendations,[186] here there was general consensus on the destination principle—ie taxation at the place of consumption. This would apply to all goods and services. The Group on Digital Economy suggested that the EU Mini One Stop Shop (MOSS) which covers business-to-consumer sales of telecommunications, television/radio broadcasting and electronic services should be expanded into a broad One Stop Shop (OSS) to cover all business-to-consumer transactions. Under the MOSS, from 1 January 2015, businesses are able to register and pay VAT for the supply of these services to non-taxable persons in their country of residence. Rather than registering in each Member State of consumption, businesses would account for VAT via a web portal of one Member State only.[187] It appears

[182] *Ibid*, p 11.

[183] *Ibid*.

[184] *Ibid*, p 24. Reference was made to the US Senate's Permanent Subcommittee on Investigations hearing on 'Offshore Profit Shifting and the US Tax Code—Part 2 (Apple Inc)': *ibid*, p 24, fn 27. The report contained, in Annexes 2A and 2B, an overview of the corporation tax charge in relation to the income and sales for a sample of the largest digital and non-digital US companies.

[185] EU Digital Economy Report, n 180 above, p 41.

[186] See Ch 2, section 2.3 of this volume.

[187] See 'Guide to the VAT Mini One Stop Shop', published by the Commission on 23 October 2013, available on: ec.europa.eu/taxation_customs/resources/documents/taxation/vat/how_vat_works/telecom/one-stop-shop-guidelines_en.pdf. This scheme is optional and it is a simplification measure following the change to the VAT place of supply rules, in that the supply takes place in the Member State of the customer and not the Member State of the supplier. MOSS mirrors the scheme in place until 2015 for supplies of electronically supplied services to non-taxable persons by suppliers not established in the EU. There is no registration threshold. This has been criticised and is likely to change. For commentary, see Paolo Centore and Maria Teresa Sutich, 'Taxation and Digital Economy: Europe is Ready' (2014) *Intertax* 784–87; Matthew Dubin, 'The EU Digital Service VAT Change and the Potential Effects on Suppliers and their Customers' (2015) 78 *Tax Notes International* 535 (9 Feb 2015); Patrick Wille, 'New Rules from 2015 Onwards for Telecommunications, Radio and Television Broadcasting, and Electronically Supplied Services' (2015) 26 *International VAT Monitor* 6–8; Marie Lamensch, 'The 2015 Rules for Electronically Supplied Services—Compliance Issues' (2015) 26 *International VAT Monitor* 11–16; Rick Minor, 'The EU's Emerging Digital Single Market' (2015) 78 *Tax Notes International* 599 (18 May 2015).

that the Group on Digital Economy views the successful introduction of MOSS as a precursor to the adoption of OSS.[188]

Furthermore, it was argued that there was no need for a new concept of digital taxable presence which would trigger taxable nexus on the collection of data over the internet, the processing and monetising of such data, 'even if this was considered reasonable from the viewpoint of an appropriate international allocation of profits'.[189] The Group on Digital Economy considered this option extensively and concluded that there was no convincing argument why the collection of data via electronic means in a country should in itself create a taxable presence in that country. It was recommended that deficiencies in the interpretation and application of the existing nexus provisions should be addressed under the BEPS project which was endorsed and the VAT system. 'Revenue concerns of the country where digital services and products are consumed should be adequately addressed via the VAT system'.[190]

As far as reviewing the PE concept was concerned, such review was justified and necessary given the business models applied in the digital economy.[191] The Group on Digital Economy suggested that the review should focus on two elements in the existing PE definition; first, remote contracting and the distinction between dependent agent and commissionaire and secondly, the definition of the 'preparatory or auxiliary activities' exemption.

As long-term policy options, it was recommended that the European Union should consider a fundamental review of international corporation tax mechanisms, including a consideration of both the allocation of the right to tax and the most appropriate base for corporation tax.[192] The emphasis was on issues related to the taxation of MNEs where problems of identifying value creation were exacerbated.

> The digitalisation and transformation of the economy suggests that IP whose value is created within highly integrated groups will be more and more the rule. It is therefore appropriate to raise the question how long transfer pricing rules based on the arm's length principle can be relied upon to give an objective outcome that is not susceptible to manipulation.[193]

One option was the CCCTB. The Group on Digital Economy also thought that given the pace of technological development and the need to avoid creating barriers to trade, more radical changes to the corporation tax system were needed. Another suggestion was a destination-based corporation tax. This would be similar to a VAT but exports would be zero-rated and imports would be taxed. Wages

188 See David D Stewart, 'Digital Economy Raises Need for Simplified Tax Regimes, EU Report Says' 2014 *WTD* 103-2 (29 May 2014). Also see Rick Minor, 'A Practical Perspective on the EU Digital Economy Expert Group's Proposals for VAT on Electronic Services', 2014 *WTD* 106-5 (3 June 2014).

189 EU Digital Economy Report, n 180 above, p 47.

190 *Ibid.*

191 *Ibid*, p 48.

192 *Ibid*, p 41.

193 *Ibid*, p 49.

would be deductible and the tax would continue to be levied on an accounting basis.[194] In the meantime, it was recommended that partial changes to the existing system such as those mentioned above would help avoid additional layers of complexity.

Given that the CCCTB has resurfaced in the Commission's Tax Transparency Package, this may accelerate the implementation of some of the Group's long-term options. Furthermore, a successful implementation of the MOSS may facilitate the application of the destination principle in this area. As such, the EU 'solution' could prove to be a precursor to an internationally-accepted solution for the purposes of Action 1 of the BEPS project too.[195]

Recently, on 6 May 2015, the Commission announced a strategy for a digital single market throughout the European Union, which includes plans to introduce legislation extending MOSS to cross-border remote sales of tangible goods.[196] A set of targeted actions are to be delivered by the end of next year and will be built on three pillars: namely, better access for consumers and businesses to digital goods and services across Europe; creating the right conditions and a level playing field for digital networks and innovative services to flourish; and maximising the growth potential of the digital economy.

5.6. The Code of Conduct Group on Business Taxation

The Code of Conduct Group (Business Taxation) has also been instrumental in the design of standards and the development of measures to tackle harmful tax competition and international tax avoidance. The Code of Conduct Group was

[194] *Ibid*, p 50. This proposal is broadly based on Michael Devereux and Alan Auerbach's research on a destination-based cash flow tax. See A Auerbach and MP Devereux, *Consumption and Cash-Flow Taxes in an International Setting* (2012) Oxford University Centre for Business Taxation Working Paper Series, WP 12/14. Also see Michael Devereux and Rita de la Feria, *Designing and implementing a destination-based corporate tax* (2014) Oxford University Centre for Business Taxation, WP 14/07. The proposal has been criticised in that, inter alia, it would lead to a significant shift of revenue between small countries and countries with a strong export business to bigger markets and countries with small export businesses. See Björn Westberg, '*Taxation of the Digital Economy—An EU Perspective*' (2014) 54 *European Taxation* 541–44.

[195] For more concrete proposals, see report recently published by the French government agency France Stratégie on taxation in the digital economy. A number of recommendations are set out based on theoretical models regarding network rents, two-sided markets, privacy protection, and fiscal competition among countries. See *Taxation and the digital economy: A survey of theoretical models—Final report*, published on 26 February 2015. The report is available on Tax Analysts, 2015 *WTD* 49-18 (26 February 2015).

[196] See Commission Communication, *A Digital Single Market Strategy for Europe*, COM(2015) 192 final (Brussels, 6 May 2015). Also see Commission Staff Working Document, *A Digital Single Market Strategy for Europe—Analysis and Evidence Accompanying the document Communication from the Commission to the European Parliament, the Council, the European Economic and Social Committee and the Committee of the Regions A Digital Single Market Strategy for Europe*, SWD(2015) 100 final (Brussels, 6 May 2015). For commentary, see William Hoke, 'EU to Propose Extending MOSS to Remote Sales of Tangible Goods', 2015 *WTD* 89-2 (8 May 2015).

established in 1998[197] under the chairmanship of UK Paymaster General Dawn Primarolo, to assess the tax measures that may fall within the scope of the Code of Conduct on Business Taxation.[198] Member States could also report harmful tax measures in other Member States.[199]

Although technically the Code of Conduct Group has no binding powers, its decisions have great political force and cannot be easily ignored. The decision-making process of the Code of Conduct Group is not based on unanimity and has been described as being far from transparent.[200] As noted in a recent report,

> the Group should maintain to aim at a (broad) consensus to reflect the positions of the Member States in the Group in its reports to ECOFIN, to avoid losing the effectiveness of the Group, while respecting the principle of unanimity as laid down in the Council conclusions of 9 March 1998 concerning the establishment of the Code Group. In the case broad consensus cannot be reached, the Group's reports can express the various views mentioned.[201]

Initially, the Code of Conduct Group's main focus was to examine potentially harmful tax measures in Member States in the context of the Code of Conduct on Business Taxation.[202] The Code of Conduct required Member States to amend existing tax measures or practices that constituted harmful tax competition (rollback) and to refrain from introducing any such measures in the future (standstill). It identified as harmful, tax measures of a legislative, regulatory and administrative nature, which had, or might have a significant impact on the location of business in the Union[203] and which departed from the benchmark system—ie which

[197] Resolution of the Council and the Representatives of the Governments of the Member States, meeting within the Council of 1 December 1997 on a code of conduct for business taxation, [1998] OJ 06.01.1998.

[198] Code of Conduct for Business Taxation, [1998] OJ C2 of 6 January 1998. For further analysis, see, inter alia, Hans Gribnau, 'The Code of Conduct for Business Taxation: An Evaluation of an EU Soft-Law Instrument' in Dennis Weber et al, *Traditional and Alternative Routes to European Tax Integration* (IBFD, 2010); William Bratton and Joseph McCahery, 'Tax Coordination and Tax Competition in the European Union: Evaluating the Code of Conduct on Business Taxation' (2001) 38 *Common Market Law Review* 677. On the work of the Code of Conduct Group in this area, which is subject to a high level of confidentiality, see Martijn Nouwen, 'The Gathering Momentum of International and Supranational Action against Aggressive Tax Planning and Harmful Tax Competition: The State of Play of Recent Work of the OECD and European Union' (2013) 53 *European Taxation* 491, at 499 et seq. Also see Carlo Pinto, *Tax Competition and EU Law* (Kluwer, 2003) 209, 217–19.

[199] As Gribnau notes, this 'informer' provision was a great success as Member States put more than 175 measures on the list. See Hans Gribnau (2010), n 198 above, p 69.

[200] Joris Luts, 'Compatibility of IP Box Regimes with EU State Aid Rules and Code of Conduct' (2014) 23 *EC Tax Review* 258–83, 276. Also see Code of Conduct Group (Business Taxation) Draft Council Conclusions (Work Packages) 26 November 2008, SN 16410/08, 5–6.

[201] Report from the EU Code of Conduct Group (Business Taxation) to the ECOFIN Council of 4 December 2012, para 4.

[202] See ch 2 in HJI Panayi (2013), n 1 above.

[203] Code of Conduct, n 198 above, para A(1).

provided for a significantly lower effective level of taxation than the general level of taxation in the Member State concerned.[204]

The first report of the Code of Conduct Group, also known as the Primarolo Report, was approved by the ECOFIN Council in Vienna on 1 December 1998. This report listed 66 preferential tax measures that had been found to be harmful. The Primarolo Report also listed six categories of harmful tax measures relating to insurance practices, financial services, transfer pricing, holding company regimes, exempt and offshore entities and miscellaneous measures. Interim draft reports had been published in 1998. Since 1999, numerous harmful tax measures in the legislation of Member States and associated or dependent territories have been revised or are being dismantled. As part of its regular work, the Code of Conduct Group monitors the standstill and rollback of harmful tax measures as agreed under the Code of Conduct.[205]

In the context of anti-abuse assessments, the Group has expanded the scope of its work to include hybrid entity and hybrid PE mismatches, patent boxes, double non-taxation, administrative practices, links to third countries and more.

In 2009, a Subgroup of the Code of Conduct Group had begun work on a general framework for hybrid mismatch rules that would apply to intra-EU mismatch arrangements involving hybrid entities. The work of the Subgroup had provided valuable guidance on a coordinated approach to addressing hybrid mismatch arrangements. In a 2010 report to the ECOFIN Council[206] the Code of Conduct Group (Business Taxation) agreed that participation exemptions should not lead to the exemption of payments that were treated as tax deductible by the country of the payer. In its 2012 Action Plan, the Commission called on the Group to provide rapid solutions to mismatches. Eventually, there was a proposal to amend the Parent–Subsidiary Directive, as discussed in section 5.3.2 above.

It was reported at the June 2014 ECOFIN meeting[207] that the Subgroup had produced a proposal for draft guidance on intra-EU hybrid entity mismatches. The Group was to continue its work for draft guidance on hybrid PEs. On 9 December 2014 the Code of Conduct Group again reported to ECOFIN as regards its work on guidance for hybrid entity mismatches. It has been reported that the guidance

[204] *Ibid*, para B(1). The Code of Conduct on Business Taxation had set out some criteria for identifying potentially harmful measures, such as ring-fencing of a beneficial tax regime in favour of non-residents, significantly lower effective levels of taxation, lack of transparency, the conferral of tax advantages in the absence of any real economic activity or the deviation from internationally accepted rules on profit determination for companies in a multinational group: *ibid*.

[205] *Ibid*. For a useful overview of the exercise of this function of the Group, see Vinod Kalloe, 'Corporate Tax Treatment of Interest: EU State Aid and the EU Code of Conduct as a Means of Combating Harmful Tax Competition' (2011) 51 *European Taxation* 504–14.

[206] Council Doc 16766/10 (7 December 2010). See also previous Code of Conduct Group Progress Report of 25 May 2010, doc 10033/10, para 31.

[207] See Doc 11227/14 FISC 102 ECOFIN 701 (Brussels, 23 June 2014), p 14. Available on: register.consilium.europa.eu/doc/srv?l=EN&f=ST%2011227%202014%20INIT.

focuses on two mismatch situations involving hybrid entities: one where a double deduction or other relief is given in two Member States for the same payment, and the other where a deduction or relief is given in one Member State without a corresponding receipt in another country. The solution put forward is for both Member States to treat the entity as non-transparent in the first situation, and as transparent in the second situation.[208] This solution seems to require joint action by two Member States, as with the BEPS linking rules under Action 2. It is not a unilateral solution, or a unilateral solution in a multilateral instrument, as with the Parent-Subsidiary Directive.[209]

The Code of Conduct Group has also been mandated to review the third criterion (economic substance) of the Code of Conduct on Business Taxation in the context of patent box regimes. On 10 December 2013 the Group was asked by ECOFIN to assess all patent boxes in the European Union, taking into account international developments. On 9 December 2014 the Code of Conduct Group reported to ECOFIN, announcing that it had come to an agreement on the interpretation of economic substance in this context. The Code of Conduct Group endorsed the modified nexus approach,[210] with a reservation from the Netherlands.[211] Overall, it was concluded that the patent box regimes in the European Union were not compatible with the nexus approach and should be amended.

It is interesting to note that the adoption of the modified nexus approach also suggests that henceforth, under patent box regimes there should be no conferral of tax benefits for intangibles developed in other Member States. This change was aimed at curbing (mainly but not only) the UK patent box regime, pursuant which benefits were broadly given irrespective of where the qualifying IP was developed.[212] Under the UK patent box, companies could apply a lower rate of corporation tax (of 10 per cent) to profits earned from its patented inventions. A company could benefit from the patent box if it owned or exclusively licensed-in patents granted by the UK Intellectual Property Office, the European Patent Office

[208] See *KPMG Euro Tax Flash*, Issue 243, 16 December 2014, available on: www.kpmg.com/Global/en/services/Tax/regional-tax-centers/european-union-tax-centre/Documents/eu-tax-flash/etf-243.pdf.

[209] See analysis in sections 5.3.2. and 6.2.

[210] See Stephanie Soong Johnston, 'EU Clarifies Position on Patent Box Inquiry', 2015 *WTD* 25-2 (6 February 2015). Also see William Hoke, 'European Commission Expands State Aid Inquiries', 2014 *WTD* 243-2 (18 December 2014).

[211] The Netherlands appeared to disagree with the limitation on the scope of the assets that would qualify for preferential treatment. For the Netherlands it was important that IP regimes were not limited to patents, but could also cover other innovations derived from R&D, provided that such activities had been certified by a competent government authority (not being the tax authorities), so that the linkage between R&D, IP-assets and profits (tracking and tracing) could be ensured. See reservation to be inserted to Council conclusions in the minutes of the ECOFIN Council on 9 December 2014 (Doc: 16846/14 FISC 233 ECOFIN 1196 (11 December 2014), para 2.

[212] On an early discussion on this topic, see Kate Alexander, 'Analysis—UK patent box: fair competition or a harmful tax practice?', *Tax Journal*, Issue 1192, 11 (8 November 2013); Carmen Aquerreta, 'The adviser Q&A: Is the UK's patent box "harmful"?', *Tax Journal*, Issue 1191, 9 (1 November 2013).

and several EEA countries.[213] Therefore, benefits were given even if the qualifying IP was developed outside of the UK.

Germany had raised objections to IP boxes and specifically objected to the UK patent box, as the number of patents obtained in the UK by German-based companies had significantly increased since the UK regime was introduced in 2011.[214] Germany had requested that the regime be investigated under the EU's Code of Conduct on Business Taxation. The Commission seemed to share the belief that the UK's patent box regime was in breach of the Code of Conduct.[215]

Germany favoured the introduction of a test limiting benefits by reference to the proportion of total R&D expenditures that a claimant company incurred.[216] This was seen as a proxy for the amount of relevant substance a claimant had. The UK had previously rejected this approach, arguing that transfer pricing rules should instead be applied to ensure that company profits properly reflect the degree of substance in the company.[217] There was also another, very important ground. Arguably, the UK position was mandated under EU law and more specifically under the fundamental freedoms of the Treaty on the Functioning of the European Union (TEFU). As shown in the next chapter, in the analysis of the compatibility of the modified nexus approach with EU law, the Court of Justice has held in the past that Member States cannot impose restrictions with respect to the location of the R&D activities giving rise to the qualifying asset.[218] This leads to the incredulous situation whereby 'a domestic (tax) legislator, by aligning his IP box regime with the fundamental freedoms of the TFEU, could fall foul of a "soft law" instrument such as the Code'.[219] It is rather unfortunate that the Code

[213] The EEA countries listed were the following: Austria, Bulgaria, the Czech Republic, Denmark, Estonia, Finland, Germany, Hungary, Poland, Portugal, Romania, Slovakia and Sweden. See HMRC guidance available on: www.gov.uk/corporation-tax-the-patent-box.

[214] See Mindy Herzfeld, 'Political Developments in BEPS and the EU' (2014) 76 *Tax Notes International* 653 (Nov 24, 2014). For an overview, see Fabian Mang, 'The (In)Compatibility of IP Box Regimes with EU Law, the Code of Conduct and the BEPS Initiatives' (2015) 55 *European Taxation* 78–87; Antonio Carlos dos Santos, 'What is Substantial Economic Activity for Tax Purposes in the Context of the European Union and the OECD Initiatives against Harmful Tax Competition?'(2015) 24 *EC Tax Review* 166–75.

[215] In a report prepared ahead of the 22 October 2013 meeting of the Code of Conduct Group, the Commission argued that the UK rules were in breach of two of the criteria of the Code of Conduct on Business Taxation. First, there was a significantly lower level of taxation on patent related income and secondly, the tax advantages were conferred notwithstanding the lack of real economic activity and substantial economic presence within the Member State. At an ECOFIN meeting on 10 December 2013, a decision on the UK patent box was postponed. Instead, as explained in the main text above, ECOFIN invited the Code of Conduct Group to assess all EU patent boxes by the end of 2014, also against the background of international developments. For commentary, see David D Stewart, 'European Commission Finds UK Patent Box in Violation of Code of Conduct', 2013 *WTD* 202-1 (18 October, 2013).

[216] See Jonathan Bridges, 'The Q&A: The UK/German proposal for preferential IP regimes', *Tax Journal*, Issue 1240, p 8 (21 November 2014).

[217] *Ibid.*

[218] See Case C-254/97 *Baxter* and Case C-39/04 *Laboratoires Fournier*, discussed in Ch 6, section 6.5 below.

[219] Joris Luts (2014), n 200 above, 280.

of Conduct Group had not considered this perspective. The point is revisited in the next chapter.

It should be noted that patent box regimes may also fall foul of the state aid prohibition. Although in 2008 the Commission approved the Spanish patent box regime as not being selective, it is now rethinking its position.[220] This was made clear in a press release in March 2014, at the beginning of an investigation in the Luxembourg tax practices.[221] The reason for the rethink was that since 2008, the Commission 'had received indications that special tax regimes seem to mainly benefit highly mobile businesses and do not trigger significant additional research and development activity'.[222] Therefore, the Commission began to gather information to assess whether the regimes grant a selective advantage to a particular group of companies, in breach of EU state aid rules. The Commission asked in total 10 Member States with patent box regimes to give information on these regimes but no formal investigation was launched.[223]

Following the December 2014 ECOFIN meeting, it was thought—though not officially confirmed—that the Commission would not be pursuing state aid investigations (or would not be pursuing any case aggressively), pending ongoing discussions at the level of the Code of Conduct Group and the OECD on this topic. Although a political compromise seems to be preferred, the Commission has not, however, excluded the possibility of taking action itself.[224]

Overall, these are the main developments that have taken place at the time of writing. As commented above, the European Union has placed a lot of emphasis on tackling tax evasion and aggressive tax planning. The Commission has seized on this unique political momentum and many legislative proposals or amendments that had been lurking for some time have now been fast-tracked at Council level. However, some of the measures that have been adopted, or aspects of them, may be incompatible with EU law. This point was made throughout the chapter. There are similar concerns as regards the compatibility of some of the BEPS deliverables with EU law. These concerns are examined in greater detail in the next chapter.

[220] Under the Spanish patent box regime notified to the Commission in August 2007, a corporate tax credit of 50% was to be given for revenues stemming from patents, designs, models, plans, secret formulas and processes. The tax credit was open to all companies, irrespective of their size or sector and there was no restriction concerning the location of the eligible activities. The public administration would have no discretion in applying the measure as the criteria were considered to be objective and defined ex-ante in the implementing regulation. The Commission concluded that the tax credit was within the logic of the Spanish tax system and that it would provide an incentive for companies to invest in R&D. See IP/08/216, dated 13 February 2008, available on: europa.eu/rapid/press-release_IP-08-216_en.htm.

[221] See IP/14/309, dated 24 March 2014. Available on: europa.eu/rapid/press-release_IP-14-309_en.htm.

[222] *Ibid*, pp 1–2.

[223] Also see Lee A Sheppard, 'Are EU Patent Boxes State Aid?' (2015) 77 *Tax Notes International* 383 (2 February 2015).

[224] See comments of Commission's spokesman, reported by Stephanie Soong Johnston, 'EU Clarifies Position on Patent Box Inquiry', 2015 *WTD* 25-2 (6 February 2015).

6

The Compatibility of the BEPS Proposals with European Union Law

This chapter examines the compatibility of some of the proposals produced under the BEPS deliverables with EU law. Where relevant, there is also a review of the compatibility of the recent EU measures taken to address aggressive tax planning. The analysis is made on the basis of several themes that arise from the BEPS deliverables. At the time of writing this book, the ambitious timeline for the delivery of the BEPS Action Plan had not yet expired. This chapter will proceed on the basis of what is already publicly available as of 1 June 2015.

6.1. Rules on the Determination and/or Allocation of Taxing Rights: BEPS Actions 1, 7–10

The proposals made under Action items 1 and 7 to 10 largely represent rules on the determination and/or allocation of taxing rights. Such rules technically fall within the exclusive competences of Member States.

As far as determination of taxing rights is concerned, the European Union cannot interfere in the tests that a Member State uses to exercise source taxation or taxation on the basis of residence (ie *when* taxing rights are to be triggered). For example, the European Union cannot interfere in the tests that a Member State uses to determine whether a permanent establishment arises in that Member State (source state jurisdiction), or when a company or an individual is tax resident (residence state jurisdiction). These fall within the exclusive competence of Member States. Technically, a Member State can determine that, notwithstanding insufficient presence for the purposes of Action 5 of the OECD Model, a permanent establishment would exist if a non-resident person is carrying on an activity in that Member State by supplying goods and services to resident customers.[1]

[1] See, for example, one of the triggers of the UK's Diverted Profits Tax, discussed in Ch 9 of this volume.

Or, a Member State can determine that a company is tax resident if it is managed and controlled in that Member State even if it is incorporated in another jurisdiction.[2]

Similarly, the European Union cannot interfere with how a Member State exercises its taxing rights vis-à-vis other countries. From a residence-state perspective, a Member State may, for example, choose to tax a resident on a worldwide basis or on a citizenship basis or on a territorial basis. It may choose to tax income earned abroad by its resident employees or not. It may choose to tax a resident on the capital gains made abroad or not. It may choose to tax the pensions of resident individuals, irrespective of where those pensions arise and/or where the place of employment was. From a source-state perspective, a Member State may, for example, choose to tax income earned in its jurisdiction by a non-resident employee or not. It may choose to tax capital gains realised in its jurisdiction (especially from immovable property) by a non-resident or not. It may choose to tax artistes and sportsmen performing in that jurisdiction or not. It may choose to tax payments made to a non-resident individual for government services rendered in the source state or not. Alternatively, Member States may coordinate with other Member States (or third countries) on how to tax certain items of income to avoid double taxation, so that in certain cases, when acting as a state of residence or a state of source they forgo their taxing rights and in other cases not. Such pre-agreed allocation of taxing rights is epitomised in tax treaties which usually follow the OECD Model. Member States' allocation of taxing rights tends to be respected by the Court of Justice.[3]

There would only be an issue of compatibility with EU law if a Member State in exercising its taxing rights *discriminates* against EU nationals or restricts their fundamental freedoms contrary to EU law. This would be the case, for example, if a permanent establishment (however defined) of a foreign company were taxed more heavily than a subsidiary of a foreign company,[4] or if a tax resident person (however defined) upon becoming non-resident were taxed more heavily than a remaining tax resident person.[5] These examples are derived from established case law of the Court of Justice, where a breach of EU law was found. In these

[2] See for example the UK test on central management and control. For a review of the issues, see Christiana HJI Panayi, 'UK Report', ch 22 in *Residence of Companies under Tax Treaties and EC Law*, EC and International Tax Law Series, vol 5 (IBFD, 2009).

[3] See section 4.3.3 in Christiana HJI Panayi, *European Union Corporate Tax Law* (Cambridge University Press, 2013). For examples of case law, see Case C-336/96 *Gilly v Directeur des services fiscaux du Bas-Rhin* [1998] ECR I-2793; and Case C-376/03 *D v Rijksbelastingdienst (D* case*)* [2005] ECR I-5821; Case C-513/03 *Heirs of MEA Van Hilten-van der Heijden v Inspecteur van de Belastingdienst/Particulieren/Ondernemingen buitenland te Heerlen* [2006] ECR I-1957; Case C-265/04 *Bouanich v Skatteverket* [2006] ECR I-923; Case C-374/04 *Test Claimants in Class IV of the ACT Group Litigation v Inland Revenue Commissioners* (*ACT GLO* case) [2006] ECR I-11673; Case C-414/06 *Lidl Belgium GmbH & Co KG/Finanzamt Heilbronn* [2008] ECR I-3601; Case C-128/08 *Damseaux v État belge* [2009] ECR I-6823.

[4] Case 270/83 *Commission v France ('Avoir Fiscal')* [1986] ECR 273.

[5] Case C-9/02 *Hughes de Lasteyrie du Saillant v Ministere de l'Economie, des Finances et de l'Industrie* [2004] ECR I-2409; Case C-470/04 *N v Inspecteur van de Belastingdienst Oost/Kantoor Almelo* [2006] ECR I-7409.

cases, the problem was not the formulation of the source or residence tests and the conditions imposed for an undertaking to be considered resident. Rather, what was problematic was the additional tax rules that, intentionally or incidentally, taxed undertakings more heavily when they engaged in cross-border activities.

Roughly speaking, two thirds of the action items of the BEPS Action Plan relate to the determination and/or allocation of taxing rights and, one way or another, their aim is to refine the application of source-based or residence-based taxation tests in some highly complex arrangements. This is notwithstanding the OECD's initial declaration that 'these actions are not directly aimed at changing the existing international standards on the allocation of taxing rights on cross-border income'.[6] Therefore, it is submitted that from an EU law perspective, there is nothing immediately objectionable, to the extent that the proposals would indeed be limited to the refinement of the rules on allocation of taxing rights. The European Union has no competence to force Member States to tax (or not to tax) commissionaire arrangements or to dictate the conditions for taxing the legal owner of intangibles and the functions that need to be performed and controlled for income allocation purposes. Nor does it have any power to force Member States to use certain methods of allocation of income (eg formulary apportionment or profit split methods) over other methods. It is very unfortunate that the Commission seems to be ignoring this very basic fact in its high-profile state aid investigations examined in the following chapter.

Nevertheless, there are a number of proposals made in the context of the rest of the BEPS deliverables that do not fall under the category of allocation of taxing rights. Very importantly, the proposals in Action items 2 to 6 deal with the application of anti-abuse rules. However legitimate from an OECD and an international tax law perspective, anti-abuse rules are still rules which potentially hinder cross-border economic activities, contrary to the fundamental freedoms of the TFEU as interpreted by the Court of Justice. As such, these proposals need to be assessed in terms of their compatibility with EU law.[7]

6.2. Unilaterally-Imposed and Mechanical Linking Rules: BEPS Action 2

One example of rules produced in the BEPS discourse which may be incompatible with EU law is the linking rules proposed under Action 2. It was shown in Chapter two that the OECD is recommending a primary rule that should be applicable in the primary jurisdiction with a defensive rule that would apply in the secondary

[6] OECD (2013), Action Plan on Base Erosion and Profit Shifting, p 11. Also see Ch 2 of this volume.

[7] For a general analysis, see Amanda Athanasiou, 'EU Perspectives on BEPS', 2014 *WTD* 182-2 (19 September 2014); Eric Kemmeren, 'Where is EU Law in the OECD BEPS Discussion?' (2014) 23 *EC Tax Review* 190–93.

jurisdiction in the absence of a primary rule in the first.[8] Specific transactions are identified and there are no exceptions for genuine commercial transactions. The rules are very mechanical.

This proposal may be problematic from an EU law perspective.

First, a Member State which applies rules that are incompatible with EU law may not be able to justify this incompatibility on the basis that there is a tax mismatch which is not 'cured' by legislation in another Member State. The Court of Justice tends to follow the per country approach. In examining whether or not a national tax measure is compatible with EU law, either under the discrimination or the restriction approach, the Court of Justice rarely takes into account the overall context in which the measure is applied.[9] The Court only considers the impugned treatment in the one Member State where the treatment is incurred. Tax benefits in the other Member State are irrelevant and cannot offset any fiscal hindrances in the Member State concerned. In the context of free movement of workers, the *Eurowings*[10] and *Danner*[11] cases unequivocally held that

> any tax advantage resulting for providers of services from the low taxation to which they are subject in the Member State in which they are established cannot be used by another Member State to justify less favourable treatment in tax matters given to recipients of services established in the latter State.[12]

Similarly, but in a factually different context, in *Denkavit*[13] and *Amurta*[14] the Court of Justice considered whether a discriminatory withholding tax in the host state could be neutralised by the provision of a unilateral tax credit in the taxpayer's home state or a treaty-based tax credit.[15] In both cases, the Court of Justice reiterated that a unilateral tax credit by the home state was not enough to neutralise the discriminatory treatment by the host state. In *Amurta*, it was emphasised that only neutralisation as a result of an underlying tax treaty was relevant. The difference between a treaty-based tax credit and a unilateral one was that the tax system resulting from the tax treaty formed part of the legal background of the proceedings and the Court of Justice had to take it into account in order to give an interpretation of EU law.[16] Therefore, a Member State could ensure compliance with its obligations under EU law through the conclusion of

[8] See section 2.4 of this volume.

[9] See HJI Panayi (2013), n 3 above, pp 165–69.

[10] Case C-294/97 *Eurowings Luftverkehrs AG v Finanzamt Dortmund-Unna* [1999] ECR I-7447.

[11] Case C-136/00 *Rolf Dieter Danner* [2002] ECR I-8147.

[12] *Ibid*, para 56; citing *Eurowings*, n 10 above, para 44. In the free movement of capital context, see Case C-35/98 *Staatssecretaris van Financiën v BGM Verkooijen*, [2000] ECR I-04071, para 61 and Case C-315/02 *Anneliese Lenz v Finanzlandesdirektion für Tirol* [2004] ECR I-7063, para 41, contain similar *dicta*. See HJI Panayi (2013), n 3 above, ch 4.

[13] Case C-170/05 *Denkavit Internationaal BV v Ministre de l'Economie, des Finances et de l'Industrie* [2006] ECR I-11949.

[14] Case C-379/05 *Amurta SGPS v Inspecteur van de Belastingdienst/Amsterdam* [2007] ECR I-9569.

[15] See Georg Kofler, 'Tax Treaty 'Neutralisation' of Source State Discrimination under the EU Fundamental Freedoms?' (2011) 65 *Bulletin for International Taxation* 684, 685.

[16] *Amurta*, n 14 above, para 80.

a tax treaty with another Member State.[17] These cases give therefore a qualified endorsement to the per country approach by suggesting that tax treaties are to be factored into the equation.

The recent *Philip Electronics*[18] case arguably presents a more direct precedent against linking rules. However, it is not clear whether the ruling should be limited to situations where a Member State applies a restrictive rule in *anticipation* of beneficial tax treatment in the other Member State or whether it also applies to situations where there is *already* beneficial treatment in the other Member State. In this case, Philips Electronics UK Ltd, a UK taxpayer, made various consortium claims for group relief in its tax returns, in respect of losses incurred by the UK permanent establishment of a Dutch company, which was also the parent company of the taxpayer. The claims were refused on the basis that the losses could have been taken into account in the Netherlands. This was found to be incompatible with freedom of establishment.

The restriction could not be justified on the basis of preserving the allocation of taxing powers, since only UK losses were to be surrendered against the profits of the UK taxpayer. Such losses as well as profits were within the scope of UK tax. Neither was the restriction justified by the need to prevent the double use of losses.[19] In any case, according to the Court of Justice the prevention of the double use of losses did not constitute an autonomous justification—it had to be combined with another justification.[20] In this case, the Court found that the restriction could not be justified by these grounds on their own or combined.[21]

Arguably, the question here was not about the ability to use losses that had already been used by an undertaking in another jurisdiction (ie double deduction) but rather the ability to use losses that *might* or *could* be used in another jurisdiction but which had not yet been used. Whether the same result would have been reached if the losses had already been used in another jurisdiction and the UK taxpayer wanted to use them again is not certain. The judgment seems to be phrased rather vaguely. For the Court of Justice, it would seem that the important point is that the UK has power to tax the permanent establishment. The losses were linked to the UK's power to impose taxes. 'That power is not at all impaired by the fact that the losses transferred might also, in appropriate circumstances, be used in the Netherlands'.[22] In any case, as already mentioned, the Court found that double use

[17] *Ibid*, para 79.

[18] Case C-18/11 *The Commissioners for Her Majesty's Revenue & Customs v Philips Electronics UK Ltd* [2012] ECR-I 532.

[19] Although there was a risk of double use of losses (both in the host state where the permanent establishment was situated and also in the Member State where the non-resident company had its seat), the host state's power of taxation was not affected: *ibid*, paras 30 and 31 (Court of Justice). The UK's tax revenue was the same irrespective of whether losses of the permanent establishment were also taken into account in the Member State of the head office.

[20] *Ibid*, para 33. Also see para 67 of the opinion of the Advocate General.

[21] *Ibid*, para 35.

[22] *Ibid*, para 31.

of losses was not enough by itself as a justification; it would have to be combined with another justification, most likely prevention of tax avoidance. This latter, more subjective justification is unlikely to be factored in mechanical rules though.

Therefore, if under the OECD proposals on Action 2, a Member State would have to disallow the interest on a hybrid loan as a deductible expense upon application of the primary rule, because the corresponding interest income was not taxed by the Member State in which the recipient is tax resident, this is likely to be incompatible with EU law.[23] The same analysis would apply vis-à-vis the secondary/defensive rule. However, case law suggests that if these linking rules are encompassed in a tax treaty between the relevant Member States, then any discriminatory tax treatment might be neutralised.

There is a further possible complication. As already mentioned in Chapter two, the OECD hybrid rules would eliminate mismatches without a distinction between intended and unintended mismatches—ie there would be no need for any 'purpose or intention test', but merely an analysis of tax outcome. This mechanical nature of the test does not factor in the commerciality or artificiality of the arrangement. Nor does it satisfy the proportionality test developed by the Court of Justice.

In the seminal case of *Cadbury Schweppes*,[24] followed by numerous cases,[25] it was held that a national measure restricting freedom of establishment (in that case) could be justified on the basis of prevention of tax avoidance and evasion only where it specifically related to wholly artificial arrangements aimed at circumventing the application of the legislation of the Member State concerned.[26] The Court of Justice also held that restrictive anti-abuse rules had to be proportional—they had to exclude from their scope situations whereby, despite the existence of tax motives, the arrangements reflected economic reality. Later cases emphasised that the taxpayer must be given the opportunity, without being subjected to undue administrative constraints, to provide evidence of any commercial justification that there may have been for that transaction. Also, where there is re-characterisation of an interest payment, this re-characterisation would be limited to the proportion of that interest which exceeds the arm's length amount.

The relevance of this case law for mainstream anti-abuse rules such as CFC (Controlled Foreign Corporation) rules and thin cap rules, also in the context of the BEPS deliverables, is considered in greater detail in the next section. What is obvious though is that, to the extent that the OECD hybrid rules apply irrespective of the artificiality of the arrangement, they are at odds with the above case law.

[23] Also see Peter Cussons, 'Analysis—BEPS: possible EU law issues', *Tax Journal*, Issue 1221, p 16 (20 June 2014). Cussons further argues that the possible carve-out from hybrid rules for certain taxpayers (eg banking regulatory capital requirements, or certain collective investment arrangements) may give rise to state aid concerns as well.

[24] Case C-196/04 *Cadbury Schweppes plc and Cadbury Schweppes Overseas Ltd v Commissioners of Customs & Excise* [2006] ECR I-7995.

[25] See ch 8 in HJI Panayi (2013), n 3 above. Also see analysis in section 6.3 immediately below.

[26] *Cadbury Schweppes*, n 24 above, para 51.

It should be noted that the same arguments and concerns which apply to the linking rules of Action 2, are equally applicable to the subject-to-tax approach suggested under the Recommendation on Aggressive Tax Planning.[27] Similarly to the linking rules, a subject-to-tax approach would apply automatically without consideration of the commerciality of the arrangement. Notwithstanding the fact that this is a clear policy paper aligned with recent international trends, the Recommendation is technically soft law and as such does not supersede the case law of the Court of Justice discussed above. It simply evinces the Commission's tax policy aspirations in this area. These should nevertheless be compatible with the principles set out in the case law of the Court of Justice.

It could be argued that the anti-hybrid amendment of the Parent-Subsidiary Directive also applies mechanically[28] and as such, it suggests an acceptance of all such mechanical rules—not just by the Commission that drafted the amendment but also by Member States that unanimously approved it. While this may be true, it does not mean that rules approved by Member States to become EU secondary legislation cannot be in breach of EU law, if they are in fact incompatible with the principles set out by the Court of Justice in its case law.

However, is an anti-hybrid rule sewn into the fabric of a multilateral instrument more compliant with EU law than any co-ordinated but effectively unilaterally imposed anti-hybrid rules? It could be argued that as the linking rule is in an instrument (here, a Directive) that forms part of the legal background of the Member State that applies it, then the tax treatment in the other Member State which has triggered the rule could be taken into account. By analogy to the *Denkavit*[29] and *Amurta*[30] cases discussed above, if discriminatory treatment by one Member State can be neutralised by a tax treaty credit given by another Member State, then there is no reason why it cannot be neutralised as a result of a provision in a Directive, such as the Parent-Subsidiary Directive. Therefore, a Member State wishing to neutralise beneficial tax treatment given in another Member State is likely to be able to do so if there is a legal agreement between these Member States—whether as a result of a tax treaty or a multilateral convention or a Directive—allowing it.

Furthermore, it could be argued that the anti-hybrid amendment of the Parent Subsidiarity Directive ultimately aims to achieve a symmetrical treatment of intra-group profit distributions on a multilateral basis—it reflects an internationally agreed allocation of taxing rights, albeit unilaterally enforced.[31] As such, it should be treated similarly to other tax treaty arrangements (on allocation of taxing rights) which, as explained elsewhere in this chapter,[32] have been tolerated

[27] See Ch 5, section 5.2.4 of this volume.

[28] See Ch 5, section 5.3.2 of this volume.

[29] *Denkavit*, n 13 above.

[30] *Amurta*, n 14 above.

[31] As the author suggested in Ch 5, section 5.3.2 of this volume, Member States seem to have discretion on whether to apply the anti-hybrid provision. If not applied consistently, there could be jurisdiction-shopping.

[32] See sections 6.1 and 6.6 of this volume.

by the Court of Justice. By contrast, the OECD hybrid rules, unless incorporated in the multilateral agreement suggested under Action 15 of the BEPS project, are likely to be presented as a single-country response to hybrid mismatches and not as part of a bilateral/multilateral treaty arrangement. In other words, the OECD hybrid rules may be a different species of rules than those derived under a tax treaty arrangement or a Directive, which would not necessarily be protected the same way under EU tax law. Therefore, adoption of the anti-hybrid rule in the Parent-Subsidiary Directive does not mean that the OECD's linking rules would be similarly welcome and, most importantly, compatible under EU law. The fact that, as shown in Chapter five, the Code of Conduct Group in its work on hybrid mismatches[33] seems to be following a similar approach to the OECD's linking rules should be a reason for concern.

6.3. Rules Targeting Wholly or Partly Artificial Arrangements: BEPS Action 3

As explained in the previous section, the proposed hybrid rules and in fact any anti-abuse rules proposed under the BEPS Action Plan, such as Actions 3 and 4, have to comply with the principles set out by the Court of Justice in its case law. *Cadbury Schweppes*[34] with its wholly artificial arrangements test is considered to be the main precedent in this area. Although this judgment was in the context of the CFC rules, the principles set out in this case have been applied in other areas dealing with anti-abuse rules.[35]

As already discussed in the previous section, in *Cadbury Schweppes* it was held that a Member State CFC regime which restricted the freedom of establishment could be justified on the basis of prevention of tax avoidance and evasion but only where it specifically related to wholly artificial arrangements aimed at circumventing the application of the legislation of the Member State concerned.[36] The Court of Justice also held that restrictive anti-abuse rules had to be proportional—they had to exclude from their scope situations whereby, despite the existence of tax motives, the arrangements reflected economic reality. In determining whether or not economic reality existed, in addition to the subjective element, which consisted of the intention to obtain a tax advantage, objective factors had to be taken into account.[37]

[33] See section 5.6 of this volume.

[34] *Cadbury Schweppes*, n 24 above.

[35] See ch 8 in HJI Panayi (2013), n 3 above.

[36] *Cadbury Schweppes*, n 24 above, para 51.

[37] *Ibid*, paras 64–65. These objective factors, which were ascertainable by third parties, included, in particular, the extent to which the CFC physically existed in terms of premises, staff and equipment. In his opinion, Advocate General Léger had explained in greater detail some relevant criteria in establishing artificiality. First, the degree of physical presence of the subsidiary, ie examining whether or not the subsidiary has the premises, staff and equipment necessary to carry out the services provided to the

In the *Thin Cap GLO*,[38] a case which examined the UK thin capitalisation rules, the proportionality requirement was further elaborated. There had to be a consideration of objective and verifiable elements which could be used to determine whether a transaction represented a purely artificial arrangement. More specifically, national legislation had to satisfy two requirements. First, the taxpayer had to be given the opportunity, without being subject to undue administrative constraints, to provide evidence of any commercial justification that there may have been for the impugned arrangement.[39] Secondly, in these circumstances, the re-characterisation of interest paid as a distribution was limited to the proportion of that interest which exceeded what would have been agreed had the relationship between the relevant parties been at arm's length.[40] In other words, compliance with the arm's length principle became part of the proportionality test, as far re-characterisation of interest was concerned.

Although in a later transfer pricing case, the *SGI* case,[41] the Court did not insist on finding wholly artificial arrangements, the proportionality test was followed.[42] More recently, in *Itelcar*[43] and *Commission v UK*,[44] the Court of Justice again placed emphasis on the wholly artificial arrangements test. It was presented as a principle of established case law, that a national measure restricting the free movement of capital (in those cases) may be justified where it specifically targets wholly

parent company. Secondly, the genuine nature of the activity provided by the subsidiary, ie considering the competence of the subsidiary's staff in relation to the services provided and the level of decision-making in carrying out those services. Thirdly, the economic value of that activity with regard to the parent company and the entire group, ie whether or not the value reflects the exercise of genuine activities in the state of the subsidiary. *Cadbury Schweppes*, n 24 above, paras 111–14 (Advocate General). Also see analysis in ch 8 in HJI Panayi (2013), n 3 above.

[38] Case C-524/04 *Test Claimants in Thin Cap Group Litigation Order* [2007] ECR I-2107. For commentary, see Christiana HJI Panayi, 'Thin Capitalisation GLO et al—a thinly concealed agenda?' (2007) 35 *Intertax* 298.

[39] *Ibid*, para 82.

[40] *Ibid*, para 83.

[41] Case C-311/08 *Société de Gestion Industrielle (SGI) v État belge* [2010] ECR I-0487.

[42] Under Belgian law, exceptional or gratuitous benefits given by a Belgian company to a non-resident company were automatically added to the taxable base of the Belgian company, if the recipient company was, directly or indirectly, in a relationship of interdependence with the Belgian company. In similar circumstances, if the recipient company was a Belgian company, such benefit was not automatically added back. The Court of Justice found that the Belgian transfer pricing rules restricted the freedom of establishment. This restriction was justified on the basis of preserving the balanced allocation of taxing powers between Member States. The Belgian legislation was also justified on the basis of preventing tax avoidance. Even though it was not specifically designed against purely artificial arrangements, the Court of Justice thought that it was justified by the objective of preventing tax avoidance, taken together with that of preserving the balanced allocation of the power to impose taxes between Member States. In subsequent paragraphs, the Court of Justice emphasised that the two justifications were to be taken together. As far as proportionality was concerned, the Court of Justice followed previous case law. The author has argued elsewhere that the *SGI* case should be interpreted as allowing Member States to apply their transfer pricing and thin capitalisation rules to a non-arm's length arrangement, notwithstanding the arrangement's otherwise commercial nature. This would help prevent a conflict with the OECD Model and the OECD Transfer Pricing Guidelines. It would also ensure more consistency with the Court's case law on thin capitalisation and transfer pricing. See HJI Panayi (2013), n 3 above, pp 363–64.

[43] Case C-282/12 *Itelcar v Fazenda Publica* [2013] ECR I-0000, para 34.

[44] Case C-112/14 *Commission v United Kingdom* [2014] ECR I-0000, para 25.

artificial arrangements which do not reflect economic reality and the sole purpose of which is to avoid the tax normally payable on the profits generated by activities carried out in the national territory. The EFTA Court used similar language in the *Fred Olsen* case.[45]

It comes, therefore, as a bit of a surprise that the OECD in its CFC Discussion Document[46] described the case law of the Court of Justice as suggesting that, on the basis of the *Thin Cap GLO* case,[47] a CFC regime may not be limited to wholly artificial arrangements. It was also argued that on the basis of the *Thin Cap GLO* case,[48] a CFC rule in a Member State that targeted income earned by a CFC that was not itself wholly artificial may be justified so long as the transaction giving rise to the income was at least partly artificial. Reference was also made to the *SGI*[49] and *Oy AA*[50] case as supporting the claim that a CFC regime may not be limited to wholly artificial arrangements if the regime explicitly ensured a balanced allocation of taxing powers.[51]

The OECD's reliance on the language of 'partly artificial arrangement' is very suspicious. First, *Cadbury Schweppes* remains the main, directly relevant authority for CFC rules and not the *Thin Cap GLO* case, which dealt with rules restricting interest deductibility.[52] Secondly, the analysis in the CFC Discussion Document ignores subsequent cases where the wholly artificial arrangements test was emphatically reiterated,[53] particularly in the context of CFC regimes.[54]

Thirdly, while there was mention once in the *Thin Cap GLO* judgment of 'the transaction in question representing, in whole or in part, a purely artificial arrangement',[55] not much importance was placed on this point by the Court of Justice—or by commentators since then. The wholly artificial arrangements test of *Cadbury Schweppes* was repeated throughout the judgment as being the guiding authority. Perhaps references to a transaction being in part a purely artificial

[45] Joined Cases E-3/13 and E-20/13 *Fred Olsen and Others and Petter Olsen and Others v The Norwegian State, represented by the Central Tax Office for Large Enterprises and the Directorate of Taxes*, [2015] OJ C68/5–6, 26.2.2015, paras 166 et seq.

[46] See Ch 2, section 2.4 of this volume.

[47] *Thin Cap GLO*, n 38 above.

[48] *Ibid*, para 76.

[49] *SGI* case, n 41 above.

[50] Case C-231/05 *Oy AA* [2007] ECR I-6373.

[51] Similar arguments were made in an article by Evgenia Kokolia and Evgenia Chatziioakeimidou, a fiscal attaché at the EU permanent representation of Greece and a member of the Legal Service of the Council of the European Union, respectively. See Evgenia Kokolia and Evgenia Chatziioakeimidou, 'BEPS Impact on EU Law: Hybrid Payments and Abusive Tax Behaviour' (2015) 55 *European Taxation* 149–56.

[52] See ch 8 in HJI Panayi (2013), n 3 above, where it is explained how there have been slight variations to the *Cadbury Schweppes* test in different areas of the anti-abuse case law, especially for transfer pricing.

[53] See *Itelcar v Fazenda Publica*, n 43 above and *Commission v UK*, n 44 above.

[54] See, for example, Case C-201/05 *Test Claimants in the CFC and Dividend Group Litigation v Commissioners of Inland Revenue (CFC GLO)* [2008] ECR I-2875.

[55] *Thin Cap GLO*, n 38 above, para 81.

arrangement were relevant to the specific transaction in question: an excessive loan interest payment. Part of this payment was at arm's length, part of this was non-arm's length. Technically, the impact of the thin cap legislation was on the non-arm's length amount. This is arguably why the Court of Justice referred to the transaction being in part a purely artificial arrangement. But the (excessive) interest payment does not arise out of nowhere—it is part of a loan agreement. While to an extent the entirety of the loan agreement could be seen as an artificial arrangement, technically, it was only a part of it—the non-arm's length part of the interest payment—that was to be re-characterised under the relevant anti-abuse legislation.

Extrapolating a new interpretation of the artificial arrangements test from a brief passing remark in a relatively old judgment is clearly aimed at eroding the importance of the *Cadbury Schweppes* test. Moreover, it seems slightly disingenuous for the OECD to argue that the relevant authority in a CFC context is a case on thin capitalisation rather than the case on CFC regimes which has hitherto been considered as the main authority. It is respectfully submitted that any proposals made under Action 3, to be compatible with EU law, should follow the established *Cadbury Schweppes* test and not the interpretation of it suggested under the CFC Discussion Draft. Whether this furthers the aims of the BEPS Action Plan is another question—very much irrelevant as far as the issue of compatibility with EU law is concerned.

6.4. Group-Wide Rules and Comparability Issues: BEPS Action 4

A few issues also arise from the Interest Deductibility Discussion Draft.[56] As shown in Chapter two, under the proposals of this Discussion Draft, there seems to be reliance on mechanical tests which do not necessarily target wholly artificial arrangements. Nor do these proposals seem to give the taxpayer an opportunity, without subjecting him to undue administrative constraints, to provide evidence of any commercial justification that there may have been for that transaction. Such tests are arguably incompatible with the case law of the Court of Justice analysed in the previous two sections—6.2 and 6.3.

Member States are well-advised to eschew mechanical tests relying on fixed benchmarking ratios. While the Interest and Royalties Directive only affects the tax position of the interest creditor and does not prevent Member States from making interest payments non-deductible at the level of the payer,[57] the thin

[56] See Ch 2, section 2.6 of this volume.

[57] See Case C-397/09 *Scheuten Solar Technology GmbH v Finanzamt Gelsenkirchen-Süd* [2011] ECR I-6455.

capitalisation case law of the Court of Justice is still relevant.[58] Any rules curbing interest deductibility must be proportional and must give the taxpayer an opportunity, without subjecting him to undue administrative constraints, to provide evidence of any commercial justification that there may have been for that transaction. Also, where there is re-characterisation of interest, this re-characterisation must be limited to the proportion of that interest which exceeds the arm's length amount.

Furthermore, it is noteworthy that under one of the suggested approaches of the Interest Deductibility Discussion Draft, the group-wide approach, a company's net interest deductions should be limited to a proportion of the group's actual net third party interest expense. While this approach may have unitary flavours and may (further) evince the OECD's shift away from strict separate entity accounting and towards group formulae, it may be problematic from an EU law perspective. As explained above, the Court of Justice in its case law tends to follow the per country approach in examining whether or not a national tax measure is compatible with EU law. Therefore, the Court of Justice may not accept a Member State rule which restricts the deductibility of an interest payment to a non-resident group company on the basis of the rest of the group's overall third party interest expenses.[59] Repeating the principles derived from the *Eurowings*[60] and *Danner*[61] cases, tax benefits in another Member State are irrelevant and cannot offset any fiscal hindrances in the Member State concerned. Although the group-wide approach aligns individual entities' interest expenses with the overall group's interest expenses and as such gives more economic substance to the structure, paraphrasing *Eurowings*, less favourable treatment in one Member State cannot be justified by any tax advantage resulting from low taxation or other tax benefits in another Member State. If the European Union is keen to go down this path, a better alternative would be to consider formulary apportionment in the context of the Common Consolidated Corporate Tax Base.

This suggestion could also lead to the odd situation where the same interest payment paid to two different non-resident group companies for the same underlying loan may be taxed differently depending on the overall leverage of their group. It might be hard to argue that the interest recipients are not in a comparable situation because of the overall leverage of a multinational group. The comparator exercise, for the purposes of finding different treatment, is likely to be undertaken

[58] See Case C-324/00 *Lankhorst-Hohorst GmbH v Finanz Steinfurt* [2002] ECR I-11779; *Thin Cap GLO*, n 38 above; Case C-105/07 *NV Lammers and Van Cleeff* [2008] ECR I-173. For an overview of the relevant case law, see ch 8, HJI Panayi (2013), n 3 above.

[59] If the whole group is resident in the Member State imposing the group-wide approach, then arguably there is no cross-border issue and no restriction of the freedom of establishment. It is an issue of domestic law. If some of the group members are resident and some are non-resident, then, arguably, taking into account the leverage of the non-resident group companies may not be consistent with the per country approach and the *Eurowings*, n 10, and *Danner*, n 11 cases discussed above and in section 6.2.

[60] *Eurowings*, n 10 above.

[61] *Danner*, n 11 above.

only in the source Member State where the interest deduction is sought. The leverage of other group companies in other jurisdictions is likely to be irrelevant.

6.5. Modified Nexus Approach and Economic Substance: BEPS Action 5

As explained in Chapter two, Action 5 aims to develop rules to counter harmful tax practices more effectively, taking into account transparency and substance. Two important components of the OECD's proposals in this area were reviewed: first, the methodology which had been developed in defining the substantial activity requirement in the context of intangible property (the nexus approach) and, secondly, the proposed framework for compulsory spontaneous exchange of tax rulings. The analysis in this chapter focuses on the first component.

The nexus approach, later on refined as the modified nexus approach,[62] has raised a few eye-brows. As discussed in Chapter five, following intense lobbying mainly from Germany, the UK agreed to change its patent box regime so as not to permit inbound transfers of IP anymore.[63] Under the UK patent box regime, acquired IP could be imported to the UK, regardless of where it was developed. With the Code of Conduct Group and the OECD agreeing to this modified approach,[64] and apparently the Commission and EU Council legal services giving their blessings,[65] the UK regime in its current form will gradually be phased out.

However, this modified nexus approach may in fact be in violation of the fundamental freedoms as, notwithstanding the availability of the 30 per cent uplift, it could still disallow most of the R&D expenses incurred in other Member States to benefit from the benefits of a domestic patent box regime. Whilst the 30 per cent uplift of the eligible R&D expenditures outsourced to related parties and IP acquisition costs does not seem to be restricted to expenditures incurred in the jurisdiction providing the patent box benefits, the mischief of this provision is to (partly) reduce the negative impact of an IP box company choosing to outsource R&D activities to group companies. It does not open the gateways for foreign R&D expenditure to be taken into account. Therefore, arguments of incompatibility with EU law persist. In the past, the Court of Justice had struck down regimes that did not extend benefits such as deductions or tax credits to expenditure incurred in other Member States, when such benefits were given for domestic expenditure.

62 See analysis in ch 2, section 2.7 of this volume which looks at the deliverables on Action 5.

63 See Ch 5, section 5.6 of this volume.

64 *Ibid.*

65 See interview of Pascal Saint Amans, where he states that the nexus approach has been agreed by the European Commission and by the Council legal services. See 'Conversations: Jeffrey Owens and Pascal Saint-Amans' (2015) 77 *Tax Notes International* 797, 2 March 2015.

In *Baxter*,[66] the Court of Justice examined French legislation which imposed a special levy on the pre-tax turnover of French undertakings that exploited proprietary medicinal products. The undertakings were allowed to deduct from the amount payable expenditure incurred during the same tax year on research carried out in France only. The legislation was found to be in breach of freedom of establishment and the free movement of capital. As the Court of Justice explained, the imposition of a levy against which only expenditure on research carried out in France was to be deducted, was such as to put the (French) secondary places of business of pharmaceutical companies whose headquarters were located in another Member State at a disadvantage in relation to pharmaceutical undertakings whose principal places of business were located in France. This was because in the majority of cases, research units were located in the same Member State as the undertaking's principal place of business.[67]

The restriction could not be justified on the basis of preserving the effectiveness of fiscal supervision. A Member State could apply measures which enabled the amount of costs deductible in that state as research expenditure to be ascertained clearly and precisely. However, national legislation which absolutely prevented the taxpayer from submitting evidence that expenditure relating to research carried out in other Member States had actually been incurred could not be justified on this basis.[68]

Similarly, in *Laboratoires Fournier*,[69] the Court of Justice struck down French rules which disallowed the deduction of R&D expenses not incurred in France. The disallowance restricted the right of companies in other Member States to provide services in the form of research. The Court rejected the French government's argument that the disallowance was justified on the basis of preserving the coherence of the tax system. Here, there was no direct link between general corporation tax, on the one hand, and a tax credit for part of the research expenditure incurred by a company, on the other hand. Therefore, the justification was inapplicable.[70]

The French government had also argued that the restriction was justified by the objective of promoting research—a justification which was rejected by the

[66] Case C-254/97 *Société Baxter, B Braun Médical SA, Société Fresenius France and Laboratoires Bristol-Myers-Squibb SA v Premier Ministre, Ministère du Travail et des Affaires sociales, Ministère de l'Economie et des Finances and Ministère de l'Agriculture, de la Pêche et de l'Alimentation* [1999] ECR I-4809.

[67] *Ibid*, para 21.

[68] *Ibid*, paras 18–19. As noted by the Court of Justice in para 20: 'The taxpayer should not be excluded *a priori* from providing relevant documentary evidence enabling the tax authorities of the Member State imposing the levy to ascertain, clearly and precisely, the nature and genuineness of the research expenditure incurred in other Member States'.

[69] Case C-39/04 *Laboratoires Fournier SA v Direction des vérifications nationales et internationals* [2005] ECR I-2057.

[70] *Ibid*, paras 20–21.

Court of Justice. Although the promotion of research and development could be an overriding reason relating to the public interest,

> the fact remains that it cannot justify a national measure such as that at issue in the main proceedings, which refuses the benefit of a tax credit for research for any research not carried out in the Member State concerned.[71]

A justification based on the effectiveness of fiscal supervision was not accepted either. While a Member State may apply measures which enable the amount of costs deductible in that state as research expenditure to be ascertained clearly and precisely,

> national legislation which absolutely prevents the taxpayer from submitting evidence that expenditure relating to research carried out in other Member States has actually been incurred and satisfies the prescribed requirements cannot be justified in the name of effectiveness of fiscal supervision.[72]

It was reiterated that the possibility of the taxpayer being able to provide relevant documentary evidence enabling the tax authorities of the Member State of taxation to ascertain, clearly and precisely, the nature and genuineness of the research expenditure incurred in other Member States could not be excluded a priori.[73]

It is difficult to see how the OECD's nexus approach, as modified following the adoption of the UK-Germany compromise, can be aligned with the above case law. More worrying is the fact that when the above arguments arose in the context of the UK patent box regime, the UK's defence—that the 'extraterritorial' element of its patent box regime was necessary under EU law—was completely ignored (or dismissed) by the Code of Conduct Group.[74] This distortion of the hierarchy between soft law and hard law, which is likely to continue in the post-BEPS world, might lead to unexpected and damaging outcomes, as explained in Chapter nine.

In any case, the need remains for an economic substance criterion to be determined for the purposes of the Code of Conduct on Business Taxation, as shown in Chapter five. How can this criterion be interpreted compatibly with EU law? Here, freedom of establishment is likely to be the relevant freedom, as the aim of the Code of Conduct is to identify potentially harmful tax measures which have a significant impact on the location of business in the European Union.[75] In other words, the mischief which the Code of Conduct tries to address is the distortion of competition by the provision of tax benefits in the absence of economic activity (leading to relocation), when such economic activity should be present. While the

[71] *Ibid*, para 23. The Court of Justice also found that the French legislation was directly contrary to the objective of the Community policy on research and technological development which was set out in ex Article 163 EC.

[72] *Ibid*, para 25.

[73] *Ibid*.

[74] See ch 5, section 5.6 of this volume.

[75] See Code of Conduct on Business Taxation, para A(1).

guidance may also have an incidental effect on the movement of capital, freedom of establishment is likely to be considered the predominantly relevant freedom.[76]

What nexus requirement could be demanded that is (more) compatible with freedom of establishment? In other words, what is the de minimis degree of nexus that triggers the protection of this freedom so that everything below that can be legitimately attacked? In order to answer this question, a prior issue has to be resolved—what type of establishment qualifies for the purposes of freedom of establishment?

The concept of establishment is broadly construed under the case law of the Court of Justice. An establishment allows

> a Community national to participate, on a stable and continuous basis, in the economic life of a Member State other than his State of origin and to profit therefrom, so contributing to economic and social interpenetration within the Community, in the sphere of activities of self-employed persons.[77]

However, in order to trigger freedom of establishment, an establishment must involve 'the actual pursuit of an economic activity through a fixed establishment in another member state for an indefinite period'.[78]

> [T]he rules of the Treaty on the free movement of persons cover only the *pursuit of effective and genuine activities* to the exclusion of activities on such a small scale as to be regarded as purely marginal and ancillary. The physical presence in the territory of the country of establishment must therefore be such as to enable such effective and genuine activities to be pursued … [P]resence in the territory of the country of establishment must be intended to be *permanent*, or at least of an indefinite duration. (emphasis added)[79]

This was reiterated by Advocate General Léger in *Cadbury Schweppes*.[80]

The EFTA Court in the *Fred Olsen* case also followed this reasoning.[81] Here, one of the issues at stake was whether a trust, whose beneficiaries were made subject to CFC taxation, fell within the scope of Article 31 of the EEA Agreement as a form of

[76] See 4.3.1 in HJI Panayi (2013), n 3 above. For recent cases confirming this point, see *Bouanich II* (Case C-375/12 *Margaretha Bouanich v Directeur des services fiscaux de la Drôme* [2014] ECR I-0000) and Case C-47/12 *Kronos International Inc v Finanzamt Leverkusen* [2014] ECR I-0000. Here, the Court of Justice reiterated established case law in that national legislation intended to apply only to those shareholdings which enable the holder to exert a definite influence on a company's decisions and to determine its activities falls within the scope of freedom of establishment. By contrast, national provisions which apply to shareholdings acquired solely with the intention of making a financial investment without any intention to influence the management and control of the undertaking must be examined exclusively in light of the free movement of capital: *Kronos*, para 31.

[77] Case C-55/94 *Gebhard v Consiglio dell'Ordine degli Avvocati e Procuratori di Milano* [1995] ECR I-4165, para 25.

[78] Case C-221/89, *The Queen v Secretary of State for Transport, ex parte Factortame Ltd and others* [1991] ECR I-3905, para 20.

[79] *Ibid*, paras 44–45 (Opinion). Also Case C-216/87, *The Queen v Ministry of Agriculture, Fisheries and Food ex parte Jaderow* [1989] ECR 4509, para 25.

[80] *Cadbury Schweppes*, n 24 above, para 42.

[81] *Fred Olsen*, n 45 above.

establishment. On this point, the EFTA Court concluded that the trust in question fell within the scope of Article 31 of the EEA Agreement provided that the trust pursued a real and genuine economic activity within the EEA for an indefinite period and through a fixed establishment. This question was for the national court to assess. If indeed that was the case, then all interested parties—here, the trust's settlors, trustees and beneficiaries—enjoyed the rights under Articles 31 and 34 of the EEA Agreement.[82]

The EFTA Court gave some useful guidance. The essential feature of real and genuine business activities that constituted an establishment was that a person or an entity carried on a business, such as by offering services, which were effected for consideration, for an indefinite period through a fixed establishment.[83] A fixed establishment may be gained and maintained by activities such as settling personally in the host state, establishing the seat of management there and/or recruiting staff to perform the services that may be required from the establishment there. In contrast, an entity not carrying out any business in another EEA State, due to the extent it exists in terms of premises, staff and equipment, and whose incorporation may thus not reflect economic reality, cannot invoke Articles 31 and 34 of the EEA Agreement because of its lack of actual economic activity.[84]

Whether there is real and genuine economic activity cannot be answered in the abstract. It depends on the actual terms of the entity's statutes, and the actual activities of that entity and its management.[85]

> If a specific assessment reveals, for example, that the trust is involved in the management of a group's companies or other activities for a group, such as managing a pool of resources, and its actual incorporation reflected its actual activities, it has to be regarded as a real and genuine economic activity, which constitutes establishment.[86]

It was not necessary for the economic activities to take effect in the EEA state of establishment, as long as they took effect in the EEA.

Provided that those conditions were fulfilled,

> neither the status under national law of the legal entity employed to that end, the income level of the establishment nor the origin of its funds can have any consequence as to whether or not there is an establishment for the purposes of EEA law.[87]

Therefore, on the basis of this case law, the concept of establishment for the purposes of freedom of establishment requires some genuine economic activity and presence intended to be permanent. It could be argued that when these factors are not present, then freedom of establishment cannot be engaged. As such,

[82] *Ibid*, para 102. Article 31 EEA sets out the general freedom of establishment and Article 34 EEA is more specific as to companies.
[83] *Ibid*, para 97.
[84] *Ibid*, para 98.
[85] *Ibid*, para 99.
[86] *Ibid.*
[87] *Ibid*, para 100.

when an economic substance criterion based on these factors is not satisfied, then the refusal of benefits would arguably be compatible with EU law.[88] This is the approach that the Code of Conduct Group ought to have taken in its analysis of the economic substance criterion. Adopting the modified nexus approach in the context of patent regimes without taking into account the particularities of the fundamental freedoms may prove to be problematic.

Further guidance can also be sought by the interpretation of the notion of 'economic activity' in the context of VAT Directives and EU competition law, which also draw some distinctions between active conduct and mere passive investment. Here, the notion of economic activity was interpreted broadly as an activity likely to be carried out on a continuing basis, by a private undertaking on a market, organised within a professional framework and generally performed in the interests of generating profit.[89] The activity must not be of a purely marginal or ancillary nature.[90] Arguably, the essence of the matter lies in whether there is some sort of active conduct or merely passive investment. For example, in *Pavlov*, a competition case, the Court of Justice found that any activity which consisted of offering goods and services to a given market was an economic activity.[91] By contrast, it was found that the mere acquisition, holding and sale of shares, did not constitute economic activities. In other words, the mere passive exploitation of the property did not qualify.[92]

It has also been found that where a transaction relating to shares or holdings in a company is carried out in order to secure a direct or indirect involvement in the management of the company in which the holding has been acquired, then there could be economic activity for the purposes of competition rules.[93] Similar guidance was given by Advocate General Léger in the *EDM* case,[94] in the context of VAT legislation. In this case, it was questioned whether for the purposes of VAT legislation the annual granting of interest-bearing loans by a holding company to the companies in which it held shares constituted an economic activity, where the

[88] Of course, there could be an issue with the free movement of capital but that is another question to be considered.

[89] See Opinion of Advocate General Maduro in Case C-08/03 *Banque Bruxelles Lambert SA v The Belgian State, Minister of Finance, Department of administration of value added tax, registration and public property* [2004] ECR I-10157, para 10.

[90] Case C-176/96 *Lehtonen et al v Fédération Royale Belge des Sociétés de Basket-ball ASBL* [2000] ECR I-2681, para 44.

[91] Cases C-180/98 to C-184/98 *Pavlov and Others* [2000] ECR I-6451, para 75.

[92] Also see Case C-80/95 *Harnas & Helm CV v Staatssecretaris van Financiën* [1997] ECR I-745, para 15; Case C-333/91 *Sofitam SA (anciennement Satam SA) v Ministre chargé du Budget* [1993] ECR I-3513, para 12; Case C-77/01 *Empresa de Desenvolvimento Mineiro SA v Fazenda Publica* (*EDM* case) [2004] ECR I-4295, para 58. For commentary, see Daniël S Smit, 'Substance Requirements for Entities Located in a Harmful Tax Jurisdiction under CFC Rules and the EU Freedom of Establishment' (2014) 16 *Derivatives & Financial Instruments* 259–65, section 3.2; Aleksandra Bal, 'Secondary Establishments in EU VAT and Treaty Law' (2015) 55 *European Taxation* 143–48.

[93] Case C-142/99 *Floridienne SA and Berginvest SA against the Belgian State* [2000] ECR I-9567, para 18; Case C-222/04 *Cassa di Risparmio di Firenze and others* [2006] ECR I-289, paras 112–13.

[94] *EDM* case, n 92 above.

holding company's principal activity was to manage those shareholdings and, to a certain extent, also to guarantee the loans taken out by them. Citing older case law, Advocate General Léger said that the activity could be an economic activity for the purposes of the VAT legislation if it was not carried out merely on an occasional basis and it was not confined to managing an investment portfolio in the same way as a private investor. It had to be carried out with a business or commercial purpose characterised, in particular, by a concern to maximise returns on capital investment.[95] According to the Advocate General, the business purpose

> involves a holding company introducing permanent human and logistical resources arranged in the same way as the resources of a credit institution and on a greater scale than the resources belonging to a private investor which are used merely for his own needs.[96]

Also, the loans must have been agreed on conditions which were comparable to the relevant market conditions—as if they had been agreed between a financial institution and its customer.[97] The Court of Justice did not go into so much detail, simply concluding that the annual granting by a holding company of interest-bearing loans to companies in which it has a shareholding constituted economic activities.[98]

Therefore, there is ample material that the Code of Conduct Group and Member States in general could resort to in interpreting economic substance, as well as the type of harmful tax practices that should not be protected under freedom of establishment. This material ought to be taken into account in reviewing any proposals under Action 5 of the BEPS Project and any proposals of the Code of Conduct Group in its work on patent regimes.

6.6. Double Non-Taxation, LOBs and PPTs: BEPS Action 6

Action 6 mandated the OECD to develop model treaty provisions and recommendations to prevent the granting of treaty benefits in inappropriate circumstances and to curb double non-taxation. The OECD proposals here also raise serious concerns as to their compatibility with EU law.

As discussed in Chapter three, the latest reports suggest that a three-pronged approach is to be adopted. First, there will be a clear indication in the OECD Model title and preamble that Contracting States, when entering into a treaty, intend to avoid creating opportunities for non-taxation or reduced taxation through tax

95 *Ibid*, para 42 (opinion).
96 *Ibid*, para 44 (opinion).
97 *Ibid*, para 45 (opinion).
98 *Ibid*, para 70 (Court of Justice).

evasion or avoidance, including through treaty-shopping arrangements. Secondly, a limitation on benefits clause based on the US Limitation of Benefits (LOB) is recommended. This is, thirdly, to be buttressed by a more general anti-abuse rule based on the principal purposes of transactions or arrangements (principal purposes test or PPT rule).[99] The preferred approach was to combine these two rules to cover the widest range of treaty abuses. However, flexibility was allowed to accommodate constitutional and EU law restrictions.

The emphasis on avoiding double non-taxation is aligned with the Commission's proposals in its Recommendation on Aggressive Tax Planning and its previous consultation on Double Non-Taxation.[100] It was argued in Chapter five that in the Recommendation on Aggressive Tax Planning the concept of aggressive tax planning as set out goes beyond the EU concept of abuse and covers also the existence of legal gaps or mismatches leading to double non-taxation. This approach is also aligned with the rationale behind the amendments to the Parent-Subsidiary Directive, as explained in Chapter five.

It should, however, be pointed out that technically, intended or unintended double non-taxation caused by national tax laws of the Member States is not incompatible with EU law, provided that the tax treatment does not constitute harmful tax competition or state aid.[101] EU law does not require Member States to levy any income taxes or corporation taxes or, if they do impose such taxes, to impose them at any level. If lack of imposition of such taxes leads to double non-taxation, so be it. Arguably, this is the reverse of juridical double taxation with which the Court of Justice has consistently refused to interfere, finding that juridical double taxation (but not economic double taxation) is a disadvantage arising from the parallel exercise of tax competences by different Member States.[102] To the extent that such an exercise is not discriminatory, juridical double taxation is not prohibited under EU law. Member States are not obliged to adapt their own tax systems to different Member State tax systems in order to eliminate this type of double taxation. By analogy, the same reasoning ought to apply to double non-taxation—if it is the result of the parallel (and non-discriminatory) exercise of tax competences by different Member States, then it is not prohibited by EU law, notwithstanding the tax advantages that might accrue to some taxpayers.

[99] See Ch 3, section 3.1 of this volume.

[100] See Ch 5, sections 5.2.2 and 5.2.4 of this volume.

[101] Marjaana Helminen, 'The Problem of Double Non-Taxation in the European Union—To What Extent Could This Be Resolved through a Multilateral EU Tax Treaty Based on the Nordic Convention?' (2013) 53 *European Taxation* 306–12, 307.

[102] See Case C-513/04 *Mark Kerckhaert and Bernadette Morres v Belgian State* [2006] ECR I-10967 and Case C-128/08 *Jacques Damseaux v Etat Belgique* [2009] ECR I-6823. For commentary, see chs 4 and 6 in HJI Panayi (2013), n 3 above; Christiana HJI Panayi 'Tax Treaties post-*Damseaux*' [2009] *Tax Journal*, 14 September 2009, 9; Luca Cerioni, 'Double Taxation and the Internal Market: Reflections on the ECJ's Decisions in Block and Damseaux and the Potential Implications' (2009) 63 *Bulletin for International Taxation* 543. The above two cases were followed by Joined Cases C-436/08 and Case C-437/08 *Haribo & Österreichische Salinen* and Case C-67/08 *Block v Finanzamt Kaufbeuren* [2009] ECR I-0883.

Furthermore, double non-taxation may not even be accepted as a justification for a restriction of fundamental freedoms. The mischief of double non-taxation is that it leads to loss of tax revenue for the Member State concerned. However, the loss of tax revenue (also called erosion of tax base in the Court's judgments) was never allowed as a justification.[103] The emphasis has always been on justifications on the basis of tax avoidance and tax evasion.[104] Obtaining a mere tax saving has never been equated to tax avoidance or evasion in the eyes of the Court of Justice.[105] Recently, in the *Felixstowe* case, the Court found that a restrictive measure might be justified by the objective of combating tax havens,[106] though at the time of writing, this justification has not featured in any later cases and in any case cannot be equated with loss of tax revenue.

Therefore, notwithstanding the Commission's initiatives to address double non-taxation examined in greater detail in the previous chapter, technically, there is no competence in the European Union to tackle double non-taxation. This is the result of lack of harmonisation of Member State laws. Arguably, only to the extent that double non-taxation can be viewed from the spectre of abuse is there some limited legal base for EU action. Otherwise, it is submitted that there is technically none.

What about LOB clauses and their compatibility with EU law? In the past decade, the compatibility of anti-treaty-shopping provisions with EU law was a topic of intense academic debate. It was argued that anti-treaty-shopping provisions and especially the LOB were in breach of the freedom of establishment and/or the free movement of capital.[107] Could Member States include anti-treaty-shopping provisions in tax treaties between themselves or with non-EU Member States?

For this argument to succeed, it has to be shown that treaty shopping, ie the activity that these anti-abuse provisions seek to curb, is an activity protected under EU law. Of course, there has to be genuine (cross-border) activity. The more abusive the structure, the less likely that the fundamental freedoms will be triggered at all. For, if the intermediary entity is a complete sham, then, arguably, there is no genuine exercise of establishment in that jurisdiction; nor is there any movement of capital. Therefore, the more economic substance there is in the intermediary

[103] See, for example, *Danner*, n 11 above; Case C-422/01 *Försäkringsaktiebolaget Skandia (publ) and Ola Ramstedt v Riksskatteverket* [2003] ECR I-6817; Case C-264/96 *Imperial Chemical Industries plc (ICI) v Kenneth Hall Colmer (Her Majesty's Inspector of Taxes)* [1998] ECR I-4695, para 28; Case C-307/97 *Compagnie de Saint-Gobain, Zweigniederlassung Deutschland v Finanzamt Aachen-Innenstadt* [1999] ECR I-6161, para 50; Case C-385/00 *FWL de Groot v Staatssecretaris van Financiën* [2002] ECR I-11819, para 103.

[104] See ch 8, HJI Panayi (2013), n 3 above.

[105] See, for example, *Eurowings*, n 10 above, paragraph 44 and other cases cited therein.

[106] See Case C-80/12 *Felixstowe Dock & Railway Co Ltd v HM Revenue & Customs* [2014] ECR I-0000, para 32.

[107] See, for example, Christiana HJI Panayi, 'Open Skies for EC Tax?' [2003] 3 BTR 189; Georg W Kofler, 'European Taxation Under an "Open Sky": LoB Clauses in Tax Treaties Between the U.S. and the EU Member States' (2004) 35 *Tax Notes International* 45; Christiana HJI Panayi, *Double Taxation, Tax Treaties, Treaty Shopping and the European Community* (Kluwer, 2007).

company itself, the more likely that the setting up of the establishment itself will be recognised as an activity that could be prima facie covered by the freedom of establishment.[108] Similarly, the more economic substance there is in the intermediary, the more likely that investment through it will be prima facie covered by the free movement of capital. Assuming this first threshold issue is satisfied and the aforementioned fundamental freedoms are prima facie engaged, is there a restriction on them?[109]

From a freedom of establishment perspective, it could be argued that treaty shopping, ie the use of the intermediary entity located in a favourable tax jurisdiction to effect the investment, is an exercise of freedom of establishment. The fact that the intermediary entity has limited economic substance (but is short of a complete sham for threshold purposes) should not prevent the arrangement from being characterised as an exercise of establishment. An analogy may be drawn with a line of non-tax related cases (*Centros*[110]/*Überseering*).[111] These cases dealt with corporate forum shopping. Here, the Court of Justice approved the formation of primary and secondary establishments, even if they lacked economic substance in one Member State and were thought to have been set up in order to circumvent the company law formation requirements applicable in another Member State.[112] Just because the undertaking was corporate forum shopping within the European Union with little economic substance in the establishment did not necessarily mean that the protection under the freedom of establishment was withdrawn. Can this strand of reasoning also apply to tax treaty shopping? Does the fact that tax treaty shopping entails tax-location shopping rather than corporate forum shopping change matters?

There is no reason why it should, at least prima facie. As emphatically held in *Cadbury Schweppes*,[113] profiting from tax advantages in force in another Member State is not per se abuse.[114] Citing the case law on corporate forum shopping, the Court of Justice reiterated that the fact that a company was established in a Member State for the purpose of benefitting from more favourable legislation did not in itself suffice to constitute abuse of that freedom—which would have *ab initio* prevented enjoyment of the freedom. The same reasoning applied to a company established in another Member State 'for the avowed purpose of benefitting

[108] On freedom of establishment and economic substance, see section 6.5 of this volume.

[109] Most of the arguments raised in this section were initially raised by the author in her PhD thesis and later on in ch 5 of HJI Panayi (2007), n 107 above. For a later analysis see also Christiana HJI Panayi and Reuven Avi-Yonah, 'Rethinking treaty-shopping: Lessons for the European Union' in M Lang et al (eds), *Tax Treaties: Building Bridges between Law and Economics* (IBFD Publications, 2010).

[110] Case C-212/97 *Centros Ltd v Erhvervs-og Selskabsstyrelsen* [1999] ECR I-1459.

[111] Case C-208/00 *Überseering BV v Nordic Construction Company Baumanagement GmbH (NCC)* [2002] ECR I-9919.

[112] See Christiana HJI Panayi, 'Corporate Mobility under Private International Law and European Community Law: Debunking Some Myths' (2009) 28 *Yearbook of European Law* 124–76.

[113] *Cadbury Schweppes*, n 24 above.

[114] *Ibid*, paras 34–38.

from the favourable tax regime which that establishment enjoyed'.[115] Such exercise of tax-forum shopping did not, according to the Court of Justice, deprive a company of the opportunity to rely on the rights conferred under freedom of establishment.[116] The arrangement had to be examined on its facts.

It would seem that just because treaty shopping entails a type of forum shopping, this does not necessarily mean it is abusive. If anything, it appeared to be encouraged by the Court of Justice in its earlier case law. As such, it could be argued that treaty shopping is an exercise of establishment, regardless of the motives behind it. What anti-treaty-shopping provisions tend to do is to disregard the intermediary entity and treat another company as the ultimate recipient of the income. Therefore, it could be argued that anti-treaty-shopping provisions restrict the freedom of establishment. Of course, this restriction could be justified, as explained below, but this is nonetheless a restriction.

From a free movement of capital perspective, it could be argued that a treaty shopper exercises its free movement of capital by investing in a company indirectly (ie through another Member State entity) and as a result receives its return from such investment indirectly. The analysis here focuses on the existence (or lack of) indirect investment rather than the use of an intermediary entity. The issue is not so much the fact of establishing a related entity through which investment is made. What is important is the fact that the treaty shopper (whether EU national or not) takes advantage of the tax treaty network of another Member State in order to invest in a third Member State, by channelling income through an intermediary entity which it does not control.

In other words, this is an instance of indirect rather than direct investment (investment through a related entity) and as such, should prima facie be protected under the free movement of capital. Anti-treaty-shopping provisions tend to disregard the intermediary entity and/or re-characterise the payment as being directly made to another company. As a result, they may ultimately make the investment of capital through an intermediary in another Member State more expensive. Therefore, it could be argued that anti-treaty-shopping provisions restrict the free movement of capital.

Of course, as under freedom of establishment, this restriction could be justified by imperative requirements in the general interest. It also has to be suitable and

[115] *Ibid*, para 38.

[116] See, similarly, the reasoning of Advocate General Léger in para 40 et seq. The Advocate General went a step further and linked the absence of economic activity in the establishment as an important factor in assessing abuse. He argued that 'as long as there is genuine and actual pursuit of an activity by the controlled subsidiary in the Member State in which it was established, the reasons for which the parent company decided to establish the subsidiary in that host State cannot call into question the rights which that company derives from the Treaty': see para 49 of the opinion. Even more in point, the Advocate General argued that 'the fact that a company centralises in another Member State with a low tax rate the carrying on of certain activities of use to the entire group and seeks by that means to reduce the group's overall tax burden does not in itself constitute abuse … as long as the subsidiary responsible for those intra-group services *is carrying on genuine economic activity in the host State*, under the tax sovereignty of which it falls, the territorial allocation of the Member States' power to impose taxes is not, *a priori*, affected' (emphasis added): see para 109 of the opinion.

proportional.[117] Not every kind of structure will ultimately be protected under EU law.

For example, the restriction could be justified on the basis of preventing tax avoidance/evasion.[118] In order for this ground to succeed, as discussed above in the context of Actions 2 to 4 of the BEPS project, the anti-treaty-shopping provisions must have the specific purpose of preventing wholly artificial arrangements. Broad anti-abuse clauses which do not distinguish between bona fide activities and abusive situations have been struck down. Prevention of tax avoidance/evasion could, therefore, exonerate a restrictive treaty provision if this is sufficiently targeted to that end. The provision must also be suitable and must not go beyond what is necessary to attain the objective pursued, whether this is prevention of tax evasion or of tax avoidance. Therefore, if less than wholly artificial arrangements are caught by an anti-treaty-shopping provision, then the restriction is unlikely to be justified. As a corollary, the more artificial the treaty-shopping arrangement, the more likely it is to have tax avoidance connotations—against which an anti-treaty-shopping provision can more readily be justified.

The restriction could also be justified on the basis of safeguarding the allocation of tax jurisdiction.[119] It could be argued that what anti-treaty-shopping provisions seek to do is restore the allocation choices of the tax treaty 'shopped'. As the original allocation choices of the relevant tax treaty are respected under EU law after the *D* case,[120] so should measures to protect and restore those allocation choices. In fact, as explained immediately below, this line of case law and the treaty allocation ground may be used to pre-empt any argument of incompatibility of the LOB with EU law altogether. Assuming though it is not so used and allocation of taxing rights is considered as a justification for a restriction, then the application of this justification has to be fine-tuned and proportional. In this context, the allocation of tax jurisdiction is less threatened by intermediary entities imbued with economic substance. The more substance there is in the treaty-shopping arrangement, the less likely it is that the allocation choices under the underlying tax treaty would be frustrated. Anti-treaty-shopping provisions have to factor that in.

Also, the applicability of this ground as an imperative requirement could depend on the actual effect of the anti-treaty-shopping provisions on the structure.

[117] *Gebhard*, n 77 above, para 37.

[118] See, for example, *ICI*, n 103 above; Case C-9/02 *Hughes de Lasteyrie du Saillant v Ministère de L'Economie des Finances et de l'Industrie* [2004] ECR I-2409. The Court of Justice, in the early cases especially, tended to use the terms 'avoidance' and 'evasion' without distinction. In some cases, it referred to the justification as being based on tax avoidance (eg *ICI*, para 26) whereas in others it referred to tax evasion (eg *Lankhorst-Hohorst*, n 58 above, para 37; Case C-436/00 *X & Y v Riksskatteverket*, [2002] ECR I-10829, para 62).

[119] See Case C-376/03 *D v Rijksbelastingdienst* (*D* case) [2005] ECR I-5821; Case C-446/03 *Marks & Spencer plc v Halsey (HM Inspector of Taxes)* [2005] ECR I-10837; *Oy AA*, n 50 above; Case C-470/04 *N v Inspecteur van de Belastingdienst Oost/kantoor Almelo* [2006] ECR I-7409l; Case C-414/06 *Lidl Belgium GmbH & Co KG/Finanzamt Heilbronn* [2008] ECR I-3601, para 51; Case C-182/08 *Glaxo Wellcome GmbH & Co KG v Finanzamt München II* [2009] ECR I-8591 para 88.

[120] See *D* case, n 119 above. Also see analysis in ch 4 in HJI Panayi (2013), n 3, and below.

Do they restore the original withholding tax rate that would have applied absent the treaty-shopping arrangement or do they impose a (penal) statutory withholding tax rate? If the former, then it could be argued that what the anti-treaty-shopping provision actually does is to restore the treaty balance. However, if the statutory withholding tax rate applies, then it is more difficult to see how the anti-treaty-shopping provision restores the treaty balance, since that balance is itself overridden.

A point to note is that under the free movement of capital, it does not matter whether the capital movement is to or from a non-Member State, so long as there is some capital movement to or from a Member State. However, this could be relevant at the justification stage.[121] A restriction may be more readily justified if it affects third-country nationals than if it affects EU nationals. Nevertheless, this has to be proven. Another point to note is that the freedom of establishment is only available to EU nationals. Therefore, if the intermediary entity is in a non-EU Member State, then an anti-treaty-shopping provision frustrating the arrangement may not be incompatible with EU law.

In conclusion, it is possible that anti-treaty-shopping provisions restrict the freedom of establishment and/or the free movement of capital. However, they could be justified, depending on how these provisions are phrased, and whether they are sufficiently targeted against wholly artificial arrangements and proportional. It also depends on whether these provisions try to curb treaty shopping through a non-EU Member State. Of course, the above discussion may simply be theoretical and/or at best academic, for the time being. If a case were to arise at the Court of Justice today, it is likely that the Court would seize on the *D* case[122] and the *ACT GLO* case[123] and avoid a clash with the LOB altogether by finding lack of comparability and non-discrimination.

The *D* case established that when dealing with tax benefits conferred to non-residents through tax treaties, there is no comparability between a non-resident of one treaty partner and a non-resident of another. Therefore, the fact that a Member State applied different treaty rates to non-residents did not mean that the Member State was discriminating between those two non-residents. In the *D* case, the Court of Justice accepted the allocation attained in the relevant tax treaties, even if this meant that some non-residents were treated more harshly than other non-residents. It was found that the Netherlands was not obliged to extend to a German resident the treaty benefits given to Belgian residents. The Germany–Netherlands tax treaty did not provide for the same allowances as the Belgium–Netherlands tax treaty. This was a question of pre-agreed allocation of tax powers between these countries. The relevant treaties were not to be interfered

[121] See, for example, Case C-446/04 *FII Group Litigation* case [2006] ECR I-11753, paras, 169–72; *Thin Cap GLO*, n 38 above; Case C-101/05 *Case A* [2007] ECR I-11531; *CFC GLO*, n 54 above; Case C-540/07 *Commission v Italy* [2009] ECR I-10983.

[122] *D* case, n 119 above.

[123] *ACT GLO* case, n 3 above.

with by extending benefits given to Belgian residents also to German residents. In other words, the tax treaty benefits given under a tax treaty were unique to that tax treaty, so an EU national not benefiting under the treaty could not demand the extension of treaty benefits.

This reasoning was followed in the *ACT GLO* case and extended to LOBs showing the Court's reluctance to interfere with anti-treaty-shopping provisions. It was found that there was no comparability between two non-residents benefiting from the *same* tax treaty, owned by residents from different treaty partners. This meant that withdrawal of tax treaty benefits on the basis of the ownership of the non-resident entity would not necessarily constitute discrimination, precisely because there would be no comparable situations being treated differently to start with. Otherwise, the 'equilibrium and reciprocity underlying the existing DTCs [double taxation conventions] would be undermined, taxpayers would be able more easily to avoid the provisions of DTCs intended to combat tax avoidance and the legal certainty of taxpayers would be affected accordingly'.[124] LOBs were considered to be a natural corollary of the bilateralism enshrined in tax treaties. They were characterised by the Court of Justice as 'an inherent consequence of bilateral double taxation conventions',[125] not precluded by Treaty provisions on freedom of establishment.

The Advocate General had similarly held that the tax treaty distinction of non-residents on the basis of the country of residence of their controlling shareholder was 'part of the equilibrium of jurisdiction and priority reached by the Contracting States in the exercise of their competence'.[126] As a result, enquiry into the reasons and justifications for this choice of equilibrium did not fall within the ambit of the non-discrimination provisions.[127]

It is noteworthy that the fact that the impugned anti-treaty-shopping provision was an LOB clause, which can be applied quite mechanically without taking into account the bona fides of the structure or the similarity of the two non-resident situations, did not concern the Court of Justice. Neither did it venture to explain the situation from the viewpoint of a restriction, for which a comparator test was not necessary. Furthermore, the Court of Justice omitted to explain the difference between *not relieving* certain double taxation as a result of tax treaty allocation and *forfeiting* relief otherwise applicable pursuant to the tax treaty allocation.[128]

The author has argued elsewhere[129] that there is a very fine distinction between the *D* case and the situation in the *ACT GLO* case. In the *D* case, no comparability was found between two non-resident individuals from *different* Member States benefiting under two *different* tax treaties. In the *ACT GLO* case, no comparability

[124] *Ibid*, para 80.
[125] *Ibid*, para 91.
[126] *Ibid*, para 101 (opinion).
[127] *Ibid.*
[128] See analysis in section 5.2.1.2 (ii) in HJI Panayi (2007), n 107 above.
[129] *Ibid*, ch 5.

Of course, it should be reminded that, irrespective of whether these tests rely on the main purpose or one of the main purposes or the sole purpose, simple tax forum shopping does not constitute abuse under the case law of the Court of Justice. As stipulated in *Cadbury Schweppes*,

> the fact that a Community national, whether a natural or legal person, sought to profit from tax advantages in force in a Member State other than his State of residence cannot in itself deprive him of the right to rely on [the fundamental freedoms].[141]

Therefore, for EU purposes, the focus of any PPT or GAAR test needs to be on the artificiality of the impugned arrangement and not (only) the purposes or intentions when entering into the arrangement.

Another difference in the various PPT clauses is the result of these anti-abuse rules being triggered. With the PPT under Action 6, tax treaty benefits are not to be given. By contrast, under the GAAR of the Recommendation on Aggressive Tax Planning, there is possibility for further action, possibly re-characterisation—'[n]ational authorities shall treat these arrangements for tax purposes by reference to their economic substance'.[142] While this possibility is not mentioned in the Parent-Subsidiary Directive's new GAAR, it cannot be excluded, as the Directive does not preclude the application of domestic or agreement-based provisions required for the prevention of tax evasion, tax fraud or abuse.

Another point of deviation is the relevance and impact of commercial justifications—ie the subjectivity of the rules. Under the amended Parent-Subsidiary Directive, an arrangement or a series of arrangements shall not be regarded as genuine to the extent that they are not put into place for valid commercial reasons which reflect economic reality. This resonates with the Court's reasoning in *Cadbury Schweppes, Thin Cap GLO* and more recently in the VAT context, the *Ocean Finance* case.[143] There is similar stipulation in the GAAR proposed in the Recommendation on Aggressive Tax Planning.[144] There is no such provision in the recommended PPT under Action 6, which suggests a more objective analysis which cannot be rebutted by commercial reasons. Arguably, valid commercial reasons could be taken into account if a discretionary relief provision is inserted in the PPT rule under Action 6, something proposed by the OECD in its latest discussion draft.[145]

Finance [2013] ECR I-0000), the Court of Justice seem to have reverted to the sole purpose test rather than 'one of the purposes' of a transaction test. Also see ch 8 in HJI Panayi (2013), n 3 above, for the pre-*Ocean Finance* case law.

[141] *Cadbury Schweppes*, n 24 above, para 36.

[142] See para 4.2 of the Recommendation on Aggressive Tax Planning.

[143] See Ch 5 of this volume.

[144] See para 4.4 of the Recommendation on Aggressive Tax Planning: 'For the purposes of point 4.2, an arrangement or a series of arrangements is artificial where it lacks commercial substance'. But also see 4.5: 'For the purposes of point 4.2, the purpose of an arrangement or series of arrangements consists in avoiding taxation where, regardless of any subjective intentions of the taxpayer, it defeats the object, spirit and purpose of the tax provisions that would otherwise apply'.

[145] See paras 87–90 in Treaty Abuse Second Revised Discussion Draft, where it is considered whether some form of discretionary relief should be provided under the PPT rule. See Ch 3, section 3.1.

It should also be noted that under the PPT proposed under Action 6, there seems to be a presumption that a tax treaty benefit is not in accordance with the object and purpose of the tax treaty, unless proven otherwise. It is stated that a benefit under a given tax treaty shall not be granted if it is reasonable to conclude, having regard to all relevant facts and circumstances, that obtaining that benefit was one of the principal purposes of any arrangement or transaction. The onus is on the taxpayer to show that 'granting that benefit in these circumstances would be in accordance with the object and purpose of the relevant provisions of this Convention'.[146] This is further illustrated in the commentaries. By contrast, there is no such presumption under the GAAR of the Recommendation on Aggressive Tax Planning and that of the Parent-Subsidiary Directive.[147]

Notwithstanding the above technical analysis of the legal credentials of the Action 6 PPT rule under EU law, it is unlikely that the Court of Justice would treat a PPT (especially if combined with an LOB) more harshly than the much more pre-emptive and mechanical LOB test. There is however another angle which needs to be considered. The PPT rule, however 'un-mechanical' and subjective, can still be problematic if deemed to be uncertain.[148] In *Itelcar*,[149] it was held that anti-abuse rules must be sufficiently clear, precise and predictable; otherwise they do not meet the requirements of legal certainty. As such, 'rules which do not meet the requirements of the principle of legal certainty cannot be considered to be proportionate to the objectives pursued'.[150] Therefore, anti-abuse rules must make it possible, at the outset, to determine their scope with sufficient precision.

Is the PPT as an anti-abuse rule sufficiently clear, precise and predictable? This would depend on how it is interpreted and applied. While the suggested wording has similarities with the GAARs under the Parent-Subsidiary Directive and the Recommendation on Aggressive Tax Planning, if the Action 6 PPT rule is applied in a way that catches both commercial and uncommercial arrangements, then arguably its ambit would not be sufficiently clear and it would risk being found in breach of EU law.[151] This point should not be ignored by Member States either in applying their GAARs or in the incorporation of the Parent-Subsidiary Directive's GAAR. The above analysis also suggests that, in the end, there might not be much scope for widely diverging—in terms of leniency or strictness—GAARs.

It is noteworthy that smaller Member States, such as Ireland, Cyprus and Malta, have expressed concerns about the application of the PPT rule in tax arrangements affecting their jurisdictions. In a report published by KPMG Ireland mentioned in

[146] See the proposed wording for the PPT rule, set out in p 12 of the September 2014 discussion draft, n 138 above. See section 3.1 of this volume.

[147] Also see Dourado, n 130 above, p 56.

[148] Eric Kemmeren, 'Where is EU Law in the OECD BEPS Discussion?' (2014) 23 *EC Tax Review* 190–93.

[149] Case C-282/12 *Itelcar v Fazenda Publica* [2013] ECR I-0000.

[150] *Ibid*, para 44. Also see Case C-318/10 *Société d'Investissement pour l'Agriculture Tropicale SA (SIAT) v Belgian State* [2013] ECR I-0000, para 58 and 59.

[151] More guidance is given on the application of the PPT rule in the latest discussion draft—see Treaty Abuse Second Revised Discussion Draft, n 145 above, paras 73–99.

Chapter three, it was argued that the proposals under Action 6 of the BEPS Action Plan were heavily biased against small countries and would potentially damage legitimate economic activity in such countries. This was because it was much easier to satisfy a main purpose test or fail to satisfy an active business/trade test in smaller countries than in larger industrial countries.[152] It was recommended that business support activities should suffice even where those activities are provided for the benefit of related group parties and where there are no or limited sales of the relevant group products or services in the small country concerned.

6.7. Country-By-Country Reporting, Dispute Resolution and Multilateralisation of Tax Treaties: Actions 13, 14 and 15

Regarding the transfer pricing deliverables and especially Action 13, there seems to be some interesting cross-fertilisation of ideas from the European Union. It has been argued that the OECD and G20 are effectively taking up some of the ideas that came out of the EU Joint Transfer Pricing Forum (JTPF).[153] The JTPF was formally set up in 2002 to assist and advise the Commission on transfer pricing tax matters. On the basis of the JTPF's work, in 2011, the Commission published a Communication setting out guidelines on technical issues related to transfer pricing taxation, including low-value-adding intra-group services and non-EU triangular services.[154] The JTPF's work on this is thought to have influenced the OECD in preparing its discussion draft on low-value-adding intra-group services.[155]

Furthermore, it would appear that in the European Union, templates and guidance for uniform country-by-country reporting long preceded the BEPS deliverables. In 2006, again as a result of the work of the JTPF, a Code of Conduct on the transfer pricing documentation for associated enterprises in the European Union

[152] See KPMG Ireland's report on Action 6 and Fairness for Small Countries, replicated in KPMG's *Response to OECD/G20 BEPS Project—Follow Up Work on BEPS Action 6: Preventing Treaty Abuse (Fairness for Smaller Economies)*, dated 9 January 2015. Available on: www.kpmg-institutes.com/content/dam/kpmg/taxwatch/pdf/2015/1-9-15-kpmg-ie-comment-letter.pdf. Also see discussion in ch 3, section 3.1.

[153] Amanda Athanasiou, 'EU Perspectives on BEPS', 2014 *WTD* 182-2 (19 September 2014).

[154] Communication setting out guidelines on technical issues related to transfer pricing taxation, including low-value-adding intra-group services and non-EU triangular services (COM(2011)16 final). Also see Council conclusions on the communication from the Commission on the work of the EU Joint Transfer Pricing Forum in the period April 2009 to June 2010 and related proposals: 1. Guidelines on low value adding intra-group services and 2. Potential approaches to non-EU triangular cases (Council of the European Union, 3088th Economic and Financial Affairs Council meeting, Brussels, 17 May 2011).

[155] *Public Discussion Draft—BEPS Action 10: Proposed Modifications to Chapter VII of the Transfer Pricing Guidelines relating to Low Value-Adding Intra-Group Services*, 3 November 2014—14 January 2015 (OECD). See Ch 3, section 3.4.1 of this volume.

was published.[156] The Code of Conduct provided a template for standardised and partially centralised transfer pricing documentation for associated enterprises in the European Union. It was addressed to Member States but was also intended to encourage MNEs to apply the standardised approach. Member States were urged to accept the standardised and partially centralised transfer pricing documentation and consider it as a basic set of information for the assessment of an MNE's transfer prices. The use of the standardised documentation was optional for a multinational group, though it provided an incentive to minimise the administrative costs of complying with several national transfer pricing documentation requirements. A multinational group adopting the standardised template had to do so in a way that was consistent throughout the European Union and from year to year.

The template for standardised documentation consisted of two main parts. First, there was one set of documentation containing common standardised information relevant for all EU group members (the 'masterfile'), and secondly, there were several sets of standardised documentation each containing country-specific information ('country-specific documentation'). The standardised documentation had to contain enough information to allow the tax administration to make a risk assessment for case selection purposes. It had to enable the tax authorities at the beginning of a tax audit, to assess the MNE's transfer pricing and the transfer prices of the inter-company transactions.

Member States retained the right to require under domestic law that a taxpayer provide more information and documents than would be contained in the documentation but only upon specific request or during a tax audit.[157] However, Member States were urged not to impose unreasonable compliance costs or administrative burden on enterprises in requesting documentation to be created or obtained, not to request documentation that had no bearing on transactions under review and to ensure that there was no public disclosure of confidential information contained in the documentation.[158]

It is generally thought that the EU approach linked country-by-country reporting with corporate social responsibility (CSR).[159] This is also aligned with the attitude taken vis-à-vis some other corporate transparency measures.[160] In the 2013 OECD White Paper on Transfer Pricing Documentation, the OECD noted

[156] See Resolution of the Council and of the representatives of the governments of the Member States, meeting within the Council, of 27 June 2006 on a code of conduct on transfer pricing documentation for associated enterprises in the European Union (EU TPD), [2006] OJ C176/1–7, 28.7.2006. Available on: eur-lex.europa.eu/legal-content/EN/TXT/?uri=CELEX:42006X0728%2801%29.

[157] See para 18 of the Annex to the Code of Conduct on Transfer Pricing Documentation for Associated Enterprises in the European Union, *ibid.*

[158] See para 6 of the Code of Conduct on Transfer Pricing Documentation for Associated Enterprises in the European Union, *ibid.*

[159] Maria A Grau Ruiz, 'Country-by-Country Reporting: The Primary Concerns Raised by a Dynamic Approach' (2014) 68 *Bulletin for International Taxation* 557–66, at 557.

[160] See the new Accounting Directive 2013/34/EU which introduces an obligation for large extractive and logging companies to report country-by-country the payments made to governments, and also on a project-basis. Also see Revised Capital Requirements Directive 2013/36/EU which improves transparency in the activities of banks and investment funds in different countries. See analysis in Ch 5, section 5.3.1 of this volume.

that the EU approach appeared to be less detailed and the information that the common template required seemed to be less extensive than the information required in some non-EU countries.[161] It is no surprise, therefore, that the OECD's country-by-country template developed under Action 13 is much more comprehensive than the template developed by the EU's JTPF. Both, however, share the same basic aim: to improve transparency and enhance compliance by MNEs, and to ensure effective supervision by tax authorities worldwide. The OECD has rightly eschewed the vague language of CSR to justify its actions.

Given recent developments and the Commission's drive for further tax transparency,[162] the EU transfer pricing reporting standards are likely to be aligned with those eventually derived from the BEPS proposals and probably supersede them in terms of strictness and comprehensiveness. Indicatively, recently, the European Parliament Development Committee has unanimously passed a resolution calling for MNEs to adopt country-by-country reporting and make beneficial ownership information publicly available.[163] More initiatives are likely to follow in this area.

As far as Action 14 of the BEPS Action Plan is concerned, it should be pointed out that arbitration (whether mandatory or not), which was not put forward as a proposal under the first discussion draft on Action 14,[164] is a route available to Member States under the Arbitration Convention.[165] Arguably, any further suggestions made to improve dispute resolution mechanisms and the tax treaty mutual agreement procedures affecting Member States ought to be aligned with the Arbitration Convention.

The Arbitration Convention seeks to establish an arbitration procedure which eliminates double taxation in the course of transfer pricing disputes between Member States.[166] Unlike a Directive or Regulation, it is merely an agreement under public international law and, as such, subject to the jurisdiction of national courts and not that of the Court of Justice. The Arbitration Convention is based on the arm's length principle. It applies when profits of an enterprise of a Member State are included or are likely to be included in the profits of an enterprise in another Member State.[167] The Arbitration Convention applies to all taxes on

[161] See White Paper on Transfer Pricing Documentation, para 30, published on 30 July 2013. Available on: www.oecd.org/ctp/transfer-pricing/white-paper-transfer-pricing-documentation.pdf. Also see literature cited therein, inter alia, Ágúst K Guðmundsson, 'Lost in Transfer Pricing: The Pitfalls of EU Transfer Pricing Documentation' [2009] 1 *International Transfer Pricing Journal* 25–28; W Nichols and L Hughes, 'EU Transfer Pricing Documentation—White Elephant or Missed Opportunity?' [2010] *Transfer Pricing International Journal*, BNA (February 2010); 'European Companies Questioning Benefits of EU Masterfile Documentation Approach', Tax Management Transfer Pricing Report, BNA (May 2006).

[162] See analysis in Ch 5 and more specifically, section 5.4 of this volume.

[163] See press release of 1 June 2015, published in Tax Analysts: 'European Parliament Committee Passes CbC Reporting Resolution', 2015 *WTD* 106-14 (1 June 2015).

[164] See analysis in Ch 4, section 4.4 of this volume.

[165] Convention 90/436/EEC of 23 July 1990 on the Elimination of Double Taxation in Connection with the Adjustment of Profits of Associated Enterprises.

[166] Croatia was the last Member State to accede to the Arbitration Convention in December 2014. For a general analysis, see Jasmin Kollmann, Petra Koch, Alicja Majdanska and Laura Turcan, 'Arbitration in International Tax Matters' (2015) 77 *Tax Notes International* 1189 (30 March 2015).

[167] Arbitration Convention, n 165 above, Art 1.

income and in particular to taxes listed therein.[168] The objective of the Arbitration Convention is to establish a procedure to eliminate double taxation arising from profit adjustments made by Contracting States because of a violation of the arm's length principle between associated enterprises; or the attribution of profits to a permanent establishment not equivalent to what it might be expected to derive if it were a distinct and separate enterprise engaged in the same or similar activities under the same or similar conditions and dealing on an arm's length basis.[169]

The Arbitration Convention sets out a three-stage procedure for eliminating double taxation. First, the Member State has to notify the affected enterprise of its intention to make a tax adjustment and to hear any objections. It must give the enterprise time to let the relevant associated party inform the other Member State, but it is not prevented from making the proposed adjustment.[170] Secondly, if the enterprise disagrees with the proposed adjustment, there is a three-year limit for it to present its case to its competent authorities, requesting a mutual agreement. This is irrespective of any remedies provided under the domestic law of the Contracting States.[171] Thirdly, if the competent authorities of the two relevant Member States fail to reach a mutual agreement within two years, they have to establish an Advisory Commission.[172] An appeal in national courts delays proceedings.

The Advisory Commission has to deliver its opinion within six months.[173] Following that, the competent authorities must make a decision which eliminates double taxation within the next six months.[174] Double taxation is regarded as eliminated if either the profits are included in the computation of taxable profits in one Member State only or the tax chargeable on those profits in one Member State is reduced by an amount equal to the tax chargeable on them in the other.[175] This three-stage procedure has to be concluded within six years. There are certain escape routes for the competent authorities of the Contracting States eg where the complaint does not appear to be well-founded,[176] or where domestic law does not permit competent authorities to derogate from the decisions of their judicial bodies or where legal or administrative proceedings have resulted in a final ruling in that, because of the transactions that gave rise to the adjustment, one of the enterprises concerned is liable to a serious administrative or criminal penalty.[177]

The JTPF has examined issues relating to the implementation of the Arbitration Convention such as the effective implementation of the Arbitration Convention and the transfer pricing documentation for associated enterprises in the

[168] *Ibid*, Art 2(2).
[169] *Ibid*, Art 4.
[170] *Ibid*, Art 5.
[171] *Ibid*, Art 6.
[172] *Ibid*, Art 7.
[173] *Ibid*, Art 9.
[174] *Ibid*, Art 10.
[175] *Ibid*, Art 14.
[176] *Ibid*, Art 6(2).
[177] *Ibid*, Art 8(1), (2).

European Union, discussed previously. The JTPF has also produced Codes of Conduct on these matters[178] and monitors compliance issues,[179] overseen by the Commission.[180] Recently, the JTPF has issued a report on improving the functioning of the Arbitration Convention.[181]

As far as Action 15 of the BEPS Action Plan is concerned, it should be pointed out that there is nothing stopping Member States from entering into multilateral agreements. Nordic countries, for example, entered into a multilateral tax treaty in 1983.[182] This multilateral tax treaty was revised several times since then but is still effective and binding on the participating countries, most of which are EU Member States as well. Member States have also entered into the Council of Europe/OECD Convention on mutual administrative assistance in tax matters in 1988. From an EU law perspective, technically, in the area in which Member States have retained exclusive competence, such as for direct taxes, there is nothing objectionable in entering into multilateral tax agreements. At least, it is not more objectionable than a bilateral tax agreement. This, however, comes with the usual caveat that established principles of EU law are to be respected.

If the multilateral tax treaty is between Member States only, then technically, the treaty cannot include any provisions that are incompatible with EU law. If the multilateral tax treaty is between Member States and third countries, then Member States may not be in a position to dictate what provisions are included and what

[178] See the Code of Conduct for the effective implementation of the Arbitration Convention. This Code of Conduct establishes common procedures concerning (a) the starting point of the three-year period which is the deadline for a company suffering double taxation to present its case to the tax administration of the relevant Member State; (b) the starting point of the two-year period during which Member States' tax administrations must attempt to reach an agreement that eliminates the double taxation that is the subject of the complaint; (c) the arrangements to be followed during this mutual agreement procedure (the practical operation of the procedure, transparency and taxpayer participation); and (d) the practical arrangements for the second phase of the dispute resolution procedure (the establishment and functioning of the Advisory Commission). This Code of Conduct also contains a recommendation to Member States to suspend the collection of taxes during the dispute resolution procedure. Also see the Revised Code of Conduct (2009/C 322/01).

[179] See, for example, the questionnaire sent regarding the implementation of the Code of Conduct on EU Transfer Pricing Documentation and the summary of the Member States' responses published by the Commission in the summer of 2010. See EU Joint Transfer Pricing Forum: *Secretariat's paper summarising MS' replies on the EUTPD questionnaire*, Meeting of 8 June 2010.

[180] For example, in September 2009, the Commission published a Communication on the work of the JTPF, including a proposal for a revised Code of Conduct, as well as a staff working paper containing a summary report on penalties in transfer pricing. See Communication on the work of the EU Joint Transfer Pricing Forum in the period March 2007 to March 2009 and a related proposal for a revised Code of Conduct for the effective implementation of the Arbitration Convention (90/436/EEC of 23 July 1990) COM(2009) 472 final.

[181] See EU Joint Transfer Pricing Forum, *Final Report on Improving the Functioning of the Arbitration Convention—Meeting of 12 March 2015* (DOC: JTPF/002/2015/EN). For the latest overview of the Arbitration Convention and suggestions for reform, see Harm Mark Pit, 'Improving the Arbitration Procedure under the EU Arbitration Convention (1)' (2015) 24 *EC Tax Review* 15–33 and Harm Mark Pit, 'Improving the Arbitration Procedure under the EU Arbitration Convention (2)' (2015) 24 *EC Tax Review* 78–95.

[182] Nordic Convention on Income and Capital entered into by Denmark, Finland, Iceland, Norway and Sweden, concluded in 1983 and replaced in 1987, 1989 and 1996.

not. This is likely to be the case with a post-BEPS multilateral tax treaty. To the extent that Member States cannot prevent multilateral treaty provisions which are incompatible with EU law,[183] then they ought to abstain from enforcing such provisions or opt out or enter reservations in the text of the treaty.

As held in the *Open Skies* cases,[184] Member States have a duty to comply with their obligations under EU law when exercising their competence to conclude international agreements. Although EU-incompatible agreements with third countries may not be automatically invalid, Member States may be forced to terminate them.[185] Notwithstanding the fact that taxation is not an area where Member States have any shared competence with the European Union, the Court of Justice might extend the *Open Skies* reasoning to a post-BEPS multilateral tax treaty containing potentially discriminatory clauses, even if the discriminatory behaviour results from a non-Member State's act or omission.[186] It has been suggested that if the compatibility issues are not clear and the Commission decides to request a legal opinion from the Court of Justice, then the OECD and EU Member States should consider awaiting such an opinion before proceeding with the signing of the multilateral agreement.[187]

Overall, any measures taken by the European Union or Member States in tackling aggressive tax planning should factor in established principles set out by the Court of Justice in its case law, considered in this and in the previous chapters. While such measures may now, more than ever, be politically appealing and feasible, both the EU institutions and Member States should resist the challenge of taking action without careful forethought and a detailed legal analysis. As shown in the next chapter in the discussion of the Commission's state aid decisions relating to several transfer pricing tax rulings, politically-motivated actions risk eroding established legal doctrines. As such, these actions generate legal uncertainty and damage the credibility of the EU institutions, with no guarantee of reciprocal actions by third countries.

[183] Eg the imposition of withholding taxes in situations in which the Parent-Subsidiary Directive would apply or contrary to the principles set out in the case law etc. See ch 6 in HJI Panayi (2013), n 3 above.

[184] The eight so-called *Open Skies* judgments are Case C-466/98 *Commission v UK* [2002] ECR I-9427; Case C-467/98 *Commission v Denmark* [2002] ECR I-9519; Case C-468/98 *Commission v Sweden* [2002] ECR I-9575; Case C-469/98 *Commission v Finland* [2002] ECR I-9627; Case C-471/98 *Commission v Belgium* [2002] ECR I-9681; Case C-472/98 *Commission v Luxembourg* [2002] ECR I-9741; Case C-475/98 *Commission v Austria* [2002] ECR I-9797; and Case C-476/98 *Commission v Germany* [2002] ECR I-9855.

[185] See the various repercussions in international law discussed in Christiana HJI Panayi, 'Exploring the Open Skies: EC-incompatible treaties between Member States and Third Countries' [2006] *Yearbook of European Law* 315–62.

[186] See analysis in Christiana HJI Panayi, 'Open Skies for European Tax?', n 107 above.

[187] See CFE Fiscal Committee, *Opinion Statement FC 15/2014 on Developing a Multilateral Instrument to Modify Bilateral Tax Treaties (BEPS Action 15)*. Available on: www.cfe-eutax.org/node/4087.

7

State Aid, Taxation and Aggressive Tax Planning

It is becoming obvious that the state aid prohibition under EU law has also been 'enlisted' as a powerful weapon in the fight against aggressive tax planning. In order to assess whether this Treaty provision is correctly applied, as well as the actual impact and limitations of this approach, it is important to examine in some detail the state aid prohibition and its procedures. The role of the Commission and of national tax authorities are considered, as well as the rights of competitors and third parties. There is a review of recent important cases in the area of tax law. In the last part of this chapter, the use of the state aid prohibition in tackling some (perceived) examples of aggressive tax planning is considered.

7.1. Introduction

Enshrined in Article 107(1) TFEU, the state aid prohibition reads as follows:

> Save as otherwise provided in this Treaty, any aid granted by a Member State or through State resources in any form whatsoever which distorts or threatens to distort competition by favouring certain undertakings or the production of certain goods shall, in so far as it affects trade between Member States, be incompatible with the common market.

Article 107(1) TFEU does not have direct effect.[1]

There has to be an aid in the sense of a benefit or advantage,[2] granted by a Member State or through Member State resources. This encompasses regional or local authorities and public bodies.[3] Very importantly, the aid must favour certain undertakings or the production of certain goods (the 'selectivity' principle),[4]

[1] Case 74/76 *Ianelli & Volpi SpA v Meroni* [1977] ECR 557. See also Case 78/76 *Steinike und Weinlig v Germany* [1977] ECR 595; Case C-354/90 *Féderation National de Commerce Extérieur des Produits Alimentaire (FNCEPA) et al v France* [1991] ECR I-5505.

[2] The salient question is whether the recipient of the advantage is receiving a benefit which it would not have otherwise received under normal market conditions. See also below.

[3] Eg Case C-323/82 *Intermills v Commission* [1984] ECR 3809; Case 177/78 *Pigs and Bacon Commission v McCarren & Co Ltd* [1979] ECR 2161.

[4] A measure can be selective even if it applies to a large number of undertakings. See, for example, Case C-143/99 *Adria-Wien Pipeline GmbH and Wietersdorfer & Peggauer Zementwerke GmbH v*

distort or threaten to distort competition, and must be capable of affecting trade between Member States.

Under Article 107(2) TFEU, certain types of aid such as aid of a social character or aid to help in case of a natural disaster are deemed to be compatible with EU law.[5] Furthermore, aid *may* be compatible with the internal market if it falls within any of the six derogations laid down in Article 107(3) TFEU.[6] Unsurprisingly, these derogations have been construed strictly.

Whether or not a given measure is state aid is a question that the courts both at European and national level have competence to decide. However, whether such state aid is compatible or not with the common market is a question that the national courts do not have legal competence to deal with.[7] There has been no attempt to formulate a precise definition of the concept of state aid, the Commission preferring a broad brush approach which examines each aid on its own merits.[8] The salient question is whether the recipient of the advantage is receiving a benefit which it would not have otherwise received under normal market conditions.[9] The benefit should improve the undertaking's financial position or reduce the costs that it would have to bear. The Commission need not prove that trade will be affected.[10] It is sufficient to show that the measure threatens competition,[11] ie that intra-EU trade may be affected and not necessarily permanently.[12] In such circumstances,

Finanzlandesdirektion für Kärnte [2001] ECR I-8365 and Case C-148/04 *Unicredito Italiano SpA v Agenzia della Entrate, Ufficio Genova 1* [2005] ECR I-11137 etc.

[5] More specifically, the following aids are encompassed in Art 107(2) TFEU:
(a) aid having a social character, granted to individual consumers, provided that such aid is granted without discrimination related to the origin of the products concerned; (b) aid to make good the damage caused by natural disasters or exceptional occurrences; (c) aid granted to the economy of certain areas of the Federal Republic of Germany affected by the division of Germany, in so far as such aid is required in order to compensate for the economic disadvantages caused by that division. Five years after the entry into force of the Treaty of Lisbon, the Council, acting on a proposal from the Commission, may adopt a decision repealing this point.

[6] Under Art 107(3) TFEU, the following may be considered to be compatible with the internal market: (a) aid to promote the economic development of areas where the standard of living is abnormally low or where there is serious underemployment, and of the regions referred to in Art 349, in view of their structural, economic and social situation; (b) aid to promote the execution of an important project of common European interest or to remedy a serious disturbance in the economy of a Member State; (c) aid to facilitate the development of certain economic activities or of certain economic areas, where such aid does not adversely affect trading conditions to an extent contrary to the common interest; (d) aid to promote culture and heritage conservation where such aid does not affect trading conditions and competition in the European Union to an extent that is contrary to the common interest; (e) such other categories of aid as may be specified by decision of the Council on a proposal from the Commission.

[7] See section 7.3 below.

[8] Conor Quigley, 'The Notion of State Aid in the EEC' [1988] *European Law Review* 242–56.

[9] Case C-39/94 *Syndicat français de l'Express international (SFEI) v La Poste* [1996] ECR I-3547, para 60; Case C-241/95P *Tiercé Ladbroke v Commission* [1997] ECR I-7007, para 35; Case T-67/94 *Ladbroke Racing v Commission* [1998] ECR II-1, para 52.

[10] See Cases T-298, 312, 313, 315 & 600–607/97 *Alzetta Mauro v Commission* [2000] ECR II-2319, paras 76–90.

[11] Case T-288/97 *Regione Autonoma Friuli Venezia Giulia v Commission* [2001] ECR II-1169, paras 49–50; Case T-35/99 *Keller SpA v Commission* [2002] ECR II-261, para 85.

[12] In Case T-211/05 *Italy v Commission* [2009] ECR II-2777, the General Court examined the compatibility of tax incentives for companies involved in initial public offering procedures with the state

distortion of competition may be easily inferred.[13] The above requirements form part of a global question.

Initially, the Commission attacked the 'paradigm' state aids such as direct grants, subsidiaries, state guarantees and loans. In the last few years, it has turned its attention to more indirect forms of state aid, with particular emphasis on social and fiscal measures. State aid has become very important in the tax field.[14] Important guidance on state aid end taxation was first given by the Commission in its 1998 Notice on the application of state aid rules to measures relating to direct business taxation (henceforth, the 1998 Notice).[15] Measures which relieve the recipients of charges that are normally borne from their budgets, such as reductions in the tax base,[16] total or partial reduction in the amount of tax (exemption or tax credit), deferral, cancellation or even special rescheduling of tax debt are, according to the Commission, examples of state aid. Such tax measures are thought to be granted by the Member State or through Member State resources. This is because a tax exemption mitigates the charge that would normally be recoverable from the undertaking. Therefore, the state loses tax revenue. This loss of tax revenue is equivalent to consumption of state resources in the form of fiscal expenditure.[17] The fact that legislation is in breach with one of the fundamental freedoms does not mean that it cannot also be incompatible with the state aid prohibition. These issues are revisited later on in this chapter.[18]

A company may be affected by the state aid prohibition whether it is the recipient of aid or the competitor of such company. Aid given to a company may

aid prohibition. The General Court argued that the Commission was not obliged to show that competition was undermined permanently, or to carry out a more detailed investigation of the substantial impact of the measures at issue on the competitive position of the recipients. The decision of the General Court was followed by the Court of Justice upon appeal. See Case C-458/09. See, inter alia, Christian Montinari, 'Italian Tax Incentives for New Companies Constitute Illegal State Aid, ECJ Confirms', 2011 *WTD* 234-4 (6 December 2011).

[13] Case C-730/79 *Philip Morris Holland BV v Commission* [1980] ECR 2671, para 11; Case C-53/00 *Ferring SA v Agence centrale des organismes de sécurité sociale (ACOSS)* [2001] ECR I-9067, para 21; Case C-234/84 *Belgium v Commission* [1986] ECR 2263, para 22. See also a more recent case: Case C-522/13 *Ministerio de Defensa and Navantia SA v Concello de Ferrol* [2014] not yet reported. Here, the Court of Justice found that a property tax exemption for state-owned land that was made available to a private company which trades goods and services within the EU constituted state aid.

[14] See Conor Quigley, *European State Aid Law*, 2nd edn (Hart Publishing, 2008); Pierpaolo Rossi-Maccanico, 'Commentary of state aid review of multinational tax regimes' [2007] 1 *European State Aid Law Quarterly* 25; Christiana HJI Panayi, 'State Aid and Tax: The Third Way?' (2004) 32 *Intertax* 287–311; Michael Rydelski, 'Distinction between State Aid and General Tax Measures' (2010) 19 *EC Tax Review* 149; Mélanie Staes, 'The Combined Application of the Fundamental Freedoms and the EU State aid Rule: In Search of a Way Out of the Maze' (2014) 42 *Intertax* 106; Conor Quigley, 'Direct Taxation and State Aid: Recent Developments Concerning the Notion of Selectivity' (2012) 40 *Intertax* 112.

[15] Commission Notice on the application of the State aid rules to measures relating to direct business taxation, [1998] OJ C384, 10 December 1998, pp 3–9, para 9. For a commentary on the 1998 Notice, see Commission, *Report on the implementation of the Commission notice on the application of the state aid rules to measures relating to direct*, COM(2004) 434.

[16] For example, by means of special deductions, special or accelerated depreciation arrangements or the entering of reserves on the balance sheet.

[17] 1998 Notice, n 15 above, para 10.

[18] See analysis in section 7.5 below.

have to be repaid if it is unlawful or has not been properly notified or approved by the Commission. If repayment is demanded, the taxpayer will have to reimburse within a period of four months the full amount of the financial benefit, including interest, for up to a maximum of 10 years prior to the start of an investigation. No recovery is necessary when the unlawful aid was paid more than 10 years before the Commission's decision.[19] Also, companies themselves may trigger investigations by lodging complaints with the Commission. In fact, when the Commission has doubts about the compatibility of a proposed aid measure, it invites interested parties to submit comments and opens a formal investigation procedure. The important role of competitors is increasingly being taken into account and is discussed further in section 7.4 below.

On 3 February 2014, the Commission released its draft notice on the notion of state aid and invited comments so as to develop practical guidance for identifying state aid measures that need approval before being implemented (henceforth, the 2014 Draft Notice).[20] The 2014 Draft Notice sets out and clarifies a number of important issues, including issues specific to taxations. The Draft Notice, once finalised, would replace the 1998 Notice, which codified the case law at the time and provided useful guidance.[21] Specific parts of the 2014 Draft Notice, especially those relating to tax law, are analysed throughout this chapter.

7.2. The Role of the Commission

The Commission has a pivotal role in the application of the state aid prohibition.[22] It keeps constant review of existing aids offered by Member States.[23] Furthermore, Member States are required to notify the Commission as to any plans to grant or alter state aid.[24] The Court of Justice has interpreted this Article as if it

[19] It has been noted that almost any communication about the aid between the Member State and the Commission, which need not be known to the beneficiary, restarts the ten year limitation period. See George Peretz, 'The Consequences of Unlawful State Aid', *Tax Journal*, Issue 1253, pp 11–13 (6 March 2015) p 11, citing Case C-276/03P *Scott SA v Commission* [2005] ECR I-8437.

[20] Draft Commission Notice on the notion of State aid pursuant to Article 107(1) TFEU, COM(2014)XXX. Available on ec.europa.eu/competition/consultations/2014_state_aid_notion/draft_guidance_en.pdf. The Notice was to be reviewed by the Commission under the 2005–2009 State Aid Action Plan but was eventually produced pursuant to the State Aid Modernisation initiative of the Commission in 2012. Also see Claire Micheau, *Tax Selectivity in European law of State Aid—Legal Assessment and Alternative Approaches*, University of Luxembourg Law Working Paper No 2014-06. Also see commentary by Timothy Lyons, 'The modernisation of EU state aid law and taxation' [2014] *British Tax Review* 113–19.

[21] 1998 Notice, n 15 above.

[22] For an excellent review of the Commission's role in reviewing tax measures, see Pierpaolo Rossi-Maccanico, 'European Commission Competence in Reviewing Direct Business Tax Measures' (2009) 18 *EC Tax Review* 221–35.

[23] See Art 108(1) TFEU.

[24] Art 108 TFEU.

imposes a standstill obligation on Member States during the period of review by the Commission.[25] The Commission must reach a decision within two months, otherwise the standstill obligation comes to an end.[26]

During the notification procedure, the Commission applies a balancing test—thought to be derived from Article 107(3) TFEU.[27] The test balances the positive effects of the aid for achieving a common interest objective and its negative effects on competition and trade.[28] This test includes an economic evaluation of the aid. If the Commission finds that the aid (whether existing or new) is incompatible with Article 107 TFEU, 'it shall decide that the State concerned shall abolish or alter such aid within a period of time to be determined by the Commission'.[29] This procedure is meant to intensify co-operation between the Commission and Member States. The Commission may also ask the Court of Justice to order a Member State to recover illegal state aid.

Furthermore, Article 109 TFEU empowers the Council, acting by qualified majority on a proposal from the Commission, and after consulting the European Parliament, to make any appropriate regulations for the application of the state aid provisions and in particular to determine the conditions under which Article 108(3) TFEU shall apply, and the categories of aid exempt from this procedure. This Article has provided the basis for Council action empowering the Commission to make regulations exempting certain categories of aid. Under the so-called General Block Exemption Regulations (GBER),[30] the Commission has declared

[25] Case C-120/73 *Gebrüder Lorenz GmbH v Germany* [1973] ECR 1471.

[26] See Art 4 of Council Regulation 659/1999 of 22 March 1999. Also see Case 120/73 *Lorenz v Germany*, n 25 above, para 4; Case 84/82 *Germany v Commission* [1984] ECR 1451, para 11.

[27] This was introduced by the State Aid Action Plan of 2005 and refined in the Staff Working Paper entitled *Common Principles for an Economic Assessment of the Compatibility of State Aid under Article 87.3* (2009). Available on: ec.europa.eu/competition/state_aid/reform/economic_assessment_en.pdf. For a review of the application of the balancing test, see Phedon Nicolaides and Ioana Eleonora Rusu, 'The "Binary" Nature of the Economics of State Aid' (2010) 37 *Issues of Economic Integration* 25–40.

[28] There are three steps to this test. (1) Is the aid measure aimed at a well-defined objective of common interest (eg economic growth, employment, cohesion, environment)? (2) Is the aid well designed to deliver the objective of common interest ie does the proposed aid address a market failure or other objective? (i) Is the aid an appropriate policy instrument to address the policy objective concerned? (ii) Is there an incentive effect, ie does the aid change the behaviour of the aid recipient? (iii) Is the aid measure proportionate to the problem tackled, ie could the same change in behaviour not be obtained with less aid? (3) Are the distortions of competition and effect on trade limited, so that the overall balance is positive? See *Common Principles for an Economic Assessment of the Compatibility of State Aid under Article 87.3* (2009), n 27 above, p 3, para 9.

[29] Art 108(2) TFEU.

[30] See, for example, Council Regulation (EC) No 994/98 of 7 May 1998 on the application of Articles 92 and 93 of the Treaty establishing the European Community to certain categories of horizontal State aid ([1998] OJ L142/1); Council Regulation No 733/2013 of 22 July 2013 amending Regulation (EC) No 994/98 on the application of Articles 92 and 93 of the Treaty establishing the European Community to certain categories of horizontal State aid ([2013] OJ L204/11, 31 July 2013); Commission Regulation (EC) No 1407/2013 of 18 December 2013 on the application of Articles 107 and 108 of the Treaty on the Functioning of the European Union to de minimis aid; and Commission Regulation (EU) No 651/2014 of 17 June 2014 declaring certain categories of aid compatible with the internal market in application of Articles 107 and 108 of the Treaty Text with EEA relevance ([2014] OJ L187/1–78, 26 June 2014).

specific categories of state aid compatible with the Treaty if they fulfil certain conditions.[31] Such categories of aid are exempt from the requirement of prior notification and Commission approval. Instead, the Member State simply informs the Commission that it has brought a scheme into place that complies with the GBER.

In May 2012, the Commission announced plans to overhaul the state aid control process.[32] In its Communication on State Aid Modernisation,[33] the Commission set out three specific objectives. The first objective was to foster growth in a strengthened, dynamic and competitive internal market.[34] To this end, the Commission would develop common principles for the compatibility assessment of national support projects and revise and streamline some existing texts.[35] Secondly, state aid enforcement would focus more on cases with the biggest impact on the internal market.[36] This would include stronger scrutiny of large and potentially distortive aid as well as enquiries by sector, across Member States.[37] Thirdly, procedures would be streamlined to deliver decisions within business-relevant timelines.[38] The Commission was also to revise the relevant regulations, seek to clarify and better explain the notion of state aid[39] and increase transparency of state aid awards.

On 17 January 2013, the European Parliament adopted a resolution supporting the initiative and its objectives.[40] The European Economic and Social Committee,[41] as well as the Committee of the Regions,[42] have also adopted an opinion in favour of modernisation. There is no specific reference to taxes in the modernisation

[31] The conditions invariably determine eligible beneficiaries, maximum aid and eligible expenses. The criteria used are thought to be derived from the Commission's market experience and decision-making practice.

[32] See ec.europa.eu/competition/state_aid/modernisation/index_en.html. For information on the 2005–2009 State Aid Reform initiative, see ec.europa.eu/competition/state_aid/reform/archive.html.

[33] Communication from the Commission to the European Parliament, the Council, the European Economic and Social Committee and the Committee of the Regions, *EU State Aid Modernisation*, (COM/2012/0209 final). For commentary, see Phedon Nicolaides, 'State Aid Modernization: Institutions for Enforcement of State Aid Rules' [2012] *World Competition* 457–69.

[34] *Ibid*, paras 10–18.

[35] For example, the Environmental, Regional or Risk Capital Guidelines, Research & Development & Infrastructure, the Guidelines for the Rescue & Restructuring of firms etc.

[36] *Ibid*, paras 19–21.

[37] See para 19: 'That outcome could be achieved by defining more proportionate and differentiated rules and by modernising State aid control procedures, with increased responsibility of Member States in designing and implementing support measures. It will require a clearer definition of the rules and an enhanced ex post monitoring by the Commission to ensure adequate compliance. It will also lower administrative burden for public authorities and for beneficiaries when smaller amounts of aid are involved'.

[38] *Ibid*, paras 22–23.

[39] See Consultation on the Notion of State Aid, which opened on 17 January 2014. Available on: ec.europa.eu/competition/consultations/2014_state_aid_notion/index_en.html

[40] European Parliament resolution of 17 January 2013 on state aid modernisation (2012/2920(RSP)).

[41] Opinion of the European Economic and Social Committee on the Communication from the Commission to the European Parliament, the Council, the European Economic and Social Committee and the Committee of the Regions, *Report on Competition Policy 2013* (COM(2014) 249 final).

[42] Opinion of the Committee of the Regions on EU State Aid Modernisation (SAM) (2013/C 17/06).

communication. However, the 2014 Draft Notice[43] deals extensively with tax and sets out the various developments of the case law.

7.3. Litigation Avenues—European Courts and National Courts

State aid cases may reach the European courts in one of the three following ways:

First, Member States may challenge a Commission decision under Article 263 TFEU. This challenge may relate to a review of the legality of the Commission's or Council's decision, or it might be an application for annulment of any binding act taken by Community institutions.

Secondly, the Commission may bring an action against a Member State under Article 108(2) TFEU when the Member State has not removed aid previously determined incompatible by the Commission (ie to enforce a negative decision). The Commission may also commence proceedings under general law for failure to act,[44] but these Articles are more cumbersome as they involve more procedural steps.

Thirdly, a person individually concerned[45] may bring an action under Article 263 TFEU against decisions prohibiting aid. The Court of Justice insists on some tangible connection between the aid and the recipient and not just for the recipient to belong to a group that could potentially benefit from the prohibited aid.[46] The decision must affect the person(s) bringing the action by reason of certain attributes which are peculiar to them, or by reason of circumstances in which they are differentiated from other persons.[47] Similarly, an action may be brought by a competitor of the recipient but the competitor needs to show that there are specific circumstances which allow them to be singled out from a potentially large group of competitors of the recipient of the aid.[48] Although initially very few cases were brought by competitors,[49] there has been an increase in the number of cases where third parties and competitors have claimed for the recovery of unlawfully granted state aid.

National courts also play an important role in the enforcement of the state aid rules.[50] The Commission has issued a Notice on the co-operation between

43 See 2014 Draft Notice, n 20 above.

44 Articles 258–260 TFEU.

45 Case 730/79 *Philip Morris*, n 13 above.

46 Case 67/85 *Van Der Kooy and others v Commission* [1988] ECR 219.

47 See the Plaumann test in Case 25/62 *Plaumann v Commission* [1963] ECR 95.

48 Case 10 and 18/68 *Eridania Zuccherifici and others v Commission* [1969] ECR 459. Also see Case C-198/91 *Cook v Commission* [1993] ECR I-2487; Case C-313/90 *CIRFS v Commission* [1993] ECR I-1125.

49 See *Application of EC State Aid Law by the Member State Courts* (Commission, 1999), at 244.

50 For an overview of the relationship of the European courts and national courts, see Malcolm Ross, 'State Aids and National Courts: Definitions and Other Problems—A case of Premature Emancipation?' (2000) 37 *Common Market Law Review* 401.

national courts and the Commission in the field of state aid.[51] In the Notice, it is acknowledged that both national courts and the Commission play essential, but distinct roles in the context of state aid enforcement.[52] Such co-operation is essential in order to guarantee the strict, effective and consistent application of EU competition law.

A national court may rule that a given aid is state aid within the meaning of Article 107(1) TFEU but it *cannot* rule on the compatibility of the aid with the common market, as this is a matter falling within the absolute discretion of the Commission.[53] However, a national court may rule aid to be illegal when it has not been properly notified. National courts have ordered interim injunctive measures in several cases to prevent or suspend the granting of unlawful aid.[54] It is noteworthy that a national court has power to assess ex officio whether the state aid rules have been infringed, even if the argument has not been brought by the parties themselves.[55] Guidance may be sought in the Commission's decision-making practice and its notices and guidelines.

When the Commission decides pursuant to Article 108(2) TFEU that an aid is incompatible with the internal market and it requires repayment of the aid, the national authorities have a duty to seek recovery without delay.[56] National courts may also order remedial action when there is unlawful aid without a Commission decision. This is, for example, where a claimant has successfully invoked the direct effect of the prohibition on the implementation of unapproved aid in Article 108(3) TFEU.

A recovery decision is addressed to the Member State that granted the unlawful aid and not to the beneficiary. However, the Member State must implement the recovery decision by seeking reimbursement of the aid from the beneficiary. Recovery of aid is limited to 10 years from the day the aid was awarded to the beneficiary. Where a beneficiary refuses to repay the aid, the Member State must commence enforcement proceedings in national courts. If national procedural

[51] Notice on Cooperation between national courts and the Commission in the State aid field, [2007] OJ C312, 23 November 1995. This was replaced by the Notice on the Enforcement of State Aid Law by National Courts, [2009] OJ C85, 9 April 2009, pp 1–22. Also see Commission Handbook on *Enforcement of EU State aid law by national courts* (2010), available on: ec.europa.eu/competition/publications/state_aid/national_courts_booklet_en.pdf. For more information on the rights of competitors, see section 7.4 below.

[52] Notice on the enforcement of State aid law by national courts (2009), n 51 above, para 19 et seq.

[53] *Ibid*, para 20.

[54] See 2009 update of the 2006 Study on the enforcement of State aid rules at national level—Final Report. Available on: ec.europa.eu/competition/state_aid/studies_reports/enforcement_study_2009.pdf.

[55] *Ibid.*

[56] See Article 14(3) of Council Regulation 659/1999, n 26 above: 'recovery shall be effected without delay and in accordance with the procedures under the national law of the Member State concerned, provided that they allow the immediate and effective execution of the Commission's decision. To this effect and in the event of a procedure before national courts, the Member States concerned shall take all necessary steps which are available in their respective legal systems, including provisional measures, without prejudice to Community law'. Also see Notice on the enforcement of State aid law by national courts (2009), n 51 above, paras 30–36.

rules do not enable the enforcement of recovery, the Member State must take steps to put the required mechanisms in place. The obligation to recover aid overrides any argument that national procedural rules preclude recovery. Therefore, national courts play a hugely important role in the enforcement of recovery decisions adopted by the Commission. There is a Commission notice providing guidance on this.[57]

National courts are under an obligation to apply all appropriate devices and remedies to protect the rights conferred on individuals under Article 108(3) TFEU. Such course of action may include setting aside any conflicting provisions of national law, repayment of aid, granting orders for interim relief, re-establishment of the pre-existing competitive position of the relevant parties and even awarding damages to parties whose interests were harmed.[58]

The amount to be recovered is calculated on the basis of a comparison between the tax actually paid and the amount that would have been paid if the generally applicable rule had applied, irrespective of the fact that a beneficiary would not have entered into the transaction absent the aid. Interest may also be ordered on the amount repayable and this could be on a compound basis.[59] In general, national courts have a duty to ensure that the *effet utile* of Article 108(3) TFEU is respected, by ensuring that state aid rules have primacy over national procedural rules.

There may be exceptional circumstances in which the recovery of unlawful state aid would not be appropriate; for example, if it is absolutely impossible or if legitimate expectations have been generated by the Commission justifying non-recovery or if it is contrary to the general principles of EU law.[60] These grounds are to be strictly construed. Statements by Member States are irrelevant, only legitimate expectations generated by the Commission or other EU institutions are relevant. Also the beneficiary must have received precise assurances from the Commission or other EU institutions to justify these expectations. This is rarely the case if the fiscal measure had not been notified to the Commission.[61] In several cases, the Commission recognised that previous decisions in which a tax scheme was approved may have created legitimate expectations for beneficiaries of similar tax schemes.[62]

[57] Notice from the Commission—*Towards an effective implementation of Commission decisions ordering Member States to recover unlawful and incompatible State aid*, [2007] OJ C272, 15 November 2007, p 4–17.

[58] Notice on the enforcement of State aid law by national courts (2009), n 51 above, paras 28–62.

[59] See Council Regulation 659/1999, n 26 above, Art 14(2); Council Regulation 794/2004 Art 11(2) and Notice on the enforcement of State aid law by national courts, n 51 above, para 41.

[60] Notice on the enforcement of State aid law by national courts (2009), n 51 above, paras 32–33. Also see Case C-354/90 *FNCEPA v France*, n 1 above; Case C-332/98 *France v Commission* [2000] ECR I-4833.

[61] See Margarida Afonso, 'Recovery of Fiscal Aid' in Alexander Rust and Claire Micheau (eds), *State Aid and Tax Law* (Kluwer, 2013) p 67. Also see George Peretz, 'The Consequences of Unlawful State Aid', n 19 above, p 11.

[62] Afonso (2013), n 61 above, p 67, citing Decision C54/2001 on Ireland's aid relief for foreign income, [2003] OJ L204/51, 13 August 2003, recitals 54–57 and Commission Decision 2011/5/EC on the tax amortisation of financial goodwill for foreign shareholding acquisitions implemented by Spain, [2011] OJ L7, 11 January 2011, recitals 158–69.

The Commission and the Member State must work together in good faith with a view to overcoming difficulties of recovery. As held in *Commission v France*

> [t]he condition that it be absolutely impossible to implement a decision is not fulfilled where the defendant Member State merely informs the Commission of the legal, political or practical difficulties involved in implementing the decision, without taking any real steps to recover the aid from the undertakings concerned, and without proposing to the Commission any alternative arrangements for implementing the decision which could have enabled those difficulties to be overcome.[63]

In applying Article 107(1) TFEU, the Commission urges national courts to refer preliminary questions to the Court of Justice under Article 267 TFEU when in doubt.[64] National courts can also ask the Commission to transmit relevant information in its possession.[65]

As stated in a 2006 Commission study on the enforcement of state aid law at national level,[66] national courts could offer claimants very effective remedies in the event of a breach of the state aid rules. However, in a later study, it was noted that national courts' powers of inquiry remained limited as far as state aid matters were concerned. This was because national courts had to judge cases on the basis of the facts presented by the parties. As state aid cases were often complex and involved economic considerations, national courts often lacked the appropriate means to establish the factual information necessary for their decision. 'The burden of proof, therefore, is often a hurdle that leads to the claimant being unsuccessful. Claimants are often unable to present sufficient evidence to support the view that the State aid criteria have been fulfilled'.[67]

7.4. The Rights of Interested Parties, Competitors and Third Parties

The Commission is entitled to set priorities in relation to state aid complaints and give differing degrees of priority.[68] Although the European courts have retained control over the concept of aid, the Commission still has substantial discretion in the overall process.

It has been argued that there are fundamental defects in the state aid procedure,[69] as there are no material procedural rights conferred on interested parties.

[63] Case C-214/07 *Commission v France* [2008] ECR I-8357, para 46.
[64] Notice on the enforcement of State aid law by national courts (2009), n 51 above, paras 89–96.
[65] *Ibid*, paras 82–88.
[66] Commission Handbook on *Enforcement of EU State aid law by national courts* (2010), n 51 above.
[67] See 2009 update of the 2006 Study on the enforcement of State aid rules at national level, Final Report, n 54 above, p 4.
[68] See Case C-119/97P *Ufex and others v Commission* [1999] ECR I-1341, para 88; Case T-475/04 *Bouygues SA v Commission* [2007] ECR II-2097, para 158.
[69] See Keith O'Donnell and Anne Muller, 'State Aid and Tax Law: Enter the Taxpayer' in *State Aid and Tax Law*, n 61 above. Also see paper (2014) by John Temple Lang, *The Charter and EU*

The procedure is essentially a bilateral one between the Commission and the Member State that has conferred the aid. The Commission is required, in the interests of sound administration, to conduct a diligent and impartial examination of the complaint, which may make it necessary for it to examine matters not expressly raised by the complainant.[70] However, interested parties have no rights at all during the preliminary examination stage. There is no right to be informed of the commencement or development of the investigation, or to have access to the evidence available to the Commission. Also, there is no right to be consulted—except on the decision to open the procedure—and there is no appointed hearing officer for state aid cases, as with other anti-trust cases. A beneficiary is very dependent on the Member State to mount a vigorous defence, even though it is the beneficiary that will ultimately suffer the brunt of a recovery decision and not the Member State. This position is not thought to change following the proposed modernisation plan.

The lack of procedural rights of interested parties has been criticised for being in breach of the Charter of Fundamental Rights; namely Article 47 of the Charter, which confers the right to an effective remedy and a fair trial (corresponding to Article 6 of the European Convention on Human Rights) and Article 41 of the Charter, which confers the right to good administration.[71] A number of suggestions have been made on how to improve the procedural rights of material parties[72] and how to make the whole procedure more transparent for companies involved and less discretionary for the Commission.

For third parties and competitors, involvement in the state aid procedure is even more problematic.[73] Locus standi remains an important hurdle. In the

State aid procedure. Available on: uksala.org/state-aid-modernisation-seminar-slides/. Also see John Temple Lang, 'Three Possibilities for Reform of the Procedure of the European Commission in Competition Cases Under Regulation 1/2003', *Centre for European Policy Studies (CEPS) Special Report*—18 November 2011. Available on: papers.ssrn.com/sol3/papers.cfm?abstract_id=1996510. See also submission of John Temple Lang to European Ombudsman, regarding the consultation on public service principles for EU civil servants. Available on: www.ombudsman.europa.eu/en/resources/otherdocument.faces/en/10447/html.bookmark. For the results of the public consultation, see: www.ombudsman.europa.eu/en/resources/otherdocument.faces/en/11069/html.bookmark.

[70] Case T-512/11 *Ryanair Ltd v European Commission*, judgment of 24 November 2014, para 105, citing Case C-367/95 *Commission v Sytraval and Brink's France* [1998] ECR I-1719, para 62.

[71] Quigley (2012), n 14 above, at p 410 mentions Case T-198/01R *Technische Glaswerke Ilmenau GmbH v Commission* [2002] ECR II-2153, para 85, where the Court of First Instance (the predecessor of the General Gourt) held that the Commission must carry out its investigations in a manner which is impartial as between all the relevant parties. There was reference to Article 41(1) of the Charter of Fundamental Rights which provides that everyone has the right to have his affairs treated impartially and without discrimination by the EU institutions. For a general overview of some of the fundamental rights of the Charter that may be relevant to taxpayers, see Eric Poelmann, 'Some Fiscal Issues of the Charter of Fundamental Rights of the European Union' (2015) 43 *Intertax* 173–78.

[72] Some of the suggestions made by Temple Lang in his 2014 paper, n 69 above, are the following: (a) access to the file for interested parties subject to confidentiality, similar to the regime for mergers, which is policed by the hearing officer; (b) imposing a legal obligation on the Commission and the Member States to act impartially throughout the investigation and to offer full and equal opportunity to interested parties to make submissions; (c) imposing an obligation to immediately publish the summary of all aid notifications and an invitation to comment; (d) having a hearing officer; (e) giving a formal right to attend settlement negotiations with Member States representatives or an oral hearing.

[73] See Lisa Paterno, 'State aid and fiscal protectionism in the European Union from the perspective of competitors' (2011) 65 *Bulletin for International Taxation* 343. For an earlier analysis of the subject

Commission Notice on enforcement of state aid law by national courts[74] there was a separate section on standing issues in tax cases.[75] In that Notice, it was reiterated that the imposition of an exceptional tax burden on specific sectors or producers can also amount to state aid in favour of other companies.[76] However, third party taxpayers may only rely on the standstill obligation where their own tax payment forms an integral part of the unlawful state aid measure.[77] If exemptions have been granted from general taxes, these criteria are usually not met. An undertaking liable to pay such taxes cannot generally claim that someone else's tax exemption is unlawful under Article 107(3) of the TFEU.[78] Extending an illegal tax exemption to the competitor is no appropriate remedy for breaches of state aid, as such a measure would not eliminate the anti-competitive effects of unlawful aid, but would on the contrary, strengthen them.[79] If a competitor can show loss or future loss as a result of the unlawful state aid, then damages may be obtained from the relevant public authorities.[80]

Many cases were alerted to the Commission as a result of complaints. For example, recently the Commission has been reviewing a complaint by the Luxembourg-based RTL Group, that an advertising tax which was implemented by Hungary was confiscatory and was contrary to the fundamental freedoms. Also, as Hungarian-based media companies paid a much lower tax rate, it was argued that there was breach of Article 107 TFEU.[81]

Another recent state aid case was also brought by competitors.[82] Here, Ryanair complained that the Irish air travel tax unfairly benefited rivals Aer Lingus and Aer Arann. The Irish air travel tax was set at €2 for any flight to a destination within

see Jan A Winter, 'The Rights of Complainants in State Aid cases: Judicial Review of Commission Decisions adopted under Article 88 (ex 93) EC' (1999) 36 *Common Market Law Review* 521–68.

[74] Notice on the enforcement of State aid law by national courts (2009), n 51 above, p 1–22.

[75] *Ibid*, section 2.4.3.

[76] *Ibid*, para 73.

[77] This is the case where, under the relevant national rules, the tax revenue is reserved exclusively for funding the unlawful state aid and has a direct impact on the amount of state aid granted. See Notice on the enforcement of State aid law by national courts (2009), n 51 above, para 74. Citing, inter alia, Joined Cases C-266/04 to C-270/04, C-276/04 and C-321/04 to C-325/04 *Casino France and Others*, [2005] ECR I-9481, para 40; and Case C-174/02 *Streekgewest Westelijk Noord-Brabant v Staatssecretaris van Financiën* [2005] ECR I-85, para 26.

[78] Notice on the enforcement of State aid law by national courts (2009), n 51 above, para 75.

[79] Joined Cases C-393/04 and C-41/05 *Air Liquide Industries Belgium SA v Ville de Seraing and Province de Liège* [2006] ECR I-5293, para 45. As Peretz, n 19 above, p 13 notes, it is only in exceptional circumstances that relief may be available to a competitor, such as when the tax paid by the competitor was levied in order to grant the advantage to the beneficiary or was hypothecated to that advantage. See Case T-473/12 *Aer Lingus Ltd* [2014] nyr, paras 67–70 and cases cited therein.

[80] See Case C-199/06 *Centre d'exportation du livre français (CELF) and Ministre de la Culture et de la Communication v Société internationale de diffusion et d'édition (SIDE)* [2008] ECR I-469, paras 53–55.

[81] William Hoke, 'European Commission Reviewing Hungarian Ad Tax', 2014 *WTD* 203-4 (21 October 2014).

[82] Case T-512/11 *Ryanair Ltd v European Commission*, judgment of 25 November 2014. For commentary, see William Hoke, 'Court Annuls EU State Aid Ruling on Ireland's Air Travel Tax', 2014 *WTD* 229-4 (28 November 2014).

300 km from Dublin and €10 for any other flight. Transfer and transit passengers were exempt from payment of the tax.

Ryanair complained in that the non-application of the tax to transit and transfer passengers was illegal state aid in favour of airlines such as Aer Lingus and Aer Arann who handled a high proportion of such passengers and flights, as well as passengers travelling to destinations located less than 300 miles from Dublin. Also, the flat-rate amount of the tax accounted for a higher proportion of the ticket price for low-cost airlines than traditional airlines.

In its decision,[83] the Commission found that the tax was not state aid because it was not selective. The General Court annulled this decision on procedural grounds, on the basis that the Commission should have initiated a formal investigation procedure to verify the selectivity of the contested measure and should not have been limited to the preliminary investigation because of the existence of serious doubts. There were various indicia for this.[84] For example the length of time it took the Commission to conduct the preliminary investigation suggests that it encountered serious difficulties in its review. Also the inconsistencies in the contents of the decision and the incomplete and insufficient nature of the overall examination '[permitted] the inference that the Commission was not able, at the date of adoption of the contested decision, to resolve all the serious difficulties identified concerning the question whether the disputed measure … was selective'.[85] The General Court concluded that in so far as the exemption for transit and transfer passengers was concerned, the decision was adopted in breach of Ryanair's procedural rights and must be annulled. There was no need to examine Ryanair's other complaints and arguments.[86]

7.5. Differences Between Fundamental Freedoms and State Aid

There are some obvious differences between fundamental freedoms and state aid.[87] Fundamental freedoms deal with inter-state differentiation between economic operators but state aid deals with intra-state differentiation. In addition, fundamental freedoms offer protection to individuals as well and not just undertakings. There are also differences in terms of remedies. Nevertheless, the

[83] Decision C(2011) 4932 final of 13 July 2011.

[84] See paras 66–105.

[85] *Ibid*, para 106.

[86] *Ibid*, para 107.

[87] For commentary, see, inter alios, Claire Micheau, 'Fundamental freedoms and state aid rules under EU law: The example of taxation' (2012) 52 *European Taxation* 210; Frank Engelen, 'State Aid and Restrictions on Free Movement: Two Sides of the Same Coin?' (2012) 52 *European Taxation* 204–9; Staes (2014), n 14 above.

Court of Justice has refrained from declaring the two courses of action mutually exclusive. It has, however, held that the Commission cannot use its state aid powers to pursue infringements of other Treaty rules, or approve infringements of fundamental freedoms.

In *Iannelli & Volpi*,[88] a case decided in the late 70s, the Court of Justice developed its so-called severability test. Here, the Court had to examine whether the tax measure at issue should be examined under the state aid rules or the free movement of goods rules. The Court recognised that sometimes a case may fall simultaneously within the field of application of both provisions. However, it applied a severability test in finding that those aspects of aid which contravene specific provisions of the Treaty other than the state aid prohibition

> may be so indissolubly linked to the object of the aid that it is impossible to evaluate them separately so that their effect on the compatibility or incompatibility of the aid viewed as a whole must therefore of necessity be determined in the light of the procedure prescribed in [ex-] Art 93.[89]

Only the aspects of an aid which are not necessary for the attainment of its object or for its functioning can be held to be incompatible with another Treaty provision. This is without prejudice to the state aid review of the measure.[90] In *Ianelli*, the Court of Justice came to the conclusion that the measure should not be regarded as falling within the scope of the free movement of goods but should rather be dealt with exclusively under the provisions of state aid.

Reference should also be made to another early case, *Hansen*.[91] In this request for a preliminary ruling, the Court was asked to consider how to deal with a dual infringement, when one Treaty rule was more specific than another. The Court of Justice argued that when a tax measure constitutes both state aid and an infringement of another specific and directly applicable Treaty rule, then the more specific infringement prevails and obliges the Court to examine the rule in light of that.[92] This approach may, however, be difficult to apply if the *lex specialis* is considered to be the state aid prohibition and the general rule is the non-discrimination provision, in cases where the Commission is inclined to authorise the state aid. The case is not mentioned in the 1998 Notice,[93] or in the 2014 Draft Notice.[94] In fact, the 2014 Draft Notice does not deal with the topic at all. It is arguably qualified by the later *Sovrapprezzo*[95] judgment which stipulated that the state aid

[88] Case 74/76 *Iannelli & Volpi SA v Meroni* [1977] ECR 557.

[89] *Ibid*, para 14.

[90] Pierpaolo Rossi-Maccanico, 'EU Review of Direct Tax Measures: Interplay between Fundamental Freedoms and State Aid Control' (2013) 22 *EC Tax Review* 19–28, 21–23. He calls this the principle of cumulative but disjoined reviews of national tax measures.

[91] Case 91/78 *Hansen GmbH & Co v Hauptzollamt Flensburg* [1979] ECR 935.

[92] See also Rossi-Maccanico (2013), n 90 above, p 24–25.

[93] 1998 Notice, n 15 above.

[94] 2014 Draft Notice, n 20 above.

[95] Case C-73/79 *Commission v Italy* [1980] ECR 1533.

procedure must never produce a result which is contrary to the specific provisions of the Treaty.[96]

Overall, it would seem that the Commission cannot exercise its discretion to authorise the granting of state aid when the measure infringes another Treaty provision. Discriminatory tax practices are not exempt by reason of the fact that they may also be a state aid.[97] This was reiterated in the 1998 Commission Notice. Here, it was stated that the Commission could not authorise aid which was in breach of both rules under the Treaty, 'particularly those relating to the ban on discrimination and to the right of establishment, and of the provisions of secondary law on taxation'.[98] It was further noted that the case law provided that those aspects of aid which are indissolubly linked to the object of the aid, and which contravene specific provisions of the Treaty other than the state aid prohibition, must nevertheless be examined in light of the procedure under the state aid provision 'as part of an overall examination of the compatibility or the incompatibility of the aid'.[99]

As state aid practices encompass, at some level, unequal treatment of undertakings of other Member States, it should not be presumed that every state aid amounts in itself to covert discrimination or restriction of fundamental freedoms. However, it has been held in a number of subsequent cases that the same tax measure could be incompatible with both rules.[100] The most recent case is the *Regione Sardegna* case.[101] In this case, the Court of Justice found that a national measure imposing a stopover tax only on passenger transport operators who were not domiciled in Sardinia could constitute both state aid and a restriction on the freedom to provide services which could not be justified on public interest grounds. Therefore, here, there was no issue of using the state aid procedure to validate a discriminatory practice.

It has been argued that it is not always the case that both state aid and fundamental freedoms apply.[102] More specifically, considering the tax that would normally be due, there cannot be both an advantage for resident undertakings and a disadvantage for non-resident undertakings. A tax rule should only be reviewed under the state aid rules when it favours resident undertakings and the free

[96] *Ibid*, para 8.

[97] See Rossi-Maccanico (2013), n 90 above, p 23.

[98] 1998 Notice, n 15 above, para 29.

[99] *Ibid.*

[100] Case 18/84, *Commission v France* [1985] ECR-1339; Case C-21/88 *Du Pont de Nemours Italiana SpA v Unità sanitaria locale No 2 di Carrara* [1990] ECR I-889, para 20.

[101] Case C-169/08 *Presidente del Consiglio dei Ministri v Regione Sardegna* [2009] ECR I-10821. Raymond Luja, 'Revisiting the balance between aid, selectivity and selective aid in respect of taxes and special levies' [2010] 1 *European State Aid Law Quarterly* 161–68.

[102] Engelen (2012), n 87 above, at p 209. 'If the measure in question reduces the tax that, in light of its object and purpose, should also have been imposed on resident undertakings and not only on non-resident undertakings, it confers a selective advantage on those resident undertakings that constitutes State aid ... However, if the legislation in question imposes a tax on non-resident undertakings that should not have been due in the light of the object and purpose of that legislation, it does not create an advantage for resident undertakings but a disadvantage for non-resident undertakings that constitutes a restriction on the fundamental freedoms but not State aid'.

movement provision should only be applied when the tax measure disadvantages non-residents. Therefore, less favourable taxation of non-resident undertakings compared to taxation of resident undertakings that are in an objectively comparable situation does not always fall under both rules. In order to find which one should apply, the benchmark practice—i.e. the norm—and the deviation from it need to be ascertained first. This may not be an easy task. Overall, the combined application of state aid rules and fundamental freedoms remains a complex matter.

7.6. State Aid and Taxes

As already explained in the introduction to this chapter, as far as taxes are concerned, state aid law began to be systematically applied in the past 20 years.[103] Reductions in the tax base,[104] tax exemptions,[105] tax credits,[106] deferment of the payment of taxes,[107] cancellation or even special rescheduling of tax debts, a favourable tax regime for the restructuring of banks,[108] the conversion of tax debt into share capital,[109] the cancellation of tax debts in bankruptcy proceedings[110] and specific tax amnesties[111] have been found to be state aid.

[103] Peter J Wattel, 'Interaction of State Aid, Free Movement, Policy Competition and Abuse Control in Direct Tax Matters' (2013) 5 *World Tax Journal* 128–44; Staes (2014) n 14 above; Wolfgang Schön, 'Taxation and State Aid Law in the European Union' (1999) 36 *Common Market Law Review* 911.

[104] For example, by means of special deductions, special or accelerated depreciation arrangements or the entering of reserves on the balance sheet. See Case C-66/02 *Italy v Commission* [2005] ECR I-10901, para 78; Case C-222/04 *Ministero dell' Economia e delle Finanze v Cassa di Risparmio di Firenze SpA* [2006] ECR I-289, para 132.

[105] See, inter alia, Case C-387/92 *Banco de Crédito Industrial SA, now Banco Exterior de España SA v Ayuntamiento de Valencia* [1994] ECR I-877; Joined cases C-465/09P to C-470/09P *Comunidad Autónoma de La Rioja v Territorio Histórico de Álava—Diputación Foral de Vizcaya and Others* [2011] ECR I-83.

[106] See Cases T-92/00 and T-103/00 *Territorio Historico de Alava—Diputacion Foral de Alava* [2002] ECR II-1385.

[107] Case C-156/98 *Germany v Commission* [2000] ECR I-6857; Case C-66/02 *Italy v Commission*, n 104 above, para 78.

[108] Case C-452/10P *BNP Paribas v Commission*, judgment of 21 June 2012, ECLI:EU:C:2012:318.

[109] Case C-124/10P *Commission v EDF*, ECLI:EU:C:2012:318.

[110] Case C-73/11P *Frucona Košice as v Commission*, ECLI:EU:C:2013:32.

[111] See Case C-417/10 *Ministero dell'Economia e delle Finanze* [2012] ECR I-0000 and Commission Decision of 11 July 2012 on the tax amnesty measure notified by Latvia, S.A. 33183, [2013] OJ C1/6, 4 January 2013. See also 2014 Draft Notice, n 20 above, paras 167–69 where, on the basis of existing case law, it is stipulated that a tax amnesty measure that applies to undertakings can be considered a general measure if the following conditions are met. First, the measure should be of an exceptional nature, provide a strong incentive for undertakings to voluntarily comply with the tax obligations and enhance tax debt collection. Secondly, it should be open to any undertaking of any sector or size without favouring any pre-defined group of undertakings. Thirdly, there should be no de facto selectivity in favour of certain undertakings or sectors. Fourthly, the tax administration's action should be limited to administering the implementation of tax amnesty without any discretionary power to intervene in the granting or intensity of the measure. Fifthly, the measure should not entail a waiver

In 1998, the Commission had issued a Notice on the application of State aid rules to measures relating to direct business taxation.[112] In the 1998 Notice, it was emphasised that tax measures which reduce a firm's tax burden in various ways[113] could be considered to be granted by the state or through state resources, as they mitigate the charge that would normally be due from the undertaking.[114] Therefore, the state loses tax revenue and this loss of tax revenue is equivalent to consumption of state resources in the form of fiscal expenditure.[115] As for the criterion of affecting competition and trade between Member States, in the 1998 Notice, it was emphasised that this 'presupposes that the beneficiary of the measure exercises an economic activity, regardless of the beneficiary's legal status or means of financing'.[116] The mere fact that the aid strengthens the firm's position compared to that of other firms which are competitors in intra-EU trade is enough to allow the conclusion to be drawn that intra-EU trade is affected. The fact that aid is relatively small in amount and the fact that the recipient is moderate in size does not alter this conclusion.[117]

The 1998 Notice also discussed the concept of selectivity. Consolidating existing case law at the time, the following test was set out.

> The main criterion in applying [Art 107(1) TFEU] to a tax measure is therefore that the measure provides in favour of certain undertakings in the Member State an exception to the application of the tax system. The common system applicable should thus first be determined. It must then be examined whether the exception to the system or differentiations within that system are justified 'by the nature or general scheme' of the tax system, that is to say, whether they derive directly from the basic or guiding principles of the tax system in the Member State concerned. If this is not the case, then State aid is involved.[118]

The application of this test has proved quite challenging at times, as shown in subsequent case law. A few years later, the Commission published an Implementation Report on the application of state aid rules to measures relating to direct business taxation.[119] As mentioned in section 7.1 above, the 1998 Notice is to be replaced by a new and more general Notice on the Notion of State Aid.[120] The 2014 Draft Notice contains very useful and 'updated' guidance on the notion of selectivity,

from verification. The limited temporal application of tax amnesties is also important. Tax amnesty measures may also be considered as general measures if they follow the national legislature's objective of ensuring compliance with a general principle of law, such as the principle that a judgment must be given within a reasonable period of time.

[112] See, generally, 1998 Notice, n 15 above.

[113] *Ibid*, para 9.

[114] *Ibid*, paras 10–11.

[115] *Ibid*, para 10.

[116] *Ibid*, para 11.

[117] *Ibid*.

[118] *Ibid*, para 16.

[119] *Report on the Implementation of the Commission Notice on the Application of the State Aid rules to measures relating to Direct Business Taxation*, C(2004)434, 9 February 2004.

[120] See 2014 Draft Notice, n 20 above.

reflecting developments in the case law. A summary of some of the important points raised is given below.

First, the distinction between material and geographical selectivity is explained.[121] Material selectivity can be established de jure or de facto.[122] De jure selectivity results directly from the legal criteria for granting a measure that is formally reserved for certain undertakings only. De facto selectivity can be established in cases where, although the formal criteria for the application of the measure are formulated in general and objective terms, the structure of the measure is such that its effects significantly favour a particular group of undertakings.[123] It was also emphasised that selectivity could arise with measures which prima facie apply to all undertakings, but are (or may be) limited by the discretionary power of administration. In such circumstances, fulfilling the given criteria does not automatically result in an entitlement to the measure. An example given is that of tax administrations varying the conditions for granting a tax concession according to the characteristics of the investment project.[124]

When measures are broad and potentially applicable to all undertakings fulfilling certain criteria, then it is more difficult to establish selectivity, compared to ad hoc measures. Here, the 2014 Draft Notice summarises the three-step test developed in the case law of the Court of Justice, as a refinement to the test set out in the 1998 Notice, which was discussed immediately above.

First, the system of reference against which the selectivity of a measure is assessed must be identified. The reference system is composed of a consistent set of rules that generally applies on the basis of objective criteria to all undertakings falling within its scope.[125] It might be necessary to evaluate whether the boundaries of the system of reference have been designed in a consistent manner or, on the contrary, in a clearly arbitrary or biased way, so as to favour certain undertakings which are in a comparable situation with regard to the underlying logic of the system in question.

Secondly, it is determined whether the measure derogates from the system 'insofar as it differentiates between economic operations who, in light of the objectives intrinsic to the system, are in a comparable factual and legal situation'.[126]

Thirdly, it is determined whether the derogatory measure is justified by the nature or the general scheme of the reference system.[127] The latter would be the

[121] *Ibid*, paras 121–56.

[122] *Ibid*, paras 122–23. Also see Andreas Bartosch, 'Is there a Need for a Rule of Reason in European State Aid Law? Or How to Arrive at a Coherent Concept of Material Selectivity?' (2010) 47 *Common Market Law Review* 729–52, 751.

[123] See, for example, the Gibraltar case, where following reform, Gibraltar tax laws de facto favoured offshore companies. Joined Cases C-106/09P and C-107/09P *Commission and Spain v Government of Gibraltar and UK* [2011] ECR I-11113.

[124] 2014 Draft Notice, n 20 above, para 125.

[125] *Ibid*, paras 132–33.

[126] *Ibid*, para 128. Also see paras 135–37.

[127] *Ibid*.

case where a measure derives directly from the intrinsic basic or guiding principles of the reference system or where it was the result of inherent mechanisms necessary for the functioning and effectiveness of the system. External policy objectives (eg environmental, industrial policy objectives) cannot be relied upon to justify differentiated treatment.[128] 'Member States should, however, introduce and apply appropriate control and monitoring procedures to ensure that derogatory measures are consistent with the logic and general scheme of the tax system'.[129]

The Draft Notice reiterates previous case law in that Article 107(1) TFEU does not distinguish between measures of state intervention in terms of their causes or aims, but defines them in relation to their effects, independently of the techniques used.[130] There has been criticism, in that case law on the notion of state aid is not always consistent.[131] Also, selectivity and general tax measures are often difficult to delineate.[132] In the Draft Notice, the Commission makes a valiant attempt to rationalise the case law. The fact that the Commission devotes a substantial part of the Draft Notice on the application of state aid law to tax shows the importance it attaches to this field.[133] In reviewing the Draft Notice, on its own and in the context of existing case law, what becomes apparent is the complexity of applying general (state aid) principles in tax law. Furthermore, for tax measures especially, whilst it is often inherently difficult to ascertain the boundaries of the reference system and as a corollary derogations and justifications, this exercise becomes more troublesome in cases of regional selectivity.

Some recent case law in this field and the themes arising therefrom, are briefly reviewed in the following section. The cases reviewed, most of which were also considered by the Commission in its 2014 Draft Notice, focus on fiscal aid in the field of direct taxation only and not indirect taxation.[134]

[128] Citing, inter alia, Joined Cases C-78/08, C-79/08 & C-80/08 *Ministero dell'Economia e delle Finanze and Agenzia delle Entrate v Paint Graphos Soc coop arl; Adige Carni Soc coop arl, in liquidation v Agenzia delle Entrate and Ministero dell'Economia e delle Finanze; Ministero delle Finanze v Michele Franchetto* [2011] ECR I-7611, paras 69–70; Case C-88/03 *Portugal v Commission* [2006] ECR I-7115, para 81; Case C-279/08 P *Commission v Netherlands (NOx)* [2011] ECR I-7671; Case C-487/06 P *British Aggregates Association v Commission* [2008] ECR I-10515.

[129] 2014 Draft Notice, n 20 above, para 140. Citing *Paint Graphos*, n 128 above, para 74.

[130] *Ibid*, para 129, citing, *inter alia, British Aggregates v Commission*, n 128 above, paras 85 and 89; Case C-279/08P *Commission v Netherlands* [2011] ECR I-7671, para 51 etc.

[131] See general, non-tax specific analysis in Andrea Biondi, 'State Aid is Falling Down, Falling Down: An Analysis of the Case Law on the Notion of Aid' (2013) 50 *Common Market Law Review* 1719–44. For a tax specific analysis, see, inter alios, Claire Micheau, 'Tax Selectivity in State Aid Review: A Debatable Case Practice' (2008) 17 *EC Tax Review* 276–84; Staes (2014), n 14 above; Quigley (2012), n 14 above.

[132] See Rydelski (2010), n 14 above.

[133] See also Lyons (2014), n 20 above, p 119.

[134] For the growing importance of the state aid prohibition in the field of indirect taxation and mainly VAT see Joachim English, 'EU State Aid Rules Applied to Indirect Tax Measures' (2013) 22 *EC Tax Review* 9.

7.7. Themes from Recent Case Law

7.7.1. Autonomous Powers and Regional Selectivity

Measures adopted by intra-state entities (decentralised, federal, regional or other) of Member States may also fall foul of the state aid provision, but the reference system need not be defined within the limits of the Member States concerned. A measure favouring undertakings active in one region of the national territory may not be selective. The conditions for assessing measures in the context of regional authorities were considered in a number of cases, the most important of which are analysed below.

In *Portugal v Commission*,[135] the Court of Justice addressed the issue of selectivity within a regional or local authority and mapped out important guidelines. In 1999 the legislative body of the Azores Region adopted detailed rules reducing income and corporation tax by 10 per cent for undertakings established in the Region. The Commission found the reduction to be selective and to be state aid. However, the aid was compatible with the common market, except in the case of undertakings carrying out financial activities or intra-group services. The Portuguese Government contested the decision arguing that the measure involved was not selective and was justified by the nature and overall structure of the tax system.

The Court upheld the Commission's decision and gave important guidance on the application of state aid rules to tax measures adopted by regions and local authorities. In order to determine whether a measure was selective, it was necessary to examine the reference framework which was not necessarily that of the territory of the Member State concerned. In the case of a measure adopted by an infra-state entity, the framework could be limited to the geographical area concerned and as such not be selective.[136] As the Court held,

> [i]t is possible that an infra-State body enjoys a legal and factual status which makes it sufficiently autonomous in relation to the central government of a Member State, with the result that, by the measures it adopts, it is that body and not the central government which plays a fundamental role in the definition of the political and economic environment in which undertakings operate.[137]

In such a case it was the area in which the infra-state body responsible for the measure exercised its powers, and not the country as a whole, which was the relevant reference framework.

[135] Case C-88/03 *Portugal v Commission* [2006] ECR I-7115. See Bruno Peeters, 'European Guidelines for Federal Member States Granting Fiscal Competences c.q. Tax Autonomy to Sub-national Authorities' (2009) 18 *EC Tax Review* 50–52; Daniel Armesto, 'The ECJ's Judgment regarding the Tax Autonomy of the Basque Country' (2009) 49 *European Taxation* 11.

[136] Case C-88/03 *Portugal v Commission*, n 135 above, para 57.

[137] *Ibid*, para 58.

As far as selectivity was concerned, in this context, three scenarios could be distinguished.

The first scenario was when the central government of a Member State unilaterally decided to apply a lower level of taxation within a defined geographical area. Here, there would be regional selectivity.[138]

The second scenario entailed a symmetrical devolution of tax powers: a model of distribution of tax competences in which all local authorities at a same level (regions, districts or others) have the autonomous power to decide, within the limit of the powers conferred on them, the applicable tax rate within their territory of competence, independently of the central government.[139] Here, there would be no selectivity 'because it is impossible to determine a normal tax rate capable of constituting the reference framework'.[140]

In the third scenario of asymmetrical devolution of tax powers, some regional or local authorities adopt tax measures applicable only to undertakings present within their territory.[141] In this situation, the legal framework appropriate to determine the selectivity of a tax measure may be limited to the geographical area concerned where the infra-state body, in particular on account of its status and powers, occupies a fundamental role in the definition of the political and economic environment in which the undertakings operate.

For this to be the case, regional authorities must satisfy cumulatively three criteria. First, the tax measures must have been taken by a regional or local authority which had, from a constitutional point of view, a political and administrative status separate from that of the central government. Secondly, the tax measures must have been adopted without the central government being able to directly intervene as regards its content. Finally, the financial consequences of a reduction of the national tax rate for undertakings in the region must not be offset by aids or subsidies from other regions or the central government.[142]

In this case, the Court of Justice concluded that the reduction of the tax burden by the Azores authorities was inextricably linked to the correction of inequalities deriving from insularity. These two aspects of the fiscal policy were dependent, from a financial point of view, on budgetary transfers managed by central government. Consequently the relevant legal framework for assessing the selective nature of the tax measures could not be limited to the geographical area of the Azores but rather must be assessed in relation to the totality of the Portuguese territory. As such, the measures appeared to be selective, and not general, measures. The scheme could not be justified by the nature of the system or its overall structure.

The Court of Justice followed this ruling in the *UGT Rioja* case.[143] Here, the Court was asked to consider whether or not a tax advantage adopted by the

[138] *Ibid*, para 64. Also see 2014 Draft Notice, n 20 above, para 144.

[139] *Ibid*. Also see 2014 Draft Notice, n 20 above, para 144.

[140] *Ibid*.

[141] *Ibid*, para 65.

[142] *Ibid*, para 67.

[143] Case C-428/06 to C-434/06 *Unión General de Trabajadores de La Rioja (UGT-Rioja) and Others v Juntas Generales del Territorio Histórico de Vizcaya and Others* [2008] ECR I-6747.

Historical Territories and the Autonomous Community of the Basque Country were state aid.[144] Reproducing the reasoning set out in *Commission v Portugal*, the Court examined the concepts of institutional, procedural and economic autonomy. However, it left it to the referring court to decide whether the relevant infra-state bodies had such autonomy. The concept of regional selectivity was further elaborated in later cases.[145]

In the *Gibraltar* case,[146] the Court of Justice found that the UK's proposed corporate tax reform in Gibraltar was incompatible with the state aid prohibition. In so doing, the Court overturned the Court of First Instance's (now General Court) earlier decision and confirmed the Commission's decision.

The UK had notified the Commission of its plans to replace profit-based taxation with general payroll tax and a business property occupation tax both capped at 15 per cent of business profits. In its decision,[147] the Commission found that the scheme was materially and regionally specific—the assumption, for the latter, being that Gibraltar is a mere UK region and not an independent territory for tax purposes.[148] The case was appealed and the decision reversed by the Court of First Instance in its entirety.[149]

The Court of First Instance had examined the role of the UK in the definition of the political and economic environment in Gibraltar as a criterion for determining the reference framework. The UK's

> residual power to legislate for Gibraltar and the various powers granted to the Governor must be interpreted as means [of] enabling the United Kingdom to assume

[144] The local authorities adopted tax legislation which set the rate of corporation tax generally at 32.5% and provided for a series of tax deductions. By contrast, the basic rate of corporation tax in Spain was 35% and did not make any provision for such deductions.

[145] See analysis in ch 4 of Claire Micheau, *State Aid, Subsidy and Tax Incentives Under EU and WTO Law* (Kluwer Law International, 2014).

[146] Joined Cases C-106/09P & C-107/09P *Commission v Gibraltar and UK* [2011] ECR I-11113. For commentary, see, inter alios, Pierpaolo Rossi-Maccanico, 'The Gibraltar Judgment and the Point on Selectivity in Fiscal Aids' (2009) 18 *EC Tax Review* 67–75; Lee Sheppard, 'Do Tax Havens Violate the TFEU?' (2011) *Tax Notes International* 52, 21 November 2011; 2011 *WTD* 224-3; Wattel (2013) n 103 above; Rossi-Maccanico (2013), n 90 above; Raymond Luja, '(Re)shaping fiscal state aid: selected recent cases and their impact' (2012) 40 *Intertax* 120–31; John Temple Lang, 'The Gibraltar State aid and taxation judgment—A "methodological revolution"' [2012] 4 *European State Aid Law Quarterly* 805–12.

[147] Commission Decision of 30/3/2004, [2005] OJ L85/1, 2/4/2005.

[148] According to the Commission's decision (see recitals 98 to 152) the proposed tax reform was both regionally and materially selective. It was regionally selective since companies in Gibraltar were taxed, in general, at a lower rate than those in the UK. Also, certain aspects of the proposed tax reform were materially selective. Also see the Court's judgment, which refers to the Commission's reasoning: 'first, the requirement to make a profit before incurring liability to payroll tax and BPOT [ie business property occupation tax], since that requirement favours companies which make no profit … and second, the cap limiting liability to payroll tax and BPOT to 15% of profits, since that cap favours companies which, for the tax year in question, have profits that are low in relation to the number of employees and occupation of business property … Third and lastly, imposition of a payroll tax and BPOT is also materially selective, since both taxes inherently favour offshore companies which have no real physical presence in Gibraltar and which as a consequence do not incur corporate tax …'. See *Commission v Gibraltar and UK* (2011) n 146 above, para 21.

[149] Joined Cases T-211/04 and T-215/04 *Government of Gibraltar and United Kingdom v Commission* [2008] ECR II-3745.

> its responsibilities towards the population of Gibraltar and to perform its obligations under international law, and not as granting an ability to intervene directly as regards the content of a tax measure adopted by the Gibraltar authorities, in particular since those residual powers have never been exercised in matters of taxation.[150]

The Court of First Instance concluded that the reference framework corresponded exclusively to the geographical limits of the territory of Gibraltar. As such, no comparison could be made between the tax regime applicable to companies established in Gibraltar and that applicable to UK companies for the purpose of establishing a selective advantage.[151] This meant that the tax reform proposals were not regionally selective, nor materially selective.

The Court of Justice reversed the Court of First Instance's judgment, on 15 November 2011. In doing so, the Court also went against Advocate General Jääskinen's opinion which agreed with the Court of First Instance. More specifically, the Court found the regime to be materially selective. Its basic features—ie the payroll tax and the business property occupation tax as the sole bases of assessment—excluded from the outset any taxation of offshore companies, since these companies had no employees and also did not occupy business properties.[152] The classification of a tax system as selective was not conditional upon that system being designed in such a way that all undertakings were liable to the same tax burden but some benefitted from derogating provisions.[153] Furthermore, for a tax system to be classified as selective, it need not be designed in accordance with a certain regulatory technique; otherwise national tax rules would fall, from the outset, outside the scope of control of state aid merely because they were adopted under a different regulatory technique although they produced the same effects.[154]

The Court of Justice held that the reference system, although founded on criteria that were of a general nature, discriminated in practice between companies which were in a comparable situation with regard to the objective of the tax reform, resulting in a selective advantage being conferred on offshore companies.[155] The measure was, therefore, de facto selective. The fact that the offshore companies were not taxed was not a random consequence of the regime. Rather, it was the inevitable consequence of the fact that the bases of assessment were specifically designed so that offshore companies, 'which by their nature have no employees and do not occupy business premises',[156] have no tax base under the bases of assessment adopted in the proposed tax reform.

> Thus, the fact that offshore companies, which constitute a group of companies with regard to the bases of assessment adopted in the proposed tax reform, avoid taxation

[150] *Ibid*, para 99.
[151] *Ibid*, para 115.
[152] *Commission v Gibraltar and UK* (2011) n 146 above, paras 100–102.
[153] *Ibid*, para 91.
[154] *Ibid*, para 92.
[155] *Ibid*, para 101.
[156] *Ibid*, para 106.

> precisely on account of the specific features characteristic of that group gives reason to conclude that those companies enjoy selective advantages.[157]

There was no need to examine whether the proposed tax reform was also regionally selective. The finding of material selectivity was sufficient to substantiate the operative part of the contested decision which found the proposed tax reform to be in breach of the state aid prohibition.[158]

The Court of Justice rejected the complaint that the Commission departed from the 1998 Notice relating to State aid in the field of taxation.[159] The Court also rejected the complaint that the Commission departed from its decision-making practice,[160] emphasising that 'the question whether a measure constitutes State aid must be assessed solely in the context of [Article 107(1) TFEU] and not in the light of an alleged earlier decision-making practice of the Commission'.[161]

Rather boldly, the Court of Justice did not follow the three-step analysis, which has traditionally been used in analysing the concept of selectivity for state aid purposes.[162] Here, even though there was no derogation from the normal tax regime, still the Court of Justice found the regime to be selective. The fact that the general tax system was effectively too narrowly defined from the outset and that it discriminated in practice between companies which were in a comparable situation was crucial to the Court. Somehow, these considerations were inserted in the analysis. As has been criticised, it was not the design of the tax system that was decisive but rather its material effect.[163]

It is interesting to note that the Commission's views that the Gibraltar tax system had an inherently discriminatory character (and the relevance of this) had been discussed and rejected by the Advocate General in his opinion.[164] As he noted:

> [T]o accept such an approach would be tantamount to triggering a methodological revolution in the application of the rules relating to State aid for the purposes of Article 87(1) EC. According to that approach, the existence of an advantage would be assessed no longer on the basis of a comparison between the measure and the generally applicable tax regime, but by virtue of a comparison between the tax regime as it exists and another—hypothetical and non-existent—system. Such an approach would require the construction of a fiscal comparator for the European Union in order to be able to assess the allegedly discriminatory effect of the choices made regarding the tax base (or tax rates) in the field of corporate taxation. However, no such common criterion exists and

[157] *Ibid*, para 107.
[158] *Ibid*, paras 184–185.
[159] *Ibid*, paras 128–134.
[160] *Ibid*, para 135–137.
[161] *Ibid*, para 136.
[162] See analysis in sections 7.1 and 7.6.
[163] Wattel (2013) n 103, p 133. Summing up his conclusions, Wattel finds that following the *Gibraltar* case '[a] main rule-exception analysis is not (always) decisive, as a State may *exclude* certain undertakings from a tax by including them in such a crafty way that they are *effectively* still *excluded* and therefore favoured': *ibid*.
[164] See paras 201–202 of the opinion.

> the application of the legal framework for State aid does not justify the de facto adoption of a tax harmonisation measure of that kind.[165]

The Advocate General also, interestingly, argued that this measure was in fact an example of harmful institutional or tax competition between Member States which

> clearly does not fall within the mechanism for controlling State aid established by the Treaty, even though there are cases where measures are liable to amount both to harmful tax competition and to State aid incompatible with the common market.[166]

In this case, the measure could only be addressed under the code of conduct on business taxation and not under the state aid provision.[167] The legitimate objective of combating harmful tax competition could not 'justify distortion of the European Union's legal framework established in the area of competition law applicable to State aid, or even the adoption of ad hoc solutions conflicting with the rule of law as enshrined in Article 2 TEU'.[168]

Although the *Gibraltar* case has been widely criticised, it has not been overruled by later case law. Nor has it been followed though, which suggests that it may be a judgment on a sui generis case. The *Gibraltar* case also deviated from another case, decided shortly before it—the *Paint Graphos* case,[169] discussed below.

7.7.2. Inherent Consistency with the Logic and General Scheme of a Tax System

In the *Paint Graphos* case, the Court of Justice clarified that as regards measures derogating from the general system, to be compatible with the state aid prohibition, they must be found inherently consistent with the logic and general scheme of the tax system and proportional to that effect. Member States should introduce and apply appropriate control and monitoring procedures to ensure that.

Here, the Italian Supreme Court asked whether incentives granted to cooperative companies through tax exemptions constituted state aid and whether the incentives could be considered proportionate. The Court of Justice found that the tax benefits granted to cooperative companies were financed through state resources and were liable to affect trade between Member States and distort competition contrary to the state aid prohibition. However, selectivity was to be determined by the referring national court. Guidance for this determination was given by the Court of Justice.

165 *Ibid*, para 202.
166 *Ibid*, para 134.
167 See para 134 of the opinion.
168 *Ibid*.
169 *Paint Graphos*, n 128 above. See Case Comment, 'State aid: ruling on Italian tax relief measures for cooperative societies' (2012) 52 *European Taxation* 27–28; Quigley (2012) n 14 above.

The Court reiterated existing case law in emphasising that aid may be selective even where it concerns a whole economic sector.[170] It was necessary to determine whether the tax exemption favoured certain undertakings or the production of certain goods by comparison with other undertakings which were in a comparable factual and legal situation, in light of the objective pursued by the corporation tax regime.[171]

In the legal context of this case, cooperative companies conformed to particular operating principles which clearly distinguished them from other economic operators.[172] For example, cooperatives were not managed in the interests of outside investors. Control was vested equally in their members, and activities were conducted for the mutual benefit of members. Reserves and assets were commonly held, non-distributable and were dedicated to the common interest of members. As a consequence, the profit margin of cooperative societies was 'considerably lower than that of capital companies, which are better able to adapt to market requirements'.[173]

Therefore, the Court of Justice concluded that cooperative companies were not in a comparable factual and legal situation to that of commercial companies,

> provided, however, that they act in the economic interest of their members and their relations with members are not purely commercial but personal and individual, the members being actively involved in the running of the business and entitled to equitable distribution of the results of economic performance.[174]

This was a question for the national court to decide.[175] If it did so decide, then it had to be examined whether the tax exemptions were justified by the nature or general scheme of the system of which they formed part.[176]

The Court of Justice reiterated that a derogation could be justified if it resulted directly from the basic or guiding principles of that tax system.

> In that context, a distinction must be made between, on the one hand, the objectives attributed to a particular tax regime and which are extrinsic to it and, on the other, the mechanisms inherent in the tax system itself which are necessary for the achievement of such objectives.[177]

Therefore, tax exemptions which were the result of an objective that was unrelated to the tax system of which they formed part could not circumvent the state aid prohibition.[178] It was necessary to ensure compliance with the requirement that a benefit must be consistent not only with the inherent characteristics of

[170] *Ibid*, para 53, citing inter alia, Case C-75/97 *Belgium v Commission* [1999] ECR I-3671, para 33.
[171] *Paint Graphos*, n 128 above, para 54.
[172] *Ibid*, paras 55–61.
[173] *Ibid*, para 60.
[174] *Ibid*, para 61.
[175] *Ibid*, para 63.
[176] *Ibid*, para 64.
[177] *Ibid*, para 69.
[178] *Ibid*, para 70.

the tax system in question but also as regards the manner in which that system was implemented.[179] Tax exemptions must also be consistent with the principle of proportionality and must not go beyond what was necessary to pursue the objective.[180] Again it was for the referring court to determine these issues.[181]

Very importantly, in its judgment, the Court of Justice stated that it was for the Member States concerned to introduce and apply appropriate control and monitoring procedures in order to ensure that the tax measures introduced were consistent with the logic and general scheme of the tax system.[182] It was also for the Member States 'to prevent economic entities from choosing that particular legal form for the sole purpose of taking advantage of the tax benefits provided for that kind of undertaking'.[183]

As for the condition relating to the effect on trade between Member States and the distortion of competition, again, the Court of Justice gave some useful guidance. Here, there was no need to show a real effect on trade and actual distortion of competition. It was enough that aid was *liable* to affect such trade and distort competition.[184] In particular, when aid granted by a Member State strengthened the position of an undertaking compared with other undertakings competing in intra-Community trade, the latter must be regarded as affected by that aid.[185] It was not necessary that the undertaking benefiting from the aid was involved in intra-Community trade.

> Where a Member State grants aid to an undertaking, internal activity may be maintained or increased as a result, so that the opportunities for undertakings established in other Member States to penetrate the market in that Member State are thereby reduced. Furthermore, the strengthening of an undertaking which, until then, was not involved in intra-Community trade may place that undertaking in a position which enables it to penetrate the market of another Member State.[186]

Some of the important dicta from this case were discussed in the Commission's 2014 Draft Notice on state aid. In discussing the point made that derogations must be justified by the inherent characteristics of a tax system, as already mentioned in section 7.6 above, the Commission finds that 'external policy objectives—such as regional, environmental or industrial policy objectives—cannot be relied upon by the Member States to justify the differentiated treatment of undertakings under a certain regime'.[187] The Commission repeats this claim by saying that 'external

[179] *Ibid*, para 73.
[180] *Ibid*, paras 74–75.
[181] *Ibid*, para 76.
[182] *Ibid*, para 74.
[183] *Ibid*.
[184] *Ibid*, para 78. Citing, inter alia, Case C-372/97 *Italy v Commission* [2004] ECR I-3679, para 44; Case C-148/04 *Unicredito Italiano v Agenzia della Entrate, Ufficio Genova 1* [2005] ECR I-11137, para 54.
[185] *Paint Graphos*, n 128 above, para 79.
[186] *Ibid*, para 80.
[187] 2014 Draft Notice, n 20 above, para 135. The Commission immediately qualifies this in paragraph 136 by stating that 'the structure of certain special-purpose levies (and in particular their tax

policy objectives which are not inherent to the system cannot be relied upon [for the purposes of justifying a derogation]'.[188] In other words, it cannot be assumed that, for example, all environmental measures would be justified, as the Court of Justice held in the *British Aggregates* case.[189]

In what follows, the Commission is perhaps opening the gateways for anti-abuse provisions to be justified by the nature or general scheme of the system, even though they could be selective and/or lead to different treatment, if the *Gibraltar* case is to be widely followed.

> The basis for a possible justification could, for instance, be the need to fight fraud or tax evasion, the need to take into account specific accounting requirements, administrative manageability, the principle of tax neutrality, the progressive nature of income tax and its redistributive purpose, the need to avoid double taxation, and the objective of optimising the recovery of fiscal debts.[190]

There is, however, also an important caveat further down, in that although the provision of anti-abuse rules might be justified by the logic of preventing tax avoidance by taxpayers, anti-abuse rules could be selective 'if they provide for a derogation (non-application of the anti-abuse rules) to specific undertakings or transactions, which would not be consistent with the logic underlying the anti-abuse rules'.[191]

To an extent, these developments and the Commission's statements in its 2014 Draft Notice seem to tie in very well with the OECD's BEPS project and the international efforts to tackle aggressive tax planning and corporate tax abuse, considered in the preceding chapters of this volume. Certainly, there was discussion in the

basis), such as environmental and health taxes imposed to discourage certain activities or products that have an adverse effect on the environment or human health, will normally integrate the policy objectives pursued. In such cases, a differentiated treatment for activities/products whose situation is different from the intrinsic objective pursued, as reflected in the structure of the tax, does not give rise to a derogatory treatment'.

[188] 2014 Draft Notice, n 20 above, para 138, citing, in addition to *Paint Graphos*, n 128 above and other cases discussed in n 128 above.

[189] *British Aggregates Association v Commission*, n 128 above. In this case, the decision of the Court of First Instance (Case T-210/02 *British Aggregates Association v Commission* [2006] ECR II-278) was reversed. The Court of Justice found that the Court of First Instance had erred in holding that Member States were free to set their own priorities with respect to the protection of the environment and the goods and services on which to impose an environmental levy. State aid, as defined in the Treaty, was a legal concept which had to be interpreted on the basis of objective factors. There was nothing to justify the Commission having a broad discretion as regards to the classification of a measure as state aid. In this case, the need to take account of environmental protection requirements could not justify the exclusion of selective measures from the scope of Article 107(1) TFEU. Account could be taken of environmental objectives in the assessment of the compatibility of a state aid measure only under Article 107(3) TFEU. For commentary, see John Temple Lang (2012) n 146 above; Gianni Lo Schiavo, 'The General Court reassesses the British Aggregates levy: selective advantages "permeated" by an exercise on the actual effects of competition?' [2013] 2 *European State Aid Law Quarterly* 384–90; Gianni Lo Schiavo, 'The role of competition analysis under article 107 paragraph 1 TFEU: the emergence of a "market analysis" assessment within the selectivity criterion?' (2013) 34 *European Competition Law Review* 400–406.

[190] 2014 Draft Notice, n 20 above, para 139.

[191] *Ibid*, para 184.

past that anti-abuse measures may be regarded as intrinsic to a general system of taxation[192] and as such, rules giving effect to such measures may not be selective. In any case, the use of the state aid prohibition to tackle aggressive tax planning or tax avoidance or tax abuse is likely to intensify. Recent Commission investigations into the tax ruling practices of several Member States corroborate this. These investigations are considered in section 7.8 below.

7.7.3. The Spanish Amortisation Case—Being Selective About Selectivity

In another important recent case, the Spanish amortisation case,[193] the Court of Justice again examined the interpretation of the selectivity requirement. According to Spanish tax laws, where a company which was taxable in Spain acquired a shareholding in a 'foreign company'[194] of at least five per cent and held it without interruption for at least one year, the goodwill resulting from that shareholding could be deducted through amortisation. This did not apply to goodwill resulting from the acquisition of a shareholding in a company established in Spain.

In two decisions,[195] the Commission found the Spanish tax regime incompatible with the state aid prohibition. Following these decisions, three undertakings established in Spain, Autogrill España, Banco Santander and Santusa Holding, asked the General Court to annul the Commission decisions. The General Court did in fact annul the Commission decisions, finding that the Commission had failed to establish the selective nature of the relevant tax measure.

The fact that a tax measure was an exception from the reference framework was not sufficient to consider that the measure was selective, particularly when the measure was potentially accessible to all undertakings. Even if to benefit from a

[192] Quigley (2012), n 14 above, p 118. One such important case is Case C-308/01 *GIL Insurance Ltd v Commissioners of Customs and Excise* [2004] ECR I-4777. Here, the introduction of a higher rate of insurance premium tax on certain contracts was not a tax scheme favouring a specified sector, since it was a system of taxation of insurance premiums intended to compensate for the fact that insurance transactions were not subject to VAT and was justified by the nature and scheme of the tax system of insurance. See, paras 70–78. This case was also cited by the Commission in its 2014 Draft Notice in discussing how anti-abuse rules may be justified by the logic of preventing tax avoidance by taxpayers. See 2014 Draft Notice, n 20 above, para 184. Also see, similarly, *R v Commissioners of Customs and Excise, ex parte Lunn Poly* [1999] EuLR 653.

[193] Joined Cases T-219/10 and T-399/11 *Autogrill España SA v Commission*, and *Banco Santander SA and Santusa Holding SL v Commission*, judgment of 7 November 2014, EULI:T:2014:939, not yet reported. The judgment was not available in English at the time of writing. See summary in Press Release No 145/14, available on: curia.europa.eu/jcms/upload/docs/application/pdf/2014-11/cp140145en.pdf.

[194] In order to qualify as a 'foreign company', a company had to be subject to a similar tax to the tax applicable in Spain and its income had to be derived mainly from business activities carried out abroad.

[195] One decision related to the acquisition of EU shareholdings and the other to the acquisition of non-EU shareholdings. See Decision 2011/5/EC of 28 October 2009 on the tax amortisation of financial goodwill for foreign shareholding acquisitions C45/07 (ex NN 51/07, ex CP 9/07) implemented by Spain ([2011] OJ L7/48) and Decision 2011/282/EU of 12 January 2011 on the tax amortisation of financial goodwill for foreign shareholding acquisitions C45/07 (ex NN 51/07, ex CP 9/07) implemented by Spain ([2011] OJ L135/1).

tax measure this required the fulfilment of certain conditions (as with the Spanish financial goodwill rules), it did not suffice to make the measure selective. It was necessary to identify a particular category of undertakings which could be differentiated from the rest of the undertakings based on their specific characteristics and not just by their eligibility for the derogation. The measure had to create a difference in treatment between undertakings in a comparable legal and factual situation. Otherwise, every tax measure the benefit of which was subject to certain conditions would be found to be selective, even though the beneficiary undertakings would not share any specific characteristics distinguishing them from other undertakings.

The General Court concluded that the Spanish regime was not aimed at any particular category of undertakings or the production of goods but, rather it was aimed at a category of economic transactions. No categories of undertakings were excluded from taking advantage of it, since the application of the rules was independent of the nature of an undertaking's activity.

Also, the fact that the Spanish rules favoured the competitive position of Spanish undertakings was of no relevance for the purposes of the selectivity analysis. It merely showed that trade between Member States was affected. The General Court emphasised that a measure which may confer an advantage on all undertakings without distinction within the state concerned did not constitute state aid as regards the criterion of selectivity. A finding of selectivity must be based, inter alia, on a difference of treatment between categories of undertakings under the legislation of the *same* Member State, not a difference in treatment between companies of a Member State and those of *other* Member States. In other words, while the effects on trade were assessed by reference to undertakings in different Member States (*inter* Member States), selectivity could only stem from a difference in treatment of undertakings within the same State (*intra* Member State).

This is an important case. It also provides a useful precedent in considering whether tax credits or exemptions conferred under tax treaties could be regarded as state aid. The author has argued in the past that tax treaty benefits, which reduce or eliminate double taxation only for certain undertakings or industries satisfying certain criteria, are a form of state aid if they are sufficiently selective.[196] Following the Spanish amortisation case, merely imposing conditions for eligibility to tax treaty benefits or conditions for negation of tax treaty benefits (eg LOBs) may not be enough to establish selectivity. There must be a particular category of undertakings which can be differentiated from the rest of the undertakings based on their specific characteristics. The measure must create a difference in treatment between undertakings in a comparable legal and factual situation. This suggests that a Member State retains some limited discretion in offering tax incentives

[196] For my earlier views on this point, see Christiana HJI Panayi, 'Limitation on Benefits and State Aid' (2004) 44 *European Taxation* 83–98 and ch 4 of Christiana HJI Panayi, *Double Taxation, Tax Treaties, Treaty Shopping and the European Community* (Kluwer Law International, EUCOTAX Series, 2007).

through tax treaties, to the extent that these are *genuinely* open to all undertakings and not just nominally open to all but in fact favouring only certain categories of undertakings or economic activities.

Although the *Gibraltar* case[197] is not overruled, the Spanish amortisation case suggests that European courts are likely to be strict in the application of the selectivity criterion henceforth, reverting back to the long-standing three-step analysis. It has recently been announced that the Commission has filed two appeals against the decision of the General Court on grounds that it had erred in law by incorrectly interpreting Article 107(1) TFEU and more specifically the concept of selectivity.[198] The main argument of the Commission is thought to be that the General Court erred by requiring, in order to demonstrate that a measure is selective, the identification of a category of undertakings with specific and inherent characteristics (identifiable ex ante).[199]

7.8. Tax Rulings, Advance Pricing Agreements and State Aid

Four recent high-profile Commission investigations appear to have formally linked state aid with the fight against aggressive tax planning and BEPS. On 11 June 2014, the Commission formally launched three separate investigations[200] to examine whether a number of MNEs had received transfer pricing tax rulings[201] leading to significant tax reductions, in violation of the state aid rules. The MNEs and jurisdictions involved were Apple in Ireland, Starbucks in the Netherlands and Fiat in Luxembourg. Another investigation looking into Luxembourg's ruling to Amazon was later launched on 7 October 2014.[202]

Broadly, all these cases dealt with tax rulings on transfer pricing arrangements between entities of the same corporate group. More specifically, the Commission

[197] *Commission v Gibraltar and UK* (2011), n 116 above.

[198] Joined Cases C-20/15 P & C-21/15 P *Commission v Autogrill España*; *Commission v Banco Santander SA and Santusa Holding SL*. Further information was not available at the time of writing.

[199] See PwC Newsalert, dated 10 March 2015.

[200] See Press Release IP/14/663 dated 11 June 2014. For commentary, see Stephanie Soong Johnston, 'EU to Investigate Apple, Starbucks and Fiat Tax Rulings', 2014 *WTD* 113-1 (12 June 2014).

[201] As explained in the Press Release: 'Tax rulings are used in particular to confirm transfer pricing arrangements. Transfer pricing refers to the prices charged for commercial transactions between various parts of the same group of companies, in particular prices set for goods sold or services provided by one subsidiary of a corporate group to another subsidiary of the same group. Transfer pricing influences the allocation of taxable profit between subsidiaries of a group located in different countries. If tax authorities, when accepting the calculation of the taxable basis proposed by a company, insist on a remuneration of a subsidiary or a branch on market terms, reflecting normal conditions of competition, this would exclude the presence of state aid. However, if the calculation is not based on remuneration on market terms, it could imply a more favourable treatment of the company compared to the treatment other taxpayers would normally receive under the Member States' tax rules. This may constitute state aid'.

[202] See Press Release IP/14/1105 dated 7 October 2014.

examined the following individual rulings: (a) the individual rulings issued by the Irish tax authorities on the calculation of the taxable profit allocated to the Irish branches of Apple Sales International and of Apple Operations Europe; (b) the individual ruling issued by the Dutch tax authorities on the calculation of the taxable basis in the Netherlands for manufacturing activities of Starbucks Manufacturing EMEA BV; (c) the individual ruling issued by the Luxembourgish tax authorities on the calculation of the taxable basis in Luxembourg for the financing activities of Fiat Finance and Trade; (d) the individual ruling issued by the Luxembourgish tax authorities on the calculation of the taxable basis in Luxembourg for Amazon EU Sàrl, especially as regards the amount of royalty payments it made which significantly lowered the taxable profits of each year.

On 30 September 2014, the Commission released letters it sent to the Irish and Luxembourg governments detailing its reasons for investigating whether the state aid rules were violated.[203] On 14 November 2014, the Commission made public a letter to the Dutch government stating its preliminary view that the Netherlands might have violated the state aid rules by entering into an advance pricing arrangement with Starbucks Manufacturing EMEA BV that granted the Starbucks subsidiary advantages not available to other companies.[204]

It is useful to consider the Commission's stance in each of these cases. The crux of the matter was whether the tax rulings under investigation allowed the MNE beneficiaries to depart from market conditions in setting the commercial conditions of intra-group transactions. As a result, the Commission argued, Member States renounced taxable revenues and as a corollary state resources. The Commission compared the transfer prices used with those of a third party prudent market operator. The premise of the Commission's decisions in all cases seemed to be that the existence of advantage and selectivity was satisfied when the arm's length principle was not complied with.

In the *Apple* investigation,[205] the Commission investigated the rulings[206] issued by the Irish tax authorities on the calculation of the taxable profit allocated to the Irish branches of the Apple group. The tax rulings under scrutiny were granted to Apple Sales International (ASI) and Apple Operations Europe (AOE) in 1991 and later on in 2007. Both ASI and AOE were incorporated in Ireland but were not tax resident there.

[203] Stephanie Soong Johnston and Kristen A Parillo, 'European Commission Outlines State Aid Cases Against Apple and Fiat', 2014 *WTD* 190-1 (1 October 2014).

[204] William Hoke, 'EU Publishes Letter Alleging Illegal Dutch State Aid to Starbucks', 2014 *WTD* 221-1 (17 November 2014).

[205] State aid SA.38373 (2014/C) (ex 2014/NN) (ex 2014/CP)—Ireland, Brussels, 11 June 2014, C(2014) 3606 final (henceforth, the *Apple* case). For commentary, see, inter alios, Mindy Herzfeld, 'What are the Goals of the EU State Aid Investigations?' 2014 *WTD* 207-2 (27 October 2014); Timothy Lyons, 'The Q&A: State aid and tax rulings', *Tax Journal*, Issue 1234, p 7 (10 October 2014).

[206] It should be noted that the Irish tax authorities do not giving binding rulings but merely non-binding guidance when advice is sought.

The Commission stated that in order to determine whether the method of assessment approved by the tax ruling conferred an advantage to the undertaking, it was necessary to compare that method to the ordinary tax system. 'Thus, where a ruling concerns transfer pricing arrangements between related companies within a corporate group, that arrangement should not depart from the arrangement or remuneration that a prudent independent operator acting under normal market conditions would have accepted'.[207] In this context, market conditions could be arrived at through transfer pricing established at arm's length.[208]

The Commission cited the *Belgium and Forum 187* case[209] as confirming that if the method of taxation for intra-group transfers does not comply with the arm's length principle and leads to a taxable base inferior to the one which would result from a correct implementation of that principle, it provides a selective advantage to the company concerned.[210] However, in this case, the Court of Justice refrained from making such radical statements but rather limited itself to a more traditional state aid analysis.[211] There were no references to prudent independent market operators (or something similar) in assessing the existence of an advantage for state aid purposes.[212] Nor were there any references to the arm's length test.

Regardless of the strength of the authority for this test, to an extent, by introducing the prudent independent operator test, the Commission is also introducing its own transfer pricing standards. This prudent independent market operator test is likely to stir controversy. It seems to be satisfied by a strict application of the arm's length principles—stricter than what the OECD Transfer Pricing Guidelines would appear to demand. The following extract makes this obvious.

> The OECD Guidelines are a reference document recommending methods for approximating an arm's length pricing outcome and have been retained as appropriate guidance for this purpose in previous Commission decisions. The different methods explained in the OECD Guidelines can result in a wide range of outcomes as regards the amount of the taxable basis. Moreover, depending on the facts and circumstances of the taxpayer, not all methods approximate a market outcome in a correct way. When accepting

[207] *Apple* case, n 205 above, para 54. The Commission cited Commission Decision 2003/757/EC of 17 February 2003, Belgian Coordination centres, OJ L282/25, 30.10.2003, recital 95. However, there is no such general assertion in the paragraph cited.

[208] *Apple* case, n 205 above, para 55.

[209] Joined Cases C-182/03 and C-217/03 *Belgium and Forum 187 v Commission* [2006] ECR I-5479.

[210] *Apple* case, n 205 above, para 55.

[211] See para 95 in *Belgium and Forum 187*, n 209 above: 'In order to decide whether a method of assessment of taxable income such as that laid down under the regime for coordination centres confers an advantage on them, it is necessary, as the Commission suggests at point 95 of the contested decision, to compare that regime with the ordinary tax system, based on the difference between profits and outgoings of an undertaking carrying on its activities in conditions of free competition'.

[212] The Court of Justice had mentioned 'a prudent and alert economic operator' in the context of legitimate expectations (ie it questions whether a prudent and alert economic operator could have foreseen the adoption of a Community measure likely to affect its interests). See *Belgium and Forum 187*, n 209 above, para 147. In the same context, see reference to a prudent economic operator in para 162.

> a calculation method of the taxable basis proposed by the taxpayer, the tax authorities should compare that method to the prudent behaviour of a hypothetical market operator, which would require a market conform remuneration of a subsidiary or a branch, which reflect normal conditions of competition. For example, a market operator would not accept that its revenues are based on a method which achieves the lowest possible outcome if the facts and circumstances of the case could justify the use of other, more appropriate methods.[213]

Similar statements were made in the other Commission preliminary decisions analysed below.[214] In all of these cases, the linkage of the prudent independent market operator test with the arm's length principle meant that the Commission had to delve into a highly technical analysis in order to verify whether the contested rulings complied with the arm's length principle, without being bound by the OECD Transfer Pricing Guidelines.

In the *Apple* case, the Commission made the following points.

First, the Commission noted that the taxable basis in the 1991 ruling was negotiated rather than substantiated by reference to comparable transactions.

> The fact that the methods used to determine profit allocation to ASI and AOE result from a negotiation rather than a pricing methodology, reinforces the idea that the outcome of the agreed method is not arm's length and that a prudent independent market operator would not have accepted the remuneration allocated to the branches of ASI and AOE.[215]

Also, no transfer pricing report was included in the documents provided by the Irish authorities to support the calculation of taxable profits as confirmed in that ruling.[216]

Secondly, the Commission had doubts as to the appropriateness of the transfer pricing method chosen for the 2007 ruling. The Commission referred to the OECD Transfer Pricing Guidelines and the transfer pricing methods set out therein to comply with the arm's length principle.[217] The method used in this case was in effect the TNMM (ie transactional net margin method), with operating costs as a net profit indicator. However, the choice of that particular net profit indicator was not explained by the tax advisor, or by the Irish Revenue.

Thirdly, the Commission noted several inconsistencies in the application of the transfer pricing method chosen to determine profit allocation to AOE and ASI. According to the Commission, it did not appear to comply with the arm's length principle.[218] Inter alia, it was argued that the mark-up of the costs attributable to

---

213 *Apple* case, n 205 above, para 56.

214 See *Fiat* decision, n 227 below, para 60; *Starbucks* decision, n 237 below, para 75; *Amazon* decision, n 245 below, para 53.

215 *Apple* case, n 205 above, para 58.

216 *Ibid*, para 59. The Commission refers to OECD Transfer Pricing Guidelines paras 5.16 to 5.27, assuming that these (as well as, to an extent, the current version of the Guidelines) were available in 1991.

217 *Apple* case, n 205 above, para 60.

218 *Ibid*, para 61.

the AOE branch appeared to be reverse engineered.[219] Furthermore, the margin on branch costs was too wide.[220] The duration of the 1991 ruling also raised eye-brows. This ruling was applied by Apple for 15 years without revision.[221] There was also disagreement with the mark-up of the 2007 ruling.[222] The Commission noted that the 2007 ruling did not factor in the evolution of sales, whereas it appeared that the sales income of ASI increased by 415 per cent over the three years 2009–12.[223]

Based on these factors, the Commission found the contested rulings to be incompatible with the arm's length principle. From this, the Commission jumps to the conclusion that the Irish authorities conferred an advantage on Apple and that the advantage was granted in a selective manner.[224] 'To the extent the Irish authorities have deviated from the arm's length principle as regards Apple, the contested rulings should also be considered selective'.[225] And, again, from this, the Commission jumps to the question whether the aid is compatible with Article 107(2) and (3) TFEU, finding that it is not.[226]

The *Fiat* case[227] followed the same format. Here, the focus of examination was the Advance Pricing Arrangement (APA) given by Luxembourg to Fiat Finance and Trade Ltd (FFT). This was considered to be state aid incompatible with the internal market. More specifically, starting from the prudent independent market operator test,[228] it was questioned 'whether the FFT APA complies with the arm's length principle or whether they give rise to a selective advantage conferred by the Luxembourgish tax authorities upon that undertaking'.[229] Again, the premise of the decision seemed to be the idea that non-compliance with the arm's length principle generated a selective advantage sufficient for the purposes of the state aid prohibition.

First, it was noted that the transfer pricing report seemed to establish a fixed tax base or a tax base which can vary only marginally. As such, the Luxembourgish tax authorities disregarded any significant increase or decrease in the activities of FFT.

> Such an approach—i.e. a virtually fixed tax base—could only reflect economic reality if it was very likely that the underlying business would remain stable throughout the duration of the APA's validity. The information submitted by the Luxembourgish authorities does

219 *Ibid*, para 62.
220 *Ibid*, para 63.
221 *Ibid*, para 65.
222 *Ibid*, para 66.
223 *Ibid*, para 67.
224 *Ibid*, paras 69–70.
225 *Ibid*, para 70.
226 *Ibid*, paras 72–78. The remaining components of the state aid test were briefly discussed in paras 46–51 and found to be satisfied.
227 State aid SA.38375 (2014/C) (ex 2014/NN) (ex 2014/CP)—Luxembourg, Brussels, 11 June 2014, C(2014) 3627 final (henceforth, the *FIAT* case).
228 *Ibid*, para 60.
229 *Ibid*, para 63.

> not, however, contain any guarantees or predictions which indicate that FFT will maintain a stable business in the period covered by the APA. Moreover, it does not follow from that APA that FFT's tax base would be modified if it doubled its underlying activities.[230]

In other words, Luxembourg permitted a fixed base while ignoring the actual performance of FFT.[231]

Secondly, the Commission doubted that the calculation of the taxable basis of FFT reflected an appropriate arm's length remuneration. The TNMM, which is one of the two indirect methods for estimating the profit level under the OECD Transfer Pricing Guidelines, was not preferred by the Commission. The CUP (ie comparable uncontrolled price) method was preferred and 'FFT could have attempted to value a number of the profit and loss items using the CUP method'.[232]

Thirdly, the Commission also had a problem with the estimation of the arm's length remuneration on the basis of CAPM (ie capital asset pricing model) in that both components where set at too low a level: the amount of capital remunerated and the level of remuneration applied to this capital amount.[233] The Commission proceeded with a lengthy technical analysis of this point.[234]

On the basis of these factors, the Commission concluded that through the APA the tax authorities had conferred an advantage on FFT. 'That advantage is obtained every year and on-going, when the annual tax liability is agreed upon by the tax authorities in view of that APA'.[235] Again, the Commission concluded that the advantage was also granted in a selective manner because the tax authorities had deviated from the arm's length principle.[236]

The Commission's preliminary decision in the *Starbucks* case was published a few weeks after the *Apple* and *Fiat* preliminary decisions.[237] Again the investigation related to the use of tax rulings concluded in 2001 on the application of transfer pricing rules affecting a Dutch Starbucks entity—Starbucks Manufacturing BV (SMBV). Here, in the APA, an arm's length remuneration was agreed for the activities performed in the Netherlands by SMBV, for the Starbucks group. The Commission argued that the ruling did not in fact comply with the arm's length principle.

230 *Ibid*, para 65.

231 Lee A Sheppard, 'EU Group Finance Subsidiaries challenged' (2014) 145 *Tax Notes* 156 (13 October 2014).

232 *Fiat* case, n 227 above, para 65.

233 *Ibid*, para 66.

234 *Ibid*, paras 67–80.

235 *Ibid*, para 81.

236 *Ibid*, para 82.

237 State aid SA.38374 (2014/C) (ex 2014/NN) (ex 2014/CP)—Netherlands, Brussels, 11 June 2014, C(2014) 3626 final (henceforth, the *Starbucks* case). See, inter alia, William Hoke, 'EU Publishes Letter Alleging Illegal Dutch State Aid to Starbucks', n 204 above; Mindy Herzfeld, 'The Case Against Starbucks', 2014 *WTD* 235-2 (8 December 2014).

Here, the Commission's decision was based on three factors. First, the Commission had doubts that SMBV was a low-risk toll manufacturer.[238] The arm's length remuneration accepted in the SMBV APA depended on SMBV being considered as a low-risk toll manufacturer, for which the Commission presented 'evidence pointing to the contrary'.[239] Secondly, the Commission questioned two adjustments which were made to the SMBV agreement in 2002 and 2004, specific elements of which were alleged to be not in line with the OECD Transfer Pricing Guidelines. Thirdly, there were doubts as to the manner in which the amount of royalties paid by SMBV was calculated. The Commission presented a number of technical arguments and made references to the OECD Transfer Pricing Guidelines to support its claims.

However, the Commission's arguments have been criticised in that there were numerous inconsistencies with the OECD Transfer Pricing Guidelines.[240]

> The Commission essentially substituted its own judgment for the business judgment of Starbucks, which the Dutch government accepted in the APA. Yet the OECD transfer pricing guidelines explicitly state that tax authorities and judges should not try to substitute their own business judgments for those of the taxpayer.[241]

The Dutch tax authorities also disagreed with the Commission's assessment and argued that they fully applied the recognised arm's length principle.[242] In a letter from the Chair of the House of Representatives, it was asserted that SMBV was

[238] See fn 1, on p 2 of the *Starbucks* case, n 237 above. 'A toll-manufacturer is a manufacturer that has been stripped of risks typically for tax planning purposes. These risks would have been transferred to another company of the group, in particular raw materials are to be acquired by another company of the group, not the manufacturer that processes them, they are put in consignment in the premises of the manufacturing company. A contract manufacturer is a manufacturer the risk[s] of which have been transferred to another company by contract but to a lesser extent than in the case of a toll-manufacturer'. Also see para 80.

[239] *Ibid*, para 81.

[240] For example, in applying the arm's length standard, a range of acceptable pricing is accepted rather than a fixed price. See para 3.55 of the OECD Transfer Pricing Guidelines. In this case, the range of acceptable mark-up was argued as being 6.6 to 20.9%. Starbucks priced its transactions in the median of this range—which it found to be 9 to 12%—and the Dutch government agreed in the APA. The Commission, conducting its own separate review, concluded that this analysis was improper and that the correct median arm's length mark-up should be 14.6%. As such, the tax liability of SMBV should have been higher. However, the median figure from the Commission's analysis was well within the original acceptable range established by Starbucks (6.6—20.9%) and ought to have been allowed on the basis of the OECD Transfer Pricing Guidelines, which recognise the enormous variability of acceptable intercompany pricing. Another criticism made was that the Commission found that the Dutch government should have conducted an adequate analysis of the economic profiles of *other* members of the group, when it agreed the intercompany pricing mark-up for SMBV. By failing to properly analyse the economics of the whole group it called into question the validity of the APA. However, this is not a pre-requisite under the OECD Transfer Pricing Guidelines. See OECD Transfer Pricing Guidelines, para 2.63. See analysis by Herzfeld, 'The Case Against Starbucks', n 237 above.

[241] See Herzfeld, 'The Case Against Starbucks', n 237 above, citing para 9.163 of the OECD Transfer Pricing Guidelines.

[242] Letter from Chair of the House of Representatives of the States-General on the Starbucks case dated 14 November 2014.

correctly characterised as a low-risk manufacturer, especially as it did not run a stock risk. The existence of arm's length remuneration was determined by means of a benchmark study employing the transactional net margin method— the most commonly used method internationally for the production function and one recognised by the OECD.

> On the basis of the OECD Guidelines and national legislation, taxpayers are in principle free to choose the transfer pricing method, provided it results in an arm's length outcome for the transaction in question. The OECD Guidelines and national legislation do not prescribe a specific method for a specific situation. So far the Commission does not seem to acknowledge this.[243]

The Dutch authorities were adamant that the APA with SMBV was aligned with international transfer pricing standards and was consistent with the policy framework applied by the government in its efforts to create an attractive business climate.[244]

This is actually a very important point. APAs and advance rulings are crucial to stimulate business investments and provide legal certainty. As a result of the Commission's state aid investigations, Member States may become reluctant to give such rulings and taxpayers may also be reluctant to seek out advance rulings from tax authorities. This would lead to increased costs to the overall system.

On 16 January 2015, the Commission published its letter to Luxembourg on its preliminary findings regarding the formal state aid investigation on the 2003 tax ruling issued to Amazon EU Sàrl, a subsidiary that recorded most of Amazon's European profits.[245] Under the ruling, which is still in force, Amazon EU Sàrl paid a tax-deductible royalty to a limited liability partnership set up in Luxembourg but not subject to corporate taxation there. The terms for calculating the royalty were set out in the ruling. Broadly, through a very complex tax structure, most of Amazon's European profits could be booked in Luxembourg but remain untaxed. As a result of an advance tax ruling given to Amazon in 2003, there was effectively a cap and a floor on profits taxable in Luxembourg, calculated at a fixed proportion of the EU revenues. The Commission had serious reservations as regards the compliance of the contested tax ruling with the state aid principle.

First, Luxembourg did not submit to the Commission any transfer pricing report prepared by Amazon in support of the arrangement in the ruling. Although there was reference to an economic analysis presented by Amazon to the Luxembourgish tax authorities, this was not made available to the Commission. Therefore, it was

[243] *Ibid*, p 2.

[244] *Ibid*, p 3.

[245] State aid SA.38944 (2014/C)—Luxembourg, Brussels, 7 October 2014 C(2014) 7156 final (henceforth, the *Amazon* case). For commentary, see William Hoke and David D Stewart, 'European Commission Details Challenge to Luxembourg's Amazon Ruling', 2015 *WTD* 12-4 (20 January 2015); Lee A Sheppard, 'EU Amazon Case: Is Transfer Pricing Really the Issue?' (2015) 77 *Tax Notes International* 291 (26 January 2015). Also see Lee A Sheppard, 'Accounting for State Aid and BEPS' (2015) 77 *Tax Notes International* 842 (9 March 2015).

'not clear whether that analysis, to the extent that it exists, constitutes a transfer pricing report with a comparability analysis for the purposes of determining arm's length pricing'.[246] In the absence of such a transfer pricing report, the Commission doubted 'whether the Luxembourgish tax authorities properly confirmed by the contested tax ruling that the transfer pricing arrangement presented in Amazon's ruling request reflected what a prudent independent operator acting under normal market conditions would have accepted'.[247] The Commission further noted that the ruling request by Amazon was assessed within 11 working days from the receipt of the first letter making the ruling request. This was a very short period of time, had a transfer pricing report been submitted and assessed.[248]

In addition, the Commission found that the method proposed by Amazon's tax advisor in the ruling request and accepted by the Luxembourgish tax authorities in the tax ruling did not seem to correspond to any of the methods listed in the OECD Transfer Pricing Guidelines. While those methods were not exhaustive, the Commission was doubtful, particularly in the absence of a transfer pricing report, whether the Luxembourgish tax authorities properly confirmed that the transfer pricing arrangement was in line with market conditions.[249]

Crucially, the Commission thought that the royalty rate might not be in line with market conditions. Referring to paragraph 6.16 of the OECD Transfer Pricing Guidelines 'a royalty would ordinarily be a recurrent payment based on the user's output, sales, or in some rare circumstances, profits'. Here, it was alleged that the royalty payment approved by the contested tax ruling was not related to output, sales, or profit. Although the royalty rate was expressed as a percentage of all revenues, the royalty payment was only presented and not calculated in the form of a royalty rate over revenue.[250] Instead, the royalty was calculated as a residual profit and not on the basis of the arm's length principle.[251] Amazon had a financial incentive to exaggerate the amount of the royalty when applying the transfer pricing arrangement approved.[252] '[I]f the royalty is exaggerated, it would unduly reduce the tax paid by Amazon in Luxembourg by shifting profits to an untaxed entity from the perspective of corporate taxation'.[253]

Another issue was that Amazon EU Sàrl's profit was capped in a range of four to six per cent of operating expenses, despite having taken numerous responsibilities. This seemed to be based on the TNMM.[254] The Commission argued that the level of that margin appeared to constitute only a part of an arm's length remuneration

[246] *Amazon* case, n 245 above, para 63.
[247] *Ibid.*
[248] *Ibid.*
[249] *Ibid*, para 64.
[250] *Ibid*, para 65.
[251] *Ibid*, para 66.
[252] *Ibid*, para 71.
[253] *Ibid*, para 71.
[254] *Ibid*, para 72.

in comparison to previous cases such as *Apple* and *Starbucks*.[255] In those cases, the Commission expressed doubts as to the level of remuneration accepted by the respective tax authorities. In both cases, the TNMM was applied using the operating costs for the pricing of activities presented as routine activities with limited risk. Nevertheless, in both cases the margin considered as arm's length by the respective tax authorities was more than double the margin accepted by the Luxembourgish tax authorities in relation to Amazon. Levels of arm's length remuneration could vary across markets and depend on economic circumstances. In this case, it could not be concluded in the absence of a complete functional analysis that the remuneration was too low. Yet, the functions of Amazon performed and the risks assumed by Amazon EU Sàrl seemed complex. They were presented as central and strategic commercial decisions concentrating the business risk of the entire European market. Therefore, the method approved (the residual profit method), did not seem appropriate, whereas the level of margin accepted seemed relatively low.[256]

The Commission also had trouble with the cap and floor mechanism, as this effectively overrode the pricing method based on operating expenses. The cap was 0.55 per cent and the floor was 0.45 per cent. This ensured Amazon EU Sàrl would only be taxed within a fixed range, no matter what it earned. The cap was also too low.[257]

Similarly to the other cases, the Commission challenged the duration of the contested tax ruling which was more than 10 years. Even if the transfer pricing arrangement was considered to comply with the arm's length principle at the time, the appropriateness of the remuneration over the years should have been called into question, given the changes to the economic environment and the required remuneration levels. Here, the ruling continued to be accepted without any revision. It was noted that the duration was much longer than the length of tax rulings currently concluded by other Member States.[258]

On the basis of these observations, the Commission found that the Amazon ruling did not comply with the arm's length principle and as such, the Luxembourgish tax authorities had conferred an advantage on Amazon.[259] That advantage was also granted in a selective manner. 'To the extent the Luxembourgish

[255] *Ibid*, para 74.

[256] *Ibid*.

[257] See, para 75: 'There is no explanation as to why such a combination of methods would be appropriate. It appears that the floor and the cap are used to ensure a relatively predictable level of taxable profit; they do not seem to be based on any arm's length reasoning. Moreover, if the overall profit of the EU business is lower than the level of the floor, the floor of 0.45% of turnover no longer applies … Therefore, the transfer pricing arrangement put in place by Amazon and accepted by the contested tax ruling effectively contains a cap on a remuneration which seems too low'.

[258] *Ibid*, para 76.

[259] *Ibid*, para 77.

authorities have deviated from the arm's length principle as regards the contested tax ruling, the measure should also be considered selective'.[260]

Arguably, in all of the above cases, the Commission appears to reject the economic rationale underlying the APAs. It also appears to be fairly confident of the way the arm's length principle and the various comparability methods ought to have applied. The Commission shows preference for some methods of finding comparables and, slightly too willingly, substitutes its own judgment and calculations. Rather worryingly, it takes today's OECD transfer pricing practice and applies it retroactively to arrangements existing and rulings given more than two decades ago. Using the state aid prohibition this way leads to the undermining of the OECD Transfer Pricing Guidelines and the various methods for finding comparables.[261]

What is remarkable is that, by introducing the concept of the prudent market operator in all these cases, the Commission seems to have created its own transfer pricing standards.

> The prudent independent market operator is the personification of the arm's length method. The hypothetical actor would never accept the lower possible return or price for a good or service. So a tax authority may have granted state aid when it accepted a multinational's intra-group pricing that deviated from market practices of prudent independent market operators.[262]

If the Court of Justice, in its judgments, follows the concept of the prudent market operator as an autonomous concept,[263] whatever the outcome of these cases, another layer of complexity would have been added for multinationals with tax structures in the European Union. Adopting a price that is within an acceptable range under the OECD Transfer Pricing Guidelines may no longer be enough. As was made clear in the *Amazon* case, even though

> the OECD Guidelines provide some flexibility with respect to the application of the arm's length principle, that flexibility is limited by the principle that the remuneration arrived at should reflect what a prudent independent operator acting under normal market conditions would have accepted.[264]

In these cases, the Commission appeared to be particularly troubled with the application of the transactional net margin method.

Furthermore, what is most disconcerting is that the Commission does not actually satisfy the five-prong test for finding state aid, and more specifically,

[260] *Ibid*, para 78.

[261] Also see Herzfeld who argues that the state aid cases may be setting up a collision course between the Commission and the OECD, which could jeopardise the future of the arm's length pricing principle. Herzfeld, 'The Case Against Starbucks', n 237 above.

[262] Sheppard, 'EU Amazon Case: Is Transfer Pricing Really the Issue?', n 245 above, p 293.

[263] See also Anna Gunn and Joris Luts, 'Tax Rulings, APAs and State Aid: Legal Issues' (2015) 24 *EC Tax Review* 119, at 124.

[264] *Amazon* case, n 245 above, para 61.

the selectivity test. It fails to examine the system of reference (ie the domestic transfer pricing rules) at the time of the relevant rulings and whether the measure derogates from the system 'insofar as it differentiates between economic operations who, in light of the objectives intrinsic to the system, are in a comparable factual and legal situation', as stipulated as recently as in the 2014 Draft Notice.[265] Rather, the OECD Transfer Pricing Guidelines seem to be treated as part of or akin to a national tax system,[266] when in fact not all Member States had adopted or followed these Guidelines (or their latest version) at the time of the relevant rulings. Also, the Commission fails to examine whether the derogation was justified by the nature or the general scheme of that *specific* reference system and *not* the general OECD Transfer Pricing Guidelines.

In other words, a crucial element in the analysis is missing: have these MNEs been treated by discretion more favourably than other taxpayers in a similar factual and legal situation in *those specific* Member States?[267] For this, there needs to be a comparison of tax rulings given to other undertakings at that time to ascertain whether there have been derogations from the reference framework. The recent Spanish amortisation case[268] suggests strict adherence to the original test. Whilst the (alleged) non-compliance with the arm's length principle may be enough to show deviation from the internationally accepted OECD standard, it does not necessarily mean deviation from the reference framework, upon which the transfer pricing analysis is premised or should be premised.

This point was made clear in the 2014 Draft Notice, which substantially elaborated on the link between discretionary practices and selectivity—something also mentioned in the 1998 Notice on state aid.[269] As was noted, treating taxpayers on a discretionary basis may indicate selectivity where the exercise of the discretionary power goes beyond the simple management of tax revenue by reference to

265 *Ibid*, para 128.

266 Gunn and Luts (2015), n 263 above, pp 122–23.

267 See also para 177 of the 2014 Draft Notice, n 20 above: 'Advance administrative rulings could be selective where the tax authorities have discretion in granting administrative rulings; the rulings are not available to undertakings in a similar legal and factual situation; the administration appears to apply a more "favourable" discretionary tax treatment compared with other taxpayers in a similar factual and legal situation; the ruling has been issued in contradiction to the applicable tax provisions and has resulted in a lower amount of tax'.

268 See Spanish amortisation case, analysed in section 7.7.3 above.

269 See paras 21–22 of the 1998 Notice, n 15 above. 'The discretionary practices of some tax authorities may also give rise to measures that are caught by [ex-]Article 92 … in particular where exercise of the discretionary power goes beyond the simple management of tax revenue by reference to objective criteria … If in daily practice tax rules need to be interpreted, they cannot leave room for a discretionary treatment of undertakings. Every decision of the administration that departs from the general tax rules to the benefit of individual undertakings in principle leads to a presumption of State aid and must be analysed in detail. As far as administrative rulings merely contain an interpretation of general rules, they do not give rise to a presumption of aid. However, the opacity of the decisions taken by the authorities and the room for manoeuvre which they sometimes enjoy support the presumption that such is at any rate their effect in some instances. This does not make Member States any less able to provide their taxpayers with legal certainty and predictability on the application of general tax rules'.

objective criteria.[270] Tax settlements might also entail state aid, in particular, where it appears that the amount of taxes due has been significantly reduced without clear justification or in a disproportionate manner to the benefit of the taxpayer.[271]

There is special reference to 'prior administrative rulings' in the 2014 Draft Notice.[272] Administrative rulings that merely contain an interpretation of the relevant tax provisions without deviating from the case law and administrative practice do not give rise to a presumption of aid.[273] While it is acknowledged that the absence of publication of tax rulings and the room for manoeuvre which tax authorities sometimes enjoy support the presumption of aid,[274] this is a mere presumption. It still has to be proved. As advised in the 2014 Draft Notice, tax rulings should only aim to provide legal certainty to the fiscal treatment of certain transactions and should not have the effect of granting the undertakings concerned lower taxation than other undertakings in a similar legal and factual situation (but which were not granted such rulings).[275] Read in the context of the Commission's recent state aid actions, this is likely to lead to very vague and general tax rulings being given out, which may not be of much use to MNEs in the future.

It is worth pointing out that there may be factual errors in the Commission's description of the national tax rulings impugned. For example, Irish tax authorities (as well as the UK's HMRC) have no power to give binding rulings but can merely give non-binding guidance. Of course, this by itself, does not absolve the Irish government. As noted, the only difference between an undertaking that did obtain a tax ruling and one that did not, is that the tax administration has looked into and accepted its tax position, whether without a challenge or following an audit.[276] What is important is not whether an advantage is embedded in a tax ruling obtained by an undertaking but whether 'this undertaking is treated selectively better than other undertakings who are in a comparable legal and factual situation'.[277]

[270] 2014 Draft Notice, n 20 above, para 170.
[271] *Ibid*, para 172.
[272] *Ibid*, para 174.
[273] *Ibid*, para 175.
[274] *Ibid*.
[275] *Ibid*, para 176. There is reference to the Commission's decisional practice which shows that rulings allowing taxpayers to use alternative methods for calculating taxable profits, eg the use of fixed margins for a cost-plus or resale-minus method for determining an appropriate transfer pricing, may involve state aid. The following Commission Decisions and cases are cited: Commission Decision 2003/438/EC of 16 October 2002 on State aid C50/2001, *Luxembourg Finance Companies*, [2003] OJ L153/40, 20 June 2003, recitals 43 and 44; Commission Decision 2003/501/EC of 16 October 2002 on State aid C49/2001, *Luxembourg Coordination centres*, [2003] OJ L170/20, 9 July 2003, recitals 46–47 and 50; Commission Decision 2003/755/EC of 17 February 2003, *Belgian Coordination centres*, [2003] OJ L282/55, 30 October 2003, recitals 89 to 95 and the related Joined Cases C-182/03 and C-217/03 *Belgium and Forum 187 v Commission* [2006] ECR I-5479, paras 96 and 97; Commission Decision 2004/76/EC of 13 May 2003, *French Headquarters and Logistic Centres*, [2004] OJ L23/1, 28 January 2004, recitals 50 and 53.
[276] See Gunn and Luts (2015), n 263 above, p 122.
[277] *Ibid*.

Another question raised from these investigations is the following: is the Commission simply applying the state aid prohibition, albeit zealously, or is it in fact pushing a political agenda? Is the Commission trying to reverse the impact of the Court of Justice's decisions which promote economic freedoms with arguably little concern for tax avoidance? Or is it trying to extend the scope of state aid into the BEPS arena? The latter appeared to be foreshadowed by Mr Pierpaolo Rossi-Maccanico from the European Commission's Legal Services department, in his article 'Fiscal Aid, Tax Competition, and BEPS', which was published on *Tax Notes International* on 8 September 2014.[278] He argued that

> state aid review should be viewed as the appropriate instrument to remedy most of the situations giving rise to inappropriate low taxation that results from the exploitation of legal or regulatory mismatches in member states' taxation of cross-border transactions, including those resulting from the application of income tax treaties.[279]

At a subsequent article,[280] the same author argued that the state aid prohibition could be used with respect to measures favouring tax arbitrage of MNEs mainly on the basis of the *Gibraltar* judgment.[281]

This proposition has been challenged in that, while it might be tempting to use the state aid provision in this way and also try to address issues which effectively fall in the scope of harmful tax competition, as has been argued, 'in the absence of comparable regimes abroad, the EU might be tying its hands when some of its main trading partners are not'.[282] Although the opening of formal state aid investigations could serve to (further) promote the BEPS project within the European Union, Article 107 TFEU is not well suited to dealing with large parts of tax avoidance in the international arena.[283] There are increased concerns among the legal community that the EU state aid investigations are going too far. To restore legal certainty for Member States and taxpayers, it has been suggested that the Commission should adopt a directive on the basis of Article 106(3) TFEU which would define the framework and procedural rules for Member State competent authorities to examine and grant tax rulings to MNEs.[284] Whilst this could help with future tax rulings and stave off a wave of Member State notifications of tax rulings, it would not reduce the uncertainty as regards existing ones.

In any case, whatever the legal conclusion of the current investigations will be, the momentum is certainly unabated. Since June 2013, the Commission has been investigating the tax ruling practices of seven Member States.[285] Information was

[278] Pierpaolo Rossi-Maccanico, 'Fiscal Aid, Tax Competition, and BEPS' (2014) 75 *Tax Notes International* 857 (8 September 2014).

[279] *Ibid*, p 868.

[280] See Pierpaolo Rossi-Maccanico, 'Fiscal State Aids, Tax Base Erosion and Profit Shifting' (2015) 24 *EC Tax Review* 63–77.

[281] *Commission v Gibraltar and UK* (2011) n 146 above.

[282] Raymond Luja, 'EU State Aid Rules and Their Limits' (2014) 76 *Tax Notes International* 353 (27 October 2014).

[283] *Ibid.*

[284] Rossi-Maccanico (2015), n 280 above, at pp 75–77.

[285] Information was requested from Cyprus, Ireland, Luxembourg, Malta, the Netherlands and the UK. Information was also requested from Belgium including on certain specific tax rulings.

also requested about intellectual property taxation regimes from 10 Member States which had such a regime at the time.[286] In December 2014, it was announced that the Commission had enlarged the enquiry on tax ruling practices to cover all Member States.[287] It was announced that all Member States would be asked to provide information about their tax ruling practices, in particular to confirm whether they provide tax rulings, and if so, to request a list of all companies that had received a tax ruling from 2010 to 2013. It was later on reported that obtaining information from Member States on tax rulings had proved to be both challenging and time-consuming.[288]

Recently, the Commission has also announced its intention to propose a new directive on the automatic exchange of information on tax rulings between EU Member States. Such exchange of rulings would certainly permit tax authorities to monitor each other's behaviour. As discussed in Chapter five, in March 2015, the Commission made several proposals in its Tax Transparency Package, including the amendment of the Mutual Assistance Directive 2011/16/EU to ensure automatic exchange of information on tax rulings.

What is certain is that many investigations are likely to be launched in Member State tax ruling regimes.[289] Also, the proposal for automatic exchange of information on tax rulings is likely to lead to some de facto peer reviewing of tax ruling practices by Member States. It could also lead to tax competition, as within the bounds of the state aid prohibition, Member States would strive not to offer comparatively disadvantageous rulings. These are very interesting times for state aid and tax lawyers.

[286] The countries were Belgium, Cyprus, France, Hungary, Luxembourg, Malta, the Netherlands, Portugal, Spain, and United Kingdom. For an excellent overview of the state aid issues arising with intellectual property taxation regimes, see Joris Luts, 'Compatibility of IP Box Regimes with EU State Aid Rules and Code of Conduct' (2014) 23 *EC Tax Review* 258–83 and Begoña Pérez Bernabeu, 'R&D&I Tax Incentives in the European Union and State Aid Rules' (2014) 5 *European Taxation* 178–91.

[287] See Press Release IP/14/2742, dated 17 December 2014. The Commission is also examining Gibraltar's tax rulings practice. For commentary, see William Hoke, 'European Commission Expands State Aid Inquiries', 2014 *WTD* 243-2 (18 December 2014).

[288] See Stephanie Soong Johnston, 'EU Delays Deadline for State Aid Tax Ruling Probes', 2015 *WTD* 87-1 (6 May 2015). It appeared at the time that the Czech Republic, Estonia and Poland were yet to comply with the Commission's information requests.

[289] See also Commission announcement IP/15/4080 on 3 February 2015, that the Commission has opened an in-depth investigation into Belgian tax rulings that allowed MNEs to reduce their Belgian taxes by claiming a deduction for excess profits that purportedly resulted from the advantage of being part of a multinational group. The deductions granted through the excess profit ruling system usually amounted to more than 50% of the profits covered by the tax ruling and could sometimes reach 90%. Benefits were only available to a limited number of MNEs and not stand-alone companies. The Commission expressed doubts that the Belgian legislation was following the OECD's arm's length principle. Also see reports that the Commission is inquiring into Luxembourg's tax ruling to McDonald's. It has been claimed that McDonald's is paying an effective tax rate of 0.48% in Europe and it has underpaid its tax obligations to European countries by more than one billion between 2009 and 2013. For commentary, see William Hoke, 'EU Begins State Aid Investigation of Belgian Excess Profits Rulings', 2015 *WTD* 23-2 (4 February 2015); William Hoke, 'EU Launches Inquiry Into Luxembourg's Tax Rulings for McDonald's', 2015 *WTD* 63-1 (2 April 2015).

8

Unanimity, Enhanced Cooperation and the Financial Transaction Tax: Challenging the European Union's Tax Traditions

Up until now, much of the analysis in this book has focused on BEPS and the efforts made by the international community and the European Union to tackle aggressive tax planning. This chapter explores another angle—the ongoing efforts by the Commission and some Member States to introduce the Financial Transaction Tax (FTT), in an attempt to make the financial sector pay its fair share for its role in the origins of the economic crisis.[1] To a large extent, this proposal fits in well with the Commission's and the EU's overall efforts to address some of the causes and effects of the financial crisis.

The focus of this chapter is on the Commission's proposal for an FTT and the current efforts to adopt it through enhanced cooperation. Before considering the development of the proposal and the suitability of the enhanced cooperation mechanism in adopting it, it is important first to understand how this mechanism works.

8.1. The Enhanced Cooperation Procedure

The existence of the fiscal veto has always been blamed for the scarcity of EU tax legislation. This is because all legislative bases used to enact direct tax legislation require unanimity in Council.[2] Overall, the fiscal veto, ie the power of even one Member State to object to a harmonising measure in direct tax law, is a fiercely

[1] European Commission—Press release, *Financial Transaction Tax: Making the financial sector pay its fair share*, IP/11/1085.

[2] The fact that Member States have retained competence in direct tax matters is a known mantra. As there is no explicit legislative base for the harmonisation of direct taxes, general legislative bases under Arts 115 and 352 TFEU have been used for direct tax legislation. These legislative bases focus on the attainment of the internal market and their use is strictly policed by the Court of Justice. Both legislative bases require unanimity by Member States.

guarded prerogative which has survived successive Treaty amendments and attempts to move to qualified majority voting. As a result, the Union has legislated in a number of limited areas, where it was deemed expedient for the proper functioning of the internal market. Therefore, 'positive integration', that is integration through proper legislative routes, *does* exist but it is scarce compared to the growing volume of case law.[3]

Recently, efforts are being made to use alternative methods to approve legislative instruments—one being the enhanced cooperation mechanism. The precursors of the enhanced cooperation rules were the closer cooperation rules introduced in the Treaty of Amsterdam,[4] which were introduced as a hybrid solution between the classical (and scarce) Community harmonisation process and intergovernmental agreements.[5] These rules enabled closer cooperation to be established amongst subsets of Member States in the framework of EU law. The procedural rules for closer cooperation were very strict and were never used in practice.[6] The rules were revised in the Treaty of Nice and renamed the enhanced cooperation rules.[7] The rules were further simplified following the ratification of the Lisbon Treaty and the procedure is now set out in Article 20 TEU and Articles 326–334 TFEU.

Currently, for enhanced cooperation to be enabled, a minimum of nine[8] Member States is needed. Under the EU Treaties, enhanced cooperation can only be used as a measure of last resort.[9] Although all Member States can participate in the Council deliberations, only participating Member States can vote on it.[10] Unanimity of the participating Member States is required.[11]

Enhanced cooperation has to comply with EU law and must not undermine the internal market, create barriers in trade or discriminate between Member States or distort competition.[12] The competences, rights and obligations of

[3] See ch 2 in Christiana HJI Panayi, *European Union Corporate Tax Law* (Cambridge University Press, 2013).

[4] Consolidated version of the Treaty on European Union (TEU) [1997] OJ C340/145; Consolidated version of the Treaty establishing the European Community (TEC) [1997] OJ C340/173. See TEU Arts 43 to 45 and TEC Art 11.

[5] Joachim Englisch, John Vella and Anzhela Yevgenyeva, 'The Financial Transaction Tax Proposal Under the Enhanced Cooperation Procedure: Legal and Practical Considerations' [2013] *British Tax Review* 221, 243.

[6] See Alexander Stubb, *Negotiating Flexibility in the European Union: Amsterdam, Nice and Beyond* (Palgrave 2002); Steve Weatherill, '"If I'd wanted you to understand I would have explained it better": What is the purpose of the provisions on closer cooperation introduced by the Treaty of Amsterdam?' in David O'Keeffe and Patrick Twomey, *Legal Issues of the Amsterdam Treaty* (Hart Publishing, 1999) p 21.

[7] The revised rules were set out in Articles 11 and 11A of the EC Treaty and Articles 40, 43–45 of the Treaty on the European Union. See Jo Shaw, 'Enhancing Cooperation After Nice: Will the Treaty do the Trick?' in Mads Andenas and John Usher (eds), *The Treaty of Nice and Beyond: Enlargement and Constitutional Reform* (Hart Publishing, 2003) p 207; José María de Areilza, 'The Reform of Enhanced Cooperation Rules: Towards Less Flexibility' in Bruno de Witte et al (eds), *The Many Faces of Differentiation in EU Law* (Intersentia, 2001) p 27.

[8] Prior to the Lisbon Treaty, eight Member States were needed to trigger enhanced cooperation.

[9] It is only considered a last resort when the Council has established that the objectives of such cooperation cannot be attained within a reasonable period by the Union as a whole. See Art 20(2) TEU.

[10] Art 20(3) TEU and Art 330 TFEU.

[11] Art 330 TFEU.

[12] Art 326 TFEU.

non-participating Member States are to be respected.[13] Acts adopted in the framework of this procedure only bind participating Member States.[14] At the same time, non-participating Member States are under an obligation not to impede the implementation of the legislation under enhanced cooperation.[15] Therefore, even though acts adopted within the framework of enhanced cooperation do not become part of EU law and cannot affect non-participating Member States, nevertheless these Member States are under an obligation not to impede the implementation of these acts. The extent of this obligation may not always be clear, or reciprocal. It should also be borne in mind that expenditure incurred from the implementation of enhanced cooperation, other than administrative costs of the institutions, is to be borne by participating Member States, unless all members of the Council acting unanimously and consulting the European Parliament, decide otherwise.[16]

Enhanced cooperation is open to all Member States satisfying the conditions of participation and, at a later time, subject to compliance with acts adopted in the framework.[17] The Commission and the participating Member States have to promote participation by as many Member States as possible.[18] The authorising decision is adopted by the Council as a measure of last resort when the objectives of cooperation cannot be attained within a reasonable period by the Union. Member States wanting to adopt legislation through enhanced cooperation have to send the request to the Commission, specifying the scope and objectives of the enhanced cooperation proposed.[19]

The Commission may submit the proposal to the Council to authorise enhanced cooperation.[20] Authorisation shall be granted by the Council after a proposal is made by the Commission and consent is obtained from the European Parliament.[21] All Member States can take part in the deliberations in Council but only those participating in enhanced cooperation can vote.[22] It is stipulated in Article 330 TFEU that unanimity has to be constituted by the votes of the participating Member States. This provision is slightly confusing. The article does not really specify what unanimity is required for. Presumably, at least nine Member States have to agree to proceed to enhanced cooperation for the proposal to be considered; otherwise it cannot be adopted. Perhaps one should interpret this provision as saying that even if the legal base used to enact legislation requires

13 Art 327 TFEU.

14 Art 20(4) TEU. In the same paragraph, it is stated that the acts shall not be regarded as part of the *acquis* which is to be accepted by candidate states for accession to the Union. However, it is not specified if they are part of the *acquis* for other purposes.

15 Art 327 TFEU.

16 Art 332 TFEU.

17 Art 328 TFEU.

18 *Ibid.*

19 Art 329(1) TFEU.

20 *Ibid.*

21 *Ibid.*

22 Art 330 TFEU.

unanimity, if adoption is through the process of enhanced cooperation, then this requirement is modified. In other words, a possible majority of non-participating Member States cannot block the minority at authorisation stage. The provision should also be read in light of Article 333 TFEU which provides that where the Treaty provision which may be applied in the context of enhanced cooperation requires unanimity, the Council acting unanimously may adopt a decision stipulating that it will act by qualified majority.

Therefore, technically, the participating Member States only have to agree between themselves on the contents of the request made to the Commission and subsequently to vote in Council for the Commission's proposal based on their request. Arguably, following the Treaty of Lisbon, it has become easier to use enhanced cooperation, as it is more flexible and depends more on participating Member States. It is obvious that the new provisions on enhanced cooperation confer on participating Member States more autonomy, both at deliberation and the subsequent implementation phase. This, however, raises potential problems in managing diversity among Member States while still preserving core values of the EU legal order.[23]

So far,[24] enhanced cooperation has been used to adopt conflict of laws rules in relation to divorce proceedings in 2010[25] and to establish the unitary patent protection system in 2012.[26] As far as the latter is concerned, the two non-participating Member States (Italy and Spain) had applied for annulment of the enhanced cooperation[27] but both the Advocate General and the Court of Justice dismissed the challenge. Notably, the Court of Justice adopted a technical, and to an extent minimalist, interpretation of the Treaty provisions on enhanced cooperation. Perhaps had it done otherwise, it would have been accused of getting embroiled in political controversies.

What was interesting in the unitary patents challenge was the Court's relative permissiveness as to the contents of the Council's authorising decision.

[23] See Editorial comments, 'Enhanced cooperation: A Union à taille réduite or à porte tournante?' (2011) 48 *Common Market Law Review* 317–27.

[24] An attempt was made in 2007 to enact rules on criminal suspects' procedural rights but there was insufficient support to go forward with the proposal on the basis of enhanced cooperation. See Framework Decision on Criminal Suspects' Procedural Rights, COM(2004) 328, 28 April 2004. Also see Steve Peers, 'Divorce, European Style: The First Authorization of Enhanced Cooperation' (2010) 6 *European Constitutional Law Review* 339–58, 342.

[25] See Council Decision of 12 July 2010 authorising enhanced cooperation in the area of the law applicable to divorce and legal separation [2010] OJ L189/12. For commentary, see Peers (2010), n 24 above.

[26] See Council Decision of 10 March 2011 authorising enhanced cooperation in the area of the creation of unitary patent protection [2011] OJ L76/53. The unitary patent system established under enhanced cooperation endeavoured to minimise complexities for the protection of patents within the European Union. It ensured that only one application would be necessary to protect a patent in the participating Member States. The patents could only be validated in one of the following languages: English, French and German. Spain and Italy objected to the use of enhanced cooperation by the other Member States on a number of grounds, all of which were rejected in the Court of Justice. For commentary, see Steve Peers, 'The Constitutional Implications of the EU Patent' (2011) 7 *European Constitutional Law Review* 229–66.

[27] See Joined Cases C-295/11 *Italy v Council of the European Union* and C-274/11 *Spain v Council of the European Union.* The Court delivered its decision on 16 April 2013. Also see Advocate General Bot's opinion delivered on 11 December 2012.

The applicants had complained that the Council disregarded the judicial system of the Union by authorising enhanced cooperation without specifying what the judicial system should be.[28] The Court of Justice noted that under Article 329(1) TFEU, Member States' requests for enhanced cooperation had to specify the scope and objectives of the enhanced cooperation proposed. According to the Court of Justice, this was done as shown in the request and the Commission proposal. The Council was not obliged to provide further information with regard to the possible content of the system adopted by the participants in the enhanced cooperation in question. The sole purpose of the decision was to authorise the request of the Member States.[29]

This judgment suggests that the amount of information that has to be provided by Member States proposing enhanced cooperation to potentially non-participating Member States does not have to be extensive, even at Council stage where enhanced cooperation is to be authorised. It is, therefore, unclear how much consultation is needed before or after making the request for enhanced cooperation. Especially as regards non-participating Member States, the lack of consultation and of opportunities to give representations, as well as the lack of clarity as to the obligations of non-participating Member States may infringe their rights and competences. This is, in fact, something that the UK complained of vis-à-vis the FTT, as explained in section 8.3 below. It is obvious from the unitary patent case that the Court of Justice was reluctant to make any general statements or give general guidelines on the parameters of reviewing compliance with the conditions for authorising enhanced cooperation. Its analysis was limited to the technical issues raised. A similarly lenient approach is apparent in the Court's dismissal of the UK action against the FTT enhanced cooperation decision, again discussed in section 8.3.

Overall, as far as taxes are concerned, although the FTT proposal is the most prominent and often mentioned example, the first time the question of enhanced cooperation was in fact raised was in the context of the proposed Common Consolidated Corporate Tax Base (CCCTB). Even before the publication of the Commission's draft CCCTB Directive,[30] it was thought that unanimity in Council was unlikely to be attained and there were suggestions to allow a few Member States to adopt the CCCTB under the enhanced cooperation procedure.[31] In fact,

[28] Under the unitary patents system, it was envisaged that a unitary patent court would be set up to decide disputes. Spain had complained that although it was not necessary to create in every instrument of secondary legislation a set of judicial rules, here, the judicial rules had to be specified in a measure authorising the creation of a new European intellectual property right. See, *ibid*, para 87.

[29] *Ibid*, paras 87–92.

[30] Brussels, COM(2011) 121/4, 2011/0058 (CNS); SEC(2011) 316 final. For more information, see Christiana HJI Panayi, *The Common Consolidated Corporate Tax Base and the UK System* (IFS, 2011) and HJI Panayi (2013), n 3 above.

[31] See HJI Panayi (2011), n 30 above, especially parts 1, 2 and 5. Also see Luca Cerioni, 'The Possible Introduction of Common Consolidated Base Taxation via Enhanced Cooperation: Some Open Issues' (2006) 46 *European Taxation* 187; Christiana HJI Panayi, 'The Common Consolidated Corporate Tax Base: Issues for Third Countries and Member States opting out' (2008) 48 *European Taxation* 114–23. The possibility of enhanced cooperation was referred to, inter alios, by Philip Baker and Ioanna Mitroyanni, 'The CCCTB Rules and Tax Treaties', and Malcolm Gammie and Christiana

in a European Parliament resolution,[32] the Commission's efforts to establish the CCCTB were supported[33] and the intention to launch it even in the framework of enhanced cooperation was welcomed.[34] It was, however, pointed out that this was 'a second-best solution as, in the absence of a comprehensive EU-wide system, the benefits of transparency and lower administrative costs may be partly mitigated'.[35]

Although the adoption of the CCCTB has been brought to light once again following the Commission's launch of the Tax Transparency Package,[36] this is likely to take time as there is still no unanimity among Member States and not sufficient Member States to trigger the enhanced cooperation mechanism. Furthermore, if the proposal is to be adopted through enhanced cooperation, there needs to be sufficient consultation with non-participating Member States as to aspects of the proposal that have to be clarified or amended to cater for the rights and obligations of these Member States. There is general concurrence that the draft CCCTB Directive, as produced by the Commission in 2011, cannot be used in case of enhanced cooperation, as a number of issues have to be resolved first.[37]

By contrast, the proposal for an FTT, although it rose to prominence much later that the CCCTB,[38] was nevertheless fast-tracked in the last few years. Following the initiatives of mainly France and Germany, it is currently being proposed to Member States via enhanced cooperation. This is examined next.

8.2. The Financial Transaction Tax

There has long been a general discussion to introduce a financial transaction tax.[39] Arguments in favour of such tax increased with the advent of the banking crisis in

HJI Panayi, 'Inbound Investment and Thin Capitalization' in Michael Lang, Pasquale Pistone, Josef Schuch and Claus Staringer, *Common Consolidated Corporate Tax Base* (Linde, 2008). For an economic analysis, see Leon Bettendorf, Albert van der Horst, Ruud A de Mooij, Handrik Vrijburg, *Corporate tax consolidation and enhanced cooperation in the European Union* (2009) Oxford University Centre for Business Taxation WP 10/01.

32 See Resolution of 15 January 2008 on Tax Treatment of Losses in Cross-Border Situations 2007/2144(INI), P6_TA(2008)0008, published in Official Journal of the European Union, C 41 E, 19 February 2009.

33 *Ibid*, paras 24–25.

34 *Ibid*, para 27.

35 *Ibid*, para 27.

36 See analysis in section 5.4 in Ch 5 of this volume.

37 The author has done extensive research which considers the possible impact of the CCCTB on non-participating Member States and the matters that ought to be resolved for enhanced cooperation to be successfully applied. These issues were explored by the author in a report commissioned by the Institute for Fiscal Studies. See HJI Panayi (2011), n 30 above.

38 The Commission had been working on the CCCTB Directive ever since the necessity for such legislation was raised in the Commission Company Tax Study published in 2001 ('Company Taxation in the Internal Market', SEC(2001) 1681). See ch 1 in HJI Panayi (2013), n 3 above.

39 See proposal for currency exchange aimed at stabilising financial markets by Nobel Laureate economics Professor James Tobin (Tobin tax). James Tobin, 'A Proposal for International Monetary Reform' (1978) 4 *Eastern Economic Journal* 153–59. Professor Tobin acknowledged the influence of

late 2007 and its impact on the world economy.[40] The ongoing discussion at the level of the G20 and the IMF[41] intensified the debate within the European Union. On 28 September 2011, the Commission published a proposal for a Council Directive introducing a common system of a Financial Transaction Tax.[42] Although the initial intention was to work towards the introduction of an FTT on a worldwide basis,[43] it was decided to attempt an EU-FTT. The proposal was accompanied by an impact assessment.[44]

Being a Directive on indirect taxes, the harmonisation base was Article 113 TFEU. The FTT was not, according to the Directive, meant to affect citizens and business. It would only apply to financial transactions between financial institutions, when at least one party to the transaction was established in a Member State and a financial institution was established in a Member State.[45] A tax of 0.1 per cent for most financial transactions other than derivatives and 0.01 per cent for derivative contracts was envisaged, as explained below.[46] These were minimum rates and participating Member States were entitled to apply higher rates.

the writings of John Maynard Keynes on his proposal. See JM Keynes, *General Theory of Employment, Interest Rates and Money* (New York, Harcourt Brace & World, 1936). For a brief overview of the proposals and subsequent developments, see, inter alios, Thornton Matheson, *Taxing Financial Transactions: Issues and Evidence*, IMF WP/11/54 (IMF, 2011); Anthony Seely, 'The Tobin tax: earlier debates', House of Commons Library Standard Note, Standard Notes SN01346, dated 16 January 2012, available on: www.parliament.uk/briefing-papers/SN01346); Pablo A Hernández González-Barreda, 'On the European Way to a Financial Transaction Tax under Enhanced Cooperation: Multi-Speed Europe or Shortcut?' (2013) 41 *Intertax* 208–9; Gerard TK Meussen, 'A New Tax Strategy for the European Union: FTT and FAT, Realistic or a Bridge too Far' (2011) 52 *European Taxation* 101–4.

[40] See Antony Seely, 'The Tobin Tax: Recent Developments', House of Commons Library, Standard Notes SN6184, dated 29 April 2013. Available on: www.parliament.uk/briefing-papers/SN06184.

[41] See G20 Saint Andrews Communique, *Meeting of Finance Ministers and Central Bank Governors*, para 6 (7/11/2009) and IMF, *A Fair and Substantial Contribution by the Financial Sector: Final Report for the G-20* (2010), cited in González-Barreda, n 39 above, p 298.

[42] Proposal for a Council Directive on a common system of financial transaction tax and amending Directive 2008/7/EC, COM(2011) 594 final, Brussels, 28 September 2011 (henceforth, the 2011 FTT Proposal). For a critical overview, see John Vella, Clemens Fuest and Tim Schmidt-Eisenlohr, 'The EU Commission's Proposal for a Financial Transaction Tax' [2011] *British Tax Review* 607; Thorsten Vogel and Benjamin Cortez, 'The Commission's Proposal to Introduce an EU Financial Transaction Tax' (2012) 52 *European Taxation* 77; Oskar Henkow, 'The Commission's Proposal for a Common System of Financial Transaction Tax: A Legal Appraisal' (2012) 21 *EC Tax Review* 5; Géry Bombeke and Evert Bleus, 'Financial Transaction Tax' (2013) 41 *Intertax* 553–56.

[43] See conclusions of European Council in its meeting on 17 June 2010 with regard to the G20 Toronto Summit that '[t]he EU should lead efforts to set a global approach for introducing systems for levies and taxes on financial institutions with a view to maintaining a world-wide level playing field and will strongly defend this position with its G-20 partners. The introduction of a global financial transaction tax should be explored and developed further in that context'. Also see the Commission's follow-up work on this: Commission Staff Working Document, *Financial Sector Taxation, accompanying the communication from the Commission to the European Parliament, the Council, the European Economic and Social Committee and the Committee of the Regions* (COM(2010) 549 final).

[44] See Commission Staff Working Paper Impact Assessment accompanying the document Proposal for a Council Directive on a common system of financial transaction tax and amending Directive 2008/7/EC (28/09/2011), SEC(2011) 1102 final (henceforth, the 2011 Impact Assessment).

[45] See Art 1(2) of the 2011 FTT Proposal, n 42 above.

[46] *Ibid*, Art 8(2).

The FTT proposal was described as a levy which would ensure that the financial sector contributes to the covering of the costs of the crisis and that it would be taxed in a fair way vis-à-vis other sectors in the future. It was also argued that a coordinated framework at EU level would help to strengthen the EU single market. At the time of the 2011 FTT proposal, 10 Member States had a type of a financial transaction tax in place. The proposal would introduce new minimum tax rates and harmonise different existing taxes on financial transactions in the European Union. This would help to reduce competitive distortions in the single market. The FTT was also meant to dis-incentivise excessively risky activities by financial institutions, to complement regulatory measures aimed at avoiding future crises and to generate additional revenue for general budgets or specific policy purposes.

The FTT would only apply if one of the two parties was a financial institution and if one of the two parties—whether the financial institution or the non-financial institution—was established in a Member State.[47] Therefore, direct transactions between non-financial institutions were not technically subject to FTT and the place where the transaction took place was not relevant.

The term 'financial transactions'[48] was defined broadly, as the close substitutability of financial transactions and instruments would increase opportunities for tax avoidance.[49] The term included the sale or purchase of financial instruments,[50] money-market instruments (with the exception of instruments of payment), units or shares in collective investment undertakings,[51] transfers of financial instruments between group entities, which are not a purchase and sale, and the conclusion or modification of derivatives (eg forwards, futures, options, swaps and financial contracts for difference). The FTT would be levied irrespective of whether or not the transaction took place through a stock exchange or over the counter.

Transactions on the primary market were exempt from the scope of the FTT.[52] Some other transactions were not included, for example, spot currency transactions, 'consumer transactions' (eg concluding insurance contracts, granting consumer credit, mortgage lending, credit card transactions, payment services,

[47] *Ibid*, Art 1(2). The financial institution may be acting either for its own account or for account of another person, or is acting in the name of a party to the transaction.

[48] *Ibid*, Art 2(1)(1).

[49] See Vella et al (2011), n 42 above, p 609.

[50] This is before netting and settlement, including repurchase and reverse repurchase and securities lending and borrowing agreements. See Art 2(1)(1)(a).

[51] See references in Art 2(3)–(6) to the definition of financial instruments in Annex I to Directive 2004/39/EC [2004] OJ L145/1, 30.4.2004. This definition covers units in collective investment undertakings. Shares and units of undertakings for collective investment in transferable securities (UCITS) as defined in Art 1(2) of Directive 2009/65/EC ([2009] OJ L302/32, 17.11.2009) and alternative investment funds (AIF) as defined in Article 4(1)(a) of Directive 2011/61/EU ([2011] OJ L174/1, 1.7.2011) are financial instruments. The subscription and redemption of these instruments are also considered financial transactions. See Explanatory Memorandum to the Proposal, p 6, fn 8. Therefore, concepts found in internal market regulation of financial services would now require a tax interpretation.

[52] Art 1(4)(a) of the 2011 FTT Proposal, n 42 above. Also excluded are Central Counter Parties (CCPs) where exercising the function of a CCP, Central Securities Depositories (CSDs) and International Central Securities Depositories (ICSDs) where exercising the function of a CSD or ICSD.

deposits), issuing of government bonds and transactions with certain bodies (eg transactions with the central banks of Member States).

'Financial institutions'[53] were broadly defined and comprised all financial institutions and SPVs, as well as certain non-financial companies where a significant part of their overall activities was financial.[54] Financial institutions would have to collect the tax and file a monthly FTT declaration. Some institutions (eg the European Financial Stability Facility and national Central Banks) were excluded from being financial institutions for the purposes of the proposed Directive.[55] The exclusion of the Central Banks was intended to guarantee that the proposed Directive would not affect the refinancing possibilities of financial institutions or the instruments of monetary policy.[56]

A financial institution would be deemed to be established in a Member State under a number of criteria set out in Article 3.[57] As a result of the rules, under certain circumstances, non-EU financial institutions would also be deemed EU-established. There was an escape clause in that no FTT would be levied where there was no link between the economic substance of the transaction and the territory of any Member State.[58]

Financial transactions other than derivatives would be taxed at 0.1 per cent and for the conclusion or modification of derivatives the tax rate would be 0.01 per cent.[59] As mentioned, both are minimum rates and Member States may increase them but cannot differentiate between financial transactions falling under the two categories. This was to mitigate the risk of tax-driven product selection of these highly mobile instruments.

[53] *Ibid*, Art 2(7).

[54] Eg credit institutions, regulated markets, investment firms, insurance/reinsurance undertakings, pension funds etc.

[55] See Art 1(3) of the 2011 FTT Proposal, n 42 above.

[56] See Explanatory Memorandum to the Proposal, p 5 and Vogel and Cortez (2012), n 42 above, p 136.

[57] Where the financial institution has been authorised to act as a financial institution, in respect of transactions covered by the authorisation (Art 3(1)(a)); where it has its registered seat (Art 3(1)(b)); where it has its permanent address or usual residence (Art 3(1)(c)); where it has a branch, in respect of transactions carried out by the branch (Art 3(1)(d)); where it is a party, acting either for its own account or for the account of another person, or is acting in the name of a party to the transaction, to a financial transaction with another financial institution established in that Member State pursuant to points (a), (b), (c) or (d), or with a party established in the territory of that Member State and which is not a financial institution (Art 3(1)(e)). This list is hierarchical so if more than one of the conditions are met, the first one takes priority. See Art 3(2) of the 2011 FTT Proposal, n 42 above. Englisch et al (2013), n 5 above, discuss the 'contagion effect' of the rules in that when a financial institution fulfils none of the criteria set out, it shall nevertheless become liable to the FTT if the other party involved in the transaction is (or is deemed to be) established in a participating Member State under the tests. See pp 236 and 240. Although the argument is made in the context of the 2013 FTT Proposal, the same applies under the 2011 FTT Proposal (see Art 3(1)(e)). However, Englisch et al point out that in the 2011 Impact Assessment, n 44 above, p 5, the Commission appears to interpret the rules as not requiring the taxation of the part of a trade that is undertaken by a non-resident buyer or seller: see Englisch et al p 240.

[58] Art 3(3) of the 2011 FTT Proposal, n 42 above.

[59] *Ibid*, Art 8(2).

The FTT liability would arise when the transaction occurred and would be payable immediately (in case of electronic transactions) or within three working days.[60] Each financial institution that was a party to the financial transaction would pay FTT[61] and there would be joint and several liability.[62] Transfers of financial instruments within a corporate group would also be subject to FTT, even if the transaction could not be characterised as a purchase or sale (cascading effect).

It was stipulated that Member States would lay down obligations as to the registration of financial institutions, accounting, reporting and other obligations to ensure effective payment, verification of correct payment of the tax, and prevention of tax evasion, avoidance and abuse.[63] The administration was left for the Member States to determine but Member States had to make use of administrative cooperation tools. It was obvious that under the proposed Directive, there would be limited coordination proposed at an EU level.

If adopted, the proposed directive would become effective on 1 January 2014. In the 2011 Impact Assessment,[64] the Commission estimated revenues of approximately €57 billion annually depending on market reactions and the effectiveness of tax collection. It was not certain how the revenue would be used. Some of it could be allocated to the EU Budget, thus reducing the contributions of Member States. To achieve harmonisation within the European Union, all Member States which already had such tax would have to abolish it and replace it with the FTT. In March 2012, the Commission proposed to split the revenues 2/3 to the EU Budget and 1/3 to Member States.

The proposed FTT Directive was not favourably seen by a number of Member States and especially the UK, Sweden, Bulgaria, the Czech Republic, Cyprus, Malta and Denmark.[65] It was criticised for having a broad field of application, potentially catching non-financial and non-EU undertakings. In February 2012, only nine Member States (Austria, Belgium, Finland, France, Germany, Greece, Italy, Portugal and Spain) had indicated their support for an EU-wide FTT.

In its opinion on the Commission's proposal, the European Parliament voted in favour of the proposal.[66] The European Parliament recommended the addition of an issuance principle to the Commission's proposal whereby non-EU financial institutions would pay the FTT if the securities traded were originally issued within

[60] *Ibid*, Arts 4 and 10(4).

[61] *Ibid*, Art 9.

[62] *Ibid*, Art 9(3).

[63] *Ibid*, Art 10.

[64] 2011 Impact Assessment, n 44 above.

[65] Thorsten Vogel and Benjamin Cortez, 'Recent Development and Resulting Implications Regarding a Financial Transaction Tax in Europe' (2013) 53 *European Taxation* 135. Also see Rebecca Christie and Jim Brunsden 'EU Transaction Tax Debate Highlights Euro-Area Disagreement' in Bloomberg, *Businessweek* (8 November 2011). Vella et al (2011), n 42 above, at p 609 describe the UK as being bitterly opposed to an FTT unless it was adopted by other G20 countries. Also see Brooke Masters, Jeremy Grant and Chris Bryant, 'Warning of unintended outcomes of Tobin tax', *Financial Times* (5/10/2011).

[66] European Parliament legislative resolution of 23 May 2012 on the proposal for a Council Directive on a common system of financial transaction tax.

the European Union. The European Parliament also stated that the FTT should be adopted even by some Member States.[67] By June 2012 at the ECOFIN meeting, it was clear that the Commission's proposal for an EU FTT had not amassed the necessary support to be unanimously adopted by all Member States. Given that unanimity was required for the proposal to be adopted as a directive under Article 113 TFEU, interested Member States had to look for alternative ways. The only option seemed to be adoption through the enhanced cooperation mechanism.

Indeed, on 28 September 2012, in a joint letter sent to the Commission and the Finance Ministers of other Member States, the German and French Finance Ministers stated their strong support in favour of the FTT and urged the Commission to trigger the enhanced cooperation mechanism in order to implement the FTT in a subset of Member States. Although France and Germany encouraged and invited other Member States to join this initiative, the letter was vague as to the detail of the actual FTT proposal, stating that it would be based on the Commission's initial proposal. As argued, this stance suggested that the 'design of the FTT is therefore still a moving target and the scope and objectives remain unclear'.[68]

Shortly thereafter, on 23 October 2012, the Commission gave the green light for the use of enhanced cooperation to adopt the FTT[69] and advised the Council to approve this. The Commission argued that enhanced cooperation on an FTT would support the EU's objective and reinforce the integration process.

> A common FTT system, shared by 11(+) Member States, would reduce the number of divergent national approaches to financial sector taxation. In doing so, it would lead to less competitive distortions, fewer tax avoidance opportunities, more transparency and information exchange amongst those taking part, and less compliance costs for businesses and operators across the EU.[70]

The Commission argued that the FTT would lead to fewer barriers and competitive distortions, as a 'common system of taxing the financial sector, even if not applied by all Member States, is preferable to the fragmentation that would result from 27 different national systems'.[71] The Commission also stated that this proposal would respect the competences and rights of non-participating Member States, giving as an example the fact that non-participating Member States would not be precluded from having their own national FTTs if they wanted to.[72]

This proposal, supported by 10 Member States at the time and eventually 11 Member States[73] was approved by the European Parliament in December

[67] See 'EU Update' (2012) 52 *European Taxation* 25–26.

[68] See PwC EU Tax Direct Group Newsflashes (Oct 2012): 'Germany and France push for EU financial transactions tax'. Available at: www.pwc.com/gx/en/tax/newsletters/eu-direct-tax-newsflashes/eudtg-newsflash-2012-4okt.jhtml.

[69] See Press Release, *Commission proposes green light for enhanced cooperation on financial transactions tax* (IP/12/1138 dated 23/10/2012).

[70] See European Commission, *Enhanced Cooperation on Financial Transaction Tax—Questions and Answers* (MEMO/12/799 dated 23/10/2012).

[71] *Ibid.*

[72] *Ibid.*

[73] Austria, Belgium, Finland, France, Germany, Greece, Italy, Portugal, Spain, Slovenia and Slovakia.

2012.[74] In the January 2013 ECOFIN Council, the adoption of the FTT through enhanced cooperation was eventually approved by qualified majority.[75] However, the UK, Luxemburg, Malta and the Czech Republic raised concerns that the Commission had not provided any analysis of the impacts that an enhanced cooperation FTT would have on individual Member States, both participating and non-participating ones. Furthermore, the UK tabled a minute statement[76] stating that it could not support the proposal as it could not take a view whether the conditions of enhanced cooperation were met.[77] The dissenting Member States abstained from voting.

Notwithstanding the disagreement of the UK and some other Member States, on 14 February 2013, the Commission published a new proposal for a Council directive implementing enhanced cooperation in the area of financial transaction tax,[78] accompanied by another Impact Assessment.[79]

The main change and perhaps the most important one compared to the 2011 FTT proposal was the issuance principle, whereby financial instruments issued in the participating Member States would be taxed when traded, even if the parties trading them were not established in FTT Member States. This principle was added as an anti-avoidance measure against the relocation of activities or establishments outside participating Member States and served as a last resort as regards the establishment of tax liability.[80] The issuance principle complimented the principle of establishment which remained the main principle. It is thought to be the most contentious recommendation as in certain circumstances it could

[74] See European Parliament/News, 'Eleven EU countries get Parliament's all clear for a financial transaction tax', Plenary Session Economic and monetary affairs—12.12.2012. Available at: www.europarl.europa.eu/news/en/pressroom/content/20121207IPR04408/html/Eleven-EU-countries-get-Parliament%27s-all-clear-for-a-financial-transaction-tax.

[75] See Council of the European Union, 'Financial transaction tax: Council agrees to enhanced cooperation', Brussels, 22 January 2013, 5555/13, PRESSE 23. Available at: register.consilium.europa.eu/pdf/en/13/st05/st05555.en13.pdf (last accessed 2 March 2013).

[76] See Written Ministerial Statement, ECOFIN 22 January 2013, www.parliament.uk/documents/commons-vote-office/January_2013/30-01-13/2.CHANCELLOR-ECOFIN-22-January.pdf.

[77] These conditions included the following: any such cooperation shall not undermine the internal market or economic, social and territorial cohesion; such cooperation shall not constitute a barrier to or discrimination in trade between Member States, nor distort competition between them; and any enhanced cooperation shall respect the competences, rights and obligations of those Member States which do not participate in it. Also see analysis of enhanced cooperation in section 8.1 above.

[78] Proposal for a Council Directive implementing enhanced cooperation in the area of financial transaction tax, COM(2013) 71 final (henceforth, the 2013 FTT Proposal). With this, the Commission withdrew the original proposal. For commentary, see Joachim Englisch et al (2013), n 5 above, p 243; Vogel and Cortez, n 65 above; Nicolas de Boynes, Andrew Thomson & Pierre-Antoine Bachellerie, 'European Commission's Revised Draft Directive on the Financial Transaction Tax' (2013) 70 *Tax Notes International* 353 (22 April 2013); Raymond Adema, 'Financial Transaction Tax: Pan-European Market for Master-Feeder Structures—or Part of It—Smothered?' (2010) 42 *Intertax* 653–61.

[79] See Commission Staff Working Document, *Impact Assessment accompanying the document Proposal for a Council Directive implementing enhanced cooperation in the area of financial transaction tax: analysis of policy options and impacts*', SWD(2013) 28 final of 14 February 2013 (henceforth, the 2013 Impact Assessment). This was meant to be read together with the impact assessment accompanying the 2011 proposal.

[80] See 2013 FTT Proposal, n 78 above, p 5.

have extraterritorial effects. For example, FTT would be due when a bank established in the USA bought shares originally issued in Germany from a bank in Singapore. Both banks would be subject to FTT as the shares had been issued in Germany.[81]

Another change was that, in the management of public debt, Member States and other public bodies were excluded from the scope of the directive.[82] Also, the European Central Bank, the European Financial Stability Facility and the European Stability Mechanism were explicitly referred to as being exempt from the FTT.[83] The issuance of shares and units in collective investment funds and restructuring operations were also excluded from the scope of taxation.[84] Also, exchanges of financial instruments were regarded as two transactions for tax purposes but repurchase and reverse agreements and securities lending and borrowing were regarded as only one transaction, as they were considered to be economically equivalent to a single credit operation.[85] Furthermore, a general anti-abuse rule was inserted whereby an artificial arrangement or an artificial series of arrangements which had been put into place for the essential purpose of avoiding taxation and led to a tax benefit would be ignored.[86]

Furthermore, the revenue estimate was adjusted and the Commission expected about €30–35 billion per year. Part of this would be added to the EU Budget directly as an own resource, reducing the contributions of participating Member States accordingly.

On 2 July 2013, the European Parliament discussed the FTT proposal, along with amendments recommended by its Committee on Economic and Monetary Affairs.[87] Opponents and supporters of the FTT aired their views.[88] The following day, the European Parliament approved the 2013 FTT Proposal.[89] However, its role in the process was only advisory. The Commission and the participating Member States were free to accept or reject any changes.

[81] For more examples, see Boynes et al (2013), n 78 above, pp 356–58; Englisch et al (2013), n 5 above.

[82] See Art 3(2)(c) of the 2013 FTT Proposal, n 78 above.

[83] *Ibid*, Art 3(4).

[84] *Ibid*, Art 3(4)(a).

[85] *Ibid*, Art 2(2).

[86] *Ibid*, Art 13(1). Pursuant to this provision, participating Member States shall treat these arrangements for tax purposes by reference to their economic substance. An arrangement was defined widely and may comprise more than one step or part (Art 13(2)). An arrangement was artificial if it lacked commercial substance. See Art 13(3). A number of situations listed were to be taken into account. The purpose of an arrangement was to avoid taxation 'where, regardless of any subjective intentions of the taxpayer, it defeats the object, spirit and purpose of the tax provisions that would otherwise apply' (see Art 13(4)).

[87] See Committee on Economic and Monetary Affairs, *Report on the proposal for a Council directive implementing enhanced cooperation in the area of financial transaction tax*, 24 June 2013 (COM(201)0071—C7, 0049/2013—2013/0045(CNS), A7-0230/2013).

[88] David D Stewart, 'FTT Opponents Air Concerns as European Parliament Takes Up Amended Proposal', 2013 *WTD* 128-1 (3 July 2013).

[89] David D Stewart, 'European Parliament Approves Amended FTT Proposal', 2013 *WTD* 129-2 (5 July 2013).

In September 2013, an internal legal opinion prepared by the EU Council Legal Service raised concerns that the proposed FTT would have an extraterritorial reach that would infringe upon the taxing rights of non-participating Member States.[90] It was also concluded that the proposed FTT breached international law norms which had to be respected under EU law, that it was discriminatory and it led to distortion of competition. However, the Commission continued to support the FTT unabated. Indicatively, on 4 February 2014, at a plenary debate at the European Parliament, EU Tax Commissioner Algirdas Šemeta spoke of the impact and future goals of the FTT. He noted: 'Europe needs to reconnect with its citizens. And the FTT is a prime example of a project which can help to achieve this'.[91] Quite how this is case—when all costs to financial institutions are expected to eventually be passed on to the consumers/citizens—is not explained.

As already mentioned, a number of Member States were against the initial proposal for the FTT and the subsequently revised proposal. The most vocal and proactive opponent has been the UK, which eventually challenged the Commission's actions at the Court of Justice. The UK Government's reaction to the FTT is considered in the next section.

8.3. The Financial Transaction Tax and Enhanced Cooperation: The UK Reaction

Broadly indicative of the UK's stance on the FTT, on 26 March 2013 the House of Lords European Union Committee published a letter that it had sent to the Financial Secretary of HM Treasury, Mr Greg Clark, urging the UK to challenge the authorising decision.[92] In this letter, the Committee criticised the 'paucity of thinking' in the FTT proposal and the lack of action by the UK Government.[93]

One criticism levied against the Commission's proposal was the lack of information given on how the tax would be collected and the costs that might

[90] David D Stewart and Stephanie Soong Johnston, 'EU Council Opinion Casts Doubt on Legality of Financial Transaction Tax', 2013 *WTD* 176-1 (11 September 2013); Adrian Cloer and Stefan Trencsik, 'Alive and Deadly—The European Financial Transaction Tax through Enhanced Cooperation: Current Progress' (2014) 54 *European Taxation* 307–12. Some authors have also expressed concerns that the FTT is in breach of the fundamental freedoms and more specifically, Art 63 TFEU. See Pablo A Hernández González-Barreda, 'On the European Way to a Financial Transaction Tax under Enhanced Cooperation: Multi-Speed Europe or Shortcut?', n 39 above; George Dietlein, 'National Approaches Towards a Financial Transaction Tax and their Compatibility with European Law' (2012) 21 *EC Tax Review* 207–11.

[91] See *Financial Transaction Tax: Time to engage, compromise and deliver—Plenary debate in Parliament*, available on Tax Analysts, 2014 *WTD* 24-10 (5 February 2014).

[92] See House of Lords, European Union Committee Letter dated 16 April 2013, p 4, available on www.parliament.uk/documents/lords-committees/eu-sub-com-a/FTTEnhancedScrutiny/260313FTT.pdf.

[93] See Stephanie Soong Johnston, 'Legal Action Possible Against EU Financial Transaction Tax, UK Lawmakers say', 2013 *WTD* 60-2 (28 March 2013).

accrue to non-participating Member States. The Committee asked for clarifications on the obligation of the UK authorities to collect the tax. Even though the UK had opted not to adopt the FTT and would not benefit from the collection of revenue, UK financial institutions entering into financial transactions with financial institutions in participating Member States would still be liable for the FTT. The FTT levy could be collected through the Mutual Assistance Directive for the Recovery of Taxes[94] or as a result of the provisions on joint and several liability set out in the proposal.[95] This is notwithstanding the fact that the Commission representative giving oral evidence to the Committee, Mr Manfred Bergmann, had said that there would be no legal obligation on UK tax authorities to collect the FTT—no greater obligation than that of non-UK financial institutions under the UK stamp duty.[96] This argument was also raised in the Commission's 2013 Impact Assessment and has been criticised. The comparison of the FTT with the Stamp Duty Reserve Tax regime is not very accurate, as the former is a tax on the financial sector rather than capital investment, which is entirely unrelated to the location of the companies whose shares are traded.[97]

[94] Council Directive 2010/24/EU of 16 March 2010 Concerning Mutual Assistance for the Recovery of Claims Relating to Taxes, Duties and Other Measures, repealing Council Directive 76/308/EEC of 15 March 1976 on Mutual Assistance for the Recovery of Claims Resulting from Operations Forming Part of the System of Financing the European Agricultural Guidance and Guarantee Fund and of Agricultural Levies and Customs Duties and in Respect of Value Added Tax and Certain Excise Duties.

[95] See House of Lords letter, n 92 above, p 2.

[96] *Ibid.* More correctly, it is the Stamp Duty Reserve Tax that the Commission representative should have mentioned. In any case, the comparison is not correct, as discussed immediately below.

[97] See Englisch et al (2013), n 5 above, pp 243–44. It is pointed out by the authors that the UK Stamp Duty has evolved historically as a tax upon the use of certain instruments needed to give effect to an agreed change in (share) ownership and its eventual registration. The Stamp Duty Reserve Tax is a tax on electronic (paperless) share transactions and was introduced when electronic settlement of share transactions began to take place in the London stock market. As explained on the HMRC website, you pay Stamp Duty Reserve Tax on paperless transactions when you buy shares in a UK company, shares in a foreign company with a share register in the UK, an option to buy shares, rights arising from shares already owned, an interest in shares, like an interest in the money made from selling them and units in unit trusts or shares in open-ended investment companies. Most paperless share transactions subject to this tax are carried out electronically through CREST, the electronic settlement and registration system administered by Euroclear. The amount of Stamp Duty Reserve Tax payable is worked out at a flat rate of 0.5 per cent (rounded up or down to the nearest penny) based on what you give for the shares, not what the shares are worth. See www.hmrc.gov.uk/sdrt/intro/basics.htm. This tax is automatically collected by CREST and sent to HMRC. Therefore, it is not collected by financial institutions or other parties trading the shares. Also, there are a number of exemptions for overseas exchange traded funds, though some foreign 'off-market' transactions of shares in UK corporations are also caught by the Stamp Duty Reserve Tax. Englisch et al (2013), n 5 above, argue that '[a] tax on capital levied by the country where the intangible representing the capital investment is "located", as determined by the issuance principle, can possibly be defended in the light of the territoriality principle, at least to the extent that it can reasonably be expected to be collected by institutions and intermediaries (e.g. stockbrokers) which are established domestically': *ibid*, pp 243–44. For more information on the UK's Stamp Duty Reserve Tax, see, inter alios, Reginald S Nock, *Monroe & Nock on the Law of Stamp Duties* (Sweet & Maxwell, loose-leaf last updated in 2012), James Mirrlees et al, *Tax By Design: The Mirrlees Review* (Oxford University Press, 2011) and John A Kay and Mervyn A King, *The British Tax System*, 5th edn (Oxford University Press, 1990).

The House of Lords Committee was of the opinion that under the FTT proposal, the UK financial institutions would be burdened with the obligation to pay the FTT tax, even if the UK was a non-participating Member State. Even more far-reaching consequences would apply in relation to the FTT tax imposed on the basis of the issuance principle. The Committee gave the example of a financial transaction involving German shares between a US and a UK financial institution. Under the issuance principle, this would give rise to an FTT on both parties which would be payable to the German tax authorities but the collection of this tax from the US financial institution might be difficult. The Committee believed that 'the proposal would enable the German tax authorities to impose joint and several liability for both instances of the FTT upon the UK financial institution and recover the whole amount using the EU mutual assistance regime'.[98] Such consequences would be serious and must be resisted, the Committee thought, especially if account is taken of the fact that a portion of the revenue would constitute a new own resource for the EU Budget.[99] This would raise 'the spectre that an FTT imposed on a financial institution resident in a non-participating Member State such as the UK would reduce the national contribution of a participating Member State'.[100] A related argument was that the issuance principle often triggered extraterritorial effects and this risked being non-compliant with customary international law. Although the UK stamp duty was based on the issuance principle, it had a much narrower scope.[101]

The uncertainty as regards the use of potential revenue from the FTT was highlighted by the House of Lords Committee. The fact that revenue collected could be used as a new own resource for the EU Budget, resulting in a corresponding reduction of the national contributions of participating Member States, would raise 'the deeply unpalatable prospect that an FTT imposed on a financial institution resident in a non-participating Member State such as the UK would reduce the national contribution of a participating Member State'.[102] There was in fact a great concern even under the original proposal in 2011 that, given London's strength as a financial centre, a disproportionate majority of the revenues would be coming from the UK, rendering a European FTT 'more of a tax on London than on the EU'.[103] A European-FTT might not even raise any additional money for the UK, as

[98] House of Lords letter, n 92 above, pp 4–5.
[99] *Ibid*, p 5.
[100] *Ibid.*
[101] See analysis in n 97 above.
[102] House of Lords letter, n 92 above, p 2.
[103] For example, the UK would lose about £3 billion per year in stamp duty, as under the 2011 FTT Proposal the UK stamp duty would be replaced by the FTT. Furthermore, there would be a reduction of corporation tax receipts from the financial sector due to the impact of the tax and a reduction of income tax receipts from the possible loss of jobs of financial sector employees etc. See letter by Stuart Fraser, Policy Chairman at the City of London Corporation, in 'Letters: How can you tax transactions that are no longer there?', *Financial Times*, 7 October 2011. Also see House of Lords EU Economic and Financial Affairs and International Trade Sub-Committee, *Financial Transaction Tax: Oral and Written Evidence*, 28 November 2011, pp 190–91 and Seely (2013), n 40 above, pp 14–17.

any gains would be offset by losses in other taxes due to the impact of the tax.[104] It is unfortunate that neither the 2011 FTT Proposal nor the provisions suggested under the 2013 FTT Proposal addressed these concerns.

The House of Lords Committee also commented on the fact that the Commission had not given much information about the implications of the proposal for non-participating Member States. There was no detailed analysis of the impact of the FTT on non-participating Member States in the 2013 Impact Assessment.

> We find this to be an unacceptable omission, suggesting that the Commission has failed in its duty to the 16 Member States who have thus far chosen not to participate in the tax, yet may be significantly affected by it.[105]

Moreover, the UK Government was accused of complacency and was criticised for not keeping the House of Lords Committee duly informed. It was warned that just because the UK will not participate in the FTT, this does not mean that 'the reverberations of an FTT would not be felt here'.[106] The Committee urged the government to cooperate with the other non-participating Member States to try and avert the worse consequences of this proposal.[107]

The Committee also voiced concerns that the 2013 Impact Assessment did not adequately address the potentially deleterious effect of the FTT on economic growth.[108] It was questioned whether the FTT would have a negative impact on economic growth and it was argued that 'at a time of ongoing financial crisis and at best fragile economic growth across the entire EU, a new tax which could have a substantial detrimental impact on EU GDP should be resisted'.[109] The Committee was also unconvinced that the FTT would curb irresponsible trading and enhance the efficiency of financial markets, an avowed purpose of the FTT proposal.[110] Given the continuous US hostility to the proposal, the Committee also remained unconvinced that an EU-wide FTT would pave the way for the introduction of a global tax.

Finally, the House of Lords Committee criticised the way the UK Government had handled the use of the enhanced cooperation procedure and emphasised the need to create alliances with non-participating Member States.[111] It was questioned whether the proposal met the criteria for the enhanced cooperation to be used and especially whether it would create a distortion of competition.[112] The Committee thought that it was 'particularly unacceptable that a full analysis of

[104] See Letter from Rt Hon George Osborne to Rt Hon Andrew Tyrie MP, Chairman, House of Commons Treasury Committee, 12 December 2011, cited by Seely (2013), n 40 above, p 17.

[105] House of Lords letter, n 92 above, p 3.

[106] *Ibid*, p 5.

[107] *Ibid*, p 5.

[108] *Ibid*, p 6.

[109] *Ibid*.

[110] *Ibid*, p 7.

[111] *Ibid*, p 8.

[112] The possibility of double taxation was conceded by the Commission. The Commission did not go into this in much detail in the 2013 Impact Assessment: House of Lords letter, n 92 above, p 8.

the impact of the proposal on non-participating Member States was not made available before the vote on enhanced cooperation took place'.[113]

This highly critical letter must have had some influence on the UK Government's policy as shortly thereafter, on 18 April 2014, an application was lodged to the Court of Justice to challenge the authorising decision to adopt the FTT through enhanced cooperation.[114] An HM Treasury spokesman emphasised that the UK was not against the principle of a global financial transactions tax, 'but think that a European-only tax would hit people's savings and pensions and hit jobs and growth'.[115] While the UK would not participate in a Europe-only tax, 'we have also said we will not stand in the way of other countries, but only if the rights of countries not taking part are respected'.[116] The UK lodged the challenge as it believed that the proposal on the table did not meet these requirements. More specifically, the UK was concerned with the extraterritorial impact of the FTT.[117]

The UK Government's challenge was welcomed by the House of Lords European Union Committee.[118] Since then, more stakeholders have expressed their support for the UK Government and disapproval of the FTT. On 17 February 2014, the Law Society commented that its chief executive had written to key European finance ministers to raise the Society's concerns that the proposal would not sufficiently respect the rights and competences of the countries that have chosen not to participate. He argued that the effects of the proposed tax would 'force a degree of participation' on countries that choose not to participate.[119] Similarly, the City of London has issued a special interest paper examining how the proposed FTT would affect European households' savings, specifically with regard to Germany, Italy, Spain, Slovakia, Luxembourg and the UK.[120]

On 30 April 2014, the Court of Justice rejected the UK's challenge to the Commission's decision to authorise the use of enhanced cooperation.[121] The request to annul the Commission's decision was rejected on the basis that its arguments were founded on the draft Directive (ie the 2013 FTT Proposal), which was not part of the decision to authorise the use of enhanced cooperation. The review of the Court of Justice was limited to the issue of whether that decision was valid as such in light of Article 20 TEU and Articles 326–334 TFEU, which defined the substantive and

[113] *Ibid*, p 9.

[114] See Case C-209/13 *United Kingdom v Council* [2015] ECR I-0000.

[115] The comments were reported in Tax Analysts on 23 April 2013. Stephanie Soong Johnston (2013) n 93 above. Also see Christiana HJI Panayi, 'The EU's Financial Transaction Tax, Enhanced Cooperation and the UK's challenge' (2013) 53 *European Taxation* 358–67.

[116] Stephanie Soong Johnston (2013) n 93 above.

[117] See statements made by the Chancellor of the Exchequer George Osborne in the press, available at: www.independent.co.uk/news/uk/politics/osborne-in-legal-challenge-to-european-commission-over-financial-transaction-tax-8581165.html.

[118] Also see Christiana HJ1 Panayi, 'The EU's Financial Transaction Tax, Enhanced cooperation and the UK's challenge', n 115 above.

[119] See Tax Analysts, Doc 2014-3586 (18 February 2014).

[120] See *The Effect of a Financial Transaction Tax on European Households' Savings*, published in Tax Analysts on 17 February 2014. See 2014 *WTD* 33-16.

[121] Case C-209/13 *United Kingdom v Council*, n 114 above.

procedural conditions relating to the granting of such authorisation. 'That review should not be confused with the review which may be undertaken, in the context of a subsequent action for annulment, of a measure adopted for the purposes of the implementation of the authorised enhanced cooperation'.[122]

Therefore, the challenge was premature. As far as the UK Government's specific arguments were concerned, the Court of Justice did not consider them. Furthermore, the Court noted that the contested decision contained no provisions relating to the issue of expenditure.[123] As such, it was

> obvious that the question of the possible effects of the future FTT on the administrative costs of the non-participating Member States cannot be examined for as long as the principles of taxation in respect of that tax have not been definitively established as part of the implementation of the enhanced cooperation authorised by the contested decision.[124]

The overtone of the Court's decision was that if and when an FTT is adopted under enhanced cooperation, it may be possible to challenge the substance of the measures at that point. Therefore, a subsequent challenge could be admissible, depending on the form and scope of any FTT.

8.4. The Future of the Financial Transaction Tax

At the May 2014 ECOFIN meeting, finance ministers from 10 of the participating Member States[125] reiterated their commitment to the FTT by issuing a joint statement. In the press release, the intention of participating Member States to work on a progressive implementation of the FTT, focusing initially on the taxation of shares and certain derivatives, was noted.[126] It was also noted that the first steps would be implemented at the latest on 1 January 2016.

Following this joint statement, it was thought that the FTT might initially involve a tax on equities and equity derivatives only, with a possible wider scoped tax at a later stage. The participating Member States would be permitted to maintain taxation of instruments that were not within the scope of the tax levied under the initial launch. Much remained to be agreed, particularly on further phases of the tax and the position of smaller Member States.

[122] *Ibid*, para 34.

[123] *Ibid*, para 37.

[124] *Ibid*, para 38.

[125] Slovakia, which was among the 11 participating Member States, did not sign the joint statement as at the time it was considering whether to withdraw from the initiative. See Stephanie Soong Johnston, 'EU Financial Transaction Tax to Take Effect in 2016 Despite Strong Opposition', 2014 *WTD* 88-1 (7 May 2014). Also see PwC bulletin available at pwc.to/1xIckFn and Ernst & Young bulletin available at: bit.ly/1zwbWtU.

[126] Press Release (PRESSE 242, PR CO 22) 3310th Council meeting, ECOFIN 6 May 2014, p 9. Available at: bit.ly/1qOX84f.

On 7 November 2014, the French Finance Minister, Michel Sapin, presented a revised, scaled-down version of the FTT to ECOFIN ministers to address concerns of smaller countries that they would be negatively affected by the FTT. Under his proposal, only transfers of shares of companies domiciled in one of the 11 participating Member States that had agreed in principle to the FTT would be subject to the tax. The FTT would not apply to all activities but credit default swaps not handled by clearinghouses would be taxed.[127] Subsequently, a document prepared by the Italian government for an ambassadors' meeting on 10 December 2014 revealed that several of the participating Member States might not be able to meet their self-imposed deadline to agree on the scope and rates of the tax by the end of 2014. More work was needed especially on the scope of the derivatives that would be taxed, how the tax would be collected, and how far-reaching the tax would be.[128]

At the ECOFIN meeting in January 2015, in another joint statement, ministers from 10 Member States reiterated their commitment to implementing the FTT in stages, adding that the tax should be based on the principle of the widest possible base and low rates.[129] It was announced that progress had been made on the scope of the FTT for transactions in shares, while the taxation of transactions in derivatives remained a key open question. Further reflection was necessary on the taxation principles to be applied for the FTT (residence principle, issuance principle) as well as on the mechanism to be used for collecting the FTT.

Therefore, despite the continuous opposition by some Member States and numerous lobbying bodies,[130] the participating Member States as well as the Commission have not abandoned the idea of launching the FTT. There were reports that the participating[131] Member States are likely to come to an agreement on the FTT by the June 2015 ECOFIN meeting, though the instrument is unlikely to be ready by 2016.[132] While there is still quite a lot of confusion as to when the FTT will be launched, what it will eventually encompass, whether it will eventually restore public confidence in the financial sector or whether it will have the opposite effect with widespread relocation from the European Union to third countries,

[127] William Hoke, 'France Proposes Scaled Down Version of Financial Transaction Tax', 2014 *WTD* 214-3 (5 November 2014).

[128] Stephanie Soong Johnston, 'EU Countries Might Miss Deadline for FTT Deal', 2014 *WTD* 234-1 (5 December 2014).

[129] Outcomes of the Meeting, 3356th Council meeting Economic and Financial Affairs, Brussels, 9 December 2014, 16603/14 (OR. en) Presse 68 PR CO 632. For commentary, see Margaret Burow, 'EU Finance Ministers Offer Up New Financial Transaction Tax Proposals', 2015 *WTD* 15-3 (23 January 2015).

[130] See, for example, the letter sent by the European Association of Cooperative Banks (EACB), the European Association of Public Banks (EAPB) and the European Banking Federation (EBF), published in Tax Analysts on 23 January 2015 (see 2015 *WTD* 21-19).

[131] Slovenia has since said it may withdraw from the initiative, reportedly because of its dissatisfaction with the tax in its current form. See Stephanie Soong Johnston, 'EU Financial Transaction Tax to Take Effect in 2016 Despite Strong Opposition', 2014 *WTD* 88-1 (7 May 2015).

[132] Stephanie Soong Johnston, 'EU FTT by 2016 Unlikely, Austrian Finance Minister Says', 2015 *WTD* 95-3 (18 May 2015).

and whether in general that is the right legislative instrument for the European Union,[133] the proposal still features high on the agenda of many Member States.

Nevertheless, it should be emphasised that linking tax legislation with enhanced cooperation could have broader constitutional implications. While the existence of the fiscal veto has always been criticised for stifling further tax integration in the EU, especially in the area of direct taxation, the perils of partial integration should not be underestimated. The developments surrounding the FTT are a good illustration of this. They show the potential of enhanced cooperation leading to a situation where non-participating Member States bear the burdens of deeper tax integration without reaping the benefits. Furthermore, as the use of the enhanced cooperation procedure is still at an embryonic stage and experience from it is almost non-existent, there are still concerns as to how it should be conducted overall—eg the level of consultation that should be undertaken during the process, how much protection should be given to non-participating Member States and built into the instrument, the cost implications, the resolution of disputes etc. It is one thing to allow flexible and coordinated action between Member States to promote further (tax) integration between them; it is another to circumvent principles of natural justice and good governance in the European Union under this pretext.

Although as argued,[134] the limits of the European Union's legislative competence are in practice imprecisely defined by the Treaty itself, enabling legislative institutions to enjoy wide discretion, as far as taxation is concerned, there is a strong and entrenched tradition of deference to Member States' sovereignty. If this is to be eroded, whether permanently or occasionally or as a one-off situation, then, arguably, this should be done gradually and in a transparent way. The FTT proposal is undeniably a very bold and controversial project. It would have been preferable if it was not introduced through enhanced cooperation—a process highly contentious itself. This combination is unlikely to yield the best possible results. It might also set a dangerous precedent as it would enable Member States pushing for more tax harmonisation to fast-track legislative proposals on the pretext of tackling aggressive tax planning.

133 There have been arguments that a Financial Activities Tax might be a preferable option. See Josephine Kaiding, 'The Financial Transaction Tax: The Way Forward for the European Union?' (2014) 23 *EC Tax Review* 30–42, and studies cited at p 41 et seq.

134 See, for example, Stephen Weatherill, 'The Limit of Legislative Harmonisation Ten Years after Tobacco Advertising: How the Court's Case Law has become a "Drafting Guide"' (2011) 12 *German Law Journal* 827. He explains that the Court of Justice has produced broad guidelines and EU legislature follows and adopts similar vague vocabulary, which is unlikely to be challenged in Court.

9

International and European Union Tax Law in the Post-BEPS World

This book set out to provide an overview of recent developments in the field of international taxation as well as in the field of EU tax law. Most of the developments were centred around the polemic against aggressive tax planning and the momentum that has been developed both internationally and in the European Union.

At the beginning of the book, there was an overview of the various factors and events that led to the launch of the BEPS project. What became apparent was that there was some sort of continuum of efforts to address the same or a similar problem, which seems to be rebranded and/or reconfigured every few years. The rhetoric against harmful tax competition and tax havens seems now to have been reconfigured to the rhetoric against aggressive tax planning. This has attracted a lot of attention by advocacy groups and NGOs, and lately the media. All these bodies have had an important role in raising public awareness on the topic. It is often claimed that the existence of tax havens has contributed to the financial crisis and has had an impact on the fiscal sustainability of countries, although there is no concrete evidence to this effect. On the other hand, the offensive against tax havens could be perceived as merely a populist measure to deflect the peoples' (essentially voters') attention from the real problems and factors that led to the financial crisis.

The strategies used by some large MNEs to benefit from low effective tax rates and/or create stateless income were then examined, mostly in light of several investigations by source states and residence states. The underlying tone of the various investigations and hearings considered was that multinationals should follow the spirit and not just the letter of the law—and pay taxes according to that. This seems to be buttressed by an overriding concept of tax morality or tax justice which trumps black-letter law.

What seems to be emerging is that due to the inadequacy of existing principles of international tax law, vague concepts of morality and fairness are increasingly becoming prevalent, to the detriment of legal certainty. The perception of taxpayers in many countries is that the system is unfair or broken—this is worsened by the global financial crisis and heightened by media scrutiny into the taxation of MNEs. It was argued in Chapter one that the injection of notions of morality into the debate has added further complexity and uncertainty to an already complicated area. It was also questioned whether standards of morality and fairness have a place in corporate taxation.

The notions of corporate social responsibility (CSR) and good governance in tax matters were analysed, with emphasis on the former. The link between CSR and aggressive tax planning was considered, both internationally and within the European Union. It was argued that it was a slippery slope for a country to expect to raise or increase corporate tax revenues from CSR. The international tax system is all about choices. A company should not be deemed socially irresponsible for benefitting from certain choices if those choices are available and there are no rules against them, either as hard law or soft law.

It was questioned whether companies that engage in aggressive tax planning are indeed socially irresponsible. While it might be difficult to justify why the payment of full (or higher) taxes is a significant act of social responsibility and even of patriotism, it was recognised that there could be business reasons for avoiding aggressive tax planning. Therefore, notwithstanding the lack of conclusive evidence on the point and the author's belief that CSR should play no role on how a company conducts its tax affairs, it was conceded that CSR implications are likely to become predominant in the whole debate.

Combined with the launch of the OECD/G20 BEPS project and the uncertainties surrounding the deliverables, it would seem that tax arrangements are being assessed on an increasingly ill-defined set of criteria.

In Chapters two to four, the reports under the BEPS project published up until 1 June 2015 were considered in greater detail. From the launch of the BEPS project, the OECD declared that it would not carry out a holistic review of the international tax regime. It was stated in the Action Plan that the project was not directly aimed at changing the existing international standards on the allocation of taxing rights on cross-border income. What it sought to do was to restore both source and residence taxation where cross-border income would otherwise go untaxed or would be taxed at very low rates. For most of the deliverables, the OECD did not make drastic recommendations but was rather limited to realistic compromises that had more chances of success and consensus.

In the Digital Economy discussion drafts produced for the purposes of Action 1, the OECD acknowledged that it would be impossible to ring-fence the digital economy for the purposes of creating separate tax rules, as the digital economy was increasingly becoming the economy itself. Some options for reform to address the broader tax challenges raised by the digital economy were made, though nothing specific recommended. As the digital economy is in a continuous state of evolution, future developments would need to be monitored to evaluate their impact on tax systems. For the time being, the tensions and disagreements remain unresolved and the fate of the digital economy deliverables remains uncertain.

Several proposals were made in the context of the rest of the Action items. As far as hybrids were concerned under Action 2, inter alia, linking rules were suggested to ensure there is no double non-taxation. The CFC discussion draft under Action 3 was not a consensus document and followed a best practices approach.

The discussion draft on interest deductibility under Action 4 also adopted a best practices approach but there were two main suggestions: a group-wide approach and a fixed ratio approach.

As far as Action 5 was concerned (countering harmful tax practices more effectively), a proposal for a modified nexus approach was made as well as a proposal for compulsory spontaneous exchange of taxpayer-specific rulings related to preferential regimes. Concrete recommendations were also made in the Treaty Abuse deliverables produced under Action 6. It was recommended to include in the title and preamble of tax treaties a clear statement that the Contracting States, when entering into a treaty, wish to prevent tax avoidance and intend to avoid creating opportunities for double non-taxation and treaty shopping. An LOB (limitation on benefits) and a PPT (principal purpose test) were also recommended as a minimum standard of protection through a flexible approach. There was a refinement of this flexible approach in follow-up discussion drafts.

In the original discussion draft under Action 7, proposals were made for changes to prevent abuse of the permanent establishment threshold through commissionaire arrangements. Several alternative options were given setting out variations in the wording of suggested paragraphs 5 and 6 of Article 5 of the OECD Model, with the aim of tackling commissionaire arrangements. Suggestions were also made as regards the specific activity exemption of the permanent establishment definition. Rules on the fragmentation of activities between related parties and on the splitting up of contracts were suggested. In the Revised PE Discussion Draft, the OECD explained which options should be followed.

The OECD's work on intangibles, under Action 8, is at the heart of the BEPS project. Taxation of intangibles has long been considered as one of the most challenging aspects of transfer pricing. The mantra used in the BEPS project is that taxable profits (and here taxable intangible returns) should correspond to value creation. There is a lot of vagueness as to what that entails and in general it is quite hard to design rules that correctly allocate intangible-related returns.

The focus of the discussion drafts under Action 8 was on value-creating functions, rather than the bearing of risk through contractual arrangements, or the implications of legal rights on remuneration. Rules would be developed for risk and capital allocation to match returns with activities rather than contractual arrangements. It was suggested that the legal owner of an intangible should be entitled to all returns attributable to the intangible only if, in substance, it performed and controlled all of the important functions related to the development, enhancement, maintenance and protection of the intangibles; it controlled other functions outsourced to independent enterprises or associated enterprises and compensated those functions on an arm's length basis; it provided all assets necessary to the development, enhancement, maintenance, and protection of the intangibles; and bore and controlled all of the risks and costs related to the development, enhancement, maintenance and protection of the intangible. To the extent that one or more members of the MNE group other than the legal owner performed the above functions, returns attributable to the intangible had to accrue to such other members through arm's length compensation reflecting their anticipated contribution to the intangible value. This could, depending on the facts and circumstances, constitute all or a substantial part of the return attributable to the intangible. Follow-up reports led to a proposal for the whole of Chapter VI of the OECD Transfer Pricing Guidelines to be redrafted in line with these recommendations and be entitled 'Special Considerations for Intangible Property'.

Similarly, the CCA Discussion Draft, again in the context of Action 8, acknowledged the need to simplify the measurement of contributions and to ensure that contributions were commensurate with the benefits received under a CCA. It reinforced the notion that the contribution of each participant to a CCA should be reflective of value contribution. The suggested revisions to the OECD Transfer Pricing Guidelines on CCAs would similarly support the use of value contributed over the costs incurred.

The rest of the transfer pricing deliverables produced guidelines in different areas. A discussion draft on low value-adding intra-group services made proposals which would fully rewrite Chapter VII of the OECD's Transfer Pricing Guidelines on intercompany services and would include an elective simplified approach. The Profit Split Discussion Draft examined several key issues related to the application of transactional profit split methods, gave illustrative scenarios for discussion purposes and posed some questions for public discussion. A proposal for clarification of the guidance in Chapter II of the OECD Transfer Pricing Guidelines was made in the Commodities Discussion Draft, as well as other suggestions.

Very importantly, the Risk and Re-characterisation Discussion Draft reduced the importance of contractual allocations of risk while raising the importance of functions such as managing and controlling risks. The draft focused on identifying the actual conduct of the parties for the purposes of delineating a controlled transaction. Attention was to be paid to the contractual terms of the transaction, the functions performed, the characteristics of the property transferred, the economic circumstances of the parties and their business strategies. The Risk and Re-characterisation Discussion Draft also added a substantially new section on non-recognition and introduced the concept of fundamental economic attributes of arrangements between unrelated parties.

Under Action 11, the discussion document sought to set out options to establish methodologies to collect and analyse data on BEPS. The options included in this discussion draft did not represent conclusions on the assessments or proposed measures, but were intended to provide stakeholders with substantive options for analysis and comment.

The Mandatory Disclosure Discussion Document produced under Action 12, examined the usefulness of disclosure initiatives in addressing the lack of comprehensive and relevant information on tax planning strategies available to tax authorities. It provided an overview of mandatory disclosure regimes, based on the experiences of countries that had such regimes, and set out recommendations for a modular design of a mandatory disclosure regime.

The country-by-country template produced under Action 13 is perhaps the proposal most likely to be followed by countries internationally without much dissent. In the CbC Revised Discussion Draft, the OECD moved from a two-tier to a three-tier approach. The three-tier approach comprised a master file, a local file, and a separate country-by-country template that had been proposed in the OECD's earlier work on this topic. The country-by-country information was to be reported to tax authorities at a very high level and for risk assessment purposes only. The amount of information being requested for risk assessment purposes was significantly curtailed. The CbC Revised Discussion Draft contained revised standards for transfer pricing documentation and a template for country-by-country reporting. In the follow-up report on Action 13, guidance was given on the implementation of country-by-country reporting, such as the timing of preparation and filing of the country-by-country report, which MNE groups should be required to file such report, etc.

In the Dispute Resolution Discussion Draft produced under Action 14, the obstacles to effective dispute resolution were discussed and various options for improving these issues with MAP (mutual agreement procedure) processes explored. However, there were no effective recommendations. The solutions proposed were primarily in the form of suggestions for amending the treaty commentary or statements regarding what different tax administrations could commit to, in order to advance dispute resolution procedures. A monitoring process within an appropriate forum was also considered. No mandatory binding arbitration was recommended, to the dissatisfaction of some stakeholders. Overall, the Dispute Resolution Discussion Draft did not recommend specific dispute resolution measures but merely outlined possibilities. As a result, the existing strained dispute resolution system is likely to come under additional pressure in the post-BEPS world.

The Multilateral Instrument Discussion Draft produced pursuant to Action 15 explored the feasibility of producing a multilateral instrument to address BEPS-related issues. It analysed the tax and public international law issues related to the development of such an instrument without infringing sovereign autonomy in tax matters. It was conceded that a multilateral instrument posed several challenges, although the OECD was positive in that legal mechanisms existed to address these challenges. The most promising approach was to have a multilateral instrument that would co-exist with bilateral tax treaties. It was emphasised that the multilateral instrument should be highly targeted, efficient but also flexible.

In Chapter four, there was also a review of the OECD's engagement with developing countries. Although the importance of developing countries in the BEPS project was mentioned many times by leading OECD figures, it was questioned whether the interests of developing countries were properly reflected in the Action Plan. In fact, there have been complaints that some of the proposals might even prejudice developing countries.

The next chapters examined the measures taken in the European Union to tackle international tax avoidance and aggressive tax planning. There was a consideration of the judicial response to the concept of tax abuse by the Court of

Justice. It was argued that, overall, recent case law suggests that EU law does not provide a general principle of abuse of rights in the field of direct taxation. Whilst a principle of abuse of rights may be deduced from some cases in the area of VAT, it does not apply in a non-harmonised area. It was noted that in the current state of the Court's jurisprudence, it was difficult to conclude that the concept of tax abuse has been de-nationalised and that there is now an EU principle of tax abuse.

The quasi-official policy of the European Union on tax abuse and aggressive tax planning that was formed in the past decade was reviewed in Chapter five. It was noted that initially, emphasis was on making sure that domestic anti-abuse rules did not restrict EU nationals from exercising their fundamental freedoms, such as the freedom of establishment and the free movement of capital. Then there was some focus on preventing double non-taxation, eventually leading to the EU Action Plan to Strengthen the Fight against Tax Fraud and Tax Evasion and the Recommendations on Aggressive Tax Planning and Good Governance. These Commission initiatives and the follow-up measures seem to form the 'new' Commission policy on international tax avoidance.

The main developments that have taken place up to the launch of the Tax Transparency Package are reviewed. What seems apparent is that the pendulum has swung and now the European Union places much more emphasis on tackling tax evasion and aggressive tax planning than it did a decade ago. What is also apparent is that the Commission has seized on this unique political momentum and, as a result, many legislative proposals or amendments that had been lurking for some time have now been fast-tracked at Council level. However, the author argued that some of the measures adopted, or aspects of them, may be incompatible with EU law, as interpreted by the Court of Justice in important cases.

This chapter set the background against which in the following chapter, there was an analysis of the compatibility of the various items of the BEPS Action Plan with EU law. In Chapter six, the analysis showed that quite a few of the BEPS Action items dealt with rules on the determination or allocation of taxing rights and were thus within the scope of Member State competences. However, most of the suggested anti-abuse rules had defects, mainly because they did not target wholly artificial arrangements or because they were applied mechanically in a way that would likely be deemed disproportional by the Court of Justice. Furthermore, proposals that were dependent on taking into account the tax treatment in another Member State might not pass muster at the Court of Justice. Concerns were also raised as regards the OECD's and the Code of Conduct Group's endorsement of a strictly territorial nexus test as regards substance. A comparison between the EU transfer pricing documentation requirements and the OECD's CbC proposal was also made, as well as a comparison of the regimes for dispute resolution. Lastly, the proposal for a multilateral instrument was reviewed and the obligations of Member States in that respect considered.

In Chapter seven, there was a detailed analysis of the state aid provision and its application to fiscal state aids. Following a comprehensive overview of the state aid prohibition and selected recent case law, there was an examination of the use of the prohibition in tackling some forms of aggressive tax planning. The Commission's state aid investigations into Apple, Fiat, Starbucks and Amazon were critically reviewed. Thoughts were offered as to the legality of the Commission's 'prudent independent market operator' test and the overall appropriateness of using the state aid prohibition in this area.

Chapter eight explored another angle of the debate by considering the ongoing efforts to introduce the Financial Transaction Tax, so as to make the financial sector pay for its role in the origins of the economic crisis. The original Commission proposal and the subsequent proposal to be adopted through enhanced cooperation were analysed. The development of the proposal and the suitability of using the enhanced cooperation procedure to adopt it were reviewed. The constitutional implications of using the enhance cooperation mechanism to promote tax legislation were also considered.

In general, the analysis suggests that while some developments were very much anticipated and long overdue, others were unexpected and took many by surprise. In fact, the developments in the European Union are short of ground-breaking. It has been questioned[1] whether the BEPS project will be the starting point for the development of new principles of international tax law or whether it will be the final failure of the OECD to gain consensus on topics, notwithstanding the unprecedented level of political support. It is widely acknowledged that BEPS is a political commitment of the OECD and the G20 countries, though as has been argued it would appear that it is a commitment to the agenda and 'not a commitment to accept whatever solutions come out of the process'.[2] It may prove impossible to reach consensus on solutions to some problems and/or some solutions agreed upon by the majority might not be implemented by all countries.[3] The need for coordination is crucial. It is not just the survival of the international tax regime at stake here but also 'the relevance of the OECD and its dominant members as the key players in the international tax world'.[4]

A review of the rules at play in the current international tax system has been long overdue. The arbitrary allocation of taxing rights, relying on a source/residence dichotomy and an active/passive income distinction first agreed in the 1920s by the League of Nations, eventually encapsulated in the OECD Model,[5] has been gravely manipulated over the years. It also proved to be ill-suited to deal with MNEs operating in today's global business environment. This is rather unequivocal given the number of corporate tax scandals that have emerged in the last few years. Stateless income and the very low effective tax rates that some MNEs enjoyed were quite provocative, especially within the context of the European

[1] Philip Baker, 'Is there a Cure for BEPS?' [2013] *British Tax Review* 605.

[2] *Ibid*, p 605.

[3] *Ibid*.

[4] Yariv Brauner, 'BEPS: An Interim Evaluation' (2014) 6 *World Tax Journal* 10, 13.

[5] See ch 1 in Christiana HJI Panayi, *Double Taxation, Tax Treaties, Treaty Shopping and the European Community* (Kluwer Law International, 2007).

Union, of which some Member States have suffered tremendously from the global financial crisis. As noted, 'the system is manipulable, distortive, often incoherent and unprincipled and encourages countries to compete with each other'.[6]

Prior to the launch of the BEPS project, it was feared that unless coordinated action had been taken at international level, countries would adopt (or would continue adopting) unilateral measures—hence the strong initial support for the BEPS project by many countries. The business sector also seemed to support the project in principle. The reputation risks faced by some MNEs and the uncertainty that had been generated by the recent tax scandals was sometimes more detrimental than higher effective tax rates. However, to an extent, it now seems that legality is taking a back seat in favour of what appears to be social justice and other vague concepts such as CSR and tax morality.

What is also noteworthy is that in the BEPS project, there is a break from tradition in the way that the proposals are presented. Instead of the OECD recommending model rules as consensus-built and definitive standards, in most discussion drafts there is a menu of options that countries may select—a series of alternative or minimum requirements. The level of support for these various options among OECD/G20 countries is not known. This is arguably attributable to the fact that the BEPS project is different from past OECD initiatives because it is not just driven by OECD countries but also non-member G20 countries. Furthermore, developing countries were strongly encouraged to participate in the process and have done so to an extent. Therefore, the divergent interests of all the participators may have eroded the OECD's traditional consensus-built model. Rather than encourage uniformity, the OECD is now offering options which could lead to more non-uniformity among country laws and could exacerbate the unilaterality problem. It could also generate more opportunities for tax arbitrage (for companies) and tax competition (for countries).

Another change is that the focus of the BEPS project is to protect tax bases and to fight stateless income. This is different from the focus of previous OECD projects which was mostly to promote trade or prevent double taxation.

In any case, while the BEPS project did not exactly go back to basics in attempting to improve the international tax regime, it has addressed some fundamental issues, and efforts were made to update the current tax system. A consideration of the source/residence taxation question was excluded from the beginning. However, to an extent, Action 1 tries to deal with the allocation of taxing rights in the context of digital economy, which has implications for the source/residence questions.

The Action items dealing with anti-abuse rules, Actions 2 to 4, mostly offer guidance in the form of best practices. In fact, most of the discussion drafts are not consensus documents. Important proposals are made in the context of Action 5—the modified nexus approach for patent boxes and the compulsory

[6] Michael P Devereux and John Vella, 'Are we Heading Towards a Corporate Tax System Fit for the 21st Century?' (2014) 35 *Fiscal Studies* 449–75, 461.

spontaneous exchange of taxpayer-specific rulings related to preferential regimes. The modified nexus approach was largely anticipated, at least among EU Member States, given the hostility shown towards the UK patent box regime and similar types of regimes. As for the exchange of tax rulings, this could reasonably be considered as a by-product of instruments dealing with exchange of information which have expanded exponentially in the past few years.

As for tax abuse and treaty shopping, the proposals clarify, consolidate and rationalise anti-treaty-shopping rules that are already in existence. A lot of these are optional to ensure that countries have maximum flexibility. These rather organic changes would likely have been made anyway. The same could also be said about the proposals under Action 7. They were likely to be developed in the normal course of affairs—the OECD Model is, after all, an ambulatory instrument.

Perhaps the most important proposals are those taken in the context of transfer pricing. The perceived deficiencies of the regime were largely attributed to the arm's length principle and its dominance. To an extent, the OECD is making an attempt to shift away from the mixed legal and economic approach in transfer pricing practice by placing a lot of emphasis on the principle that profits should follow value creation. Such an approach, interestingly, resembles the traditional approach of the United Nations to transfer pricing, which has not been followed by the OECD.

Notwithstanding this very perceptible shift of emphasis, the OECD does not seek to replace the arm's length principle, however much some of the BEPS discussion drafts seem to transform it from a pricing standard to a behavioural standard.[7] In any case, replacing the arm's length principle is not currently an option because even though some countries have shown some willingness to move beyond the arm's length principle, other countries are strongly resisting it. This also partly explains the failure to obtain a complete consensus on many of the Action items. As shown in Chapter three, there is a refinement of the application of the arm's length principle in specific areas and in very rare cases, deviations from it.[8] Profit split methods are mentioned in Action 10 but there is strong resistance by some countries. The same goes for the proposals made under the Risk and Re-characterisation Discussion Draft it remains to be seen if the final scope of this discussion draft will be limited. Nevertheless, the fact that the OECD has, for the first time, shown some willingness to divert from the exclusive application of the arm's length principle, even in limited circumstances, could be seen as a small victory for those advocating change.

What does seem to emerge from the BEPS project, though again, to an extent, this could have resulted anyway, are increased reporting requirements for MNEs. Under Action 13, the OECD recommended that MNEs prepare master files and

[7] See Jens Wittendorff, 'More Black Smoke From the OECD's Chimney—Third Draft on Intangibles' (2015) 77 *Tax Notes International* 167 (12 January 2015) p 172.

[8] Yariv Brauner, 'Transfer Pricing in BEPS: First Round—Business Interests Win (But, Not in Knock-Out)' (2015) 43 *Intertax* 72–84, 73–74.

local files for transfer pricing documentation purposes, as well as the country-by-country report. Action 11 raises the possibility that tax authorities may require MNEs to provide additional firm-level information to assist authorities in analysing the extent of base erosion and profit shifting. Action 12 makes several recommendations for mandatory disclosure rules. Action 5 provides for spontaneous exchange of taxpayer-specific rulings related to preferential regimes. All these are in addition to the US-led FATCA reporting system and its accompanying intergovernmental agreements, as well as in addition to the OECD's Common Reporting Standard for automatic exchange of financial account information, aimed primarily at financial institutions. Moreover, for MNEs doing business in the European Union, there are likely to be additional reporting standards, on the basis of other corporate transparency initiatives discussed in Chapter five.

Which begs the question—if the OECD refuses to properly address the basics such as the source/residence dichotomy or the role of tax competition in generating stateless income, does the BEPS project have any chances of success? Or will it also lead to a reconfiguration of the old solutions? Can there be any rational evolution of the transfer pricing rules without a clearer articulation of the principle of value creation? Can the anti-abuse rules in the problematic areas considered in the BEPS project be improved and streamlined without some sort of uniformity of standards? One could argue that some of the proposals shaping up the BEPS deliverables are likely to generate more tax competition rather than less.

It is not, therefore, surprising, that some countries that have been at the core of nations leading the BEPS project are actually considering taking unilateral action or have already done so. The UK's Diverted Profits Tax (DPT) is the best example.[9] The DPT, also misleadingly called the Google Tax, seems to be based on the idea that the volume of sales of an entity in a particular country should determine the tax paid in that country, ie it should be a connecting factor for exercising tax jurisdiction.[10]

The DPT was introduced in the UK Finance Act 2015.[11] It was intended to apply to large MNEs with business activities in the UK who entered into contrived arrangements to divert profits from the UK by avoiding a UK taxable permanent establishment and/or by other contrived arrangements between connected entities. Broadly, the DPT applies in two situations: when a foreign company artificially

[9] For commentary, see Sol Picciotto, 'The UK's Diverted Profits Tax: Admission of Defeat or Pre-Emptive Strike?', 2015 *WTD* 12-12 (20 January 2015); David Stewart and Stephanie Soong Johnston, 'The UK Government reveals Details of Diverted Profits Tax', 2014 *WTD* 238-1 (11 December 2014); Amanda Athanasiou, 'U.K. Diverted Profits Tax Remains a Work in Progress', 2015 *WTD* 29-4 (12 February 2015); Heather Self, 'Diverted Profits Tax: Give BEPS a chance', *Tax Journal*, Issue 1244 (15 December 2014).

[10] Luca Cerioni, 'The New "Google Tax": The "Beginning of the End" for Tax Residence as a Connecting Factor for Tax Jurisdiction?' (2015) 55 *European Taxation* 185–95. For a criticism of the DPT and the haste with which the UK government had adopted it, see Heather Self, 'The UK's New Diverted Profits Tax: Compliance with EU Law' (2015) 43 *Intertax* 333–36.

[11] See Kristen A Parillo, 'UK Diverted Profits Tax Legislation Both Narrowed and Broadened', 2015 *WTD* 57-2 (25 March 2015).

avoids having a UK permanent establishment (essentially where a person is carrying on activity in the UK in connection with the supply of goods and services by a non-UK resident company to customers in the UK) and when a UK company, or a foreign company with a UK permanent establishment, creates a tax advantage by using entities or transactions that lack economic substance. The tax is at a rate of 25 per cent of the diverted profits relating to the UK activity. The DPT is unlikely to arise where there is sufficient substance in offshore asset-owning companies, or arm's length transfer pricing through the international value chain, or a taxable presence in the UK eg through a permanent establishment. There are also exemptions for small and medium sized enterprises.

Under the DPT legislation, non-resident companies have a duty to notify HMRC under rather vague and subjective circumstances. Broadly, a non-resident company must notify HMRC within three months of the end of an accounting period if it was *reasonable* for the company to assume that diverted profits might arise for that period (ie if it is potentially within the scope of the DPT legislation).[12] Where the designated HMRC officer determines that the DPT should apply, a preliminary notice is issued.[13]

As a policy choice, the DPT arguably reduces the pressure on the OECD to adopt a more wholesale change to global permanent establishment and transfer pricing rules in the BEPS project. The DPT is a more targeted approach than that so far proposed by the OECD. It also appears to address one of the main criticisms on the OECD proposals on Action 7, namely, that they would create a huge number of permanent establishments and associated compliance burden but no significant additional tax in many circumstances. From that perspective, the DPT could be viewed as a more attractive option.

Nevertheless, there is concern that the DPT is likely to give rise to considerable uncertainty in its application in the short-term. Although the intention is for the DPT to only narrowly target cases of 'contrived' avoidance of UK tax, the drafting of the provisions is very broad. The DPT applies to a large range of transactions across all industry sectors, even though it has been widely reported as targeting the digital sector.

There are also concerns in how the DPT would be applied and whether it would give rise to double taxation if more jurisdictions implement a similar tax. It has been announced that HMRC is sharing information with five other tax authorities

[12] There is no duty to notify if HMRC has confirmed there is no need to do so or if it is reasonable for the company to assume that it has provided sufficient information to HMRC to enable the agency to decide whether to give a preliminary notice for that period and that HMRC has examined that information (either as part of an inquiry into a return or otherwise); or if it is reasonable for the company to conclude that no DPT charge will arise.

[13] The recipient of the notice has 30 days to make representations and the designated HMRC officer may consider certain specified matters within a further 30 day period before either issuing a charging notice on the original or a revised amount, or confirming that no charge arises. The charging notice requires the payment of the DPT within 30 days. Penalties apply for late payment.

on how digital multinationals might be shifting their profits to tax havens.[14] This is the E6 project which started in August 2013 and is expected to feed into the DPT regime. The Australian government has also recently announced that it would set up a joint working party with the UK to further consider and develop initiatives in relation to diverted profits by MNEs.[15] Australia is expected to pursue a similar measure as the DPT and other countries may follow suit. In fact on 11 May 2015, the Australian government announced that it would propose a 100 per cent penalty on multinational companies engaging in tax avoidance. This has been coined as the 'Netflix tax'.[16]

Incidentally, it has been recently reported that Amazon has changed its EU business structure so that from 1 May 2015 it would record retail sales made to customers in the UK and some other EU jurisdictions in those jurisdictions rather than Luxembourg.[17] With this move, Amazon might also avoid the UK's DPT which is higher than the normal tax due. To the extent that the UK is the only country to have a diverted profits tax so far, this seems logical and appropriate. It may prove more problematic for MNEs once other countries adopt their own overlapping versions of a diverted profits tax, leading to a need for coordination as with the current BEPS Action Plan.

The OECD/G20's BEPS project is certainly not panacea. There is a risk that the compliance costs generated from some of the actions might be out of line with any additional revenue that the governments might collect. In fact, the BEPS project may not even help reduce unilateral actions, as the enactment of the UK's DPT and other initiatives suggest. According to data compiled by PwC, more than 30 unilateral BEPS-focused measures were introduced by at least 19 countries in 2014 alone.[18] The measures included guidance and legislation or proposed legislation on hybrids, interest deductibility, CFC rules, harmful tax practices, artificial avoidance of permanent establishments etc.

It is obvious that several countries are not waiting for a consensus approach.[19] In fact, it would seem that countries have started using BEPS as an excuse for unilateral actions. There is definitely political pressure to take swift action. However, the unilateral actions of developing countries and BRICS countries such as

[14] See HMRC Press Release of 25 March 2015, available on: www.gov.uk/government/news/government-ramps-up-efforts-to-tackle-digital-multinational-tax-risks.

[15] Also see Teri Sprackland, 'Australia to Work with UK on its Own Diverted Profits Solution', 2015 *WTD* 76-3 (21 April 2015).

[16] See William Hoke, 'Australian Budget to Include 100 Percent Tax Avoidance Fine, "Netflix Tax"', 2015 *WTD* 91-2 (12 May 2015).

[17] Stephanie Soong Johnston, 'Amazon Changes EU Structure to Book Profits in Local Countries', 2015 *WTD* 101-1 (27 May 2015).

[18] PwC TaxTalk Monthly, 'The forces and tensions shaping BEPS', 1 April 2014. Available on: www.pwc.com.au/tax/taxtalk/assets/alerts/TaxTalk-Alert-BEPS-Apr14.pdf.

[19] See Amanda Athanasiou, 'Jumping the Gate on BEPS: Unilateral Actions Weaken OECD's Plan', 2015 *WTD* 49-2 (13 March 2015); Amanda Athanasiou, 'The Cost of BEPS', 2015 *WTD* 9-1 (14 January 2015); Margaret Burow, 'Countries Aren't Waiting on OECD to Implement BEPS', 2014 *WTD* 218-2 (12 November, 2014).

India and China might be more radical than the unilateral actions of the UK or Australia, given their wider divergence of interests from the traditional OECD paradigm. In any case, it is likely to be harder to gain consensus if countries have already locked in their positions though unilateral actions. Furthermore, even post-BEPS there is likely to be unilateral action by some countries, mostly in the areas where the deliverables offered a menu of options rather than made specific recommendations for amendments to the OECD Model, the Commentary or the Transfer Pricing Guidelines.

There may well be dissentients to the final product. US Treasury officials have expressed their frustration with the direction of some parts of the BEPS project. It was emphasised that the US would not commit to substantive changes in existing laws without a commitment from other countries. The US Congress is likely to be hostile to the idea of new transfer pricing documentation requirements that would subject US companies to greater foreign taxation, while limiting the ability of the US to tax their profits.[20] There is an overall feeling that in committing to the BEPS project, the US is effectively signing up to provide indirect aid to other jurisdictions by reallocating its rights to tax global profits.[21] It has even been argued that the primary objective of the US involvement in the BEPS project is not to avoid double non-taxation but to minimise the impact of the project on the US and its MNEs and to ensure that *if* any double non-taxed income of US MNEs is to be taxed, then it should be taxed by the US Government.[22]

Nevertheless, there are reports that the next US Model Tax Treaty, which is expected to be released by the end of 2015, reflects some of the BEPS policy concerns such as double non-taxation, stateless income via treaty shopping, etc.[23] In fact, some of the recommendations expressed by the US delegates in the BEPS consultation process—thought to be based on the forthcoming version of the US Model Tax Treaty—have been incorporated in the latest version of the Treaty Abuse discussion draft (the Treaty Abuse Second Revised Discussion Draft), examined in Chapter three. Therefore, notwithstanding the initial and to an extent on-going US recalcitrance on some of the BEPS proposals, there has been cross-fertilisation of ideas and confluence of actions. The status quo is unlikely to remain the same.

In any case, the OECD is moving fast to keep whatever level of consensus has been preserved among countries and to prevent them from acting unilaterally to tackle BEPS, as much as possible.[24] There is also a hurry to benefit from the

[20] Mindy Herzfeld, 'Making Bets on CbC Reporting' (2015) 78 *Tax Notes International* 595 (18 May 2015).

[21] Ibid.

[22] Antony Ting, 'The Politics of BEPS—Apple's International Tax Structure and the US attitude towards BEPS' (2015) 69 *Bulletin for International Taxation* 410–15. Also see Manal Corwin, *Sense and Sensibility: The Policy and Politics of BEPS*, 19th Annual Tillinghast Lecture (30 September, 2014).

[23] See Kristen A Parillo, 'Model Treaty Proposals Reflect Dramatic Change in US Policy', 2015 *WTD* 99-1 (22 May 2015).

[24] See Stephanie Soong Johnston, 'Pascal Saint-Amans—the Face of BEPS' (2014) 76 *Tax Notes International* 1051 (22 December 2014).

political momentum. This is certainly the case in the European Union, where a lot of emphasis was placed on tackling tax avoidance, tax evasion and aggressive tax planning. The Commission has fast-tracked many legislative proposals or amendments at Council level, which are questionable from an EU law perspective. It has also launched state aid investigations on tax rulings enjoyed by several high-profile MNEs, which are again dubious from a pure state aid perspective. And more behind the scenes, it has been facilitating the adoption of an important tax instrument—the Financial Transaction Tax—through enhanced cooperation, without really addressing the serious and detrimental impact of this instrument on non-participating Member States. These concerns were examined in greater detail throughout the book.

There certainly needs to be coordination with the principles set out by the Court of Justice in established case law, otherwise legal certainty is being jeopardised. Nevertheless, one should question whether in the absence of harmonisation the European Union is currently going too far by restricting options for tax competition. To an extent, much of the criticism directed at MNEs or their legal advisors or accountants might be misdirected because individual countries themselves engage in tax competition, offering a wide choice of alternative strategies from which to choose.[25] This type of forum shopping was until recently condoned and to an extent protected under EU law. Attempts for harmonisation were very much resisted by Member States. A good example is the proposal for the Common Consolidated Corporate Tax Base, which is still pending since it was released in 2011.

Furthermore, Member States such as Ireland and Luxembourg have long been associated with some of the low-substance aggressive tax planning practices now criticised (but previously partly copied) by other Member States and attacked by the Commission in its state aid investigations. In fact, the current president of the Commission, Jean-Claude Juncker, who is so fervently pushing for reform to fight tax evasion and to instil 'some morality, some ethics, into the European tax landscape',[26] was the Prime Minister of Luxembourg at the time these practices thrived and has been accused of turning Luxembourg into a major European centre of corporate tax avoidance during his premiership. Following the Luxembourg leaks considered in Chapter one, Juncker was embroiled in political controversy but still survived a vote of confidence in the European Parliament in November 2014.

In any case, this traditionalist anti-harmonisation mindset is likely to change as BEPS is not just about the loss of revenue for countries—it also affects tax competition between countries and the ability to confer tax incentives to attract capital. The European Union is likely to adopt some BEPS policies, or variations of them, in the near future. In fact, it has already adopted elements of the BEPS proposals such as the amendments to the Parent-Subsidiary Directive considered in

[25] William Hoke, 'Big 4 Defend MNE Tax Advice to EU Parliament and Urge Reform', 2015 *WTD* 88-2 (7 May 2015).

[26] See speech in Brussels, in July 2014, reported by several media outlets. See, eg www.theguardian.com/business/2014/nov/05/-sp-luxembourg-tax-files-tax-avoidance-industrial-scale.

Chapter five. These measures are binding on Member States, irrespective of their stance on the BEPS project, their attitudes and expectations. Therefore, the BEPS deliverables are likely to have an impact on EU law, whether directly or indirectly. In any case, the widely anticipated Action Plan on Corporate Taxation is expected to change the EU tax landscape in a more defined way than some of the mosaic of proposals under BEPS.

Nevertheless, an EU strategy focusing only on the fight against tax avoidance and aggressive tax planning runs the risk of hindering the single market and reducing its efficiency and potential.[27] In the absence of a single *fiscal* market, such an ad hoc strategy can only do more damage than good in the long term. The recent state aid litigation on tax rulings shows the problematic nature of an ad hoc approach. Whilst the enthusiasm to grasp the opportunity to increase tax revenues by closing some loopholes and to 'punish' MNEs for their aggressive tax planning is understandable, a holistic approach to tax reform and an acceptance of the absolute necessity for some partial tax harmonisation are essential if the EU efforts are to succeed.

It is undeniable that the international tax community and especially the EU tax community are moving to a new direction. There are many unresolved issues and the post-BEPS tax world is likely to be very challenging. The abundance of vague concepts embedded in the pre-BEPS discourse, such as CSR, good tax governance, morality and fairness, are likely to remain and as such amplify the legal uncertainty. How will this story end? None knows but at least from a European Union perspective, a new and possibly irreversible era has begun with much wider implications than originally thought.

[27] Michel Aujean, 'Plea for a New Tax Package' (2015) 24 *EC Tax Review* 60–62, 61.

INDEX

Lightning Source UK Ltd.
Milton Keynes UK
UKHW02f0004160318
319551UK00003B/116/P

9 781509 921096